Glickman's
Clinical
Periodontology

SIXTH EDITION

Fermin A. Carranza, Jr., Dr. Odont.

Professor and Chairman, Section of Periodontology
School of Dentistry, Center for the Health Sciences
Member, Dental Research Institute
University of California
Los Angeles, California

W.B. Saunders Company

Philadelphia   London   Toronto   Mexico City   Rio de Janeiro   Sydney   Tokyo

W. B. Saunders Company: West Washington Square
Philadelphia, PA 19105

1 St. Anne's Road
Eastbourne, East Sussex BN21 3UN, England

1 Goldthorne Avenue
Toronto, Ontario M8Z 5T9, Canada

Apartado 26370—Cedro 512
Mexico 4, D.F., Mexico

Rua Coronel Cabrita, 8
Sao Cristovao Caixa Postal 21176
Rio de Janeiro, Brazil

9 Waltham Street
Artarmon, N.S.W. 2064, Australia

Ichibancho, Central Bldg., 22-1 Ichibancho
Chiyoda-Ku, Tokyo 102, Japan

Library of Congress Cataloging in Publication Data

Glickman, Irving.

Glickman's Clinical periodontology.

Includes bibliographies and index.

1. Periodontics.   I. Carranza, Fermin A.   II. Title.
III. Title: Clinical periodontology. [DNLM: 1. Periodontal
diseases. WU 240 G559c]

RK361.G58 1984   617.6′32   83–7868

ISBN 0–7216–2441–3

Listed here is the latest translated edition of this book
together with the language of the translation and the publisher.

Italian (2nd Edition)—Editrice Scientifica, Milan, Italy

French (4th Edition)—Julien Prelat, Paris, France

Spanish (5th Edition)—Nueva Editorial Interamericana, Mexico City, Mexico

Portuguese (5th Edition)—Interamericana, Rio de Janeiro, Brazil

Glickman's Clinical Periodontology   ISBN   0-7216-2441-3

Last digit is the print number: 9   8   7   6   5   4

To Rita

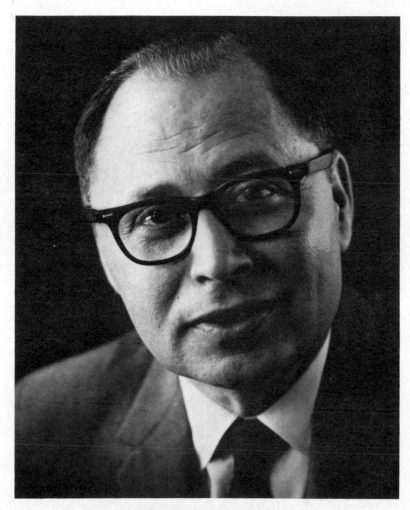

Irving Glickman (1914–1972)
Brilliant researcher, inspired teacher, dear friend

CONTRIBUTORS

E. BARRIE KENNEY, B.D.Sc., D.D.S., M.S.
Professor of Periodontics and
Director of Postdoctoral Periodontics
School of Dentistry
University of California, Los Angeles

ROBERT L. MERIN, D.D.S., M.S.
Lecturer in Periodontics
School of Dentistry
University of California, Los Angeles

MICHAEL G. NEWMAN, D.D.S.
Adjunct Professor of Periodontics
School of Dentistry
University of California, Los Angeles

RUSSELL J. NISENGARD, D.D.S., Ph.D.
Professor of Periodontology and Microbiology
Schools of Dentistry and Medicine
State University of New York at Buffalo

JOAN ANN OTOMO, B.A., M.P.H., D.D.S.
Assistant Professor of Periodontics
School of Dentistry
University of California, Los Angeles
Staff Periodontist
Veterans Administration Medical Centers at Wadsworth and Sepulveda
Los Angeles, California

ANNA MATSUISHI PATTISON, R.D.H., M.S.
Associate Professor of Dental Hygiene and Periodontics
School of Dentistry
University of Southern California, Los Angeles

GORDON L. PATTISON, D.D.S.
Assistant Professor of Periodontics
School of Dentistry
University of California, Los Angeles

F. REINALDO SAGLIE, Dr. Odont., Ph.D.
Associate Professor of Periodontics
School of Dentistry
University of California, Los Angeles

MAX O. SCHMID, B.A., D.M.D.
Private Practice
Arrau, Switzerland
Former Associate Professor of Periodontics
School of Dentistry
University of California, Los Angeles

GERALD SHKLAR, D.D.S., M.S.
Charles A. Brackett Professor of Oral Pathology and
Head of the Department of Oral Medicine and Oral Pathology
Harvard University School of Dental Medicine
Boston, Massachusetts

THOMAS N. SIMS, B.S., D.D.S.
Assistant Professor of Periodontics
School of Dentistry
University of California, Los Angeles
Director of the Periodontal Residency Program
Veterans Administration Wadsworth Medical Center
Los Angeles, California

WILLIAM K. SOLBERG, D.D.S., M.S.D.
Professor of Restorative Dentistry,
Chairman of the Section of Gnathology and Occlusion
School of Dentistry
University of California, Los Angeles

VLADIMIR W. SPOLSKY, B.S., D.M.D., M.P.H.
Associate Professor of Preventive Dentistry and Public Health
School of Dentistry
University of California, Los Angeles

HENRY H. TAKEI, D.D.S., M.S.
Clinical Professor of Periodontics
School of Dentistry
University of California, Los Angeles

ALFRED WEINSTOCK, D.D.S., Ph.D.
Clinical Professor of Periodontics and
Clinical Professor of Anatomy
School of Dentistry and
School of Medicine
University of California, Los Angeles

PREFACE

This is a textbook for practitioners of general dentistry and students preparing to become general practitioners. It is predicated on the premise that the periodontal care of the American public is primarily the concern of the general dentist. The general practitioner can never disregard his responsibility to provide periodontal care for all his patients. The extremely high incidence of periodontal problems in the population makes it impossible for the necessarily small number of specialists in periodontics to cope with them; in addition, the close relationship between periodontal and restorative dental therapies makes it very important for the general dentist to have a thorough knowledge of periodontics. The availability of a well-trained group of periodontists for the diagnosis and treatment of severe or unusual problems should serve only to supplement the general dental care available to our population.

In the experience of the author the type of preparation which dental students and dentists need most for the clinical management of periodontal problems is an understanding of the clinical phenomena in terms of underlying tissue changes and a comprehension of the biologic nature of the periodontal responses. Once this aspect is mastered, the treatment techniques can be performed with the degree of skill possessed by every qualified general dentist.

A great amount of information regarding the nature of periodontal disease and its treatment has resulted from the efforts of clinicians and researchers. A considerable portion of this information is applicable to the practice of dentistry. It is the purpose of this textbook to present existing knowledge regarding periodontal problems in such a manner that it can be incorporated in the practice of dentistry. It has been the desire of the author to create an analytic text that would provide answers to the fundamental and the clinical questions regarding periodontal disease and its modern treatment.

The first four editions of this book were authored by Dr. Irving Glickman. Dr. Glickman died on October 2, 1972. He was a distinguished researcher and teacher whose dynamic personality, clear judgment, and profound knowledge of all areas of periodontics and related fields marked him as a leader in the progress of our discipline for three decades. This new edition of *Clinical Periodontology* is dedicated to his memory.

The present edition incorporates all the major advances that have taken place in periodontics in recent years. Most of the book has been brought up to date and rewritten, and several new chapters have been introduced. It remains, however, a standard textbook with exhaustive coverage of past and present basic and clinical developments in periodontics and related fields.

The author has been very fortunate to be able to obtain the valuable help of a group of scientists with remarkable expertise and knowledge in different clinical and research areas of periodontics. Their important collaboration is gratefully acknowledged.

I am particularly indebted to Drs. E. Barrie Kenney, Michael G. Newman, and Henry H. Takei for their constructive criticism and constant support. I also gratefully acknowledge the following colleagues who have contributed unpublished information or illustrations: R. Barbanell, M. Barnett, J. M. Baty, S. Bernick, A. Brendel, R. L. Cabrini, R. G. Caffesse, J. Cane, J. J. Carraro, A. Chaudhry, N. Chilton, E. S. Cohen, M. M. Cohen, J. Flocken, R. Frank, M. Goodson, B. Gratt, A. Haffajee, A. G. Hannum, T. Hansson, L. Hirschfeld, J. Hsiou, J. Ingle, J. Klingsberg, S. Levine, J. Lindhe, M. Listgarten, I. Logan, H. Lundeen, C. Martin, M. Massler, I. Meyer, D. F. Mitchell, C. F. Moorrees, T. Öberg, R. G. Oliver, R. Page, C. A. Palioca, B. Patur, R. E. Robinson, M. Ruben, Z. Skobe, J. Smulow, S. Socransky, J. Sottosanti, S. Toll, A. Ubios, V. Vandersloot, D. Weisberger, S. White, S. Woolfe, and J. Yee. Dr. Dorothy Perry read many chapters and offered helpful suggestions.

I am also indebted to Ms. Irene Petravicius for her excellent artwork and untiring efforts to follow our ideas; to Ms. Catherine Boris and Mr. Richard A. Friske for their photographic expertise; to Ms. Rhoda Freeman and the UCLA Word Processing Center (Ms. Michele Kirsch, Ms. Barbara Mersini, and Ms. Roseanna Espinoza) for their excellent typing assistance; to Ms. Helene Redmond and Ms. Susan Morris for their invaluable secretarial help; and to Ms. Sue Nelson and Ms. Ana Hyde for their assistance in the clinic, where many book-related activities took place.

Special appreciation goes to Dr. Violeta Arboleda for her confidence and support; and to Mr. Robert Reinhardt, Mr. Raymond Kersey, Ms. Laura Tarves, Ms. Joan Vandegrift, and the W. B. Saunders Company for their trust and expertise.

Finally, I wish to acknowledge the constant support of my family, who have been so tolerant and understanding.

FERMIN A. CARRANZA, JR.

CONTENTS

The Historical Background of Periodontology

Gingival and periodontal diseases, in their various forms, have afflicted mankind since the dawn of history, and studies in paleopathology have indicated that destructive periodontal disease, as evidenced by bone loss, has affected early man in such diverse cultures as ancient Egypt and early pre-Columbian America.[25] Our earliest historical records dealing with medical topics reveal an awareness of periodontal disease and the need for treating it. Almost all of the early writings that have been preserved have several sections or chapters dealing with oral diseases, and periodontal problems take up a significant amount of space. The relationship of calculus to periodontal disease was often considered, and underlying systemic disease was often postulated as a cause of periodontal disease, but methodical, carefully reasoned, therapeutic discussions did not exist until the Arabic surgical treatises of the Middle Ages; and modern treatment, with illustrated texts and sophisticated instrumentation, did not develop until the time of Pierre Fauchard.

Oral hygiene was practiced by the Sumerians of 3000 B.C., and elaborately decorated gold toothpicks found in the excavations at Ur in Mesopotamia suggest an interest in cleanliness of the mouth. The Babylonians and Assyrians following the earlier Sumerian civilization apparently suffered from periodontal problems, and a clay tablet of the period tells of treatment by gingival massage combined with various herbal medications.[15]

Medicinal mouthwashes were also used, and Jastrow[18] refers to a tablet in which six different drugs are suggested for treatment of "sickness of the mouth."

Periodontal disease was the commonest of all diseases of which there is evidence in the embalmed bodies of the ancient Egyptians. It is thus not surprising that the problem received attention in medical and surgical writings of the time. The Ebers papyrus contains many references to gingival disease and offers a number of prescriptions for strengthening the teeth and gums. These remedies were made from various plants and minerals and were applied to the gums in the form of a paste, with honey, vegetable gum, or residue of beer as a vehicle.[11]

Among the various medical papyri that have been preserved, the most sophisticated, in terms of modern medical practice, is the Edwin Smith surgical papyrus.[5] This remnant of a larger work presents 48 cases and discusses diagnosis, prognosis, and appropriate therapy. Mandibular fractures and mandibular dislocations are considered, but periodontal problems are not mentioned as diseases requiring surgical therapy.

The medical works of ancient India devote a significant amount of space to oral and periodontal problems. In the *Susruta Samhita* there are numerous descriptions of severe periodontal disease with loose teeth and purulent discharge from the gingiva.[27] In a later treatise, the *Charaka Samhita*, toothbrushing and oral hygiene are stressed: "The stick for brushing the teeth should be either astringent or pungent or bitter. One of its ends should be chewed into the form of a brush. It should be used twice a day, taking care that the gums not be injured."[8]

Ancient Chinese medical works also discuss periodontal disease. In the oldest book, written by Hwang-Ti about 2500 B.C., there is a chapter devoted to dental and gingival diseases. Oral diseases were divided into three types: (1) "Fong Ya," or inflammatory conditions; (2) "Ya Kon," or diseases of the soft investing tissues of the teeth; and (3) "Chong-Ya," or dental caries.[9]

Gingival inflammations, periodontal abscesses, and gingival ulcerations are described in accurate detail. One gingival condition is described as follows: "The gingivae are pale or violet red, hard and lumpy, sometimes bleeding: the toothache is continuous." Herbal remedies, "Zn-hine-tong," are mentioned for the treatment of these conditions. The Chinese were among the earliest people to use the "chew stick" as a toothpick and toothbrush to clean the teeth and massage the gingival tissues.

The importance of oral hygiene was recognized by the early Hebrews. Many pathologic conditions of the teeth and their surrounding structures are described in the Talmudic writings. Artifacts of the Phoenician civilization include a specimen of wire splinting apparently constructed to stabilize teeth loosened by chronic destructive periodontal disease.[15]

With the development of Greek culture and science came one of the golden ages of Western civilization. The Greeks were to attain preeminence in almost every field or discipline they touched. Architecture, painting, sculpture, pottery, poetry, drama, philosophy, and history reached a degree of perfection rarely surpassed in succeeding ages. This was the age of Homer, Plato, and Aristotle, of Euripides, Aeschylus, and Sophocles, of Herodotus and Xenophon, of Phidias and Praxiteles. Modern science also had its birth in Greece, and medicine developed in terms of diagnostic approach and technical skill. Greek medicine continued into the succeeding Roman civilization and the early Byzantine Age.

Among the ancient Greeks, Hippocrates of Cos (460–335 B.C.) was the father of modern medicine, the first to institute a systematic examination of the patient's pulse, temperature, respiration, excreta, sputum, and pains.[6, 19] He discussed the function and eruption of the teeth and also the etiology of periodontal disease. He believed that inflammation of the gums could be caused by accumulations of pituita or calculus, with gingival hemorrhage occurring in cases of persistent disease. He described different varieties of splenic maladies, to one of which he assigned the following symptoms: "The belly becomes swollen, the spleen enlarged and hard, the patient suffers from acute pain. The gums are detached from the teeth and smell bad."[16]

The Etruscans, much before 735 B.C., were adept in the art of constructing artificial dentures, but there is no evidence that they were aware of the existence of periodontal disease or its treatment.

Among the Romans, Aulus Cornelius Celsus (first century A.D.) referred to diseases which affect the soft parts of the mouth and their treatment as follows: "If the gums separate from the teeth, it is beneficial to chew unripe pears and apples and keep their juices in the mouth." He described looseness of the teeth caused by the weakness of their roots or by flaccidity of the gums and noted that in these cases it is necessary to touch the gums lightly with a red-hot iron and then smear them with honey.[7] The Romans were very interested in oral hygiene. Celsus believed that stains on

the teeth should first be removed and the teeth then rubbed with a dentifrice. The use of the toothbrush is mentioned in the writings of many of the Roman poets. Gingival massage was an integral part of oral hygiene. Paul of Aegina during the seventh century differentiated between epulis, a fleshy excrescence of gums in the area of a tooth, and parulis, which he described as an abscess of the gums. He wrote that tartar incrustations must be removed with either scrapers or a small file and that the teeth should be carefully cleansed after the last meal of the day.[22]

While the decline and eventual fall of the Roman Empire plunged Europe into an age of darkness, the rise of Islam and the golden age of Arabic science and medicine occurred. The astonishing attainments of Islam are not only of interest in the history of medicine; they provided, to a very large extent, the impetus for the rise of European medicine in the late Middle Ages and Renaissance. In the early medical schools of Salerno and Montpellier, the available texts were primarily the renowned Arabic treatises in adequate, but far from accurate, Latin translations.

Much of medieval and Renaissance stomatology and dentistry was derived directly from Arabic writings, particularly the treatises of Ibn Sina (Avicenna) and Abu'l-Qasim (Albucasis). The Arabic treatises derived much of their information from Greek medical treatises, but many refinements and novel approaches were added, particularly in the surgical specialties.[26] Many of the Greek classics translated into Arabic in Baghdad during the Abbassid Caliphate were eventually to be rehabilitated in Latin translations following the destruction and virtual disappearance of scholarship in Europe during the Dark Ages. Baghdad shared with Córdoba in Spain both intellectual and medical eminence, with the two cities representing the greatness of the Eastern and Western Caliphates. Hunayn ibn-Ishaq (809–873) and his associates translated into Arabic the Greek originals of Galen, Oribasius, Paul of Aegina, Dioscorides, and the Hippocratic corpus, as well as the philosophy of Plato and Aristotle and the mathematics of Archimedes. Abu Bakr Muhammed ibn Zakariya al Razi (Rhazes) (841–926) wrote an encyclopedic work on medicine and surgery in 25 books. He was also physician-in-chief at the great Baghdad hospital and taught medicine in terms of clinical cases. Ali ibn Abbas al Majousi (Haly Abbas) (930–944) described many dermatologic diseases and recommended such surgical advances as the suturing of blood vessels prior to the removal of tumors. He also wrote extensively on dental subjects.

Ibn Sina (Avicenna) (980–1037) was possibly the greatest of the Arabic physicians. His *Canon,* a comprehensive treatise on medicine, is probably the most famous medical text of all time, in continuous use for almost 600 years. Ibn Sina used an extensive materia medica for oral and periodontal diseases and rarely resorted to surgery. Various headings in the *Canon* on gingival disease include "Bleeding Gums," "Fissures of the Gums," "Ulcers of the Gums," "Separation of the Gums," "Recession of the Gums," "Looseness of the Gums," and "Epulis."[3]

Abu'l-Qasim (Albucasis, in Latin translation) (936–1013) was the pre-eminent physician and surgeon of the Western Caliphate at Córdoba. His contributions to dentistry and periodontology were among his outstanding achievements. He had a clear understanding of the major etiologic role of calculus deposits and described in detail the technique of scaling the teeth, using a sophisticated set of instruments that he developed. He also wrote in detail on the extraction of teeth, on splinting loose teeth with gold wire, and on filing gross occlusal abnormalities. The fame of his treatise spread throughout the Arab world and beyond. It was translated into Latin by Gerard

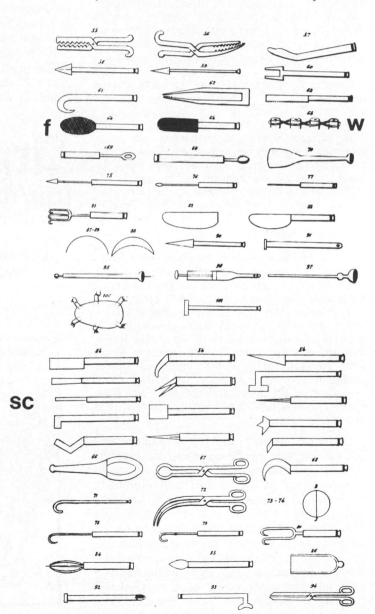

Figure 1 Illustration of Abu'l-Qasim's periodontal instruments, showing scalers (*sc*), files (*f*), and the wiring of loose teeth (*w*).

of Cremona in 1497 and greatly influenced the surgeons William of Saliceto,[23] in the thirteenth century, Guy de Chauliac,[24] in the thirteenth century, and Fabricius of Aquapendente, in the sixteenth century. Two brief chapters offer a clear picture of Abu'l-Qasim's knowledge and skill.[1]

Chapter 28—Excision of Superfluous Growths on the Gums

The gums are frequently the site of superfluous growths which the ancients named "epulis." It is necessary to raise them with hooks or to grasp them with forceps and excise them at the base. One should let the blood or pus flow and then place on the surface pulverized green vitriol or other astringent or drying powders. If the lesions recur after the operation, something that frequently happens, it is necessary to excise them a second time and to cauterize. They will not recur after cauterization.

Chapter 29 —On Scraping the Teeth with an Iron Instrument

Occasionally there is deposited in the inner and outer surfaces of the teeth or between the gums, large and rough ugly concretions: the teeth take on a black, yellow, or green color, following which the gums are altered and the teeth become unsightly.

To treat this disease, seat the patient in front of you, placing the head in your lap. Scale (scrape) the teeth and molars that present the concretions or the gritty deposits until nothing remains. Scrape also throughout where the teeth are black, yellow, green or otherwise colored, until they (the calculus deposits) are gone. It is possible that one scaling will suffice. If not, begin a second, third or fourth time, until your purpose is completely attained.

You should know that the scaling of teeth is done with instruments of various shapes (forms) according to the use that is required for them. The scalers that one uses for scaling the inner surfaces of the teeth are different than those employed for the scaling of the exterior surfaces, and those that are used to scale the interdental surfaces. Here is an assortment of scalers all of which you have at your disposition. *(Fig. 1)*

In the Renaissance, with a rebirth of classical scholarship and the development of scientific thought and medical knowledge in addition to the flowering of art, music, and literature, there were significant contributions to anatomy and surgery. Vesalius studied from human dissection and wrote a magnificent book on anatomy, with excellent illustrations throughout, which were drawn by a student of Titian's.[29] Eustachius was another outstanding anatomist and wrote a small book on dentistry, *Libellus de Dentibus*, in 30 chapters. He describes the firmness of the teeth in the jaws as

follows: "there exists besides a very strong ligament, principally attached to the roots by which these latter are tightly connected with the alveoli." "The gums also contribute to their firmness." Eustachius compares this with the joining of the skin to the fingernails.[12]

Ambroise Paré (1517–1590) was the outstanding surgeon of the Renaissance, and his contributions to dental surgery were substantial. He developed obturators for palatal defects and described many oral surgical procedures in detail, including gingivectomy for hyperplastic gingival tissues.[21] He also understood the etiologic significance of calculus and had a set of scalers to remove the hard deposits on the teeth. Paré wrote in French rather than in Latin; therefore his works could be widely read and understood.

In 1530 the first book specifically devoted to dental practice and written in a common language (German) was published in Leipzig by Blum. It was entitled *Artzney Buchlein* (Fig.

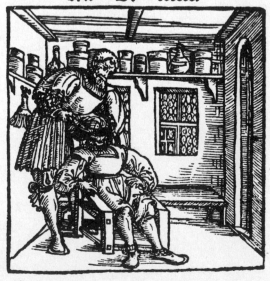

Figure 2 Frontispiece of *Artzney Buchlein* of 1530.

2). Later editions were published by Egenolff in Frankfurt.[2] It was essentially a compendium of previous writings on oral and dental diseases and their management. Three chapters are devoted specifically to periodontal problems. In Chapter 7, entitled "Concerning Yellow and Black Teeth," the author describes "tartar . . . a white, yellow and black slime that settles on the lower part of the teeth and over the gums." He suggests that a natural appearance of the teeth may be retained or restored by medicines which "dry up and cleanse, which have the power to rub away the uncleanness and to make clean, as pumice-stone and common salt, etc." He also suggests scraping black teeth and the use of toothpastes or powders to rub against the teeth. The composition of several pastes and powders is offered. In Chapter 9, "Of Loose Teeth," there is a description of periodontitis "which happens either through negligence or weakness or disease of the gums, or through the separation of those substances that hold the teeth in their places which happens when humors from the head drop down upon the gums or roots of the teeth and loosen them by their noxious action." Thus a crude concept was presented of both systemic and local factors in the etiology of periodontal disease. The presence of local infective agents or "worms" was also mentioned. A variety of ointments are suggested, often astrigent in nature, and it is recommended that loose teeth be bound to sound ones, using silk or gold thread. Cauterizing the gingiva with a hot iron is mentioned, but "this burning is dangerous and needs an expensive skilled master." In Chapter 11, entitled "Ulceration, Bad Smell and Decay of the Gums," the management of necrotizing gingivitis with medicines containing vinegar and alum is discussed.

Anton van Leeuwenhoek (1632–1723) of Delft contributed more to the development of modern biologic science than any classically trained scholar of his age. A layman with an inquisitive mind and a hobby of grinding lenses, he developed the microscope and used it to discover microorganisms, cellular structure, blood cells, sperm, and various other microscopic structures, including the tubular structure of dentin.[10] Using material from his gingival tissues, he first described the oral bacterial flora, and his drawings offered a reasonably good presentation of oral spirochetes and bacilli (Fig. 3). "I didn't clean my teeth (on purpose) for three days and then took the material that had lodged in small amounts on the gums above my front teeth. . . . I found a few living animalcules." He

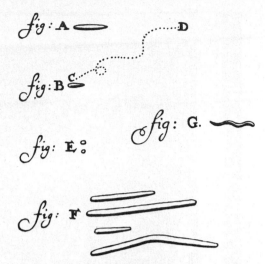

Figure 3 Leeuwenhoek's drawing of oral spirochetes, bacilli, and other microorganisms.

described a great amount of bacteria in a man who had never cleaned his mouth.

Modern dentistry essentially developed in eighteenth-century Europe, particularly France and England. Pierre Fauchard, born in Brittany in 1678, is rightly regarded as the father of the profession as we know it. Although he was self-educated in dentistry, he was able to develop a systematized approach to dental practice based on the knowledge of his age. He significantly improved the instruments and the technical skills required for dental treatment, and his book, *The Surgeon Dentist*, published in 1728 (Fig. 4), gave respectability to the profession and developed a wide appreciation for the technical and surgical skills of the dental practitioner.[13] Fauchard became the leading dentist in Paris and died in 1761 after a long life of service and achievement. His book not only transformed dental practice, but served to educate the succeeding generation of dentists, some of whom emigrated to America and practiced in the early years of the Republic. Some of George Washington's dentures were made with springs similar to those in the design illustrated by Fauchard. All aspects of dental practice are presented in his book— restorative dentistry, prosthodontics, oral surgery, periodontics, and orthodontics. Preventive dentistry is described in Chapter 4 ("The Regimen and Care Required for the Preservation of the Teeth") and Chapter 5 ("How to Keep the Teeth White and Strengthen the Gums"). Fauchard wrote that confections and sweets destroy the teeth by sticking to their surfaces and producing an acid. His clear de-

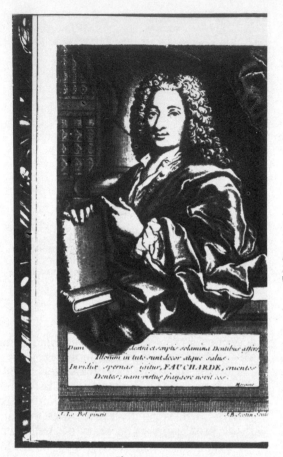

Figure 4 Frontispiece of *The Surgeon Dentist* of Fauchard (1746).

scriptions of his periodontal instruments and scaling technique are worth quoting in detail.

Chapter 2—Description of Instruments Appropriate for Detaching Hard Matter or Tartar from the Teeth *(Fig. 5)*

Some of those who clean the teeth ordinarily have an assortment of instruments of all kinds and try to persuade by this that they cannot be properly cleaned without all these instruments, which are useless for operating, but necessary to impress the public. I use for cleaning the teeth only five types of instruments, a rabbet chisel (number 1), a parrot beak (number 2), a three-faced graver (number 3), a small knife with convex blade (number 4) and a Z shaped hook (number 5). These five instruments are sharp and used like files or rasps. They suffice me for the removal of tartar from any place where it is found. As most of the instruments used for cleaning the teeth seem to me very unsuitable and even clumsy, I have been obliged to invent others which are very simple and to reshape certain others which are in common use.

Chapter 3—Manner of Operating Methodically to Clean the Mouth by Detaching, Taking Off and Removing the Tartar Without Affecting the Enamel of the Teeth

When a person presents himself to us for treatment of his mouth, the first thing that we perceive in opening it is the tartar, when it is present. In that case one should begin to remove it, after having examined all the teeth with an explorer to assure whether some of them are carious or not; for in the case of caries, one would treat them after having cleaned them; and if it were necessary to file them, cauterize or fill with lead one should not defer these operations.

To operate comfortably, the patient should be seated in a chair or a stable armchair which should be neither too high nor too low, the head gently placed against the back. One begins by removing the tartar from those teeth that are the most covered, and one does this with a rabbet (donkey beak) chisel which one holds in the right hand with the thumb, index finger and middle finger: one holds it somewhat like a writing pen, while its extremity and cutting edge act successively. Then the dentist places himself on the right side, passing his left arm over the head of the person upon whom he will operate: the thumb of the left hand is placed on the lower incisors and the index finger on the lip to depress it.

One begins the operation with the incisors of the lower jaw because they are usually the most covered with tartar. In operating, one places the back of the instrument on the index finger of the left hand which serves to support it: it is with the cutting edges of this instrument that one easily removes the tartarous matter by short, light repeated movements from below upwards. One follows the same method during the whole operation without changing the position previously indicated. One should not change it nor should one place oneself in front of the patient except to clean the right side of the mouth. Then one places the index finger of the left hand on the commissure of the lips on the right side to separate the cheek from the teeth. Then one places the cutting edge of the instrument against the tooth which should be cleaned first, and one removes the tartar from below upwards as lightly as possible. The teeth which are loose should be supported by the finger which is nearest and the tartar removed from above downwards or from the side.

After one removes that which is on the outside of the teeth one takes off that which is on the inside. It is necessary for the dentist to continue to be situated in the same way. Having lowered the lip with the index finger he places the thumb on the incisors if they are not firm, and, to begin with them, he holds the instrument as described; he presses on the neighboring teeth which serve as a fulcrum and facilitate his movement. He continues to act in the same manner until the last tooth of the left side. Then changing his position to clean the other side of the teeth, he passes from the right of the patient to the left. He brings the index finger of

the left hand onto the teeth that he wishes to clean first, and, successively, he carries the instrument onto the teeth situated after those where he started. He operates on this side as he has done on the other; with this difference, that he brings the end of the index finger of the left hand to the side of the last molar so that the instrument passes from one tooth to the next.

When the dentist has finished with the chisel (donkey beak) all that can be removed by it, he takes the parrot beak, places himself in front of the patient and pulls down the lower lip with the index finger of the left hand. He then brings the point of this instrument between the interior spaces that the teeth form between them. He holds it similarly to the preceding; with this difference, that the hollow of its point should face towards the hand which holds it and that the handle is raised upwards to remove the tartar. As he passes from one tooth to the other, he continues to support the adjacent teeth with the index finger of the left hand.

After he has used the parrot beak in operating in the interdental spaces he takes the graver with three faces to remove towards the outside whatever matter is between these spaces. He places himself on the right side of the patient, he pulls down the lower lip and inserts the point of the instrument which he holds in the same way as the two preceding instruments and he works it in these spaces. It must be observed that the bevel which is at its end should be turned upwards so as to facilitate the removal of the tartar. One follows the same method for all the spaces as required, separating the lips and cheeks as much as necessary and taking the most comfortable positions.

When he has finished with the three-faced graver, he takes the small knife with the convex blade. He holds it in the same way as before and he turns its cutting edge upwards, so that being on the right side of the patient he inserts this instrument successively in the interdental space between each tooth to remove whatever the other instruments did not remove.

When one has finished with the small knife, one shall use, if necessary, the Z shaped hook, to remove from the interior surface of the teeth that which the others could not reach. The dentist places himself for this on the right side or in front of the patient, he holds the instrument in his right hand, and lowering the end of the hook which should face the hand and approaching there, he passes it onto the inner surfaces of the teeth to detach everything that he wishes to remove.

After having used this last instrument for the inner surfaces of the teeth, it can also be used to remove the material attached to their crowns. The lips and cheeks again should be adjusted with the index finger of the left hand, while the right holds the instrument to remove all that is present on the crowns of the teeth.

The same instruments used for cleaning the teeth of the lower jaw are also used for cleaning those of the upper, being equally convenient for one or the other jaw.

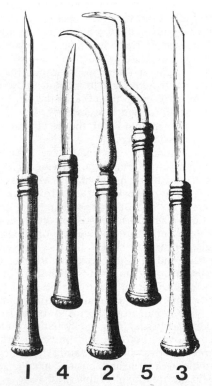

Figure 5 The five types of instruments used by Fauchard for detaching tartar from the teeth: *1,* chisel; *2,* parrot beak; *3,* graver; *4,* convex blade; *5,* Z-shaped hook.

xxii   The Historical Background of Periodontology

John Hunter (1728–1793), the most distinguished anatomist, surgeon, and pathologist of
eighteenth-century England, wrote an excellent treatise on dentistry entitled *The Natural
History of the Human Teeth*.[17] He offered
remarkably clear illustrations of the anatomy
of the teeth and their supporting structures.
He described the features of periodontal diseases and enunciated the concept of active and
passive eruption of teeth. "Though the wasting
of the alveoli at their mouths, and the filling
up at their bottoms, are to be considered as
diseases, when they happen early in life, yet it
would appear to be only on account of a
natural effect taking place too soon."

A contemporary of Hunter, Thomas Berdmore (1740–1785), was considered the outstanding dentist in England and was known as
"Dentist to His Majesty." He published a
*Treatise on the Disorders and Deformities of
the Teeth and Gums* in 1770, with several
chapters devoted to periodontal problems.[4] In
Chapter 7, "Of Tartar of the Teeth, and the
Recess of the Gums, and Toothache Occa-
sioned by Tartarous Concretions Long Neglected," he offers detailed descriptions of
instrumentation for tartar removal, but stresses
prevention. He also uses surgery, when necessary, to remove hyperplastic gingival tissue
once the tartar is removed. "for without this,
the gums will not closely embrace a tooth
which has been made smaller at the collar by
the removal of its tartar."

The first qualified American dentists were,
essentially, trained in England or France.[30]
Robert Woffendale was trained by Berdmore
and wrote one of the early dental books in
America. In an advertisement in the *New York
Weekly Journal* of 1766 he "begs Leave to
inform the Public that he performs all Operations upon the Teeth, Gums, Sockets and
Palate." Similar advertisements were placed
by many contemporary dentists. John Baker
was one of George Washington's dentists and
had a very successful career. He imparted his
dental knowledge to Paul Revere, Isaac
Greenwood, and Josiah Flagg. In an advertisement in the *New York Weekly Journal* of 1768,
he tells the public that he

cures the scurvy in the gums, be it ever so bad;
first cleans and scales the teeth from that corrosive
tartarous gritty substance, which hinders the gums
from growing, infects the breath and is one of the
principle causes of the scurvy, and, if not timely
prevented, eats away the gums so that many people's teeth fall out fresh. . . . His dentifrice, with
proper directions for preserving the teeth and gums
is to be had at his lodgings.

The best-known French dentists in Revolu-
tionary America were Jean Pierre LeMayeur,
who became a close friend of Washington, and
Jacques Gardette, who practiced in Philadelphia and knew Rush, Shippen, and the other
eminent physicians of the time.

In the nineteenth century, John W. Riggs
(1811–1885) offered a comprehensive discussion of periodontal disease and its treatment.[24]
For many years afterward periodontitis, or
"alveolar pyorrhea," was known in America
as Riggs' disease. Riggs was an associate of
Horace Wells in Hartford, and it is of interest
that he performed the first surgical operation
under anesthesia, extracting a tooth of Dr.
Wells under nitrous oxide in 1844. His description of periodontal therapy in his paper of 1876
is worth quoting.[24]

The teeth in perfect polish and cleanliness, at and
under the margin of the gums, whether of animals
or man, produce no inflamed action in that tissue.
It can be artificially produced, however, by inserting
a foreign body into or beneath its substance. If then
diseased action can be set up by a foreign body,
artificially introduced, it can be arrested and cured
by withdrawing the same. And, therefore, if the
tooth becomes an extraneous body by reason of the
accretions and concretions upon it, near and under
the free margin of the gum, and inflammation
ensues, as it certainly will, the true prophylactic and
pathologic treatment surely would be to thoroughly
and carefully remove said concretion, tartar or
roughness—polish the tooth and let nature take
care of the rest. In two hours time the inflamed and
bleeding gum will assume a lighter color, its swollen
tissue will begin to shrink to its normal thickness,
will grow more tense and firm, and in twenty to
thirty hours will grasp the neck of the tooth to the
exclusion of all foreign substances.
I have thus pointed out the treatment of the
disease in the first stage.
The treatment of the second stage is the same,
only being careful to reach the extreme limits of the
disease action, breaking up the diseased tissue and
removing every particle of tartar from the tooth,
and necrosed bone from edge or margin of process.
The third stage presents greater difficulties from
the greater depth of the active line of disease, and
demands a firm and skilled hand, a delicate and
nice touch, and, I might add, the transfer of the
sense of sight to the fingerends. The sense of touch
must be so trained and cultivated that all foreign
bodies can be readily distinguished from tooth substance—live bone from necrosed bone—healthy
from diseased tissue. This manipulation cannot be
attained at once, but time and practice, with close
and earnest study, will qualify and school the hand,
and embolden the true and sensitive mind to achieve
success in the treatment of this third stage.
Of the treatment of the fourth and last stage,
little can be said, except that the loss of the tooth
or teeth is inevitable.

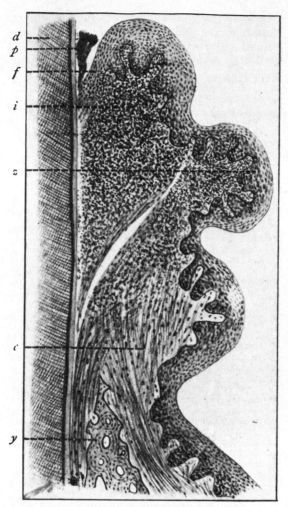

Figure 6 Microscopic features of periodontal disease as presented by Znamensky.

The major advance in the nineteenth century was an understanding of the pathogenesis of periodontal disease, based upon histopathologic studies.

Znamensky, in Moscow, understood the complex interaction of local and systemic factors in the etiology of periodontal disease[31] (Fig. 6). His observations and concepts were summarized in 1902 in a classic paper, "Alveolar Pyorrhoea—Its Pathological Anatomy and Its Radical Treatment."

The microscopical examination of a series of preparations has given very interesting results. By examining them one could follow, degree by degree, the progressive development of the pathological process, beginning by the very first step, when the irritation of the gum margin is only commencing. Upon every preparation there exists a deposit of tartar under the gum. A very hard, swollen rim of the gum resembling a fungus excrescence appears strongly infiltrated, but not having yet lost its epithelial coat upon its free surface. The infiltration

with white blood corpuscles is still not deep, it embraces almost exclusively the papillary layer of the gum; the bone of the socket is yet normal. In Fig. 2 one sees a further expansion of the disease; the swollen and infiltrated rim of the gum loses its epithelial covering and a sore surface is formed. The infiltration with white blood corpuscles is getting deeper, and well nigh comes up to the free edge of the socket. . . . The socket loses lime salts and gets transformed into an osteoid tissue and afterwards into a fibrous intervening (uniting) tissue. Directly this is done the infiltration with white blood corpuscles begins. Those places of the thin socket which began to lose lime, when magnified by the aid of a microscope, present a uniform, homogeneous, semi-lucid mass, in which no bony laminae are to be seen; and the bone corpuscles, lessened in their number, have lost their characteristic forms and have become more and more like the cells of an intervening tissue. But the destructive process has here another peculiarity, namely, besides the bone losing its salts, the so-called lacunar absorption of bone is here more acutely expressed than in the marrowless part of the socket. The absorption proceeds from the side of the periosteum of the socket, and also from the Haversian canals. Here near to the surface of the laminae appear large multi-nucleated cells (osteoclasts), in consequence of which there are some hollow places formed in the bone, which bear the name of Howship's lacunae.

Znamensky treated pyorrhea with removal of calculus and also deep curettage of the sockets, using cocaine anesthesia.

In all, the work with each socket took from five to fifteen minutes, according to the degree the bone was affected. In cases of deeply affected bones, when the acting instrument went too deep into the thickness of the bone—more than a centimetre from the upper front teeth—one could not, of course, succeed in scraping out the whole diseased area to perfect smoothness at once, so in these cases, sometimes a few months after, the operation around those teeth was repeated.

The scraped-out particles present a granular tissue, wherein there are to be found some fragments of dead bone sensible to the touch when rubbed between the fingers, just as in a rarefying osteitis.

This work was extended by Fleischmann and Gottlieb in Vienna in the early twentieth century. They offered clear photomicrographic illustrations of a variety of cases of periodontal disease and stressed the importance of histopathology in gaining a better understanding of the nature of the disease[14] (Fig. 7).

Without belittling the significance of the clinic for the investigation of a disease, we are still forced to insist on the most exact regard for the pathological anatomy as an obvious and urgent prerequisite. All authors who have left this condition unfulfilled have been building only upon sand. This holds good

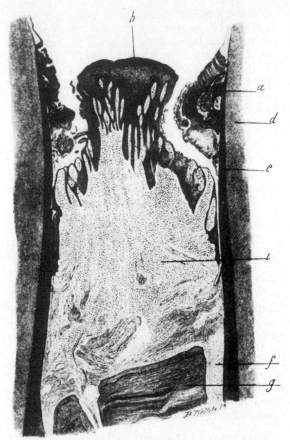

Figure 7 Histopathology of periodontitis, as illustrated by Fleischmann and Gottlieb.

especially for the decision of the long-contested question of the etiological relationship of the two chief symptoms of pyorrhea alveolaris—the absorption of the bone and the suppurative exudate from the gingival pocket. Is the absorption of the bony alveolus the primary causal factor, followed secondarily by the suppuration, or is the suppuration (i.e., the inflammation responsible therefor) the primary factor which secondarily induces the alveolar absorption?

Other contemporary investigators who broadened the etiologic concepts of periodontal disease by pathologic studies were Talbot, Hopewell-Smith, Orban, Box, Becks, Weski, and Simonton.

The major advances of the twentieth century, however, have been in the field of experimental pathology. Animal models of periodontal disease, involving both local and systemic factors, were developed and studied by many investigators. Irving Glickman was a prominent researcher of this period.

The microbiology of periodontal disease has also received considerable attention in recent years, with advances in germ-free research, antibiotic therapy, and immunologic concepts.

Much of the exciting current and recent research in the field of periodontology is presented and discussed in this book.

REFERENCES

1. Albucasis: La Chirurgie. Translated by Lucien LeClerc. Paris, Balliere, 1861.
2. Artzney Buchlein. Leipzig, Michael Blum, 1530. English translation in Dent. Cosmos, *29*:1, 1887.
3. Avicenna: Liber Canonis. Venice, 1507. Reprinted, Hildesheim, Georg Olms, 1964.
4. Berdmore, T.: A Treatise on the Disorders and Deformities of the Teeth and Gums. London, B. White, 1786.
5. Breasted, J. H.: The Edwin Smith Surgical Papyrus. 2 vols. Chicago, University of Chicago Press, 1930.
6. Castiglione, A.: History of Medicine. 2nd ed. New York, Alfred A. Knopf, 1941.
7. Celsus, A.: De Medicina. 3 vols. Translated by W. G. Spencer. London, Heinemann, 1935–1938.
8. Charaka Samhita. Edited, translated, and published by A. C. Kaviratna. Calcutta, 1892–1905.
9. Dabry, P.: La Medicine chez les Chinois. Paris, Plon, 1863.
10. Dobell, C.: Antony van Leeuwenhoek and His "Little Animals." New York, Harcourt, 1932. Reprinted, New York, Dover Publications, 1960.
11. Ebbel, B.: The Papyrus Ebers. Copenhagen, Levin and Munksgaard, 1937.
12. Eustachius, B.: Libellus de Dentibus. Venice, 1563. Reprinted in facsimile, Vienna, Urban and Schwarzenberg, 1951.
13. Fauchard, P.: Le Chirurgien Dentiste, ou Traite des Dents. 2 vols. Paris, J. Mariette, 1728. Reprinted in facsimile, Paris, Prélat, 1961. *(An English translation by Lillian Lindsay appeared in 1946, published by Butterworth & Company, London.)*
14. Fleischmann, L., and Gottlieb, B.: A contribution to the histology and pathogenesis of pyorrhea alveolaris. Dent. Cosmos, *63*:215, 1921.
15. Guerini, V.: History of Dentistry. Philadelphia, Lea & Febiger, 1909.
16. Hippocrates: Works. 4 vols. Edited and translated by W. H. S. Jones and E. T. Withington. London, Heinemann, 1923–1931.
17. Hunter, J.: The Natural History of the Human Teeth. London, J. Johnson, 1771. Reprinted as Treatise on the Natural History and Diseases of the Human Teeth. *In* Bell, T. (ed.): Collected Works. 4 vols. London, Longman Rees, 1835.
18. Jastrow, N.: The medicine of the Babylonians and Assyrians. Proc. Soc. Med., London, *7*:109, 1914.
19. Major, R. H.: A History of Medicine. 2 vols. Springfield, Ill., Charles C Thomas, 1954.
20. Nicaise, E.: La Grande Chirurgie de Guy de Chauliac. Paris, Alean, 1890.
21. Paré, A.: Oeuvres completes. 3 vols. Edited by J. F. Malgaigne. Paris, Bailliere, 1840–1841.
22. Paul of Aegina: The Seven Books. 3 vols. Translated by F. Adams. London, Sydenham Society, 1844–1847.
23. Pifteau, P.: Chirurgie de Guillaume de Salicet: Traduition et Commentaire. Toulouse, St. Cyprien, 1898.
24. Riggs, J. W.: Suppurative inflammation of the gums and absorption of the gums and alveolar process. Pa. J. Dent. Sci., *3*:99, 1876. Reprinted in Arch. Clin. Oral Pathol., *2*:423, 1938.
25. Ruffer, M. A.: Studies in the Palaeopathology of Egypt. Chicago, University of Chicago Press, 1921.
26. Shklar, G.: Stomatology and dentistry in the golden age of Arabian medicine. Bull. Hist. Dent., *17*:17, 1969.
27. Susruta Samhita. 3 vols. Edited, translated, and published by K. K. L. Bhishagratna. Calcutta, 1907–1916.
28. Van Leeuwenhoek, A.: Arcana Naturae. Delphis Batavorum, 1695. Reprinted in facsimile, Brussels, Culture et Civilisation, 1966.
29. Vesalius, A.: De Humani Corporis Fabrica. Basle, 1542. Reprinted in facsimile, Brussels, Culture et Civilisation, 1964.
30. Weinberger, B. W.: An Introduction to the History of Dentistry. 2 vols. St. Louis, C. V. Mosby Company, 1948.
31. Znamensky, N.: Alveolar pyorrhoea—its pathological anatomy and its radical treatment. J. Br. Dent. Assoc., *23*:585, 1902.

THE TISSUES OF THE PERIODONTIUM

The periodontium consists of the investing and supporting tissues of the tooth *(gingiva, periodontal ligament, cementum,* and *alveolar bone)*. The cementum is considered a part of the periodontium because, with the bone, it serves as the support for the fibers of the periodontal ligament. The periodontium is subject to morphologic and functional variations, as well as changes associated with age. This section deals with the normal features of the tissues of the periodontium, knowledge of which is necessary for an understanding of periodontal disease.

The Gingiva

The *oral mucosa* consists of three zones: the gingiva and the covering of the hard palate, termed the **masticatory mucosa;** the dorsum of the tongue, covered by **specialized mucosa;** and the oral mucous membrane lining the remainder of the oral cavity. *The gingiva is the part of the oral mucosa that covers the alveolar processes of the jaws and surrounds the necks of the teeth.*

NORMAL CLINICAL FEATURES

The gingiva is divided anatomically into the marginal, attached, and interdental areas.

The Marginal Gingiva (Unattached Gingiva)

The marginal (unattached) gingiva is the terminal edge or border of the gingiva surrounding the teeth in collar-like fashion (Figs. 1–1 and 1–2). In about 50 per cent of cases it is demarcated from the adjacent attached gingiva by a shallow linear depression, the **free gingival groove.**[3] Usually about 1 mm wide, it forms the soft tissue wall of the gingival sulcus. It may be separated from the tooth surface with a periodontal probe.

The Gingival Sulcus

The gingival sulcus is the shallow crevice or space around the tooth bounded by the surface of the tooth on one side and the epithelium lining the free margin of the gingiva on the other. It is V-shaped and barely permits the entrance of a periodontal probe. The clinical determination of the depth of the gingival sulcus is an important diagnostic parameter. Under absolutely normal conditions, the depth of the gingival sulcus is 0 or about 0.[53, 115] These strict conditions of normalcy can be produced experimentally only in germ-free animals[5] or after intense, prolonged plaque control.[8, 78]

However, in clinically healthy gingiva in man or animals a sulcus of some depth can be found. The depth of this sulcus as determined in histologic sections has been reported as 1.8 mm, with variations from 0 to 6 mm[105]; other studies have reported 1.5 mm[154] and 0.69 mm.[46] The clinical maneuver used to determine the depth of the sulcus is the introduction of a metallic instrument and the estimation of the distance it penetrates. It should be clearly understood that the **histologic depth** of a sulcus need not be and is not exactly equal to the depth of penetration of the probe. The so-

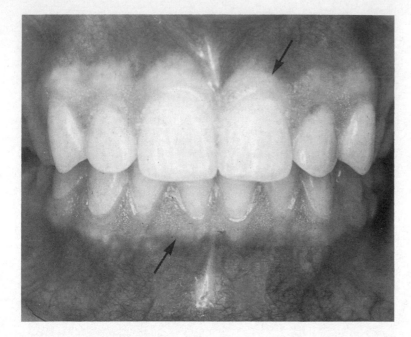

Figure 1–1 Normal Gingiva in Young Adult. Note the demarcation (mucogingival line) (*arrows*) between the attached gingiva and darker alveolar mucosa.

called **probing depth** of a clinically normal gingival sulcus in man is 2 to 3 mm.

The Attached Gingiva

The attached gingiva is continuous with the marginal gingiva. It is firm, resilient, and tightly bound to the underlying periosteum of alveolar bone. The facial aspect of the attached gingiva extends to the relatively loose and movable alveolar mucosa, from which it is demarcated by the *mucogingival junction* (Fig. 1–2).

The **width of the attached gingiva** is an important clinical parameter. *It is the distance between the mucogingival junction and the projection on the external surface of the bottom of the gingival sulcus or the periodontal pocket.* It should not be confused with the width of the keratinized gingiva because the latter also includes the marginal gingiva (Fig. 1–2).

The width of the attached gingiva on the facial aspect differs in different areas of the mouth.[19] It is generally greatest in the incisor region (3.5 to 4.5 mm in the maxilla and 3.3 to 3.9 mm in the mandible) and less in the posterior segments, with the least width in the first premolar area (1.9 mm in the maxilla and 1.8 mm in the mandible)[3] (Fig. 1–3).

Because the mucogingival junction remains stationary throughout adult life,[1] changes in

gingival sulcus
FREE OR MARGINAL GINGIVA
marginal groove

ATTACHED GINGIVA

mucogingival junction

ALVEOLAR MUCOSA

Figure 1–2 Diagram showing anatomic landmarks of the gingiva.

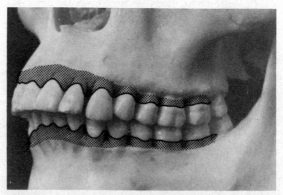

Figure 1–3 Mean width of attached gingiva in human permanent dentition. (Data from Ainamo, A., and Löe, H.: J. Periodontol., *37*:5, 1966.)

the width of the attached gingiva are due to modifications in the position of its coronal end. The width of the attached gingiva increases with age[4] and in supraerupted teeth.[2] On the lingual aspect of the mandible, the attached gingiva terminates at the junction with the lingual alveolar mucosa, which is continuous with the mucous membrane lining the floor of the mouth. The palatal surface of the attached gingiva in the maxilla blends imperceptibly with the equally firm, resilient palatal mucosa.

The Interdental Gingiva

The interdental gingiva occupies the **gingival embrasure,** which is the interproximal space beneath the area of tooth contact. It usually consists of two papillae, one facial and one lingual, and the *col*.[32] The latter is a *valley-like depression which connects the papillae and conforms to the shape of the interproximal contact area* (Figs. 1–4 and 1–5). When teeth are not in contact, the col is often absent. Even when teeth are in contact, the col may be absent in some individuals (Fig. 1–6).

Each interdental papilla is pyramidal; the facial and lingual surfaces are tapered toward the interproximal contact area, and the mesial and distal surfaces are slightly concave. The lateral borders and tip of the interdental papillae are formed by a continuation of the marginal gingiva from the adjacent teeth. The

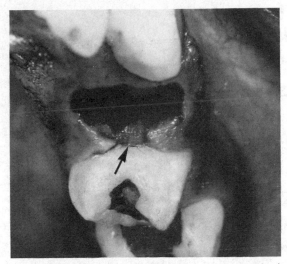

Figure 1–4 Site of extraction showing the facial and palatal interdental papillae and the intervening col (*arrow*).

intervening portion consists of attached gingiva (Fig. 1–7).

In the absence of proximal tooth contact, the gingiva is firmly bound over the interdental bone and forms a smooth rounded surface without interdental papillae (Fig. 1–8).

NORMAL MICROSCOPIC FEATURES

The gingiva consists of a central core of connective tissue covered by stratified squa-

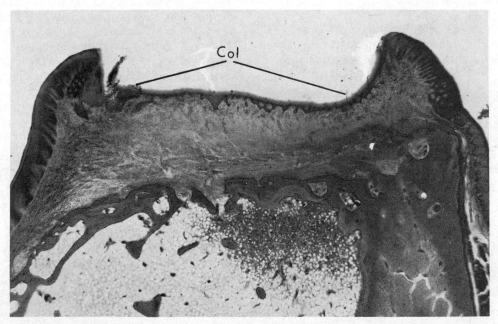

Figure 1–5 Faciolingual Section (Monkey) Showing Col Between the Facial and Lingual Interdental Papillae. The col is covered with nonkeratinized stratified squamous epithelium.

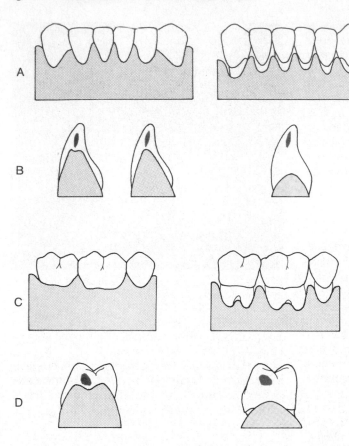

Figure 1–6 Diagram comparing anatomic variations of the interdental col in the normal gingiva (left side) and after gingival recession (right side). *A* and *B,* Mandibular anterior segment, facial and buccolingual views, respectively. *C* and *D,* Mandibular posterior region, facial and buccolingual views, respectively. Tooth contact points are shown in *B* and *D.*

mous epithelium. These two tissues will be considered separately.

Gingival Epithelium

Three areas of epithelium exist in the gingiva: the oral or outer epithelium, the sulcular epithelium, and the junctional epithelium.

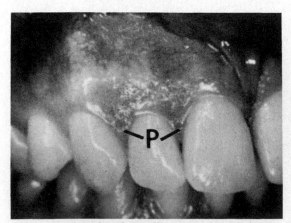

Figure 1–7 Interdental Papillae with Central Portion Formed by Attached Gingiva. The shape of the papillae (P) varies according to the dimension of the gingival embrasure.

ORAL OR OUTER EPITHELIUM. The oral or outer epithelium covers the crest and outer surface of the marginal gingiva and the surface of the attached gingiva. *It consists of keratinized or parakeratinized stratified squamous epithelium.* As such, it has a cuboidal or columnar basal layer, a spinous layer composed of polygonal cells, sometimes a granular layer consisting of flattened cells with basophilic keratohyaline granules and a somewhat shrunken hyperchromic nucleus, and a superficial layer that may be keratinized or parakeratinized (Fig. 1–9).

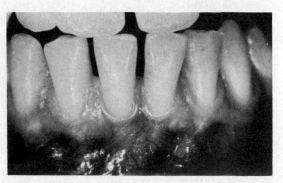

Figure 1–8 Absence of interdental papillae and col where proximal tooth contact is missing.

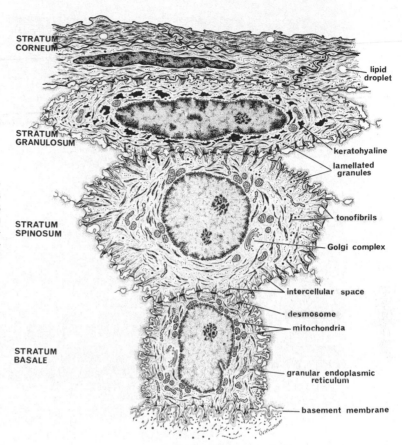

STRATUM
CORNEUM

lipid
droplet

STRATUM
GRANULOSUM

keratohyaline

lamellated
granules

STRATUM
SPINOSUM

tonofibrils

Golgi complex

intercellular space

desmosome

mitochondria

STRATUM
BASALE

granular endoplasmic
reticulum

basement membrane

Figure 1–9 Diagram showing representative cells from the various layers of stratified squamous epithelium as seen by electron microscopy. (From A. Weinstock. *In* Ham, A. W.: Histology, 7th ed. Philadelphia, J. B. Lippincott Company, 1974.)

The gingival epithelium is similar in structure to epidermis. In the female, a large Feulgen-positive particle has been found adjacent to the nuclear membrane in 75 per cent of the examined cells; in the male, a similar but smaller particle is present in 1 to 2 per cent of the cells.[90]

Electron microscopy reveals that the cells of the gingival epithelium are connected to each other by structures along the cell periphery called *desmosomes*.[80] These desmosomes have a typical structure consisting of two dense *attachment plaques* into which tonofilaments insert and an intermediate electron-dense line in the extracellular space. Tonofibrils radiate in brush-like fashion from the attachment plaques into the cytoplasm of the cells. The space between the cells shows cytoplasmic projections resembling microvilli that extend into the intercellular space and often interdigitate.

Less frequently observed forms of epithelial cell connections[135, 150, 155] have been reported to represent *tight junctions* (zonulae occludens), areas where the membranes of adjoining cells are believed to be fused; nevertheless, experimental evidence to verify this hypothesis for gingival epithelium is lacking. It is possible that these structures represent either patches of membrane fusion (rather than a zonula) or gap junctions. There is evidence suggesting that these structures allow ions and small molecules to pass from one cell to another.

The epithelium is joined to the underlying connective tissue by a *basal lamina* 300 to 400 Å thick which lies approximately 400 Å beneath the basal epithelial layer.[75, 117, 127] The basal lamina consists of lamina lucida and lamina densa. The lamina densa is composed in part of glycoprotein.[73] Hemidesmosomes of the basal epithelial cells abut the lamina lucida.

The basal lamina is synthesized by the basal epithelial cells and consists of a polysaccharide-protein complex and collagen (reticulin) fibers.[101] Anchoring fibrils (also a component of what is believed to be reticulin) extend from the underlying connective tissue into the basal lamina, and some penetrate through the lamina densa and lamina lucida to the membrane of the basal epithelial cells.[131] The basal lamina is permeable to fluids but acts as a barrier to particulate matter (Fig. 1–10).

SULCULAR EPITHELIUM. The sulcular epithelium lines the gingival sulcus (Figs. 1–11

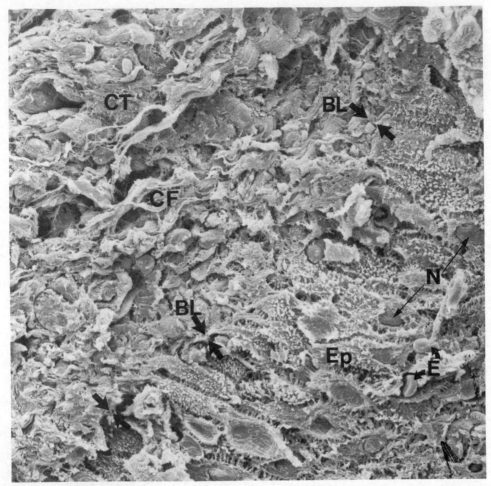

Figure 1–10 Scanning electron microscopic view of sectioned normal human gingiva. The lower right portion of the photograph shows the epithelium (Ep), and the upper right region shows the connective tissue (CT). The basement lamina (BL) can be seen between arrows. Note the intercellular spaces of the epithelium and the collagen fibers (CF). N, nucleus of epithelial cell; E, erythrocytes, ×3000.

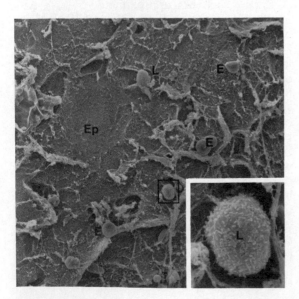

Figure 1–11 Scanning electron microscopic view of epithelial surface facing the tooth in a normal human gingival sulcus. The epithelium (Ep) shows desquamating cells, some scattered erythrocytes (E), and a few emerging leukocytes (L). ×1000. Inset shows leukocyte, probably a lymphocyte. ×6000.

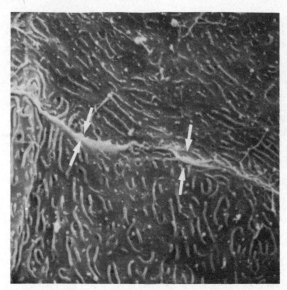

Figure 1–12 Scanning electron microscopic view of boundary (*arrows*) between two epithelial cells in normal human gingival sulcus. × 20,000.

and 1–12). It is a thin, nonkeratinized stratified squamous epithelium without rete pegs (Fig. 1–13) and extends from the coronal limit of the junctional epithelium to the crest of the gingival margin. This epithelium does not keratinize under normal circumstances, probably owing to continuous irritation by subclinical amounts of plaque. When everted into the oral cavity,[26] or after intensive antibacterial therapy,[27] it regains its keratinized surface.

The sulcular epithelium is extremely important, because it may act as a semipermeable membrane through which injurious bacterial products pass into the gingiva and tissue fluid from the gingiva seeps into the sulcus.[134]

JUNCTIONAL EPITHELIUM. The junctional epithelium consists of a collar-like band of stratified squamous nonkeratinizing epithelium. It is three to four layers thick in early life, but the number of layers increases with age to 10 or even 20; its length ranges from 0.25 to 1.35 mm (Fig. 1–14).

Figure 1–13 An Epon-embedded human biopsy specimen showing a relatively normal gingival sulcus. The soft tissue wall of the gingival sulcus is made up of the oral sulcular epithelium (ose) and its underlying connective tissue (ct), whereas the base of the gingival sulcus is formed by the sloughing surface of the junctional epithelium (je). The enamel space is delineated by a dense cuticular structure (dc). There is a relatively sharp line of demarcation between the junctional epithelium and the oral sulcular epithelium (*arrow*), and several polymorphonuclear leukocytes (pmn) can be seen traversing the junctional epithelium. The sulcus contains red blood cells resulting from the hemorrhage occurring at the time of biopsy. × 391; inset × 55. (From Schluger, S., Youdelis, R., and Page, R. C.: Periodontal Disease. Philadelphia, Lea & Febiger, 1977.)

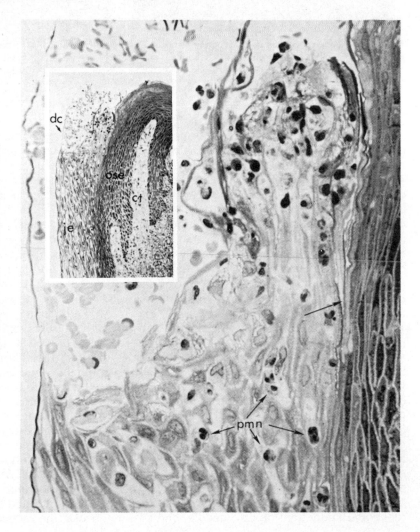

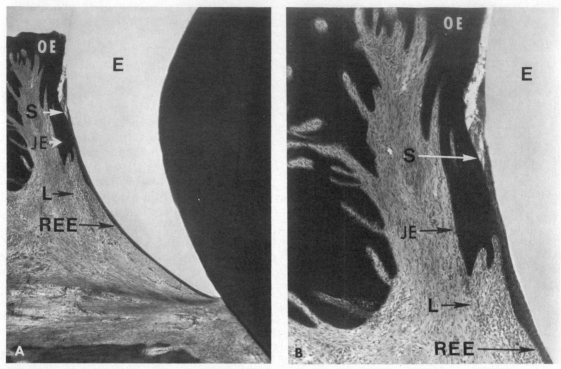

Figure 1–14 Gingival Sulcus in an Erupting Monkey Tooth. *A,* Gingival sulcus (S), the enamel (E), and the junctional epithelium (JE). Note the oral epithelium (OE), the reduced enamel epithelium (REE), and the leukocytic infiltration (L). *B,* High-power section showing the base of the sulcus (S), the enamel (E), and the junctional epithelium (JE). Leukocytic infiltration (L) usually present in clinically normal gingiva is shown beneath the base of the sulcus. Tissues within the sulcus are artifact and debris.

The epithelial attachment of the junctional epithelium consists of a basal lamina (basement membrane)[81] that is comparable to that which attaches epithelium to connective tissue elsewhere in the body. The basal lamina consists of a lamina densa (adjacent to the enamel) and a lamina lucida to which hemidesmosomes are attached (Fig. 1–15). Organic strands from the enamel appear to extend into the lamina densa.[129] The junctional epithelium attaches to afibrillar cementum when it is present on the crown (usually restricted to an area within 1 mm of the cemento-enamel junction)[116] (Fig. 1–15) and to root cementum in a similar manner.

Cell layers not juxtaposed to the tooth exhibit numerous free ribosomes and prominent membrane-bound structures such as Golgi complexes, lysosome-like bodies, and cytoplasmic vacuoles, presumably phagocytic.[158] Similar morphology has been described in germ-free rats. Polymorphonuclear neutrophil leukocytes are found routinely in the junctional epithelium of both conventional and germ-free rats.[158]

Three zones have been described in the junctional epithelium: apical, middle, and co-ronal. The apical zone shows cells with germinative characteristics, the middle zone is one of major adhesiveness, and the coronal zone is one of greater permeability[112] (Fig. 1–16).

Histochemical evidence for the presence of neutral polysaccharides in the zone of the epithelial attachment has been reported.[139] Data have also shown that the basal lamina of the junctional epithelium resembles that of endothelial and epithelial cells in its glycoprotein content, and it has been suggested that it plays a key role in the adhesion mechanism.[71–73]

The attachment of the junctional epithelium to the tooth is reinforced by the gingival fibers, which brace the marginal gingiva against the tooth surface. For this reason the junctional epithelium and the gingival fibers are considered a functional unit, referred to as the **dentogingival unit.**

DEVELOPMENT OF THE GINGIVAL SULCUS. After enamel formation is complete, the enamel is covered with reduced enamel epithelium which is attached to the tooth by a basal lamina. Hemidesmosomes can be seen on the apical plasma membrane of the reduced ameloblasts.[82, 128] When the tooth penetrates the oral mucosa, the reduced enamel epithelium unites

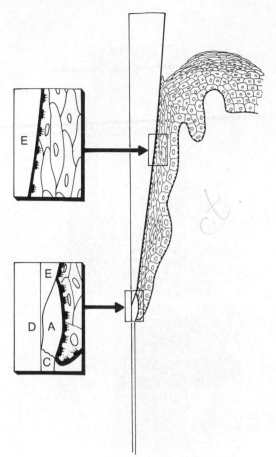

Figure 1–15 Diagram of the dentogingival junction showing the junctional epithelium adhering to the tooth surface. At upper left, an enlarged view of epithelial cells showing hemidesmosomes in those cells along the enamel (E) surface. Intervening between the epithelial cells and the enamel are the basal lamina and dental cuticle, respectively; both of these structures are represented by the single, thick line along the enamel. At lower left, an enlarged view of the cemento-enamel junction showing a small area of afibrillar cementum (A). C, cementum; D, dentin.

with the oral epithelium to form what Gottlieb termed the **epithelial attachment**[51, 52] and described as being organically attached to the enamel. According to current terminology,[116] the united epithelium is called the **"junctional epithelium,"** whereas the *epithelial attachment refers to the union of the epithelial cells with the tooth surfaces.* As the tooth erupts, this united epithelium condenses along the crown. The reduced (shortened) ameloblasts, which form the inner layer of the reduced enamel epithelium (see Fig. 1–13), disappear and are gradually replaced by squamous epithelial cells. The junctional epithelium forms a collar around the fully erupted tooth, which is attached to the enamel in the same manner as the ameloblasts it displaced.

The junctional epithelium is a continually *self-renewing structure* with mitotic activity occurring in all cell layers.[92] The regenerating epithelial cells move toward the tooth surface and along it in a coronal direction to the gingival sulcus, where they are shed[13] (Fig. 1–17). The migrating daughter cells provide a continuous attachment to the tooth surface. Although the epithelial attachment, composed of hemidesmosomes and the basal lamina, represents the biologic bond of the junctional epithelium to the tooth surface, the strength of the attachment has not been measured.

The gingival sulcus is formed when the tooth erupts into the oral cavity. At that time the junctional epithelium and reduced enamel epithelium together form a broad band that is attached to the tooth surface from near the tip of the crown to the cemento-enamel junction.

The gingival sulcus is the shallow V-shaped space or groove between the tooth and gingiva that encircles the newly erupted tip of the crown. In the fully erupted tooth, only the junctional epithelium persists. *The sulcus consists of the shallow space that is coronal to the attachment of the junctional epithelium and is bounded by the tooth on one side and the sulcular epithelium on the other.* The coronal extent of the gingival sulcus is the gingival margin.

Historical Note. A brief description of the historical evolution of our concepts of the gingival sulcus and the junctional epithelium appears to be in order owing to the great controversies that the subject has aroused and its great biologic and clinical importance. The prevailing theory until the 1960s described a virtual space between the epithelium and the tooth surface and therefore located the bottom of the gingival sulcus at the apical end of the junctional epithelium. This theory was advocated initially by Bödecker,[18] Black,[17] and many others[103, 130] and was given additional impetus in the 1950s by Waerhaug[145] and others.[32, 85] It was challenged in 1921 by Gottlieb[51] who thought that the epithelium was attached to the tooth and the bottom of the sulcus situated in the coronal end of the junctional epithelium. Gottlieb's idea was supported by others,[12, 88, 137, 144] and considerable controversy developed (Fig. 1–18). Several authors presented different variants of Gottlieb's ideas. Weski,[154] Gross[57] and Wodehouse[157] contended that the gingival sulcus was formed by a split in the epithelial attachment (intraepithelial split) rather than by separation from the tooth. Becks[14] and Skillen[123] maintained that the reduced enamel epithelium degenerated and dis-

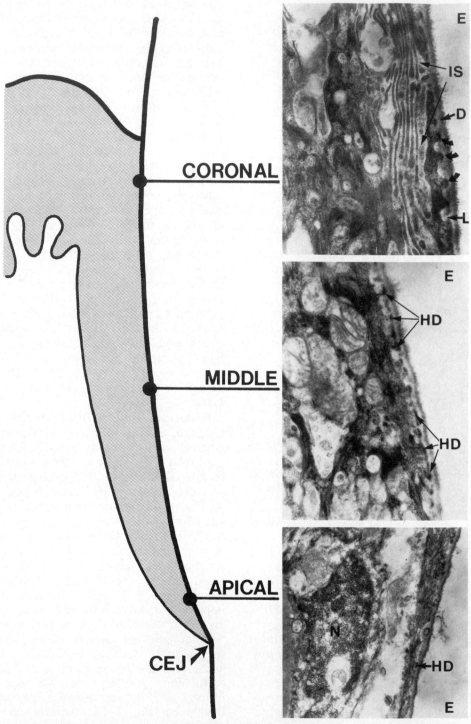

Figure 1–16 Electron microscopic view of human junctional epithelium attached to enamel (E). *Top,* Coronal region. Area of greater permeability characterized by numerous intercellular spaces (IS), some of which open directly to the internal basement lamina. D, lamina densa; L, lamina lucida. Curved arrows point to hemidesmosomes. × 20,000. *Middle,* Area of greater attachment with a greater number of hemidesmosomes (HD). × 20,000. *Bottom,* Apical region. This area contains fewer hemidesmosomes and cells with germinative characteristics. N, cell nucleus. × 14,000.

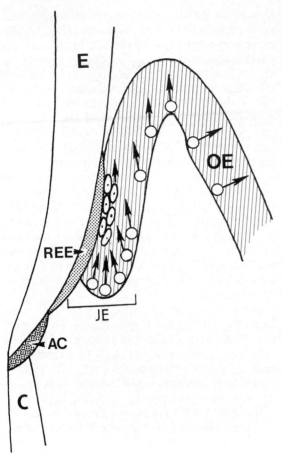

Figure 1–17 Junctional epithelium on an erupting tooth. The junctional epithelium (JE) is formed by the joining of the oral epithelium (OE) and the reduced enamel epithelium (REE). Afibrillar cementum, sometimes formed on enamel after degeneration of the reduced enamel epithelium, is shown at AC. The arrows indicate the coronal movement of the regenerating epithelial cells, which multiply more rapidly in the junctional epithelium than in the oral epithelium. E, enamel; C, root cementum. (From Listgarten, M. A.: J. Can. Dent. Assoc., 36:70, 1970.)

A similar cell turnover pattern exists in the fully erupted tooth.

The process involves progressive flattening of the cell, with an increasing prevalence of tonofilaments and intercellular junctions, as well as disappearance of the nucleus and production of keratohyaline granules. For a more detailed description of the process of keratinization, see the review by Bye and Caffesse.[22]

Three types of surface differentiation can occur in gingival epithelium.[25] (1) **Keratinization,** in which the surface cells form scales of keratin and lose their nuclei. Keratohyaline granules appear in the subsurface layer (granular layer or stratum granulosum). (2) **Parakeratinization,** in which the cells of the superficial layers retain their nuclei, albeit pyknotic, but show some signs of being keratinized; the granular layer is absent. (3) **Nonkeratinization,** in which the cells of the surface layers are nucleated and no signs of keratinization are present.

The epithelium covering the outer surface of the marginal gingiva and the attached gingiva

appeared when the gingival sulcus was formed and that it did not persist as an epithelial attachment.

The problem was resolved when electron microscopic techniques to analyze soft and hard tissues together were developed. Listgarten,[81-83] Schroeder,[116] Stern,[127-129] and others clarified this important area of gingival biology and their views are reflected in this chapter.

KERATINIZATION. The process of keratinization involves a sequence of biochemical and morphologic events that occur in the cell as it migrates from the basal layer toward the keratinized surface (Figs. 1–19 and 1–20).

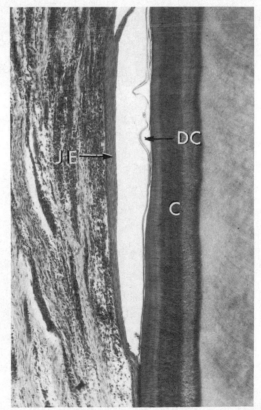

Figure 1–18 "Secondary" cuticle or dental cuticle. In this paraffin section the dental cuticle (DC) consists of both the amorphous, homogeneous layer seen in the electron microscope and surface epithelial cells torn away from the sulcus epithelium. This structure is similar to that which Gottlieb described. C, cementum; JE, junctional epithelium.

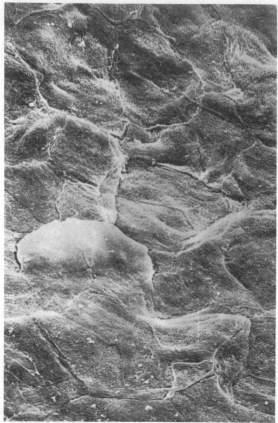

Figure 1–19 Scanning electron micrograph of keratinized gingiva showing the flattened keratinocytes and their boundaries on the surface of the gingiva. × 1000. (From Kaplan, G. B., Pameijer, C. H., and Ruben, M. P.: J. Periodontol., *48*:446, 1977.)

is keratinized or parakeratinized or presents varied combinations of both conditions.[113] The most prevalent type of surface in this area is parakeratinization.[16, 148] The degree of gingival keratinization is not necessarily correlated with the different phases of the menstrual cycle,[67, 98] but it diminishes with age and the onset of menopause.[107] Keratinization of the oral mucosa varies in different areas in the following order: palate (most keratinized), gingiva, tongue, and cheek (least keratinized).[97]

The gingival sulcular epithelium is normally nonkeratinized and usually shows numerous cells with hydropic degeneration.[16] This epithelium, however, has the potential to keratinize if (1) it is reflected and exposed to the oral cavity[20, 26] or (2) the bacterial flora of the sulcus is eliminated.[27] These findings suggest that the *local irritation of the sulcus prevents sulcular keratinization.*

Furthermore, research on free gingival grafts (see Chapter 56) has shown that when connective tissue is transplanted from a keratinized area to a nonkeratinized area it becomes covered by keratinized epithelium.[69] This finding suggests a *connective tissue–based genetic determination of the type of epithelial surface.*

RENEWAL OF GINGIVAL EPITHELIUM. The oral epithelium undergoes continuous renewal. Its thickness is maintained by a balance between new cell formation in the basal and spinous layers and the shedding of old cells at the surface. The mitotic activity exhibits a 24-

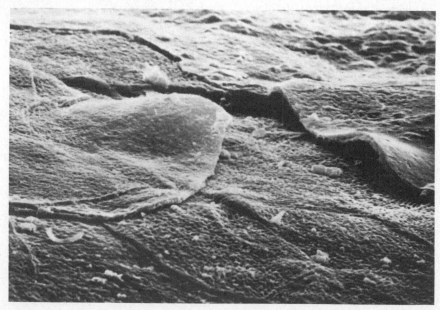

Figure 1–20 Scanning electron micrograph of gingival margin at edge of gingival sulcus showing at close-up view several keratinocytes about to be exfoliated. × 3000. (From Kaplan, G. B., Pameijer, C. H., and Ruben, M. P.: J. Periodontol., *48*:446, 1977.)

hour periodicity, with highest and lowest rates occurring in the morning and evening, respectively.[141] The mitotic rate is higher in nonkeratinized areas and is increased in gingivitis, without significant sex differences. Opinions differ as to whether the mitotic rate is increased[87, 95] or decreased[11] with age.

The mitotic rate in experimental animals varies in different areas of the oral epithelium in the following descending order: buccal mucosa, hard palate, sulcular epithelium, junctional epithelium, outer surface of the marginal gingiva, and attached gingiva.[6, 58, 86, 141] The following have been reported as the turnover times for different areas of the oral epithelium in experimental animals: palate, tongue, and cheek, 5 to 6 days; gingiva, 10 to 12 days, with the same or more time required with age; and junctional epithelium, 1 to 6 days.[13, 124]

CUTICULAR STRUCTURES ON THE TOOTH. The term *cuticle* is used to describe a thin acellular structure with a homogeneous matrix, sometimes enclosed within clearly demarcated linear borders.

Listgarten has classified cuticular structures into coatings of developmental origin and acquired coatings.[84]

The **acquired coatings** include those of exogenous origin, such as saliva, bacteria, calculus, surface stains, and so forth. They will be discussed in Chapters 25 and 32.

The **coatings of developmental origin** are those normally formed as part of tooth development. They include the reduced enamel epithelium, the coronal cementum, the dental cuticle, and the subsurface enamel matrix.

After enamel formation is completed, the ameloblastic epithelium becomes reduced to one or two layers of cells that remain attached to the enamel surface by hemidesmosomes and a basal lamina. This *reduced enamel epithelium* consists of postsecretory ameloblasts and cells from the stratum intermedium of the enamel organ.

In some animal species the reduced enamel epithelium disappears entirely very rapidly, thereby placing the enamel surface in contact with the connective tissue. Connective tissue cells then deposit a thin layer of cementum, known as *coronal cementum,* on the enamel. In man, thin patches of afibrillar cementum may sometimes be seen in the cervical half of the crown.

Electron microscopy has shown a *dental cuticle* consisting of a layer of homogeneous organic material of variable thickness (approximately 0.25 micron) overlying the enamel surface. It is nonmineralized and is not always present. In some instances near the cementoenamel junction, it is deposited over a layer of afibrillar cementum which, in turn, overlies enamel. The cuticle may or may not be present between the junctional epithelium and the tooth. It is believed to be deposited, at least in part, by reduced ameloblasts (see Fig. 1–16), but its origin is still uncertain.[116] Studies have shown that reduced ameloblasts have a secretory function.[149] Some investigators believe that the dental cuticle is a pathologic product of inflamed gingiva[96] or a pathologic conglutination of erythrocytes.[61] Ultrastructural histochemistry has shown it to be of proteinaceous nature.[72]

Listgarten has further described the dental cuticle as a not yet completely mineralized enamel surface, a layer of residual enamel matrix which persists between the densely packed hydroxyapatite crystallites. This material has been called *subsurface enamel matrix.*

Historical Note. The following films on teeth have been described, although at present both the names and the concepts are obsolete.

Nasmyth's Membrane. Described as the "persistent dental capsule" that floats off the surface of enamel dissolved by acids.[102, 133] It may have included several or all of the abovementioned cuticular structures.

Primary Cuticle. Described by Gottlieb as the final secretory product of the ameloblasts, before they degenerate and disappear. It covered only the crown and may have included the coronal cementum, or it may have been an optical image produced by the basal lamina, which is below the resolution limits of the light microscope.

Secondary Cuticle or Dental Cuticle (Cuticula Dentis, Transposed Crevicular Cuticle).[51] This cuticle was believed to be deposited upon the enamel (external to the primary enamel cuticle, with which it supposedly combined) and on the nearby cementum. It was thought to be deposited by the epithelial attachment as it migrated along the tooth and separated from crown and root during eruption stages (see Fig. 1–18). It was not present on cementum to which the periodontal ligament is attached. The secondary cuticle was originally described as keratinized,[53, 74] but this observation has not been supported by subsequent histochemical studies.[152, 153]

GINGIVAL FLUID (SULCULAR FLUID). The gingival sulcus contains a fluid which seeps into it from the gingival connective tissue through the thin sulcular wall.[21, 30, 89] The gingival fluid is believed to (1) cleanse material from the sulcus, (2) contain plasma proteins which may improve adhesion of the epithèlial attachment to the tooth, (3) possess antimicrobial properties, and (4) exert antibody activity in defense of the gingiva.

The gingival fluid and its significance in health and disease will be discussed in detail in Chapter 7.

Gingival Connective Tissue

The connective tissue of the gingiva is known as the *lamina propria.* It is densely collagenous with few elastic fibers. Argyrophilic reticulin fibers ramify between the collagen fibers and are continuous with reticulin in the blood vessel walls.[87] The lamina propria consists of two layers: (1) a *papillary layer* subjacent to the epithelium which consists of papillary projections between the epithelial rete pegs and (2) a *reticular layer* contiguous with the periosteum of the alveolar bone.

GINGIVAL FIBERS. The connective tissue of the marginal gingiva is densely collagenous, containing a prominent system of collagen fiber bundles called the gingival fibers. The gingival fibers have the following functions: to brace the marginal gingiva firmly against the tooth, to provide the rigidity necessary to withstand the forces of mastication without being deflected away from the tooth surface, and to unite the free marginal gingiva with the cementum of the root and the adjacent attached gingiva. The gingival fibers are arranged in three groups: gingivodental, circular, and transseptal.[7, 74]

Gingivodental Group. These are the fibers of the facial, lingual, and interproximal surfaces. They are embedded in the cementum just beneath the epithelium at the base of the gingival sulcus. On the facial and lingual surfaces they project from the cementum in fanlike conformation toward the crest and outer surface of the marginal gingiva and terminate short of the epithelium (Figs. 1–21 and 1–22). They also extend external to the periosteum of the facial and lingual alveolar bone and terminate in the attached gingiva or blend with the periosteum of the bone. Interproximally, the gingivodental fibers extend toward the crest of the interdental gingiva.

Circular Group. These fibers course through the connective tissue of the marginal and interdental gingiva and encircle the tooth in ring-like fashion.

Transseptal Group. Located interproximally, the transseptal fibers form horizontal bundles that extend between the cementum of

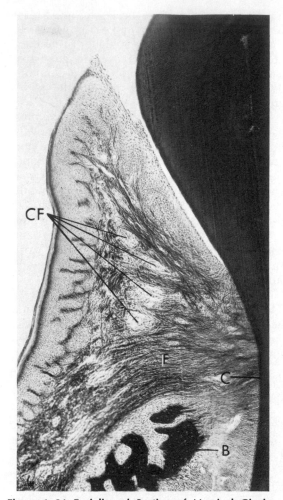

Figure 1–21 Faciolingual Section of Marginal Gingiva, showing gingival fibers (F) extending from the cementum (C) to the crest of the gingiva, to the outer gingival surface, and external to the periosteum of the bone (B). Circular fibers (CF) are shown in cross section between the other groups. (Courtesy of Dr. Sol Bernick.)

approximating teeth into which they are embedded. They lie in the area between the epithelium at the base of the gingival sulcus and the crest of the interdental bone and are sometimes classified with the principal fibers of the periodontal ligament.

CONNECTIVE TISSUE CELLULAR ELEMENTS. The preponderant cellular element in the gingival connective tissue is the *fibroblast.* Numerous fibroblasts are found between the fiber bundles. As in connective tissue elsewhere in the body, fibroblasts synthesize and secrete the collagen fibers, as well as elastin, the noncollagenous proteins, glycoproteins, and glycosaminoglycans. The renewal of collagen fibers and other chemical constituents, and possibly their degradation, is regulated by fibroblasts. Wound healing following gingival surgery or

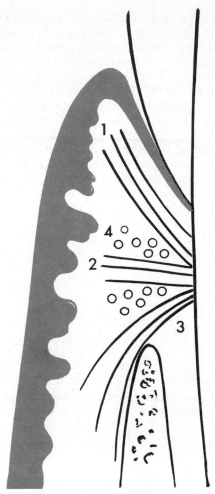

Figure 1–22 Diagrammatic Illustration of the Gingivodental Fibers extending from the cementum (1) to the crest of the gingiva, (2) to the outer surface, and (3) external to the periosteum of the labial plate. Circular fibers (4) are shown in cross section.

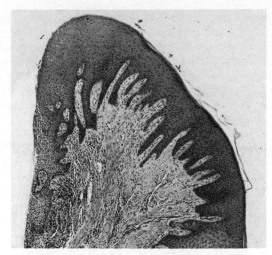

Figure 1–23 Section of Clinically Normal Gingiva, showing inflammation which is almost always present near the base of the sulcus. Keratin strands are visible on the outer surface, where they have been displaced owing to artifact.

frequency of their occurrence, the inflammatory infiltrate cells are not a normal component of the gingival tissue.

BLOOD SUPPLY, LYMPHATICS, AND NERVES. There are three sources of blood supply to the gingiva: (1) **Supraperiosteal arterioles** along the facial and lingual surfaces of the alveolar bone, from which capillaries extend along the sulcular epithelium and between the rete pegs of the external gingival surface.[40, 70] Occasional branches of the arterioles pass through the alveolar bone to the periodontal ligament or run over the crest of the alveolar bone (Fig. 1–24). (2) **Vessels of the**

as a result of injury or pathologic processes is also regulated by gingival fibroblasts.

Mast cells, which are distributed throughout the body, are numerous in the connective tissue of the oral mucosa and the gingiva.[28, 151]

In clinically normal gingiva, small foci of *plasma cells* and *lymphocytes* are found in the connective tissue near the base of the sulcus. *Neutrophils* can be seen in relatively high numbers in both the gingival connective tissue and the sulcus. These inflammatory cells are usually present in small amounts in clinically normal gingiva. Their presence is believed to be related to the penetration of antigenic substances from the oral cavity via the sulcular and junctional epithelia (Fig. 1–23) (see Chapters 7 and 8). They are not present, however, if gingival normalcy is judged by very strict clinical criteria.[104] Therefore, *in spite of the*

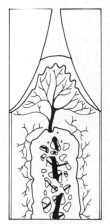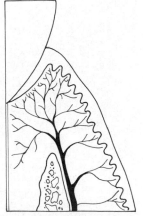

Figure 1–24 Diagrammatic representation of arteriole penetrating the interdental alveolar bone to supply the interdental tissues (*left*), and a supraperiosteal arteriole overlying the facial alveolar bone, sending branches to the surrounding tissue (*right*).

periodontal ligament, which extend into the gingiva and anastomose with capillaries in the sulcus area. (3) **Arterioles, which emerge from the crest of the interdental septa**[43] and extend parallel to the crest of the bone to anastomose with vessels of the periodontal ligament, with capillaries in the gingival crevicular areas, and with vessels which run over the alveolar crest.

Beneath the epithelium on the outer gingival surface, capillaries extend into the papillary connective tissue between the epithelial rete pegs in the form of terminal hairpin loops with efferent and afferent branches, spirals, and varices[29, 65] (Fig. 1–25). The loops are sometimes linked by cross-communications,[44] and there are also flattened capillaries which serve as reserve vessels when the circulation is increased in response to irritation.[48] Along the sulcular epithelium, capillaries are arranged in a flat anastomosing plexus which extends parallel to the enamel from the base of the sulcus to the gingival margin.[29] In the col area there is a mixed pattern of anastomosing capillaries and loops.

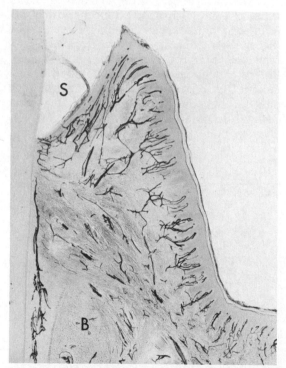

Figure 1–25 Blood Supply and Peripheral Circulation of the Gingiva. Tissues perfused with India ink. Note the capillary plexus parallel to the sulcus (S) and the capillary loops in the outer papillary layer. Note also the supraperiosteal vessels external to the bone (B) which supply the gingiva and a periodontal ligament vessel anastomosing with the sulcus plexus. (See also Fig. 2–5.) (Courtesy of Dr. Sol Bernick.)

The **lymphatic drainage of the gingiva** brings in the lymphatics of the connective tissue papillae. It progresses into the collecting network external to the periosteum of the alveolar process and then to the regional lymph nodes (particularly the submaxillary group).[130] In addition, lymphatics just beneath the junctional epithelium extend into the periodontal ligament and accompany the blood vessels.

Gingival innervation is derived from fibers arising from nerves in the periodontal ligament and from the labial, buccal, and palatal nerves.[15] The following nerve structures are present in the connective tissue: a meshwork of terminal argyrophilic fibers, some of which extend into the epithelium; Meissner-type tactile corpuscles; Krause-type end bulbs, which are temperature receptors; and encapsulated spindles.[9]

CORRELATION OF THE NORMAL CLINICAL AND MICROSCOPIC FEATURES

To understand the normal clinical features of the gingiva, one must be able to interpret them in terms of the microscopic structures they represent.

Color

The color of the attached and marginal gingivae is generally described as *coral pink* and is produced by the *vascular supply, the thickness and degree of keratinization of the epithelium, and the presence of pigment-containing cells.* The color varies in different persons and appears to be correlated with the cutaneous pigmentation. It is lighter in blond individuals with a fair complexion than in swarthy brunettes (Plate I).

The attached gingiva is demarcated from the adjacent alveolar mucosa on the buccal aspect by a clearly defined mucogingival line. The alveolar mucosa is red, smooth, and shiny rather than pink and stippled. Comparison of the microscopic structure of the attached gingiva and alveolar mucosa affords an explanation for the difference in appearance. The epithelium of the alveolar mucosa is thinner, nonkeratinized, and contains no rete pegs (Fig. 1–26). The connective tissue of the alveolar mucosa is loosely arranged, and the blood vessels are more numerous.

PHYSIOLOGIC PIGMENTATION (MELANIN). Melanin, a non–hemoglobin-derived brown pigment, is responsible for the normal pigmentation of the skin, gingiva, and remainder of

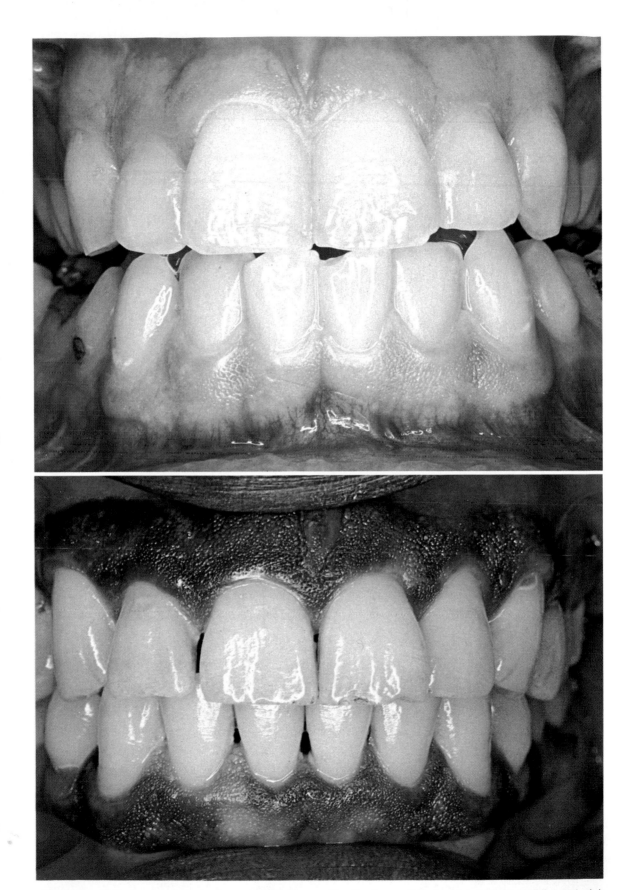

Plate I *Top,* Clinically normal gingiva in young adult. *Bottom,* Heavily pigmented (melanotic) gingiva in middle-aged adult. (From Glickman, I., and Smulow, J. B.: Periodontal Disease: Clinical, Radiographic, and Histopathologic Features. Philadelphia, W. B. Saunders Company, 1974.)

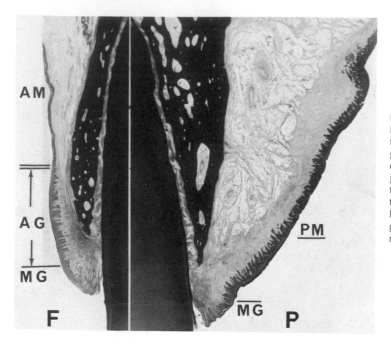

Figure 1–26 Oral Mucosa, Facial and Palatal Surfaces. *F,* Facial surface showing the marginal gingiva (MG), attached gingiva (AG), and alveolar mucosa (AM). The double line (=) marks the mucogingival junction. Note the differences in the epithelium and connective tissue in the attached gingiva and alveolar mucosa. *P,* Palatal surface showing the marginal gingiva (MG) and thick keratinized palatal mucosa (PM).

the oral mucous membrane. It is present in all normal individuals, often not in sufficient quantities to be detected clinically, but is absent or severely diminished in albinos. Melanin pigmentation in the oral cavity is prominent in blacks (Plate I).

Melanin is formed by dendritic melanocytes in the basal and spinous layers of the gingival epithelium (Fig. 1–27). It is synthesized in organelles within the cells called *premelanosomes* or *melanosomes*.[33, 114, 126] These contain tyrosinase, which hydroxylates tyrosine to dihydroxyphenylalanine (dopa), which in turn is progressively converted to melanin. Melanin

granules are phagocytosed by and contained within other cells of the epithelium and connective tissue called *melanophages* or *melanophores.*

According to Dummett,[38] the distribution of oral pigmentation in blacks is as follows: gingiva, 60 per cent; hard palate, 61 per cent; mucous membrane, 22 per cent; and tongue, 15 per cent. *Gingival pigmentation occurs as a diffuse, deep purplish discoloration or as irregularly shaped brown and light brown patches.* It may appear in the gingiva as early as 3 hours after birth and often is the only evidence of pigmentation.[38]

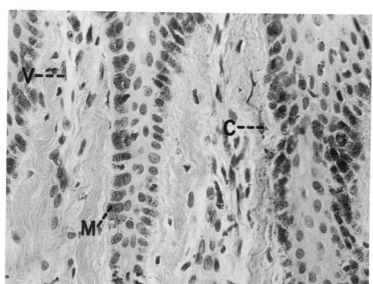

Figure 1–27 Pigmented Gingiva, showing melanocytes (M) in the basal epithelial layer and melanophores (C) in the connective tissue. Also shown is a capillary (V) in the papillary connective tissue.

Size

The size of the gingiva corresponds to the sum total of the bulk of cellular and intercellular elements and their vascular supply. Alteration in size is a common feature of gingival disease.

Contour

The contour or shape of the gingiva varies considerably and depends upon the shape of the teeth and their alignment in the arch, the location and size of the area of proximal contact, and the dimensions of the facial and lingual gingival embrasures. The marginal gingiva envelops the teeth in collar-like fashion and follows a scalloped outline on the facial and lingual surfaces. It forms a straight line along teeth with relatively flat surfaces. On teeth with pronounced mesiodistal convexity (e.g., maxillary canines) or teeth in labial version, the normal arcuate contour is accentuated and the gingiva is located farther apically. On teeth in lingual version the gingiva is horizontal and thickened (Fig. 1–28).

The **shape of the interdental gingiva** is governed by the contour of the proximal tooth surfaces and the location and shape of gingival embrasures. When the proximal surfaces of the crowns are relatively flat faciolingually, the roots are close together, the interdental bone is thin mesiodistally, and the gingival embrasures and interdental gingiva are narrow me-

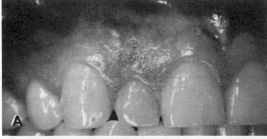
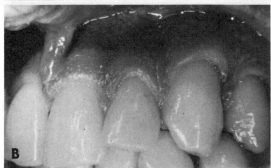

Figure 1–29 Shape of interdental gingival papillae correlated with shape of teeth and embrasures. *A,* Broad interdental papillae; *B,* narrow interdental papillae.

siodistally. Conversely, with proximal surfaces that flare away from the area of contact, the mesiodistal diameter of the interdental gingiva is broad (Fig. 1–29). The height of the interdental gingiva varies with the location of the proximal contact.

Consistency

The gingiva is *firm and resilient* and, with the exception of the movable free margin, *tightly bound to the underlying bone.* The collagenous nature of the lamina propria and its contiguity with the mucoperiosteum of the alveolar bone determine the firm consistency of the attached gingiva. The gingival fibers contribute to the firmness of the gingival margin.

Surface Texture

The gingiva presents a textured surface like an orange peel and is referred to as being **stippled.** Stippling is best viewed by drying the gingiva (Fig. 1–30). *The attached gingiva is stippled; the marginal gingiva is not.* The central portion of the interdental papillae is usually stippled, but the marginal borders are smooth. The pattern and extent of stippling vary from person to person and in different

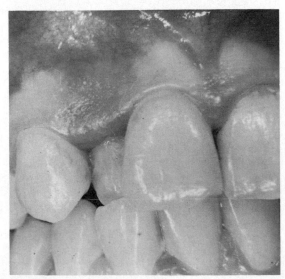

Figure 1–28 Thickened shelf-like contour of gingiva on tooth in lingual version aggravated by local irritation caused by plaque accumulation.

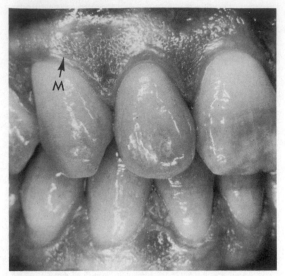

Figure 1–30 Stippling of attached gingiva and central portions of interdental papillae. The gingival margin (M) is smooth.

cavity, the margin and sulcus are at the tip of the crown; as eruption progresses, they are seen closer to the root. During this eruption process, as described earlier, the junctional epithelium, oral epithelium, and reduced enamel epithelium undergo extensive alterations and remodeling, while at the same time maintaining the shallow physiologic depth of the sulcus. Without this remodeling of the epithelia, an abnormal anatomic relationship between the gingiva and tooth would result.

CONTINUOUS TOOTH ERUPTION. According to the concept of continuous eruption,[54] erup-

areas of the same mouth.[55, 111] It is less prominent on lingual than on facial surfaces and may be absent in some persons.

Stippling varies with age. It is absent in infancy, appears in some children at about 5 years of age, increases until adulthood, and frequently begins to disappear in old age.

Microscopically, stippling is produced by alternate rounded protuberances and depressions in the gingival surface. The papillary layer of the connective tissue projects into the elevations, and both the elevated and the depressed areas are covered by stratified squamous epithelium (Fig. 1–31). The degree of keratinization and the prominence of stippling appear to be related.

Scanning electron microscopy has shown considerable variation in shape but a relatively constant depth; at low magnification a rippled surface is seen, interrupted by irregular depressions 50 microns in diameter. At higher magnification cell micropits are seen.[31]

Stippling is a form of adaptive specialization or reinforcement for function. It is a feature of healthy gingiva, and reduction or loss of stippling is a common sign of gingival disease. When the gingiva is restored to health following treatment, the stippled appearance returns.

Position

The position of the gingiva refers to the level at which the *gingival margin is attached to the tooth*. When the tooth erupts into the oral

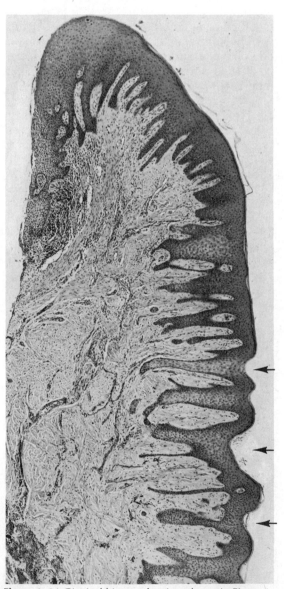

Figure 1–31 Gingival biopsy of patient shown in Figure 1–30, demonstrating alternate elevations and depressions (*arrows*) in the attached gingiva responsible for stippled appearance.

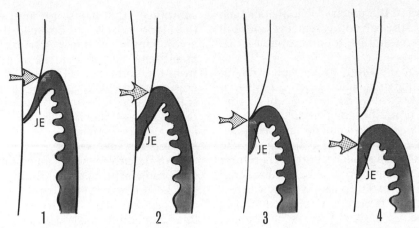

Figure 1–32 Diagrammatic representation of the four steps in passive eruption according to Gottlieb and Orban.[54] 1, Base of the gingival sulcus (*arrow*) and the junctional epithelium (JE) are on the enamel. 2, Base of the gingival sulcus (*arrow*) is on the enamel, and part of the junctional epithelium is on the root. 3, Base of the gingival sulcus (*arrow*) is at the cemento-enamel line, and the entire junctional epithelium is on the root. 4, Base of the gingival sulcus (*arrow*) and the junctional epithelium are on the root.

tion does not cease when teeth meet their functional antagonists, but continues throughout life. It consists of an active and a passive phase. *Active eruption is the movement of the teeth in the direction of the occlusal plane, whereas passive eruption is the exposure of the teeth by separation of the junctional epithelium from the enamel and migration onto the cementum.*

Inherent in the concept is the distinction between the *anatomic crown* (the portion of the tooth covered by enamel) and the *anatomic root* (the portion of the tooth covered by cementum) and the clinical crown and clinical root. The *clinical crown* is the part of the tooth that has been denuded of epithelium and projects into the oral cavity; the *clinical root* is that portion of the tooth covered by periodontal tissues.

When the teeth reach their functional antagonists, the gingival sulcus and junctional epithelium are still on the enamel, and the clinical crown is approximately two thirds of the anatomic crown.

Active and passive eruption were believed by Gottlieb to proceed together. Active eruption is coordinated with attrition. The teeth erupt to compensate for tooth substance worn away by attrition. Attrition reduces the clinical crown and prevents it from becoming disproportionately long in relation to the clinical root, thus avoiding excessive leverage on the periodontal tissues. Ideally, the rate of active eruption keeps pace with tooth wear, preserving the vertical dimension of the dentition.

As the teeth erupt, cementum is deposited at the apices and furcations of the roots, and

bone is formed along the fundus of the alveolus and at the crest of the alveolar bone. In this way part of the tooth substance lost by attrition is replaced by lengthening of the root, and socket depth is maintained to support the root.

Passive eruption is divided into four stages (Fig. 1–32). Although this was originally thought to be a normal physiologic process, it is now recognized to be a pathologic process.

Stage One: The teeth reach the line of occlusion. The junctional epithelium and base of the gingival sulcus are on the enamel.

Stage Two: The junctional epithelium proliferates so that part is on the cementum and part on the enamel. The base of the sulcus is still on the enamel.

Stage Three: The entire junctional epithelium is on the cementum, and the base of the sulcus is at the cemento-enamel junction. As the junctional epithelium proliferates from the crown onto the root, it remains no longer at the cemento-enamel junction than at any other area of the tooth.

Stage Four: The junctional epithelium has proliferated farther on the cementum. The base of the sulcus is on the cementum, a portion of which is exposed.

Proliferation of the junctional epithelium onto the root is accompanied by degeneration of gingival and periodontal ligament fibers and their detachment from the tooth. The cause of this degeneration is not understood. At present, however, it is believed to be the result of chronic inflammation, and therefore a pathologic process.

As noted above, apposition of bone accompanies active eruption. The distance between the apical end of the junctional epithelium and the crest of the alveolus remains constant throughout continuous tooth eruption (1.07 mm).[46]

Exposure of the tooth by the apical migration of the gingiva is called *gingival recession,* or *atrophy.* According to the concept of continuous eruption, the gingival sulcus may be located on the crown, cemento-enamel junction, or root, depending upon the age of the patient and the stage of eruption. Therefore, some root exposure with age is considered normal and is referred to as physiologic recession; excessive exposure is termed pathologic recession (see Chapter 9). As mentioned above, this concept is not accepted at present.

HISTOCHEMICAL ASPECTS OF NORMAL GINGIVA

Cellular and Intercellular Substances

Histochemical techniques provide useful information regarding the chemical components and enzyme systems of normal gingiva. In addition to improving our understanding of physiologic processes in the gingiva, this information may provide guidelines for interpreting the changes which occur in gingival disease.

The connective tissue of normal gingiva contains a **periodic acid–Schiff (PAS)–positive stain heteropolysaccharide intercellular ground substance**[41] that is also present in the walls of the blood vessels and between the cells of the epithelium.[119] A thin PAS-positive basement membrane demarcates the connective tissue from the epithelium (Fig. 1–33). Electron microscopy reveals this to be a band of thin collagen fibers (reticulin) on the connective tissue side of the lamina densa of the basal lamina, rather than the basal lamina itself, which is not involved in the PAS reaction.[132]

PAS-negative acid mucopolysaccharides, hyaluronic acid, and chondroitin sulfate A, C, and B[138] demonstrated between the epithelial cells are considered by some[136] to be intercellular cementing substances and by others[49] to be stained portions of the intercellular attachment apparatus. **Neutral mucopolysaccharides** also occur intercellularly in the epithelium.

Glycogen, which is PAS-positive, is an intracellular component seen throughout the connective tissue and in the smooth muscle of the arterioles.[140, 143] In the epithelium, glycogen occurs intracellularly, in concentrations inversely related to the degree of keratinization. Some consider it a normal component of epithelium[118, 148]; others find it only in acanthosis, usually associated with inflammation.[37] **Phosphorylase activity** generally occurs in the epithelium where glycogen is located.[110]

RNA is found in large quantities in the basal cells of normal gingival epithelium, decreasing toward the superficial layers, and in lowest

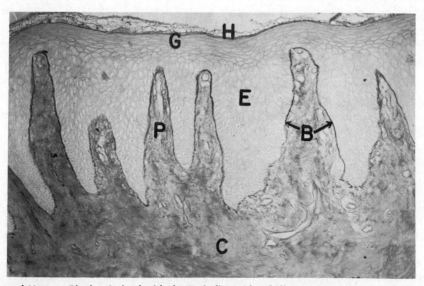

Figure 1–33 Normal Human Gingiva Stained with the Periodic Acid–Schiff (PAS) Histochemical Method. The basement membrane (B) is seen between the epithelium (E) and underlying connective tissue (C). In the epithelium there is glycoprotein material between the cells and in the cell membrane of the superficial hornified (H) and underlying granular layers (G). The connective tissue presents a diffuse amorphous ground substance and collagen fibers. The blood vessel walls stand out clearly in the papillary projections of the connective tissue (P).

concentration in the crevicular epithelium. **DNA**, normally present in the nucleus of all gingival cells, is increased in gingival hyperplasia. The DNA and RNA activity of the epithelium at the gingival margin and junctional epithelium is greater than in the remaining oral mucosa.[47, 56]

Sulfhydryls and **disulfides** are normal components of the gingival epithelium and connective tissue.[142] In the keratinization process sulfhydryls are oxidized to disulfides, and both are significant in a wide range of biologic activities such as enzymatic and antibody reactions, cell growth and division, and cell permeability and detoxification. Sulfhydryls and disulfides are present throughout the gingival epithelium; the former are increased in keratinized and parakeratinized layers,[142] the latter in the surface keratinized cells.[91] In the connective tissue, sulfhydryls and disulfides occur intercellularly and in the fibroblasts and endothelial cells. The **phospholipid** and **cholesterol** content of the gingiva is comparable to that of skin,[60] and lipids have been demonstrated in keratohyaline granules in the epithelium.[35]

Enzymes

Alkaline phosphatase is present in the endothelial cells, in the capillary walls, and possibly in the fibers of the connective tissue.[159] It has been described in keratinized and parakeratinized surface layers,[36] but there is some doubt that it occurs in epithelium.[24]

Acid phosphatase, found in the epithelium in greatest concentration in the surface and prickle cell layers,[147] is related to keratinization.[23] It is not present in the junctional epithelium or sulcus lining. Different patterns of distribution have been described in different animal species for acid and alkaline phosphatases.[63]

Diphospho- and **triphosphopyridine nucleotide reductases**, present in all epithelial cells except keratin and parakeratin layers, and in desmosomes, tonofibrils, and nucleoli, suggest an oxidative metabolic pathway for the formation of the keratin precursor substance and keratin.[40]

Acetylcholinesterase and **nonspecific cholinesterase** are present in gingival connective tissue.[10] **Endogenous reducing enzymes, succinic dehydrogenase, glucose-6-phosphate dehydrogenase, lactic dehydrogenase,**[41] **beta D-glucuronidase, beta-glucosidase, beta-galactosidase,**[79] **and aminopeptidase**[100, 110] have

been observed in gingiva. **Esterase**[64, 79] occurs in the basal and granular layers of the epithelium and in the connective tissue near periodontal pockets.

In a quantitative histochemical study of human gingival epithelium,[65] glucose-6-phosphate dehydrogenase was found to have its maximum content in epithelium of marginal gingiva and lower content in oral mucosal epithelium, sulcular epithelium, and junctional epithelium. Succinic dehydrogenase content was found to be greater in attached gingiva. Glucose-6-phosphate dehydrogenase increased its concentration from the basal to the superficial layers in attached and marginal gingiva, remained stable in all strata of oral mucosal epithelium and sulcular epithelium, and reduced its activity toward the surface in junctional epithelium. Succinic dehydrogenase decreased its concentration from the basal to the superficial layers in all zones. These findings have suggested that the *basal layer has an oxidative activity of the Krebs'-cycle type that tends to switch to the pentose shunt as it approaches the surface*.

Collagenase is produced in epithelium and connective tissue of normal gingiva as well as in the periodontal ligament and alveolar bone.[45] **Cytochrome oxidase** activity occurs in the sulcular and junctional epithelium, in the basal layers of marginal and attached gingiva, and in the connective tissue.[108] **5-Nucleotidase** occurs in the blood vessels and surface epithelial cells of keratinized gingiva and only in the blood vessels of nonkeratinized and parakeratinized gingiva.[34, 64] **Lysosomes** have been demonstrated in exfoliated cells of the junctional epithelium.[77]

The **oxygen consumption** of normal gingiva (QO_2 1.6 ± 0.37) is comparable to that of skin (QO_2 1.48 ± 0.48).[50] The respiratory activity of the epithelium is approximately three times greater than that of the connective tissue,[99] and that of the sulcular epithelium is approximately twice that of the whole gingiva.[76]

REFERENCES

1. Ainamo, A.: Influence of age on the location of the maxillary mucogingival junction. J. Periodont. Res., *13*:189, 1978.
2. Ainamo, A., and Ainamo, J.: The width of attached gingiva on supraerupted teeth. J. Periodont. Res., *13*:194, 1978.
3. Ainamo, J., and Löe, H.: Anatomical characteristics of gingiva. A clinical and microscopic study of the free and attached gingiva. J. Periodontol., *37*:5, 1966.
4. Ainamo, J., and Talari, A.: The increase with age of the width of attached gingiva. J. Periodont. Res., *11*:182, 1976.
5. Amstad-Jossi, M., and Schroeder, H. E.: Age-related alterations of periodontal structures around the cemento-enamel

junction and of the gingival connective tissue composition in germ-free rats. J. Periodont. Res., *13*:76, 1978.

6. Anderson, G. S., and Stern, I.: The proliferation and migration of the attachment epithelium on the cemental surface of the rat incisor. Periodontics, *4*:115, 1966.

7. Arnim, S. S., and Hagerman, D. A.: The connective tissue fibers of the marginal gingiva. J. Am. Dent. Assoc., *47*:271, 1953.

8. Attström, R. M., Graf-de Beer, M., and Schroeder, H. E.: Clinical and histologic characteristics of normal gingiva in dogs. J. Periodont. Res., *10*:115, 1975.

9. Avery, J. K., and Rapp, R.: Pain conduction in human dental tissues. Dent. Clin. North Am., July 1959, p. 489.

10. Avery, J. K., and Rapp, R.: Presence of acetylcholinesterase in human gingiva. J. Periodontol., *30*:152, 1959.

11. Barakat, M. H., Toto, P. D., and Choukas, N. C.: Aging and cell renewal of oral epithelium. J. Periodontol., *40*:599, 1969.

12. Baume, J. L.: The structure of the epithelial attachment revealed by phase contrast microscopy. J. Periodontol., *24*:99, 1953.

13. Beagrie, G. S., and Skougaard, M. R.: Observations on the life cycle of the gingival epithelial cells of mice as revealed by autoradiography. Acta Odontol. Scand., *20*:15, 1962.

14. Becks, H.: Normal and pathologic pocket formation. J. Am. Dent. Assoc., *16*:2167, 1929.

15. Bernick, S.: Innervation of the teeth and periodontium. Dent. Clin. North Am., July 1959, p. 503.

16. Biolcati, E. L., Carranza, F. A., Jr., and Cabrini, R. L.: Variaciones y alteraciones de la queratinización en encias humanas clinicamente sanas. Rev. Asoc. Odontol. Argent., *41*:446, 1953.

17. Black, G. V.: Special Dental Pathology. Chicago, Medico-Dental Publishing Co., 1915.

18. Bödecker, C. F.: The Anatomy and Pathology of the Teeth. Philadelphia, White Manufacturing Co., 1894.

19. Bowers, G. M.: A study of the width of the attached gingiva. J. Periodontol., *34*:210, 1963.

20. Bral, M. M., and Stahl, S. S.: Keratinizing potential of human crevicular epithelium. J. Periodontol., *48*:381, 1977.

21. Brill, N., and Björn, H.: Passage of tissue fluid into human gingival pockets. Acta Odontol. Scand., *17*:11, 1959.

22. Bye, F. L., and Caffesse, R. G.: The process of keratinization of the gingival epithelium. J. Western Soc. Periodontol., *27*:72, 1979.

23. Cabrini, R. L., and Carranza, F. A., Jr.: Histochemical distribution of acid phosphatase in human gingiva. J. Periodontol., *29*:34, 1958.

24. Cabrini, R. L., and Carranza, F. A., Jr.: Histochemistry of periodontal tissues. A review of the literature. Int. Dent. J., *16*:476, 1966.

25. Cabrini, R., Cabrini, R. L., and Carranza, F. A., Jr.: Estudio histológico de la queratinización del epitelio gingival y de la adherencia epitelial. Rev. Asoc. Odontol. Argent., *41*:212, 1953.

26. Caffesse, R. G., Karring, T., and Nasjleti, C. E.: Keratinizing potential of sulcular epithelium. J. Periodontol., *48*:140, 1977.

27. Caffesse, R. G., Korman, K. S., and Nasjleti, C. E.: The effect of intensive antibacterial therapy on the sulcular environment in monkeys. II. Inflammation, mitotic activity and keratinization of the sulcular epithelium. J. Periodontol., *51*:155, 1980.

28. Carranza, F. A., Jr., and Cabrini, R. L.: Mast cells in human gingiva. Oral Surg., *8*:1093, 1955.

29. Carranza, F. A., Jr., Itoiz, M. E., Cabrini, R. L., and Dotto, C. A.: A study of periodontal vascularization in different laboratory animals. J. Periodont. Res., *1*:120, 1966.

30. Cimasoni, G.: The crevicular fluid. Monographs in Oral Science. Vol. 3. Basel, S. Karger, 1974.

31. Cleaton-Jones, P., Buskin, S. A., and Volchansky, A.: Surface ultrastructure of human gingiva. J. Periodont. Res., *13*:367, 1978.

32. Cohen, B.: Morphological factors in the pathogenesis of periodontal disease. Br. Dent. J., *107*:31, 1959.

33. Cohen, L.: ATPase and dopa oxidase activity in human gingival epithelium. Arch. Oral Biol. *12*:1241, 1967.

34. Cohen, L.: Presence of 5-nucleotidase in human gingiva. J. Dent. Res., *46*:757, 1967.

35. Cohen, L.: Presence of lipids in keratohyaline granules of human gingiva. J. Dent. Res., *46*:630, 1967.

36. Cohen, L.: Alkaline phosphatase activity in human gingival epithelium. Periodontics, *6*:23, 1968.

37. Dewar, M. R.: Observations on the composition and metabolism of normal and inflamed gingivae. J. Periodontol., *26*:29, 1955.

38. Dummett, C. O.: Physiologic pigmentation of the oral and cutaneous tissues in the Negro. J. Dent. Res., *25*:422, 1946.

39. Egelberg, J.: The topography and permeability of blood vessels at the dentogingival junction in dogs. J. Periodont. Res., *2*(Suppl. 1), 1967.

40. Eichel, B., Shahrik, H. A., and Lisanti, V. F.: Cytochemical demonstration and metabolic significance of reduced diphospho-pyridine-nucleotide and triphospho-pyridine-nucleotide reductases in human gingiva. J. Dent. Res., *43*:92, 1964.

41. Engel, M. B.: Water-soluble mucoproteins of the gingiva. J. Dent. Res., *32*:779, 1953.

42. Engler, W. O., Ramfjord, S. P., and Hiniker, J. J.: Development of epithelial attachment and gingival sulcus in Rhesus monkeys. J. Periodontol., *36*:44, 1965.

43. Folke, L. E. A., and Stallard, R. E.: Periodontal microcirculation as revealed by plastic microspheres. J. Periodont. Res., *2*:53, 1967.

44. Forsslund, G.: Structure and function of capillary system in the gingiva in man. Development of stereophotogrammetric method and its application for study of the subepithelial blood vessels in vivo. Acta Odontol. Scand., *17*(Suppl. 26):9, 1959.

45. Fullmer, H. M., et al.: The origin of collagenase in periodontal tissues of man. J. Dent. Res., *48*:636, 1969.

46. Gargiulo, A. W., Wentz, F. M., and Orban, B.: Dimensions and relations of the dentogingival junction in humans. J. Periodontol., *32*:261, 1961.

47. Gimenez, I. B., and Carranza, F. A., Jr.: Microspectrophotometric study of DNA in gingival epithelium. J. Dent. Res., *52*:1345, 1973.

48. Glickman, I., and Johannessen, L.: Biomicroscopic (slit-lamp) evaluation of the normal gingiva of the albino rat. J. Am. Dent. Assoc., *41*:521, 1950.

49. Glickman, I., and Smulow, J. B.: Histopathology and histochemistry of chronic desquamative gingivitis. Oral Surg., *21*:325, 1966.

50. Glickman, I., Turesky, S., and Hill, R.: Determination of oxygen consumption in normal and inflamed human gingiva using the Warburg manometric technic. J. Dent. Res., *28*:83, 1949.

51. Gottlieb, B.: Der Epithelansatz am Zahne. Dtsch. Monatschr. Zahnhk., *39*:142, 1921.

52. Gottlieb, B.: Zur Biologie des Epithelansatzes und des Alveolarrandes. Dtsch. Zahnärztl. Wochenschr., *25*:434, 1922.

53. Gottlieb, B.: What is a normal pocket? J. Am. Dent. Assoc., *13*:1747, 1926.

54. Gottlieb, B., and Orban, B.: Active and passive eruption of the teeth. J. Dent. Res., *13*:214, 1933.

55. Greene, A. H.: A study of the characteristics of stippling and its relation to gingival health. J. Periodontol., *33*:176, 1962.

56. Greulich, R. C.: Epithelial DNA and RNA synthetic activities of the gingival margin. J. Periodontol., *40*:682, 1961.

57. Gross, H.: Zur Genese der vertieften Zahnfleischtasche. Paradentium, *3*:69, 1930.

58. Hansen, E. R.: Mitotic activity of the gingival epithelium in colchicinized rats. Odont. T., *74*:229, 1966.

59. Hansson, B. O., Lindhe, J., and Branemark, P. I.: Microvascular topography and function in clinically healthy and chronically inflamed dentogingival tissues—a vital microscopic study in dogs. Periodontics, *6*:265, 1968.

60. Hodge, H. C.: Gingival tissue lipids. J. Biol. Chem., *101*:55, 1933.

61. Hodson, J.: The distribution, structure, origin, and nature of the dental cuticle of Gottlieb. Periodontics, *5*:295, 1967.

62. Ito, H., Enomoto, S., and Kobayashi, K.: Electron microscopic study of the human epithelial attachment. Bull. Tokyo Med. Dent. Univ., *14*:267, 1967.

63. Itoiz, M. E., Carranza, F. A., Jr., and Cabrini, R. L.: Histotopographic distribution of alkaline and acid phosphatase in periodontal tissues of laboratory animals. J. Periodontol., *35*:470, 1964.

64. Itoiz, M. E., Carranza, F. A., Jr., and Cabrini, R. L.: Histotopographic study of esterase and 5-nucleotidase in periodontal tissues of laboratory animals. J. Periodontol., *38*:130, 1967.
65. Itoiz, M. E., Carranza, F. A., Jr., Gimenez, I., and Cabrini, R. L.: Microspectrophotometric analysis of succinic dehydrogenase and glucose-6-phosphate dehydrogenase in human oral epithelium. J. Periodont. Res., 7:14, 1972.
66. Itoiz, M. E., Carranza, F. A., Jr., Neira, V., and Cabrini, R. L.: Fine structural localization of thiamine pyrophosphatase in normal human gingiva. J. Periodontol., *45*:579, 1974.
67. Iusem, R.: A cytological study of the cornification of the oral mucosa in women. Oral Surg., 3:1516, 1950.
68. Kaplan, G. B., Pameijer, C. H., and Ruben, M. P.: Scanning electron microscopy of sulcular and junctional epithelia correlated with histology (Part 1). J. Periodontol., *48*:446, 1977.
69. Karring, T., Lang, N. P., and Löe, H.: The role of gingival connective tissue in determining epithelial differentiation. J. Periodont. Res., *10*:1, 1975.
70. Kindlova, M.: The blood supply of the marginal periodontium in Macaccus Rhesus. Arch. Oral Biol., *10*:869, 1965.
71. Kobayashi, K., and Rose, G. G.: Ultrastructural histochemistry of the dentoepithelial junction. II. Colloidal thorium and ruthenium red. J. Periodont. Res., *13*:164, 1978.
72. Kobayashi, K., and Rose, G. G.: Ultrastructural histochemistry of the dentoepithelial junction. III. Chloramine T-silver methenamine. J. Periodont. Res., *14*:123, 1979.
73. Kobayashi, K., Rose, G. G., and Mahan, C. J.: Ultrastructural histochemistry of the dentoepithelial junction. I. Phosphotungstic acid periodic acid–silver methenamine and periodic acid–thiosemicarbazide-silver proteinate. J. Periodont. Res., *12*:351, 1977.
74. Kronfeld, R.: Histopathology of the Teeth and Their Surrounding Structures. Philadelphia, Lea & Febiger, 1939.
75. Kurahashi, Y., and Takuma, S.: Electron microscopy of human gingival epithelium. Bull. Tokyo Dent. Col., *3*:29, 1962.
76. Lainson, P. A., and Fisher, A. K.: Endogenous oxygen consumption rates of bovine attached gingiva. J. Periodont. Res., *3*:132, 1968.
77. Lange, D., and Camelleri, G. E.: Cytochemical demonstration of lysosomes in the exfoliated epithelial cells of the gingival cuff. J. Dent. Res., *46*:625, 1967.
78. Lindhe, J., and Rylander, H.: Experimental gingivitis in young dogs. Scand. J. Dent. Res., *83*:314, 1975.
79. Lisanti, V. F.: Hydrolytic enzymes in periodontal disease. Ann. N.Y. Acid. Sci., *85*:461, 1960.
80. Listgarten, M. A.: The ultrastructure of human gingival epithelium. Am. J. Anat., *114*:49, 1964.
81. Listgarten, M. A.: Electron microscopic study of the gingivodental junction of man. Am. J. Anat., *119*:147, 1966.
82. Listgarten, M. A.: Phase contrast and electron microscopic study of the junction between reduced enamel epithelium and enamel in unerupted human teeth. Arch. Oral Biol., *11*:999, 1966.
83. Listgarten, M. A.: Changing concepts about the dentoepithelial junction. J. Can. Dent. Assoc., *36*:70, 1970.
84. Listgarten, M. A.: Structure and surface coatings on teeth. A review. J. Periodontol., *47*:139, 1976.
85. Löe, H.: The structure and physiology of the dento-gingival junction. *In* Miles, A. E. W. (ed.): Structural and Chemical Organization of Teeth. Vol. 2. New York, Academic Press, 1967.
86. Löe, H., and Karring, T.: Mitotic activity and renewal time of the gingival epithelium of young and old rats. J. Periodont. Res., *4*(Suppl.):18, 1969.
87. Löe, H., and Karring, T.: A quantitative analysis of the epithelium–connective tissue interface in relation to assessments of the mitotic index. J. Dent. Res., *48*:634, 1969.
88. Macapanpan, L. C.: Union of the enamel and gingival epithelium. J. Periodontol., *25*:243, 1954.
89. Mandel, J. I., and Weinstein, E.: The fluid of the gingival sulcus. Periodontics, *2*:147, 1964.
90. Marwah, A. S., and Weinmann, J. P.: A sex difference in epithelial cells of human gingiva. J. Periodontol., *26*:11, 1955.
91. McHugh, W. D.: Keratinization of gingival epithelium in laboratory animals. J. Periodontol., *35*:338, 1964.
92. McHugh, W. D., and Zander, H. A.: Cell division in the periodontium of developing and erupted teeth. Dent. Pract., *15*:451, 1965.
93. Meckel, A. H.: The formation and properties of organic fibers on teeth. Arch. Oral Biol., *10*:585, 1965.
94. Melcher, A. H.: Gingival reticulin: identification and role in histogenesis of collagen fibers. J. Dent. Res., *45*:426, 1966.
95. Meyer, J., Marwah, A. S., and Weinmann, J. P.: Mitotic rate of gingival epithelium in two age groups. J. Invest. Dermatol., *27*:237, 1956.
96. Meyer, W.: Controversial questions regarding the histology of the enamel cuticle. Vierteljahrschr. Zahnheilk., *46*:42, 1930.
97. Miller, S. C., Soberman, A., and Stahl, S.: A study of the cornification of the oral mucosa of young male adults. J. Dent. Res., *30*:4, 1951.
98. Montgomery, P. W.: A study of exfoliative cytology of normal human oral mucosa. J. Dent. Res., *30*:12, 1951.
99. Morgan, R. E., and Wingo, W. J.: The oxygen consumption of gingival crevicular epithelium. Oral Surg., *22*:257, 1966.
100. Mori, M., and Kishiro, A.: Histochemical observation of aminopeptidase activity in the normal and inflamed oral epithelium. J. Osaka Univ. Dent. Sch., *1*:39, 1961.
101. Moss, M. L.: Phylogeny and comparative anatomy of oral ectodermal-ectomesenchymal inductive interactions. J. Dent. Res., *48*:732, 1969.
102. Nasmyth, A.: On the structure, physiology, and pathology of the persistent capsular investments and pulp of the tooth. Med.-Chir. Trans. Roy. Med. Chir. Soc. Lond., *22*:310, 1839.
103. Noyes, F. B.: Dental Histology and Embryology. Philadelphia, Kimpton, 1921.
104. Oliver, R. C., Holm-Pedersen, P., and Löe, H.: The correlation between clinical scoring, exudate measurements and microscopic evaluation of inflammation in the gingiva. J. Periodontol., *40*:201, 1969.
105. Orban, B., and Kohler, J.: The physiologic gingival sulcus. Z. Stomatol., *22*:353, 1924.
106. Orban, R., et al.: The epithelial attachment (the attached epithelial cuff). J. Periodontol., *27*:167, 1956.
107. Papic, M., and Glickman, I.: Keratinization of the human gingiva in the menstrual cycle and menopause. Oral Surg., *3*:504, 1950.
108. Person, P., Felton, J., and Fine, A.: Biochemical and histochemical studies of aerobic oxidative metabolism of oral tissues. III. Specific metabolic activities of enzymatically separated gingival epithelium and connective tissue components. J. Dent. Res., *44*:91, 1965.
109. Quintarelli, G.: Histochemistry of the gingiva. III. The distribution of aminopeptidase in normal and inflammatory conditions. Arch. Oral Biol., *2*:271, 1960.
110. Quintarelli, G., and Cheraskin, E.: Histochemistry of the gingiva. VI. Distribution and localization of phosphorylase. J. Periodontol., *32*:339, 1961.
111. Rosenberg, H., and Massler, M. J.: Gingival stippling in young adult males. J. Periodontol., *38*:473, 1967.
112. Saglie, R., Sabag, N., and Mery, C.: Ultrastructure of the normal human epithelial attachment. J. Periodontol., *50*:544, 1979.
113. Schilli, W.: The most superficial zone of the stratum corneum of the gingiva. Oral Surg., *25*:896, 1968.
114. Schroeder, H. E.: Melanin containing organelles in cells of the human gingiva. J. Periodont. Res., *4*:1, 1969.
115. Schroeder, H. E.: Histopathology of the gingival sulcus. *In* Lehner, T. (ed.): The Borderland Between Caries and Periodontal Disease. London, Academic Press, 1977.
116. Schroeder, H. E., and Listgarten, M. A.: Fine structure of the developing epithelial attachment of human teeth. Monographs in Developmental Biology. Vol. 2. Basel, S. Karger, 1971.
117. Schroeder, H. E., and Theilade, J.: Electron microscopy of normal human gingival epithelium. J. Periodont. Res., *1*:95, 1966.
118. Schultz-Haudt, S. D., and From, S.: Dynamics of periodontal tissues. I. The epithelium. Odont. T., *69*:431, 1961.
119. Schultz-Haudt, S. D., Paus, S., and Assev, S.: Periodic acid–Schiff reactive components of human gingiva. J. Dent. Res., *40*:141, 1961.
120. Schweitzer, G.: Lymph vessels of the gingiva and teeth. Arch. Mik., Anat. Ent., *69*:807, 1907.

121. Shapiro, S., Ulmansky, M., and Scheuer, M.: Mast cell population in gingiva affected by chronic destructive periodontal disease. J. Periodontol., *40*:276, 1969.

122. Shelton, L., and Hall, W.: Human gingival mast cells. J. Periodont. Res., *3*:214, 1968.

123. Skillen, W. G.: The morphology of the gingivae of the rat molar. J. Am. Dent. Assoc., *17*:645, 1930.

124. Skougaard, M. R., and Beagrie, G. S.: The renewal of gingival epithelium in marmosets *(Callithrix jacchus)* as determined through autoradiography with thymidine-H_3. Acta Odontol. Scand., *20*:467, 1962.

125. Soni. N. N., Silberkweit, M., and Hayes, R. L.: Pattern of mitotic activity and cell densities in human gingival epithelium. J. Periodontol., *36*:15, 1965.

126. Squier, C. A., and Waterhouse, L. P.: The ultrastructure of the melanocyte in human gingival epithelium. J. Dent. Res., *46*:112, 1967.

127. Stern, I. B.: Electron microscopic observations of oral epithelium. I. Basal cells and the basement membrane. Periodontics, *3*:224, 1965.

128. Stern, I. B.: The fine structure of the ameloblast-enamel junction in rat incisors, epithelial attachment and cuticular membrane. 5th International Congress for Electron Microscopy. Vol. 2, p. 6, 1966.

129. Stern, I. B.: Further electron microscopic observations of the epithelial attachment. International Association for Dental Research Abstracts, 45th General Meeting, 1967, p. 118.

130. Stillman, P. R., and McCall, J. O.: Textbook of Clinical Periodontics. New York, Macmillan, 1922.

131. Susi, F.: Histochemical autoradiographic and electron microscopic studies of keratinization in oral mucosa. Ph.D. thesis. Tufts University, 1967.

132. Swift, J. A., and Saxton, C. A.: The ultrastructural location of the periodate-Schiff reactive basement membrane of the dermoepidermal junctions of human scalp and monkey gingiva. J. Ultrastruct. Res., *17*:23, 1967.

133. Talbot, E.: Histopathology of the jaws and apical dental tissues: the so-called Nasmyth's membrane. Dent. Cosmos, *69*:929, 1920.

134. Thilander, H.: Permeability of the gingival pocket epithelium. Int. Dent. J., *14*:416, 1964.

135. Thilander, H., and Bloom, G. D.: Cell contacts in oral epithelia. J. Periodont. Res., *3*:96, 1968.

136. Thonard, J. C., and Scherp, H. W.: Histochemical demonstration of acid mucopolysaccharides in human gingival epithelial intercellular spaces. Arch. Oral Biol., *7*:125, 1962.

137. Toller, J. R.: The organic continuity of the dentine, the enamel and the epithelial attachment in dogs. Br. Dent. J., *67*:443, 1939.

138. Toto, P. D., and Grundel, E. R.: Acid mucopolysaccharides in the oral epithelium. J. Dent. Res., *45*:211, 1966.

139. Toto, P. D., and Sicher, H. J.: Mucopolysaccharides in the epithelial attachment. J. Dent. Res., *44*:451, 1965.

140. Trott, J. R.: An investigation into the glycogen content of the gingivae. Dent. Pract., *7*:234, 1957.

141. Trott, J. R., and Gorenstein, S. L.: Mitotic rates in the oral and gingival epithelium of the rat. Arch. Oral Biol., *8*:425, 1963.

142. Turesky, S., Crowley, J., and Glickman, I.: A histochemical study of protein-bound sulfhydryl and disulfide groups in normal and inflamed human gingiva. J. Dent. Res., *36*:225, 1957.

143. Turesky, S., Glickman, I., and Litwin, T.: A histochemical evaluation of normal and inflamed human gingivae. J. Dent. Res., *30*:792, 1951.

144. Ussing, M. J.: The development of the epithelial attachment. Acta Odontol. Scand., *13*:123, 1956.

145. Waerhaug, J.: The gingival pocket. Odont. T. *60*(Suppl. 1), 1952.

146. Waerhaug, J.: Current views on the epithelial cuff. Periodontics, *4*:278, 1966.

147. Waterhouse, J. P.: The gingival part of the human periodontium. Its ultrastructure and the distribution in it of acid phosphatase in relation to cell attachment and the lysosome concept. Dent. Pract., *15*:409, 1965.

148. Weinmann, J. P., and Meyer, J.: Types of keratinization in the human gingiva. J. Invest. Dermatol., *32*:87, 1959.

149. Weinstock, A.: Secretory function of "postsecretory" ameloblasts as shown by electron microscope radioautography. J. Dent. Res., *50*:82, 1971.

150. Weinstock, A., and Albright, J. T.: Electron microscopic observations on specialized structures in the epithelium of the normal human palate. J. Dent. Res. *45*(Suppl.):79, 1966.

151. Weinstock, A., and Albright, J. T.: The fine structure of mast cell in normal human gingiva. J. Ultrastruct. Res., *17*:245, 1967.

152. Wertheimer, F. W.: A histologic comparison of apical cuticles, secondary dental cuticles and hyaline bodies. J. Periodontol., *37*:5, 1966.

153. Wertheimer, F. W., and Fullmer, H. M.: Morphologic and histochemical observations on the human dental cuticle. J. Periodontol., *33*:29, 1962.

154. Weski, O.: Die chronischen marginalen Entzündungen des Alveolar-fortsatzes mit besonderer Berücksichtigung der Alveolarpyorrhoe. Vierteljahrschr. Zahnheilk., *38*:1, 1922.

155. Wilgram, G. F., and Weinstock, A.: Advances in genetic dermatology: acantholysis, hyperkeratosis, and dyskeratosis. Arch. Dermatol., *94*:456, 1966.

156. Wislocki, G. B., and Sognnaes, R. F.: Histochemical reactions of normal teeth. Am. J. Anat., *87*:239, 1950.

157. Wodehouse, W. B.: The gingival trough—its early development. Aust. J. Dent., *33*:139, 1929.

158. Yamasaki, A., et al.: Ultrastructure of the junctional epithelium of germ-free rat gingiva. J. Periodontol., *50*:641, 1979.

159. Zander, H. A.: The distribution of phosphatase in gingival tissue. J. Dent. Res., *20*:347, 1941.

The Periodontal Ligament

The periodontal ligament is the connective tissue structure that surrounds the root and connects it with the bone. It is continuous with the connective tissue of the gingiva and communicates with the marrow spaces through vascular channels in the bone.

NORMAL MICROSCOPIC FEATURES

Principal Fibers

The most important elements of the periodontal ligament are the principal fibers, which are collagenous, arranged in bundles, and follow a wavy course when viewed in longitudinal section (Fig. 2–1). Electron microscopy has shown an intimate relationship between the collagen fibers and fibroblasts.[49] Terminal portions of the principal fibers that insert into

cementum (Fig. 2–2) and bone are termed Sharpey's fibers.

PRINCIPAL FIBER GROUPS OF THE PERIODONTAL LIGAMENT. The principal fibers are arranged in the following groups: transseptal, alveolar crest, horizontal, oblique, and apical (Figs. 2–3 and 2–4).

Transseptal Group. These fibers extend interproximally over the alveolar crest and are embedded in the cementum of adjacent teeth (Fig. 2–5). The transseptal fibers are a remarkably constant finding. They are reconstructed even after destruction of the alveolar bone has occurred in periodontal disease.

Alveolar Crest Group. These fibers extend obliquely from the cementum just beneath the junctional epithelium to the alveolar crest. Their function is to counterbalance the coronal thrust of the more apical fibers, thus helping to retain the tooth within its socket[12] and resist

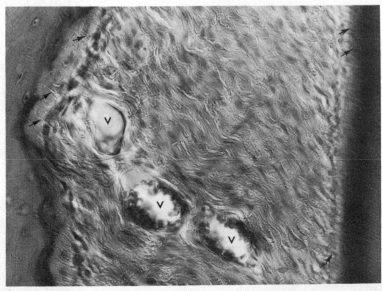

Figure 2–1 Principal Fibers of the Periodontal Ligament Follow a Wavy Course When Sectioned Longitudinally. The formative function of the periodontal ligament is illustrated by the newly formed osteoid and osteoblasts along a previously resorbed bone surface (*left*) and the cementoid and cementoblasts (*right*). Note the fibers embedded in the forming calcified tissues (*arrows*). V, vascular channels.

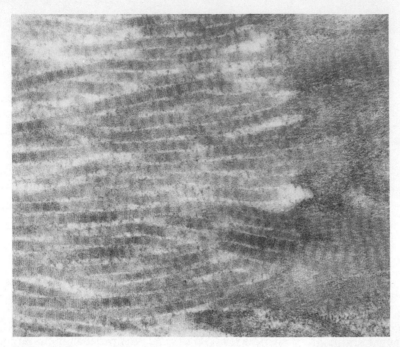

Figure 2–2 Electron Micrograph of Attachment of Periodontal Ligament Collagen Fibers to Cementum as seen in longitudinal section at high power. The collagen fibers generally run parallel and insert at varying angles into the electron-opaque cementum matrix (*far right*). The fibers have a periodic cross-banding pattern typical of collagen. Rat molar. × 66,250. (Courtesy of Dr. Jack Yee.)

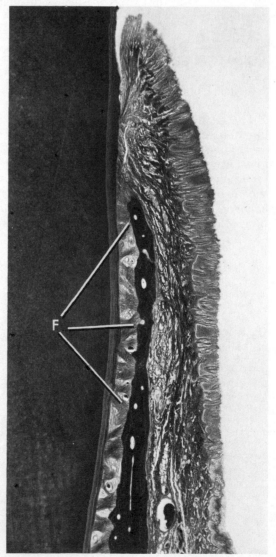

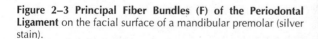

Figure 2–3 Principal Fiber Bundles (F) of the Periodontal Ligament on the facial surface of a mandibular premolar (silver stain).

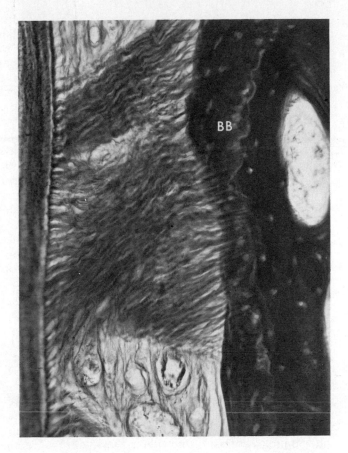

Figure 2–4 Detailed View of Figure 2–3 showing continuous collagen fibers embedded in the cementum (*left*) and bone (*right*) (silver stain). Note the Sharpey's fibers within the bundle bone (BB) overlying lamellar bone.

lateral tooth movements. However, their incision does not significantly increase the mobility of a normal premolar.[28]

Horizontal Group. These fibers extend at right angles to the long axis of the tooth from the cementum to the alveolar bone. Their function is similar to that of the alveolar crest fibers.

Oblique Group. These fibers, the largest group in the periodontal ligament, extend from the cementum in a coronal direction obliquely to the bone. They bear the brunt of vertical masticatory stresses and transform them into tension on the alveolar bone.

Apical Group. The apical fibers radiate from the cementum to the bone at the fundus of the

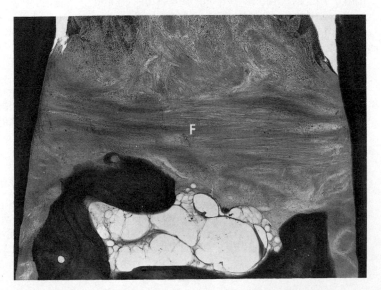

Figure 2–5 Transseptal Fibers (F) at the Crest of the Interdental Bone.

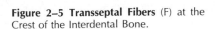

socket. They do not occur on incompletely formed roots.

Other Fibers

Other well-formed fiber bundles interdigitate at right angles or splay around and between regularly arranged fiber bundles.

Less regularly arranged *collagen fibers* are found in the interstitial connective tissue between the principal fiber groups which contains the blood vessels, lymphatics, and nerves. Other fibers of the periodontal ligament are the *elastic fibers*,[61] which are relatively few, and the so-called *oxytalan*[24, 29] *(acid-resistant) fibers*, which are distributed mainly around the blood vessels and embedded in cementum in the cervical third of the root. Their function is not understood, but many investigators believe that they represent an immature form of elastin. Under the electron microscope, mature elastin has a homogeneous, amorphous appearance, whereas immature elastin appears as bundles of microfilaments.

Small collagen fibers have been detected in association with the larger principal collagen fibers. These fibers appear to form a plexus and have been termed "indifferent" fibers.[50]

THE INTERMEDIATE PLEXUS. The principal fiber bundles consist of individual fibers which form a continuous anastomosing network between tooth and bone.[14, 55] It has been suggested that instead of being continuous the individual fibers consist of two separate parts spliced together midway between cementum and bone in a zone called the *intermediate plexus.* The plexus has been reported in the periodontal ligament of continuously growing incisors of animals,[34, 41, 51] but not in the posterior teeth,[68] and in actively erupting human and monkey[31] teeth, but not after they reach occlusal contact. Rearrangement of the fiber ends in the plexus is supposed to accommodate tooth eruption, without necessitating the embedding of new fibers into tooth and bone.[41] There are doubts regarding the existence of such a plexus[6, 62]; some consider it a microscopic artifact,[25] and no evidence of its existence has been found when collagen fiber formation is traced with radioactive proline.[18]

Cellular Elements

The cellular elements of the periodontal ligament are fibroblasts, endothelial cells, cementoblasts, osteoblasts, osteoclasts, tissue macrophages, and strands of epithelial cells termed the "epithelial rests of Malassez" or "resting epithelial cells."[65] Using scanning electron microscopy Roberts and Chamberlain[49] have identified four types of cells in the rat molar periodontal ligament: irregular oblong cells oriented along the principal fibers, smaller stellate-shaped cells located in lacunar spaces between the principal fibers, spheroid-type cells in perivascular areas, and, occasionally, elongated, stellate-shaped large cells (Fig. 2–6).

Investigations have shown that *fibroblasts* synthesize collagen by first producing a precursor molecule called procollagen. Procollagen is believed to be carried within the cell in small, elongated secretory granules.[67] Upon discharge from the cell, the procollagen molecules become chemically modified, and collagen fibers then arise. Periodontal ligament fibroblasts have been shown to possess the capacity to phagocytose "old" collagen fibers and degrade them[20, 59] by enzyme hydrolysis. Thus, collagen turnover appears to be regulated by the same cell type.

The *epithelial rests* form a latticework in the periodontal ligament and appear as either isolated clusters of cells or interlacing strands, depending on the plane in which the microscopic section is cut. Continuity with the junctional epithelium in experimental animals has been suggested.[30] They are considered to be remnants of the Hertwig root sheath, which disintegrates during root development after cementum is formed on the dentin surface, but this concept has been questioned.[21]

Epithelial rests are distributed close to the cementum throughout the periodontal ligament of most teeth and are most numerous in the apical[47] and cervical areas.[66] They diminish in number with age[52] by degenerating and disappearing or undergoing calcification to become cementicles. They are surrounded by a periodic acid–Schiff (PAS)–positive, argyrophilic, fibrillar, sometimes hyaline capsule from which they are separated by a distinct basement lamina or membrane. Epithelial rests proliferate when stimulated[56, 63] and participate in the formation of periapical cysts and lateral root cysts.

The periodontal ligament may also contain calcified masses called cementicles which are adherent to, or detached from, the root surfaces.

Vascular Supply

The blood supply is derived from the *inferior* and *superior alveolar arteries* and reaches the periodontal ligament from three sources: *apical vessels, penetrating vessels from the alveolar bone,* and *anastomosing vessels from the gin-*

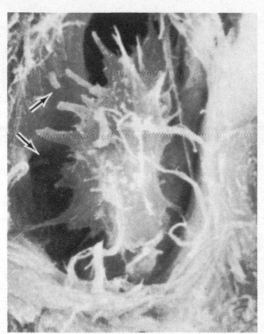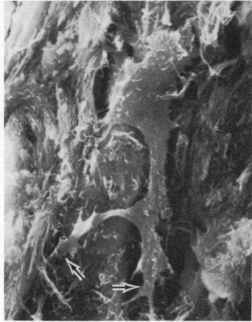

Figure 2–6 *Left,* Stellate-shaped cell with abundant cellular processes and enclosed in a lacunar structure formed by primary collagen fibers of the periodontal ligament. Broken cell processes (*arrows*) are probably dehydration artifacts. × 8157. *Right,* Large (60 microns long) fibroblast-like periodontal ligament cell with multiple cellular processes and pseudopodia-like structures (*arrows*). × 3062. (From Roberts, W. E., and Chamberlain, J. G.: Arch. Oral Biol., 23:587, 1978.)

giva.[15] The apical vessels enter the periodontal ligament at the apical region and extend to the gingiva, giving off lateral branches in the direction of the cementum and bone. The vessels within the periodontal ligament are connected in a net-like plexus which runs closer to the bone than to the cementum.[13] The plexus receives its principal supply from alveolar perforating arteries and small vessels which penetrate through channels in the alveolar bone[22] (Figs. 2–7 and 2–8). The blood supply from this source increases from the incisors to the molars; is greatest in the gingival third of single-rooted teeth, less in the apical third, and least in the middle; is equal in the apical and middle thirds of multirooted teeth; is slightly greater on the mesial and distal surfaces than on the facial and lingual; and is greater on the mesial surfaces of mandibular molars than on the distal.[8] The vascular supply from the gingiva is derived from branches of deep vessels in the lamina propria. The venous drainage of the periodontal ligament accompanies the arterial supply.

Lymphatics

Lymphatics supplement the venous drainage system. Those draining the region just beneath the junctional epithelium pass into the perio-

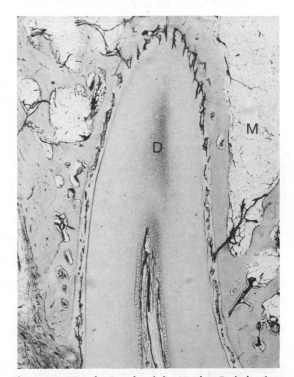

Figure 2–7 Vascular Supply of the Monkey Periodontium (perfused with India ink). Note the longitudinal vessels in the periodontal ligament and alveolar arteries passing through channels between the bone marrow (M) and periodontal ligament. D, dentin. (Courtesy of Dr. Sol Bernick.)

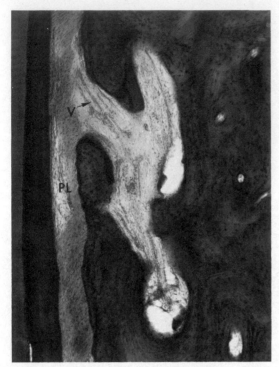

Figure 2–8 Small Vessels (V) in Channel connecting the periodontal ligament (PL) and alveolar bone.

nective tissue surrounding the tooth bud. On the basis of histologic,[23] histochemical, embryologic, and transplantation studies,[60] Ten Cate[57] has suggested that the dental follicle be defined as only the zone immediately in contact with the dental organ and continuous with the ectomesenchyme of the dental papilla. This investing layer (for which Ten Cate reserves the name "dental follicle") consists of undifferentiated fibroblasts that give rise to cementoblasts and fibroblasts of the ligament. In addition, undifferentiated perivascular mesenchymal cells of vessels close to the alveolar bone surface also give rise to periodontal ligament fibroblasts.[60] Alveolar bone deposition occurs simultaneously with periodontal ligament organization.[58]

Studies on the squirrel monkey[31] have shown that during eruption cemental fibers are observed first, followed by Sharpey's fibers emerging from bone. When the tooth reaches occlusal function, fiber bundles become thicker and soon become organized into classic principal fiber arrangements. Nevertheless, the transseptal and alveolar crest fibers develop upon emergence of the tooth into the oral cavity.

FUNCTIONS OF THE PERIODONTAL LIGAMENT

The functions of the periodontal ligament are *physical, formative, nutritional,* and *sensory.*

Physical Function

The physical functions of the periodontal ligament entail the following[42]: transmission of occlusal forces to the bone; attachment of the teeth to the bone, maintenance of the gingival tissues in their proper relationship to the teeth, resistance to the impact of occlusal forces (shock absorption), and provision of a "soft tissue casing" to protect the vessels and nerves from injury by mechanical forces.

RESISTANCE TO THE IMPACT OF OCCLUSAL FORCES (SHOCK ABSORPTION). Three theories relative to the mechanism of tooth support have been considered:

1. **The tensional theory** of tooth support ascribes to the principal fibers of the periodontal ligament the major responsibility in supporting the tooth and transmitting forces to the bone. When a force is applied to the crown, the principal fibers first unfold and straighten,

dontal ligament and accompany the blood vessels into the periapical region.[9] From there they pass through the alveolar bone to the inferior dental canal in the mandible, or the infraorbital canal in the maxilla, and to the submaxillary group of lymph nodes.

Innervation

The periodontal ligament is abundantly supplied with sensory nerve fibers capable of transmitting *tactile, pressure,* and *pain* sensations by the trigeminal pathways.[2, 5] Nerve bundles pass into the periodontal ligament from the periapical area and through channels from the alveolar bone. The nerve bundles follow the course of the blood vessels and divide into single myelinized fibers, which ultimately lose their myelin sheaths and terminate as either free nerve endings or elongate spindle-like structures. The latter are *proprioceptive receptors* that account for the sense of localization when a tooth is touched.

Development of the Periodontal Ligament

The periodontal ligament develops from the *dental sac* or *follicle,* a circular layer of con-

then transmit forces to the alveolar bone, causing an elastic deformation of the bony socket; finally, when the alveolar bone has reached its limit, the load is transmitted to the basal bone. Many investigators find this theory insufficient to explain available experimental evidence.

2. **The viscoelastic system theory** considers the displacement of the tooth to be largely controlled by fluid movements, and fibers having only a secondary role.[7, 10] When forces are transmitted to the tooth, the extracellular fluid passes from the periodontal ligament into the marrow spaces of bone through foramina in the cortical layer. Following the depletion of tissue fluids, the fiber bundles absorb the slack and tighten. This leads to blood vessel stenosis; arterial back pressure causes ballooning of the vessels and the passage of blood ultrafiltrates into the tissues, thereby replenishing the tissue fluids.[7]

3. **The thixotropic theory**[36] claims that the periodontal ligament has the rheologic behavior of a thixotropic gel.* The physiologic response of the periodontal ligament may be explained by changes in the viscosity of the biologic system.

TRANSMISSION OF OCCLUSAL FORCES TO THE BONE. The arrangement of the principal fibers is similar to a suspension bridge or a hammock. When an axial force is applied to a tooth, there is a tendency toward displacement of the root into the alveolus. The oblique fibers alter their wavy untensed pattern, assume their full length, and sustain the major part of the axial force.

When a horizontal or tipping force is applied, there are **two characteristic phases** of tooth movement: the first is **within the confines of the periodontal ligament,** and the second

---

*Thixotropy: the property, exhibited by certain gels, of becoming fluid when shaken or stirred, and then becoming semisolid again (Dorland's Illustrated Medical Dictionary, 26th ed. Philadelphia, W. B. Saunders Company, 1981).

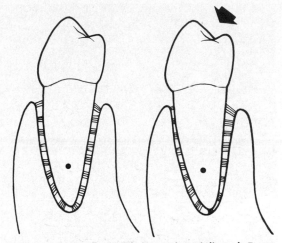

Figure 2–9. *Right,* **Distribution of Faciolingual Forces** *(arrow)* **Around the Axis of Rotation** *(black circle on root)* in a mandibular premolar. The periodontal ligament fibers are compressed in areas of pressure and tension. *Left,* The same tooth in a resting state.

produces a **displacement of the facial and lingual bony plates**.[19] The tooth rotates about an axis which may change as the force is increased. The apical portion of the root moves in a direction opposite to the coronal portion. In areas of tension the principal fiber bundles are taut rather than wavy. In areas of pressure the fibers are compressed, the tooth is displaced, and there is a corresponding distortion of bone in the direction of root movement.[45]

In single-rooted teeth the axis of rotation is located slightly apical to the middle third of the root (Fig. 2–9). The root apex[42] and the coronal half of the clinical root have been suggested as other locations of the axis of rotation. The periodontal ligament, shaped like an hourglass, is narrowest in the region of the axis of rotation[17, 38] (Table 2–1). In multirooted teeth the axis of rotation is located in the bone between the roots.

In compliance with the physiologic mesial migration of the teeth, the periodontal ligament is thinner on the mesial root surface than on the distal surface (Figs. 2–10 and 2–11).

TABLE 2–1 THICKNESS OF PERIODONTAL LIGAMENT OF 172 TEETH FROM 15 HUMAN JAWS*

	Average of Alveolar Crest	Average of Midroot	Average of Apex	Average of Tooth
Ages 11–16 83 teeth from 4 jaws	0.23	0.17	0.24	0.21
Ages 32–50 36 teeth from 5 jaws	0.20	0.14	0.19	0.18
Ages 51–67 35 teeth from 5 jaws	0.17	0.12	0.16	0.15
Age 24 (1 case) 18 teeth from 1 jaw	0.16	0.09	0.15	0.13

*From Coolidge, E. D.: J. Am. Dent. Assoc., *24*:1260, 1937.

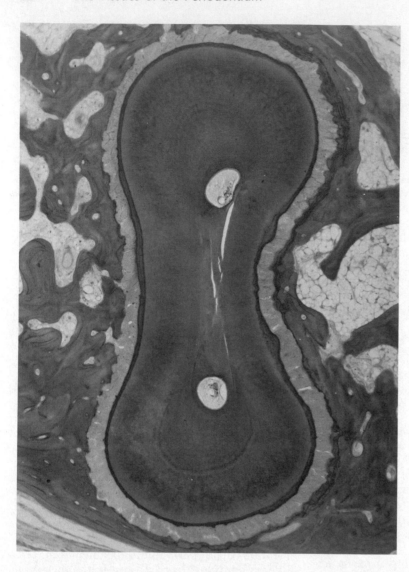

Figure 2–10 Physiologic Mesial Migration. Horizontal section through molar root. The periodontal ligament is thinner on the side toward which the tooth is migrating (mesial surface, *left*) than on the distal surface (*right*). The distal fibers are taut.

OCCLUSAL FUNCTION AND THE STRUCTURE OF THE PERIODONTAL LIGAMENT. Just as the tooth depends upon the periodontal ligament to support it during function, so does the periodontal ligament depend upon stimulation provided by occlusal function to preserve its structure. Within physiologic limits the periodontal ligament can accommodate increased function by an increase in width (Table 2–2), a thickening of the fiber bundles, and an increase in diameter and number of Sharpey's fibers. Occlusal forces which exceed what the periodontal ligament can withstand produce injury called *trauma from occlusion* (see Chapter 19).

When function is diminished or absent, the periodontal ligament atrophies. It is thinned, and the fibers are reduced in number and density, become disoriented,[1, 48] and ultimately are arranged parallel to the root surface (Fig.

2–12). In addition, the cementum is either unaffected[16] or thickened, and the distance from the cemento-enamel junction to the alveolar crest is increased.[46]

Destruction of the periodontal ligament and alveolar bone by periodontal disease disrupts the balance between the periodontium and occlusal forces. When supporting tissues are reduced by disease, the burden upon the tissue which remains is increased. Occlusal forces which were beneficial to the intact periodontal ligament may now become injurious.

Formative Function

The periodontal ligament serves as the periosteum for cementum and bone. Cells of the periodontal ligament participate in the formation and resorption of these tissues, which

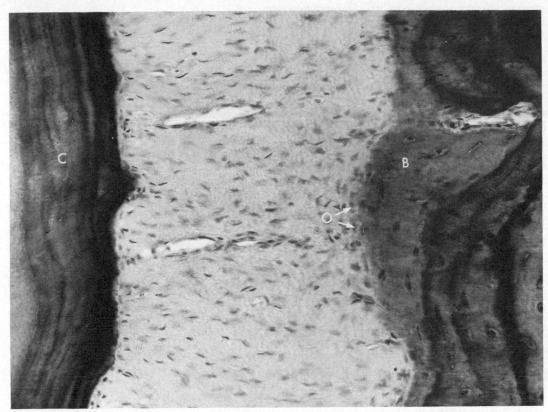

Figure 2–11 High-Power View of Figure 2–10. Distal surface, showing cementum (C), periodontal ligament, and bone. The tooth is migrating mesially (toward the left). Note the osteoblasts (O) and new bone formation (B) (*right*).

occur in physiologic tooth movement, in the accommodation of the periodontium to occlusal forces, and in the repair of injuries. Variations in cellular enzyme activity (certain dehydrogenases[25] and nonspecific esterase[27]) are correlated with the remodeling process. In areas of bone formation, osteoblasts, fibroblasts, and cementoblasts stain intensely, suggesting the presence of nonspecific alkaline phosphatase, glucose-6-phosphatase, and thiamine pyrophosphatase.[26] In areas of bone resorption, osteoclasts, fibroblasts, osteocytes, and cementocytes show a staining reaction for nonspecific acid phosphatase. Cartilage for-

mation in the periodontal ligament, although unusual, may represent a metaplastic phenomenon in the repair of this ligament following injury.[3]

Like all structures of the periodontium, the periodontal ligament is constantly undergoing remodeling. Old cells and fibers are broken down and replaced by new ones, and mitotic activity can be observed in the fibroblasts and endothelial cells.[43] Fibroblasts form the collagen fibers and may also develop into osteoblasts and cementoblasts. The rate of formation and differentiation of fibroblasts affects the rate of formation of collagen cementum

TABLE 2–2 COMPARISON OF PERIODONTAL WIDTH OF FUNCTIONING AND FUNCTIONLESS TEETH IN A MALE AGED 38*

	Heavy Function Left Upper 2nd Bicuspid	Light Function Left Lower 1st Bicuspid	Functionless Left Upper 3rd Molar
Average width of periodontal space at entrance of alveolus	0.35 mm	0.14 mm	0.10mm
Average width of periodontal space at middle of alveolus	0.28 mm	0.10 mm	0.06 mm
Average width of periodontal space at fundus of alveolus	0.30 mm	0.12 mm	0.06 mm

*From Kronfeld, R.: J. Am. Dent. Assoc., *18*:1242, 1931.

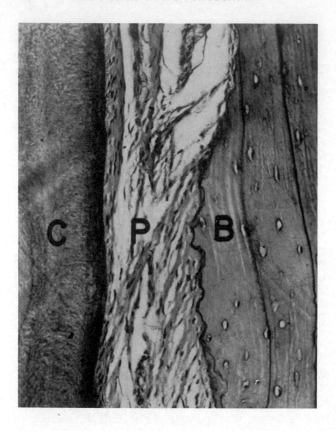

Figure 2–12 Atrophic Periodontal Ligament (P) of Tooth Devoid of Function. Note the scalloped edge of the alveolar bone (B), suggesting that resorption has occurred. C, cementum.

and bone. Collagen formation increases with the rate of eruption.[53, 54]

Radioautographic studies with radioactive thymidine, proline, and glycine indicate a high rate of collagen metabolism in the periodontal ligament. Formation of new fibroblasts and collagen is most active adjacent to the bone and in the middle of the ligament and least active on the cementum side.[18, 53] Collagen turnover is greatest at the crest and apex, according to one study,[11] and less in the crestal region than in other areas, according to another investigation.[48] There is also rapid turnover of sulfated mucopolysaccharides in the cells and amorphous ground substance of the periodontal ligament.[4]

Nutritional and Sensory Functions

The periodontal ligament supplies nutrients to the cementum, bone, and gingiva by way of the blood vessels and provides lymphatic drainage. The innervation of the periodontal ligament provides *proprioceptive* and *tactile sensitivity*,[37, 64] which detects and localizes external forces acting upon the individual teeth and serves an important role in the neuromuscular mechanism controlling the masticatory musculature.

REFERENCES

1. Anneroth, G., and Ericsson, S. G.: An experimental histological study of monkey teeth without antagonist. Revy, *18*:345, 1967.
2. Avery, J. K., and Rapp, R.: Pain conduction in human dental tissues. Dent. Clin. North Am., July 1959, p. 489.
3. Bauer, W. H.: Effect of a faulty constructed partial denture on a tooth and its supporting tissue, with special reference to formation of fibrocartilage in the periodontal membrane as a result of disturbed healing caused by abnormal stresses. Am. J. Orthod. Oral Surg., *27*:640, 1941.
4. Baumhammers, A., and Stallard, R.: S35-sulfate utilization and turnover by connective tissues of the periodontium. J. Periodont. Res., *3*:187, 1968.
5. Bernick, S.: Innervation of the teeth and periodontium. Dent. Clin. North Am., July 1959, p. 503.
6. Bevelander, G., and Nakara, H.: The fine structure of the human periodontal ligament. Anat. Rec., *162*:313, 1968.
7. Bien, S. M.: Hydrodynamic damping of tooth movement. J. Dent. Res., *45*:907, 1966.
8. Birn, H.: The vascular supply of the periodontal membrane. J. Periodont. Res., *1*:51, 1966.
9. Box, K. F.: Evidence of lymphatics in the periodontium. J. Can. Dent. Assoc., *15*:8, 1949.
10. Boyle, P. E.: Tooth suspension. A comparative study of the paradental tissues of man and of the guinea pig. J. Dent. Res., *17*:37, 1938.
11. Carneiro, J., and Fava de Moraes, F.: Radioautographic visualization of collagen metabolism in the periodontal tissues of the mouse. Arch. Oral Biol., *10*:833, 1955.
12. Carranza, F. A., Sr., and Carranza, F. A., Jr.: The management of the alveolar bone in the treatment of the periodontal pocket. J. Periodontol., *27*:29, 1956.
13. Carranza, F. A., Jr., Itoiz, M. E., Cabrini, R. H., and Dotto, C. A.: A study of periodontal vascularization in different laboratory animals. J. Periodont. Res., *1*:120, 1966.
14. Ciancio, S. C., Neiders, M. E., and Hazen, S. P.: The principal fibers of the periodontal ligament. Periodontics, *5*:76, 1967.

15. Cohen, L.: Further studies into the vascular architecture of the mandible. J. Dent. Res., *39*:936, 1960.
16. Cohn, S. A.: Disuse atrophy of the periodontium in mice. Arch. Oral Biol., *10*:909, 1965.
17. Coolidge, E. D.: The thickness of the human periodontal membrane. J. Am. Dent. Assoc., *24*:1260, 1937.
18. Crumley, P. J.: Collagen formation in the normal and stressed periodontium. Periodontics, *2*:53, 1964.
19. Davies, R., and Picton, D. C. A.: Dimensional changes in the periodontal membrane of monkey's teeth with horizontal thrusts. J. Dent. Res., *46*:114, 1967.
20. Deporter, D. A., and Ten Cate, A. R.: Fine structural localization of acid and alkaline phosphatase in collagen-containing vesicles of fibroblasts. J. Anat. (Lond.), *114*:457, 1973.
21. Diab, M. A., and Stallard, R. E.: A study of the relationship between epithelial root sheath and root development. Periodontics, *3*:10, 1965.
22. Folke, L. E. A., and Stallard, R. E.: Periodontal microcirculation as revealed by plastic microspheres. J. Periodont. Res., *2*:53, 1967.
23. Freeman, E., and Ten Cate, A. R.: Development of the periodontium: An electron microscopic study. J. Periodontol., *42*:387, 1971.
24. Fullmer, H. M.: A critique of normal connective tissues of the periodontium and some alterations with periodontal disease. J. Dent. Res., *41*(Suppl. to No. 1):223, 1962.
25. Gibson, W., and Fullmer, H.: Histochemistry of the periodontal ligament. I. The dehydrogenases. Periodontics, *4*:63, 1966.
26. Gibson, W., and Fullmer, H.: Histochemistry of the periodontal ligament. II. The phosphatases. Periodontics, *5*:226, 1967.
27. Gibson, W., and Fullmer, H.: Histochemistry of the periodontal ligament. III. The esterases. Periodontics, *6*:71, 1968.
28. Gillespie, B. R., Chasens, A. F., Brownstein, C. N., and Alfano, M. C.: The relationship between the mobility of human teeth and their supracrestal fiber support. J. Periodontol., *50*:120, 1979.
29. Goggins, J. F.: The distribution of oxytalan connective tissue fibers in periodontal ligaments of deciduous teeth. Periodontics, *4*:182, 1966.
30. Grant, D., and Bernick, S.: A possible continuity between epithelial rests and epithelial attachment in miniature swine. J. Periodontol., *40*:87, 1969.
31. Grant, D., and Bernick, S.: The formation of the periodontal ligament. J. Periodontol., *43*:17, 1972.
32. Griffin, J. C.: Fine structure of the synthetizing periodontal fibroblasts and the maturation of periodontal collagen. J. Dent. Res., *46*:1311, 1967.
33. Grupe, H. E., Ten Cate, A. R., and Zander, H. A.: A histochemical and radiobiological study of *in vitro* and *in vivo* human epithelial cell rest proliferation. Arch. Oral Biol., *12*:1321, 1967.
34. Hindle, M. C.: Quantitative differences in periodontal membrane fibers. J. Dent. Res., *43*:953, 1964.
35. Inoue, M., and Akiyoshi, M.: Histologic investigation on Sharpey's fibers in cementum of teeth in abnormal function. J. Dent. Res., *41*:503, 1962.
36. Kardos, T. B., and Simpson, L. D.: A theoretical consideration of the periodontal membrane as a collagenous thixotropic system and its relationship to tooth eruption. J. Periodont. Res., *14*:444, 1979.
37. Kizior, J. E., Cuozzo, J. W., and Bowman, D. C.: Functional and histologic assessment of the sensory innervation of the periodontal ligament of the cat. J. Dent. Res., *47*:59, 1968.
38. Kronfeld, R.: Histologic study of the influence of function on the human periodontal membrane. J. Am. Dent. Assoc., *18*:1242, 1931.
39. Levy, B. M., and Bernick, S.: Studies on the biology of the periodontium of marmosets. II. Development and organization of the periodontal ligament of deciduous teeth in marmosets *(Callithrix jacchus)*. J. Dent. Res., *47*:27, 1968.
40. Levy, G., and Mailland, M. L.: Étude quantitative des effets de l'hypofonction occlusale sur la largeur desmodontale et la resorption osteoclastique alveolaire chez le rat. J. Biol. Buccale, *8*:17, 1980.

41. Melcher, A. H.: Remodelling of the periodontal ligament during eruption of the rat incisor. Arch. Oral Biol., *12*:1649, 1967.
42. Muhlemann, H. R.: The determination of tooth rotation centers. Oral Surg., *7*:392, 1954.
43. Muhlemann, H. R., Zander, H. A., and Halberg, F.: Mitotic activity in the periodontal tissues of the rat molar. J. Dent. Res., *33*:459, 1954.
44. Parfitt, G. H.: The physical analysis of tooth supporting structures. *In* The Mechanism of Tooth Support. Bristol, J. Wright and Sons, Ltd., 1967, p. 154.
45. Picton, D. C. S., and Davies, W. I. R.: Dimensional changes in the periodontal membrane of monkeys (*Macaca irus*) due to horizontal thrusts applied to the tooth. Arch. Oral Biol., *12*:1635, 1967.
46. Pihlstrom, B. L., and Ramfjord, S. P.: Periodontal effects of nonfunction in monkeys. J. Periodontol., *42*:748, 1971.
47. Reeve, C. M., and Wentz, F. J.: The prevalence, morphology and distribution of epithelial rests in the human periodontal ligament. Oral Surg., *15*:785, 1962.
48. Rippin, J. W.: Collagen turnover in the periodontal ligament under normal and altered functional forces. II. Adult rat molars. J. Periodont. Res., *13*:149, 1978.
49. Roberts, W. E., and Chamberlain, J. G.: Scanning electron microscopy of the cellular elements of rat periodontal ligament. Arch. Oral Biol., *23*:587, 1978.
50. Shackleford, J. M.: The indifferent fiber plexus and its relationship to principal fibers of the periodontium. Am. J. Anat., *131*:427, 1971.
51. Sicher, H.: The axial movement of continuously growing teeth. J. Dent. Res., *21*:201, 1942.
52. Simpson, H. E.: The degeneration of the rests of Malassez with age as observed by the apoxestic technique. J. Periodontol., *36*:288, 1965.
53. Stallard, R. E.: The utilization of H₃-proline by the connective tissues of the periodontium. Periodontics, *1*:185, 1963.
54. Stallard, R. E.: The effect of occlusal alterations on collagen formation within the periodontal ligament. Periodontics, *2*:49, 1964.
55. Stern, I. B.: An electron microscopic study of the cementum, Sharpey's fibers and periodontal ligament in the rat incisor. Am. J. Anat., *115*:377, 1964.
56. Ten Cate, A. R.: The histochemical demonstration of specific oxidative enzymes and glycogen in the epithelial cell of Malassez. Arch. Oral Biol., *10*:207, 1965.
57. Ten Cate, A. R.: The development of the periodontium. *In* Melcher, A. H., and Bowen, W. H. (eds.): Biology of the Periodontium. New York, Academic Press, 1969.
58. Ten Cate, A. R.: Formation of supporting bone in association with periodontal ligament organization in the mouse. Arch. Oral Biol., *20*:137, 1975.
59. Ten Cate, A. R., and Deporter, D. A.: The degradative role of the fibroblast in the remodelling and turnover of collagen in soft connective tissue. Anat. Rec., *182*:1, 1975.
60. Ten Cate, A. R., Mills, C., and Solomon, G.: The development of the periodontium. A transplantation and autoradiographic study. Anat. Rec., *170*:365, 1971.
61. Thomas, N. G.: Elastic fibers in periodontal membrane and pulp. J. Dent. Res., *7*:325, 1927.
62. Troth, J. R.: The development of the periodontal attachment in the rat. Acta Anat., *51*:313, 1962.
63. Trowbridge, H. O., and Shibata, F.: Mitotic activity in epithelial rests of Malassez. Periodontics, *5*:109, 1967.
64. Tryde, G., Frydenberg, O., and Brill, N.: An assessment of the tactile sensibility in human teeth. An evaluation of a quantitative method. Acta Odontol. Scand., *20*:233, 1962.
65. Valderhaug, J. P., and Nylen, M. U.: Function of epithelial rests as suggested by their ultrastructure. J. Periodont. Res., *1*:69, 1966.
66. Valderhaug, J. P., and Zander, H.: Relationship of "epithelial rests of Malassez" to other periodontal structures. Periodontics, *5*:254, 1967.
67. Weinstock, M.: Collagen formation—observations on its intracellular packaging and transport. Z. Zellforsch., *129*:455, 1972.
68. Zwarych, P. D., and Quigley, M. B.: The intermediate plexus of the periodontal ligament: history and further observations. J. Dent. Res., *44*:383, 1965.

The Cementum

NORMAL MICROSCOPIC FEATURES

Cementum is the calcified mesenchymal tissue that forms the outer covering of the anatomic root. It may exert a far more critical role in the development of periodontal disease than has thus far been demonstrated.

There are two main forms of root cementum: *acellular* (primary) and *cellular* (secondary). Both consist of a calcified interfibrillar matrix and collagen fibrils. Afibrillar cementum was discussed in Chapter 1 and will be mentioned briefly below. The cellular type contains cementocytes in individual spaces (lacunae) which communicate with each other through a system of anastomosing canaliculi. There are two sources of collagen fibers in cementum: (1) Sharpey's fibers, the embedded portion of the principal fibers of the periodontal ligament,[31, 42] which are formed by the fibroblasts; and (2) a group of fibers, belonging to the cementum matrix per se, produced by the cementoblasts.[36] Cementoblasts also form the glycoprotein interfibrillar ground substance.

Both acellular and cellular cementum are arranged in *lamellae* separated by incremental lines parallel to the long axis of the root (Figs. 3–1 and 3–2). These lines represent rest periods in cementum formation and are more mineralized than the adjacent cementum.[48] Sharpey's fibers make up most of the structure of *acellular cementum,* which has a principal role in supporting the tooth. Most of the fibers are inserted at approximately right angles into the root surface and penetrate deep into the cementum (Fig. 3–3; see also Fig. 2–2), but others enter from several different directions. Their size, number, and distribution increase

with function.[15] Sharpey's fibers are completely calcified, with the mineral crystals oriented parallel to the fibrils as they are in dentin and bone, except in a 10- to 50-micron-wide zone near the cemento-dentinal junction where they are partly calcified. The peripheral portions of Sharpey's fibers in actively mineralizing cementum tend to be more calcified than the interior regions according to evidence obtained

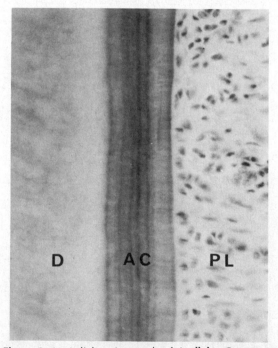

Figure 3–1 A light micrograph of **Acellular Cementum (AC)** showing incremental lines running parallel to the long axis of the tooth. These lines represent the appositional growth of cementum. Note the thin light lines running into the cementum perpendicular to the surface; these represent Sharpey's fibers of the periodontal ligament (PL). D, dentin. ×300.

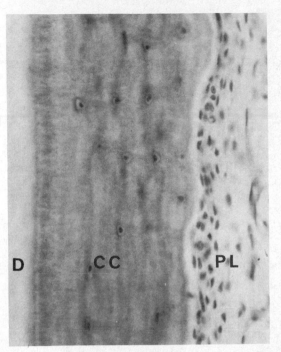

Figure 3–2 Cellular Cementum (CC) showing cemento-cytes lying within lacunae. Cellular cementum is thicker than acellular cementum (cf. Fig. 3–1). There is also evidence of incremental lines, but they are less distinct than in acellular cementum. The cells adjacent to the surface of the cementum in the periodontal ligament (PL) space are cementoblasts. D, dentin. ×300.

by scanning electron microscopy.[18] Acellular cementum also contains other collagen fibrils which are calcified and irregularly arranged or parallel to the surface.[35]

Cellular cementum is less calcified than the acellular type.[16] Sharpey's fibers occupy a smaller portion of cellular cementum and are separated by other fibers which are arranged either parallel to the root surface or at random (Fig. 3–4). Some of Sharpey's fibers are completely calcified, others are partially calcified, and in some there is a central uncalcified core surrounded by a calcified border.[18, 36]

The distribution of acellular and cellular cementum varies. The coronal half of the root is usually covered by the acellular type, and cellular cementum is more common in the apical half. With age, the greatest increase in cementum is of the cellular type in the apical half of the root and in the furcation areas.

Intermediate cementum is an ill-defined zone near the cemento-dentinal junction of certain teeth which appears to contain cellular remnants of Hertwig's sheath embedded in calcified ground substance.[7, 22]

The *inorganic content* of cementum [hydroxyapatite, $Ca_{10}(PO_4)_6(OH)_2$] is 45 to 50 per cent, which is less than that of bone (65 per cent), enamel (97 per cent), or dentin (70 per cent).[51] The calcium and magnesium–phospho-

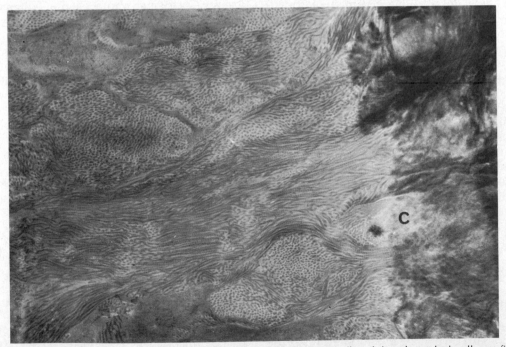

Figure 3–3 Electron Micrograph of the Surface of Acellular Cementum. Bundles of densely packed collagen fibrils of the periodontal ligament *(left)* are inserted into the cementum (C) surface. ×10,000. (From Dr. Knut A. Selvig: Studies on the Genesis, Composition, and Fine Structure of Cementum. Berlin-Oslo-Tromsö, Universitetsforlaget, 1967.)

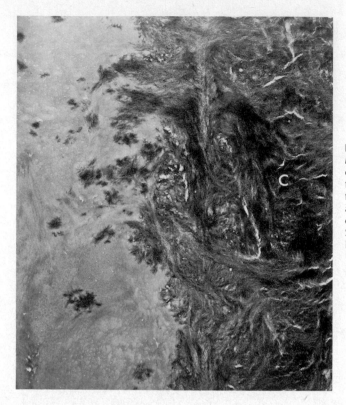

Figure 3–4   Electron Micrograph of the Surface of Mineralized Cellular Cementum. The cementum (C) contains irregularly arranged bundles of collagen fibrils covered with apatite crystals. Calcification foci are present in the precementum (*left*, unmineralized) within a 5-micron-wide zone at the surface of the cementum. × 10,000. (From Dr. Knut A. Selvig: Studies on the Genesis, Composition, and Fine Structure of Cementum. Berlin-Oslo-Tromsö, Universitetsforlaget, 1967.)

rus ratio is higher in apical than in cervical areas.[40] Opinions differ as to whether the microhardness increases[25] or decreases with age,[46] and no relationship has been established between aging and the mineral content of cementum.

Histochemical studies indicate that the *matrix of cementum* contains a *carbohydrate-protein complex. Neutral and acid mucopolysaccharides* are present in the matrix and cytoplasm of some cementoblasts. The lining of the lacunae, the incremental lines, and the precementum are rich in *acid mucopolysaccharides, possibly chondroitin sulfate B.*[34] Precementum stains metachromatically,[12] and the ground substance of acellular and cellular cementum is orthochromatic.

The reader is referred to the excellent review by Selvig[39] for further information on the chemical composition of cementum.

The Cemento-enamel Junction

The cementum at and immediately subjacent to the cemento-enamel junction is of particular clinical importance in root scaling procedures.[30] Three types of relationships involving the cementum may exist at the cemento-enamel junction.[26] Cementum *overlaps the en-amel* in about 60 to 65 per cent of the cases (Fig. 3–5). In about 30 per cent there is an *edge-to-edge butt joint,* and in 5 to 10 per cent the *cementum and enamel fail to meet.* In the last instance gingival recession may be accompanied by an accentuated sensitivity because the dentin is exposed.

A layer of *afibrillar cementum* sometimes extends a short distance onto the enamel at the cemento-enamel junction (see Chapter 1). It contains acid mucopolysaccharides and possibly a nonfibrillar form of collagen, in contrast with root cementum, which is rich in collagen fibers. It has been hypothesized that this material is deposited on the enamel by connective tissue following degeneration and shrinkage of the reduced enamel epithelium.[23] The afibrillar cementum may be partially covered by root cementum.

Cementum occurs on the crown of the tooth overlying the enamel in swine, covering more of the surface than in humans,[23] and over the entire enamel of bovine teeth.[9, 38]

Thickness of Cementum

The thickness of cementum on the coronal half of the root varies from 16 to 60 microns, or about the thickness of a hair. It attains its

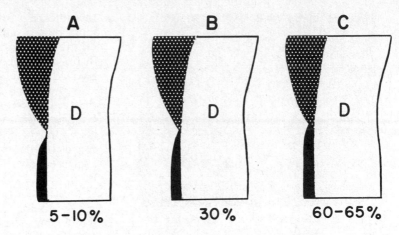

Figure 3–5 Statistical Representation of Normal Variations in Tooth Morphology at the Cemento-Enamel Junction. *A,* Space between enamel and cementum with dentin (D) exposed. *B,* End-to-end relationship of enamel and cementum. *C,* Cementum overlapping the enamel. (After Hopewell-Smith.)

greatest thickness, up to 150 to 200 microns, in the apical third, and also in the bifurcation and trifurcation areas.[29] Between the ages of 11 and 70 the average thickness of the cementum increases threefold, with the greatest increase in the apical region. Average thicknesses of 95 microns at age 20 and 215 microns at age 60 have been reported.[49]

Permeability of Cementum

In very young animals, both cellular and acellular cementum are very permeable and permit the diffusion of dyes from the pulp canal and from the external root surface. In cellular cementum the canaliculi in some areas are contiguous with the dentinal tubuli. Devitalized teeth take up about one tenth as much radioactive phosphorus (^{32}P) through the cementum as vital teeth.[47]

With age, the permeability of cementum diminishes.[5] There is also a relative diminution in the contribution of the pulp to the nutrition of the tooth, which increases the importance of the periodontal ligament as a pathway for metabolic exchange.[45] In the very aged, the phosphate exchange in the tooth by way of the periodontal ligament and cementum increases to 50 per cent of the total.[44]

CEMENTOGENESIS

Cementum formation starts, as does formation of bone and dentin, with the deposition of a meshwork of irregularly arranged collagen fibrils sparsely distributed in an interfibrillar ground substance or matrix called *precementum* or *cementoid.*[37, 38] It increases in thickness by the apposition of the matrix by cemento-

blasts. The progressive mineralization of the matrix begins at the cemento-dentinal junction and advances in the direction of the cementoblasts. Hydroxyapatite crystals are deposited first within and on the surface of the fibers and then in the ground substance. Periodontal ligament fibers being incorporated into the cementum at approximately right angles to the surface (Sharpey's fibers) become mineralized and appear under the scanning electron microscope as a series of mineralized spurs from which a fiber projects into the periodontal ligament.[18] Cementoblasts, initially separated from the cementum by uncalcified cementoid, sometimes become enclosed within the matrix and become trapped. Once enclosed they are referred to as cementocytes, and they remain viable in a fashion similar to osteocytes. Cementum formation is a continuous process which proceeds at a varying rate, but it is usually much slower than bone or dentin formation.

Continuous Deposition of Cementum

Cementum deposition continues after the teeth have erupted into contact with their functional antagonists and throughout life. Cementum formation is most rapid in the apical regions where it compensates for tooth eruption, which itself compensates for attrition.

An uncalcified surface layer of precementum, part of the process of continuous cementum deposition, was considered by Gottlieb[10] to be the natural barrier to excessive apical migration of the junctional epithelium. Impaired cementum formation ("cementopathia") was thought to be a cause of pathologic periodontal pocket formation because it reduced the restraint on epithelial migration.

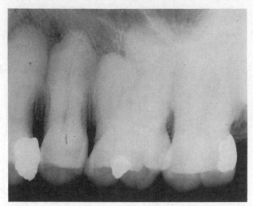

Figure 3–6   Hypercementosis in Paget's Disease.

Function and Cementum Formation

No clear-cut correlation has been established between occlusal function and cementum deposition.[21] From the findings of well-developed cementum on the roots of teeth in dermoid cysts and from the presence of thicker cementum on embedded teeth than on functional teeth,[11] it has been inferred that function is not necessary for cementum formation.

The biologic role of afibrillar cementum and its clinical implications are not understood at present.

Hypercementosis

The term *hypercementosis* (cementum hyperplasia) refers to a prominent thickening of the cementum. It may be localized to one tooth or may affect the entire dentition. Because of considerable physiologic variation in the thickness of cementum among different teeth of the same person and among teeth of different persons, it is sometimes difficult to distinguish between hypercementosis and physiologic thickening of cementum.

Hypercementosis occurs as a generalized thickening of the cementum, with nodular enlargement of the apical third of the root. It also appears in the form of spike-like excrescences (cemental spikes) created by either the coalescence of cementicles that adhere to the root[11] or the calcification of periodontal fibers at the sites of insertion into the cementum.[20]

The etiology of hypercementosis varies and is not completely understood. The spike-like type of hypercementosis generally results from excessive tension from orthodontic appliances or occlusal forces. The generalized type occurs in a variety of circumstances. In teeth without antagonists, it is interpreted as an effort to keep pace with excessive tooth eruption. In teeth subject to low-grade periapical irritation arising from pulp disease, it is considered compensation for the destroyed fibrous attachment to the tooth. The cementum is deposited adjacent to the inflamed periapical tissue. Hypercementosis of the entire dentition may be hereditary[50]; it also occurs in Paget's disease[33] (Fig. 3–6). Localized hypercementosis occurs at the insertion of the transseptal fibers in experimental lathyrism.[8]

Cementicles

Cementicles are globular masses of cementum arranged in concentric lamellae that lie free in the periodontal ligament or adhere to

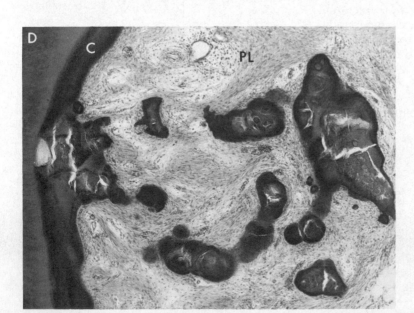

Figure 3–7   Cementicles free in the periodontal ligament (PL) and adherent to the root surface. C, cementum; D, dentin.

the root surface (Fig. 3–7). Cementicles may develop from calcified epithelial rests, around small spicules of cementum or alveolar bone traumatically displaced into the periodontal ligament, from calcified Sharpey's fibers, and from calcified thrombosed vessels within the periodontal ligament.[24]

Cementoma

Cementomas are masses of cementum generally situated apical to the teeth, to which they may or may not be attached. They are considered either odontogenic neoplasms or developmental malformations. Cementomas occur more frequently in females than in males, more often in the mandible than in the maxilla,[3] and may occur singly or multiply.[35] Usually harmless, they are generally discov-ered upon radiographic examination. In some cases they produce deformity of jaw contour.

The microscopic structure of the cementoma varies with regard to the proportions of connective tissue and cementum. The cementum may be arranged either as numerous coalescent cementicles or as an irregular meshwork of trabeculae separated by fibrous connective tissue.[10]

The surface of the cementoma is generally formed by a layer of newly formed, incompletely calcified cementoid lined by cementoblasts and surrounded by a connective tissue capsule. With continued deposition of cementum, the proportion of connective tissue within the lesion is reduced.

The radiographic appearance of the cementoma varies, depending upon the proportion

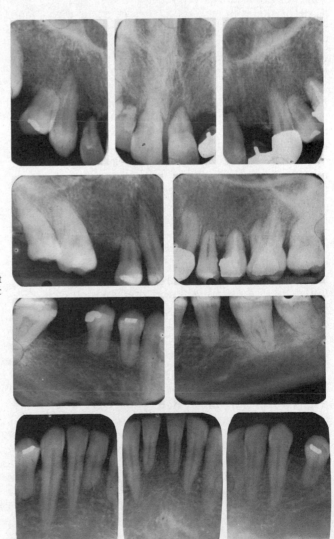

Figure 3–8 Idiopathic Root Resorption without unusual medical findings or history of orthodontic treatment.

of calcified cementum and fibrous connective tissue in the lesion. When composed principally of cementum, the lesion appears as a discrete, circumscribed, dense, radiopaque mass within which isolated radiolucent markings may be seen.

CEMENTUM RESORPTION AND REPAIR

The cementum of erupted as well as of unerupted teeth is subject to resorption. The resorptive changes may be of microscopic proportion or sufficiently extensive to present a radiographically detectable alteration in the root contour. Cementum resorption is extremely common. In a microscopic study of 261 teeth it occurred in 236 (90.5 per cent).[14] The average number of resorption areas per tooth was 3.5. Of the 922 areas of resorption, 708 (76.8 per cent) were located in the apical third of the root, 177 (19.2 per cent) in the middle third, and 37 (4.0 per cent) in the gingival third. Seventy per cent of all resorption areas were confined to the cementum without involving the dentin.

Cementum resorption may be due to local or systemic causes or may occur without the etiology being apparent (idiopathic) (Fig. 3–8). Among the local conditions in which it occurs are trauma from occlusion[28] (Fig. 3–9), orthodontic movement,[13, 19, 27, 32] pressure from malaligned erupting teeth, cysts and tumors,[21] teeth without functional antagonists, embedded teeth, replanted and transplanted teeth,[1] periapical disease, and periodontal disease. The peculiar susceptibility of the cervical area to resorption has been attributed to the absence of either uncalcified precementum or reduced enamel epithelium.[41] Among the systemic conditions suspected as predisposing to or inducing cemental resorption are deficiencies of calcium,[17] vitamin D, and vitamin A;[6] hypothyroidism;[2] hereditary fibrous osteodystrophy;[43] and Paget's disease.[33]

Cementum resorption appears microscopically as bay-like concavities in the root surface (Fig. 3–10). Multinucleated giant cells and large mononuclear macrophages are generally found adjacent to cementum undergoing active resorption (Fig. 3–11). Several sites of resorption may coalesce to form a large area of destruction. The resorptive process may extend into the underlying dentin and even into the pulp, but it is usually painless.

Cementum resorption is not necessarily continuous and may alternate with periods of **repair and the deposition of new cementum. The newly formed cementum is demarcated from the root by a deeply staining irregular line, termed a reversal line, which designates the border of the previous resorption (Fig. 3–12). Embedded fibers of the periodontal ligament re-establish a functional relationship in the new cementum. Cementum repair requires the presence of viable connective tissue. If epithelium proliferates into an area of resorption, repair will not take place. Cementum repair can occur in devitalized as well as in vital teeth.**

Fusion of the cementum and alveolar bone with obliteration of the periodontal ligament is termed **ankylosis.** Ankylosis occurs in teeth with cemental resorption, which suggests that it may represent a form of abnormal repair. Ankylosis may also develop following chronic periapical inflammation, tooth replantation, and occlusal trauma and around embedded teeth.

INJURIES TO CEMENTUM

Fracture

When a tooth is subjected to a severe external force, such as a blow or biting on a hard object, fracture of the root (Fig. 3–13) or "tearing" of the cementum may occur. Complete horizontal or oblique fractures may be followed by repair, which includes the deposition of calcified tissues and the embedding of new periodontal fibers. Several factors influence the likelihood of such repair. Exposure of the site of fracture to the oral cavity with subsequent infection will interfere with repair. Even in unexposed fractures, the deposition of calcified tissue is reduced upon *proximity of the fracture to the oral cavity.*[4] The distance between the fractured root ends and the inherent reparative capacity of the individual also influence repair of complete horizontal or oblique root fractures.

Cemental Tear

Detachment of a fragment of cementum from the root surface is known as a *cemental tear.* The separation of cementum may be complete, with displacement of a fragment into the periodontal ligament, or it may be incomplete, with the cementum fragment remaining

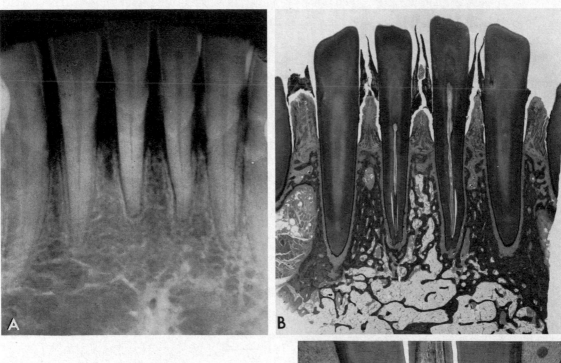

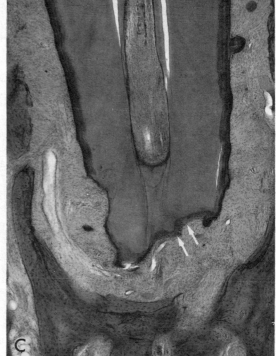

Figure 3–9　Cemental Resorption Associated with Excessive Occlusal Forces. *A,* Radiograph of mandibular anterior teeth. Note the thickening of the periodontal ligament space and lamina dura, with blunting of the apices of the central incisors. *B,* Low-power histologic section of the mandibular anterior teeth. *C,* Higher-power micrograph of left central incisor shortened by resorption of cementum and dentin. Note partial repair of the eroded areas *(arrows)* and cementicle at upper right.

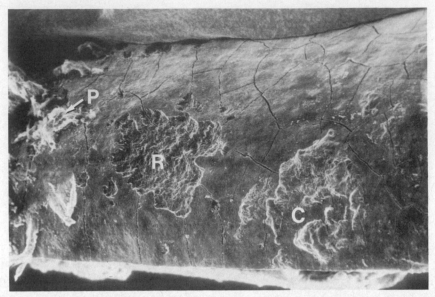

Figure 3–10   Scanning elecron micrograph of root exposed by periodontal disease showing large resorption bay (R). Remnants of the periodontal ligament are seen at P and calculus at C. Cracking of the tooth surface occurs as a result of the preparation technique. ×160. (Courtesy Dr. John Sottosanti.)

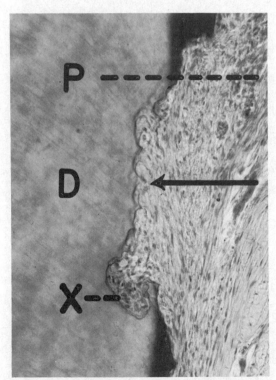

Figure 3–11   Resorption of Cementum and Dentin. A multinuclear osteoclast is seen at X. The direction of resorption is indicated by the arrow. Note the scalloped resorption front in the dentin (D). The cementum is the darkly stained band at upper and lower right. P, periodontal ligament.

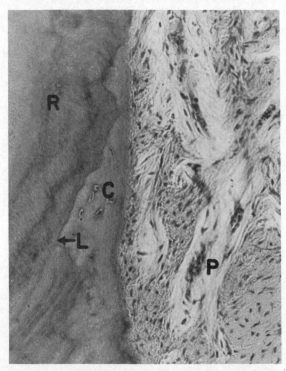

Figure 3–12   Section Showing Repair of Previously Resorbed Root. The defect is filled in with cellular cementum (C), which is separated from the older cementum (R) by an irregular line (L) that indicates the pre-existent outline of the resorbed root. P, periodontal ligament.

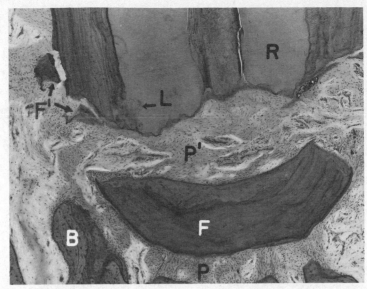

Figure 3–13   Root Repair After Traumatic Fracture. Detached fragments of cementum are shown at F′ at upper left. The apical section of cementum (F) is separated from the remainder of the root (R) by dense connective tissue (P′) and attached to the bone (B) by the periodontal ligament (P). A filled-in root defect is indicated by L.

partially attached to the roots (Figs. 3–14 and 3–15).

Cementum fragments displaced into the periodontal ligament may undergo a variety of changes. New cementum may be deposited at the periphery, and periodontal fibers may become embedded in it, so as to establish a functional relationship between the tooth on one aspect and alveolar bone on the other. The detached cementum may be reunited to the root surface by new cementum. Detached cementum fragments may be completely resorbed or may undergo partial resorption followed by addition of new cementum and embedding of collagen fibers.

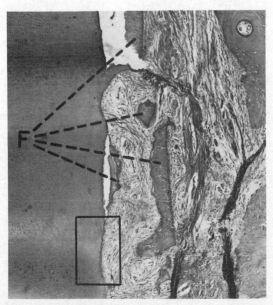

Figure 3–14   Traumatic "Cemental Tear" with fragments of cementum (F) free in the periodontal ligament.

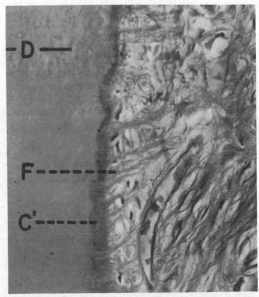

Figure 3–15   High-power section of area within rectangle in Figure 3–14. New cementum (C′) is shown along dentin (D). Collagen fibers (F) are embedded in the new cementum.

REFERENCES

1. Agnew, R. G., and Fong, C. C.: Histologic studies on experimental transplantation of teeth. Oral Surg., *9*:18, 1956.
2. Becks, H.: Root resorptions and their relation to pathologic bone formation. Int. J. Orthod. Oral Surg., *22*:445, 1936.
3. Bernier, J. L., and Thompson, H. C.: The histogenesis of the cementoma. Am. J. Orthod., *32*:543, 1946.
4. Bevelander, G.: Tissue reactions in experimental tooth fracture. J. Dent. Res., *21*:481, 1942.
5. Blayney, J. R., Wasserman, F., Groetzinger, G., and DeWitt, T. F.: Further studies on mineral metabolism of human teeth by the use of radioactive isotopes. J. Dent. Res., *29*:559, 1941.
6. Burn, C. G., Orten, A. I., and Smith, A. H.: Changes in the structure of the developing tooth in rats maintained on a diet deficient in vitamin A. Yale J. Biol. Med., *13*:817, 1940–41.
7. El Mostehy, M. R., and Stallard, R. E.: Intermediate cementum. J. Periodont. Res., *3*:24, 1968.
8. Gardner, A. F.: Alterations in mesenchymal and ectodermal tissues during experimental lathyrism. Apposition and calcification of cementum. Parodontologie, *20*:111, 1966.
9. Glimcher, M., Friberg, U., and Levine, P.: The identification and characterization of a calcified layer of coronal cementum in erupted bovine teeth. J. Ultrastruct. Res., *10*:76, 1964.
10. Gottlieb, B.: Biology of the cementum. J. Periodontol., *17*:7, 1942.
11. Gottlieb, B., and Orban, B.: Biology and Pathology of the Tooth and Its Supporting Mechanism. Trans. by M. Diamond. New York, The Macmillan Company, 1938, p. 70.
12. Haim, G.: Histochemische Untersuchungen des Zementgewebes. Dtsch. Zahnärtzl. Z., *16*:71, 1962.
13. Hemley, S.: The incidence of root resorption of vital permanent teeth. J. Dent Res., *20*:133, 1941.
14. Henry, J. L., and Weinmann, J. P.: The pattern of resorption and repair of human cementum. J. Am. Dent. Assoc., *42*:271, 1951.
15. Inoue, M., and Akiyoshi, M.: Histological investigation on Sharpey's fibers in cementum of teeth in abnormal function. J. Dent. Res., *41*:503, 1962.
16. Ishikawa, J., Yamamoto, H., Ito, K., and Masuda, M.: Microradiographic study of cementum and alveolar bone. J. Dent. Res., *43*:936, 1964.
17. Jones, M. R., and Simonton, F. V.: Mineral metabolism in relation to alveolar atrophy in dogs. J. Am. Dent. Assoc., *15*:881, 1928.
18. Jones, S. J., and Boyde, A.: A study of human root cementum surfaces as prepared for and examined in the scanning electron microscope. Z. Zellforsch., *130*:318, 1972.
19. Ketcham, A. H.: A progress report of an investigation of apical root resorption of permanent teeth. Int. J. Orthod., *15*:310, 1929.
20. Kronfeld, R.: Cementum and Sharpey's fibers. Z. Stomatol., *26*:714, 1928.
21. Kronfeld, R.: Biology of the cementum. J. Am. Dent. Assoc., *25*:1451, 1938.
22. Lester, K.: The incorporation of epithelial cells by cementum. J. Ultrastruct. Res., *27*:63, 1969.
23. Listgarten, M. A.: A light and electron microscopic study of coronal cementogenesis. Arch. Oral Biol., *13*:93, 1968.
24. Mikola, O. J., and Bauer, W. H.: Cementicles and fragments of cementum in the periodontal membrane. Oral Surg., *2*:1063, 1949.
25. Nihei, I.: A study of the hardness of human teeth. J. Osaka Univ. Dent. Soc., *4*:1, 1959.
26. Noyes, F. B., Schour, I., and Noyes, H. J.: A Textbook of Dental Histology and Embryology, 5th ed. Philadelphia, Lea & Febiger, 1938, p. 113.
27. Oppenheim, A.: Human tissue response to orthodontic intervention of short and long duration. Am. J. Orthod. Oral Surg., *28*:263, 1942.
28. Orban, B.: Tissue changes in traumatic occlusion. J. Am. Dent. Assoc., *15*:2090, 1928.
29. Orban, B.: Oral Histology and Embryology, 2nd ed. St. Louis, C. V. Mosby Company, 1944, p. 161.
30. Riffle, A. B.: Cemento-enamel junction. J. Periodontol., *23*:41, 1952.
31. Romaniuk, K.: Some observations of the fine structure of human cementum. J. Dent. Res., *46*:152, 1967.
32. Rudolph, C. E.: An evaluation of root resorption occurring during orthodontic therapy. J. Dent. Res., *19*:367, 1940.
33. Rushton, M. A.: Dental tissues in osteitis deformans. Guys Hosp. Rep., *88*:163, 1938.
34. Sasso, W.: Histochemical study of human dental cementum. Rev. Fac. Odont., *4*:189, 1966.
35. Scannell, J. M.: Cementoma. Oral Surg., *2*:1169, 1949.
36. Selvig, K.: The fine structure of human cementum. Acta Odontol. Scand., *23*:423, 1965.
37. Selvig, K. A.: Electron microscopy of Hertwig's epithelial sheath and early dentin and cementum formation in the mouse incisor. Acta Odontol. Scand., *21*:175, 1963.
38. Selvig, K. A.: An ultrastructural study of cementum formation. Acta Odontol. Scand., *22*:105, 1964.
39. Selvig, K. A.: Structure and metabolism of the normal periodontium. International Conference on Research in the Biology of Periodontal Diseases. Chicago, 1977.
40. Selvig, K. A., and Selvig, S. K.: Mineral content of human and seal cementum. J. Dent. Res., *41*:624, 1962.
41. Southam, J.: Clinical and histological aspects of peripheral cervical resorption. J. Periodontol., *38*:534, 1967.
42. Stern, I. B.: An electron-microscopic study of the cementum, Sharpey's fibrils and periodontal ligament in the rat incisor. Am. J. Anat., *115*:377, 1964.
43. Thoma, K. H., Sosman, M. C., and Bennett, G. A.: An unusual case of hereditary fibrous osteodystrophy (fragilitas ossium) with replacement of dentine by osteocementum. Am. J. Orthod. Oral Surg., *29*:1, 1943.
44. Volker, J. F.: The phosphate metabolism of the erupted tooth as indicated by studies utilizing the radioactive isotope. Tufts Outlook, *16*:3, 1942.
45. Volker, J. F., Gilda, J. E., and Ginn, J. T.: Radiophosphorus metabolism of pulpless teeth. J. Dent. Res., *21*:322, 1942.
46. Warren, E. B., et al.: Effects of periodontal disease and of calculus solvents on microhardness of cementum. J. Periodontol., *35*:505, 1964.
47. Wasserman, F., Blayney, J. R., Groetzinger, G., and DeWitt, T. G.: Studies on the different pathways of exchange of minerals in teeth with the aid of radioactive phosphorus. J. Dent. Res., *20*:389, 1941.
48. Yamamoto, H., et al.: Microradiographic and histopathological study of the cementum. Bull. Tokyo Dent. Univ., *9*:141, 1962.
49. Zander, H. A., and Hurzeler, B.: Continuous cementum apposition. J. Dent. Res., *37*:1035, 1958.
50. Zemsky, J. L.: Hypercementosis and heredity: An introduction and plan of investigation. Dent. Items Int., *53*:355, 1931.
51. Zipkin, I.: The inorganic composition of bones and teeth. *In* Schraer, H. (ed.): Biological Calcification. New York, Appleton-Century-Crofts, 1970.

chapter four

The Alveolar Bone

NORMAL MICROSCOPIC FEATURES

The **alveolar process** is the bone which forms and supports the tooth sockets (alveoli). It consists of the inner socket wall of thin compact bone called the **alveolar bone proper (cribriform plate),** the **supporting alveolar bone** which consists of cancellous trabeculae, and the facial and lingual plates of compact bone. The interdental septum consists of cancellous supporting bone enclosed within a compact border (Fig. 4–1).

The alveolar process is divisible into separate areas on an anatomic basis, *but it functions as a unit. All parts are interrelated in the support of the teeth.* Occlusal forces which are transmitted from the periodontal ligament to the inner wall of the alveolus are supported by the cancellous trabeculae, which in turn are buttressed by the labial and lingual cortical plates.

Cells and Intercellular Matrix

Alveolar bone is formed during fetal growth by intramembranous ossification and consists of a calcified matrix with **osteocytes** enclosed within spaces called lacunae. The osteocytes extend processes into canaliculi which radiate from the lacunae. The canaliculi form an anastomosing system through the intercellular matrix of the bone, which brings oxygen and nutrients via the blood to the osteocytes and removes metabolic waste products. Blood vessels branch extensively and travel through the periosteum. The endosteum lies adjacent to the marrow vasculature. Bone growth occurs by apposition of an organic matrix that is deposited by osteoblasts. For a detailed account of bone histology the reader is referred to any current standard textbook of histology.

Bone is composed principally of the minerals calcium and phosphate, along with hydroxyl, carbonates, citrate, and trace amounts of other ions, such as sodium, magnesium, and fluorine. The mineral salts are in the form of hydroxyapatite crystals of ultramicroscopic size and constitute approximately 65 to 70 per cent of

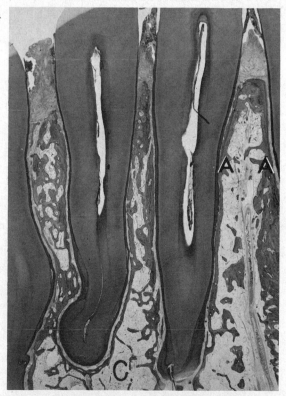

Figure 4–1 Mesiodistal Section Through Mandibular Canine and Premolars Showing Interdental Bony Septa. The dense bony plates (A) represent the alveolar bone proper (cribriform plates) and are supported by cancellous bony trabeculae (C). Note the vertical blood vessels within a nutrient canal in the interdental septum at the right.

the bone structure. The organic matrix[6] consists mainly (90 per cent) of collagen (Type I),[19] with small amounts of noncollagenous proteins, glycoproteins, phosphoproteins, lipids and proteoglycans. The apatite crystals are generally aligned with their long axes parallel to the long axes of collagen fibers and appear to be deposited upon and within the collagen fibers. In this fashion bone matrix is able to withstand heavy mechanical stresses applied to it during function.

Although the alveolar bone tissue is constantly changing in its internal organization, it retains approximately the same form from childhood through adult life. Bone deposition by osteoblasts is balanced by resorption by osteoclasts during the processes of tissue remodeling and renewal.

The bone matrix that is laid down by osteoblasts is not mineralized and is referred to as **prebone** or **osteoid.** While new prebone is being deposited, the older prebone located below the surface becomes mineralized as the mineralization front advances.

Prior to becoming mineralized, bone matrix collagen becomes coated or associated with a glycoprotein (or proteoglycan) material which, in the electron microscope, appears as an opaque granular substance. It is conceivable that this glycoprotein has an important role in the mineralization process. Osteoblasts produce this material together with other matrix constituents. A similar series of events is believed to occur during dentin matrix production and mineralization.[31]

Osteoclasts are large, multinucleated cells that are often seen on the surface of bone within eroded bony depressions referred to as *Howship's lacunae* (Fig. 4–2). The main function of these cells is considered to be resorption of bone. When they are active, as opposed to resting, they possess an elaborately developed ruffled border from which hydrolytic enzymes are believed to be secreted. These enzymes digest the organic portion of bone. The activity of osteoclasts and the morphology of the ruffled border can be modified and regulated by hormones such as parathormone and calcitonin.[14] The origin of osteoclasts is still a matter of speculation and controversy.

Small mononucleated cells have also been described as bone-resorbing cells.[30]

The Socket Wall

The principal fibers of the periodontal ligament which anchor the tooth in the socket are embedded for a considerable distance into the alveolar bone, where they are referred to as **Sharpey's fibers.** Some Sharpey's fibers are completely calcified, but most contain an un-

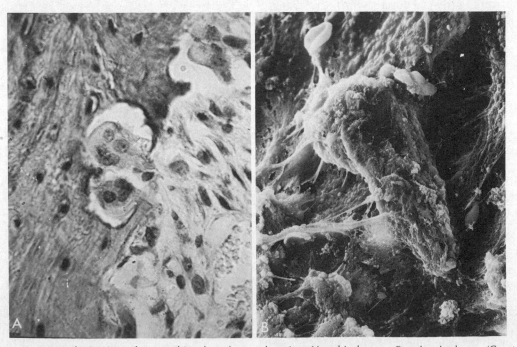

Figure 4–2   *A,* Histologic view of two multinucleated osteoclasts in a Howship lacuna. Rat alveolar bone. (Courtesy of Dr. Angela Ubios.) *B,* Scanning electron microscopic view of osteoclast on bone surface. Rat alveolar bone. (Courtesy of Drs. Angela Ubios and C. Martin.)

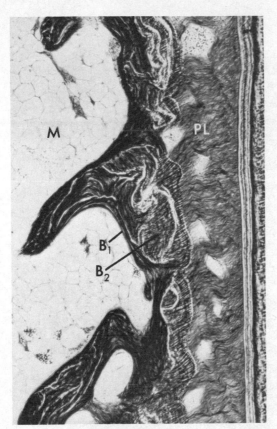

Figure 4–3 Deep Penetration of Sharpey's Fibers into Bundle Bone. The darkly stained bone (B₁) is lamellar bone. Bundle bone (B₂) takes up less stain and shows numerous white lines running more or less parallel to each other; these lines correspond to Sharpey's fibers. M, fatty marrow; PL, periodontal ligament.

calcified central core within a calcified outer layer.[8, 25] The socket wall consists of dense lamellated bone, some of which is arranged in haversian systems, and **bundle bone.** Bundle bone is the term given to bone adjacent to the periodontal ligament because of its content of Sharpey's fibers[29] (Fig. 4–3). It is arranged in layers with intervening appositional lines, parallel to the root (Fig. 4–4). Bundle bone is not unique to the jaws; it occurs throughout the skeletal system where ligaments and muscles are attached. Bundle bone is gradually resorbed on the side of the marrow spaces and replaced by lamellated bone.

The **cancellous portion of the alveolar bone** consists of trabeculae which enclose irregularly shaped marrow spaces lined with a layer of thin, flattened endosteal cells. There is wide variation in the trabecular pattern of the cancellous bone,[21] which is affected by occlusal forces. The matrix of the cancellous trabeculae consists of irregularly arranged lamellae separated by deeply staining incremental and re-

sorption lines indicative of previous bone activity, with an occasional haversian system.

Vascular Supply, Lymphatics, and Nerves

The cribriform plate of the tooth socket appears radiographically as a thin, radiopaque line, termed the **lamina dura.** However, it is perforated by numerous channels, containing blood, lymph vessels, and nerves, which link the periodontal ligament with the cancellous portion of the alveolar bone (Fig. 4–5). The vascular supply of the bone is derived from blood vessels branching off of the superior or inferior alveolar arteries. These arterioles enter the interdental septa within nutrient canals together with veins, nerves, and lymphatics. Dental arterioles, also branching off of the alveolar arteries, send tributaries through the periodontal ligament, and some small branches enter the narrow spaces of the bone via the perforations in the cribriform plate. Small vessels emanating from the facial and lingual compact bone also enter the marrow and spongy bone.

The Interdental Septum

The interdental septum consists of cancellous bone bordered by the socket walls of approximating teeth and the facial and lingual cortical plates (Fig. 4–6).

The mesiodistal angulation of the crest of the interdental septum usually parallels a line drawn between the cemento-enamel junctions of the approximating teeth.[23] The average distance between the crest of the alveolar bone and the cemento-enamel junction in the mandibular anterior region of young adults varies between 0.96 mm and 1.22 mm.[12] With age, the distance between the bone and the cemento-enamel junction increases throughout the mouth (1.88 mm to 2.81 mm).[9] However, this phenomenon may not be as much a function of age as of periodontal disease.

The Marrow

In the embryo and newborn, the cavities of all the bones are occupied by red hematopoietic marrow. The red marrow gradually undergoes a physiologic change to the fatty or yellow inactive type of marrow. In the adult, the marrow of the jaw is normally of the latter type, and red marrow is found only in the ribs,

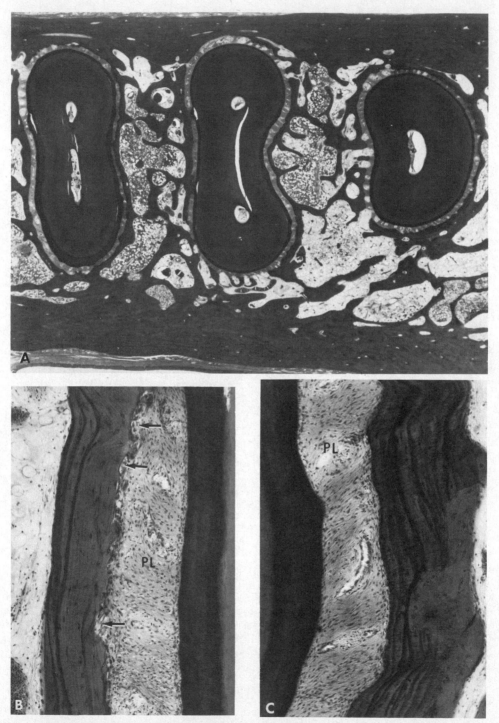

Figure 4–4   Bundle Bone Associated with Physiologic Mesial Migration of the Teeth. *A,* Horizontal section through molar roots in the process of mesial migration (mesial, *left;* distal, *right*). *B,* Mesial root surface showing osteoclasis of bone *(arrows). C,* Distal root surface showing bundle bone which has been partially replaced with dense bone on the marrow side. PL, periodontal ligament.

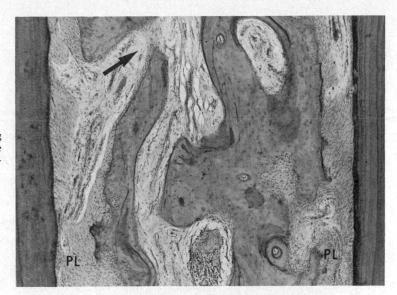

Figure 4–5   Interdental Bone showing vessel channel *(arrow)* connecting the marrow spaces with the periodontal ligament (PL).

sternum, vertebrae, skull, and humerus. However, foci of red bone marrow are occasionally seen in the jaws, often accompanied by resorption of bony trabeculae.[3] Common locations are the maxillary tuberosity (Fig. 4–7) and the maxillary and mandibular molar and premolar areas, which may be visible radiographically as zones of radiolucency. It has been suggested that they may be (1) remnants of the original marrow that has not undergone physiologic change to the fatty state, (2) localized manifestations of a generalized increase in red blood cell formation or of systemic disease such as tuberculosis,[4] or (3) the response to local injury or dental infection.

Bone is the calcium reservoir of the body, and the alveolar bone participates in the maintenance of the body calcium balance. *Calcium is constantly being deposited and withdrawn from the alveolar bone to provide for the needs of other tissues and to maintain the calcium level of the blood.* The calcium in the cancellous trabeculae is more readily available than that in compact bone. Conversely, easily mobilizable calcium is deposited in the trabeculae rather than in the cortex of adult bone. The hormonal control of calcium metabolism is complex, and information may be obtained from textbooks specifically on this subject.

So persistent is the effort to maintain a normal calcium level in the blood that even in cases of skeletal osteoporosis the blood calcium level may be normal. In experimental animals the rate of metabolism of alveolar bone is more rapid than that of the diaphysis of the femur, but it is slower than that of the metaphysis or "growth zone."[24]

THE EXTERNAL CONTOUR OF ALVEOLAR BONE

The bone contour normally conforms to the prominence of the roots, with intervening vertical depressions which taper toward the margin (Fig. 4–8). For a detailed anatomic account of the structure and relations of the alveolar processes, the reader is referred elsewhere.[23, 27] Alveolar bone anatomy varies from patient to patient and has important clinical implications.

The height and thickness of the facial and lingual bony plates are affected by the alignment of the teeth and angulation of the root to the bone and by occlusal forces. On teeth in labial version, the margin of the labial bone is located farther apically than on teeth in proper alignment. The bone margin is thinned to a knife edge and presents an accentuated arc in the direction of the apex (Fig. 4–9). On teeth in lingual version, the facial bony plate is thicker than normal. The margin is blunt and rounded, and horizontal rather than arcuate. The effect of the *root-to-bone angulation* upon the height of alveolar bone is most noticeable on the palatal roots of maxillary molars. *The bone margin is located farther apically on the roots, which form relatively acute angles with the palatal bone.*[13] The cervical portion of the alveolar plate is sometimes considerably thickened on the facial surface, apparently as reinforcement against occlusal forces (Fig. 4–10).

Fenestrations and Dehiscences

Isolated areas in which the root is denuded of bone and the root surface is covered only

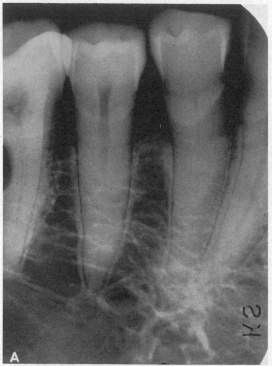

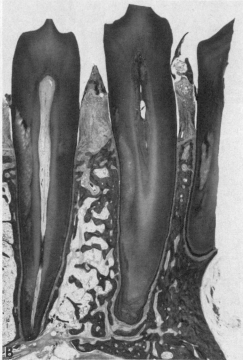

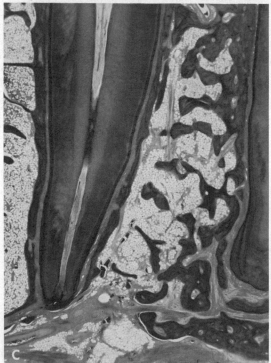

Figure 4–6 Interdental Septa. A, Mandibular premolar area. Note the prominent lamina dura. B, Interdental septa between the canine (right) and premolars. The central cancellous portion is bordered by the dense bony cribriform plates of the socket. (This forms the lamina dura around the teeth in the radiograph.) C, Interdental septum between the premolars, showing central cancellous bone and dense cribriform plate around the roots.

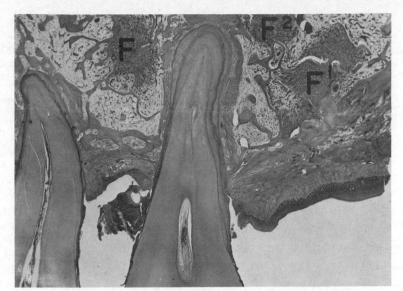

Figure 4–7   Mesiodistal section in the molar area of the maxilla of a 59-year-old male, showing foci of hematopoiesis in the marrow (F, F¹, F²).

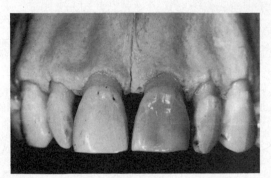

Figure 4–8   Normal Bone Contour conforms to the prominence of the roots.

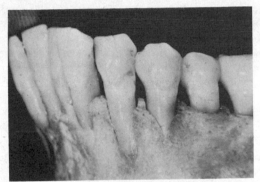

Figure 4–9   Apical location of bone on the labially placed mandibular canine and first premolar. Compare with higher level and thicker margin of the bone on the second premolar.

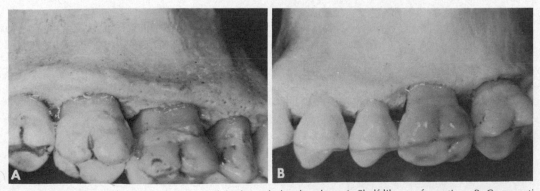

Figure 4–10   Variation in the cervical portion of the buccal alveolar plate. *A,* Shelf-like conformation. *B,* Comparatively thin buccal plate.

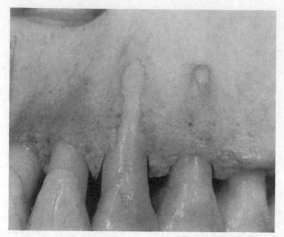

Figure 4–11 **Dehiscence** on the canine and **Fenestration** of the first premolar.

by periosteum and overlying gingiva are termed *fenestrations.* In this instance the marginal bone is intact. When the denuded areas extend through the marginal bone, the defect is called a *dehiscence* (Fig. 4–11). Such defects occur on approximately 20 per cent of the teeth; they occur more often on the facial bone than on the lingual, are more commonly on anterior teeth than on posterior teeth, and are frequently bilateral. There is microscopic evidence of lacunar resorption at the margins. The cause is not clear, but trauma from occlusion may be suspected.[28] Prominent root contours, malposition, and labial protrusion of the

root combined with a thin bony plate are predisposing factors.[7] Fenestration and dehiscence are important because they may complicate the outcome of periodontal surgery.

THE LABILITY OF ALVEOLAR BONE

In contrast to its apparent rigidity, alveolar bone is the least stable of the periodontal tissues; its structure is in a constant state of flux.[17] The physiologic lability of alveolar bone is maintained by a sensitive balance between bone formation and bone resorption, regulated by local and systemic influences (Fig. 4–12). Bone is resorbed in areas of pressure and formed in areas of tension. The cellular activity which affects the height, contour, and density of alveolar bone is manifested in three areas: (1) *adjacent to the periodontal ligament,* (2) *in relation to the periosteum of the facial and lingual plates,* and (3) *along the endosteal surface of the marrow spaces.*

Mesial Migration of the Teeth and Reconstruction of Alveolar Bone

With time and wear the proximal contact areas of the teeth are flattened and the teeth tend to move mesially. This is referred to as **physiologic mesial migration,** a gradual process with intermittent periods of activity, rest, and repair. By age 40, it effects a reduction of 0.5

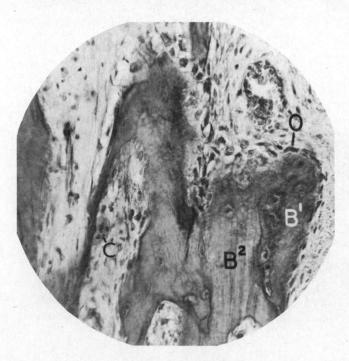

Figure 4–12 **Bone Formation and Bone Resorption in Close Proximity in Alveolar Bone.** Osteoblast (O) at the periphery of new bone (B¹) formed on older lamellated bone (B²) at site of previous resorption, indicated by irregular reversal line. Note osteoclast (C) along adjacent partially resorbed trabecula.

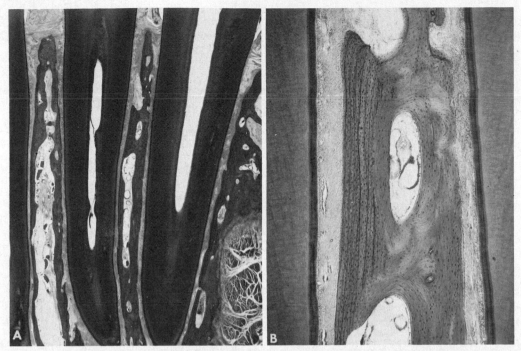

Figure 4–13   Bone Response to Physiologic Mesial Migration. *A,* Interdental septa between the canine *(left)* and first and second premolars. *B,* Interdental septum between the first and second premolars, showing lamellae of newly apposed bone opposite the distal of the first premolar *(left)* and resorption opposite the mesial of the second *(right).*

cm in the length of the dental arch from the midline to the third molars.[2] *Alveolar bone is reconstructed in compliance with the physiologic mesial migration of the teeth.* Bone resorption is increased in areas of pressure along the mesial surfaces of the teeth, and new layers of bundle bone are formed in areas of tension on the distal surfaces (Fig. 4–13; see also Fig. 4–4).

Occlusal Forces and Alveolar Bone

There are two aspects to the relationship between occlusal forces and alveolar bone. **The bone exists for the purpose of supporting teeth during function** and, in common with the remainder of the skeletal system, **depends upon the stimulation it receives from function for the preservation of its structure**. There is therefore a constant and sensitive balance between occlusal forces and the structure of alveolar bone.[16]

Alveolar bone undergoes constant physiologic remodeling in response to occlusal forces. Osteoclasts and osteoblasts redistribute bone substance to meet new functional demands most efficiently. Bone is removed from where it is no longer needed and added where new needs arise.

When an occlusal force is applied to a tooth either through a food bolus or by contact with opposing teeth, several things happen, depending upon the direction, intensity, and duration of the force. The tooth is displaced against the resilient periodontal ligament, in which it creates areas of tension and compression. The facial and lingual walls of the socket stretch somewhat in the direction of the force.[23] When the force is released, the tooth, ligament, and bone spring back to their original positions.

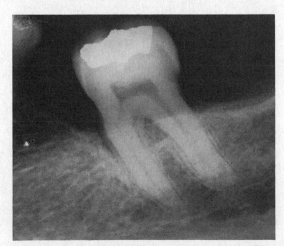

Figure 4–14   Bony Trabeculae realigned perpendicular to the mesial root of tilted molar.

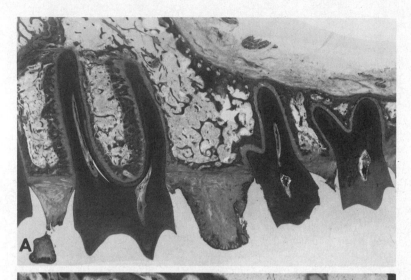

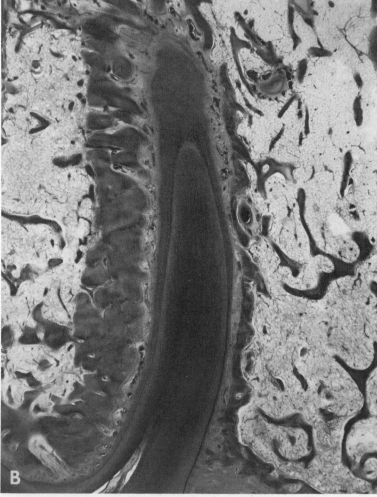

Figure 4–15   Bone Response to In-creased Occlusal Forces. *A,* Mesio-distal section through maxillary molar and premolars subjected to increased occlusal forces in a monkey. *B,* Me-siobuccal root of the second molar, showing thickening of bone along the distal surface in response to increased tension and thinning of the bone on the mesial aspect caused by increased pressure.

The socket wall reflects the responsiveness of alveolar bone to traumatic occlusal forces. Osteoblasts and newly formed osteoid line the socket in areas of tension; osteoclasts and bone resorption occur in areas of pressure.[2, 20]

The number, density, and alignment of cancellous trabeculae are also influenced by occlusal forces (Fig. 4–14). Experimental systems utilizing photoelastic analysis indicate alterations in stress patterns in the periodontium created by changes in the direction and intensity of occlusal forces.[11] The bony trabeculae are aligned in the path of the tensile and compressive stresses so as to provide maximum resistance to the occlusal force with a minimum of bone substance (Fig. 4–15).[26] Forces which exceed the adaptive capacity of the bone produce injury called trauma from occlusion (see Chapter 19).

When occlusal forces are increased, the cancellous trabeculae are increased in number and thickness, and bone may be added to the external surface of the labial and lingual plates (see Fig. 4–10). When occlusal forces are reduced, bone is resorbed, bone height is diminished, and the number and thickness of the trabeculae are reduced.[15] This is termed **disuse** or **afunctional atrophy.** Although occlusal forces are extremely important in determining the internal architecture and external contour of alveolar bone, other factors such as local physiochemical conditions, vascular anatomy, and the individual systemic condition are also involved.[1]

REFERENCES

1. Anderson, B. G., Smith, A. H., Arnim, S. S., and Orten, A. V.: Changes in molar teeth and their supporting structures in rats following extraction of the upper right first and second molars. Yale J. Biol. Med., *9*:189, 1936.
2. Black, C. V.: Pathology of the Hard Tissues of the Teeth. Oral Diagnosis. 8th ed. Woodstock, Ill., Medico-Dental Publishing Company, 1948, p. 389.
3. Box, H. K.: Bone resorption in red marrow hyperplasia in human jaws. Bull. 21, Can. Dent. Res. Found., 1936.
4. Cahn, L. R.: Red marrow in the jaws. J. Am. Dent. Assoc., *27*:1056, 1940.
5. Cohn, S. A.: Disuse atrophy of the periodontium in mice. Arch. Oral Biol., *10*:909, 1965.
6. Eastoe, J. E.: The organic matrix of bone. *In* Bourne, G. H. (ed.): The Biochemistry and Physiology of Bone. New York, Academic Press, 1956, p. 81.
7. Elliot, J. R., and Bowers, G. M.: Alveolar dehiscence and fenestration. Periodontics, *1*:245, 1963.
8. Frank, R., Lindemann, G., and Vedrine, J.: Structure submicroscopique de l'os alveolaire des maxillaires á l'etat normal. Rev. Franc. Odont., *5*:1507, 1958.
9. Gargiulo, A. W., Wentz, F. M., and Orban, B.: Dimensions and relations of the dentogingival junction in humans. J. Periodontol., *32*:216, 1961.
10. Glickman, I., and Wood, H.: Bone histology in periodontal disease. J. Dent. Res., *21*:35, 1942.
11. Glickman, I., Roeber, F. W., Brion, M., and Pameijer, J. H. N.: Photoelastic analysis of internal stresses in the periodontium created by occlusal forces. J. Periodontol., *41*:30, 1970.
12. Herulf, G.: On det marginala alveolarbenet hos ungdom i studiealder-nenrontgenstudie. Svensk Tandklakare-Tidsskrift., *43*:42, 1950.
13. Hirschfeld, I.: A study of skulls in the American Museum of Natural History in relation to periodontal disease. J. Dent. Res., *5*:241, 1923.
14. Holtrop, M. E., Raisz, L. G., and Simmons, H. A.: The effects of parathyroid hormone, colchicine and calcitonin on the ultrastructure and the activity of osteoclasts in organ culture. J. Cell Biol., *60*:346, 1974.
15. Kellner, E.: Histologic findings on teeth without antagonists. Z. Stomatol., *26*:271, 1928.
16. MacMillan, H. W.: A consideration of the structure of the alveolar process, with special reference to the principle underlying its surgery and regeneration. J. Dent. Res., *6*:251, 1924–1926.
17. Manson, J. D.: Age Changes in Bone Activity in the Mandible. Proceedings of the First European Bone and Tooth Symposium. Oxford, Pergamon Press, 1964, pp. 343–349.
18. McLean, F. C., and Urist, M. R.: Bone. 2nd ed. Chicago, University of Chicago Press, 1961, p. 38.
19. Miller, E. J.: A review of biochemical studies on the genetically distinct collagens of the skeletal system. Clin. Orthop., *92*:260, 1973.
20. Orban, B.: Tissue changes in traumatic occlusion. J. Am. Dent. Assoc., *15*:2090, 1928.
21. Parfitt, G. J.: An investigation of the normal variations in alveolar bone trabeculation. Oral Surg., *15*:1453, 1962.
22. Picton, D. A.: On the part played by the socket in tooth support. Arch. Oral Biol., *10*:945, 1965.
23. Ritchey, B., and Orban, B.: The crests of the interdental alveolar septa. J. Periodontol., *24*:75, 1953.
24. Rogers, H. J., and Weidman, S. M.: Metabolism of alveolar bone. Br. Dent. J., *90*:7, 1951.
25. Selvig, K. A.: The fine structure of human cementum. Acta Odontol. Scand., *23*:423, 1965.
26. Sepel, C. M.: Trajectories of jaws. Acta Odontol. Scand., *8*:81, 191, 1948.
27. Sicher, H.: Oral Anatomy. St. Louis, C. V. Mosby Company, 1949, p. 385.
28. Stahl, S. S., Cantor, M., and Zwig, E.: Fenestrations of the labial alveolar plate in human skulls. Periodontology, *1*:99, 1963.
29. Stein, G., and Weinmann, J. P.: The physiologic movement of the teeth. Z. Stomatol., *23*:733, 1925.
30. Vilmarin, H.: Characteristics of growing bone surfaces. Scand. J. Dent. Res., *87*:65, 1979.
31. Weinstock, A., Bibb, C., Burgeson, R. E., Fessler, L. I., and Fessler, J. H.: Intracellular transport and secretion of procollagen in chick bone as shown by E. M. radioautography and biochemical analysis. *In* Slavkin, H. C., and Greulich, R. C. (eds.): Extracellular Matrix Influence on Gene Expression. New York, Academic Press, 1975, p. 101.

Masticatory Function

Recognition and correction of occlusal relationships that are injurious to the periodontium and that may be associated with disorders of the masticatory musculature and temporomandibular joints require an understanding of the principles of occlusion and masticatory function. Fundamentals of occlusal function are presented here; clinical application is described in other chapters.

DEFINITION OF FUNCTIONAL OCCLUSION

The term occlusion *refers to the contact relationships of the teeth resulting from neuromuscular control of the masticatory system (musculature, temporomandibular joints, mandible, and periodontium).*[65] **In the functional sense, normality or abnormality of an individual occlusion is determined by the manner in which it functions and by its effect upon the periodontium, musculature, and temporomandibular joints rather than by the alignment of the teeth in each arch and the static relationship of the arches to each other.**

Three classes of functional occlusion are identified:

PHYSIOLOGIC OCCLUSION. *An occlusion that exists in an individual in whom the signs of occlusion-related pathosis are absent is a physiologic occlusion.* This implies a range of morphologic variability in occlusion of the teeth and, in addition, a sense of psychologic and physical comfort. In fact, no occlusion can be considered more ideal than that which exists in a given mouth free of disease and dysfunction.[78] Under conditions of physiologic occlusion, there is a controlled adaptive response characterized by minimal muscle hyperactivity and limited stress to the system.

TRAUMATIC OCCLUSION. *A traumatic occlusion is an occlusion judged to be a causal factor in the formation of traumatic lesions or disturbances in the supporting structures of the teeth, muscles, and temporomandibular joints.* **The criterion that determines whether an occlusion is traumatic is whether it produces injury, not how the teeth occlude.** Actually, almost every dentition has supracontacts that have traumatic potential under states of altered muscle tonus and stress.

THERAPEUTIC OCCLUSION. *A treatment occlusion employed to counteract structural interrelationships related to traumatic occlusion is called a therapeutic occlusion.* The term is also used to describe an occlusal scheme employed in restoring or replacing occlusal surfaces so that minimum adaptation is required of the individual and compensatory tissue changes are minimized.

Terminology

The terminology of occlusion was developed by workers in several biologic and dental specialties, resulting in a richly heterogeneous and confusing terminology. The interpretation of the word *centric* has contributed to the controversy.[29] Owing to the confusion concerning the terms for the various "centrics," alternative terms are used in this text. The following terms are advocated in an attempt at clarity[39, 79] and in response to research[79] regarding various jaw positions and recording methods:

Intercuspal position (ICP): (1) The position of the mandible with maximum intercuspation of the teeth; (2) the most cranial point of all functional contact movement. Synonyms: centric occlusion (CO), habitual occlusion, acquired centric, habitual centric.

Muscular contact position (MCP): The position of the mandible when it has been lifted from its resting posture to the very first occlusal contact by a minimum of muscular effort.

Retruded position (RP): Any position of the mandible on the terminal hinge path. Synonyms: centric relation (CR), terminal hinge position.

Retruded contact position (RCP): The end point of terminal hinge closure. Synonym: centric relation contact (CRC).

Excursive movement*: Movement occurring when

---

*The movement of the mandible can be related to the direction in which the mandibular teeth move from ICP during excursion. The Latin word *trudere,* meaning "to thrust," is used with appropriate prefixes denoting the direction of movement.

the mandible moves away from the intercuspal position (Fig. 5–1).

Protrusion: Movement occurring when the mandible moves anteriorly from the intercuspal position.

Retrusion: Movement occurring when the mandible moves posteriorly from the intercuspal position.

Laterotrusion: Movement occurring when the mandible moves away from the midline. Synonym: working movement.

Functional segments: (See Figure 5–1).

Laterotrusive side: The side that moves away from the midline in laterotrusion. Synonyms: working side, functional side.

Mediotrusive side: The side that moves toward the midline in laterotrusion. Synonyms: nonworking side, balancing side, nonfunctional side, idling side.

Intercuspal Contacts

The teeth make contact in a variety of patterns, with fewer contacts than frequently believed. This suggests that ideal tooth contact relationships in natural dentitions are not common.[2]

Studies of Australian aborigines show that the anterior teeth should make very light contact or no contact.[9] However, in young American adults, firm contacts on the incisor teeth have been observed in many functionally

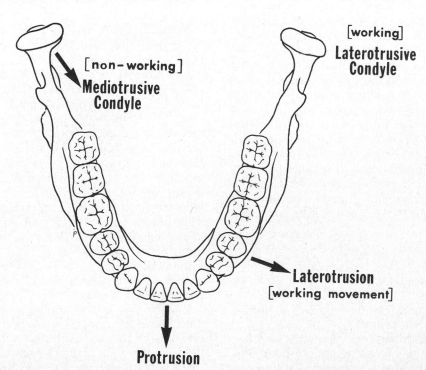

Figure 5–1 Mandibular movement is named after the direction of movement the mandible takes when it moves away from the intercuspal position. Functional parts of the mandible can also be identified by reference to the movement to which they are related.

asymptomatic individuals.[61] Therefore, a variety of interincisal contact schemes appear acceptable. In occlusal therapy, however, heavy anterior interincisal contact should be avoided because of the increased risk of creating bite discomfort, avoidance of certain muscles, mandibular instability, and trauma from occlusion.

In almost all asymptomatic individuals, simultaneous posterior contacts on the existing posterior teeth are the norm during firm ICP closure. Deviations from this pattern should arouse the attention of the clinician. There are significantly more contacts with hard pressure than with light pressure.[69] Although individual posterior supporting cusps occlude with variable stability on marginal ridges and in fossae, total arch stability is rendered by the combined effect of multiple, simultaneous contacts having an overall horizontal vector of zero at the ICP. Objective reporting of the frequency and distribution of ICP contact should include documentation of the results of ultrathin feeler gauge testing in the molar, premolar, canine, and incisal zones of each half of the dental arch.[61]

Supracontacts and Occlusal Interferences

Supracontact is a general term for any contact that hinders the remaining occlusal surfaces in achieving a many-pointed, stable contact. A supracontact is a *morphologic relationship* and does not necessarily imply a dysfunctional situation. Moreover, a supracontact in relation to one mandibular contact situation is not necessarily a supracontact in relation to others.[39] *Occlusal interferences* are supracontacts capable of injuring the supporting periodontal tissues or complicating mandibular movement. Interferences that deflect closure in the retruded position are referred to as *retrusive prematurities;* those that interfere with closure in ICP are called *intercuspal prematurities.*

MANDIBULAR MOVEMENT

Jaw movement can be classified as **border, intraborder,** and **contact.**

Border movements are the limits to which the mandible can move in any direction. Posselt, in a classic study,[59] developed a rhomboid figure that represents border movement of the mandible (Fig. 5–2).

Contact movement is the movement of the mandible with one or more of the opposing occlusal surfaces in contact (Fig. 5–3). The difference between ICP and RCP is about 1.0 mm measured at the incisors and 0.5 mm measured at the mandibular condyles.[31, 32, 80, 81] Moreover, ICP lies in a symmetrical, forward position relative to RCP in about 85 per cent of young adults (see Fig. 5–2).[81] In a small but significant percentage of individuals (10 to 30 per cent), RCP and ICP are coincident or nearly coincident. Although muscular effort is necessary to reach RCP, most individuals with coincident RCP-ICP relationships show no discomfort when closing to full contacts. One of the characteristics of a physiologic occlusion is that the teeth normally contact in ICP when they are closed with a minimum muscular effort from rest position. "Touch and slide" from MCP to ICP is a sign often found in patients with traumatic or uncomfortable occlusions.

Intraborder movement is any mandibular movement within the perimeter of border movement. Intraborder movement is chiefly associated with free movement, chewing, and phonation.

Condyle Positions and Movements

Retruded position **(RP)** refers to a position of the mandible and is synonymous with the term *centric relation* **(CR).** The term *intercuspal position* **(ICP)** is synonymous with the term *centric occlusion* **(CO)** and refers to the position of the teeth. When the mandible is in the retruded position (RP), the condyles are in their most retruded, superior position against the posterior slope of the articular eminence. Restraint on retrusive jaw movement is imposed by the lateral ligaments[3] and to some degree by the muscles.[44] During jaw movements from RCP to ICP, the condyles undergo slight anterior and inferior movement. In some individuals RCP and ICP are identical; hence, the position of the condyle does not change. When the mandible is in rest position, the condyles are usually anterior and inferior to their position in ICP.[32, 68]

In opening and closing the jaw, the condyles are capable of rotation or translation or combinations of the two motions. On full opening, the condyles glide along the posterior slope of the articular eminence to an average of 1 mm anterior to the inferior crest of the eminence.[68]

With the jaw opened wide there may be a

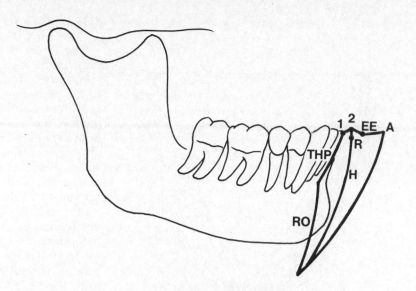

Figure 5–2 Rhomboid Figure of Mandibular Movements in the Sagittal Plane (Posselt). 1, Retruded contact position. 2, Intercuspal position. THP, Terminal hinge path. EE, Edge-to-edge position. RO, retruded path beyond terminal hinge opening. The condyles undergo both rotation and translation at this point. A, Border movement with maximum protrusion. H, Habitual (functional) pathway of the mandible. R, The rest (postural) position of the mandible.

slight reduction (approximately 0.09 mm) in the width of the mandible in the molar area.[67] The jaws ordinarily open and close into ICP, rather than into RCP. Opening involves simultaneous rotation and downward translation of the condyle.

Movements of the mandible with the teeth in contact, which are termed *excursions,* may be *laterotrusive, protrusive, lateroprotrusive,* or *retrusive* (see Fig. 5–1). Laterotrusive (side-to-side) contacts of the mandibular posterior teeth along the buccal cusps of the maxillary teeth (lateral excursions) occur occasionally in chewing and swallowing; they occur often in bruxism. Protrusive excursions are also part of the opening chewing cycle but similarly, are more extensive in bruxism.

In the lateral movements of the mandible, the laterotrusive side either rotates about a vertical axis or combines lateral movement with rotation (Fig. 5–4). The lateral shift of the condyle (average, 0.2 mm)[8, 20] is called the **Bennett movement** (Fig. 5–4*B*). The term *side shift* is misleading because the condyles rarely move purely horizontally, but instead translate and rotate in curvilinear paths in three planes

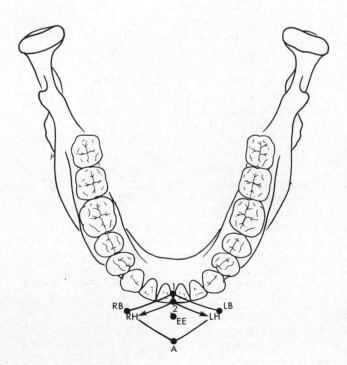

Figure 5–3 Movements of the Mandible at the Incisal Point (Infradentale). 1, Retruded contact position. 2, Intercuspal position. EE, Edge-to-edge position. A, Contact at maximal protrusin. RH and LH, Right and left habitual movement positions. RB and LB, Right and left border positions. Jaw undergoes maximum lateral movement at RB and LB.

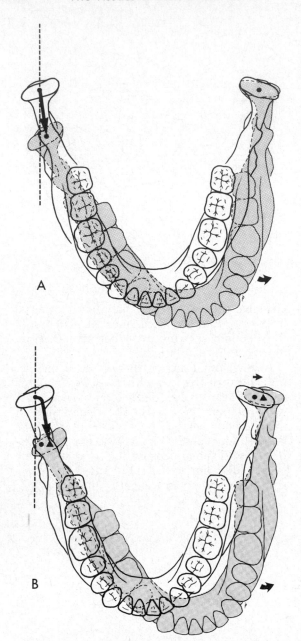

Figure 5–4 *A*, Pure left lateral rotation of the mandible (no Bennett movement). *B*, Lateral movement of the jaw incorporating Bennett movement.

of space simultaneously.[42] The condyle on the mediotrusive (nonworking) side moves downward, forward, and inward and describes the **Bennett angle** with respect to a sagittal line, when viewed in the horizontal plane (Fig. 5–4). To make the distinction between the two terms, it should be noted that the Bennett *angle* is always present, but the Bennett *movement* may not be present.

THE FORCES OF OCCLUSION

The forces of occlusion are created by the musculature in chewing, swallowing, and speech and are transmitted through the teeth to the periodontium. These forces function in synchronized balance. They guide the alignment of the teeth as they erupt and participate in maintaining the position of the teeth in the arches. Tooth position and arch form are not static; they are maintained by the balance among the various forces of occlusion. Disturbance of this balance may lead to altered tooth positions and changes in the functional environment that may be injurious to the periodontium.

The following factors are involved in the creation and distribution of the forces of occlusion:

1. *The forces of the muscles of mastication and the counteracting oral musculature.* The balance between the antagonistic forces of occlusion is shown in Table 5–1.[11]

2. *Inclined planes of the teeth and the anterior component of force.* The forces exerted by the muscles on closure of the mandible are distributed in several directions by the inclined planes of the teeth. *The resultant of the occlusal forces gives rise to an anterior force, which tends to move the teeth mesially and is termed the anterior component of force* (Fig. 5–5).

The anterior component of force pushes the teeth mesially in their sockets. When the force is released, the teeth move back to their previous position because of the resilience of the periodontal ligament. With time, that areas of proximal contact are flattened by wear, permitting mesial movement of the teeth, referred to as physiologic mesial migration. The overall effect is a reduction of 0.5 cm in the length of the dental arch from the third molars to the midline by the age of 40 years.

3. *Proximal contacts.* The anterior component of force is transmitted through intact proximal contacts. Contacts malpositioned in a cervicoincisal or faciolingual direction deflect the forces of occlusion and may cause displacement of the teeth (Fig. 5–6) and create abnormal forces on the periodontium.

4. *Design and inclination of the teeth.* Certain features of tooth design affect the transmission of occlusal forces. For example, the maxillary central incisor is shaped so that it is inclined mesially to provide maximum efficiency of its cutting edge. In function, the maxillary incisors tend to be driven mesially and buttress each other. The root of the max-

TABLE 5–1   BALANCE BETWEEN ANTAGONISTIC OCCLUSAL FORCES[11]

Lips ————————————————→	←——Tongue
Cheeks————————————————→	←——Tongue
Eruption (growth of teeth)————————→	←——Masticatory muscles (masseter, temporalis, internal pterygoid)
Air pressure on skin and nasal cavity———→	←——Tongue in closed mouth, air pressure in open mouth
Masseter————————————————→	←——Elasticity of periodontal ligament, particularly of molars, and suprahyoid muscles
Internal pterygoid	
in vertical movement ———→	←——Same as masseter
in lateral movement———→	←——Internal pterygoid of other side
External pterygoid	
in anterior movement———→	←——Posterior third of temporalis, suprahyoid group, digastricus, muscles of the neck
in lateral movement———→	←——External pterygoid of other side

illary incisors is shaped so that there is a greater area of attachment of periodontal fibers on the palatal and distal sides, which counteracts the tendency toward facial and mesial displacement during function. The molars are inclined mesially so as to transmit a component of the vertical occlusal forces to the premolars and canines.

5. *Atmospheric equilibrium during breathing and swallowing.*

THE MUSCULOSKELETAL SYSTEM

The Temporomandibular Joints

The temporomandibular joint (TMJ) differs from other synovial joints in many structural and functional aspects (Fig. 5–7). The articulating surfaces are not hyaline, as in other weight-bearing joints, but consist of a dense, well-organized collagen tissue very sparse in actual cartilage cells. Factors of embryology and the TMJ's need to withstand twisting, turning, compressive forces are the most common explanations for this structural difference. The joint is freely movable and has two compartments separated by an intact *articular disc*. The functional unit of the lower compartment is termed the *disc-condyle complex.*[7] This functional arrangement allows gliding in the upper compartment. Lower compartment movement between the articulating surface of the condyle and the inferior surface of the disc involves rotation only, except under states of increased laxity when the disc is displaced bodily from the condyle. The investing capsular tissues are inserted widely over the temporal bone to allow adequate gliding. In the lower compartment the disc is attached more securely to the

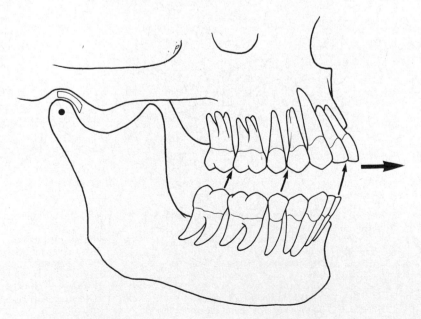

Figure 5–5 Anterior component of force (*large arrow*) is developed as a result of contact along the occlusal plane. The forces are anteriorly directed because of the orientation and placement of the occlusal plane below the level of the axis of rotation.

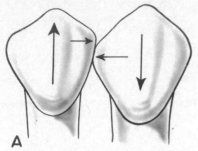

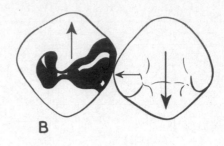

Figure 5–6 *A,* **Improper Proximal Contact Relationship** (*horizontal arrows*). This relationship is a potential source of excessive force in the directions indicated by the vertical arrows. *B,* Improper contact relationship in the faciolingual plane (*horizontal arrows*). This relationship is a potential cause of displacement of the teeth facially and lingually as indicated by the vertical arrows. (After R. A. Jentsch.)

lateral poles of the condyle to allow antero-posterior hinge gliding of the disc about the condyle. With these structural features, the joint is adequately protected to withstand sudden changes in the open-close movements, but it is subject to injury during sudden or repetitive lateral thrusts. Under active opening, both a hinge and a glide are observed, whereas in passive opening under retrusive jaw manipulation a hinge motion is produced.

Although the joint structures are mainly housed in the mandibular fossa, the functional activity occurs over the biconvex surfaces between the anterosuperior aspect of the mandibular condyle and the posteroinferior aspect of the articular eminence of the temporal bone. The inclination of the posterior surface of the articular eminence is correlated with that of the lingual surface of the maxillary anterior teeth (incisal guidance) but not necessarily with the cuspal inclines of the posterior teeth[38]

(Fig. 5–8). The flexible articular disc is the equalizer among these incongruous surfaces. It can be divided into two major parts (see Fig. 5–7). The *disc proper* is composed of firmly woven avascular fibrous tissue. The *posterior attachment (bilaminar zone)* is composed of soft, open-textured tissue containing various amounts of elastin.[16] The extent and nature of innervation suggest that nociception from compression of the posterior attachment or from inflammatory conditions of the joint could give rise to painful joint symptoms. The articular disc attaches anteriorly to the upper head of the lateral pterygoid muscle. Posteriorly, the posterior attachment fuses with the capsular wall, which in turn attaches to the tympanic plate with its uppermost insertion terminating in the area of the squamotympanic fissure (see Fig. 5–7).

The biomechanics of the TMJ is best conceptualized by considering the articular disc

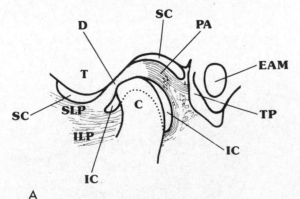

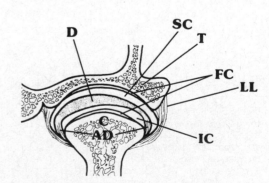

Figure 5–7 Parts of the Temporomandibular Joint. *A,* Lateral view (anterior to left of illustration). *B,* Frontal view. lateral to right of illustration.

AD	attachments of the articular disc	ILL	lateral capsular wall and lateral ligament
C	condyle	PA	posterior attachment of disc
D	articular disc	SC	superior compartment
EAM	external auditory meatus	SLP	superior head of lateral pterygoid muscle
FC	fibrocartilage	T	temporal bone (articular eminence)
IC	inferior compartment	TP	tympanic plate
ILP	inferior head of lateral pterygoid muscle		

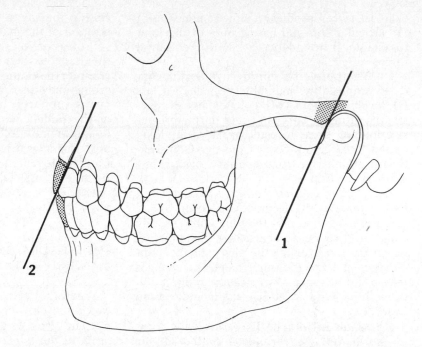

Figure 5–8 Correlation of the Plane of the Articular Eminence (1) with the Lingual Surface of the Maxillary Incisors (2).

and the condyle as one unit, the *disc-condyle complex*.[7] During opening, the *disc rotates posteriorly relative to the condyle*, as the disc-condyle complex simultaneously glides along the articular eminence; the posterior attachment, equipped with elastin, helps bring about backward disc rotation. Reported inactivity in the superior lateral pterygoid muscles during wide opening allows for backward rotation of the disc at full opening.[7] As a result, the often-described recoil action of the posterior attachment during jaw closing may be less important than its recoil effect on the disc during the jaw-opening cycle.

Jaw mobility would be markedly limited without a disc. True fibrous tissue discs occur only where two separate movements occur[40]; hence, the disc facilitates the hinge and glide functions. Together with the capsular ligaments, the disc allows for *stabilization* of the mandibular condyle against the articular eminence. This stability is maintained even though the interarticular curvature varies with condyle movement. This stabilizing function could not be served by a stiff, cartilaginous articular disc.

Wherever fibrous discs are found, they do not withstand pressure very well.[40] It has been shown that the condyles and the TMJs are loaded during function. These loads are normally of short duration and appear adapted to varied light forces rather than to unidirectional severe forces. *Under loading conditions, the presence of a disc acts as a "buffer" in the transmission of stress to the articular eminence.* Further, discs serve a *spreading function* which facilitates lubrication within the joint.[40] Although rupture and degeneration of the disc may create symptoms which make it necessary to remove the disc, this procedure has the potential to compromise long-term joint function.

The temporomandibular *capsule* surrounds the joint and unites its parts (see Fig. 5–7). It is composed of (1) an outer dense fibrous layer attached around the periphery of the articular disc and (2) a loose inner vascularized synovial layer. The fibrous capsule of the TMJ is rather thin, but the lateral surface of the fibrous capsule is strengthened by the *lateral (temporomandibular) ligament,* which arises from the articular tubercle and inserts on the lateral pole of the condyle. The lateral ligament is structured into two separate layers, both of which act as a strong "checkrein" limiting joint movement.[77] The superficial *oblique band* prevents downward condyle displacement during protrusion. The deep *horizontal band* prevents posterior displacement further into the mandibular fossa. There is no comparable reinforcement of the medial capsule, since the right and left TMJs function as one articulation. The sphenomandibular and the stylomandibular ligaments are accessory ligaments of the TMJ and have little influence on the movements of the mandible.[77]

ADAPTIVE REMODELING OF THE TEMPOROMANDIBULAR JOINTS. Throughout life, mechanical forces produce a slow remodeling of the articular soft and hard tissues of the joint to enable it to adapt to changing occlusal forces.[10, 13, 28, 49, 56, 58]

During transverse shifting of the disc-condyle complex, the mandible becomes a Class III lever and the TMJ components become stress bearing.[85] This can occur during protrusive loading or as a result of lateral wedging of the TMJ components from maxillomandibular instability or from repetitive loading during parafunction.

Remodeling is a rebuilding of adult soft and hard tissue layers. Remodeling occurs in all soft and hard tissues of the joint and is usually considered to be a subarticular phenomenon which does not affect the shape of the joint components. On the other hand, the changes may be so advanced as to cause an alteration of the joint surfaces, which is termed **deviation in form.**[27]

Deviation in form (DIF) *is deviation from the normally slightly rounded contour of the articular surface: e.g., condyle flattening or enlargement, thickening of the soft tissue layers of the articular components, surface unevenness, or scalloping* (Fig. 5–9A). Continuation of these changes with diminution in the proliferative ability of the articular tissues leads to breakdown of the articulating surfaces of the joints, a process which is termed **degenerative joint disease (DJD)** (Fig. 5–9B). Degenerative joint disease is *primarily a noninflammatory joint disease characterized by wear and tear of the articular soft tissues and by remodeling of the underlying hard tissues. Synonyms are osteoarthrosis and arthrosis.*[27] DIF can cause disturbances of movement and clicking and, with continued unfavorable loading, may gradually lead to DJD (arthrosis) with crepitation (grating) as a clinical symptom.[27]

Muscles of Mastication*

The **inferior division of the lateral pterygoid muscle** is the main trigger muscle in opening the jaw[44]; it is coordinated with the activities of the **suprahyoid muscles** (the **digastric,** the **mylohyoid,** and the **geniohyoid**), which assist in retracting and depressing the mandible and also in fixing and elevating the hyoid bone. The **masseter, medial pterygoid, superior division of the lateral pterygoid,** and **temporal muscles** are the principal muscles involved in

closing the jaw and in the regulation of the position of the mandible in space.

Protrusion of the jaw is accomplished by simultaneous bilateral contraction of the **lateral pterygoid muscles;** the jaw-closing muscle groups may also participate. Retrusion of the jaw is produced by simultaneous contraction of the **middle and posterior portions of the temporal muscles,** assisted by the **masseter, posterior digastric,** and **geniohyoid muscles.** Lateral movements are achieved by the contraction of the **lateral and medial pterygoid muscle** on one side and the contralateral **temporal muscle.**

THE POSTURAL POSITION OF THE MANDIBLE AND THE FREE WAY SPACE

When the teeth are not in contact in mastication, swallowing, or speech, the lips are at rest and the jaws are apart. This is termed the *postural position* of the mandible. It is often referred to as the *"physiologic rest position,"*[87] but *"postural position"* is more appropriate.[57] In order to maintain the mandible in this position, it is necessary to support it against the force of gravity; the muscles are in a mild state of contraction, especially the temporal muscle.[53] The postural position is not constant; it varies with the position of the head and body and is affected by proprioceptive stimuli from the dentition and by emotional factors.[60] Thus, there is no single, constant position of the mandible when the subject is at rest.[47]

The space between the mandibular and maxillary teeth when the mandible is in the postural position is called the free way space or the vertical dimension of rest. The postural position and free way space are fairly stable and reproducible but are not necessarily constant throughout life. They vary from individual to individual, and even within the same individual with changes in the dentition.[64] A large free way space has been observed in subjects with a deep overbite. Furthermore, a large sagittal difference between postural positions and ICP has been observed in subjects with marked overjet.[86] The average normal space is thought to be 1.7 mm,[19] but it has also been reported to be somewhat greater.[88] Generally, it ranges between 0 and 3 mm. Aging, malocclusion, tooth mobility, periodontal disease, unreplaced posterior teeth, improperly constructed dental restorations, excessive occlusal wear, and unilateral chewing, which change the teeth and their functional relationships, may also change the muscle tonus, which in turn may

---

*For a review of the biomechanics of masticatory function, see Sicher and Du Brul.[77]

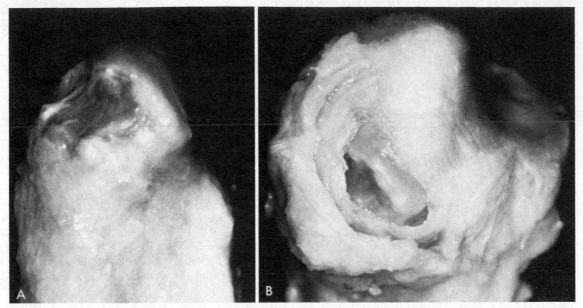

Figure 5–9 *A*, **Right Mandibular Condyle Dissected Free at Autopsy.** Lateral view showing flattening and soft tissue lipping, predominantly in the lateral third of the condyle. Even though there are marked changes in the shape of the condyle the articular surfaces are shiny and intact; hence, this condition is classified as a deviation in form. *B*, **Lateral View of Articular Disc Showing Large Perforation Localized Directly Over the Deviation in Form on the Mandibular Condyle.** By definition, a disc perforation is classified as degenerative joint disease. (Courtesy of T. Öberg and T. Hansson.)

alter the postural position and the free way space.[43]

The relationship between the clinical rest position and the jaw position occurring at minimal electromyographic activity the (electromyographic rest position or EMG rest) has been compared.[17, 19] The clinical rest position was always superior to the point of minimal muscle activity by an average distance of 8 mm. Of interest is the finding by Rugh and Drago[71a] that there is a significant difference in EMG rest between men (10.4 mm) and women (6.8 mm). Clinical norms for the free way space should not be applied using the values obtained at EMG rest.

Vertical Dimension of Occlusion

The term vertical dimension of occlusion designates the distance between the maxilla and mandible when the teeth are in occlusion. The vertical dimension is maintained by a balance between the rates of occlusal wear and continuous tooth eruption. Whereas the vertical dimension of occlusion should not be changed without a definite biomechanical reason, small changes in the course of dental therapy are usually accommodated by a re-establishment of the free way space.[14] There is no evidence to suggest that the vertical dimension of occlu-

sion should be changed in the presence of a large free way space, since there is considerable normal variation in this space. One serious problem in increasing the vertical dimension of occlusion could be the intrusion of teeth or a rapid resorption of alveolar bone under dentures. In this respect, it may be wise to err on the side of a wider-than-average interocclusal space if no other means are available to assess the proper vertical dimension of occlusion.[63]

NEUROMUSCULAR CONTROL OF MANDIBULAR MOVEMENTS

Knowledge of the neuromuscular control of mandibular movements has developed tremendously through active worldwide research in the area of oral physiology. As a result, dental practitioners have been increasingly interested in the application of these concepts to their daily practice. At this point, however, much information is available but not directly applicable to the complex clinical picture of occlusion in daily practice. The reader is referred to other sources for a detailed presentation of this subject.[34–36, 47, 64, 76] Clinical observations supported by research investigations have suggested that the following principles should be applied in the consideration of occlusal contact relationships:

Most occlusal contact relationships are harmonious in nature (they do not produce inappropriate, guarded, or painful responses in the masticatory muscles). Tooth guidances are likewise passive and unlabored. If a noxious response occurs following occlusal contact, it may be generated from the sensory receptors in the dentition as well as those in the joints, the muscles, or the ligaments of the masticatory system.[84]

There are many factors which influence reactions to noxious responses (producing a reflex response in the masticatory muscles), among them the magnitude, direction, and duration of the force, the age of the dentition, pulpal and periodontal health, muscle and joint health, and central nervous system effects.[62]

Various effects have been observed after placement of experimental occlusal interferences.[66, 70, 74] In one study,[70] the placement of a silver amalgam supracontact was followed after a short period by spontaneous postural hyperactivity. This effect was thought to be an attempt to shift the position of the mandible to avoid the interference. Apparently, normal oral reflex systems prevent damage through the increased inhibition of muscle activity at the most closed position in these circumstances.[55] Randow et al.[66] observed that mild temporomandibular signs and symptoms occurred in individuals after the insertion of one high filling. Simultaneous electromyographic changes were observed and were judged to be indications of poor muscle coordination.[66]

The silent period has been claimed to be important in diagnosis because it is of longer duration in patients with masticatory problems. However, documentation of large variations in this parameter make it difficult to set criteria for a healthy or a pathologic silent period.[30] Clinical history and examination appear to be more reliable approaches in the diagnosis of masticatory muscle disorders.[30]

Not enough is known about occlusal interferences to predict accurately which type is most active in masticatory dysfunction. *All occlusal therapy should be directed at preventing and eliminating factors which perpetuate noxious or inappropriate reflex responses.*[84]

ELECTROMYOGRAPHY

The electrical activity of muscles is assessed by electromyography, which is the recording of action potentials from motor units.[52] The significance of the electrical activity in the muscles of mastication springs from its relation to both sensorimotor coordination and motor performance.[52] Electromyography can disclose motor patterns at various levels: coordination of groups of muscles and activity in individual muscles and even in individual motor units,[23] which allows a more definitive recording of the factors regulating motor neuron function.[52, 54]

The duration, timing, and amplitude of muscle activity have been documented for the normally functioning occlusion through the use of surface electrodes on the skin.[51] Surface recordings are relatively simple to make, but the record so obtained cannot always be attributed with certainty to one particular muscle,[47] nor can the biomechanical action of the muscles be determined, be it shortening, holding, or lengthening under contraction. Deep muscles (e.g., lateral pterygoids) are particularly difficult to monitor with this method. As a result, studies of the deep muscles must be conducted with an intramuscular needle or fine wire electrodes.[44] Integrated EMG can give a reliable indication of muscle tension provided that the electrode is centered over the active muscle fibers in question and that the muscle contraction is causing no movement but merely a build-up in tension (isometric contraction).[47]

More recently, electromyography has been combined with the measurement of jaw displacement during natural oral function (Fig. 5–10).[26] Moreover, the action of specific muscles has been investigated. Both parts of the lateral pterygoid muscle have been studied in monkeys, using fine wire electrode techniques.[48] This study and others[44, 50] in humans suggest that the lateral pterygoid muscle is functionally separated into two parts; there is increased activity in the superior lateral pterygoid on closing, whereas the inferior pterygoid is active on opening and in lateral movements. During hard closure to ICP, both muscles are active.[44]

Occlusal and psychologic factors have been shown to affect muscular activity measured electromyographically. Occlusal interferences were observed to have caused a synchronous and hypertonic muscular activity that returned to normal after the occlusion was corrected.[62] Other studies[18, 37, 74] have demonstrated that occlusal interferences created a disturbance among the jaw muscles, manifested as an altered EMG activity. Psychologic stress, in both the experimental and the natural environments, has been reported to increase the activity of the jaw-closing muscles.[72, 89]

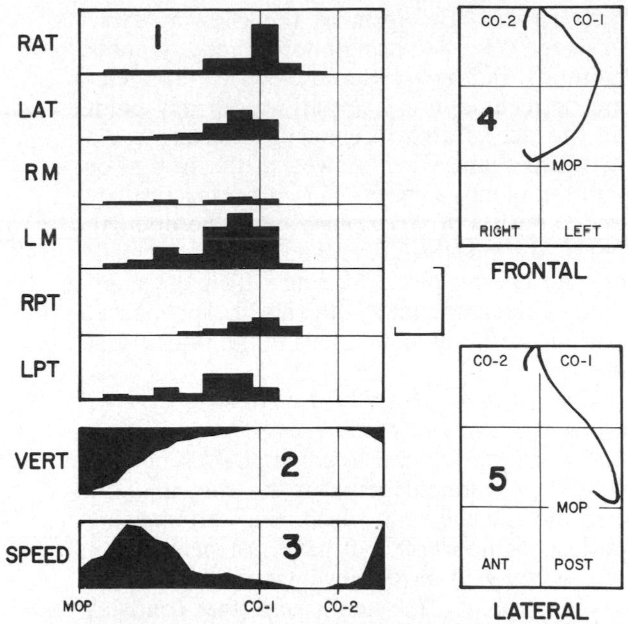

Figure 5–10 Muscle Activity and Jaw Displacement During a Single Chewing Stroke. Data from the closing phase of single, left-sided stroke during a gum-chewing sequence. Electromyographic signals recorded from the right and left anterior temporal (RAT, LAT), posterior temporal (RPT, LPT), and right and left masseter (RM, LM) muscles have been rectified and averaged over continuous 50-msec periods and appear as histograms (1). Jaw displacement, measured as movement of an incisor point on the mandible, is shown in three different ways: in time, as the vertical separation of the jaws from the position of maximum intercuspation (2); in time, as the resultant of the speed of jaw movement in three dimensions (3); and as envelopes of jaw displacement seen from frontal (4) and lateral (5) viewpoints. Maximum jaw opening is indicated by MOP and the points marking the beginning and ending of the intercuspal phase by CO-1 and CO-2. In the frontal and lateral views, this phase is represented by the small flattened area between CO-1 and CO-2. The vertical calibration bar represents 400 µV, 20 mm, and 200 mm per second in sections 1, 2, and 3, respectively. The horizontal bar represents 100 msec.

Each square in sections 4 and 5 measures 10 mm × 10 mm. In this instance the planes are referenced to the Frankfort Horizontal plane or at right angles to it.

The speed of jaw movement reaches its maximum early in the closing phase and begins to decline well before the food bolus is crushed by any major muscle contraction. It falls toward zero during the phase when the teeth dwell in maximum intercuspation (2 and 3). Peak muscle activity differs from muscle to muscle both in amplitude (RM, LM) and in time (Rpt, Lpt) and is related to the side chewed upon and the form of the chewing stroke. Activity in all muscles continues well into the intercuspal position (1), and although no vertical movement of the jaw occurs in this area (2), a small anterolateral shift has occurred (3, 4, and 5). Electrical activity in these muscles probably precedes their resultant development of interocclusal force by approximately 7 msec. (Courtesy of A. G. Hannum.)

Although it seems clear that muscle hyperactivity is initiated by both central and peripheral stimuli induced by stress and structural abnormalities, the relationship of muscle hyperactivity to orofacial pain and mandibular dysfunction is not well understood. One of the difficulties is that muscle hyperactivity may exert only a transient effect, followed by structural adaptations such as tooth movement and remodeling of the TMJs. Thus, the etiologic association may be masked.[70]

THE PHYSIOLOGY OF MASTICATION*

Mastication consists of the coordinated function of various parts of the oral cavity to prepare food for swallowing and digestion. Although the teeth are the most essential unit in mastication, there are other important related factors, such as the lubricating and enzymatic action of the saliva, the lips, the cheeks, the tongue, the hard palate and the gingiva, the muscles of mastication, and the temporomandibular articulation.

Mastication involves a definite pattern characterized by lateral closing movements, tooth gliding contact, and a period of high force at ICP.[20]

Incision

Incision reduces the food to sizes suitable for mastication. It involves coordinated action of the hand, arm, head, neck, and shoulders, as well as the teeth and masticatory musculature.

Once a bolus has been introduced into the mouth, mastication is automatic and practically involuntary, but it can readily be brought under voluntary control. The very act of establishing voluntary control implies a difference between masticatory function under ordinary conditions and parafunctional jaw movements with the teeth either together or separated.[4]

The Masticatory Cycle

The pathway of the mandible in chewing is referred to as the chewing cycle or the masti-

---

*For a comprehensive review of this subject, see Bates et al.[4-6] and Matthews.[47]

catory cycle. The form of the chewing cycle has been observed using photography, graphic methods, radiography, and electrical and telemetric techniques.[6] The pathway of any point on the dental arch in chewing typically has a teardrop shape when viewed in the frontal or sagittal plane[1] (Fig. 5–11). The masticatory cycle consists of three phases: (1) the opening phase, during which the mandible is depressed; (2) the closing phase, during which the mandible is elevated; and (3) the intercuspal phase, during which the mandible is in the intercuspal position (ICP).

The teardrop shape of the chewing cycle is more or less consistent for a given individual but is unique for every person. Differences in condyle movement between the chewing side and the nonchewing side during the chewing cycle are important and have not been taken into account in most chewing studies.[20] In the opening phase, the teeth and the condyles begin movement immediately downward and forward. Early in the closing phase, the entire mandible moves laterally. The chewing-side condyle moves to an upward and rearward position well in advance of the intercuspal phase (SRP in Fig. 5–12A, B, and C). During the remainder of final closure to ICP, the chewing-side condyle usually demonstrates a slight forward (0.33 mm) and medial (Bennett) movement (0.2 mm). The nonchewing-side condyle lags somewhat behind as it moves a considerable distance upward and backward to a condyle position dictated by ICP (Fig. 5–12C).[20]

Subjects chew on the side where there is the most stable intercuspal contact. Where occlusal conditions are similar on both sides, chewing takes place on the right and left alternately, and the food is passed from side to side regularly and consistently according to the individual's particular pattern.[6] The chewing pattern is influenced by the consistency, shape, size, and taste of the bolus of food.

The chewing patterns of the adult and the child differ in the opening movement. In the adult, the opening stroke is medial to the closing stroke. In the child, the opening stroke is typically lateral to the closing stroke. The change from the chewing pattern of the child to that of the adult appears to be related mostly to the eruption of the anterior teeth.[20]

The occlusion of the teeth is of significant importance for the development of masticatory movements.[1] In general, those individuals with normal occlusion have regular and coordinated chewing movements. Subjects with malocclu-

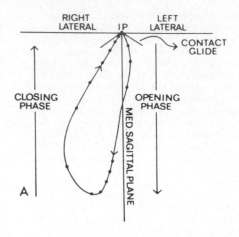

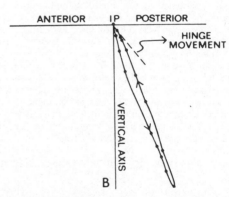

Figure 5–11 Incisal Points During One Chewing Cycle. *A,* Frontal projection. *B,* Sagittal projection. (From Ahlgren, J.: *In* Anderson, D. J., and Mathews, B. [eds.]: Mastication. Bristol, J. Wright and Sons, 1976.)

sion have an irregular chewing pattern.[1] The most consistent difference between the two groups appeared in the pause in ICP (shorter in malocclusion groups). Clinical experience has shown that individuals with continuous, habitual one-sided chewing often display latent or obvious masticatory problems.[20] In addition, occlusal alterations or treatments cause changes in the chewing pattern.[6, 20] The occurrence of a deep overbite is associated with chopping chewing strokes, whereas in reduced lateral cuspal guidance, the chewing stroke assumes a more horizontal component.[1]

There are about 15 chews in a series from the time of food entry until swallowing. Jaw opening is greatest when food first enters the mouth and decreases in a somewhat linear fashion as chewing continues. The average jaw opening during chewing is between 16 and 20 mm,[1] and the average lateral displacement on chewing is between 3 and 5 mm.[1] The duration of the masticatory cycle varies be-

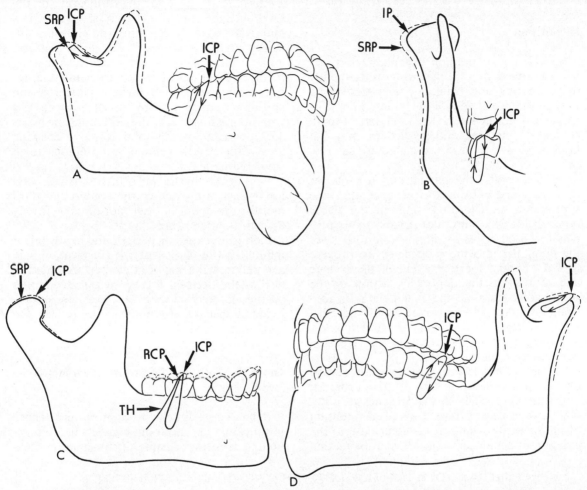

Figure 5–12 Masticatory Cycle. *A,* Seen from the chewing side during one chewing cycle. The chewing-side condyle moves upward and rearward and reaches a superior, rearward position (SRP() before the teeth reach the intercuspal phase. The teeth then close along the lateroretrusive cusp inclines on the path to the intercuspal position (ICP). *B,* Frontal view of chewing side, as in *A. C,* Sagittal component of the masticatory cycle (chewing side) seen in relation to the terminal hinge path (TH), the retruded contact position (RCP), and the intercuspal position (ICP). Note the retrusive component of the masticatory cycle on the chewing side. *D,* The masticatory cycle seen from the nonchewing side. The nonchewing-side condyle (mediotrusive condyle) moves a considerable distance upward and rearward to close directly to the intercuspal position (ICP). Note that closure is along the medioprotrusive maxillary cusp inclines on a path to the inter-cuspal position. The differences between the condyle paths and the paths of the cusps during the chewing cycle for the chewing side and the nonchewing side are significant and have not been taken into account in most chewing studies. (Courtesy of Dr. Harry Lundeen, after Gibbs.)

tween 0.6 and 1.0 second. Different test materials have a significant influence on the duration of the masticatory cycle, with sticky and tough foods increasing it.[1] The duration is decreased and the chewing forces are increased when the subject is stressed or in a hurry to eat.[71]

Deglutition

Swallowing occurs approximately 600 times in a 24-hour period.[41] It occurs most frequently during eating and drinking, at a lesser rate during the usual indoor activities, and least frequently during sleep. The total time of tooth contact in chewing and swallowing in a 24-hour period has been estimated to be 17½ minutes[25] (Table 5–2).

In swallowing, the palatal muscles seal off the oropharynx from the nasopharynx, the suprahyoid muscles raise and tilt the hyoid bone and larynx, and the tongue forcibly propels the food bolus or liquid posteriorly over the epiglottis into the esophagus. To provide firm anchorage for the action of the tongue and to oppose the depressing action of the suprahyoid muscles, the mandible is braced against the maxilla and cranium by the masseter, temporal, and medial pterygoid muscles. A *normal swallow, therefore, generally occurs with the teeth together.*

The act of swallowing may have a profound effect on the development of the orofacial structures, especially in the presence of a deviant swallowing pattern. Prolonged retention of the infantile swallow may contribute to the creation of a malocclusion.[43] It is probable that abnormal swallowing behavior is due to many factors, some of which are habitual, genetic, mechanical, or neurologic.

Masticatory Efficiency

The size of the food platform area, or the total available functional contact surface, is a major factor in determining the chewing efficiency of the dentition.[91] The food platform area is diminished by such factors as missing teeth,[46] cuspal interferences, incomplete eruption, tilting, and other forms of malocclusion and may be increased by attrition. In mouths with no missing teeth, the first molar provides 36.7 per cent of the total effective chewing area, with the other molar and premolar teeth contributing less.[45]

Loss of the first molar is often compensated for by mesial drifting of the second and third molars; the dentition then performs as if only the third molars were absent.

Pain from caries or periodontal involvement influences the choice of the mastication side and reduces the masticatory performance, as well as the occlusal force that can be exerted on the affected side. Severe bone loss in periodontal disease also appears to reduce the maximum occlusal force.

Tooth Contacts and Forces in Chewing and Swallowing

It has been difficult to capture and record jaw movements and tooth contacts in the functioning dentition, despite the imaginative tech-

TABLE 5–2   TOTAL DURATION OF TOOTH CONTACTS IN A 24-HOUR PERIOD*

Chewing:		
Actual chewing time per meal	450 sec.	
4 meals a day	1800 sec.	
Each second 1 chewing stroke	1800 strokes	
Duration of each stroke	0.3 sec.	
Total chewing forces per day	540 sec. = 9.0 min.	
Swallowing:		
1. Meals		
Duration of 1 deglutition movement	1 sec.	
During chewing 3 × per minute		
⅓ of movements with occlusal force only	30 sec.	0.5 min.
2. Between meals		
Daytime 25 per hour (16 hrs.)	400 sec.	6.6 min.
Sleep 10 per hour (8 hrs.)	80 sec.	1.3 min.
TOTAL	1050 sec. ca. 17.5 min.	

*From Graf, H.: Dent. Clin. North Am., *13*:659, 1969.

niques used for this purpose (e.g., visual studies of attrition facets, photography, graphic methods, radiography, and electrical and telemetric techniques).[4, 12] A review of these studies has been published by Bates et al.[4-6]

There is some variation in the findings of photographic, graphic, and electronic techniques investigating tooth contact in chewing and swallowing, but the preponderance of evidence indicates the following: **(1) Tooth contacts occur in chewing and swallowing in the majority of chewing cycles. The retruded contact position is rarely a terminal occlusal position in chewing or swallowing.** Chewing cycles without tooth contact occur mainly at the beginning of the chewing sequence, i.e., the crushing strokes.[1] When full closure to ICP is attained, stoppage of movement for about 0.1 to 0.2 second occurs for the subject with good occlusion, but the total contact time, which includes the gliding aspects of the feature, may be double this time.[6] Subjects with pathologic occlusions, especially those with mobile teeth, are less likely to reach ICP and less likely to demonstrate stoppage of jaw movement even when ICP is reached.[21] The chewing force is greatest during the short pause in ICP.[1, 21] **(2) Almost all chewing contacts and most swallowing contacts involve contact in ICP, and this position is the terminal functional position during the masticatory act.**[1, 21] Chewing contacts in ICP are brief compared with the duration of swallowing contacts, and forces during swallowing have been found to be greater than those during chewing.[20] **(3) Gliding contact to and from ICP occurs frequently during mastication, the average glide length being 1 mm at the incision point in both the opening and the closing strokes** (Fig. 5–12). These glides are less on the molar teeth because of cusp morphology and their proximity to the axes of jaw motion. The working-side molar closes from a rear and lateral direction with a small anterior component. The nonworking-side molar closes from an anterior and medial direction with no anterior component. According to Gibbs and Lundeen,[20] "steep anterior guidance does not appear to expose the teeth to extreme lateral forces. The tooth gliding contacts while entering and leaving the intercuspal position have been known to be of short duration and low magnitude when compared to the forces generated in the intercuspal position." In some individuals there is no tooth gliding contact at all, but merely a chopping stroke.

The occurrence of lateral tooth contact during the closing phase depends upon the type of food and occlusion. The glide is significantly longer in aborigines chewing tough food. As the attrition proceeds and the cuspal guidance is reduced, the closing stroke assumes a more horizontal direction when moving into ICP.[1]

The angle of approach to and from ICP is steeper than the cuspal inclination; thus the angle within the masticatory cycle always lies within the confines of the cuspal inclines. The teeth are a major guiding factor in the closing phases of the masticatory cycle but exert little influence in the opening phases.[6]

The Retruded Position and Intercuspal Position in Function

Clinicians have placed an enormous emphasis on the significance of the relationship between the retruded contact position (RCP) and the intercuspal position (ICP). This controversial topic has been recently reviewed by Møller[55] and Gibbs and Lundeen.[20] Møller[55] has characterized ICP as a *"working position"* in view of its importance as an entry and exit position in chewing and because it represents a position selected by the central nervous system primarily to withstand the exertion of strong force. Regardless of where ICP is located with respect to RCP, this force can be supplied as long as there are stable contact relationships at ICP. Instability at ICP causes reflex inhibition of the elevators and promotes increased neuromuscular control over mandibular positioning.[3] The positioning of the jaws at ICP can therefore be thought of as a morphofunctional reflex adaptation. Whether this adaptation is successful depends upon the positional tolerances of the masticatory muscles and the ability of the TMJs to resist destabilizing forces.[55]

The term *"structural position"* (after Møller[55]) is used to signify the position of the mandible in which the muscles and joints are best suited to work. Because the working position (ICP) is selected by the central nervous system with the goal of providing the most stable and most cranial contact possible, *ICP need not necessarily coincide with the structural position* to permit purposeful function. The concept of muscle hyperactivity and untoward adaptive responses in the TMJ is based upon the understanding of the ICP in its role as both a working position and a structural position.[55] A discrepancy between the working position and an optimal structural position can induce muscular hyperactivity, ischemic pain,[55] and altered responses in the TMJs.[81] The degree to which these problems are expressed clinically depends on muscle strength and coordination and on TMJ integrity, among other factors. In treatment, the establishment of superior stability in the structural position immediately transfers the work to this position, as in the case of an occlusal splint.[55] The action of the splint is to permit this transfer temporarily (or permanently) while at the same time causing neurophysiologic engrams of the inadequately located working position to dissipate.[55]

The above concepts are supported by the studies of Gibbs and Lundeen,[20] as it appears, at least, that the neuromuscular system exerts fine control during chewing to avoid particular occlusal interferences. In subjects with good occlusions such fine control does not appear to be necessary. This concept also applies to the anterior teeth if they encroach upon chewing and speaking motion. Therefore, occlusal form should be harmonious with the envelope of jaw movement during chewing.[20]

On the basis of jaw tracking and EMG studies it seems reasonable to suggest that RCP is a useful reference position from which to judge the alignment and positional requirements for an optimal structural position. The alignment is most physiologic if the disc and the condyle are stable in their relationship to each other. From a practical standpoint this would involve establishing a compatible relationship between RCP and ICP (less than 0.5 mm) with bilateral posterior contact in both positions.[64] The presence of a symmetrical occlusal glide from RCP to ICP is compatible with a favorable RCP-ICP relationship. The concept of utilizing RCP analysis does not necessarily apply to joints having TMJ derangements involving chronic clicking near the closed position and arrested jaw motion due to locking of the articular disc. After the entire dentition is reconstructed so that RCP is stable and on the same horizontal plane as ICP, a patient may persist in using ICP.[22]

Occlusion, like other physiologic body processes, changes with age. The therapist should consider the needs of the individual occlusion at the patient's age, rather than attempt a standard occlusion for all ages.

CONCEPTS OF ARTICULATION

Balanced Occlusion

The term *balanced occlusion* refers to simultaneous contact between the right and left posterior segments of the arch in lateral excursion of the mandible and simultaneous contact between the posterior and anterior segments of the arch in protrusive excursion. Although at one time considered to be an ideal type of functional relationship, balanced occlusion is rarely encountered in the natural dentition.[33] Balancing tooth contacts introduces a risk of damage to the periodontium which outweighs the ostensible benefits of attempting to create bilateral balance by occlusal adjustment or prosthetic restorations.[75, 82] In patients with periodontal disease, molars with nonworking-side contact showed significantly greater mobility, bone loss, and pocket depth than teeth which did not contact on the nonworking side.[90]

Canine-protected Occlusion

According to the concept of a canine-protected occlusion,[15] the maxillary canines act to guide the mandible so that the posterior teeth come into closure with a minimum of horizontal forces (Fig. 5–13A). In lateral and protrusive excursions, the mandibular canines and first premolars engage the lingual surface of the maxillary canines so as to disclude the incisors, premolars, and molars and protect them from undesirable horizontal forces. This concept hypothesizes that the maxillary canines are especially equipped to absorb lateral forces because of the size of the root and radicular bone and because of an especially sensitive proprioceptive mechanism which reflexly reduces muscle forces when the canines make occlusal contact. In a recent study, the teeth of persons having canine-protected occlusions had significantly lower mean Periodontal Disease Index scores than those of individuals having progressive disclusion (Fig. 5–13B) or group function (Fig. 5–13C).

Group Function

"Group function" is the simultaneous gliding contact of teeth on the laterotrusive side during laterotrusion (Fig. 5–13C). Although group function is physiologically acceptable as a disclusion system, it is not a requirement in restorative therapy.

None of the above concepts fulfills the needs of the clinician who must evaluate cuspal guidance in individual patients presenting with a variety of dental and skeletal malocclusions. Individualization is ultimately necessary.

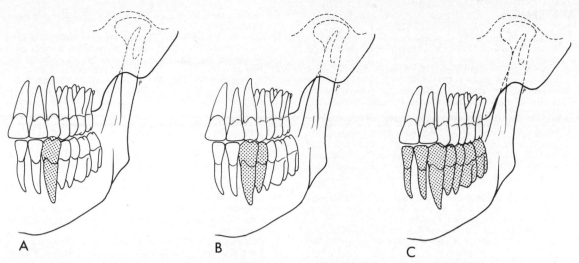

Figure 5–13 Types of Occlusion. *A,* Canine-protected occlusion. The canine teeth act as the discluders of the other teeth. *B,* Canine-premolar disclusion as found in normal young adults.[33] *C,* Group function occlusion.

ORTHOFUNCTION AND DYSFUNCTION

Trauma-producing oral activity has been called **dysfunction;** this is a descriptive term for the *forces* causing a wide variety of trauma throughout the stomatognathic system.[73] A more specific term describes dysfunction in the periodontium: namely, **traumatic occlusion.** Dysfunction (traumatic occlusion) is not a pure expression of behavior. It involves both structure (teeth, jaws) and behavior (neuromuscular force). Like two sides of a coin, they can be observed separately, but they are not independent.[39] *Using this concept, trauma generated in the teeth, supporting structures, muscles, or temporomandibular joints may be viewed as different manifestations of an adverse loading phenomenon termed* dysfunction.

Orthofunction *is defined as purposeful,* *adaptive, noninjurious function. The patient's adaptive ability appears to be the key determinant in tipping the balance in favor of orthofunction or dysfunction at any point in his or her life* (Fig. 5–14). The effects of dysfunction may be presumed to focus at the site where the greatest forces are exerted and the host resistance is the least.[39] Although not easily observed, the lesions resulting from dysfunction are usually expressed through inflammatory, proliferative, or degenerative tissue responses. In the initial stages, these lesions are largely *reversible* if the stresses that caused them to occur are normalized. Broadly viewed, the adaptive response has far-reaching implications not only as a determinant of injury production and localization, but also in terms of the psychologic host reaction to the symptom itself.[73]

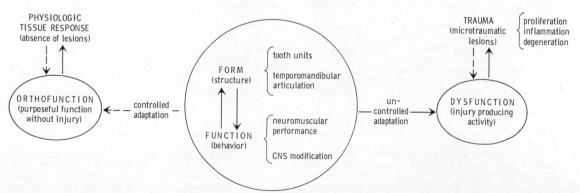

Figure 5–14 The Spectrum of Morphofunctional Harmony and Disharmony. Dysfunction is the immediate cause by which any functional disturbance or microtrauma may arise, including temporomandibular disorders. The most important determinant of orthofunction is the extent of the individual's adaptive ability, which is determined by host resistance and other nonspecific psychologic and physical factors. (From Melcher, A., and Zarb, G. [eds.]: Oral Sciences Reviews, 7, 1976.)

REFERENCES

1. Ahlgren, J.: Masticatory movements in man. *In* Anderson, D. J., and Mathews, B. (eds.): Mastication. Bristol, John Wright and Sons, 1976, p. 119.
2. Anderson, J. R., and Myers, G. E.: Natural contacts in centric occlusion in 32 adults. J. Dent. Res., *50*:7, 1971.
3. Bakke, M., and Møller, E.: Distortion of maximal elevator activity by unilateral premature contact. Scand. J. Dent. Res., *88*:67, 1980.
4. Bates, J. F., Stafford, G. D., and Harrison, A.: Masticatory function—a review of the literature. I. The form of the masticatory cycle. J. Oral Rehabil., 2:281, 1975.
5. Bates, J. F., Stafford, G. D., and Harrison, A.: Masticatory function—a review of the literature. II. Speed of movement of the mandible, rate of chewing. J. Oral Rehabil., *2*:349, 1975.
6. Bates, J. F., Stafford, G. D., and Harrison, A.: Masticatory function—a review of the literature. III. Masticatory performance and efficiency. J. Oral Rehabil., *3*:57, 1976.
7. Bell, W. E.: Clinical Management of Temporomandibular Disorders. Chicago, Yearbook Medical Publishers, 1982, 231 pp.
8. Bellanti, N. D., and Martin, K. R.: The significance of articular capability. Part II: The prevalence of immediate sideshift. J. Prosthet. Dent., *42*:255, 1979.
9. Beyron, H. L.: Occlusal changes in the adult dentition. J. Am. Dent. Assoc., *48*:674, 1954.
9a. Beyron, H. L.: Occlusal relations and mastication in Australian aborigines. Acta Odontol. Scand., *22*:597, 1964.
10. Blackwood, H. J. J.: Adaptive changes in the mandibular joints with function. Dent. Clin. North Am., *10*:559, 1966.
11. Breitner, C.: The tooth-supporting apparatus under occlusal changes. J. Priodontol., *13*:72, 1942.
12. Butler, J. H.: Recent research on physiology of occlusion. Dent. Clin. North Am., *13*:555, 1969.
13. Carlsson, G. E., and Oberg, T.: Remodelling of the temporomandibular joints. Oral Sci. Rev., *6*:53, 1974.
14. Carlsson, G. E., Ingevall, B.,and Kocak, G.: Effect of increasing vertical dimension on the masticatory system in subjects with natural teeth. J. Prosthet. Dent., *410*:284, 1979.
15. D'Amico, A.: The canine teeth:normal functional relation of the natural teeth of man. J. South Calif. Dent Assoc., *26*:6, 49, 127, 175, 194, 239, 1958.
16. Dixon, A. D.: Structure and functional significance of the intra-articular disc of the human temporomandibular joint. Oral Surg., *15*:48, 1962.
17. Drago, C. J., and Rugh, J. D.: Measurement of vertical jaw relationship. *In* Lundeen, H. C., and Gibbs, C. H. (eds.): Advances in Occlusion. Postgraduate Dental Handbook Series, Vol. 14, Bristol, John Wright and Sons, 1982, p. 158.
18. Funakoshi, M., Fujita, N., and Takehana, S.: Relations between occlusal interference and jaw muscle activities in responses to changes in head position. J. Dent. Res., *55*:684, 1976.
19. Garnick, J., and Ramfjord, S. P.: Rest position. An electromyographic and clinical investigation. J. Prosthet. Dent., *12*:895, 1962.
20. Gibbs, C. H., and Lundeen, H. C.: Jaw movements and forces during chewing and swallowing and their clinical significance. *In* Lundeen, H. C., and Gibbs, C. H. (eds.): Advances in Occlusion. Postgraduate Dental Handbook Series, Vol. 14, Bristol, John Wright and Sons, 1982, p. 7.
21. Gibbs, C. H., Messerman, T., Reswick, J. B., and Derda, H. J.: Functional movements of the mandible. J. Prosthet. Dent., *26*:604, 1971.
22. Glickman, I., Haddad, A. W., Martignoni, M., Mehta, N., Roeber, F. W., and Clark, R. E.: Telemetric comparison of centric relation and centric occlusion reconstructions. J. Prosthet. Dent., *31*:527, 1974.
23. Goldberg, L. J.: Masseter muscle excitation induced by stimulation of periodontal and gingival receptors in man. Brain Res., *32*:369, 1971.
24. Goldstein, G. R.: The relationship of canine-protected occlusion to a periodontal index. J. Prosthet. Dent., *41*:277, 1979.
25. Graf, H.: Bruxism. Dent. Clin. North Am., *13*:659, 1969.
26. Hannum, A. G., De Gou, J. D., Scott, J. D., and Wood, W. W.: The relationship between dental occlusion, muscle activity and jaw movement in man. Arch. Oral Biol., *22*:25, 1977.
27. Hansson, T.: Temporomandibular joint changes: occurrence and development. Doctoral dissertation, University of Lund, Sweden, 1978.
28. Hansson, T., and Oberg, T.: Arthrosis and deviation in form in the temporomandibular joint. A microscopic study on a human autopsy material. Acta Odontol Scand., *35*:167, 1977.
29. Helkimo, M.: Various centric positions and methods of recording them. *In* Zarb, G. A., Bergman, B., Clayton, J. A., and MacKay, H. F. (eds.): Prosthodontic Treatment for Partially Edentulous Patients. St. Louis, C. V. Mosby Company, 1978.
30. Hellsing, G., and Klineberg, I.: The masseter muscle: the silent period and its clinical implications. J. Prosthet. Dent., *49*:106, 1983.
31. Ingervoll, B.: Retruded contact position of the mandible. A comparison between children and adults. Odontol. Revy, *15*:130, 1964.
32. Ingervoll, B.: Studies of mandibular positions in children. Odontol. Revy, *19*(Suppl.):15, 1968.
33. Ingervoll, B.: Tooth contacts on the functional and nonfunctional side in children and young adults. Arch. Oral Biol., *17*:191, 1972.
34. Kawamura, Y.: Physiology of mastication. *In* Kawamura, Y. (ed.): Frontiers of Oral Physiology. Vol. 1. Basel, S. Karger, 1974.
35. Kawamura, Y.: Physiology of oral tissues. *In* Frontiers of Oral Physiology. Vol. 2. Basel, S. Karger, 1976.
36. Kawamura, Y., and Dubner, R. (eds.): Oral-Facial Sensory and Motor Functions. Tokyo, Quintessence Publishing Company, 1981, 354 pp.
37. Kloprogge, M. J., and van Griethysen, A. M.: Disturbances in contraction and coordination pattern of the masticatory muscles due to dental restoration. J. Oral Rehabil., *3*:207, 1976.
38. Koyourndjisky, E.: The correlation of the inclined planes of the articular surface of the glenoid fossa with the cuspal and palatal slopes of the teeth. J. Dent. Res., *35*:890, 1956.
39. Krogh-Poulsen, W. G., and Olsson, A.: Management of the occlusion of the teeth. *In* Schwarz, L., and Chayes, C. (eds.): Facial Pain and Mandibular Dysfunction. Philadelphia, W. B. Saunders Company, 1968.
40. Last, R. J.: Personal communication, 1977.
41. Lear, C. S. C., Flanagan, J. B., Jr., and Moorees, C. F. A.: The frequency of deglutition in man. Arch. Oral Biol., *10*:83, 1965.
42. Lee, R. L.: Anterior guidance. *In* Lundeen, H. C., and Gibbs, C. H. (eds.): Advances in Occlusion. Postgraduate Dental Handbook Series, Vol. 14, Bristol, John Wright and Sons, 1982, p. 62.
43. Lous, I., Sheik-Ol-Eslam, A., and Møller, E.: Postural activity in subjects with functional disorders of the chewing apparatus. Scand. J. Dent. Res., *78*:404, 1970.
44. Mahan, P. A., Gibbs, C. J., and Mauderli, A.: Superior and inferior lateral pterygoid activity. J. Dent. Res., *61*:272, 1982 (abstract).
45. Manly, R. S., and Braley, L. C.: Masticatory performance and efficiency. J. Dent. Res., *29*:448, 1950.
46. Manly, R. S., and Shiere, F. R.: The effect of dental deficiency on mastication and food preference. Oral Surg., *3*:674, 1950.
47. Matthews, B.: Mastication. *In* Lavelle, C. L. B. (ed.): Applied Physiology of the Mouth. Bristol, John Wright and Sons, 1975, p. 199.
48. McNamara, J. A.: The independent functions of the two heads of the lateral pterygoid muscle. Am. J. Anat., *138*:197, 1973.
49. Moffett, B. C., Johnson, L. C., McCabe, J. B., and Askew, H. C.: Articular remodeling in the adult human temporomandibular joint. Am. J. Anat., *115*:119, 1964.
50. Molin, C.: An electromyographic study of the function of the lateral pterygoid muscle. Swed. Dent. J., *66*:203, 1973.
51. Møller, E.: The chewing apparatus. Acta Physiol. Scand., *69*(Suppl.): 280, 1966.
52. Møller, E.: Quantitative features of masticatory muscle activity. *In* Rowe, N. H. (ed.): Occlusion: Research in Form and Function. Proceedings of Symposium, University of Michigan School of Dentistry, 1975, p. 54.
53. Møller, E.: Evidence that the rest position is subject to servo-control. *In* Anderson, D. J., and Mathew, B. (eds.): Mastication. Bristol, John Wright and Sons, 1976, pp. 72–80.
54. Møller, E.: Human muscle patterns. *In* Sessle, B., and Hannam, A. (eds.): Mastication and Swallowing, Toronto, University of Toronto Press, 1976, p. 128.

55. Møller, E.: The myogenic factor in headache and facial pain. *In* Kawamura, Y., and Dubner, R. (eds.): Oral-Facial Sensory and Motor Functions. Tokyo, Quintessence Publishing Company, 1981, pp. 225–239.

56. Mongini, F.: Anatomic and clinical evaluation of the relationship between the temporomandibular joint and occlusion. J. Prosthet. Dent., *38*:539, 1977.

57. Moyers, R. E.: Some physiologic considerations of centric and other jaw relations. J. Prosthet. Dent., *6*:183, 1956.

58. Öberg, T., Carlsson, G. E., and Fajers, C. M.: The temporomandibular joint. A morphological study on a human autopsy material. Acta Odontol. Scand., *29*:349, 1971.

59. Posselt, V.: Studies in the mobility of the human mandible. Acta Odontol. Scand., *10*(Suppl. 10):1, 1952.

60. Preiskel, H. W.: Some observations on the postural position of the mandible. J. Prosthet Dent., *15*:625, 1965.

60a. Pruzansky, S.: Applicability of electromyographic procedures as a clinical aid in the detection of occlusal disharmony. Dent. Clin. North Am., *4*:117, 1960.

61. Pullinger, A. G., Solberg, W. K., and Xu, Y.-H.: Epidemiological studies of occlusal contact in young adults. (Unpublished data.)

62. Ramfjord, S. P.: Bruxism, a clinical and electromyographic study. J. Am. Dent. Assoc., *62*:21, 1961.

63. Ramfjord, S. P.: Occlusion. Indent, *1*:19, 1973.

64. Ramfjord, S. P., and Ash, M. M.: Occlusion Philadelphia, W. B. Saunders Company, 3rd Ed., 1983, 544 pp.

65. Ramfjord, S. P., Kerr, D. A., and Ash, M. M.: World Workshop in Periodontics. Ann Arbor, University of Michigan Press, 1966.

66. Randow, K., Carlsson, K., Edlund, J., and Oberg, T.: The effect of an occlusal interference on the masticatory system. Odontol. Revy, *27*:245, 1976.

67. Regli, C. P., and Kelly, E. K.: The phenomenon of decreased mandibular arch width in opening movements. J. Prosthet. Dent., *17*:49, 1967.

68. Ricketts, R. M.: Variations of the temporomandibular joint as revealed by cephalometric laminagraphy. Am. J. Orthod., *36*:877, 1950.

69. Riise, C.: A clinical study of the number of occlusal tooth contacts in the intercuspal position at light and hard pressure in adults. J. Oral Rehabil., *9*:469, 1982.

70. Riise, C., and Sheikholeslan, A.: The influence of experimental interfering occlusal contacts on the postural activity of the anterior temporal and masseter muscles in young adults. J. Oral Rehabil., *9*:419, 1982.

71. Rugh, J. D.: Variation in human masticatory behavior under temporal constraints. J. Compar. Physiol. Psychol., *80*:169, 1972.

71a. Rugh, J. D., and Drago, C. J.: Vertical dimension: a study of clinical rest position and jaw muscle activity. J. Prosthet. Dent., *45*:670, 1981.

72. Rugh, J. D., and Solberg, W. K.: Electromyographic studies of bruxist behavior before and after treatment. Calif. Dent. Assoc. J., *3*:56, 1975.

73. Rugh, J. D., and Solberg, W. K.: Psychological implications in temporomandibular pain and dysfunction. *In* Melcher, A. H., and Zarb, G. A. (eds.): Oral Sciences Reviews: Temporomandibular Joint Function and Dysfunction. III. Copenhagen, Munksgaard, 1976.

74. Schärer, P.: Bruxism. Front. Oral Physiol., *1*:293, 1974.

75. Schuyler, C. H.: Factors contributing to traumatic occlusion. J. Prosthet. Dent., *11*:708, 1961.

76. Sessle, B. J., and Hannam, A. G. (eds.): Mastication and Swallowing, Toronto, University of Toronto Press, 1976.

77. Sicher, H., and DuBrul, E. L. Oral Anatomy, 6th ed. St. Louis, C. V. Mosby Company, 1975.

78. Sochat, P., and Schwarz, M. S.: Individualized occlusal adjustment. Part I. Rationale. J. South Cal. Dent. Assoc., *40*:827, 1972.

79. Solberg, W. K.: Terminology in occlusion. *In* Abou-Rass, M. (ed.): Workshop in Occlusion Education. University of Southern California, 1975.

80. Solberg, W. K., Flint, R. T., and Branter, J. P.: Temporomandibular joint pain and dysfunction. A clinical study of emotional and occlusal components. J. Prosthet. Dent., *28*:412, 1972.

81. Solberg, W. K., Woo, M., and Houston, J. B.: Prevalence of mandibular dysfunction in young adults. J. Am. Dent. Assoc., *98*:25, 1979.

82. Stallard, H., and Stuart, C. E.: Eliminating tooth guidance in natural dentitions. J. Prosthet. Dent., *11*:47, 1961.

83. Standlee, J. P., Caputo, A. A., and Ralph, J. P.: Stress trajectories within the mandible under occlusal loads. J. Dent. Res., *56*:1297, 1977.

84. Storey, A. T.: Physiology of occlusion. *In* Rowe, N. H. (ed.): Occlusion: Research in Form and Function. Proceedings of Symposium. University of Michigan School of Dentistry, 1975, p. 38.

85. Storey, A. T.: Neurologic aspects of TM disorders. President's Conference on the Examination, Diagnosis, and Management of Temporomandibular Disorders. June, 1982. American Dental Association monograph, in press.

86. Talgren, A.: Muscle activity relative to changes in occlusal jaw relationship: cephalometric and electromyographic correlation. *In* Rowe, N. H. (ed.): Occlusion: Research in Form and Function. Proceedings of Symposium, University of Michigan School of Dentistry, 1975, p. 21.

87. Thompson, J. R.: The rest position of the mandible and its significance to dental science. J. Am. Dent. Assoc., *33*:151, 1946.

88. Wessberg, G. A., Epker, B. N., and Elliott, A. C.: Comparison of mandibular rest positions induced by phonetics, transcutaneous electrical stimulation, nd masticatory electromyography. J. Prosthet. Dent., *49*:100, 1983.

89. Yemm, R.: Neurophysiological studies of temporomandibular joint dysfunction. *In* Melcher, A. H., and Zarb, G. A. (eds.): Oral Sciences Reviews: Temporomandibular Joint—Function and Dysfunction. III. Copenhagen, Munksgaard, 1976.

90. Yuodelis, R. A., and Mann, W. V., Jr.: The prevalence and possible role of nonworking contacts in periodontal disease. Periodontics, *3*:219, 1965.

91. Yurkstas, A. A.: The masticatory act. J. Prosthet. Dent., *15*:248, 1965.

AGING AND THE PERIODONTIUM

Disease of the periodontium occurs in childhood, adolescence, and early adulthood, but the prevalence of periodontal disease and the tissue destruction and tooth loss it causes increase with age. Many tissue changes occur with aging, some of which may affect the disease experience of the periodontium. *It is sometimes difficult to draw a sharp line between physiologic aging and the cumulative effects of disease.*

Aging is a slowing down of natural function, a disintegration of the balanced control and organization that characterize the young.[34] It is a process of physiologic and morphologic disintegration, as distinguished from infancy, childhood, and adolescence, which are processes of integration and coordination. Aging is described in detail in texts devoted to the subject. Some general age changes and alterations in the periodontium will be considered here.

GENERAL EFFECTS OF AGING

Aging is manifested to a different degree and in a different manner in various tissues and organs, but it includes general changes[42, 45, 46] such as tissue desiccation, reduced elasticity, diminished reparative capacity, and altered cell permeability.

In the **skin**, the dermis and epidermis are thinned, keratinization is diminished,[21] the blood supply is decreased, and there is degeneration of the nerve endings. Capillaries appear to become more fragile with age, which may result in large hematomas from small traumas. Tissue elasticity is reduced with aging,[23] and there is degeneration of the elastic tissue fibers of the corium. The atrophic skin changes are less marked in females and may be reversed in local areas by application of estrogen.

Bone undergoes osteoporosis with aging. The bone is rarified, trabeculae are reduced in number, the cortical plates are thinned, vascularity is reduced, lacunar resorption is more prominent, and susceptibility to fracture is increased. Generalized osteoporosis occurs in aged females more commonly than in aged males and has been associated with sex hormone dysfunction.[22] With age, water content of bone is reduced, the mineral crystals are increased in size, and collagen fibrils are thickened.[18]

AGE CHANGES IN THE PERIODONTIUM

Gingiva and Other Areas of the Oral Mucosa. In the gingiva the following changes have been identified with aging: diminished keratinization in both males[45] and females,[36] stippling reduced[16] or unchanged,[38] increased width of attached gingiva[2] with constant location of the mucogingival junction throughout adult life,[1] decreased connective tissue cellularity, increased intercellular substances,[50] and reduced oxygen consumption, a measure of metabolic activity.[49] In menopausal patients the gingiva is less keratinized than in patients of comparable age with active menstrual cycles.

Both thinning of the oral epithelium[41] and no change in width[30] have been reported to occur with age. The keratinizing potential of the hard palate epithelium does not change with age.[33] An increased keratinization of lip and cheek mucosa with age has been reported;[41] this might, however, be related to smoking.[33] Other changes reported in the oral mucosa include atrophy of the connective tissue with loss of elasticity,[40] decrease in protein-bound hexoses and mucoproteins,[6] and increase in mast cells.[7]

Periodontal Ligament. In the periodontal ligament aging results in an increase in elastic fibers[17]; decreases in vascularity, mitotic activity,[47] fibroplasia,[20, 29] collagen fibers, and mucopolysaccharides;[37, 43, 48] and increases

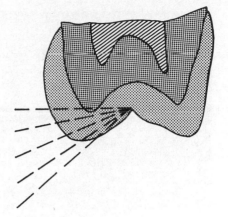

Figure 6–1   Diminution in Cuspal Inclination with increasing age.

in arteriosclerotic changes.[14] Both an increase[24] and a decrease[9] in width have been described in aging. In instances where there is a decrease in width, it may be accounted for by a lower functional demand due to the decrease in strength of the masticatory musculature. The decreased width may also result from encroachment upon the ligament by continuous deposition of cementum and bone.[27]

ALVEOLAR BONE AND CEMENTUM. Changes occur in alveolar bone with aging that are similar to changes in the remainder of the skeletal system. These include osteoporosis,[3, 27] decreased vascularity, and a reduction in metabolism and healing capacity.[46] Resorption activity is increased,[32] bone formation is decreased,[13, 44] and bone porosity may result.

Bone density may increase or decrease depending on location and animal species.[25, 31]

There is an increased irregularity in the surfaces of both the cementum and the alveolar bone facing the periodontal ligament with increasing age.[15, 19] A continuous increase in the amount of cementum also occurs with age.[19]

TOOTH-PERIODONTIUM RELATIONSHIPS. The most obvious change in the teeth with aging is a loss of tooth substance caused by attrition. Occlusal wear reduces cusp height and inclination (Fig. 6–1), with a resultant increase in the food table area and loss of sluiceways. The degree of attrition is influenced by the musculature, consistency of the food, tooth hardness, occupational factors, and habits such as bruxism and clenching.[26, 39]

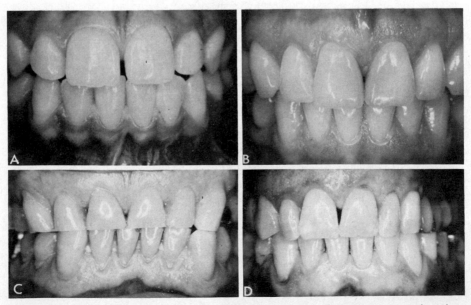

Figure 6–2   Tooth-Periodontium Relationships at Different Ages. *A,* Age 12. The gingiva is located on the enamel, and the clinical crown is shorter than the anatomic crown. *B,* Age 25. The gingiva is attached close to the cemento-enamel junction. *C,* Age 50. Slight occlusal wear and slight recession. *D,* Age 72. Moderate attrition and slight to moderate recession. These variations may be due not to an aging process but to the cumulative effect of injurious factors.

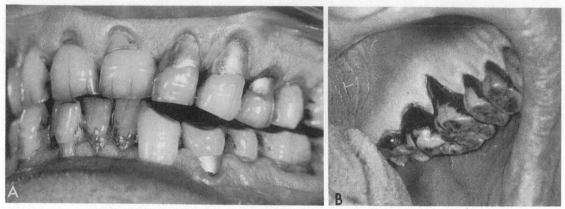

Figure 6–3   *A,* **Attrition of the Teeth** and gingival recession in a 65-year-old male. Note the elliptical contour of the tooth wear associated with biting the stem of a pipe while smoking. *B,* Lingual view showing accentuated recession on the first molar.

The rate of attrition may be coordinated with other age changes such as continuous tooth eruption and gingival recession (Fig. 6–2). As the tooth erupts, cementum is usually deposited in the apical region of the root. Reduction in bone height which occurs with aging is not necessarily related to occlusal wear.[5] In those cases in which bone support is reduced, the clinical crown tends to become disproportionately long and creates excessive leverage upon the bone. *By reducing the clinical crowns, attrition appears to preserve the balance between the teeth and their bony support.*

Wear of teeth also occurs on the proximal surfaces, accompanied by mesial migration of the teeth.[35] Proximal wear reduces the anteposterior length of the dental arch by approximately 0.5 cm by age 40.[51] Anteroposterior narrowing from proximal wear is greater in teeth that taper toward the cervical, such as the incisors.[51] Progressive attrition and proximal wear result in a reduced maxillary-mandibular overjet in the molar area and an edge-to-edge bite anteriorly.

MASTICATORY EFFICIENCY. Slight atrophy of the buccal musculature has been described as a physiologic feature of aging.[11] However,

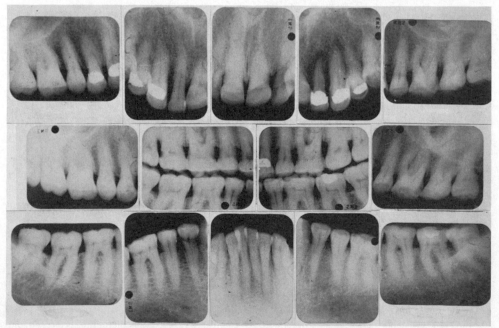

Figure 6–4   Radiographs of the patient shown in Figure 6–3. Aside from a few localized areas of bone loss there is little evidence of reduced bone height, which is considered by some to be a physiologic feature of aging.

reduction in masticatory efficiency in aged individuals is more likely to be the result of unreplaced missing teeth, loose teeth, poorly fitting dentures, or an unwillingness to wear dentures. Reduced masticatory efficiency leads to poor chewing habits and the possibility of associated digestive disturbances. Aged persons select carbohydrates and foods requiring less chewing effort when masticatory efficiency is impaired.

Avitaminosis is common in aged persons, but the extent to which it results from impaired masticatory efficiency has not been established. The vitamin requirement of older persons may be increased because of their dietary habits. Long-standing calcium deficiency has been considered by some to be a causative factor in senile osteoporosis.[11] The advisability of increased calcium intake in aged individuals is doubtful, but a diet high in protein and vitamins and comparatively low in carbohydrates and fat may be beneficial.

AGING AND THE CUMULATIVE EFFECTS OF ORAL DISEASE

With time, chronic disease can produce many oral changes, and it is difficult to determine how much physiologic aging contributes to the total picture. Some contend that gingival recession, attrition, and reduction in bone height in the aged result more from disease and factors in the oral environment than from physiologic aging.[4] Although gingival recession, attrition, and bone loss commonly occur with age, they are not present in all patients and vary considerably in the same age group. An aged individual with marked attrition may present relatively little alveolar bone loss (Figs. 6–3 and 6–4). Marked attrition may also be

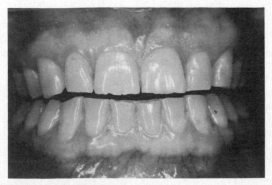

Figure 6–5 Bruxing Habit and Marked Attrition in a 25-year-old woman.

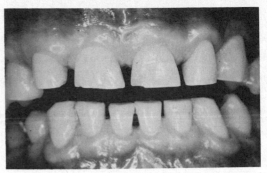

Figure 6–6 Bruxing Habit and Marked Attrition in 43-year-old man.

produced in young and middle-aged adults by bruxing and clenching habits (Figs. 6–5 and 6–6).

Increased alveolar bone loss in the aged has been related to less efficient oral hygiene.[41] Bone loss, pathologic migration of the teeth, and loss of vertical dimension in the aged may be the results of periodontal disease and failure to replace missing teeth.

A decline in the cellular immune response to bacterial plaque with increasing age has been considered of significance in the natural history of periodontal disease.[8]

REFERENCES

1. Ainamo, A.: Influence of age on the location of the maxillary mucogingival junction. J. Periodont. Res., *13*:189, 1978.
2. Ainamo, J., and Talari, A.: The increase with age of the width of attached gingiva. J. Periodont. Res., *11*:182, 1976.
3. Atkinson, P. J., and Woodhead, C.: Changes in human mandibular structure with age. Arch. Oral Biol., *13*:1453, 1968.
4. Baer, P. N., and Bernick, S.: Age changes in the periodontium of the mouse. Oral Surg., *10*:430, 1957.
5. Baer, P. N., et al.: Alveolar bone loss and occlusal wear. Periodontics, *1*:45, 1963.
6. Burzynski, N. J.: Relationship between age and palatal tissue and gingival tissue in the guinea pig. J. Dent. Res., *46*:539, 1967.
7. Carranza, F. A., Jr., and Cabrini, R. L.: Age variations in the number of mast cells in oral mucosa and skin of albino rats. J. Dent. Res., *38*:631, 1959.
8. Church, H., and Dolby, A. E.: The effect of age on the cellular immune response to dento-gingival plaque extract. J. Periodont. Res., *13*:120, 1978.
9. Coolidge, E.: The thickness of the periodontal membrane. J. Am. Dent. Assoc., *24*:1260, 1937.
10. Flieder, D. E.: Cytochemistry of human oral mucosa: determination of phospholipids, protein-bound hexoses, mucoproteins, collagenous and non-collagenous proteins. J. Dent. Res., *41*:112, 1962.
11. Freeman, J. T.: The basic factors of nutrition in old age. Geriatrics, *2*:41, 1947.
12. Froehlich, E.: Periodontal changes in aging. Dtsch. Zahnärztl. Z., *9*:1005, 1965.
13. Gilmore, N., and Glickman, I.: Some age changes in the periodontium of the albino mouse. J. Dent. Res., *38*:1195, 1959.
14. Grant, D., and Bernick, S.: Arteriosclerosis in periodontal vessels of aging humans. J. Periodontol., *41*:170, 1970.

15. Grant, D., and Bernick, S.: The periodontium of aging humans. J. Periodontol., *43*:660, 1972.
16. Greene, A. J.: Study of the characteristics of stippling and its relation to gingival health. J. Periodontol., *33*:176, 1962.
17. Haim, G., and Baumgartel, R.: Alterations in the periodontal ligament due to age. Dtsch. Zahnärtzl. Z., *23*:340, 1968.
18. Hall, D. A.: The Aging of Connective Tissue. London, Academic Press, 1976.
19. Ive, J. C., Shapiro, P. A., and Ivey, J. L.: Age-related changes in the periodontium of pigtail monkeys. J. Periodont. Res., *15*:420, 1980.
20. Jensen, J. L., and Toto, P. D.: Radioactive labeling index of the periodontal ligament in aging rats. J. Dent. Res., *47*:149, 1968.
21. Joseph, N. R., Molimard, R., and Bourliere, F.: Aging of skin. I. Titration curves of human epidermis in relation to age. Gerontologia, *1*:18, 1957.
22. Kesson, C. M., Morris, N., and McCutcheon, A.: Generalized osteoporosis in old age. Ann. Rheum. Dis., *6*:146, 1947.
23. Kirk, E., and Kvorning, S. A.: Quantitative measurements of the elastic properties of the skin and subcutaneous tissue in young and old individuals. J. Gerontol., *4*:273, 1949.
24. Klein, A.: Systemic investigations concerning the thickness of the periodontal membrane. Z. Stomatol., *26*:417, 1928.
25. Klingsberg, J., and Butcher, E. O.: Comparative histology of age changes in oral tissues of rat, hamster and monkey. J. Dent. Res., *39*:158, 1960.
26. Kronfeld, R.: Structure, function, and pathology of the human periodontal membrane. N.Y. J. Dent., *6*:112, 1936.
27. Kronfeld, R.: Biology of cementum. J. Am. Dent. Assoc., *25*:1451, 1938.
28. Lansing, A. I.: Calcium growth in aging and cancer. Science, *106*:187, 1947.
29. Lavelle, C. L. B.: The effect of age on the proliferative activity of the periodontal membrane of the rat incisor. J. Periodont. Res., *3*:48, 1968.
30. Löe, H., and Karring, T.: The three-dimensional morphology of the epithelium–connective tissue interface of the gingiva as related to age and sex. Scand. J. Dent. Res., *79*:315, 1971.
31. Lopez Otero, R., Carranza, F. A., Jr., and Cabrini, R. L.: Histometric study of age changes in interradicular bone of Wistar rats. J. Periodont. Res., *2*:40, 1967.
32. Manson, J. D., and Lucas, R. B.: A microradiographic study of age changes in the human mandible. Arch. Oral Biol., *7*:761, 1962.
33. Mosadomi, A., Shklar, G., Loftus, D. R., and Chauncey, H. H.: Effects of tobacco smoking and age on the keratinization of palatal mucosa. A cytological study. Oral Surg., *46*:413, 1978.
34. Muller, H. S., Little, C. C., and Snyder, L. H.: Genetics, Medicine and Man. Ithaca, N.Y., Cornell University Press, 1947. Chapter IV, Growth and Individuality, by C. C. Little, p. 104.
35. Murphy, T. R.: Reduction of the dental arch by approximal attrition. Br. Dent. J., *116*:483, 1964.
36. Papic, M., and Glickman, I.: Keratinization of the human gingiva in the menstrual cycle and menopause. Oral Surg., *3*:504, 1950.
37. Paunio, K.: The age change of acid mucopolysaccharides in the periodontal membrane of man. J. Periodont. Res., *32*(Suppl. 4), 1969.
38. Riethe, P.: Surface changes in the attached gingiva in young and old people. Dtsch. Zahnärztl. Z., *9*:1028. 1965.
39. Robinson, H. B. G.: Some clinical aspects of intraoral age change. Geriatrics, *2*:9, 1947.
40. Schei, O., Waerhaug, J., Lovdal, A., and Arno, A.: Alveolar bone loss as related to oral hygiene and age. J. Periodontol., *30*:7, 1959.
41. Shklar, G.: The effects of aging upon oral mucosa. J. Invest. Dermatol., *47*:115, 1966.
42. Simms, H. S., and Stolman, A.: Changes in human tissue electrolytes in senescence. Science, *86*:269, 1937.
43. Skougaard, M. R., Levy, B. M., and Simpson, J.: Collagen metabolism in skin and periodontal membrane of the marmoset. J. Periodont. Res., *28* (Suppl. 4), 1969.
44. Soni, N. N.: Quantitative study of bone activity in alveolar and femoral bone of the guinea pig. J. Dent. Res., *47*:584, 1968.
45. Stone, A.: Keratinization of human oral mucosa in the aged male. J. Dent. Med., *8*:69, 1953.
46. Thomas, B. O. A.: Gerodontology. The study of changes in oral tissue associated with aging. J. Am. Dent. Assoc., *33*:207. 1946.
47. Toto, P. D., and Borg, M.: Effect of age changes on the premitotic index in the periodontium of mice. J. Dent. Res., *47*:70, 1968.
48. Toto, P. D., Jensen, J., and Sawinski, J.: Sulfate uptake and cell kinetics in teeth and bone of aging mice. Periodontics, *5*:292, 1967.
49. Volpe, A. R., Manhold, J. H., and Manhold, B. S.: Effect of age and other factors upon normal gingival tissue respiration. J. Dent. Res., *41*:1060, 1962.
50. Wentz, F. W., Maier, A. W., and Orban, B.: Age changes and sex differences in the clinically normal gingiva. J. Periodontol., *23*:13, 1952.
51. Wood, H. E.: Causal factors in shortening tooth series with age. J. Dent. Res., *17*:1, 1938.

PERIODONTAL PATHOLOGY

Part I

Gingival Disease

chapter seven

Defense Mechanisms of the Gingiva

The gingival tissue is constantly subjected to mechanical and bacterial aggressions. Resistance to these actions is provided by the saliva, the epithelial surface, and the initial stages of the inflammatory response. The role of the epithelium, through its degree of keratinization and turnover rate, has been considered in Chapter 1. The permeability of the junctional and sulcular epithelia and the role of sulcular fluid, leukocytes, and saliva will be described here.

SULCULAR FLUID

Although the presence of sulcular fluid (gingival fluid) was noted in the nineteenth century, interest in its detailed study was triggered only in 1958 by Brill and Krasse.[12] These authors introduced filter paper into the gingival sulci of dogs that had previously been injected intramuscularly with fluorescein; within 3 minutes the fluorescent material was recovered on the paper strips.

In subsequent papers Brill[10] confirmed the presence of sulcular fluid in humans and considered it to be a transudate. However, it was shown by others that *sulcular fluid is an inflammatory exudate, not a continuous transudate.* This difference of opinion was in part based on the different methods of collection of the fluid.

Methods of Collection

Sulcular fluid can be collected by means of (1) absorbing paper strips, (2) microcapillary pipets, and (3) gingival washings. The **absorbing paper strips** are placed within the sulcus (intrasulcular method) or at its entrance (extrasulcular method) (Fig. 7–1). The placement of the filter paper strip in relation to the sulcus/pocket is very important. The Brill technique placed it into the pocket until resistance was felt (Fig. 7–1A). This method introduces a degree of irritation of the sulcular epithelium that can, by itself, trigger the oozing of fluid.

In order to minimize this irritation, Löe and Holm-Pedersen[52] placed the filter paper strip just at the entrance of the pocket or over the pocket entrance (Fig. 7–1B and C). In this way fluid seeping out will be picked up by the strip, but the sulcular epithelium will not be contacted by the paper.

The use of **micropipets** permits the absorption of fluid by capillarity. Capillary tubes of standardized length and diameter are placed in the pocket, and their content is later centrifuged and analyzed.[8, 10, 11, 15]

The method of **gingival washings** uses a special plastic appliance that covers the hard palate and the vestibulum. Fluid is obtained by rinsing the sulci from one side to the other through palatal and facial channels with syringes or a pump.[15]

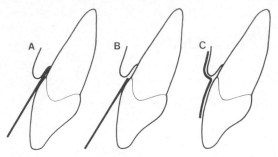

Figure 7–1 Placement of filter strip in gingival sulcus for collection of fluid. *A,* Intrasulcular method. *B* and *C,* Extrasulcular methods.

Permeability of Junctional and Sulcular Epithelia

The initial studies by Brill and Krasse with fluorescein, later confirmed for substances such as India ink[12] and saccharated iron oxide,[15] showed that there is *a passage of materials from the blood vessels into the connective tissue and through the epithelium to the sulcus.* Substances which have been shown to penetrate the sulcular epithelium include albumin,[70, 75, 93] endotoxin,[69, 73, 74, 80] thymidine,[39] histamine,[19] phenytoin,[90] and horseradish peroxidase.[59, 60] These findings indicate permeability to substances of molecular weight up to 1 million.[81]

The mechanisms of penetration through an intact epithelium have been reviewed by Squier and Johnson.[89] Intercellular movement of molecules and ions along intercellular spaces appears to be a possible mechanism. Substances taking this route do not traverse the cell membranes.

Amount

The amount of fluid collected in a paper strip can be evaluated in a variety of ways. The wetted area can be made more visible by staining with ninhydrin; it is then measured planimetrically on an enlarged photograph or with the help of a magnifying glass or a microscope.

An electronic method has been devised for measuring the fluid collected in a "blotter" (periopaper), employing an electronic transducer* (Fig. 7–2). The wetness of the paper strip affects the flow of an electronic current and gives a digital read-out. A comparison between the ninhydrin-stained method and the

---

*Harco Electronics, Dental Products Division, Winnipeg, Manitoba, Canada.

electronic method ("Periotron") performed in vitro revealed no significant differences between the two techniques.[91]

The amount of fluid collected is extremely small. Measurements performed by Cimasoni[15] have shown that a strip of paper 1.5 mm wide, inserted 1 mm within the gingival sulcus of a slightly inflamed gingiva, absorbs about 0.1 mg of fluid in 3 minutes.

As mentioned before, initial investigations concluded that sulcular fluid is present in the sulci of normal gingiva,[12, 96] suggesting that it is a physiologic filtration product from the blood vessels that is modified as it seeps through the sulcular epithelium. However, it was later shown that gingival fluid is an inflammatory exudate.[52] Its presence in normal sulci is considered an artefact caused by the increased permeability of capillaries that are damaged when the fluid is collected by inserting filter paper strips to the base of the sulcus instead of confining them to the crest of the gingival margin.[20] The question of whether gingival fluid is a product of normal gingiva is complicated by the fact that, with few exceptions, gingiva which appears normal clinically invariably exhibits inflammation when examined microscopically.

The amount of gingival fluid increases with inflammation,[25, 82] sometimes proportionally to its severity.[66] Gingival fluid is also increased by chewing coarse foods, by toothbrushing and massage, by ovulation,[49] and by hormonal contraceptives.[50] Gingival fluid is not increased by trauma from occlusion.[57]

Composition

CELLULAR ELEMENTS. Cellular elements found in the gingival fluid are bacteria, des-

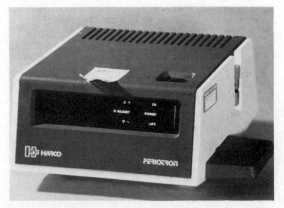

Figure 7–2 Electronic machine for measuring the amount of fluid collected on filter paper.

quamated epithelial cells, and leukocytes (polymorphonuclear leukocytes [PMNs], lymphocytes, and monocytes) which migrate through the sulcular epithelium.[19, 22, 87]

ELECTROLYTES. The following electrolytes have been studied in gingival fluid: potassium, sodium, and calcium. Most studies have shown a positive correlation of calcium, sodium, and the sodium:potassium ratio with inflammation (see Cimasoni[15]).

ORGANIC COMPOUNDS. Carbohydrates and proteins have been investigated. Glucose hexosamine and hexuronic acid have been found in gingival fluid.[35] Glucose blood levels do not correlate with glucose gingival fluid levels; glucose concentration in gingival fluid is three to four times higher than that in serum. This is interpreted to be a result not only of metabolic activity of adjacent tissues but also of local microbial flora.

The total protein content of gingival fluid was found to be much lower than that of serum.[11] No significant correlations were found between the concentration of proteins in the gingival fluid and the following periodontal parameters: gingival index, pocket depth, and bone loss.[6]

Identification of the proteins in the gingival fluid by immunoelectrophoresis and other methods has been attempted by several investigators.[64] The following have been identified: IgG, IgA, IgM, C3, C4, and plasma proteins (albumin, fibrinogen, and so forth).

The following metabolic and bacterial products have been identified in gingival fluid: lactic acid,[36] urea,[30] hydroxyproline,[68] endotoxins,[84, 85] cytotoxic substances, hydrogen sulfide,[88] and antibacterial factors.[16] Several enzymes have also been identified: acid phosphatase, beta-glucuronidase, lysozyme, cathepsin D, proteases, alkaline phosphatase, and lactic dehydrogenase.[15]

Antibacterial Action

The gingival fluid plays a protective role. Several mechanisms have been suggested: (1) cleansing action, based on the flushing out of bacteria and particulate matter; (2) antibacterial properties, based on its content of viable leukocytes that can engulf and destroy bacteria and of antibodies against plaque bacteria; and (3) adhesive properties, based on the presence of sticky plasma proteins which may improve adhesion of the junctional epithelium to the tooth.

Clinical Significance

Several investigators have found a positive correlation between the amount of gingival fluid and/or some of its components and the severity of gingival inflammation.[85] This correlation can be modified by the experimental methods used for collection and evaluation of the fluid and by other factors such as circadian periodicity, hormonal and mechanical influences, and periodontal therapy.

INFLUENCE OF CIRCADIAN PERIODICITY. There is a gradual increase in gingival fluid from 6:00 A.M. to 10:00 P.M. and a decrease afterward.[7]

INFLUENCE OF SEX HORMONES. Female sex hormones increase the gingival fluid flow, probably because these hormones increase vascular permeability.[51] For example, pregnancy, ovulation,[49] and hormonal contraceptives[50] all increase gingival fluid.

INFLUENCE OF MECHANICAL STIMULATION. Chewing[10] and vigorous gingival brushing stimulate the oozing of gingival fluid. Even the minor stimuli represented by intrasulcular placement of paper strips increase the production of fluid.

INFLUENCE OF PERIODONTAL THERAPY. It has been shown that there is an increase in gingival fluid during the healing period after periodontal surgery.[2, 78]

Drugs in the Sulcular Fluid

Drugs that are excreted through the gingival fluid may be used very advantageously in periodontal therapy. Bader and Goldhaber[5] have demonstrated in dogs that tetracyclines are excreted through the gingival fluid, and this finding triggered an extensive wave of research exploring this area[31] (see Chapter 45).

LEUKOCYTES IN THE DENTOGINGIVAL AREA

Leukocytes have been found in clinically healthy gingival sulci in humans and experimental animals. The leukocytes found are predominantly neutrophils. They appear in small numbers extravascularly in the connective tissue adjacent to the bottom of the sulcus; from there they travel across the epithelium[14, 32] to the gingival sulcus, where they are expelled (Figs. 7–3 and 7–4).

Leukocytes are present in sulci, even when histologic sections of adjacent tissue are free

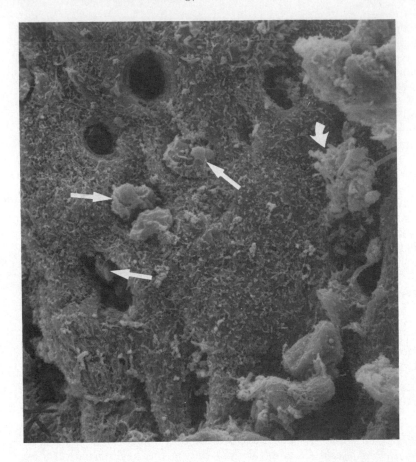

Figure 7–3 Scanning electron microscope view of periodontal pocket wall. Several leukocytes are emerging *(arrows)*, some partially covered by bacteria *(curved arrow)*. Empty holes correspond to "tunnels" through which leukocytes have emerged.

of inflammatory infiltrate.[3] Differential counts of leukocytes from clinically healthy human gingival sulci have shown 91.2 to 91.5 per cent PMNs and 8.5 to 8.8 per cent mononuclear cells.[86, 98]

Mononuclear cells were identified as 58 per cent B-lymphocytes, 24 per cent T-lymphocytes, and 18 per cent mononuclear phagocytes.[98]

The ratio of T-lymphocytes to B-lymphocytes was found to be reversed from the normal ratio of about 3:1 found in peripheral blood to about 1:3 in crevicular fluid.

Leukocytes are attracted by different plaque bacteria[40, 97] but can also be found in the dentogingival region of adult germ-free animals.[55, 77] Leukocytes have been reported in the gingival sulcus in nonmechanically irritated (resting) healthy gingiva, indicating that their migration may be independent of an increase in vascular permeability.[4, 92]

The majority of these cells are viable and have been found to have phagocytic and killing capacity.[45, 67, 72] *Therefore, they constitute a ma-*

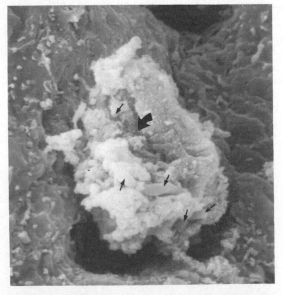

Figure 7–4 Higher magnification, scanning electron microscopy. A leukocyte emerging from the pocket wall is covered with bacteria *(small arrows)*. Curved arrow points at phagosomal vacuole through which bacteria are being engulfed.

jor protective mechanism against the extension of plaque into the gingival sulcus.

Leukocytes are also found in saliva (see next section). The main port of entry of leukocytes into the oral cavity is the gingival sulcus.[79]

SALIVA

Salivary secretions are protective in nature because they maintain the oral tissues in a physiologic state (Table 7–1). Saliva exerts a major influence on plaque by mechanically cleansing the exposed oral surfaces, by buffering acids produced by bacteria, and by controlling bacterial activity.

Antibacterial Factors

Saliva contains numerous antibacterial factors such as lysozyme, lactoperoxidase, and antibodies.

Lysozyme is a hydrolytic enzyme which cleaves the linkage between structural components of the glycopeptide muramic acid–containing region of the cell wall of certain bacteria in vitro. The concentration of lysozyme appears to be higher in sublingual and submandibular saliva than in parotid saliva. The antibacterial effect in vivo is poorly understood and probably plays a minor role. It probably serves to repel certain transient bacterial invaders of the mouth.[1]

The *lactoperoxidase-thiocyanate* system in saliva has been shown to be antibacterial to some strains of *Lactobacillus* and *Streptococcus*.[61, 76] It is present in submandibular and parotid saliva. The system prevents the accumulation of lysine and glutamic acid, both essential for bacterial growth, by susceptible bacteria.

Salivary Antibodies

Saliva, like sulcular fluid, contains antibodies reactive with indigenous oral bacterial species. Although IgG and IgM are present, the predominant immunoglobulin found in saliva is IgA, whereas IgG predominates in sulcular fluid.[53, 94]

Salivary antibodies appear to be synthesized locally, for they will react with strains of bacteria indigenous to the mouth but not with organisms characteristic of the intestinal tract.[26, 28] Many bacteria found in saliva have been shown to be coated with IgA, and the bacterial deposits on teeth contain both IgA and IgG in quantities greater than 1 per cent of their dry weight.[27] It has been shown that IgA antibodies present in parotid saliva can inhibit the attachment of oral *Streptococcus* species to epithelial cells.[23, 97]

Gibbons and co-workers suggest that antibodies in secretions may react with bacteria while they are proliferating on the surfaces of mucosal epithelial cells;[26–28] hence, when the organisms become dislodged, they would have an impaired ability to reattach. It is possible that this mechanism may play a major role in determining the course of bacterial diseases such as cholera, dental caries,[9, 47, 53] and periodontitis in which bacterial adhesion and colonization of mucosal or dental tissues may be a necessary step in pathogenesis. Inhibition of bacterial adherence has not been found to require accessory factors such as complement in the systems so far studied. Secretory IgA has a valence of 4, which may lead to multivalent binding to cell surfaces, thereby increasing the efficiency of secretory IgA antibodies.

The antibacterial activities of secretory IgA antibodies are not very well understood. There is conflicting evidence regarding the ability of secretory IgA antibodies to function in bacterial opsonization and bactericidal activities. These conflicting results may be resolved by

TABLE 7–1 ROLE OF SALIVA IN ORAL HEALTH

Function	Salivary Components	Probable Mechanism
Lubrication	Glycoproteins, mucoids	Coating similar to gastric mucin
Physical protection	Glycoproteins, mucoids	Coating similar to gastric mucin
Cleansing	Physical flow	Clearance of debris and bacteria
Buffering	Bicarbonate and phosphate	Antacids
Tooth integrity	Minerals	Maturation, remineralization
	Glycoprotein pellicle	Mechanical protection
Antibacterial	IgA	Control of bacterial colonization
	Lysozyme	Breaks bacterial cell walls
	Lactoperoxidase	Oxidation of susceptible bacteria

further studies defining the assay systems and accessory factors in more detail.

The **enzymes** normally found in the saliva are derived from the salivary glands, bacteria, leukocytes, oral tissues, and ingested substances; the major enzyme is parotid amylase. Certain salivary enzymes have been reported to increase in the periodontal disease; these are hyaluronidase and lipase,[13] beta-glucuronidase and chondroitin sulfatase,[17] amino acid decarboxylases,[8] catalase, peroxidase, and collagenase.[34, 38]

A mixture of glycoprotein components of saliva appears to make up salivary mucin. Mucin concentration is primarily responsible for the control of salivary viscosity. The glycoproteins are produced by the mucous cells of all salivary glands; however, some are produced exclusively by individual glands.

The high molecular weight mucinous glycoproteins in saliva bind specifically to many plaque-forming bacteria. The glycoprotein-bacterial interactions facilitate bacterial accumulation on the exposed tooth surface.[23, 26–28, 97]

The specificity of these interactions has been demonstrated. The interbacterial matrix of human plaque appears to contain polymers similar to salivary glycoproteins, which may aid in maintaining the integrity of plaque. In addition, these glycoproteins selectively adsorb to the hydroxyapatite to make up part of the acquired pellicle. Other salivary glycoproteins inhibit the sorption of some bacteria to the tooth surface and to oral mucosa epithelial cells.[9] This activity appears to be associated with the glycoproteins which possess blood group reactivity.[1, 23, 26, 28, 97] Glycoproteins and a glycolipid present on mammalian cell surfaces appear to serve as receptors for the attachment of some viruses and bacteria. Thus the close similarity between glycoproteins of salivary secretions and components of the epithelial cell surface suggests that the secretions can competitively inhibit antigen sorption and therefore may limit pathologic alterations.

Salivary Buffers, Coagulation Factors, and Vitamins

The maintenance of physiologic hydrogen ion concentration (pH) at the mucosal epithelial cell surface and tooth surface is an important function of **salivary buffers.** Its primary effect has been studied in relationship to dental caries.

In saliva the most important salivary buffer is the bicarbonate–carbonic acid system.[56] Bi-carbonate concentration increases with increased flow rate, providing greater salivary buffering capacity. The system acts by the loss of carbon dioxide, which tends to raise the pH. In addition, the pK of saliva is 6.1, which is similar to that of whole plaque and therefore would be more effective in maintaining a physiologic pH. Urea and phosphate buffers also occur in saliva and contribute to the maintenance of a physiologic pH.

Saliva also contains **coagulation factors** (VIII, IX, X, PTA, and the Hageman factor) that hasten blood coagulation and protect wounds from bacterial invasion.[48] The presence of an active fibrinolytic enzyme has also been suggested.

The following **vitamins** are found in saliva: thiamine, riboflavin, niacin, pyridoxine, pantothenic acid, biotin, folic acid, and vitamin B_{12}.[58] Vitamin C and vitamin K have also been reported.[62] Suggested sources of the vitamins are microbial synthesis and secretion by salivary glands, food debris, degenerating leukocytes, and exfoliated epithelial cells.

Leukocytes

In addition to desquamated epithelial cells, the saliva contains all forms of **leukocytes,** of which the principal cells are polymorphonuclear leukocytes. The number of leukocytes varies from person to person and at different times of the day and is increased in gingivitis. Leukocytes reach the oral cavity by migrating through the lining of the gingival sulcus. Living polymorphonuclear leukocytes in saliva are sometimes referred to as orogranulocytes and their rate of migration into the oral cavity as the **orogranulocytic migratory rate.** Some feel that the rate of migration is correlated with the severity of gingival inflammation and is therefore a reliable index for assessing gingivitis.[87]

Role in Periodontal Pathology

Saliva exerts a major influence on plaque initiation, maturation, and metabolism. Calculus formation, periodontal disease, and caries are also influenced by salivary flow and composition. The removal of the salivary glands in experimental animals significantly increases the incidence of dental caries[29] and of periodontal disease[33] and delays the healing of gingivectomy wounds.[83]

An inverse relationship has been reported

between the amount of calculus and the pyrophosphate content of parotid saliva. This finding, however, has been disputed.[44]

In humans an increase in inflammatory gingival diseases, dental caries, and rapid tooth destruction associated with cervical or cemental caries is partially a consequence of decreased salivary gland secretion (xerostomia). Xerostomia may be a result of a variety of factors, among them sialolithiasis, sarcoidosis, Sjögren's syndrome, Mikulicz's disease, irradiation, and surgical removal of the salivary glands.

REFERENCES

1. Adinolfi, M., Mollison, P. L., Polley, M. J., and Rose, J. M.: A blood group antibodies. J. Exp. Med., *123*:951, 1966.
2. Arnold, R., et al.: Alterations in crevicular fluid flow during healing following gingival surgery. J. Periodont. Res., *1*:303, 1966.
3. Attstrom, R.: Presence of leukocytes in the crevices of healthy and clinically inflamed gingiva. J. Periodontol., *5*:42, 1970.
4. Attstrom, R., and Egelberg, J.: Emigration of blood neutrophils and monocytes into the gingival crevices. J. Periodont. Res., *5*:48, 1970.
5. Bader, H. J., and Goldhaber, P.: The passage of intravenously administered tetracycline in the gingival sulcus of dogs. J. Oral Ther., *2*:324, 1966.
6. Bang, J., and Cimasoni, G.: Total protein in human crevicular fluid. J. Dent. Res., *50*:1683, 1971.
7. Bissada, N. F., Schaffer, E. M., and Haus, E.: Circadian periodicity of human crevicular fluid. J. Periodontol., *38*:36, 1967.
8. Bjorn, H. L., Koch, G., and Lindhe, J.: Evaluation of gingival fluid measurements. Odont. Rev., *16*:300, 1965.
9. Brandtzaeg, P., Tjellanger, I., and Gjeruldsen, S. I.: Human secretory immunoglobulin. I. Salivary secretions from individuals with normal or low levels of serum immunoglobulins. Scand. J. Haematol. [Suppl.], *12*:1, 1970.
10. Brill, N.: Effect of chewing on flow of tissue fluid into gingival pockets. Acta Odontol. Scand., *17*:277, 1959.
11. Brill, N., and Bronnestam, R.: Immuno-electrophoretic study of tissue fluid from gingival pockets. Acta Odontol. Scand., *18*:95, 1960.
12. Brill, N., and Krasse, B.: The passage of tissue fluid into the clinically healthy gingival pocket. Acta Odontol. Scand., *16*:223, 1958.
13. Carlsson, J., and Egelberg, J.: Local effect of diet on plaque formation and development of gingivitis in dogs. II. Effect of high carbohydrate versus high protein-fat diets. Odont. Rev., *16*:42, 1965.
14. Cattoni, M.: Lymphocytes in the epithelium of healthy gingiva. J. Dent. Res., *30*:627, 1951.
15. Cimasoni, G.: The Crevicular Fluid. Monographs in Oral Science. Vol. 3. Basel, S. Karger, 1974.
16. Cobb, C. M., and Brown, L. R.: The effects of exudate from the periodontal pocket on cell culture. Peridontics, *5*:5, 1967.
17. Dawes, C.: The chemistry and physiology of saliva. *In* Shaw, J. H., Sweeney, E. A., Cappuccino, C. C., and Meller, S. M. (eds.): Textbook of Oral Biology. Philadelphia, W. B. Saunders Company, 1978.
18. Dawes, C., Jenkins, G. M., and Tonge, C. H.: The nomenclature of the integuments of the enamel surface of teeth. Br. Dent. J., *115*:65, 1963.
19. Egelberg, J.: Cellular elements in gingival pocket fluid. Acta Odontol. Scand., *21*:283, 1963.
20. Egelberg, J.: Gingival exudate measurements for evaluation of inflammatory changes of the gingiva. Odont. Rev., *15*:381, 1964.
21. Egelberg, J.: Permeability of the dento-gingival vessels. II. Clinically healthy gingiva. J. Periodont. Res., *1*:276, 1966.
22. Egelberg, J., and Attstrom, R.: Presence of leukocytes within crevices of healthy and inflamed gingiva and their immigration from the blood. J. Periodont. Res. *4*(Suppl.):23, 1969.
23. Ellen, R. P., and Gibbons, R. J.: M-Protein associated adherence of *Streptococcus pyogenes* to epithelial surfaces: prerequisite for virulence. Infect. Immun., *5*:826, 1972.
24. Fitzgerald, R. J., and Jordan, H. V.: Polysaccharide producing bacteria and dental caries. *In* Harris, R. S. (ed.): The Art and Science of Dental Caries Research. New York, Academic Press, 1968.
25. Garnick, J. J., Pearson, R., and Harrell, D.: The evaluation of the periotron. J. Periodontol., *50*:424, 1979.
26. Gibbons, R. J., and van Houte, J.: Selective bacterial adherence to oral epithelial surfaces and its role as an ecological determinant. Infect. Immun., *3*:567, 1971.
27. Gibbons, R. J., and van Houte, J.: On the formation of dental plaques. J. Periodontol., *44*:347, 1973.
28. Gibbons, R. J., van Houte, J., and Liljemark, W. F.: Some parameters that effect the adherence of *S. salivarius* to oral epithelial surfaces. J. Dent. Res., *51*:424, 1972.
29. Gilda, J. E., and Keyes, P. H.: Increased dental caries activity in the Syrian hamster following desalivation. Proc. Soc. Exp. Biol. Med., *66*:28, 1947.
30. Golub, L. M., Borden, S. M., and Kleinberg, K.: Urea content of gingival crevicular fluid and its relation to periodontal disease in humans. J. Periodont. Res., *6*:243, 1971.
31. Gordon, J. M., et al.: Sensitive assay for measuring tetracycline levels in gingival crevice fluid. Antimicrob. Agents Chemother., *17*:193, 1980.
32. Grant, D. A., and Orban, B. J.: Leukocytes in the epithelial attachment. J. Periodontol., *31*:87, 1960.
33. Gupta, O. N., Blechman, H., and Stahl, S. S.: The effects of desalivation on periodontal tissues of the Syrian hamster. Oral Surg., *13*:470, 1960.
34. Hampar, B., Mandel, I. D., and Ellison, S. A.: The carbohydrate components of supragingival calculus. J. Dent. Res., *40*:752, 1961 (abstract).
35. Hara, K., and Löe, H.: Carbohydrate components of the gingival exudate. J. Periodont. Res., *4*:202, 1969.
36. Hasegawa, K.: Biochemical study of gingival fluid. Lactic acid in gingival fluid. Bull. Tokyo Med. Dent. Univ., *14*:359, 1967.
37. Jacoby, R., and Ketterl, W.: Quantitative measurements of gingival pocket exudate in normal and inflamed gingiva. Dtsch. Zahnärztl. Z., *27*:485, 1972.
38. Jensen, A. T., and Dano, M.: Crystallography of dental calculus and precipitation of certain calcium phosphates. J. Dent. Res., *33*:741, 1954.
39. Jensen, R. L., and Folke, L. E. A.: The passage of exogenous tritiated thymidine into gingival tissues. J. Periodontol., *45*:786, 1974.
40. Kahnberg, K.-E., Lindhe, J., and Helden, J.: Initial gingivitis induced by topical application of plaque extract. A histometric study in dogs with normal gingiva. J. Periodont. Res., *11*:218, 1976.
41. Kaslick, R. S., et al.: Concentration of inorganic ions in gingival fluid. J. Dent. Res., *49*:887, 1970.
42. Kaslick, R. S., et al.: Quantitative analysis of sodium, potassium and calcium in gingival fluid from gingiva in varying degrees of inflammation. J. Periodontol., *41*:93, 1970.
43. Kaslick, R. S., et al.: Sodium, potassium and calcium in gingival fluid. A study of the relationship of the ions to one another, to circadian rhythms, gingival bleeding, purulence, and to conservative periodontal therapy. J. Periodontol., *41*:442, 1970.
44. Kiroshita, J. J., and Mühlemann, H. R.: Effect of sodium ortho- and pyrophosphate on supragingival calculus. Helv. Odont. Acta, *10*:46, 1966.
45. Kowolik, M. J., and Raeburn, J. A.: Functional integrity of gingival crevicular neutrophil polymorphonuclear leucocytes as demonstrated by nitroblue tetrazolium reduction. J. Periodont. Res., *5*:483, 1980.
46. Krasse, B., and Egelberg, J.: The relative proportions of sodium, potassium and calcium in gingival pocket fluid. Acta Odontol. Scand., *20*:143, 1962.
47. Lehner, J., Cardwell, J. E., and Clarry, E. D.: Immunoglobulins in saliva and serum in dental caries. Lancet, *2*:1294, 1967.

48. Leung, S. W., and Jensen, A. T.: Factors controlling the deposition of calculus. Int. Dent. J., *8*:613, 1958.
49. Lindhe, J., and Attstrom, R.: Gingival exudation during the menstrual cycle. J. Periodont. Res., *2*:194, 1967.
50. Lindhe, J., and Bjorn, A. L.: Influence of hormonal contraceptives on the gingiva of women. J. Periodont. Res., *2*:1, 1967.
51. Lindhe, J., Attstrom, R., and Bjorn, A. L.: Influence of sex hormones on gingival exudate of gingivitis-free female dogs. J. Periodont. Res., *3*:273, 1968.
52. Löe, H., and Holm-Pedersen, P.: Absence and presence of fluid from normal and inflamed gingiva. Periodontics, *3*:171, 1965.
53. Lo Grippo, G. A., Hayashi, H., and Perry, M.: Immunoglobulins in serum and saliva in health and diseases. Fed. Proc., *28*:553, 1969.
54. Lovdal, A., Arno, A., and Waerhaug, J.: Incidence of clinical manifestations of periodontal disease in light of oral hygiene and calculus formation. J. Am. Dent. Assoc., *56*:21, 1958.
55. Magnusson, B.: Mucosal changes at erupting molars in germfree rats. J. Periodont. Res., *4*:181, 1969.
56. Mandel, I.: Relation of saliva and plaque to caries. J. Dent. Res., *53*(Suppl.):246, 1974.
57. Martin, L. P., and Noble, W. H.: Gingival fluid in relation to tooth mobility and occlusal interferences. J. Periodontol., *45*:444, 1974.
58. Matt, M. M., Stout, F. W., and Swancar, J. R.: Deposition curves of in vivo calculus formation. I.A.D.R. Abstracts, No. 705, 1970, p. 225.
59. McDougall, W. A.: Pathways of penetration and effects of horseradish peroxidase in rat molar gingiva. Arch. Oral Biol., *15*:621, 1970.
60. McDougall, W. A.: The effect of topical antigen on the gingiva of sensitized rabbits. J. Periodont. Res., *9*:153, 1974.
61. Mühlemann, H. R., and Schroeder, H.: Dynamics of supragingival calculus formation. Adv. Oral Biol., *1*:175, 1964.
62. Mühlemann, H. R., and Villa, P. R.: The marginal line calculus index. Helv. Odont. Acta, *11*:175, 1967.
63. Nagao, M.: Influence of prosthetic appliances upon the flow of crevicular tissue fluid. I. Relation between crevicular tissue fluid and prosthetic appliances. Bull. Tokyo Med. Dent. Clin., *14*:241, 1967.
64. Novaes, A. B., Jr., Ruben, M. P., and Kramer, G. M.: Proteins of the gingival exudate: a review and discussion of the literature. J. Western Soc. Periodontol., *27*:12, 1979.
65. Oppenheim, F. G.: Preliminary observations on the presence and origin of serum albumin in human saliva. Helv. Odont. Acta, *14*:10, 1970.
66. Orban, J. E., and Stallard, R. E.: Gingival crevicular fluid: a reliable predictor of gingival health? J. Periodontol., *40*:231, 1969.
67. Passo, S. A., et al.: Interaction of inflammatory cells and oral microorganisms. IX. The bacterial effect of human PMN leukocytes on isolated plaque microorganisms. J. Periodont. Res., *5*:470, 1980.
68. Paunio, K.: On the hydroxyproline-containing components in the gingival exudate. J. Periodont. Res., *6*:115, 1971.
69. Ranney, R. R., and Montgomery, E. H.: Vascular leakage resulting from topical application of endotoxin to the gingiva of the beagle dog. Arch. Oral Biol., *18*:963, 1973.
70. Ranney, R. R., and Zander, H. A.: Allergic periodontal disease in sensitized squirrel monkeys. J. Periodontol., *41*:12, 1970.
71. Ratcliff, P.: Permeability of healthy gingival epithelium by microscopically observable particles. J. Periodontol., *37*:291, 1966.
72. Renggli, H. H.: Phagocytosis and killing by crevicular neutrophils. *In* Lehner, T. (ed.): The Borderland Between Caries and Periodontal Disease. New York, Grune & Stratton, 1977.
73. Rizzo, A. A.: Absorption of bacterial endotoxin into rabbit gingival pocket tissue. Periodontics, *6*:65, 1968.

74. Rizzo, A. A.: Histologic and immunologic evaluation of antigen penetration with oral tissues after topical application. Periodontics, *41*:210, 1970.
75. Rizzo, A. A., and Mitchell, C. T.: Chronic allergic inflammation induced by repeated deposition of antigen in rabbit gingival pockets. Periodontics, *4*:5, 1966.
76. Rosebury, R., and Karshan, M.: Salivary Calculus: Dental Science and Dental Art. Philadelphia, Lea & Febiger, 1938.
77. Rovin, S., Costich, E. R., and Gordon, H. A.: The influence of bacteria and irritation in the initiation of periodontal disease in germfree and conventional rats. J. Periodont. Res., *1*:193, 1966.
78. Sandalli, P., and Wade, A. B.: Alterations in crevicular fluid flow during healing following gingivectomy and flap procedures. J. Periodont. Res., *4*:314, 1969.
79. Schiott, C. R., and Löe, H.: The origin and variation in the number of leukocytes in the human saliva. J. Periodont. Res., *4*(Suppl.):24, 1969.
80. Schwartz, J., Stinson, F. L., and Parker, R. B.: The passage of tritiated bacterial endotoxin across intact gingival crevicular epithelium. J. Periodontol., *43*:270, 1972.
81. Selvig, K.: Structure and metabolism of the normal periodontium. Position paper. International Conference on Research in the Biology of Periodontal Disease, 1977.
82. Shapiro, L., Goldman, H., and Bloom, A.: Sulcular exudate flow in gingival inflammation. J. Periodontol., *50*:301, 1979.
83. Shen, L. S., Ghavamzadeh, G., and Shklar, G.: Gingival healing in sialadenectomized rats. J. Periodontol., *50*:533, 1979.
84. Simon, B., et al.: The role of endotoxin in periodontal disease. II. Correlation of the amount of endotoxin in human gingival exudate with the clinical degree of inflammation. J. Periodontol., *42*:81, 1970.
85. Simon, B., et al.: The role of endotoxin in periodontal disease. III. Correlation of the amount of endotoxin with the histologic degree of inflammation. J. Periodontol., *42*:210, 1971.
86. Skapski, H., and Lehner, T.: A crevicular washing method for investigating immune components of crevicular fluid in man. J. Periodont. Res., *11*:19, 1976.
87. Skougaard, M. R., Bay, I., and Klinkhammer, J. M.: Correlation between gingivitis and orogranulocytic migratory rate. J. Dent. Res., *48*:716, 1969.
88. Solis-Gaffar, M. C., Rustogi, K. N., and Gaffar, A.: Hydrogen sulfide production from gingival crevicular fluid. J. Periodontol., *51*:603, 1980.
89. Squier, C. A., and Johnson, N. W.: Permeability of oral mucosa. Br. Med. Bull., *31*:169, 1975.
90. Steinberg, A. D., et al.: The effect of alteration in the sulcular environment upon the movement of ^{14}C-diphenylhydantoin through rabbit sulcular tissues. J. Periodont. Res., *11*:47, 1976.
91. Suppipat, W., and Suppipat, N.: Evaluation of an electronic device for gingival fluid quantitation. J. Periodontol., *48*:388, 1977.
92. Theilade, J., Egelberg, J., and Attstrom, R.: Vascular permeability to colloidal carbon in clinically inflamed gingiva. J. Periodont. Res., *6*:100, 1971.
93. Tolo, K.: Transport across stratified nonkeratinized epithelium. J. Periodont. Res., *6*:237, 1971.
94. Tomasi, T. B., and Bienenstock, J.: Secretory immunoglobulins. Adv. Immunol., *9*:1, 1968.
95. Vogel, J. J., and Amdur, B. H.: Inorganic pyrophosphate in parotid saliva. Arch. Oral Biol., *12*:159, 1967.
96. Weinstein, E., et al.: Studies on gingival fluid. Periodontics, *5*:161, 1967.
97. Williams, R. W., and Gibbons, R. G.: Inhibition of bacterial adherence by secretory immunoglobulin A: a mechanism of antigen disposal. Science, *177*:697, 1972.
98. Wilton, J. M. A., Renggli, H. H., and Lehner, T.: The isolation and identification of mononuclear cells from the gingival crevice in man. J. Periodont. Res., *11*:243, 1976.

chapter eight

Gingival Inflammation

PATHOLOGY OF GINGIVITIS

It is generally agreed that the pathologic changes that accompany gingivitis are associated with the presence of oral microorganisms in the gingival sulcus (see Chapter 25). These organisms are capable of synthesizing potentially harmful products that cause damage to epithelial and connective tissue cells, as well as to intercellular constituents, i.e, collagen, ground substance, glycocalyx (cell coat), and so forth. The resulting widening of the intercellular spaces between the junctional epithelial cells during early gingivitis may permit injurious agents derived from bacteria, or bacteria themselves,[31] to gain access to the connective tissue.

The sequence of events in the development of gingivitis will be analyzed in three different stages. Clearly, one stage evolves into the next, with no clear-cut dividing lines.

Stage I Gingivitis

Vascular changes have been described as the first response to initial gingival inflammation. *Clinically,* the initial response of the gingiva to bacterial plaque is not apparent (subclinical gingivitis[18]). This vascular response is essentially the dilation of capillaries and increased blood flow.

Histologically, Stage I gingivitis shows some classic features of acute inflammation in the connective tissue beneath the junctional epithelium. **Changes in blood vessel morphology, such as widening of small capillaries or venules and adherence of neutrophils to vessel walls, occur within 1 week and sometimes as early as 2 days after plaque has been allowed to accumulate**[13, 27] (Fig. 8–1). **Leukocytes, mainly polymorphonuclear neutrophils (PMNs), leave the capillaries by migrating through the walls**[30] (Figs. 8–2*B* and 8–3). **They can be seen in increased quantities in the connective tissue, junctional epithelium, and gingival sulcus.**[1, 18, 24, 27, 34] Several microorganisms which

have been associated with gingival inflammation and periodontitis, such as *Treponema denticola, Actinomyces viscosus,* and *Bacteroides melaninogenicus,* have been shown to promote neutrophil chemotaxis and vascular exudation.[19, 40]

Subtle changes can also be detected in the junctional epithelium and perivascular connective tissue at this early stage of development. Lymphocytes soon begin to accumulate (Fig. 8–2*D*). The increase in the migration of leukocytes and their accumulation within the gingival sulcus can be correlated with an increase in the flow of gingival fluid into the sulcus.[2]

Page and Schroeder[25] call this stage the *"initial lesion"* and describe in it "classic vasculitis of vessels subjacent to the junctional epithelium and gingival sulcus; presence of serum proteins, especially fibrin, extracellularly; alteration of the most coronal portion of the junctional epithelium; and loss of perivascular collagen."

The nature and character of the host response determine whether this initial lesion resolves rapidly, with the tissue restored to normal, or evolves into a chronic inflammatory lesion. If the latter occurs, an infiltrate of macrophages and lymphoid cells appears in a few days.[26]

Stage II Gingivitis

As time goes on, clinical signs of erythema may appear, mainly owing to the proliferation of capillaries and increased formation of capillary loops between rete pegs or ridges. Bleeding upon probing may also be evident.

Histologic examination of the gingiva reveals a leukocyte infiltration in the connective tissue beneath the junctional epithelium, consisting mainly of lymphocytes (75 per cent)[34] **but also of some migrating neutrophils, as well as macrophages, plasma cells, and mast cells** (Fig. 8–4). There is an intensified overall inflammatory cell response as compared with the Stage I initial lesion.[12, 15, 19, 21, 27, 35] **The junctional epi-**

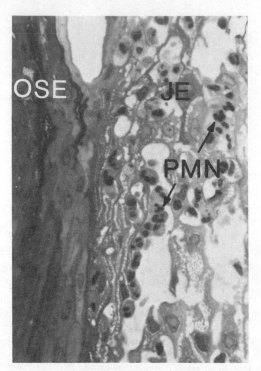

Figure 8–1 Biopsy from a human subject in an experimental gingivitis study specimen. After 4 days of plaque accumulation the blood vessels immediately adjacent to the junctional epithelium (JE) are distended and contain polymorphonuclear neutrophils (PMN). Neutrophils have also migrated between the cells of the junctional epithelium. OSE, oral sulcular epithelium. × 500. (From Payne, W. A., Page, R. C., Ogilvie, A. L., et al.: J. Periodont. Res., *10*:51, 1975.)

thelium becomes densely infiltrated with neutrophils, as does the gingival sulcus, and the junctional epithelium may begin to show development of rete pegs or ridges. There is an increase in the amount of collagen destruction as determined both histologically[35] and biochemically[8]; 70 per cent of the collagen is destroyed around the cellular infiltrate. The main fiber groups that are affected appear to be the circular and dentogingival fiber assemblies. Alterations in blood vessel morphology and vascular bed patterns have also been described.[13, 14] Page and Schroeder[25] call this stage the *"early lesion."*

PMNs that have left the blood vessels in response to chemotactic stimuli from plaque components travel to the epithelium, cross the basement lamina, and are found in the epithelium and emerging in the pocket area (Fig. 7–3). PMNs are attracted to bacteria and engulf them in a process of phagocytosis (Fig. 8–5). PMNs release their lysosomes in association with the ingestion of bacteria[15] and also in response to plaque in the absence of bacteria.[3]

Stage III Gingivitis

In chronic gingivitis (Stage III), the blood vessels become engorged and congested, venous return is impaired, and the blood flow becomes sluggish. The result is localized gingival anoxemia, which superimposes a somewhat bluish hue upon the reddened gingiva. Extravasation of red blood cells into the connective tissue and breakdown of hemoglobin into its component pigments can also deepen the color of the chronically inflamed gingiva.

The Stage III lesion can be described as moderately to severely inflamed gingiva. In histologic sections of this tissue an intense, chronic inflammatory reaction is observed. Several detailed cytologic studies have been carried out on chronically inflamed gingiva.[9, 11, 12, 26, 32, 36, 38] A key feature that differentiates this lesion from the Stage II lesion is the **increase in the number of plasma cells, which become the predominant inflammatory cell type. Plasma cells invade the connective tissue not only immediately below the junctional epithelium, but also deep into the connective tissue, around blood vessels, and between bundles of collagen fibers. The junctional epithelium reveals widened intercellular spaces filled with granular cellular debris, lysosomes derived from disrupted neutrophils, lymphocytes, and monocytes** (Fig. 8–6). The lysosomes contain acid hydrolases that can destroy tissue components. **The junctional epithelium develops rete pegs or ridges that protrude into the connective tissue, and the basal lamina is destroyed in some areas. In the connective tissue, collagen fibers are destroyed around the infiltrate of intact and disrupted plasma cells, neutrophils, lymphocytes, monocytes, and mast cells.** There appears to be an inverse relationship between the number of intact collagen bundles and the number of inflammatory cells.[36] Collagenolytic activity is increased in inflamed gingival tissue[10] by the enzyme collagenase. Collagenase is normally present in gingival tissues[4] and is produced by some oral bacteria and by polymorphonuclear neutrophils.

Enzyme histochemistry has shown that chronically inflamed gingiva has elevated levels of acid and alkaline phosphatase,[40] beta-glucuronidase, beta-glucosidase, beta-galactosidase, esterases,[20] aminopeptidase,[22, 28] and cytochrome oxidase.[5] Neutral mucopolysaccharides are decreased,[39] presumably as a result of degradation of the ground substance.

This stage has been called the *"established*

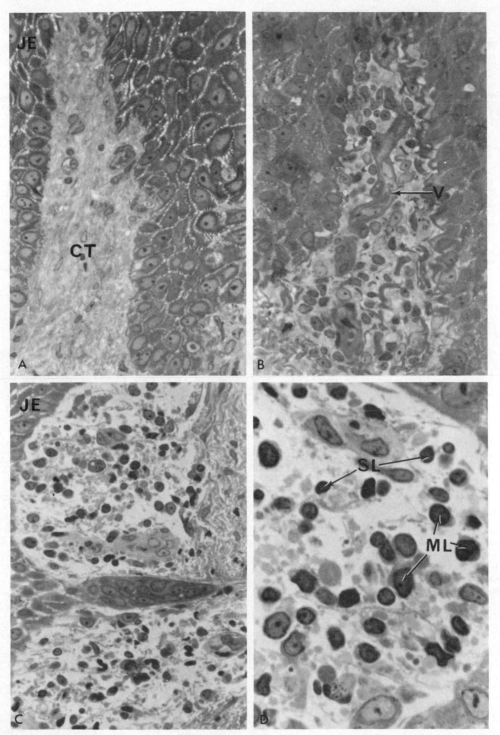

Figure 8–2 Biopsy specimens from human subjects in an experimental gingivitis study. *A,* Control biopsy specimen from a patient with good oral hygiene and no detectable plaque accumulation. The junctional epithelium (JE) is at the left. The connective tissue (CT) shows few cells other than fibroblasts, blood vessels, and a dense background of collagen fibers. × 500. *B,* Biopsy specimen taken after 8 days of plaque accumulation. The connective tissue is infiltrated with inflammatory cells, which displace the collagen fibers. A distended blood vessel (V) is seen in the center. × 500. *C,* After 8 days of plaque accumulation the connective tissue next to the junctional epithelium (JE) at the base of the sulcus shows a mononuclear cell infiltrate and evidence of collagen degeneration (clear spaces around cellular infiltrate). × 500. *D,* The inflammatory cell infiltrate at higher magnification. After 8 days of plaque accumulation numerous small (SL) and medium size (ML) lymphocytes are seen within the connective tissue. Most of the collagen fibers around these cells have disappeared, presumably as a result of enzymatic digestion. × 1250. (From Payne, W. A., Page, R. C., Ogilvie, A. L., et al.: J. Periodont. Res., *10*:51, 1975.)

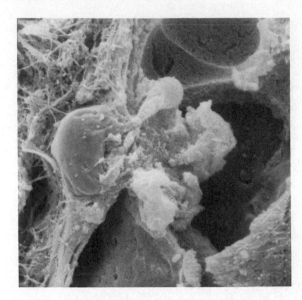

Figure 8–3   Scanning electron micrograph showing a leukocyte traversing the vessel wall to enter into the gingival connective tissue.

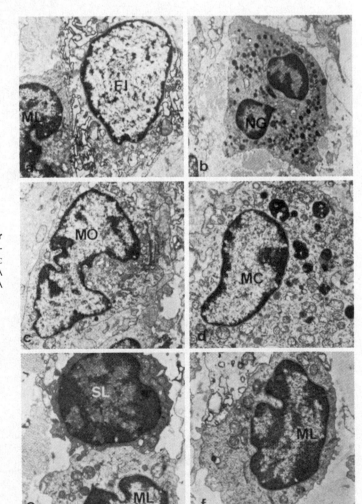

Figure 8–4   Morphologic Features of Cellular Constituents. *Above, a,* A typical pathologically altered fibroblast (FI). *b,* A neutrophilic granulocyte (NG). *c,* A monocyte (MO). *d,* A macrophage (MC). *e,* A small (SL) and *f,* A medium-sized (ML) lymphocyte.

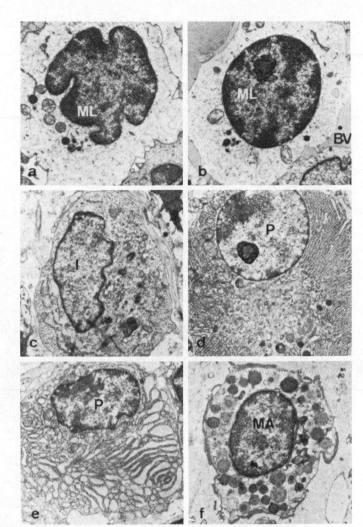

Figure 8–4 *Continued a,* Medium-sized (ML) lymphocytes outside and *b,* Inside blood vessel (BV). *c,* An immunoblast (I). *d* and *e,* Plasma cells (P) in varying stages of maturation. *f,* A mast cell. (From Schroeder, H. E., and Münzel-Pedrazzoli, S.: J. Microsc., *99*:301, 1973.)

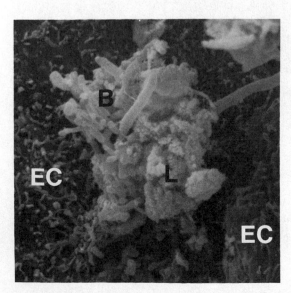

Figure 8–5 Scanning electron micrograph of leukocyte (L) emerging to pocket wall and covered with bacteria (B) and extracellular lysosomes. EC, epithelial cells.

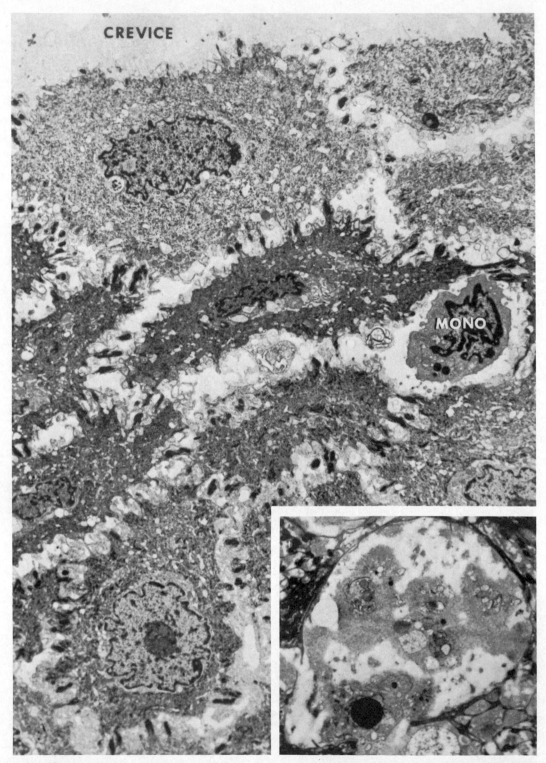

Figure 8–6 Chronic Gingivitis—Crevicular Epithelium. The crevice is at the top. The intercellular spaces are dilated and contain a granular precipitate and cellular fragments. An emigrating monocyte (MONO) is shown between the eipthelial cells. × 4400. *Inset*, Cellular fragments and precipitated material in a dilated intercellular space of the crevicular epithelium. Bacteria are not present. × 4036. (From Freedman, H. L., Listgarten, M. A., and Taichman, N. S.: J. Periodont. Res., *3*:313, 1968.)

lesion" by Page and Schroder.[25] The extension of the lesion into alveolar bone characterizes a fourth stage that Page and Schroeder have named the *"advanced lesion"*[25] and that Lindhe et al. term the *"phase of periodontal breakdown."*[18] It will be described in detail in Chapters 15 and 16.

REFERENCES

1. Attstrom, R.: Studies on neutrophil polymorphonuclear leukocytes at the dento-gingival junction in gingival health and disease. J. Periodont. Res., 6(Suppl. 8), 1971.
2. Attstrom, R., and Egelberg, J.: Emigration of blood neutrophils and monocytes into the gingival crevices. J. Periodont. Res., 5:48, 1970.
3. Baehni, P., Tsai, C. C., Taichman, N. S., and McArthur, W.: Interaction of inflammatory cells and oral microorganisms. V. E. M. and biochemical study on the mechanisms of release of lysosomal constituents of human PMN leukocytes exposed to dental plaque. J. Periodont. Res., 13:333, 1978.
4. Beutner, E. H., Triftshauser, C., and Hazen, S. P.: Collagenase activity of gingival tissue from patients with periodontal disease. Proc. Soc. Exp. Biol. Med., 121:1082, 1966.
5. Burstone, M. S.: Histochemical study of cytochrome oxidase in normal and inflamed gingiva. Oral Surg., 13.1501, 1960.
6. Egelberg, J.: Permeability of the dento-gingival blood vessels. III. Chronically inflamed gingivae. J. Periodont. Res., 1:287, 1966.
7. Egelberg, J.: The topography and permeability of vessels at the dento-gingival junction in dogs. J. Periodont. Res., 2(Suppl. 1), 1967.
8. Flieder, D. E., and Sun, C. N.: Chemistry of normal and inflamed human gingival tissues. Periodontics, 4:302, 1966.
9. Freedman, H. L., Listgarten, M. A., and Taichman, N. S.: Electron microscopic features of chronically inflamed human gingiva. J. Periodont. Res., 3:313, 1968.
10. Fullmer, H., and Gibson, W.: Collagenolytic activity in gingivae of man. Nature, 209:728, 1966.
11. Garant, P. R., and Mulvihill, J. E.: The fine structure of gingivitis in the beagle. III. Plasma cell infiltration of the subepithelial connective tissue. J. Periodont. Res., 7:161, 1971.
12. Gavin, J. R.: Ultrastructural features of chronic marginal gingivitis. J. Periodont. Res., 5:19, 1970.
13. Hock, J., and Nuki, K.: A vital microscopy study of the morphology of normal and inflamed gingiva. J. Periodont. Res., 6:81, 1971.
14. Kindlova, M.: Changes in the vascular bed of the marginal periodontium in periodontitis. J. Dent. Res., 44:456, 1965.
15. Lange, D., and Schroeder, H. E.: Cytochemistry and ultrastructure of gingival sulcus cells. Helv. Odontol. Acta, 15(Suppl. 6):65, 1971.
16. Levy, B. M., Taylor, A. C., and Bernick, S.: Relationship between epithelium and connective tissue in gingival inflammation. J. Dent. Res., 48:625, 1969.
17. Lindhe, J., and Socransky, S. S.: Chemotaxis and vascular permeability produced by human periodontopathic bacteria. J. Periodont. Res., 14:138, 1979.
18. Lindhe, J., Hamp, S. E., and Löe, H.: Experimental periodontitis in the beagle dog. J. Periodont. Res., 8:1, 1973.
19. Lindhe, J., Schroeder, H. E., Page, R. C., Munzel-Pedrazzoli, S., and Hugoson, A.: Clinical and stereologic analysis of the course of early gingivitis in dogs. J. Periodont. Res., 9:314, 1974.
20. Lisanti, V. F.: Hydrolytic enzymes in periodontal tissues. Ann. N.Y. Acad. Sci., 85:461, 1960.
21. Listgarten, M. A., and Ellegaard, B.: Experimental gingivitis in Rhesus monkeys. J. Periodont. Res., 8:199, 1973.
22. Mori, M., and Kishiro, A.: Histochemical observation of aminopeptidase activity in the normal and inflamed oral epithelium. J. Osaka Univ. Dent. Sch., 1:39, 1961.
23. Newman, M. G., Socransky, S., Savitt, E. D., Propas, E. D., and Crawford, A.: Studies of the microbiology of periodontosis. J. Periodontol., 47:373, 1976.
24. Oliver, R. C., Holm-Pedersen, P., and Löe, H.: The correlation between clinical scoring, exudate measurements, and microscopic evaluation of inflammation of the gingiva. J. Periodontol., 40:201, 1969.
25. Page, R. C., and Schroeder, H. E.: Pathogenic mechanisms. In Schluger, S., Youdelis, R., and Page, R. C. (eds.): Periodontal Disease: Basic Phenomena, Clinical Management and Restorative Interrelationships. Philadelphia, Lea & Febiger, 1977.
26. Page, R. C., Ammons, W. F., and Simpson, D. M.: Host tissue response in chronic inflammatory periodontal disease. IV. The periodontal and dental status of a group of aged great apes. J. Periodontol., 46:144, 1975.
27. Payne, W. A., Page, R. C., Ogilvie, A. L., and Hall, W. B.: Histopathologic features of the initial and early stages of experimental gingivitis in man. J. Periodont. Res., 10:51, 1975.
28. Quintarelli, G.: Histochemistry of gingiva. III. The distribution of amino-peptidase in normal and inflammatory conditions. Arch. Oral Biol., 2:271, 1960.
29. Rizzo, A. A., and Mergenhagen, S. E.: Host responses in periodontal disease. Proceedings of the International Conference on Research on the Biology of Periodontal Disease. Chicago, 1977.
30. Saglie, R., Newman, M. G., and Carranza, F. A., Jr.: Scanning electron microscopy study of the interaction of leukocytes and bacteria in human periodontitis. J. Periodontol., 53:752, 1982.
31. Saglie, R., Newman, M. G., Carranza, F. A., Jr., and Pattison, G. L.: Bacterial invasion of gingiva in advanced periodontitis in humans. J. Periodontol., 53:217, 1982.
32. Schectman, L. R., Ammons, W. F., Simpson, D. M., and Page, R. C.: Host tissue response in chronic periodontal disease. II. Histologic features of the normal periodontium, and histopathologic and ultrastructural manifestations of disease in the marmoset. J. Periodont. Res., 7:195, 1972.
33. Schroeder, H. E.: Transmigration and infiltration of leucocytes in human junctional epithelium. Helv. Odontol. Acta, 17:6, 1973.
34. Schroeder, H. E., Graf-de Beer, M., and Attstrom, R.: Initial gingivitis in dogs. J. Periodont. Res., 10:128, 1975.
35. Schroeder, H. E., Munzell-Pedrazzoli, S., and Page, R. C.: Correlated morphological and biochemical analysis of gingival tissue in early chronic gingivitis in man. Arch. Oral Biol., 18:899, 1973.
36. Simpson, D. M., and Avery, B. E.: Histopathologic and ultrastructural features of inflamed gingiva in the baboon. J. Periodontol., 45:500, 1974.
37. Soderholm, G., and Egelberg, J.: Morphological changes in gingival blood vessels during developing gingivitis in dogs. J. Periodont. Res., 8:16, 1973.
38. Thilander, H.: Epithelial changes in gingivitis. An electron microscopic study. J. Periodont. Res., 3:303, 1968.
39. Wennstrom, J., Heijl, L., Lindhe, J., and Socransky, S.: Migration of gingival leukocytes mediated by plaque bacteria. J. Periodont. Res., 15:363, 1980.
40. Winer, R. A., et al.: Enzyme activity in periodontal disease. J. Periodontol., 41:449, 1970.

chapter nine

Clinical Features of Gingivitis

THE ROLE OF INFLAMMATION IN GINGIVAL DISEASE

Gingivitis, inflammation of the gingiva, is the most common form of gingival disease. Inflammation is almost always present in all forms of gingival disease because bacterial plaque, which causes inflammation, and irritational factors, which favor plaque accumulation, are very often present in the gingival environment. The inflammation caused by dental plaque gives rise to associated degenerative, necrotic, and proliferative changes in the gingival tissues. There is a tendency to designate all forms of gingival disease as gingivitis, as if inflammation were the only disease process involved. However, pathologic processes not caused by local irritation, such as atrophy, hyperplasia, and neoplasia, also occur in the gingiva. All cases of gingivitis are not necessarily the same because they present inflammatory changes, and it is often necessary to differentiate between inflammation and other pathologic processes that may be present in gingival disease.

The *role of inflammation* in individual cases of gingivitis varies as follows:

1. Inflammation may be the *primary* and *only* pathologic change. This is by far the most prevalent type of gingival disease.

2. Inflammation may be a *secondary* feature, superimposed upon systemically caused gingival disease. For example, inflammation commonly complicates gingival hyperplasia caused by the systemic administration of phenytoin.

3. Inflammation may be the precipitating factor responsible for clinical changes in pa-

tients with systemic conditions that of themselves do not produce clinically detectable gingival disease. Gingivitis in pregnancy is an example.

TYPES OF GINGIVAL DISEASES

The most common type of gingival disease is the simple inflammatory involvement caused by bacterial plaque attached to the tooth surface. This type of gingivitis, sometimes called chronic marginal gingivitis or simple gingivitis, may remain stationary for indefinite periods of time or may proceed to destruction of the supporting structures (periodontitis). The reasons for these different behaviors are not clearly understood.

In addition, the gingiva can be involved in other diseases, sometimes but not always related to the usual periodontal problems. An attempt to classify these diseases is difficult and its usefulness doubtful. We prefer to list some of the other types of gingival diseases.

1. Acute necrotizing ulcerative gingivitis (see Chapter 11).

2. Acute herpetic gingivostomatitis (see Chapter 11) and other viral diseases (see Chapter 21).

3. Allergic gingivitis, caused by different allergies (see Chapter 12).

4. Many dermatoses will attack the gingival tissues, inducing characteristic types of gingival disease, such as that seen in lichen planus, pemphigus, erythema multiforme, and so forth. They are described in detail in Chapter 12.

5. Some gingivitis may be initiated by bac-

terial plaque, but the tissue response may be conditioned by systemic factors. Such is the case in pregnancy, puberty gingivitis (see Chapter 29), and vitamin C deficiency (see Chapter 28).

6. The gingival response to a variety of pathogenic agents may include an increase in volume, termed gingival enlargement. This is described in Chapter 10.

7. Different benign and malignant tumors may appear in the gingiva, either as primary tumors or as metastatic ones. They are discussed in Chapter 10.

COURSE, DURATION, AND DISTRIBUTION OF GINGIVITIS

Course and Duration

ACUTE GINGIVITIS. A painful condition which comes on suddenly and is of short duration.

SUBACUTE GINGIVITIS. A less severe phase of the acute condition.

RECURRENT GINGIVITIS. Disease that reappears after having been eliminated by treatment or that disappears spontaneously and reappears.

CHRONIC GINGIVITIS. Disease which comes on slowly, is of long duration and is painless unless complicated by acute or subacute exacerbations. Chronic gingivitis is the type most commonly encountered (Fig. 9–1). Patients seldom recollect having had any acute symptoms. Chronic gingivitis is a fluctuating disease in which inflamed areas persist or become normal and normal areas become inflamed.[11, 12]

Distribution

LOCALIZED GINGIVITIS. Confined to the gingiva in relation to a single tooth or group of teeth.

GENERALIZED GINVIGITIS. Involving the entire mouth.

MARGINAL GINGIVITIS. Involving the gingival margin, but may include a portion of the contiguous attached gingiva.

PAPILLARY GINGIVITIS. Involving the interdental papillae and often extending into the adjacent portion of the gingival margin. Papillae are more frequently involved than is the gingival margin, and the earliest signs of gingivitis most often occur in the papillae.

DIFFUSE GINGIVITIS. Involving the gingival margin, attached gingiva, and interdental papillae.

The distribution of gingival disease in individual cases is described by combining the above terms as follows:

LOCALIZED MARGINAL GINGIVITIS. Confined to one or more areas of the marginal gingiva (Fig. 9–2).

LOCALIZED DIFFUSE GINGIVITIS. Extending from the margin to the mucobuccal fold, but limited in area (Fig. 9–3).

PAPILLARY GINGIVITIS. Confined to one or more interdental spaces in a limited area (Fig. 9–4).

GENERALIZED MARGINAL GINGIVITIS. Involvement of the gingival margin in relation to all the teeth. The interdental papillae are usually also involved in generalized marginal gingivitis (Fig. 9–5).

GENERALIZED DIFFUSE GINGIVITIS. Involving the entire gingiva. The alveolar mucosa is usually also affected, so the demarcation between it and the attached gingiva is obliterated (Fig. 9–6). Systemic conditions are involved in the etiology of generalized diffuse gingivitis except in cases caused by acute infection or generalized chemical irritation.

CLINICAL FEATURES OF GINGIVITIS

In evaluating the clinical features of gingivitis, it is necessary to be systematic. Attention should be focused on very subtle tissue alterations from the norm, since these may be of great diagnostic significance. A systematic clinical approach requires an orderly examination of the gingiva for the following features: color, size and shape, consistency, surface texture and position, ease of bleeding, and pain. These

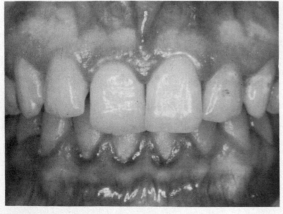

Figure 9–1 Chronic Gingivitis. The marginal and interdental gingivae are smooth, edematous, and discolored.

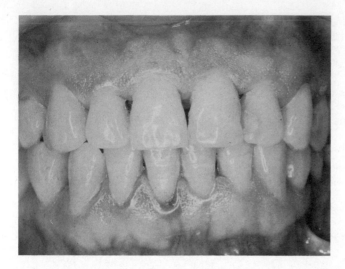

Figure 9–2 Localized Marginal Gingivitis in the mandibular anterior region.

Figure 9–3 Localized Diffuse Gingivitis involving both the marginal and attached gingiva.

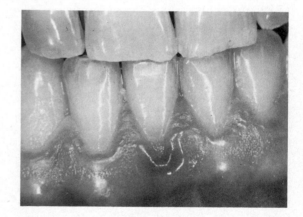

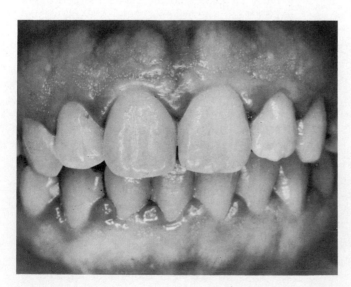

Figure 9–4 Papillary Gingivitis.

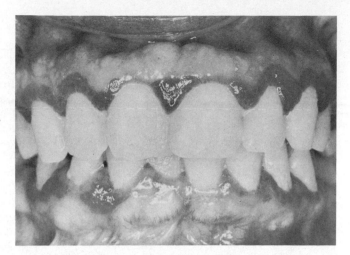

Figure 9–5 Generalized Marginal Gingivitis. The interdental papillae are also involved.

clinical characteristics and the microscopic changes responsible for each are discussed in the sections that follow.

Gingival Bleeding

The two earliest symptoms of gingival inflammation preceding established gingivitis are (1) increased gingival fluid rate and (2) bleeding from the gingival sulcus upon gentle probing (Fig. 9–7). Gingival fluid has been dealt with in detail in Chapter 7.

Bleeding upon probing is clinically easily detectable and therefore of great value for the early diagnosis and prevention of more advanced gingivitis. It has been shown that bleeding upon probing appears earlier than change in color or other visual signs of inflammation[12, 13, 16]; moreover, the use of bleeding rather than color changes to diagnose early gingival inflammation has the advantage that bleeding is a more objective sign, requiring less subjective estimation by the examiner. Several gingival indices based on bleeding have been developed[1, 5, 22] and are described in Chapter 23. Although observing the presence or absence of gingival bleeding is a very objective maneuver, these indices also have a subjective component: the force with and manner in which the probe is inserted into the sulcus. See Chapter 32 for further considerations on probing.

Gingival bleeding varies in severity, duration, and the ease with which it is provoked.

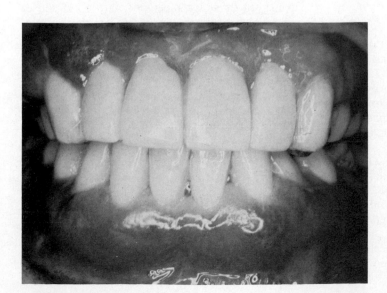

Figure 9–6 Generalized Diffuse Gingivitis. The marginal, interdental, and attached gingivae are involved in chronic desquamative gingivitis.

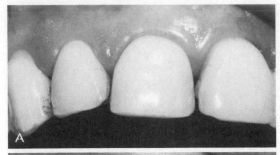
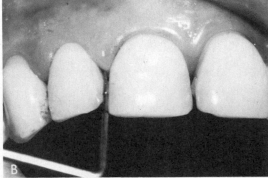
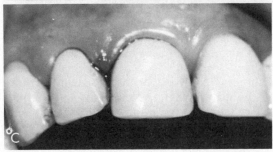

Figure 9–7   Bleeding upon Probing. *A,* Mild gingivitis with slight edema. *B,* Introduction of the periodontal probe to the bottom of the gingival sulcus. *C,* Bleeding appears after a few seconds. (Courtesy of Dr. Joseph Hsiou.)

Gingival Bleeding Caused by Local Factors

CHRONIC AND RECURRENT BLEEDING. *The most common cause of abnormal gingival bleeding is chronic inflammation.*[19] The bleeding is chronic or recurrent and is provoked by mechanical trauma such as that from toothbrushing, toothpicks, or food impaction, by biting into solid foods such as apples, or by grinding the teeth (bruxism).

Histopathology. The blood vessels of the gingiva are contained in the papillary connective tissue. On the outer surface they are protected from injury by a considerable thickness of keratinized or parakeratinized stratified squamous epithelium. Adjacent to the tooth a plexus of capillaries lies close to the sulcus space, separated from it by a thin layer of semipermeable epithelium.

In gingival inflammation the following alterations result in abnormal gingival bleeding.

Dilation and engorgement of the capillaries increase the susceptibility to injury and bleeding. Injurious agents which initiate the inflammation increase the permeability of the sulcular epithelium by degrading the intercellular cement substance and widening the intercellular spaces. As the inflammation becomes chronic, the sulcular epithelium undergoes ulceration. The cellular and fluid exudate and the proliferation of new blood vessels and connective tissue cells create pressure upon the epithelium on the crest and external surface of the marginal and interdental gingivae. The epithelium is thinned and presents varying degrees of degeneration (Fig. 9–8). Because the capillaries are engorged and closer to the surface and the thinned, degenerated epithelium is less protective, stimuli that are ordinarily innocuous cause rupture of the capillaries and gingival bleeding.

The severity of the bleeding and the ease with which it is provoked depend upon the intensity of the inflammation. After the vessels rupture, a complex of mechanisms induces hemostasis.[31] The vessel walls contract and blood flow is diminished; blood platelets adhere to the edges of the tissue; and a fibrous clot is formed, which contracts and results in approximation of the edges of the injured area. Bleeding recurs, however, when the area is irritated.

ACUTE BLEEDING. *Acute episodes of gingival bleeding* are caused by injury or occur spontaneously in acute gingival disease. Laceration of the gingiva by aggressive toothbrushing or sharp pieces of hard food causes gingival bleeding even in the absence of gingival disease. Gingival burns from hot foods or chemicals increase the ease of gingival bleeding.

Spontaneous bleeding or bleeding upon slight provocation occurs in *acute necrotizing ulcerative gingivitis.* **In this condition, engorged blood vessels in the inflamed connective tissue are exposed by desquamation of necrotic surface epithelium.**

Gingival Bleeding Associated with Systemic Disturbances

There are systemic disorders in which gingival hemorrhage, unprovoked by mechanical irritation, occurs spontaneously, or in which gingival bleeding following irritation is exces-

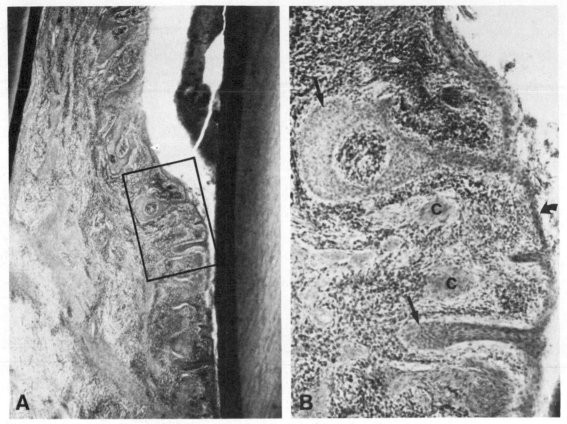

Figure 9–8 *A,* Microscopic view of interdental space in human autopsy specimen. *B,* Higher magnification of rectangle in *A.* Note the dense inflammatory infiltrate, the thinned epithelium *(curved arrow),* the extension of rete pegs *(straight arrows),* and the remnants of collagen fibers (C).

sive and difficult to control. These are called **hemorrhagic diseases** and represent a wide variety of conditions that vary in etiology and clinical manifestations. Such conditions have one feature in common: namely, abnormal bleeding in the skin, internal organs, and other tissues as well as the oral mucous membrane.

In individual patients the hemorrhagic tendency may be due to failure of one or more of the hemostatic mechanisms.[29] *Hemorrhagic disorders in which abnormal gingival bleeding is encountered include the following:* vascular abnormalities (vitamin C deficiency or allergy such as Schönlein-Henoch purpura), platelet disorders (idiopathic thrombocytopenic purpura or thrombocytopenic purpura secondary to diffuse injury to the bone marrow), hypoprothrombinemia (vitamin K deficiency resulting from liver disease or sprue), other coagulation defects (hemophilia, leukemia, Christmas disease), deficient platelet thromboplastic factor (PF_3) secondary to uremia,[17] and postrubella purpura.[9] Bleeding may follow the administration of excessive amounts of drugs such as salicylates and the administration

of anticoagulants such as dicumarol and heparin. (Periodontal involvement in hematologic disorders is considered in Chapter 30.)

Cyclic episodes of abnormal gingival bleeding occasionally occur associated with the menstrual period (Chapter 29), and comparatively poor general health and nutritional status have been associated with gingival bleeding following toothbrushing.[27]

Color Changes in the Gingiva

Color Changes in Chronic Gingivitis

Change in color is a very important clinical sign of gingival disease. The normal gingival color is "coral pink," owing to the tissue's vascularity, modified by the overlying epithelial layers. For this reason, the gingiva will become redder when (1) there is an increase in vascularization or (2) the degree of epithelial keratinization becomes reduced or disappears. The color will become paler when (1) vascularization is reduced (associated with fibrosis

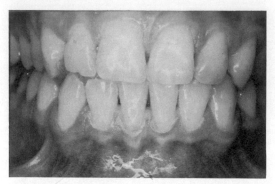

Figure 9–9 **"Traumatic Crescents."** Crescent-shaped marginal areas of gingival erythema in the mandibular anterior region. Vascular changes produced by trauma from occlusion are the suspected but not proven cause.

of the corium) or (2) epithelial keratinization increases. Therefore, chronic inflammation will intensify the red or bluish-red color owing to vascular proliferation and to reduction of keratinization due to epithelial compression by the inflamed tissue. Venous stasis will add a bluish hue. Originally a light red, the color changes through varying shades of red, reddish blue, and deep blue with increasing chronicity of the inflammatory process. The changes start in the interdental papillae and gingival margin and spread to the attached gingiva (see Fig. 9–1). Proper diagnosis and treatment require an understanding of the tissue changes which alter the color of the gingiva at the clinical level.

"TRAUMATIC CRESCENTS." These are small, crescent-shaped, bluish-red areas in the marginal gingiva attributed to trauma from occlusion (Fig. 9–9). *They are chronic inflammatory lesions caused by local irritants.* The suspected contributory role of excessive occlusal forces has not been demonstrated.

Color Changes in Acute Gingivitis

Color changes in acute gingival inflammation differ somewhat from those in chronic gingivitis in nature and distribution. The color changes may be marginal, diffuse, or patch-like, depending upon the acute condition. In *acute necrotizing ulcerative gingivitis* the involvement is marginal, in *herpetic gingivostomatitis* it is diffuse, and in *acute reactions to chemical irritation* it is patch-like or diffuse.

Color changes vary with the intensity of the inflammation. In all instances there is an initial bright red erythema. If the condition does not worsen, this is the only color change until the gingiva reverts to normal. In severe acute inflammation, the red color changes to a shiny slate gray, which gradually becomes a dull whitish gray. The gray discoloration produced by tissue necrosis is demarcated from the adjacent gingiva by a thin, sharply defined erythematous zone. Detailed descriptions of the clinical features and pathology of the various forms of acute gingivitis are found in Chapter 11.

Metallic Pigmentation

Heavy metals absorbed systemically from therapeutic use or occupational environments may discolor the gingiva and other areas of the oral mucosa.[15] This is different from tattooing produced by the accidental embedding of amalgam[4] or other metal fragments (Fig. 9–10). *Bismuth, arsenic,* and *mercury* produce a black line in the gingiva which follows the contour of the margin (Fig. 9–11). The pigmentation may also appear as isolated black blotches involving the marginal, interdental, and attached gingivae. *Lead* results in a bluish-red or deep blue linear pigmentation of the

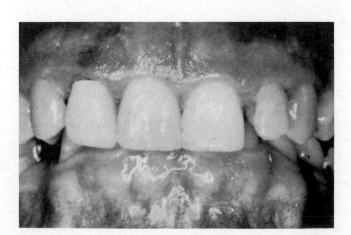

Figure 9–10 **Discoloration of Gingiva** over lateral incisor caused by embedded metal particles.

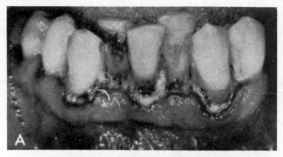

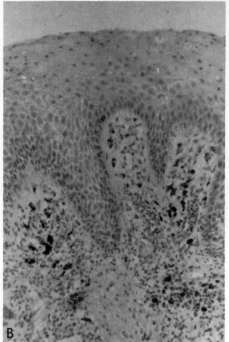

Figure 9–11   Bismuth Line. *A,* Linear discoloration of the gingiva in relation to local irritation in a patient receiving bismuth therapy. *B,* Biopsy specimen showing bismuth particles engulfed by macrophages.

gingival margin (burtonian line)[6] and *silver* (argyria) in a violet marginal line, often accompanied by a diffuse bluish-gray discoloration throughout the oral mucosa.[26]

Gingival pigmentation from systemically absorbed metals results from **perivascular precipitation of metallic sulfides in the subepithelial connective tissue.** Gingival pigmentation is not an effect of systemic toxicity. It occurs only in areas of inflammation, where the increased permeability of irritated blood vessels permits seepage of the metal into the surrounding tissue. In addition to inflamed gingiva, mucosal areas irritated by biting or abnormal chewing habits, such as the inner surface of the lips, the cheek at the level of the occlusal line, and the lateral border of the tongue, are common pigmentation sites.

Gingival or mucosal pigmentation is eliminated by **removing the local irritating factors and restoring tissue health,** without necessarily discontinuing the metal-containing drugs required for therapeutic purposes. *Temporary correction* is obtained by topical application of concentrated peroxide or by insufflating the gingiva with oxygen to oxidize the dark metallic sulfides. The discoloration reappears unless the procedures are repeated.

Color Changes Associated With Systemic Factors

Many systemic diseases may cause color changes in the oral mucosa, including the gingiva.[7] In general, these abnormal pigmentations are nonspecific in nature and should stimulate further diagnostic efforts or referral to the proper specialist.[28]

Endogenous oral pigmentations can be due to melanin, bilirubin, or iron.[26]

Melanin oral pigmentations can be normal physiologic pigmentations which are commonly found in darker races (see Chapter 1), including Caucasian brunettes. Diseases that increase melanin pigmentation include the following: *Addison's disease,* which is caused by adrenal dysfunction and produces isolated patches of discoloration varying from bluish black to brown (Fig. 9–12 and 9–13); *Peutz-Jeghers syndrome,* which produces intestinal polyposis and melanin pigmentation in the oral mucosa and lips; and *Albright's syndrome* (polyostotic fibrous dysplasia) and *von Recklinghausen's disease* (neurofibromatosis), both of which produce areas of oral melanin pigmentation.

Skin and mucous membranes can also be stained by bile pigments. *Jaundice* is best detected by examination of the sclera, but the oral mucosa may also acquire a yellowish color. The deposition of iron in *hemochromatosis* may produce a blue-gray pigmentation of the oral mucosa. Several endocrine and metabolic disturbances may produce color changes: these include diabetes and pregnancy. Blood dyscrasias such as anemia, polycythemia, and leukemia may also induce color changes.

Exogenous factors capable of producing color changes in the gingiva include atmospheric irritants, such as coal and metal dust, and coloring agents in food or lozenges. Tobacco causes a gray hyperkeratosis of the gingiva. Localized bluish-black areas of pigment are commonly due to amalgam implanted in the mucosa (Fig. 9–14).

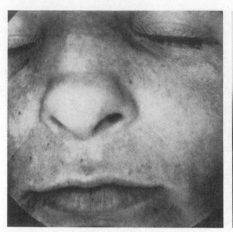

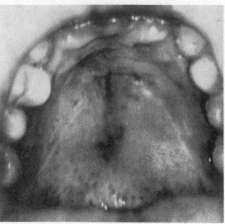

Figure 9–12   **Figure 9–13**

Figure 9–12   Addison's Disease. Diffuse pigmentation of the skin.

Figure 9–13   Addison's Disease. Palate of patient shown in Figure 9–12 with spotty distribution of pigment.

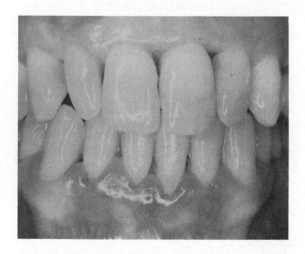

Figure 9–14   Vertical Discoloration of marginal and attached gingivae associated with periodontal pockets.

Figure 9–15   Chronic Gingivitis, showing swelling and discoloration produced when inflammatory exudate and tissue degeneration are the predominant microscopic changes. The gingiva is soft, friable, and bleeds easily. Note the mottled teeth.

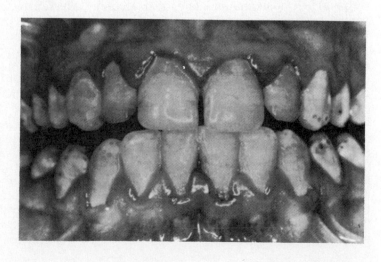

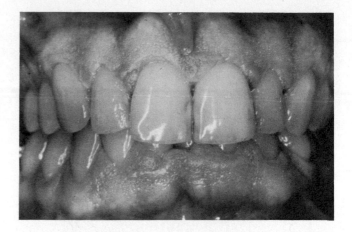

Figure 9–16 Chronic Gingivitis, showing firm gingiva with minutely nodular surface produced when fibrosis predominates in the inflammatory process.

Changes in the Consistency of the Gingiva

Both chronic and acute inflammations produce changes in the normal firm resilient consistency of the gingiva. As noted earlier, chronic gingivitis is a conflict between destructive and reparative changes, with the consistency of the gingiva determined by the relative balance between the two (Figs. 9–15 and 9–16). *The clinical alterations in the consistency of the gingiva and the microscopic changes which produce them are summarized in Table 9–1.*

Calcified Masses in the Gingiva

Calcified microscopic masses are frequently seen in the gingiva.[3] They occur singly or in groups and vary in size, location, shape, and structure. Such masses may be calcified material removed from the tooth and traumatically displaced into the gingiva during scaling,[21] root remnants, cementum fragments, or cementicles (Fig. 9–17). Chronic inflammation and fibrosis and occasionally foreign body giant cell activity occur in relation to these masses. They are sometimes enclosed in an osteoid-

---

TABLE 9–1   CLINICAL AND HISTOPATHOLOGIC CHANGES IN GINGIVAL CONSISTENCY

Chronic Gingivitis	
Clinical Changes	*Underlying Microscopic Features*
1. Soggy puffiness that pits on pressure	1. Infiltration by fluid and cells of the inflammatory exudate
2. Marked softness and friability, with ready fragmentation upon exploration with a probe and pinpoint surface areas of redness and desquamation	2. Degeneration of connective tissue and epithelium associated with injurious substances which provoke the inflammation and the inflammatory exudate. Change in the connective tissue–epithelium relationship, with the inflamed, engorged connective tissue expanding to within a few epithelial cells of the surface. Thinning of the epithelium and degeneration associated with edema and leukocytic invasion, separated by areas in which the rete pegs are elongated into the connective tissue
3. Firm, leathery consistency	3. Fibrosis and epithelial proliferation associated with long-standing chronic inflammation
Acute Gingivitis	
Clinical Changes	*Underlying Microscopic Features*
1. Diffuse puffiness and softening	1. Diffuse edema of acute inflammatory origin; fatty infiltration in xanthomatosis
2. Sloughing with grayish flake-like particles of debris adhering to the eroded surface	2. Necrosis with the formation of a pseudomembrane composed of bacteria, polymorphonuclear leukocytes and degenerated epithelial cells in a fibrinous meshwork
3. Vesicle formation	3. Inter- and intracellular edema with degeneration of the nucleus and cytoplasm and rupture of the cell wall

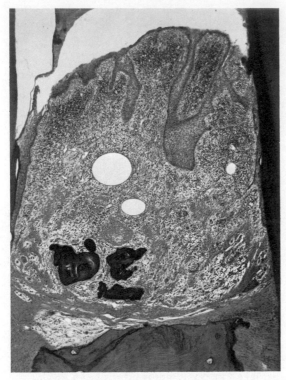

Figure 9–17   Cementicles in the gingiva.

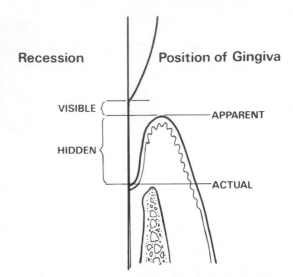

Figure 9–18   Diagram illustrating **Apparent and Actual Position of the Gingiva** and **Visible and Hidden Recession.**

like matrix. Crystalline foreign bodies have also been described in the gingiva, but their origin has not been determined.[25]

Changes in the Surface Texture of the Gingiva

Loss of surface stippling is an early sign of gingivitis. In chronic inflammation the surface is either smooth and shiny or firm and nodular, **depending upon whether the dominant changes are exudative or fibrotic.** Smooth surface texture is also produced by epithelial atrophy in *senile atrophic gingivitis,* and peeling of the surface occurs in *chronic desquamative gingivitis. Hyperkeratosis* results in a leathery texture, and noninflammatory gingival hyperplasia produces a minutely nodular surface.

Changes in the Position of the Gingiva (Recession, Gingival Atrophy)

"Actual" and "Apparent" Positions of the Gingiva

Recession is the *exposure of the root surface by an apical shift in the position of the gingiva.*

To understand what is meant by recession one must distinguish between the "actual" and "apparent" positions of the gingiva. The **actual position** is the level of the epithelial attachment on the tooth (Fig. 9–18), whereas the **apparent position** is the level of the crest of the gingival margin. **It is the actual position of the gingiva, not the apparent position, which determines the severity of recession.** *There are two types of recession: visible, which is clinically observable; and hidden, which is covered by gingiva*

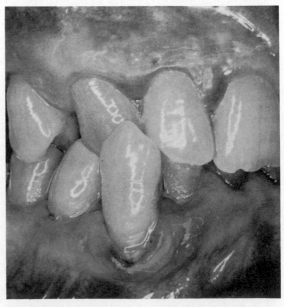

Figure 9–19   Recession on Prominent Canine. Note the severe inflammatory reaction to local irritation.

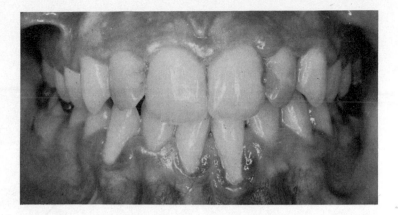

Figure 9–20 **Recession** around malposed anterior teeth. The gingiva is markedly inflamed.

and can only be measured by inserting a probe to the level of epithelial attachment (Fig. 9–18). For example, in periodontal disease part of the denuded root is covered by the inflamed pocket wall; thus, some of the recession is hidden, and some is visible (Fig. 9–18). The total amount of recession is the sum of the two.

Recession refers to the location of the gingiva, not its condition. Receded gingiva is often inflamed (Figs. 9–19 and 9–20) but may be normal except for its position (Fig. 9–21). Recession may be localized to a tooth (Fig. 9–22) or group of teeth or generalized through the mouth (Fig. 9–23).

Etiology of Recession

Gingival recession increases with age; the incidence varies from 8 per cent in children to 100 per cent after the age of 50.[36] This has led some authors to assume that recession may be a physiologic process related to aging. Convincing evidence for a physiologic shift of the gingival attachment has never been pre-

sented.[14] The gradual apical shift is most probably the result of the cumulative effect of minor pathologic involvement and/or repeated minor direct trauma to the gingiva.

The following factors have been implicated in the etiology of gingival recession: faulty toothbrushing (gingival abrasion), tooth malposition, friction from soft tissues (gingival ablation),[30] gingival inflammation, and high frenum attachment. Trauma from occlusion has also been suggested, but its mechanism of action has never been demonstrated. Orthodontic movement in a labial direction has been shown in monkeys to result in loss of marginal bone and connective tissue attachment, as well as in gingival recession.[32]

Although toothbrushing is important for gingival health, **faulty toothbrushing may cause gingival recession.** Recession tends to be more frequent and severe in patients with comparatively healthy gingiva, little bacterial plaque, and good oral hygiene.[8, 23, 24]

Susceptibility to recession is influenced by the position of teeth in the arch,[35] the angle of the root in the bone, and the mesiodistal

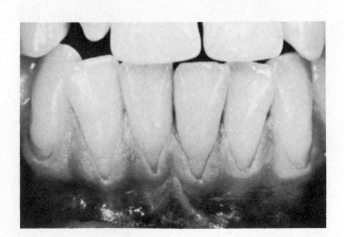

Figure 9–21 **Recession** on malposed teeth. Note excellent condition of the gingiva.

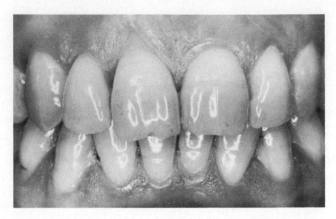

Figure 9–22 Localized Recession on maxillary central incisor associated with aggressive toothbrushing.

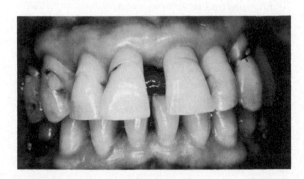

Figure 9–23 Generalized Recession resulting from chronic periodontal disease.

Figure 9–24 Accentuated Recession on a maxillary first molar aggravated by the angulation of the prominent palatal root in the bone.

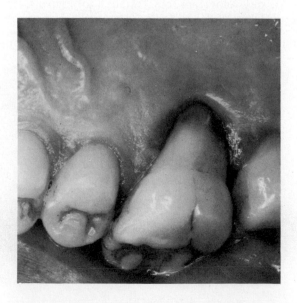

curvature of the tooth surface.[20] On rotated, tilted, or facially displaced teeth, the bony plate is thinned or reduced in height. Pressure from mastication or moderate toothbrushing wears away the unsupported gingiva and produces recession. The effect of the angle of the root in the bone upon recession is often observed in the maxillary molar area (Fig. 9–24). If the lingual inclination of the palatal root is prominent or the buccal roots flare outward, the bone in the cervical area is thinned or shortened and recession results from wear of the unsupported marginal gingiva (Fig. 9–25). On maxillary molars with flared roots, recession is aggravated by occlusal wear. Occlusal wear is accompanied by eruption of the tooth and accentuation of its normal buccal inclination. This increases the angulation of the lingual root in the palate, reduces the bone level, and furthers recession by lessening the gingival support (Fig. 9–25).

The effect of cheek and lip muscle action on the gingival tissue may also lead to gingival recession. Sognnaes has described this effect on artificial dentures and on natural dentitions and has coined the term "dento-alveolar ablation" to describe it.[30]

The role of inflammation in the production of gingival recession in rats has been investigated by Baker and Seymour.[2] They suggest that gingival recession involves a localized inflammatory process which causes the breakdown of connective tissue and proliferation of the epithelium into the site of connective tissue destruction. Proliferation of epithelial cells into the connective tissue brings about a subsidence of the epithelial surface which is manifested clinically as recession.[2]

Clinical Significance

Several aspects of gingival recession make it clinically significant. Exposed root surfaces are susceptible to caries. Wearing away of the cementum exposed by recession leaves an underlying dentinal surface that is extremely sensitive, particularly to the touch. Hyperemia of the pulp and associated symptoms may also result from exposure of the root surface.[18] Interproximal recession creates spaces in which plaque, food, and bacteria accumulate.

Changes in Gingival Contour

Changes in gingival contour are for the most part associated with gingival enlargement (see

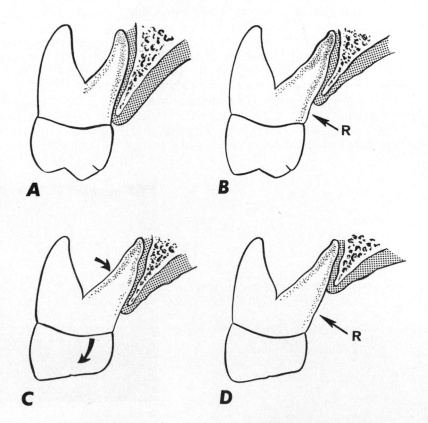

Figure 9–25 Prominent Palatal Root and Occlusal Wear Aggravating Gingival Recession. *A,* Maxillary first molar with gingiva close to the cervical line. *B,* Maxillary molar with prominent palatal root. The altered root–bone angle results in shortened bone support and gingival recession (R). *C,* Occlusal wear is accompanied by tooth eruption with increase in the normal occlusofacial inclination of the tooth *(lower* arrow) and worsening of the palatal root–bone angle *(upper arrow). D,* Altered palatal root–bone angle following occlusal wear lessens bone support and aggravates gingival recession (R).

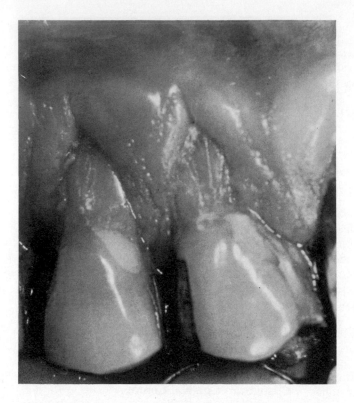

Figure 9–26 **Stillman's Clefts** in the gingiva.

Chapter 10), but such changes may also occur in other conditions.

STILLMAN'S CLEFTS. Stillman's clefts are apostrophe-shaped indentations extending from and into the gingival margin for varying distances. The clefts generally occur on the facial surface (Fig. 9–26). One or two may be present in relation to a single tooth. The margins of the clefts are rolled underneath the linear gap in the gingiva, and the remainder of the gingival margin is blunt instead of knife-edged. Originally described by Stillman[33] and considered to be the result of occlusal trauma,

these clefts were subsequently described by Box[3] as pathologic pockets in which the ulcerative process had extended through to the facial surface of the gingiva. The clefts may repair spontaneously or persist as surface lesions of deep periodontal pockets that penetrate into the supporting tissues. Their association with trauma from occlusion has not been substantiated.

The clefts are divided into: *simple,* cleavage in a single direction (most common); and *compound,* cleavage in more than one direction (Tishler[34]). The length of the clefts varies from

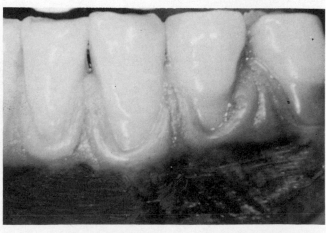

Figure 9–27 **McCall's Festoons** showing characteristic rim-like enlargement of the gingival margin.

a slight break in the gingival margin to a depth of 5 to 6 mm or more.

McCall's Festoons. McCall's festoons are life saver–shaped enlargements of the marginal gingiva that occur most frequently in the canine and premolar areas on the facial surface. In the early stages, the color and consistency of the gingiva are normal. Accumulation of food debris leads to secondary inflammatory changes (Fig. 9–27). Trauma from occlusion and mechanical stimulation are suggested etiologic factors. However, festoons occur on teeth without occlusal antagonists.

REFERENCES

1. Ainamo, J., and Bay, I.: Problems and proposals for recording gingivitis and plaque. Int. Dent. J., *25*:229, 1975.
2. Baker, D. L., and Seymour, G. J.: The possible pathogenesis of gingival recession. J. Clin. Periodontol., *3*:208, 1976.
3. Box, H. K.: Gingival clefts and associated tracts. N.Y. State Dent. J., *16*:3, 1950.
4. Buchner, A., and Hansen, L. A.: Amalgam pigmentation (amalgam tattoo) of the oral mucosa. A clinicopathologic study of 268 cases. Oral Surg., *49*:139, 1980.
5. Carter, H. G., and Barnes, G. P.: The gingival bleeding index. J. Periodontol., *45*:801, 1974.
6. Dummett, C. O.: Abnormal color changes in gingivae. Oral Surg., *2*:649, 1949.
7. Dummett, C. O.: Oral tissue color changes. Ala. J. Med. Sci., *16*:274, 1979.
8. Gorman, N. J.: Prevalence and etiology of gingival recession. J. Periodontol., *38*:316, 1967.
9. Haeb, H. P.: Post-rubella thrombocytopenic purpura. A report of cases with discussion of hemorrhagic manifestations of rubella. Clin. Pediatr. (Phila.), *7*:350, 1968.
10. Hirschfeld, I.: A study of skulls in the American Museum of Natural History in relation to periodontal disease. J. Dent. Res., *5*:241, 1923.
11. Hoover, D. R., and Lefkowitz, W.: Fluctuation in marginal gingivitis. J. Periodontol., *36*:310, 1965.
12. Larato, D., et al.: The effect of a prescribed method of toothbrushing on the fluctuation of marginal gingivitis. J. Periodontol., *40*:142, 1969.
13. Lenox, J. A., and Kopczyk, R. A.: A clinical system for scoring a patient's oral hygiene performance. J. Am. Dent. Assoc., *86*:849, 1973.
14. Löe, H.: The structure and physiology of the dentogingival junction. *In* Miles, A. E. (ed.): Structural and Chemical Organization of Teeth. Vol. 2. New York, Academic Press, 1967.
15. McCarthy, F. P., and Dexter, S. O., Jr.: Oral manifestations of bismuth. N. Engl. J. Med., *213*:345, 1935.
16. Meitner, S. W., et al.: Identification of inflamed gingival surfaces. J. Clin. Periodontol., *6*:93, 1979.
17. Merril, A., et al.: Gingival hemorrhage secondary to uremia. Review and report of a case. Oral Sug., *29*:530, 1970.
18. Merritt, A. A.: Hyperemia of the dental pulp caused by gingival recession. J. Periodontol., *4*:30, 1933.
19. Milne, A. M.: Gingival bleeding in 848 army recruits. An assessment. Br. Dent. J., *122*:111, 1967.
20. Morris, M. L.: The position of the margin of the gingiva. Oral Surg., *11*:969, 1958.
21. Moskow, B. S.: Calcified material in human gingival tissues. J. Dent. Res., *40*:644, 1961.
22. Mühlemann, H. R., and Son, S.: Gingival sulcus bleeding, a leading symptom in initial gingivitis. Helv. Odontol. Acta, *15*:107, 1971.
23. O'Leary, T. J., Drake, R. V., Crump, P., and Allen, N. F.: The incidence of recession in young males—a further study. J. Periodontol., *42*:264, 1971.
24. O'Leary, T. J., Drake, R. V., Jividen, G. J., and Allen, N. F.: The incidence of recession in young males: relationship to gingival and plaque scores. U.S.A.F. School Aerosp. Med., SAM-TR-67–97:1, November, 1967.
25. Orban, B.: Gingival inclusions. J. Periodontol., *16*:16, 1945.
26. Prinz, H.: Pigmentations of oral mucous membrane. Dent. Cosmos, *74*:554, 1932.
27. Ringsdorf, W., Cheraskin, E., and Clark, J.: Gingival bleeding and general health. Dent. Survey, *44*:49, 1968.
28. Shklar, G., and McCarthy, P. L.: The Oral Manifestations of Systemic Disease. Boston, Butterworth, 1976.
29. Sodeman, W. A., Jr. and Sodeman, W. A.: Pathologic Physiology: Mechanisms of Disease. 6th ed. Philadelphia, W. B. Saunders Company, 1979.
30. Sognnaes, R. F.: Periodontal significance of intra-oral frictional ablation. J. Western Soc. Periodontol., *25*:112, 1977.
31. Stefanini, M., and Dameshek, W.: The Hemorrhagic Disorders. 2nd ed. New York, Grune & Stratton, 1962, p. 78.
32. Steiner, G. G., Person, J. K., and Ainamo, J.: Changes of the marginal periodontium as a result of labial tooth movement in monkeys. J. Periodontol., *52*:314, 1981.
33. Stillman, P. R.: Early clinical evidence of disease in the gingiva and the pericementum. J. Dent. Res., *3*:25, 1921.
34. Tishler, B.: Gingival clefts and their significance. Dent. Cosmos, *49*:1003, 1927.
35. Trott, J. R., and Love, B.: An analysis of localized gingival recession in 766 Winnipeg high school students. Dent. Pract. (Bristol), *16*:209, 1966.
36. Woofter, C.: The prevalence and etiology of gingival recession. Periodont. Abstracts, *17*:45, 1969.

Gingival Enlargement

Gingival enlargement, increase in size, is a common feature of gingival disease. There are many types of gingival enlargement which vary according to the etiologic factors and pathologic processes that produce them.[31]

The term *hypertrophic gingivitis* is not appropriate for pathologic increases in the size of the gingiva. Hypertrophy means an increase in the size of cells resulting in an increase in the size of the organ. This is not what happens in gingival enlargement.

CLASSIFICATION OF GINGIVAL ENLARGEMENT

Gingival enlargement is classified according to etiology and pathology as follows:

I. Inflammatory enlargement
  A. Chronic inflammatory enlargement
    1. Localized or generalized
    2. Discrete (tumor-like)
  B. Acute inflammatory enlargement
    1. Gingival abscess
    2. Periodontal (lateral) abscess
II. Noninflammatory hyperplastic enlargement (gingival hyperplasia)
  A. Gingival hyperplasia associated with phenytoin therapy
  B. Familial, hereditary, or idiopathic hyperplastic enlargement
III. Combined enlargement
IV. Conditioned enlargement
  A. Hormonal enlargement
    1. Enlargement in pregnancy
    2. Enlargement in puberty
  B. Leukemic enlargement
  C. Enlargement associated with vitamin C deficiency
  D. Nonspecific conditioned enlargement (granuloma pyogenicum)
V. Neoplastic enlargement (gingival tumors)
  A. Benign tumors of the gingiva
  B. Malignant tumors of the gingiva
VI. Developmental enlargement

Location and Distribution

Using the criteria of location and distribution, gingival enlargement is designated as follows:

Localized: Limited to the gingiva adjacent to a single tooth or group of teeth.

Generalized: Involving the gingiva throughout the mouth.

Marginal: Confined to the marginal gingiva.

Papillary: Confined to the interdental papilla.

Diffuse: Involving the marginal and attached gingivae and papillae.

Discrete: An isolated sessile or pedunculated "tumor-like" enlargement.

I. INFLAMMATORY ENLARGEMENT

Gingival enlargement may result from chronic or acute inflammatory changes. The former is by far the more common cause.

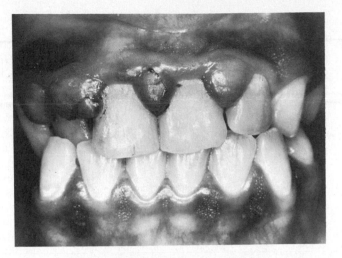

Figure 10–1 **Chronic Inflammatory Gingival Enlargement** localized to the anterior region, associated with irregularity of teeth.

Chronic Inflammatory Enlargement

Localized or Generalized

Chronic inflammatory gingival enlargement originates as a slight ballooning of the interdental papilla, marginal gingiva, or both. In the early stages it produces a life saver–like bulge around the involved teeth. This bulge increases in size until it covers part of the crowns. The enlargement is generally papillary or marginal and may be localized (Fig. 10–1) or generalized (Fig. 10–2). It progresses slowly and painlessly unless it is complicated by acute infection or trauma.

Discrete (Tumor-Like)

Occasionally, chronic inflammatory gingival enlargement occurs as a discrete sessile or pedunculated mass resembling a tumor. It may be interproximal or on the marginal or attached gingiva (Fig. 10–3). The lesions are slow growing and usually painless. They may undergo spontaneous reduction in size, followed by reappearance and continued enlargement. Painful ulceration in the fold between the mass and the adjacent gingiva sometimes occurs.

HISTOPATHOLOGY. The following features produce chronic inflammatory gingival enlargement (Figs. 10–4 and 10–5): inflammatory fluid and cellular exudate, degeneration of epithelium and connective tissue, new capillary formation, vascular engorgement, hemorrhage, proliferation of epithelium and connective tissue, and new collagen fibers.

The microscopic components determine clinical features of the enlargement such as color, consistency, and texture. Lesions that consist of a preponderance of inflammatory cells and fluid with associated degenerative changes are deep red or bluish red, soft, and friable, with a smooth, shiny surface; they bleed easily. Lesions that are predominantly fibrotic, with an abundance of fibroblasts and collagen bundles, are relatively firm, resilient, and pink.

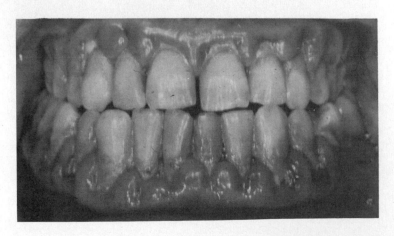

Figure 10–2 **Generalized Chronic Inflammatory Gingival Enlargement.**

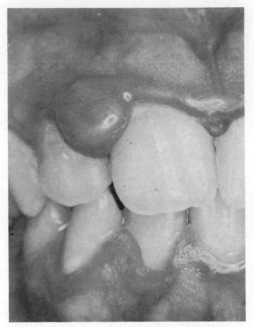

Figure 10–3   Discrete Tumor-like Gingival Enlargement.

ETIOLOGY. Chronic inflammatory gingival enlargement is caused by prolonged local irritation. The following are typical etiologic factors:[40] poor oral hygiene (Fig. 10–6), abnormal relationships of adjacent teeth (Fig. 10–7) and opposing teeth, lack of tooth function, cervical cavities (Fig. 10–8), overhanging margins of dental restorations, improperly contoured dental restorations or pontics, food impaction (Fig. 10–9), irritation from clasps or saddle areas of removable prostheses, mouth breath-ing, nasal obstruction, repositioning of teeth by orthodontic therapy, and habitual pressing of the tongue against the gingiva.

Gingival Changes Associated with Mouth Breathing. Gingivitis and gingival enlargement are often seen in mouth breathers.[56] The gingiva appears red and edematous, with a diffuse surface shininess of the exposed area. The maxillary anterior region is the common site of such involvement. In many cases the altered gingiva is clearly demarcated from the adjacent unexposed normal gingiva (Fig. 10–10). The exact manner in which mouth breathing affects gingival changes has not been demonstrated. Its harmful effect is generally attributed to irritation from surface dehydration. However, comparable changes could not be produced by "air drying" the gingiva of experimental animals.[53]

Acute Inflammatory Enlargement

Gingival Abscess

A gingival abscess is a localized, painful, rapidly expanding lesion that is usually of sudden onset. It is generally limited to the marginal gingiva or interdental papilla (Fig. 10–11). In its early stages it appears as a red swelling with a smooth, shiny surface. Within 24 to 48 hours, the lesion is usually fluctuant and pointed, with a surface orifice from which a purulent exudate may be expressed. The adjacent teeth are often sensitive to percussion. If permitted to progress, the lesion generally ruptures spontaneously.

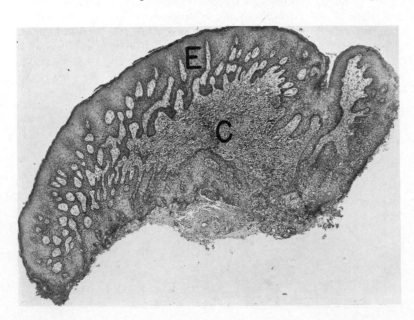

Figure 10–4 Survey Section of Chronic Inflammatory Gingival Enlargement showing the central connective tissue core (C) and thickened epithelium at the periphery (E). Note the ulceration of the epithelial surface at the lower border of the mass that was adjacent to the tooth surface.

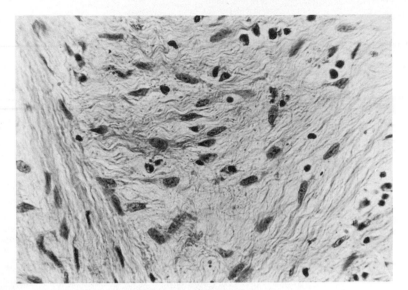

Figure 10–5 High-Power Study Showing Young Fibroblasts and collagen fibrils that contribute to the increase in size in chronic inflammatory gingival enlargement.

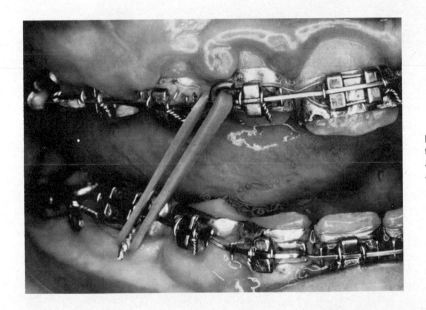

Figure 10–6 Chronic Inflammatory Gingival Enlargement associated with plaque accumulation around orthodontic appliance.

Figure 10–7 Chronic Inflammatory Gingival Enlargement Associated with Irregularity in Tooth Alignment. The difference in the color intensity of the enlarged gingiva and the adjacent comparatively uninvolved attached gingiva is shown in the mandible.

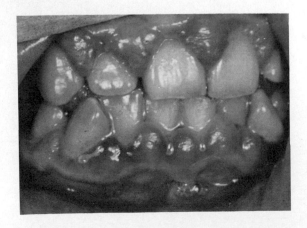

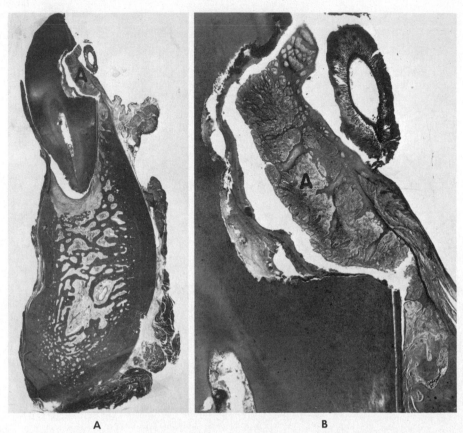

A   B

Figure 10–8   *A,* Survey section of mandibular canine in situ with cervical carious lesion (A). *B,* Detail of Figure 10–8*A* showing a **Chronic Inflammatory Enlargement** of the gingiva (A) in the carious lesion. Note the continuity between the enlarged mass and the facial gingiva at the lower right.

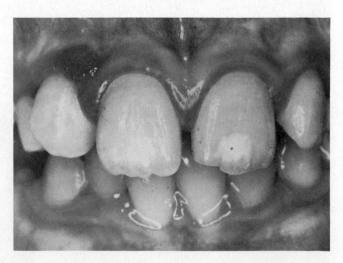

Figure 10–9 Chronic Inflammatory Enlargement Associated with Impaction and Retention of Food in Relation to Malposed Lateral Incisor. Note the extreme vascularity of the lesion.

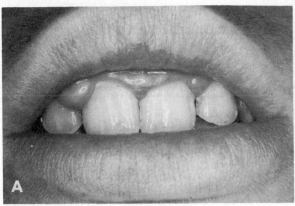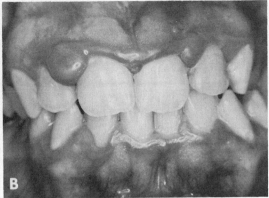

Figure 10–10   Gingivitis in Mouth Breather. *A,* High lip line in mouth breather. *B,* Gingivitis and inflammatory gingival enlargement in exposed area of gingiva.

HISTOPATHOLOGY. The gingival abscess consists of a purulent focus in the connective tissue surrounded by a diffuse infiltration of polymorphonuclear leukocytes, edematous tissue, and vascular engorgement. The surface epithelium presents varying degrees of intra- and extracellular edema, invasion by leukocytes, and ulceration.

ETIOLOGY. Acute inflammatory gingival enlargement is a response to irritation from foreign substances such as a toothbrush bristle, a piece of apple core, or lobster shell fragment forcefully embedded into the gingiva. The lesion is confined to the gingiva and should not be confused with periodontal or lateral abscesses.

Periodontal (Lateral) Abscess

Periodontal abscesses generally produce enlargement of the gingiva, but they also involve the supporting periodontal tissues. For a detailed description of periodontal abscesses, see Chapter 18.

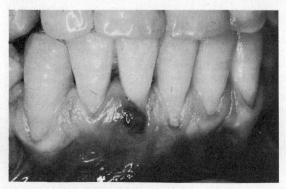

Figure 10–11   Acute Gingival Abscess.

II. NONINFLAMMATORY HYPERPLASTIC ENLARGEMENT (GINGIVAL HYPERPLASIA)

The term hyperplasia refers to an increase in the size of tissue or an organ produced by an increase in the number of its component cells. Noninflammatory gingival hyperplasia is produced by factors other than local irritation. It is not common and occurs most often in association with phenytoin therapy.

Gingival Hyperplasia Associated with Phenytoin Therapy

Enlargement of the gingiva caused by phenytoin,* an anticonvulsant used in the treatment of epilepsy, occurs in some of the patients receiving the drug. Its reported incidence varies from 3 to 84.5 per cent,[3, 32, 66] with the greater frequencies in younger patients.[4] Its occurrence and severity are not necessarily related to the dosage, concentration of phenytoin in serum or saliva, or duration of drug therapy, although some reports indicate a definite relation between dosage of the drug and degree of gingival hyperplasia.[46, 52]

CLINICAL FEATURES. The primary or basic lesion starts as a painless, bead-like enlargement of the facial and lingual gingival margin and interdental papillae (Figs. 10–12 to 10–14). As the condition progresses, the marginal and papillary enlargements unite; they may develop into a massive tissue fold covering a considerable portion of the crowns, and they may interfere with occlusion (Fig. 10–15). When uncomplicated by inflammation, the le-

---

*Commonly known in the United States by its trade name, Dilantin; in other countries, Epanutin.

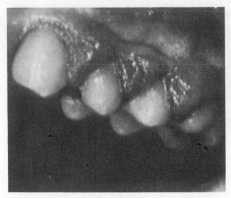

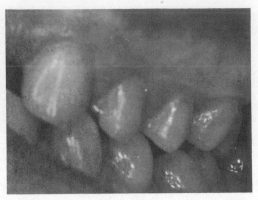

Figure 10–12   **Figure 10–13**

Figure 10–12   Gingival Enlargement Associated with Phenytoin Therapy. Note the minutely lobulated surface of the enlarged gingiva.

Figure 10–13   Same patient as in Figure 10–12 showing disappearance of the gingival enlargement 1 month after the cessation of the phenytoin therapy.

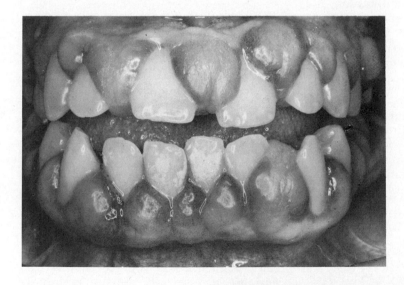

Figure 10–14 Gingival Enlargement Associated with Phenytoin Therapy. Note the prominent papillary lesions. The gingiva is firm and nodular. There is marginal inflammation along the crevices deepened by the gingival overgrowth.

Figure 10–15 Massive Hyperplasia Associated with Phenytoin Therapy. The teeth are completely covered. The gingiva is firm and dense with a nodular surface.

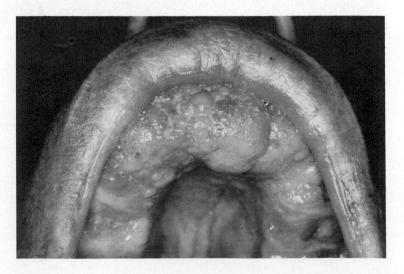

sion is mulberry-shaped, firm, pale pink, and resilient, with a minutely lobulated surface and no tendency to bleed. The enlargement characteristically appears to project from beneath the gingival margin, from which it is separated by a linear groove.

Phenytoin-induced hyperplasia may occur in mouths devoid of local irritants and may be absent in mouths in which local irritants are profuse.

The hyperplasia is usually generalized throughout the mouth but is more severe in the maxillary and mandibular anterior regions. It occurs in areas in which teeth are present—not in edentulous spaces—and the enlargement disappears in areas from which teeth are extracted. Hyperplasia of the mucosa in edentulous mouths has been reported, but it is rare.[23, 24]

The enlargement is chronic and slowly in-

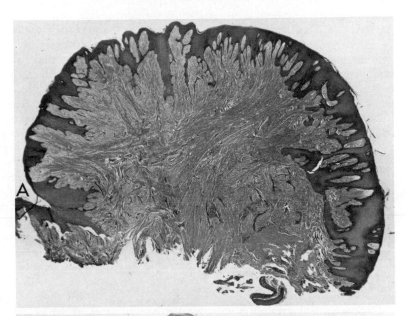

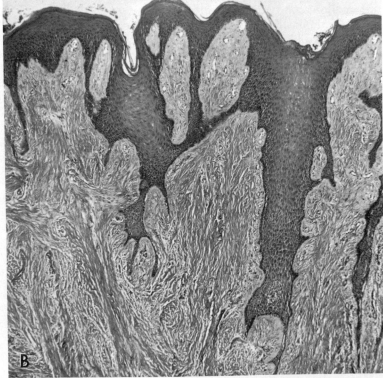

Figure 10–16 Gingival Enlargement Associated with Phenytoin Therapy. *A,* Survey section, showing bulbous gingival enlargement. *B,* Detailed view, showing hyperplasia and acanthosis of the epithelium with extension of deep rete pegs into the connective tissue. The connective tissue is densely collagenous. There is little evidence of inflammation.

creases in size until it interferes with occlusion or becomes unsightly. When surgically removed, it recurs. Spontaneous disappearance occurs within a few months after the drug is discontinued.

Local irritants (e.g., materia alba, calculus, overhanging margins of restorations, and food impaction) favor plaque accumulation, thereby causing inflammation which often complicates gingival hyperplasia caused by the drug. *It is important to distinguish between the increase in size caused by the phenytoin-induced hyperplasia and the complicating inflammation caused by local irritation.* Secondary inflammatory changes add to the size of the lesion caused by phenytoin, produce red or bluish-red discoloration, obliterate the lobulated surface demarcations, and create an increased tendency toward bleeding.

HISTOPATHOLOGY. The enlargement presents pronounced hyperplasia of the connective tissue and epithelium (Fig. 10–16). There is acanthosis of the epithelium, and elongated rete pegs extend deep into the connective tissue, which presents densely arranged collagen bundles with an increase in fibroblasts and new blood vessels. Oxytalan fibers are numerous beneath the epithelium and in areas of inflammation.[7] Inflammation is common along the sulcular surfaces of the gingiva.

Recurrent enlargements appear as granulation tissue composed of numerous young capillaries and fibroblasts and irregularly arranged collagen fibrils with occasional lymphocytes (Figs. 10–17 and 10–18).

NATURE OF THE LESION. The enlargement is basically a hyperplastic reaction initiated by the drug, with inflammation a secondary complicating factor. Some feel that inflammation is a prerequisite for development of the hyperplasia and that it can be prevented by the removal of local irritants and fastidious oral hygiene.[35, 54, 65] Others find that oral hygiene by means of toothbrushing[25] or the use of a chlorhexidine toothpaste[72] reduces the inflammation but does not lessen the hyperplasia or prevent it.[25]

Except in one study,[41] tissue-culture experiments indicate that phenytoin stimulates proliferation of fibroblast-like cells[76] and epithelium.[63] Two analogues of Dilantin (1-allyl,5-phenylhydantoinate and 5-methyl,5-phenylhydantoinate) have a similar effect on fibroblast-like cells.[75] Stimulation by phenytoin is inhibited in irradiated cells.[77]

Experimental attempts to induce phenytoin enlargement in laboratory animals have been successful only in the cat,[44] the ferret, and the *Macaca speciosa* monkey.[82] In experimental animals, phenytoin causes gingival enlargement independent of local inflammation. **It starts as hyperplasia of the connective tissue core of the marginal gingiva, which is followed by proliferation of the epithelium.[44] The enlargement increases by proliferation and expansion of the central core beyond the crest of the gingival margin.**

In cats, one of the metabolic products of phenytoin is 5-(parahydroxyphenyl)-5-phenylhydantoin; administration of this metabolite to cats also induces gingival enlargement in some cases.[38] This has led Hassell and Page to hypothesize that gingival hyperplasia may result from the genetically determined ability or inability of the host to deal effectively with prolonged administration of phenytoin.[38]

Phenytoin occurs in the saliva. There is no consensus, however, on whether the severity of the hyperplasia is related to the levels of phenytoin in plasma or saliva.[3, 5, 92]

Systemic administration of phenytoin accelerates the healing of gingival wounds in nonepileptic humans[79] and increases the tensile strength of healing abdominal wounds in rats.[78] The administration of phenytoin may precipi-

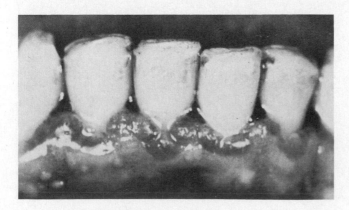

Figure 10–17 Early Recurrence following surgical removal of enlarged gingiva in patient receiving phenytoin therapy.

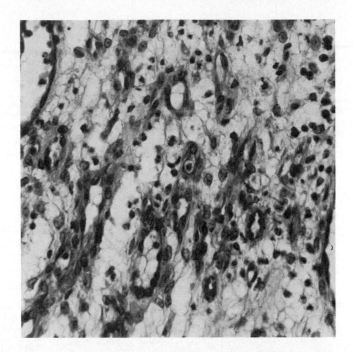

Figure 10–18 Biopsy Specimen of Recurrent Gingival Enlargement shown in Figure 10–17. Note the abundance of new blood vessels.

tate a megaloblastic anemia[58] and a folic acid deficiency.[84] For further information on this topic the reader is referred to the excellent monograph by Hassell.[37]

Recently, a gingival enlargement induced by cyclosporin-A, an immunosuppressive drug used for kidney transplant patients, has been described.[69a]

Familial, Hereditary, or Idiopathic Hyperplastic Enlargement

This is a rare condition of undetermined etiology which has been designated by such terms as gingivomatosis elephantiasis,[6, 48] diffuse fibroma,[18] familial elephantiasis, idiopathic fibromatosis,[94] hereditary or idiopathic hyperplasia,[71, 89] hereditary gingival fibromatosis,[93] and congenital familial fibromatosis.

CLINICAL FEATURES. The enlargement affects the attached gingiva as well as the gingival margin and interdental papillae, in contrast with phenytoin-induced hyperplasia, which is often limited to the gingival margin and interdental papillae. The facial and lingual surfaces of the mandible and maxilla are generally affected, but the involvement may be limited to either jaw. The enlarged gingiva is pink, firm, almost leathery in consistency, and presents a characteristic minutely "pebbled" surface (Fig. 10–19). In severe cases the teeth are almost completely covered and the enlargement projects into the oral vestibule. The jaws appear distorted because of the bulbous enlargement of the gingiva. Secondary inflammatory changes are common at the gingival margin.

HISTOPATHOLOGY. There is a bulbous increase in the amount of connective tissue (Fig.

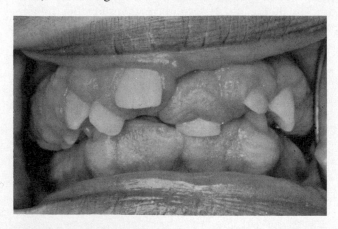

Figure 10–19   Idiopathic Hyperplastic Gingival Enlargement. The gingiva is firm with a nodular pebbled surface. The hyperplastic gingiva deflects the erupting teeth from proper alignment. (From Ball, E. I.: J. Periodontol., *12*:96, 1941.)

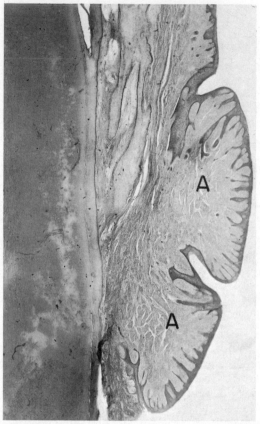

Figure 10–20 Nodular Noninflammatory Hyperplastic Gingival Enlargement (A) involving the attached gingiva.

10–20) that is relatively avascular and consists of densely arranged collagen bundles and numerous fibroblasts. The surface epithelium is thickened and acanthotic, with elongated rete pegs.

ETIOLOGY. Some cases have been explained on a hereditary basis,[26, 93-95] but the etiology is unknown, and the hyperplasia is appropriately designated as *idiopathic*. The genetic mechanisms involved are not well understood. A study of several families has found the mode of inheritance to be autosomal recessive in some cases and autosomal dominant in others.[47, 69] In some families the gingival hyperplasia may be linked with retardation of physical development.[51] The enlargement usually begins with the eruption of the primary or secondary dentition and may regress after extraction, suggesting the possibility that the teeth (or the plaque attached to them) may be initiating factors. Nutritional and hormonal etiologies have been explored but have not been substantiated.[64] Local irritation is a complicating factor. Gingival hyperplasia has been described in tuberous sclerosis, which is an inherited condition characterized by a triad of

epilepsy, mental deficiency, and cutaneous angiofibromas.[85]

Diffuse gingival hyperplasia should be differentiated from the bulbous distortion in the contour of the jaws associated with marked malocclusion. In the latter condition, the gingiva may be essentially unaltered or may present chronic inflammation of the gingival margin in relation to the malposed teeth (Figs. 10–21 and 10–22). The combination of inflamed marginal gingiva and unaltered attached gingiva on the deformed bone creates the erroneous impression of diffuse gingival enlargement. The dense fibrous consistency and accentuated stippling seen in diffuse hyperplastic enlargement are absent.

III. COMBINED ENLARGEMENT

This condition results when gingival hyperplasia is complicated by secondary inflammatory changes. The development of the combined type of gingival enlargement is depicted in Figure 10–23. Gingival hyperplasia creates conditions favorable for the accumulation of plaque and materia alba by accentuating the depth of the gingival sulcus, by interfering with effective hygienic measures, and by deflecting the normal excursive pathways of food. The secondary inflammatory changes (Fig. 10–23*B*) increase the size of the pre-existing gingival hyperplasia (Fig. 10–23*A*) and produce combined gingival enlargement (Fig. 10–23*C*). In many instances, secondary inflammation obscures the features of the pre-existent noninflammatory hyperplasia to the extent that the entire lesion appears to be inflammatory (Fig. 10–24).

It is essential that the nature of combined gingival enlargement be understood. It consists of two components: **a primary or basic hyperplasia of connective tissue and epithelium— the origin of which is unrelated to inflammation—and a secondary complicating inflammatory component.** The removal of local irritation eliminates the secondary inflammatory component and reduces the size of the lesion proportionately, but the noninflammatory hyperplasia remains (see Fig. 10–23*A*). Elimination of the noninflammatory hyperplasia requires correction of the causative factors.

IV. CONDITIONED ENLARGEMENT

This type of enlargement occurs when the systemic condition of the patient is such as to

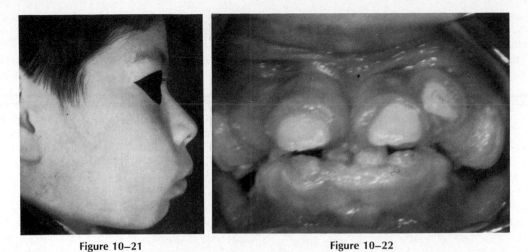

Figure 10–21   **Figure 10–22**

Figure 10–21 Prominent contour of the mouth in a patient with malocclusion.
Figure 10–22 Bulbous distortion of the maxilla and mandible in patient shown in Figure 10–21, aggravated by chronic inflammatory gingival enlargement.

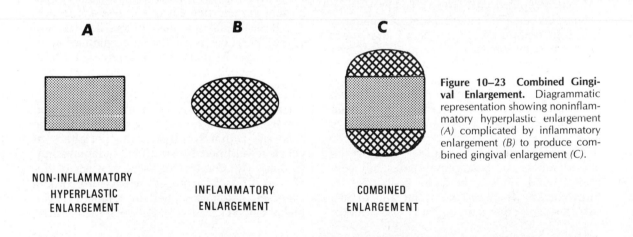

A **B** **C**

NON-INFLAMMATORY
HYPERPLASTIC
ENLARGEMENT

INFLAMMATORY
ENLARGEMENT

COMBINED
ENLARGEMENT

Figure 10–23 Combined Gingival Enlargement. Diagrammatic representation showing noninflammatory hyperplastic enlargement *(A)* complicated by inflammatory enlargement *(B)* to produce combined gingival enlargement *(C)*.

Figure 10–24 Combined Gingival Enlargement in a patient receiving phenytoin therapy. The basic hyperplasia is complicated by secondary inflammatory involvement. Note the edema and discoloration produced by the inflammation.

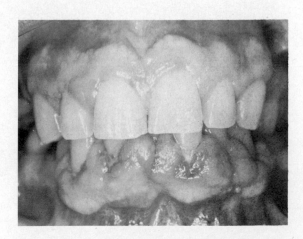

exaggerate or distort the usual gingival response to local irritation and produces a corresponding modification of the usual clinical features of chronic gingivitis. The specific manner in which the clinical picture of conditioned gingival enlargement differs from chronic gingivitis depends upon the nature of the modifying systemic influence. *Local irritation is necessary for the initiation of this type of enlargement.* The irritation does not, however, solely determine the nature of the clinical features.

There are three types of conditioned gingival enlargement: hormonal, leukemic, and that associated with vitamin C deficiency.

Hormonal Enlargement

Enlargement in Pregnancy

In pregnancy, gingival enlargement may be marginal and generalized or occur as single or multiple tumor-like masses.

MARGINAL ENLARGEMENT. The prevalence of marginal gingival enlargement in pregnancy has been reported as 10 per cent[19] and 70 per cent.[95] It results from the aggravation of previously inflamed areas. However, the gingival enlargement does not occur without clinical evidence of local irritation. *Pregnancy does not cause the condition; the altered tissue metabolism in pregnancy accentuates the response to local irritants.*[42]

Clinical Features. The clinical picture varies considerably. The enlargement is usually generalized and tends to be more prominent interproximally than on the facial and lingual surfaces. The enlarged gingiva is bright red or magenta, soft, and friable and has a smooth, shiny surface. Bleeding occurs spontaneously or upon slight provocation.[74]

TUMOR-LIKE GINGIVAL ENLARGEMENT. *The so-called pregnancy tumor is not a neoplasm; it is an inflammatory response to local irritation* and is modified by the patient's condition. It usually appears after the third month of pregnancy, but may occur earlier,[55] and has a reported incidence of 1.8 to 5 per cent.[59]

Clinical Features. The lesion appears as a discrete, mushroom-like, flattened spherical mass protruding from the gingival margin or, more frequently, from the interproximal space, attached by a sessile or pedunculated base (Figs. 10–25 and 10–26). It tends to expand laterally, and pressure from the tongue and cheek perpetuates its flattened appearance. Generally dusky red or magenta, it has a smooth, glistening surface that frequently presents numerous deep-red pinpoint markings. It is a superficial lesion and ordinarily does not invade the underlying bone. The consistency varies; the mass is usually semifirm, but it may present varying degrees of softness and friability. It is usually painless unless its size and shape are such as to foster accumulation of debris under its margin or interfere with occlusion, in which cases painful ulceration may occur.

HISTOPATHOLOGY. Both the marginal and tumor-like enlargements consist of a central mass of connective tissue, the periphery of which is outlined by stratified squamous epithelium. The connective tissue consists of numerous diffusely arranged, newly formed, and engorged capillaries lined by cuboidal endothelial cells (Fig. 10–27). Between the capillar-

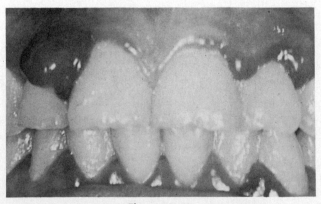

Figure 10–25

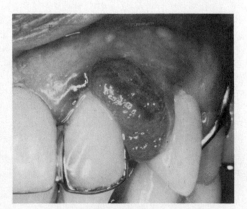

Figure 10–26

Figure 10–25   **Conditioned Gingival Enlargement** in pregnancy.
Figure 10–26   **Conditioned Gingival Enlargement** in pregnancy associated with local irritation and food impaction.

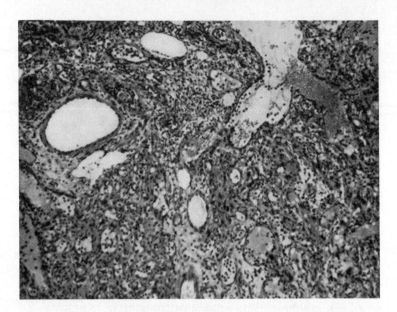

Figure 10–27 Conditioned Gingival Enlargement in pregnancy showing abundance of blood vessels and interspersed inflammatory cells.

ies there is a moderately fibrous stroma that presents varying degrees of edema and leukocytic infiltration. The stratified squamous epithelium is thickened, with prominent rete pegs. The basal epithelium presents some degree of intra- and extracellular edema; there are prominent intercellular bridges and leukocytic infiltration. The surface of the epithelium is generally keratinized. There is generalized chronic inflammatory involvement, usually with a surface zone of acute inflammation.

Gingival enlargement in pregnancy is termed angiogranuloma, which avoids the implication of neoplasm implicit in such terms as fibrohemangioma or pregnancy tumor. Prominent endothelial proliferation with capillary formation and associated inflammation are its characteristic features. The capillary formation exceeds the usual gingival response to chronic irritation and accounts for the enlargement. Although the microscopic findings are characteristic of gingival enlargement in pregnancy, they are not pathognomonic in the sense that they cannot be used to differentiate between pregnant and nonpregnant patients.[59]

Most gingival disease during pregnancy can be prevented by the removal of local irritants and the institution of fastidious oral hygiene at the outset. In pregnancy, treatment of the gingiva that is limited to the removal of tissue, without complete elimination of local irritants, is followed by recurrence. Although spontaneous reduction in the size of gingival enlargement commonly follows the termination of pregnancy, the complete elimination of the residual inflammatory lesion requires the removal of all forms of local irritation.

Enlargement in Puberty

Enlargement of the gingiva is frequently seen during puberty. It occurs in both males and females and appears in areas of local irritation.

CLINICAL FEATURES. The size of the gingival enlargement is far in excess of that usually seen associated with comparable local factors. It is marginal and interdental and is characterized by prominent bulbous interproximal papillae (Fig. 10–28). Frequently, only the facial gingivae are enlarged; the lingual surfaces are relatively unaltered. This occurs because the mechanical action of the tongue and the excursion of food prevent a heavy accumulation of local irritants on the lingual surface.

In addition to an increase in size, gingival enlargement during puberty presents all of the clinical features generally associated with chronic inflammatory gingival disease. *It is the degree of enlargement and the tendency toward massive recurrence in the presence of relatively little local irritation that distinguish the gingival enlargement of puberty from uncomplicated chronic inflammatory gingival enlargement.* After puberty, the enlargement undergoes spontaneous reduction, but it does not disappear until local irritants are removed.

A longitudinal study of 127 children, 11 to 17 years of age, showed a high initial prevalence of gingival enlargement that tended to decline with age.[86] When the mean number of inflamed gingival sites per child are arranged according to the time of maximum number of inflamed sites observed and superimposed on the oral hygiene index at the time, it can be clearly seen that a pubertal peak in gingival

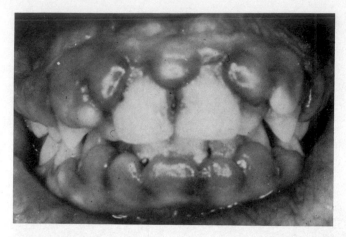

Figure 10–28   Conditioned Gingival Enlargement in puberty in a 13-year-old male.

inflammation occurs and that it is unrelated to oral hygiene.[86]

HISTOPATHOLOGY. Because the enlargement is predominantly inflammatory in nature, it is difficult to discern the conditioning systemic influence in terms of specific histologic changes. The microscopic picture is that of chronic inflammation with prominent edema and associated degenerative changes.

Leukemic Enlargement

CLINICAL FEATURES. *Leukemic gingival enlargement may represent an exaggerated response to local irritation manifested by a dense infiltration of immature and proliferating leukocytes or a neoplastic lesion.* The clinical picture is more severe than that of simple chronic inflammation. In some leukemic patients gingival enlargement results from chronic inflammation without the involvement of leukemic cells and presents the same clinical and microscopic features as in nonleukemic patients.

True leukemic enlargement occurs in acute or subacute leukemia, seldom in chronic leukemia. Clinically, true leukemic enlargement may be diffuse or marginal, localized or generalized. It may appear as a diffuse enlargement of the gingival mucosa (Fig. 10–29), an oversized extension of the marginal gingiva, or a discrete tumor-like interproximal mass. In true leukemic enlargement the gingiva is generally bluish red and has a shiny surface. The consistency is moderately firm, but there is a tendency toward friability and hemorrhage, either spontaneously or upon slight irritation. Acute painful necrotizing ulcerative inflammatory involvement frequently occurs in the crevice formed at the junction of the enlarged gingiva and the contiguous tooth surfaces.

HISTOPATHOLOGY. The connective tissue is infiltrated with a dense mass of immature and proliferating leukocytes, the specific nature of which varies with the type of leukemia. Mature leukocytes associated with chronic inflammation are also seen. The capillaries are engorged; the connective tissue is for the most part edematous and degenerated. The epithelium presents varying degrees of leukocytic infiltration with edema. Isolated surface areas of acute necrotizing inflammation with a pseudomembranous meshwork of fibrin, necrotic epithelial cells, polymorphonuclear leukocytes, and bacteria are frequently seen.

Enlargement Associated with Vitamin C Deficiency

Enlargement of the gingiva is generally included in classic descriptions of scurvy. It is important to recognize that such enlargement is essentially a conditioned response to local irritation. *Acute vitamin C deficiency does not of itself cause gingival inflammation, but it does cause hemorrhage, collagen degeneration, and edema of the gingival connective tissue.* These changes modify the response of the gingiva to local irritation to the extent that the normal defensive delimiting reaction is inhibited and the extension of the inflammation exaggerated.[30] The combined effect of acute vitamin C deficiency and inflammation produces the massive gingival enlargement in scurvy (Fig. 10–30A).

CLINICAL FEATURES. Gingival enlargement in vitamin C deficiency is marginal; the gingiva is bluish red, soft, and friable and has a smooth, shiny surface. Hemorrhage, either spontaneous or upon slight provocation, and surface necrosis with pseudomembrane formation are common features.

Figure 10–29 Leukemic Gingival Enlargement. *Top,* Leukemic gingival enlargement in a patient with acute myelocytic leukemia. Note that the enlargement is more prominent in the maxilla, associated with greater local irritation. *Bottom,* Lingual view of gingival enlargement in a patient with subacute monocytic leukemia, showing bulbous increase in size with discoloration and smooth shiny surface. Note the difference between the enlarged gingiva and the adjacent palatal mucosa.

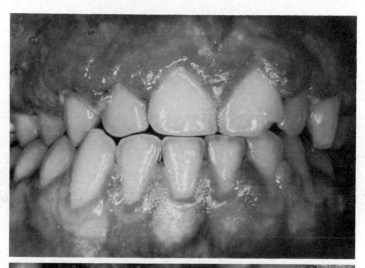

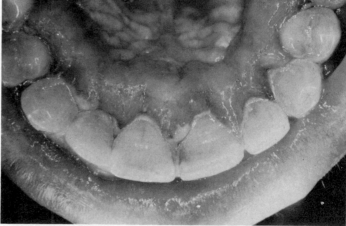

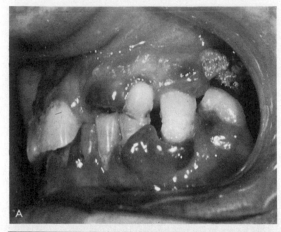

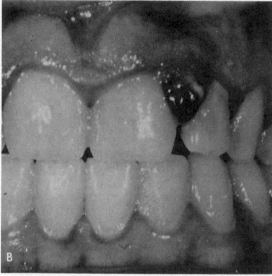

Figure 10–30 *A*, **Conditioned Gingival Enlargement** in vitamin C deficiency. Note the prominent hemorrhagic areas. *B*, **Pyogenic Granuloma** in a young adult female.

HISTOPATHOLOGY. The gingiva presents a chronic inflammatory cellular infiltration with a superficial acute response. There are scattered areas of hemorrhage, with engorged capillaries. Marked diffuse edema, collagen degeneration, and scarcity of collagen fibrils or fibroblasts are striking findings.

Nonspecific Conditioned Enlargement (Granuloma Pyogenicum)

Granuloma pyogenicum is a tumor-like gingival enlargement considered to be an exaggerated conditioned response to minor trauma (Fig. 10–30*B*). The exact nature of the systemic conditioning factor has not been identified.[50]

CLINICAL FEATURES. The lesion varies from a discrete spherical tumor-like mass with a pedunculated attachment to a flattened keloid-like enlargement with a broad base. It is bright red or purple and either friable or firm, depending upon its duration; in the majority of cases it presents surface ulceration and purulent exudation. The lesion tends to involute spontaneously to become a fibroepithelial papilloma or persists relatively unchanged for years. Treatment consists of removal of the lesions plus the elimination of irritating local factors. The recurrence rate is about 15 per cent.[13] Granuloma pyogenicum is similar in clinical and microscopic appearance to the conditioned gingival enlargement seen in pregnancy.[55] Differential diagnosis depends upon the patient's history.

HISTOPATHOLOGY. Granuloma pyogenicum appears as a mass of granulation tissue with chronic inflammatory cellular infiltration. Endothelial proliferation and the formation of numerous vascular spaces are the prominent features. The surface epithelium is atrophic in some areas and hyperplastic in others. Surface ulceration and exudation are common features.

V. NEOPLASTIC ENLARGEMENT (GINGIVAL TUMORS)

Benign Tumors of the Gingiva

Epulis is a generic term used clinically to designate all tumors of the gingiva. It serves to locate the tumor, but not to describe it. (Most lesions referred to as epulis are inflammatory rather than neoplastic.) Neoplasms account for a comparatively small proportion of gingival enlargements and make up a small percentage of the total number of oral neoplasms. In a survey of 257 oral tumors,[61] approximately 8 per cent occurred on the gingiva. In another study[10] of 868 growths of the gingiva and palate, of which 57 per cent were neoplastic and the remainder inflammatory, the following incidence of tumors was noted: carcinoma, 11.0 per cent; fibroma, 9.3 per cent; giant cell tumor, 8.4 per cent; papilloma, 7.3 per cent; leukoplakia, 4.9 per cent; mixed tumor (salivary gland type), 2.5 per cent; angioma, 1.5 per cent; osteofibroma, 1.3 per cent; sarcoma, 0.5 per cent; melanoma, 0.5 per cent; myxoma, 0.45 per cent; fibropapilloma, 0.4 per cent; adenoma, 0.4 per cent; and lipoma, 0.3 per cent.

Fibroma

Fibromas of the gingiva arise from the gingival connective tissue or from the periodontal ligament. They are slow-growing, spherical tumors that tend to be firm and nodular but may be soft and vascular. Fibromas are usually pedunculated. Hard fibromas of the gingiva are very rare; most of the lesions diagnosed clinically as fibromas are inflammatory hyperplasias.[73]

HISTOPATHOLOGY. The hard fibroma is composed of densely arranged bundles of well-formed collagen fibers with a scattering of flattened elliptical fibrocytes. It is a relatively avascular tumor. In the soft fibroma, fibroblasts are comparatively more numerous and stellate in shape. Collagen is present but is less densely arranged. Varying degrees of vascularity are also seen. Bone formation within fibromas is a frequent finding. The bone appears as irregularly arranged trabeculae with osteoblasts and osteoid along the margins. Lipofibroma[60] and myxofibroma[11] of the gingiva and alveolar mucosa have also been described.

Nevus

The nevus may be pigmented or nonpigmented. It commonly occurs on the skin, but a few cases of gingival nevus have been reported. The lesion is benign and slow growing, varying in color from pale gray to dark brown. It may be flat or raised slightly above the gingival surface, sessile or nodular.[12]

HISTOPATHOLOGY. The tumor presents discrete clumps of nevus cells in the submucosa directly beneath the basal cell layer of epithelium and separated from it by connective tissue. The cells may contain melanin or may be pigment-free. In either instance, the nevus cells are demonstrable when stained with dihydroxyphenylalanine (DOPA).

Myoblastoma

Myoblastoma is a benign lesion that is nodular and slightly raised above the gingival surface.[34, 49]

HISTOPATHOLOGY. The lesion appears as a mass of polyhedral or spindle-shaped cells with prominent acidophilic granular cytoplasm. There is a marked pseudoepitheliomatous hyperplasia of the covering epithelium. Congenital myoblastoma is sometimes referred to as congenital epulis.

Hemangioma

These are benign blood vessel tumors occasionally seen on the gingiva. They occur as a *capillary* or *cavernous* type, more commonly the former. These tumors are soft, sessile or pedunculated, and painless. They may be smooth or irregularly bulbous in outline. The color varies from deep red to purple, and the tumor blanches on the application of pressure. These lesions often appear to arise from the interdental gingival papilla and spread laterally to involve the adjacent teeth.[9] They may give rise to hemorrhagic episodes, producing secondary ferropenic anemia.[87] A flat, irregularly outlined, diffuse *congenital form of hemangioma* is also seen, either with or without comparable involvement of the face. Hematomas sometimes occur on the gingiva as the result of trauma (Fig. 10–31).

Papilloma

Papilloma of the gingiva appears as a hard, wart like protuberance from the gingival surface (Fig. 10–32). The lesion may be small and discrete or may appear as a broad, hard elevation of the gingiva with minutely irregular surfaces.

HISTOPATHOLOGY. The lesion presents a central core of connective tissue with a marked proliferation and hyperkeratosis of the epithelium.

Peripheral Giant Cell Reparative Granuloma

Giant cell lesions of the gingiva arise interdentally or from the gingival margin, occur most frequently on the labial surface, and may be sessile or pedunculated. They vary in appearance from a smooth, regularly outlined mass to an irregularly shaped, multilobulated protuberance with surface indentations (Fig. 10–33). Ulceration of the margin is occasionally seen. The lesions are painless, vary in size, and may cover several teeth. They may be firm or spongy, and the color varies from pink to deep red or purplish blue. There are no pathognomonic clinical features whereby these lesions can be differentiated from other forms of gingival enlargement. Microscopic examination is required for definitive diagnosis (Figs. 10–34 to 10–37).

In the past, giant cell lesions of the gingiva have been referred to as *giant cell epulis* or *peripheral giant cell tumor*. Most often, however, these gingival lesions are essentially responses to local injury and not neoplasms.

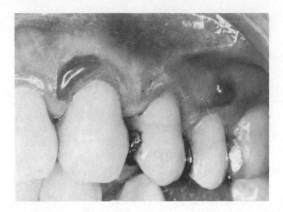

Figure 10–31   **Hematomas** produced by trauma.

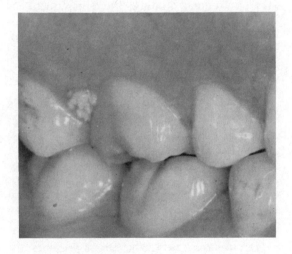

Figure 10–32   **Papilloma** of the gingiva appears as a hard wart-like mass. (Courtesy of Dr. Neal Chilton.)

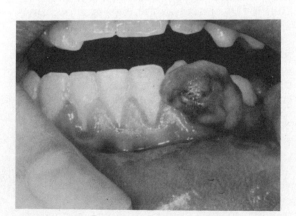

Figure 10–33   **Peripheral Giant Cell Reparative Granuloma.** Comparison of this lesion with the one shown in Figure 10–36 indicates the importance of biopsy for definitive diagnosis.

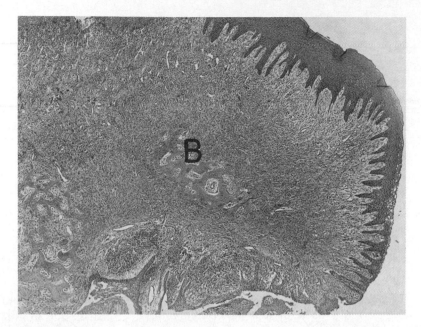

Figure 10–34 Microscopic survey of lesion shown in Figure 10–33. Trabeculae of newly formed bone (B) are contained within the mass.

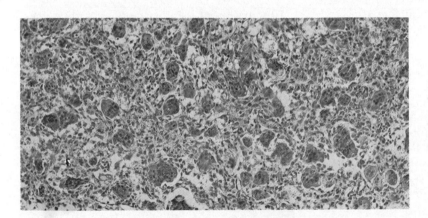

Figure 10–35 High-power study of the lesion shown in Figure 10–33 demonstrating the giant cells and intervening stroma which make up the major portion of the mass.

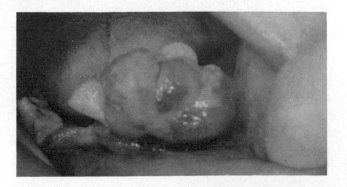

Figure 10–36 Localized gingival enlargement. Microscopic examination reveals it to be a chronic inflammatory lesion. (Compare with Fig. 10–33.)

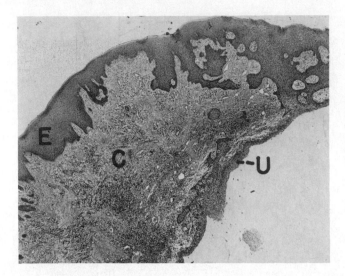

Figure 10–37 Survey section of lesion shown in Figure 10–36. The lesion consists of connective tissue (C) surrounded by stratified squamous epithelium (E). The connective tissue presented marked chronic inflammatory involvement. The surface of the lesion that was in apposition with the teeth is ulcerated (U).

When they occur on the gingiva, they should be referred to as *peripheral giant cell reparative granulomas*[68, 71] to differentiate them from comparable lesions that originate within the jaw bone (central giant cell reparative granulomas).[45]

In some instances, the giant cell reparative granuloma of the gingiva is locally invasive and causes destruction of the underlying bone (Fig. 10–38). Complete removal leads to uneventful recovery.

HISTOPATHOLOGY. The giant cell reparative granuloma presents numerous foci of multinuclear giant cells and hemosiderin particles in a connective tissue stroma. Areas of chronic inflammation are scattered throughout the lesion, with acute involvement at the surface. The overlying epithelium is usually hyperplastic, with ulceration at the base. Bone formation occasionally occurs within the lesion.

Central Giant Cell Reparative Granuloma

These lesions arise within the jaws and produce central cavitation. They occasionally create deformity of the jaw such that the gingiva appears enlarged (Fig. 10–39).

Mixed tumors, salivary gland–type tumors, eosinophilic granulomas, and *plasmacytomas* of the gingiva have also been described but are not often seen.

Plasma Cell Granuloma

This is a benign lesion of the marginal, interdental, or attached gingiva.[15] It usually occurs as a localized mass but may be generalized. It is red, friable, sometimes granular, bleeds easily, and is accompanied by focal distribution of adjacent bone.

Microscopically, it appears as a dense almost exclusively plasma cell accumulation in solid sheets or a lobular pattern.

Elimination of local irritants by scaling usually suffices as treatment, but surgical removal may be necessary.

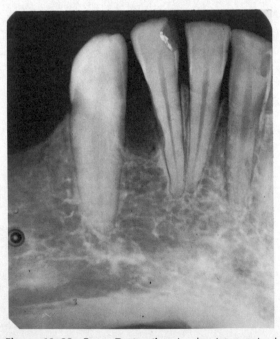

Figure 10–38 Bone Destruction in the interproximal space between the canine and lateral incisor caused by the extension of a peripheral giant cell reparative granuloma of the gingiva. (Courtesy of Dr. Sam Toll.)

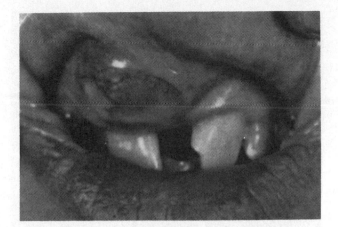

Figure 10–39 Localized Bone Deformity in relation to the maxillary central incisor *(left)* produced by a central giant cell reparative granuloma.

Leukoplakia

Leukoplakia of the gingiva varies in appearance from a grayish-white, flattened, scaly lesion to a thick, irregularly shaped, keratinous plaque (Fig. 10–40).

HISTOPATHOLOGY. Leukoplakia presents thickening of the epithelium with hyperkeratosis, acanthosis, and some degree of dyskeratosis. Inflammatory involvement of the underlying connective tissue is a commonly associated finding. Leukoplakia is caused by chronic irritation. Its capacity for malignant transformation must be borne in mind.

Gingival Cyst

Gingival cysts of microscopic proportions are common, but they seldom reach a clinically significant size.[62] When they do, they appear as localized enlargements that may involve the marginal and attached gingivae.[70] They occur in the mandibular canine and premolar areas, most often on the lingual surface. They are painless but with expansion may cause erosion of the surface of the alveolar bone. The cysts develop from odontogenic epithelium or from surface or sulcular epithelium traumatically implanted in the area. Removal is followed by uneventful recovery.

Microscopically, they present a cyst cavity lined by a thin, flattened epithelium with or without localized areas of thickening. Less frequently, the following types of epithelium can be found: unkeratinized stratified squamous epithelium, keratinized stratified squamous epithelium, and parakeratinized epithelium with palisading basal cells.[17]

Mucus-secreting cysts (mucoceles)[90] have been described as rare findings in the gingiva.

Malignant Tumors of the Gingiva

Carcinoma

The gingiva is not a frequent site of oral malignancy. *Squamous cell carcinoma is the most common malignant tumor of the gingiva.* Only 1.9[28] to 5.4 per cent[2] of oral carcinomas occur on the gingiva, with the mandible, usually the molar area, being the most common site. There is often an associated leukoplakia. In patients with multiple primary oral carcinomas, 25 per cent of the tumors were present on the gingiva.[81]

Carcinomas may be *exophytic* or *verrucous*, both of which are outgrowths from the gingival surface, or *ulcerative*, which appear as flat, erosive lesions. They are locally invasive, involving the underlying bone and adjacent mucosa. Often symptom-free, they are frequently unnoticed until complicated by painful inflammation. The inflammatory changes may mask the neoplasm. Metastasis is usually confined to the region above the clavicle; however, more extensive involvement may include the lung,

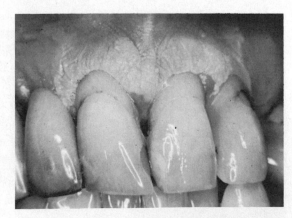

Figure 10–40 Leukoplakia of the Gingiva.

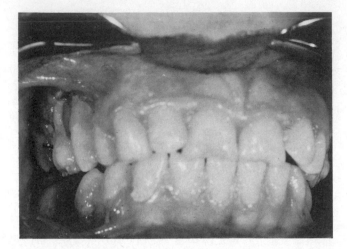

Figure 10–41 Malignant Lymphoma of the Gingiva in a Young Female. The tumor appears as bead-like masses of granulation tissue in the maxillary molar area *(left)*.

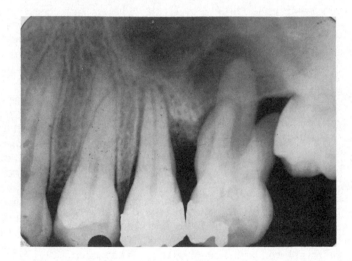

Figure 10–42 Radiograph of patient with malignant lymphoma shown in Figure 10–41. There is extensive loss of bone in relation to the molar and premolar as a result of progressive invasion of the tumor. Note the thickening of the periodontal space around the premolar.

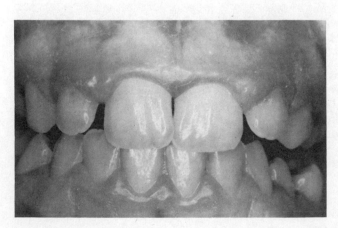

Figure 10–43 Developmental Gingival Enlargement. The normal bulbous contour of the gingiva around the incompletely erupted anterior teeth is accentuated by chronic inflammation.

liver, or bone. A 5-year survival rate of 24 per cent has been reported for gingival carcinomas.[80]

Malignant Melanoma

Malignant melanoma is a rare oral tumor that tends to occur in the gingiva of the anterior maxilla.[8] The malignant melanoma is usually darkly pigmented and is often preceded by the occurrence of localized pigmentation.[20] It may be flat or nodular and is characterized by rapid growth and early metastasis. It arises from melanoblasts in the gingiva, cheek, or palate. An unpigmented malignant melanoma of the gingiva has been reported.[57] Infiltration into the underlying bone and metastasis to cervical and axillary lymph nodes are common.

HISTOPATHOLOGY. The malignant melanoma shows some resemblance to the benign nevus; however, the malignant cells vary in morphology. The distribution is irregular and invasive, lacking the clear-cut grouping of the benign lesions, and in some areas the malignant cells are continuous with the surface epithelium. The connective tissue stroma is more often delicate and relatively scarce.

Sarcoma

Fibrosarcoma, lymphosarcoma, and *reticulum cell sarcoma* of the gingiva are rare; only isolated cases have been described in the literature[22, 33, 88] (Figs. 10–41 and 10–42).

Metastasis

Tumor metastasis to the gingiva is not common. Cases of metastasis to the gingiva have been reported from the following tumors: *adenocarcinoma from the colon,*[43] *carcinoma from the lung, chondromyxosarcoma from the axilla, hypernephroma,*[67, 83] *primary hepatocellular carcinoma,*[91] *testicular tumor,*[27] *and renal cell carcinoma.*[16]

One must not be misled by the low incidence of malignancy of the gingiva. Ulcerations that do not respond to therapy in the usual manner and all gingival tumors and tumor-like lesions must be biopsied (see Chapter 32) and submitted for microscopic diagnosis.

VI. DEVELOPMENTAL ENLARGEMENT

CLINICAL FEATURES. This type of enlargement appears as a bulbous distortion of the labial and marginal contours of the gingiva of teeth in various stages of eruption. It is caused by superimposition of the bulk of the gingiva upon the normal prominence of the enamel in the gingival half of the crown. The enlargement often persists until the junctional epithelium has migrated from the enamel to the cemento-enamel junction.

In a strict sense, developmental gingival enlargement is physiologic, and it ordinarily presents no problem. However, when it is complicated by marginal inflammation, the composite picture gives the impression of extensive gingival enlargement (Fig. 10–43). Treatment to alleviate the marginal inflammation, rather than resection of the enlargement, is sufficient in these cases.

HISTOPATHOLOGY. When uncomplicated by inflammation, developmental enlargement presents no notable pathologic changes. A zone of chronic inflammation at the gingival margin is, however, a common finding.

REFERENCES

1. Aas, E.: Hyperplasia gingivae diphenylhydantoinea. Universitetsforlaget, 1963.
2. Ackerman, L. V., and del Regato, J. A.: Cancer: Diagnosis, Treatment and Prognosis. St. Louis, C. V. Mosby Company, 1947.
3. Angelopoulos, A. P., and Goaz, P. W.: Incidence of diphenylhydantoin gingival hyperplasia. Oral Surg., 34:898, 1972.
4. Babcock, J. R.: Incidence of gingival hyperplasia associated with dilantin therapy in a hospital population. J. Am. Dent. Assoc., 71:1447, 1965.
5. Babcock, J. R., and Nelson, G. H.: Gingival hyperplasia and dilantin content of saliva. J. Am. Dent. Assoc., 68:195, 1964.
6. Ball, E. I.: Case of gingivomatosis or elephantiasis of the gingiva. J. Periodontol., 12:96, 1941.
7. Baratieri, A.: The oxytalan connective tissue fibers in gingival hyperplasia in patients treated with sodium diphenylhydantoin. J. Periodont. Res., 2:106, 1967.
8. Baxter, H. A., Brown, J. B., and Byars, L. T.: Malignant melanomas. Am. J. Orthod., 27:90, 1941.
9. Bellinger, D. H.: Blood and lymph vessel tumors involving the mouth. J. Oral Surg., 2:141, 1944.
10. Bernick, S.: Growth of the gingiva and palate. II. Connective tissue tumors. Oral Surg., 1:1098, 1948.
11. Bernier, J. L., and Ash, J. E.: Atlas of dental and oral pathology. Washington, D.C., Registry Press, 1948.
12. Bernier, J. L., and Tiecke, R. W.: Nevus of the gingiva. J. Oral Surg., 8:165, 1950.
13. Bhaskar, S. N., and Jacoway, J. R.: Pyogenic granuloma—clinical features, incidence, histology and result of treatment. J. Oral Surg., 24:391, 1966.
14. Bhaskar, S. N., Bernier, J. L., and Godby, F.: Aneurysmal bone cyst and other giant cell lesions of the jaws. Report of 104 cases. J. Oral Surg., 17:30, 1959.
15. Bhaskar, S. N., Levin, M. P., and Frisch, J.: Plasma cell granuloma of periodontal tissues. Report of 45 cases. Periodontics, 6:272, 1968.
16. Buchner, A., and Begleiter, A.: Metastatic renal cell carcinoma in the gingiva mimicking a hyperplastic lesion. J. Periodontol., 51:413, 1980.
17. Buchner, A., and Hansen, A. S.: The histomorphologic spectrum of the gingival cyst in the adult. Oral Surg., 48:532, 1979.
18. Buckner, H. J.: Diffuse fibroma of the gums. J. Am. Dent. Assoc., 24:2003, 1937.

19. Burket, L. W.: Oral Medicine. Philadelphia, J. B. Lippincott Company, 1946, p. 295.
20. Chaudry, A. P., Hampel, A., and Gorlin, R. J.: Primary malignant melanoma of the oral cavity: a review of 105 cases. Cancer, *11*:923, 1958.
21. Ciancio, S. G., Yaffe, S. J., and Catz, C. C.: Gingival hyperplasia and diphenylhydantoin. J. Periodontol., *7*:411, 1972.
22. Cook, H. P.: Oral lymphomas. Oral Surg., *14*:690, 1961.
23. Dallas, B. M.: Hyperplasia of the oral mucosa in an edentulous epileptic. N.Z. Dent. J., *59*:54, 1963.
24. Dreyer, W. P., and Thomas, C. J.: DPH-induced hyperplasia of the masticatory mucosa in an edentulous epileptic patient. Oral Surg., *45*:701, 1978.
25. Elzay, R. P., and Swenson, H. M.: Effect of an electric toothbrush on dilantin sodium induced gingival hyperplasia. N.Y. J. Dent., *34*:13, 1964.
26. Emerson, T. G.: Hereditary gingival hyperplasia. A family pedigree of four generations. Oral Surg., *19*:1, 1965.
27. Fantasia, J. E., and Chen, A.: A testicular tumor with gingival metastasis. Oral Surg., *48*:64, 1979.
28. Gardner, A. F., Schwartz, F. L., and Pallen, H. S.: Carcinoma of the oral regions. Ann. Dent., *21*:80, 1962.
29. Glickman, I.: The periodontal tissues of the guinea pig in vitamin C deficiency. J. Dent. Res., *27*:9, 1948.
30. Glickman, I.: The effect of acute vitamin C deficiency upon the response of the periodontal tissues of the guinea pig to artificially induced inflammation. J. Dent. Res., *27*:201, 1948.
31. Glickman, I.: A basic classification of gingival enlargement. J. Periodontol., *21*:131, 1950.
32. Glickman, I., and Lewitus, M.: Hyperplasia of the gingiva associated with dilantin (sodium diphenyl hydantoinate) therapy. J. Am. Dent. Assoc., *28*:199, 1941.
33. Goldman, H. M.: Sarcoma. Am. J. Orthod., *30*:311, 1944.
34. Hagen, J. D., Soule, E. H., and Gores, R. J.: Granular-cell myoblastoma of the oral cavity. Oral Surg., *14*:454, 1961.
35. Hall, W. B.: Dilantin hyperplasia: a preventable lesion. J. Periodont. Res., *4*(Suppl.):36, 1969.
36. Hardman, F. G.: Secondary sarcoma presenting clinical appearance of fibrous epulis. Br. Dent. J., *86*:109, 1949.
37. Hassell, T. M.: Epilepsy and the Oral Manifestations of Phenytoin Therapy. Monographs in Oral Science. Vol. 9. New York, S. Karger, 1981.
38. Hassell, T. M., and Page, R. C.: The major metabolite of phenytoin (Dilantin) induces gingival overgrowth in cats. J. Periodont. Res., *13*:280, 1978.
39. Henefer, E. P., and Kay, L. A.: Congenital idiopathic gingival fibromatosis in the deciduous dentition. Oral Surg., *24*:65, 1967.
40. Hirschfeld, I.: Hypertrophic gingivitis—its clinical aspect. J. Am. Dent. Assoc., *19*:799, 1932.
41. Hoess, T.: The effect of 5,5 diphenylhydantoin (Dilantin) on fibroblast-like cells in culture. J. Periodont. Res., *4*:163, 1969.
42. Hugoson, A.: Gingival inflammation and female sex hormones. J. Periodont. Res., *5*(Suppl.), 1970.
43. Humphrey, A. A., and Amos, N. H.: Metastatic gingival adenocarcinoma from primary lesion of colon. Am. J. Cancer, *28*:128, 1936.
44. Ishikawa, J., and Glickman, I.: Gingival response to the systemic administration of sodium diphenyl hydantoinate (Dilantin) in cats. J. Periodontol., *32*:149, 1961.
45. Jaffe, H. L.: Giant cell reparative granuloma, traumatic bone cyst, and fibrous (fibro-osseous) dysplasia of the jaw bones. Oral Surg., *6*:159, 1953.
46. Kapur, R. N., Grigis, S., Little, T. M., and Masotti, R. E.: Diphenylhydantoin-induced gingival hyperplasia: its relation to dose and serum level. Dev. Med. Child Neurol., *15*:483, 1973.
47. Jorgenson, R. J., and Cocker, M. E.: Variation in the inheritance and expression of gingival fibromatosis. J. Periodontol., *45*:472, 1974.
48. Kerageorgis, B. P.: Elephantiasis of the gingivae (Elephantiasis des Gengives). Rev. Chir. Par., *68*:308, 1949. Abst. Surg. Gynecol. Obstet, *90*:461, 1950.
49. Kerr, D. A.: Myoblastic myoma. Oral Surg., *2*:41, 1949.
50. Kerr, D. A.: Granuloma pyogenicum. Oral Surg., *4*:155, 1951.
51. Kilpinen, E., Raeste, A.-M., and Collan, Y.: Hereditary gingival hyperplasia and physical maturation. Scand. J. Dent. Res., *86*:118, 1978.

52. Klar, L. A.: Gingival hyperplasia during dilantin therapy: a survey of 312 patients. J. Public Health Dent., *33*:180, 1973.
53. Klingsberg, J., Cancellaro, L. A., and Butcher, E. O.: Effects of air drying in rodent oral mucous membrane. A histologic study of simulated mouth breathing. J. Periodontol., *32*:38, 1961.
54. Larmas, L. A., Mackinen, K. K., and Paunio, K. U.: A histochemical study of amylaminopeptidase in hydantoin induced hyperplastic, healthy and inflamed human gingiva. J. Periodont. Res., *8*:21, 1973.
55. Lee, K. W.: The fibrous epulis and related lesions. Granuloma pyogenicum, "pregnancy tumor," fibro-epithelial polyp and calcifying fibroblastic granuloma. A clinico-pathological study. Periodontics, *6*:277, 1968.
56. Lite, T., et al.: Gingival patterns in mouth breathers. A clinical and histopathologic study and a method of treatment. Oral Surg., *8*:382, 1955.
57. Loscalzo, L. J.: Unpigmented melanocarcinoma of the gingivae. Report of a case. Oral Surg., *11*:646, 1958.
58. Lustberg, A., Goldman, D., and Dreskin, O. H.: Megaloblastic anemia due to dilantin therapy. Ann. Int. Med., *54*:153, 1961.
59. Maier, A. W., and Orban, B.: Gingivitis in pregnancy. Oral Surg., *2*:334, 1949.
60. Marfino, N. R.: Developing fibrolipoma of the free gingiva. Oral Surg., *12*:489, 1959.
61. McCarthy, F. P.: A clinical and pathological study of oral disease. J.A.M.A., *116*:16, 1941.
62. Moskow, B. S.: The pathogenesis of the gingival cyst. Periodontics, *4*:23, 1966.
63. Nease, W. J.: Effect of sodium diphenylhydantoinate on tissue cultures of human gingiva. J. Periodontol., *36*:22, 1965.
64. Newby, C. D.: A report on a case of hypertrophied gum tissue. J. Can. Dent. Assoc., *6*:183, 1940.
65. Nuki, K., and Cooper, S. H.: The role of inflammation in the pathogenesis of gingival enlargement during the administration of diphenylhydantoin sodium in cats. J. Periodont Res., *7*:91, 1972.
66. Panuska, H. J., Gorlin, R. J., Bearman, J. E., and Mitchell, D. F.: The effect of anticonvulsant drugs upon the gingiva. A series of 1048 patients. II. J. Periodontol., *32*:15, 1961.
67. Persson, P. A., and Wallenino, K.: Metastatic renal carcinoma (hypernephroma) in the gingiva of the lower jaw. Acta Odontol. Scand., *19*:289, 1961.
68. Phillips, R. L., and Shafer, W. G.: An evaluation of the peripheral giant cell tumor. J. Periodontol., *26*:216, 1955.
69. Raeste, A.-M., Collan, Y., and Kilpinen, E.: Hereditary fibrous hyperplasia of the gingiva with varying penetrance and expressivity. Scand. J. Dent. Res., *86*:357, 1978.
69a. Rateitschak-Plüss, E. M., Hefti, A., Lörtscher, R., and Thiel, G.: Initial observation that cyclosporin-A induces gingival enlargement in man. J. Clin. Periodontol., *10*:237, 1983.
70. Rickles, N. H., and Everett, F. G.: Gingival and lateral periodontal cysts. Parodontologie, *14*:41, 1960.
71. Rushton, M. A.: Hereditary or idiopathic hyperplasia of the gums. Dent. Prac., *7*:136, 1957.
72. Russell, B. J., and Bay, L. M.: Oral use of chlorhexidine gluconate toothpaste in epileptic children. Scand. J. Dent. Res., *86*:52, 1978.
73. Schneider, L. C., and Weisinger, E.: The true gingival fibroma—an analysis of 129 fibrous gingival lesions. J. Periodontol., *49*:423, 1978.
74. Setia, A. P.: Severe bleeding from a pregnancy tumor. Oral Surg., *36*:192, 1973.
75. Shafer, W. G.: Effect of dilantin sodium analogues on cell proliferation in tissue culture. Proc. Soc. Exp. Biol. Med., *106*:205, 1960.
76. Shafer, W. G.: Effect of dilantin sodium on various cell lines in tissue culture. Proc. Soc. Exp. Biol. Med., *108*:694, 1961.
77. Shafer, W. G.: Response of radiated human gingival fibroblast-like cells to dilantin sodium in tissue culture. J. Dent Res., *44*:671, 1965.
78. Shafer, W. G., Beatty, R. E., and Davis, W. B.: Effect of dilantin sodium on tensile strength of healing wounds. Proc. Soc. Exp. Biol. Med., *98*:348, 1958.
79. Shapiro, M.: Acceleration of gingival wound healing in nonepileptic patients receiving diphenylhydantoin sodium. Exp. Med. Surg., *16*:41, 1958.

80. Sharp, G. S.: Carcinoma of the gingivae. J. Tenn. State Dent. Assoc., *29*:236, 1959.

81. Sharp, G. S., Bullock, W. K., and Helsper, J. T.: Multiple oral carcinomas. Cancer, *14*:512, 1961.

82. Staple, P. H., and Reed, M. J.: Diphenylhydantoin gingival hyperplasia in *Macaca speciosa:* a new human model. J. Dent. Res., *54A*:146, 1975 (abstract).

83. Stein, G.: Hypernephrometastase als Epulis. Dtsch Ztschr. Chir., *219*:318, 1929.

84. Stein, G. M., and Lewis, H.: Oral changes in a folic acid deficient patient precipitated by anticonvulsant drug therapy. J. Periodontol., *44*:645, 1973.

85. Stirrups, D., and Inglis, J.: Tuberous sclerosis with nonhydantoin gingival hyperplasia. Report of a case. Oral Surg., *49*:211, 1980.

86. Sutcliffe, P.: A longitudinal study of gingivitis and puberty. J. Periodont. Res., *7*:52, 1972.

87. Sznajder, N., Dominguez, F. V., Carraro, J. J., and Lis, G.: Hemorrhagic hemangioma of the gingiva: report of a case. J. Periodontol., *44*:579, 1973.

88. Thoma, K. H., Holland, D. J., Woodbury, H. W., Burrow, J. G., and Sleeper, E. I.: Malignant lymphoma of the gingiva. Oral Surg., *1*:57, 1948.

89. Thukral, P. P.: Idiopathic gingival hyperplasia. J. Indian Dent. Assoc., *44*:109, 1972.

90. Traeger, K. A.: Cyst of the gingiva (mucocele): report of a case. Oral Surg., *14*:243, 1961.

91. Wedgwood, D., Rusen, D., and Balk, S.: Gingival metastases from primary hepatocellular carcinoma. Oral Surg., *47*:263, 1979.

92. Westphal, P.: Salivary secretion and gingival hyperplasia in diphenylhydantoin-treated guinea pigs. Svensk Tandlak. T., *62*:505, 1969.

93. Zackin, S. J., and Weisberger, D.: Hereditary gingival fibromatosis. Oral Surg., *14*:828, 1961.

94. Ziskin, D. E., and Zegarelli, E.: Idiopathic fibromatosis of the gingivae. Ann. Dent., *2*:50, 1943.

95. Ziskin, D. E., Blackberg, S. M., and Stout, A. P.: The gingivae during pregnancy. Surg. Gynecol. Obstet., *57*:719, 1933.

chapter eleven

Acute Gingival Infections

ACUTE NECROTIZING ULCERATIVE GINGIVITIS

Acute necrotizing ulcerative gingivitis (ANUG) is an inflammatory destructive disease of the gingiva which presents characteristic signs and symptoms. Other terms by which this condition is known are Vincent's infection, acute ulceromembranous gingivitis, trench mouth, trench gums, phagedenic gingivitis, acute ulcerous gingivitis, acute ulcerative gingivitis, ulcerative gingivitis, ulcerative stomatitis, Vincent's stomatitis, Plaut-Vincent stomatitis, stomatitis ulcerosa, stomatitis ulceromembranacea, fusospirillary gingivitis, fusospirillary marginal gingivitis, fusospirillary periodontal gingivitis, fusospirillary peridental gingivitis, fusospirillary periodontitis, fetid stomatitis, putrid stomatitis, putrid sore mouth, stomatocace, stomacace, acute septic gingivitis, pseudomembranous angina, and spirochetal stomatitis.

Acute necrotizing ulcerative gingivitis was recognized as far back as the fourth century B.C. by Xenophon, who mentioned that Greek soldiers were affected with "sore mouth" and foul-smelling breath. John Hunter in 1778 described the clinical findings and differentiated it from scurvy and chronic destructive periodontal disease. Acute necrotizing ulcerative gingivitis occurred in epidemic form in the French army in the nineteenth century, and in 1886 Hersch discussed some of the features associated with the disease, such as enlarged lymph nodes, fever, malaise, and increased salivation. In the 1890s Plaut[34] and Vincent[54] described the disease and attributed its origin to fusiform and spirochete bacteria. It was commonly known as *Vincent's infection* during the first half of the twentieth century, but the current designation is acute necrotizing ulcerative gingivitis.

Clinical Features

CLASSIFICATION. Necrotizing ulcerative gingivitis most often occurs as an *acute* disease. Its relatively mild and more persistent form is referred to as *subacute*. *Recurrent* disease is marked by periods of remission and exacerbation. Reference is sometimes made to *chronic* necrotizing ulcerative gingivitis. However, it is difficult to justify this designation as a separate entity because most periodontal pockets with ulceration and destruction of gin-

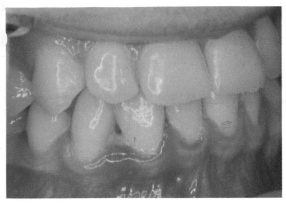

A

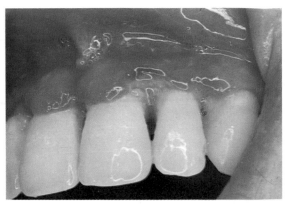

B

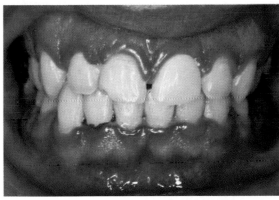

C

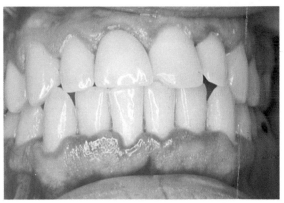

D

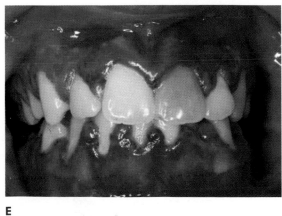

E

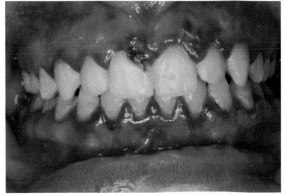

F

Plate II

A, **Acute necrotizing ulcerative gingivitis:** typical punched out interdental papilla between mandibular canine and lateral incisor.

B, **Acute necrotizing ulcerative gingivitis:** typical lesions with progressive tissue destruction.

C, **Acute necrotizing ulcerative gingivitis:** typical lesions with spontaneous hemorrhage.

D, **Acute necrotizing ulcerative gingivitis:** typical lesions have produced irregular gingival contour.

E, **Acute herpetic gingivostomatitis:** typical diffuse erythema.

F, **Acute herpetic gingivostomatitis:** vesicles on the gingiva.

gival tissue present comparable microscopic and clinical features.

HISTORY. Acute necrotizing ulcerative gingivitis is characterized by *sudden onset,* frequently following an episode of debilitating disease or acute respiratory infection. Change in living habits, protracted work without adequate rest, and psychologic stress are frequent features of the patient's history.

ORAL SIGNS. *Characteristic lesions are punched-out, crater-like depressions at the crest of the gingiva that involve the interdental papillae, the marginal gingiva, or both.* The surface of the gingival craters is covered by a gray, pseudomembranous slough demarcated from the remainder of the gingival mucosa by a pronounced linear erythema (Plate IIA). In some instances, the lesions are denuded of the surface pseudomembrane, exposing the gingival margin, which is red, shiny, and hemorrhagic. The characteristic lesions progressively destroy the gingiva and underlying periodontal tissues (Plate IIB).

A fetid odor, increased salivation, and spontaneous gingival hemorrhage or pronounced bleeding upon the slightest stimulation are additional characteristic clinical signs (Plate IIC).

Acute necrotizing ulcerative gingivitis can

occur in otherwise disease-free mouths or superimposed upon chronic gingivitis (Plate IID) or periodontal pockets. Involvement may be limited to a single tooth or group of teeth (Fig. 11–1) or be widespread throughout the mouth. It is rare in edentulous mouths, but isolated spherical lesions occasionally occur on the soft palate.

ORAL SYMPTOMS. The lesions are extremely sensitive to the touch, and the patient complains of a constant radiating, gnawing pain that is intensified by spicy or hot foods and mastication. There is a metallic foul taste, and the patient is conscious of an excessive amount of "pasty" saliva.

EXTRAORAL AND SYSTEMIC SIGNS AND SYMPTOMS. Patients are usually ambulatory, with a minimum of systemic complications. *Local lymphadenopathy and a slight elevation in temperature* are common features of the mild and moderate stages of the disease. In severe cases there are marked systemic complications such as high fever, increased pulse rate, leukocytosis, loss of appetite, and general lassitude. Systemic reactions are more severe in children. *Insomnia, constipation, gastrointestinal disorders, headache, and mental depression sometimes accompany the condition.*

In very rare cases severe sequelae such as

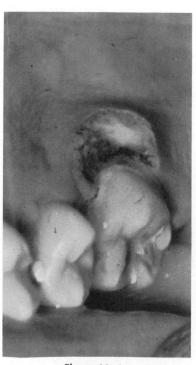

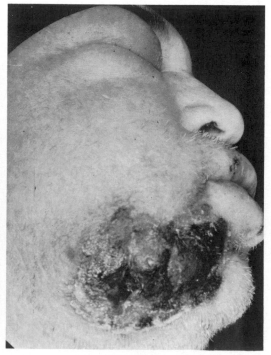

Figure 11–1   **Figure 11–2**

Figure 11–1   Localized Zone of Acute Necrotizing Ulcerative Gingivitis.
Figure 11–2   Noma Following Acute Necrotizing Ulcerative Gingivitis in a 50-year-old male with severe anemia.

the following may occur: noma or gangrenous stomatitis[2, 3, 12] (Fig. 11–2), fusospirochetal meningitis and peritonitis, pulmonary infections,[31] toxemia, and fatal brain abscess.[49]

CLINICAL COURSE. The clinical course is indefinite. If untreated, acute necrotizing ulcerative gingivitis may result in progressive destruction of the periodontium and denudation of the roots, accompanied by an increase in the severity of toxic systemic complications. It often undergoes a diminution in severity, leading to a subacute stage with varying degrees of clinical symptomatology. *The disease may subside spontaneously without treatment.* Such patients generally present a history of repeated remissions and exacerbations. Recurrence of the condition in previously treated patients is also frequent.

Acute Necrotizing Ulcerative Gingivitis and Chronic Destructive Periodontal Disease

It is important to understand the relationship between acute necrotizing ulcerative gingivitis and chronic destructive periodontal disease. As pointed out earlier, acute necrotizing ulcerative gingivitis may occur in a mouth devoid of pre-existing gingival disease or it may be superimposed upon underlying chronic gingivitis and periodontal pockets. **However, it does not usually lead to periodontal pocket formation.** It causes rapid destruction of tissue, in contrast to the chronic inflammatory and proliferative changes which give rise to pocket formation.

Histopathology of the Characteristic Lesion

Microscopically, the lesion appears as a nonspecific acute necrotizing inflammation at the gingival margin, involving both the stratified squamous epithelium and the underlying connective tissue. The surface epithelium is destroyed and replaced by a pseudomembranous meshwork of fibrin, necrotic epithelial cells, polymorphonuclear leukocytes, and various types of microorganisms (Fig. 11–3). This is the zone that appears clinically as the surface pseudomembrane. The underlying connective tissue is markedly hyperemic, with numerous engorged capillaries and a dense infiltration of polymorphonuclear leukocytes. This acutely inflamed hyperemic zone appears clinically as the linear erythema beneath the surface pseudomembrane. Numerous plasma cells may appear in the periphery of the infiltrate; this is interpreted as being an area of established chronic marginal gingivitis upon which the acute lesion became superimposed.[20]

The epithelium and connective tissue present alterations in appearance as the distance from the necrotic gingival margin increases. There is a gradual blending of the epithelium from the uninvolved gingiva to the necrotic lesion. At the immediate border of the necrotic pseudomembrane, the epithelium is edematous and the individual cells present varying degrees of hydropic degeneration. In addition, there is an infiltration of polymorphonuclear leukocytes in the intercellular spaces. The inflammatory involvement in the connective tissue diminishes as the distance from the necrotic lesion increases until the involved tissue blends in appearance with the uninvolved connective tissue stroma of the normal gingival mucosa.

It is noteworthy that the microscopic appearance of acute necrotizing ulcerative gingivitis is nonspecific. Comparable changes result from trauma, chemical irritation, or the application of escharotic drugs.

The Relation of Bacteria to the Characteristic Lesion

Both the light microscope and the electron microscope have been used to study the relationship of bacteria to the characteristic lesion of ANUG. With the former it appears that the exudate on the surface of the necrotic lesion contains microorganisms which morphologically resemble cocci, fusiform bacilli, and spirochetes.[52] The layer between the necrotic and the living tissue contains enormous numbers of fusiform bacilli and spirochetes, in addition to leukocytes and fibrin. Spirochetes invade the underlying living tissue[3, 10, 52]; however, the other organisms seen on the surface are not found there.

Electron microscopic examination reveals that in acute necrotizing ulcerative gingivitis the gingiva is divisible into the following four zones, which blend with each other and may not all be present in every case:[25]

Zone 1: *Bacterial zone*, most superficial, consists of varied bacteria, including a few spirochetes of the small, medium, and large types.

Zone 2: *Neutrophil-rich zone*, contains numerous leukocytes, predominantly neutrophils, with bacteria, including many spirochetes of various types, between the leukocytes.

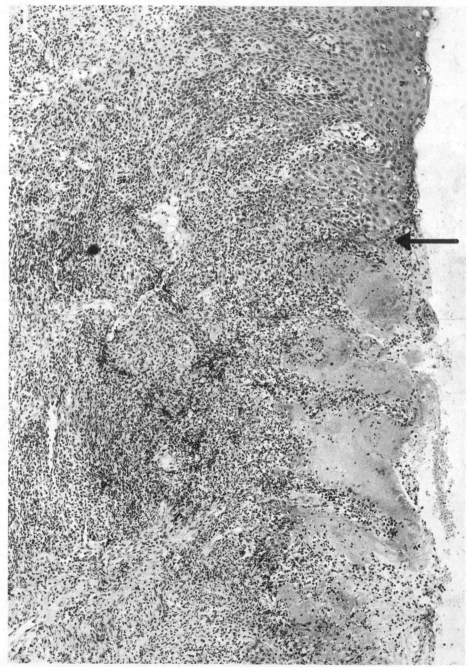

Figure 11–3 Survey Section of the Gingiva in Acute Necrotizing Ulcerative Gingivitis. The portion of the section below the arrow is the accumulation of leukocytes, fibrin, and necrotic tissue which form the gray marginal pseudomembrane.

Zone 3: *Necrotic zone,* **consists of disintegrated tissue cells, fibrillar material, remnants of collagen fibers, and numerous spirochetes of the intermediate and large types, with few other organisms.**

Zone 4: *Zone of spirochetal infiltration,* **consists of well-preserved tissue infiltrated with intermediate and large spirochetes, without other organisms.**

Spirochetes have been found as deep as 300 microns from the surface. The majority of spirochetes in the deeper zones are morphologically different from cultivated strains of *Treponema microdentium.* They occur in nonnecrotic tissue ahead of other types of bacteria and may be present in high concentrations intercellularly in the epithelium adjacent to the ulcerated lesion and in the connective tissue.

The Bacterial Flora

Smears taken of the lesions (Fig. 11–4) present scattered bacteria, predominantly spirochetes and fusiform bacilli, desquamated epithelial cells, and occasional polymorphonuclear leukocytes. A smear containing only spirochetes and fusiform bacilli is rarely seen. Usually these two organisms are seen with other oral spirochetes, vibrios, streptococci, and filamentous organisms. The spirochetal organisms form a light-staining, conspicuous, interlacing network throughout the microscopic field.

Electron microscopic studies indicate that **the spirochetes may be classified into three morphologic groups: "small,"** 7 to 39 per cent of the total spirochetes present; **"intermediate,"** 43.9 to 90 per cent, and **"large,"** 0 to 20 per cent.[26] It was also suggested that intermediate spirochetes are present in greater numbers in pooled scrapings from lesions of acute necrotizing ulcerative gingivitis and are found in greater percentages in the deeper portion of the lesions.

The mean fusiform bacillus count in the saliva of patients with acute necrotizing ulcerative gingivitis is higher than that in the saliva of "normal" persons. *Fusobacterium* species

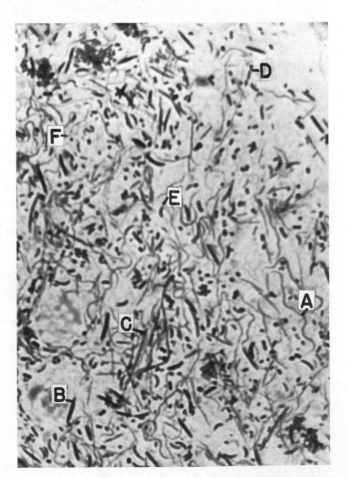

Figure 11–4   Bacterial Smear from Lesion in Acute Necrotizing Ulcerative Gingivitis. A, Spirochete; B, *Bacillus fusiformis;* C, filamentous organism (*Actinomycetes* or *Leptotrichia*); D, *Streptococcus;* E, *Vibrio;* F, *Treponema microdentium.*

account for the majority of the total fusiform bacilli in both groups.

Diagnosis

Diagnosis is based upon clinical findings. A bacterial smear may be used to corroborate the clinical diagnosis, but it is not necessary or definitive because the bacterial picture is not appreciably different from that in marginal gingivitis, periodontal pockets, pericoronitis, or herpetic gingivostomatitis.[39] Bacterial studies are useful, however, in the differential diagnosis between acute necrotizing ulcerative gingivitis and specific infections of the oral cavity such as diphtheria, thrush, actinomycosis, and streptococcal stomatitis.

Microscopic examination of the biopsied tissue is not sufficiently specific to be diagnostic. It can be used to differentiate acute necrotizing ulcerative gingivitis from specific infections such as tuberculosis or from neoplastic disease, but it does not differentiate between acute necrotizing ulcerative gingivitis and other acute necrotizing conditions of nonspecific origin such as those produced by trauma or escharotic drugs.

Differential Diagnosis

Necrotizing ulcerative gingivitis should be differentiated from other conditions that resemble it in some respects, such as acute herpetic gingivostomatitis (Table 11–1), chronic periodontal pockets, desquamative gingivitis (Table 11–2), streptococcal gingivostomatitis, aphthous stomatitis, gonococcal gingivostomatitis, diphtheritic and syphilitic lesions (Table 11–3), tuberculous gingival lesions, moniliasis, agranulocytosis, dermatoses (pemphigus, erythema multiforme, lichen planus), and stomatitis venenata.

Streptococcal gingivostomatitis[29] is a rare condition characterized by a diffuse erythema of the gingiva and other areas of the oral mucosa. In some instances it is confined as a marginal erythema with marginal hemorrhage. Necrosis of the gingival margin is not a feature of this disease, nor is there a notably fetid odor. Bacterial smears show a predominance of streptococcal forms, which upon culture appear as *Streptococcus viridans.*

Gonococcal stomatitis is rare and is caused by *Neisseria gonorrhoeae.* The oral mucosa is covered with a grayish membrane that sloughs off in areas to expose an underlying raw, bleeding surface.[29] It is most common in the newborn and is caused by infection from the maternal passages, but cases in adults caused by direct contact have been described.

Agranulocytosis is characterized by ulceration and necrosis of the gingiva, which resemble that of acute necrotizing ulcerative gingivitis. The oral condition in agranulocytosis is primarily necrotizing. Because of the diminished defense mechanism in agranulocytosis, the clinical picture is not marked by the severe inflammatory reaction seen in acute necrotizing ulcerative gingivitis. Blood studies serve to differentiate between necrotizing ulcerative gingivitis and the gingival necrosis in agranulocytosis.

Vincent's angina is a fusospirochetal infection of the oropharynx and throat, as distinguished from acute necrotizing ulcerative gingivitis, which affects the marginal gingiva. In Vincent's angina there is a painful membranous ulceration of the throat, with edema and hyperemic patches breaking down to form ulcers covered with pseudomembranous material. The process may extend to the larynx and middle ear.

Other conditions to be considered in the differential diagnosis of acute necrotizing ulcerative gingivitis include erythema multiforme, erosive lichen planus, lupus erythematosus, pemphigus, tuberculous ulcer, moniliasis, stomatitis venenata, and chemical burns (see Chapter 12).

ACUTE NECROTIZING ULCERATIVE GINGIVITIS IN LEUKEMIA. Leukemia, per se, does not produce acute necrotizing ulcerative gingival inflammation. However, acute necrotizing ulcerative gingivitis may occur superimposed upon gingival tissues altered by leukemia.

The differential diagnosis consists not in distinguishing between acute necrotizing ulcerative gingivitis and leukemic gingival changes, but rather in determining whether leukemia is a *predisposing factor* in a mouth in which acute necrotizing ulcerative gingivitis is present. For example, if a patient with acute necrotizing involvement of the gingival margin also presents generalized diffuse discoloration and edema of the attached gingiva, the possibility of an *underlying, systemically induced gingival change* should be considered. Leukemia is one of the conditions which would have to be ruled out.

Etiology

THE ROLE OF BACTERIA. Plaut[34] and Vincent,[54] in 1894 and 1896, respectively, intro-

TABLE 11–1 DIFFERENTIATION BETWEEN ACUTE NECROTIZING ULCERATIVE GINGIVITIS AND ACUTE HERPETIC GINGIVOSTOMATITIS

Acute Necrotizing Ulcerative Gingivitis	Acute Herpetic Gingivostomatitis
Etiology: interaction between host and bacteria, most probably fusospirochetes	Specific viral etiology
Necrotizing condition	Diffuse erythema and vesicular eruption
Punched-out gingival margin. Pseudomembrane that peels off leaving raw areas. Marginal gingiva affected, other oral tissues rarely	Vesicles rupture and leave slightly depressed oval or spherical ulcer
	Diffuse involvement of gingiva, may include buccal mucosa and lips
Relatively uncommon in children	Occurs more frequently in children
No definite duration	Duration of 7 to 10 days
No demonstrated immunity	An acute episode results in some degree of immunity
Contagion not demonstrated	Contagious

TABLE 11–2 DIFFERENTIATION BETWEEN ACUTE NECROTIZING ULCERATIVE GINGIVITIS, CHRONIC DESQUAMATIVE GINGIVITIS, AND CHRONIC PERIODONTAL DISEASE

Acute Necrotizing Ulcerative Gingivitis	Desquamative Gingivitis	Chronic Destructive Periodontal Disease
Bacterial smears show fusospirochetal complex	Bacterial smears reveal numerous epithelial cells, few bacterial forms	Bacterial smears are variable
Marginal gingiva affected	Diffuse involvement of the marginal and attached gingiva and other areas of the oral mucosa	Marginal gingiva affected
Acute history	Chronic history	Chronic history
Painful	May or may not be painful	Painless if uncomplicated
Pseudomembrane	Patchy desquamation of the gingival epithelium	No desquamation generally but purulent material may appear from pockets
Papillary and marginal necrotic lesions	Papillae do not undergo necrosis	Papillae do not undergo notable necrosis
Affects adults of both sexes, occasionally children	Affects adults, most often females	Generally in adults, occasionally in children
Characteristic fetid odor	None	Some odor present but not strikingly fetid

TABLE 11–3 DIFFERENTIATION BETWEEN ACUTE NECROTIZING ULCERATIVE GINGIVITIS, DIPHTHERIA, AND SECONDARY STAGE OF SYPHILIS

Acute Necrotizing Ulcerative Gingivitis	Diphtheria	Secondary Stage of Syphilis (Mucous Patch)
Etiology: interaction between host and bacteria, possibly fusospirochetes	Specific bacterial etiology: *Corynebacterium diphtheriae*	Specific bacterial etiology: *Treponema pallidum*
Affects marginal gingiva	Very rarely affects marginal gingiva	Rarely affects marginal gingiva
Membrane removal very easy	Membrane removal difficult	Membrane not detachable
Painful condition	Less painful	Not very painful
Marginal gingiva affected	Throat, fauces, tonsils affected	Any part of mouth affected
Serology negative	Serology negative	Serology positive (Wassermann, Kahn, VDRL)
Immunity not conferred	Immunity conferred by an attack	Immunity not conferred
Doubtful contagiousness	Very contagious	Only direct contact will communicate the disease
Antibiotic therapy relieves symptoms	Antibiotic treatment has little effect	Antibiotic therapy has excellent results

duced the concept that acute necrotizing ulcerative gingivitis is caused by specific bacteria, namely, a fusiform bacillus and a spirochetal organism.

Opinions still differ regarding whether bacteria are the primary causative factors in acute necrotizing ulcerative gingivitis. Several observations encourage the concept of primary etiology: **spirochetal organisms and fusiform bacilli are always found in the disease;** other organisms are also involved. Rosebury et al.[39] described a fusospirochetal complex consisting of *Treponema microdentium,* intermediate spirochetes, vibrios, fusiform bacilli, and filamentous organisms in addition to several species termed *Borrelia.* The fact that necrotizing ulcerative gingivitis occurs in groups, suggesting contagion, supports the concept of bacterial origin. The pathogenic mechanism of bacteria, however, remains unclear. An immune pathogenesis has been postulated on the basis of differences in cell-mediated immunity between patients and controls (as measured by the lymphocyte transformation test)[56] and the decreased salivary immunoglobulin concentration in patients with acute necrotizing ulcerative gingivitis as compared with normal persons.[19]

Acute necrotizing ulcerative gingivitis has not been produced experimentally in humans or animals by inoculation of bacterial exudates from the lesions. Exudates from acute necrotizing ulcerative gingivitis produce fusospirochetal abscesses when inoculated subcutaneously in experimental animals, and the infection is freely transmissible in series.[38] Local intracutaneous injection of a hyaluronidase- and chondroitinase-containing cell-free filtrate of oral microaerophilic diphtheroid bacilli aggravated spirochetal lesions produced by oral treponemes.[18] Only in one animal exeriment has the transmission of lesions comparable to those seen in man been reported.[2]

The specific etiology of acute necrotizing ulcerative gingivitis has not been established. The prevalent opinion is that it is caused by a complex of bacterial organisms but requires underlying tissue changes to facilitate the pathogenic activity of the bacteria. In addition to fusiform bacilli, spirochetes, vibrios, and streptococci are invariably included in the complex of bacteria isolated from the lesions in this group of diseases. The other diseases in the group are Vincent's angina, cancrum oris, genital fusospirochetosis, pulmonary fusospirochetosis, tropical ulcer, gangrenous stomatitis, and noma.

LOCAL PREDISPOSING FACTORS. Pre-existing gingivitis, injury to the gingiva, and smoking are important predisposing factors. Although necrotizing ulcerative gingivitis may appear in an otherwise disease-free mouth, it most often occurs *superimposed upon pre-existing chronic gingival disease and periodontal pockets.* Chronic inflammation entails circulatory and degenerative alterations that increase the susceptibility to infection. Any local factors capable of inducing chronic gingival inflammation may predispose to acute necrotizing ulcerative gingivitis. Deep periodontal pockets and pericoronal flaps are particularly vulnerable areas for the occurrence of the disease because they offer a favorable environment for the proliferation of the anaerobic fusiform bacilli and spirochetes. Box[3] refers to such locations as *"incubation zones."*

Areas of the gingiva traumatized by opposing teeth in malocclusion, such as the palatal surface behind the maxillary incisors and the labial gingival surface of the mandibular incisors, are frequent sites of acute necrotizing ulcerative gingivitis.

SYSTEMIC PREDISPOSING FACTORS. Acute necrotizing ulcerative gingivitis is often superimposed upon gingiva altered by severe systemic disease.

Nutritional Deficiency. Necrotizing gingivitis has been produced by placing animals on nutritionally deficient diets.[16, 22, 31, 45, 50, 53] Animals on diets deficient in vitamin B complex in particular developed severe oral ulcerating lesions.[6] Several authors found an increase in the fusospirochetal flora in the mouths of the experimental animals, but the bacteria were regarded as opportunists, proliferating only when the tissues were altered by the vitamin deficiency. Clinical observations have been presented that suggest that low vitamin intake[24] or vitamin C deficiency[36] predisposes to acute necrotizing ulcerative gingivitis.

The Conditioning Effect of Nutritional Deficiency upon Bacterial Pathogenicity. Nutritional deficiencies (vitamin C deficiency) accentuate the severity of the pathologic changes induced when the fusospirochetal bacterial complex is injected into animals.[45] Necrotizing lesions have been produced by injecting fusospirochetal organisms into vitamin B_2–deficient rats.[23] A correlation between vitamin C deficiency and intestinal fusospirochetosis has been reported in humans and animals.[57] Fusospirochetes may gain a foothold in the intestines in small breaks in the mucosa caused by vitamin C deficiency–induced mucosal hemorrhages.

Debilitating Disease. Debilitating systemic disease may predispose the gingiva to acute necrotizing ulcerative gingivitis. Included among such systemic disturbances are metallic intoxication, cachexia caused by such chronic diseases as syphilis and cancer, severe gastrointestinal disorders such as ulcerative colitis, blood dyscrasias such as the leukemias and anemia, influenza, and the common cold.[7] Nutritional deficiency secondary to debilitating disease may be an additional predisposing factor. Fusospirochetal abscesses and gingival bleeding have been produced in experimental animals by injecting scillaren B, a mixture of glucosides derived from squill, which lowers tissue resistance by reducing the leukocytes.[48, 51] An ulcerative gangrenous stomatitis occurred in animals with experimentally induced leukopenia.[31, 47] Necrotizing gingivitis and stomatitis occurred in 74 per cent of animals with experimentally produced renal insufficiency.[17] Mayo et al.[28] have produced ulceronecrotic lesions in the gingival margin of hamsters exposed to total body irradiation; these lesions could be prevented by systemic antibiotics.[27]

PSYCHOSOMATIC FACTORS. Psychologic factors appear to be important in the etiology of acute necrotizing ulcerative gingivitis. The disease often occurs under stress situations such as induction into the army and school examinations.[11, 15] Psychologic disturbances are common in patients with the disease,[17] along with increased adrenocortical secretion.[42] Significant correlation between disease incidence and two personality traits, dominance and abasement, suggests the presence of an acute necrotizing ulcerative gingivitis–prone personality.[13] The mechanisms whereby psychologic factors create or predispose to gingival damage have not been established, but alterations in digital and gingival capillary responses suggestive of increased autonomic nervous activity have been demonstrated in patients with acute necrotizing ulcerative gingivitis.[14]

Epidemiology and Prevalence

Acute necrotizing ulcerative gingivitis often occurs in groups in an epidemic pattern. At one time it was considered contagious, but this has not been substantiated.[40]

The prevalence of acute necrotizing ulcerative gingivitis appears to have been rather low in the United States and Europe prior to 1914. In World Wars I and II there were numerous "epidemics" among the Allied troops, but Germans did not seem to be similarly affected. There have also been epidemic-like outbreaks among civilian populations. In individuals attending a dental clinic, the following prevalence was reported: 0.08 per cent between 15 and 19 years of age, 0.05 per cent between 20 and 24 years, and 0.02 per cent between 25 and 29 years.[44]

Acute necrotizing ulcerative gingivitis occurs at all ages,[8] with the highest prevalence reported between ages 20 and 30[9, 46] and between ages 15 and 20.[25] It is not common in children in the United States, Canada, and Europe, but it has been reported in children from low socioeconomic groups in underdeveloped countries.[21] In India 54 per cent[30] and 58 per cent[33] of the patients in two studies were under 10 years old. In a random school population in Nigeria acute necrotizing ulcerative gingivitis occurred in 11.3 per cent of children between the ages of 2 and 6 years,[43] and in a Nigerian hospital population it was present in 23 per cent of children under 10 years old.[11] In low socioeconomic groups it has been reported in several members of the same family. It is more common in children with Down's syndrome than in other retarded children.[4]

Opinions differ as to whether it is more common during the winter,[32, 35] summer, or fall,[23, 44] or whether there are no peak seasons.[9, 55]

COMMUNICABILITY. A distinction must be made between communicability and transmissibility when referring to the characteristics of disease. The term *transmissible* denotes a capacity for the maintenance of an infectious agent in successive passage through a susceptible animal host.[37] The term *communicable* signifies a capacity for the maintenance of infection by natural modes of spread such as direct contact through drinking water, food, and eating utensils; via the airborne route; or by means of arthropod vectors. A disease that is communicable is described as contagious. It has been demonstrated that disease associated with the fusospirochetal bacterial complex is transmissible; *however, it has not been shown to be communicable or contagious.*

Attempts have been made to spread acute necrotizing ulcerative gingivitis from human to human, without success.[41] King[22] traumatized an area in his gingiva and introduced debris from a patient with a severe case of acute necrotizing ulcerative gingivitis. There was no response until he happened to fall ill shortly thereafter; and subsequent to his illness, he observed the characteristic lesion in the experimental area. It may be inferred with reservation from this experiment that systemic debility is a prerequisite for the contagion of acute necrotizing ulcerative gingivitis.

It is a common impression that, because acute necrotizing ulcerative gingivitis often occurs in groups using the same kitchen facilities, the disease is spread by bacteria on eating utensils. Growth of fusospirochetal organisms requires extremely carefully controlled conditions and an anaerobic environment; they do not ordinarily survive on eating utensils.[18]

The occurrence of the disease in epidemic-like outbreaks does not necessarily mean that it is contagious. The affected groups may be afflicted by the disease because of common predisposing factors rather than because of its spread from person to person. In all likelihood both a predisposed host and appropriate bacteria are necessary for the production of this disease.

REFERENCES TO ACUTE NECROTIZING ULCERATIVE GINGIVITIS

1. Barnes, G. P., Bowles, W. F., III, and Carter, H. G.: Acute necrotizing ulcerative gingivitis: a survey of 218 cases. J. Periodontol., *44*:35, 1973.
2. Berke, J. D.: Experimental study of acute ulcerative stomatitis. J. Am. Dent. Assoc., *63*:86, 1961.
3. Box, H. K.: Necrotic Gingivitis. Toronto, University of Toronto Press, 1930.
4. Brown, R. H.: Necrotizing ulcerative gingivitis in mongoloid and non-mongoloid retarded individuals. J. Periodont. Res., *8*:290, 1973.
5. Cahn, L. R.: The penetration of the tissue by Vincent's organisms. A report of a case. J. Dent. Res., *9*:695, 1929.
6. Chapman, O. D., and Harris, A. E.: Oral lesions associated with dietary deficiencies in monkeys. J. Infect. Dis., *69*:7, 1941.
7. Coutley, R. L.: Vincent's infection. Br. Dent. J., *74*:34, 1943.
8. Daley, F. H.: Studies of Vincent's infection at the clinic of Tufts College Dental School from October, 1926 to February, 1928. J. Dent. Res., *8*:408, 1928.
9. Dean, H. T., and Singleton, J. E., Jr.: Vincent's infection—a wartime disease. Am. J. Public Health, *35*:433, 1945.
10. Ellerman: Vincent's organisms in tissue. Z. Hyg. Infekt. Pr.. *56*:453, 1907.
11. Emslie, R. D.: Cancrum oris. Dent. Pract., *13*:481, 1963.
12. Enwonwu, C. O.: Epidemiological and biochemical studies of necrotizing ulcerative gingivitis and noma (cancrum oris) in Nigerian children. Arch. Oral Biol., *17*:1357, 1972.
13. Formicola, A. J., Witte, E. T., and Curran, P. M.: A study of personality traits and acute necrotizing ulcerative gingivitis. J. Periodontol., *41*:36, 1970.
14. Giddon, D. B.: Psychophysiology of the oral cavity. J. Dent. Res., *45*(Suppl. 6):1627, 1966.
15. Giddon, D. B., Zackin, S. J., and Goldhaber, P.: Acute necrotizing gingivitis in college students. J. Am. Dent. Assoc., *68*:381, 1964.
16. Goldberger, J., and Wheeler, G. A.: Experimental black tongue of dogs and its relation to pellagra. U.S. Public Health Rep., *43*:172, 1928.
17. Goldhaber, P., and Giddon, D. B.: Present concepts concerning the etiology and treatment of acute necrotizing ulcerative gingivitis. Int. Dent. J., *14*:468, 1964.
18. Hampp, E. G., and Mergenhagen, S. E.: Experimental infection with oral spirochetes. J. Infect. Dis., *109*:43, 1961.
19. Harding, J., Berry, W. C., Marsh, C., and Jolliff, C. R.: Salivary antibodies in acute gingivitis. J. Periodontol., *51*:63, 1980.
20. Hooper, P. A., and Seymour, G. J.: The histopathogenesis of acute ulcerative gingivitis. J. Periodontol., *50*:419, 1979.
21. Jimenez, M., and Baer, P. N.: Necrotizing ulcerative gingivitis in children: a 9 year clinical study. J. Periodontol., *46*:715, 1975.
22. King, J. D.: Nutritional and other factors in trench mouth with special reference to the nicotinic acid component of vitamin B complex. Br. Dent. J., *74*:113. 1943.
23. Kirkpatrick, R. M., and Clements, F. W.: Diet in relation to Vincent's infection. Dent. J. Aust., *6*:371, 1934.
24. Lapira, E.: Ulcerative stomatitis associated with avitaminosis in Malta. Br. Dent. J., *74*:257, 1943.
25. Listgarten, M. A.: Electron microscopic observations on the bacterial flora of acute necrotizing ulcerative gingivitis. J. Periodontol., *36*:328, 1965.
26. Listgarten, M. A., and Lewis, D. W.: The distribution of spirochetes in the lesion of acute necrotizing ulcerative gingivitis: an electron microscopic and statistical survey. J. Periodontol., *38*:379, 1967.
27. Mayo, J., Carranza, F. A., Jr., and Cabrini, R. L.: Comparative study of the effect of antibiotics, bone marrow and cysteamine on oral lesions produced in hamsters by total body irradiation. Experientia, *20*:403, 1964.
28. Mayo, J., Carranza, F. A., Jr., Epper, C. E., and Cabrini, R. L.: The effect of total-body irradiation on the oral tissues of the Syrian hamster. Oral Surg., *15*:739, 1962.
29. McCarthy, P. L., and Shklar, G.: Diseases of the Oral Mucosa. 2nd ed. Philadelphia, Lea & Febiger, 1980.
30. Miglani, D. C., and Sharma, O. P.: Incidence of acute necrotizing gingivitis and periodontosis among cases seen at the government hospital, Madras. J. All India Dent. Assoc., *37*:183, 1965.
31. Miller, D. K., and Rhoads, C. P.: The experimental production in dogs of acute stomatitis associated with leukopenia and a maturation defect of the myeloid elements of the bone marrow. J. Exp. Med., *61*:173, 1935.
32. Pedler, J. A., and Radden, B. G.: Seasonal influence of acute ulcerative gingivitis. Dent. Pract., *8*:23, 1957.
33. Pindborg, J. J., et al.: Occurrence of acute necrotizing gingivitis in South Indian children. J. Periodontol., *37*:14, 1966.
34. Plaut, H. C.: Studien zur bakteriellen Diagnostik der Diphtherie und der Anginen. Dtsch. Med. Wochnschr., *20*:920, 1894.
35. Proske, H. O., and Sayers, R. R.: Pulmonary fusospirochetal infection. U.S. Public Health Rep., *49*:839, 1934.
36. Radusch, D. F.: Nutrition and dental health. J. Periodontol., *17*:27, 1946.
37. Rosebury, T.: Is Vincent's infection a communicable disease? J. Am. Dent. Assoc., *29*:823, 1942.
38. Rosebury, T., and Foley, G.: Experimental Vincent's infection. J. Am. Dent. Assoc., *26*:1978, 1939.
39. Rosebury, T., MacDonald, J. B., and Clark, A.: A bacteriologic survey of gingival scrapings from periodontal infections by direct examination, guinea pig inoculation and anaerobic cultivation. J. Dent. Res., *29*:718, 1950.
40. Schluger, S.: Necrotizing ulcerative gingivitis in the army. Incidence, communicability, and treatment. J. Am. Dent. Assoc., *38*:174, 1949.
41. Schwartzman, J., and Grossman, L.: Vincent's ulceromembranous gingivostomatitis. Arch. Pediatr., *58*:515, 1941.
42. Shannon, I. L., Kilgore, W. G., and Leary, T. J.: Stress as a predisposing factor in necrotizing ulcerative gingivitis. J. Periodontol., *40*:240, 1969.
43. Sheiham, A.: An epidemiological study of oral disease in Nigerians. J. Dent. Res., *44*:1184, 1965.
44. Skach, M., Zabrodsky, S., and Mrklas, L.: A study of the effect of age and season on the incidence of ulcerative gingivitis. J. Periodont. Res., *5*:187, 1970.
45. Smith, D. T.: Spirochetes and related organisms in fusospirochetal disease. Baltimore, Williams & Wilkins Company, 1932.
46. Stammers, A. F.: Vincent's infection. Br. Dent. J., *76*:171, 1944.
47. Swenson, H. M.: Induced Vincent's infection in dogs. J. Dent. Res., *23*:190, 1944.
48. Swenson, H. M., and Muhler, J. C.: Induced fusospirochetal infection in dogs. J. Dent. Res., *26*:161, 1947.
49. Thompson, L. E.: A fatal case of brain abscess from Vincent's angina. Dent. Digest, *35*:821, 1929.
50. Topping, N. H., and Fraser, H. F.: Mouth lesions associated with dietary deficiencies in monkeys. U.S. Public Health Rep., *54*:431, 1939.
51. Tunnicliff, R., and Hammond, C.: Abscess production by fusiform bacilli in rabbits and mice by the use of Scillaren–B or Mucin, J. Dent. Res., *16*:479, 1937.

52. Tunnicliff, R., Fink, E. B., and Hammond, C.: Significance of fusiform bacilli and spirilla in gingival tissue. J. Am. Dent. Assoc., *23*:1959, 1936.
53. Underhill, F. P., and Mendel, L. B.: Further experiments on the pellagra-like syndrome in dogs. Am. J. Physiol., *83*:589, 1928
54. Vincent, H.: Sur l'étiologie et sur les lésions anatomopathologiques, de la pourriture d'hôpital. Ann. de l'Inst. Pasteur, *10*:448, 1896.
55. Wilkie, R.: An etiology of Vincent's gingivitis. Br. Dent. J., *78*:65, 1945.
56. Wilton, J. M. A., Ivanyi, A., and Lehner, T.: Cell-mediated immunity and humoral antibodies in acute ulcerative gingivitis. J. Periodont. Res., 6:9, 1971.
57. Woolsey, F. M., and Black, S. R.: Vitamin C deficiency and intestinal fusospirochetoses. Arch. Pathol., *28*:503, 1939.

ACUTE HERPETIC GINGIVOSTOMATITIS

Etiology

Acute herpetic gingivostomatitis is an infection of the oral cavity caused by the herpes simplex virus.[6, 13, 17] Secondary bacterial infection frequently complicates the clinical picture. Acute herpetic gingivostomatitis occurs most frequently in infants and children below the age of 6 years,[17] but it is also seen in adolescents and adults. It occurs with equal frequency in males and females.

Clinical Features

ORAL SIGNS. The condition appears as a diffuse, erythematous, shiny involvement of the gingiva and the adjacent oral mucosa, with varying degrees of edema and gingival bleeding (Plate II*E*). In its initial stage, it is characterized by the presence of discrete spherical gray vesicles (Plate II*F*), which may occur on the gingiva, the labial and buccal mucosa, the soft palate, the pharynx, the sublingual mucosa, and the tongue (Fig. 11–5). After approximately 24 hours the vesicles rupture and form painful small ulcers with a red, elevated, halo-like margin and a depressed yellowish or grayish-white central portion. These occur either in widely separated areas or in clusters where confluence occurs (Fig. 11–6).

Occasionally, acute herpetic gingivitis may occur without overt vesiculation. Diffuse, erythematous, shiny discoloration and edematous enlargement of the gingivae with a tendency toward bleeding make up the clinical picture.

The course of the disease is limited to 7 to 10 days. The diffuse gingival erythema and edema that appear early in the disease persist for several days after the ulcerative lesions have healed. Scarring does not occur in the areas of healed ulcerations.

Acute herpetic gingivostomatitis may appear in a *localized* form following operative procedures in the oral cavity. Surfaces of the oral mucosa traumatized by cotton rolls or vigorous application of digital pressure in the course of operative procedures are the sites of predilection. The condition appears 1 or 2 days after the trauma, and the involvement presents a diffuse, shiny erythema with numerous pinpoint vesicles confined to an area that can be clearly demarcated from the adjacent uninvolved mucosa (Fig. 11–7). The vesicles rupture and form painful ulcerations. The duration of the involvement is 7 to 10 days, followed by uneventful healing.

ORAL SYMPTOMS. The disease is accompanied by generalized "soreness" of the oral cavity, which interferes with eating and drinking. The ruptured vesicles are the focal sites of pain and are particularly sensitive to touch, thermal changes, condiments, fruit juices, and the excursive action of coarse foods. In infants the disease is marked by irritability and refusal to take food.

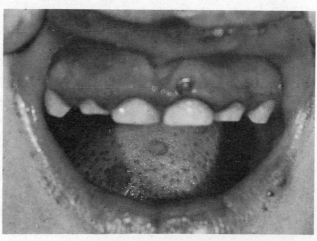

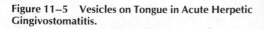
Figure 11–5   Vesicles on Tongue in Acute Herpetic Gingivostomatitis.

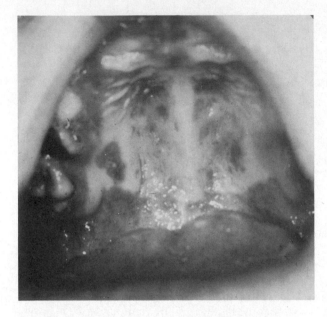

Figure 11–6   Involvement of the Palate in Acute Herpetic Gingivostomatitis.

EXTRAORAL AND SYSTEMIC SIGNS AND SYMPTOMS. Herpetic involvement of the lips or face (herpes labialis, "cold sore"), with vesicles and surface scab formation, may accompany the intraoral disease (Fig. 11–8). Cervical adenitis, fever as high as 101 to 105° F (38.3 to 40.6° C), and generalized malaise are common.

HISTORY. Recent acute infection is a common feature of the history of patients with acute herpetic gingivostomatitis.[6] The condition frequently occurs during and immediately after an episode of such febrile diseases as pneumonia, meningitis, influenza, and typhoid. It also tends to occur in periods of anxiety, strain, or exhaustion and during menstruation. A history of exposure to patients with herpetic infection of the oral cavity or lips may also be elicited. Acute herpetic gingivostomatitis often occurs in the early stage of infectious mononucleosis.[14]

Histopathology

The discrete ulcerations of herpetic gingivostomatitis that result from rupture of the vesicles present a central portion of acute inflammation, with ulceration and varying degrees of purulent exudate, surrounded by a zone rich in engorged blood vessels. The microscopic picture of the vesicles is characterized by extra- and intracellular edema and degeneration of the epithelial cells. The cell

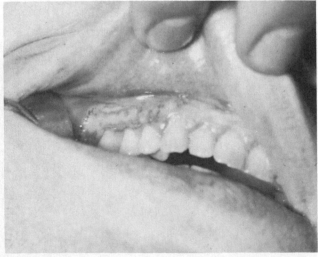
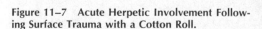

Figure 11–7   Acute Herpetic Involvement Following Surface Trauma with a Cotton Roll.

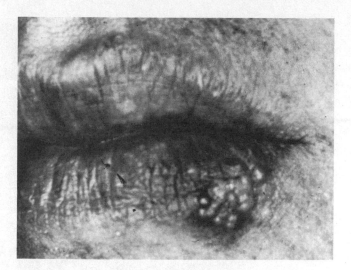

Figure 11–8   Cluster of Hepetic Vesicles ("Cold Sore").

cytoplasm appears liquefied and clear; the cell membrane and nucleus stand out in relief. The nucleus later degenerates, loses its affinity for stain, and finally disintegrates. The vesicle formation results from fragmentation of the degenerated epithelial cells.

The fully developed vesicle is a cavity in the epithelial cells with occasional polymorphonuclear leukocytes. The base of the vesicle is formed by edematous epithelial cells of the basal and prickle cell layers. The superficial surface of the vesicle is formed by compressed upper layers of prickle cells of the stratum granulosum and the stratum corneum. Occasionally, rounded eosinophilic inclusion bodies[12] are found in the nuclei of epithelial cells bordering vesicles. Inclusion bodies may be a colony of virus particles, degenerated protoplasm remnants of the affected cell, or a combination of both.[15]

Diagnosis

The diagnosis is usually established from the patient's history and the clinical findings.[11] Material may be obtained from the lesions and submitted to the laboratory for confirmatory tests.

DIRECT SMEARS. If the vesicle is intact, the top is removed and the fluid allowed to escape. The base of the lesion is scraped with a sharp instrument, and the material obtained is smeared on a glass, allowed to dry, and stained. The finding of multinuclear cells with swelling, ballooning, and degeneration is adequate for diagnosis; negative findings due to too early or too late sampling constitute a

serious limitation.[4] Electron microscopy of fresh or formalin-fixed material can also be used for diagnosis of herpetic infections.[16] Immunofluorescent antibody techniques have also been used successfully.[8]

ISOLATION OF THE VIRUS. This can be done in tissue culture or in the chorioallantoic membrane of a chick embryo. For the analysis in *tissue culture*, material obtained from the lesion on a sterile cotton-tipped applicator is sent to the laboratory in skimmed milk. This is then inoculated into cultures of susceptible cells and incubated for 24 hours. Degenerative cellular changes preventable by antibody to herpes simplex constitute a positive finding.

For the analysis in *chick embryo*, the material removed from the suspected lesion is placed in salivary solution or thioglycolate medium. Small amounts of the material are injected into 10-day-old embryonated eggs; after 48 hours the egg is opened and the chorioallantoic membrane is inspected for pocks or viral colonies.

ANTIBODY TITRATIONS. If a specimen of blood is collected when the patient is first seen and examined for neutralizing antibodies, none will be found. Successive specimens taken during the convalescent period will show a rising titer of neutralizing antibodies that will remain high permanently.

BIOPSY. Stained sections of the vesicles of acute herpetic gingivostomatitis, herpes zoster, and varicella (chicken pox) reveal eosinophilic intranuclear inclusion bodies in the peripheral cells (Fig. 11–9).

HEMATOLOGIC STUDIES. It has not been possible to demonstrate alterations in the hematologic picture of patients with acute herpetic gingivostomatitis.

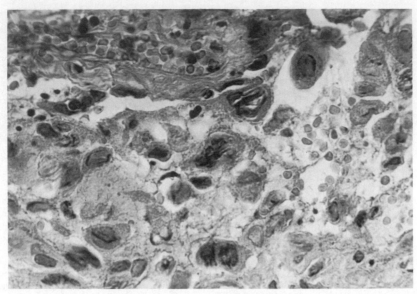

Figure 11–9   Biopsy Showing Giant Cells with Inclusion Bodies at Base of Herpetic Lesion.

Differential Diagnosis

Acute herpetic gingivostomatitis should be differentiated from the following conditions:

ACUTE NECROTIZING ULCERATIVE GINGIVITIS. (See page 146.)

ERYTHEMA MULTIFORME. The vesicles in erythema multiforme are generally more extensive than those in acute herpetic gingivostomatitis and upon rupture present a tendency toward pseudomembrane formation. In addition, the tongue in the former condition usually is markedly involved, with infection of the ruptured vesicles resulting in varying degrees of ulceration. Oral involvement in erythema multiforme may be accompanied by skin lesions. The duration of erythema multiforme may be comparable to that of acute herpetic gingivostomatitis, but prolonged involvement for a period of weeks is not uncommon.

The Stevens-Johnson Syndrome. This is a comparatively rare form of erythema multiforme, characterized by vesicular hemorrhagic lesions in the oral cavity, hemorrhagic ocular lesions, and bullous skin lesions.

BULLOUS LICHEN PLANUS. This painful condition, characterized by large blisters on the tongue and cheek that rupture and undergo ulceration, runs a prolonged, indefinite course. Patches of linear gray lace-like lesions of lichen planus are often interspersed among the bullous eruptions. Coexistent involvement of the skin in the former affords a basis for differentiation between bullous lichen planus and acute herpetic gingivostomatitis.

DESQUAMATIVE GINGIVITIS. This condition is characterized by diffuse involvement of the gingiva, with varying degrees of "peeling" of the epithelial surface and exposure of the underlying tissue. It is a chronic condition.

APHTHOUS STOMATITIS (CANKER SORE). This is a condition characterized by the appearance of discrete spherical vesicles that rupture after 1 or 2 days and form depressed spherical ulcers. The ulcers consist of a saucer-like red or grayish-red central portion and an elevated rim-like periphery (Fig. 11–10). The lesions may occur anywhere in the oral cavity, the mucobuccal fold and the floor of the mouth being common sites. Aphthous stomatitis is

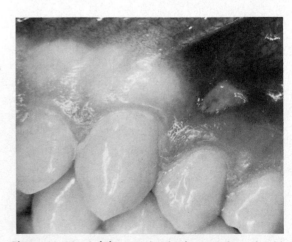

Figure 11–10   Aphthous Lesion in the Mucobuccal Fold. The depressed gray center is surrounded by an elevated red border.

painful. It may occur as a single lesion or as lesions scattered throughout the mouth. The duration of each lesion is 7 to 10 days. As a rule, the lesions are larger than those seen in acute herpetic gingivostomatitis.

Aphthous stomatitis occurs in the following forms:

Occasional Aphthae. In this condition a single lesion occurs occasionally, at intervals that vary from months to years. Healing of the lesion is followed by uneventful recovery.

Acute Aphthae. This condition is characterized by an acute episode of aphthae, which may persist for weeks. During this period, lesions appear in different areas of the mouth, replacing others that are healing or healed. Such acute episodes are often seen in children with acute gastrointestinal disorders and may also occur in adults under comparable conditions. Remission of the gastrointestinal disturbance is generally accompanied by cessation of the acute episode of aphthae.

Chronic Recurrent Aphthae. This is a perplexing condition in which one or more oral lesions are always present. The involvement may extend over a period of years. In rare instances, lesions on the genital, anal, and conjunctival mucosa accompany the oral aphthae. One or more oral lesions are always present. The duration of involvement with chronic aphthae may be a period of years.

The etiology of aphthous stomatitis is unknown. Herpes simplex virus was suspected to be the cause, but antibody[20] and tissue-culture[18] studies discourage this opinion. Other factors suggested as causing or predisposing to aphthous stomatitis include hormonal disturbances, allergic phenomena,[2] gastrointestinal disorders, and psychosomatic factors.[1]

Aphthous stomatitis is a different clinical entity from acute herpetic gingivostomatitis.[7, 21] The ulcerations may look the same in the two conditions, but diffuse erythematous involvement of the gingiva and acute toxic systemic symptoms do not occur in aphthous stomatitis.

Communicability

Acute herpetic gingivostomatitis is contagious.[5, 12] Most adults have developed immunity to herpes simplex virus as the result of infection during childhood,[3] which in most instances is subclinical. For this reason acute herpetic gingivostomatitis occurs most often in infants and children. Although recurrent herpetic gingivostomatitis has been reported,[10] it does not ordinarily recur unless immunity is destroyed by debilitating systemic disease. Herpetic infection of the skin, such as herpes labialis, does recur.[19]

REFERENCES TO ACUTE HERPETIC GINGIVOSTOMATITIS

1. Alexander, F., and French, W.: Studies in Psychosomatic Medicine, Chicago, University of Chicago Press, 1948.
2. Brinck, O.: Clinical observations on the etiology of stomatitis aphthosa. Paradentium, *11*:192, 1939.
3. Burnet, F. M., and Williams, S. W.: Herpes simplex: new point of view. Med. J. Aust., *1*:637, 1939.
4. Cawson, R. A.: Infections of the oral mucous membrane. *In* Cohen, B., and Kramer, I. R. H. (eds.): Scientific Foundations of Dentistry. Chicago, Year Book Medical Publishers, 1976.
5. Chilton, N. W.: Herpetic stomatitis. Am. J. Orthod. Oral Surg., *30*:335, 1944.
6. Dodd, K., Johnston, L. M., and Buddingh, G. J.: Herpetic stomatitis. J. Pediatr., *12*:95, 1938.
7. Dodd, R., and Ruchman, J.: Herpes simplex virus not the etiologic agent of recurrent stomatitis. Pediatrics, *5*:833, 1950.
8. Gardner, P. S., McQuillin, J., Black, M. M., and Richardson, J.: Rapid diagnosis of herpesvirus hominis infections in superficial lesions by immunofluorescent antibody techniques. Br. Med. J., *4*:89, 1968.
9. Greenberg, M. S., Brightman, V. J., and Ship, I. I.: Clinical and laboratory differentiation of recurrent intraoral herpes simplex virus infections following fever. J. Dent. Res., *48*:385, 1969.
10. Griffin, J. W.: Recurrent intraoral herpes simplex virus infection. Oral Surg., *19*:209, 1965.
11. Grinspan, D.: Enfermedades de la Boca, Vol. 2: Patologia Clínica y Terapeutica de la Mucosa Bucal. Buenos Aires, Ed. Mundi, 1972.
12. Levine, H. D., et al.: Vesicular pharyngitis and stomatitis. J.A.M.A., *112*:2020, 1939.
13. McNair, S. T.: Herpetic stomatitis. J. Dent. Res., *29*:647, 1950.
14. Nathanson, I., and Morin, G. E.: Herpetic stomatitis. An aid in the early diagnosis of infectious mononucleosis. Oral Surg., *6*:1284, 1953.
15. Nicolau, S., and Kopciowska, L.: Inclusion bodies in experimental herpes. Ann. Inst. Pasteur, *60*:401, 1938.
16. Roy, S., and Wolman, L.: Electron microscopic observations on the virus particles in herpes simplex encephalitis. J. Clin. Pathol., *22*:51, 1969.
17. Scott, T. F. M., Steigman, A. S., and Convey, J. H.: Acute infectious gingivostomatitis: etiology, epidemiology, and clinical picture of common disorders caused by virus of herpes simplex. J.A.M.A., *117*:999, 1941.
18. Ship, I. I., Ashe, W. K., and Scherp, H. W.: Recurrent "fever blister" and "canker sore": test for herpes simplex and other viruses with mammalian cell cultures. Arch. Oral Biol., *3*:117, 1961.
19. Ship, I. I., Brightman, V. J., and Laster, L. L.: The patient with recurrent aphthous ulcers and the patient with recurrent herpes labialis: a study of two population samples. J. Am. Dent. Assoc., *75*:645, 1967.
20. Stark, M. M., Kibbrick, S., and Weisberger, D.: Studies on recurrent aphthae. Evidence that herpes simplex is not the etiologic agent with further observations on the immune responses in herpetic infection. J. Lab. Clin. Med., *44*:261, 1954.
21. Weathers, D. R., and Griffin, J. W.: Intraoral ulcerations of recurrent herpes simplex and recurrent aphthae: two distinct clinical entities. J. Am. Dent. Assoc., *81*:81, 1970.

PERICORONITIS

The term *pericoronitis* refers to inflammation of the gingiva in relation to the crown of an incompletely erupted tooth (Fig. 11–11). It

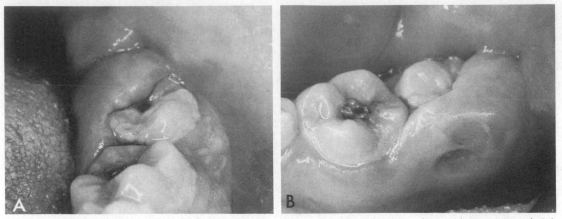

Figure 11–11   Pericoronitis. *A,* Third molar partially covered by infected flap. *B,* Lingual view showing sinus draining from infected flap.

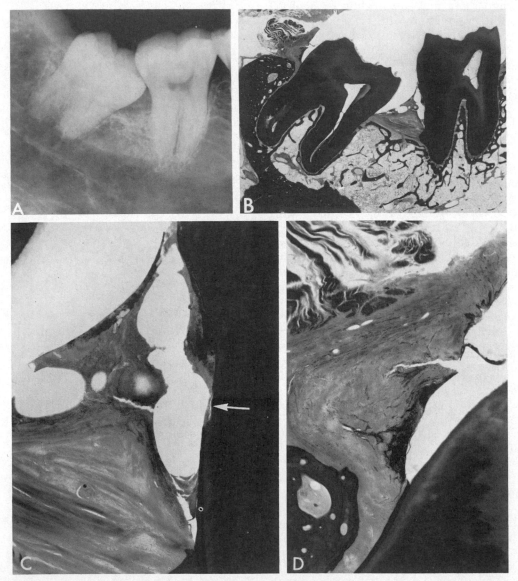

Figure 11–12   Pericoronitis Around Impacted Third Molar. *A,* Radiograph of impacted mandibular third molar. *B,* Survey section of molar area. *C,* Plaque, bacteria, and calculus between the second and third molars. Note the resorption of cementum and dentin on the distal surface of the second molar *(arrow). D,* Inflamed gingiva on the distal surface of the third molar.

occurs most frequently in the mandibular third molar area.[1, 4, 5] Pericoronitis may be acute, subacute, or chronic.

Clinical Features

The partially erupted or impacted mandibular third molar is the most common site of pericoronitis. The space between the crown of the tooth and the overlying gingival flap is an ideal area for the accumulation of food debris and bacterial growth (Fig. 11–12). Even in patients with no clinical signs or symptoms, the gingival flap is often chronically inflamed and infected and presents varying degrees of ulceration along its inner surface. Acute inflammatory involvement is a constant possibility.

Acute pericoronitis is identified by varying degrees of involvement of the pericoronal flap and adjacent structures, as well as systemic complications. An influx of inflammatory fluid and cellular exudate results in an increase in the bulk of the flap, which interferes with complete closure of the jaws. The flap is traumatized by contact with the opposing jaw and the inflammatory involvement is aggravated. **The resultant clinical picture is that of a markedly red, swollen, suppurating lesion that is exquisitely tender, with radiating pains to the ear, throat, and floor of the mouth.** In addition to the pain, the patient is extremely uncomfortable because of a foul taste and an inability to close the jaws. Swelling of the cheek in the region of the angle of the jaw and lymphadenitis are common findings. The patient may also present toxic systemic complications such as fever, leukocytosis, and malaise.

Complications

The involvement may become localized in the form of a pericoronal abscess. It may spread posteriorly into the oropharyngeal area and medially to the base of the tongue, making it difficult for the patient to swallow. Depending upon the severity and extent of the infection, there is involvement of the submaxillary, posterior cervical, deep cervical, and retropharyngeal lymph nodes.[2, 3] Peritonsillar abscess formation, cellulitis, and Ludwig's angina are infrequent but nevertheless potential sequelae of acute pericoronitis.

REFERENCES TO PERICORONITIS

1. Blair, V. P.: The gingival operculum and the erupting lower third molar. Arch. Clin. Oral Pathol., *4*:283, 1940.
2. Jacobs, M. H.: Pericoronal and Vincent's infections: bacteriology and treatment. J. Am. Dent. Assoc., *30*:392, 1943.
3. Perkins, A. E.: Acute infections around erupting mandibular third molar. Br. Dent. J., *76*:199, 1944.
4. Robinson, R. A.: Clinical aspects of diseases associated with impacted mandibular third molars. Arch. Clin. Oral Pathol., *4*:348, 1940.
5. Salman, I.: Pericoronal infection. Dent. Outlook, *26*:460, 1939.

chapter twelve

Desquamative Gingivitis and Oral Mucous Membrane Diseases

A variety of oral mucous membrane diseases are capable of producing erosive or vesiculobullous lesions of the gingiva, with either localized or relatively extensive involvement. Occasionally, the gingival erosive or desquamating lesions may represent the initial expression of a specific mucosal disease, such as lichen planus or pemphigus. In other instances, the disease may be confined to the gingiva, and diagnosis may be more difficult. Gingival involvement may be accompanied by involvement of other areas, but this might be relatively insignificant and could go unobserved unless the gingival pathology alerted the clinician to examine the remainder of the oral mucosa carefully and to obtain an adequate medical history with emphasis on the skin and mucosal sites other than the mouth.

For many years, erosive and desquamating lesions of the gingiva were termed "desquamative gingivitis" and a specific disease entity was postulated. It is now understood that so-called desquamative gingivitis encompasses a variety of different conditions requiring different types of management. An extensive literature on so-called desquamative gingivitis has resulted in considerable confusion over the years; however, since the term is so common, we will continue to use it in this chapter as well.

Desquamative gingivitis will be discussed, followed by a review of the various oral mucosal diseases that can result in erosive, desquamating, or vesiculobullous lesions of the gingiva. These include dermatoses, drug reactions, and chronic bacterial and mycotic infections.

CHRONIC DESQUAMATIVE GINGIVITIS

Chronic desquamative gingivitis is a term that has been used in dental medicine for many years to describe a unique condition of the gingiva characterized by intense redness and desquamation of the surface epithelium. The cause of the condition was unknown, and a variety of etiologic influences were suggested, particularly some form of endocrine imbalance, since most cases were described in postmenopausal females. McCarthy et al.[9] in 1960 reconsidered the literature on desquamative gingivitis and from a study of 40 cases concluded that desquamative gingivitis was not a specific disease entity but, rather, a nonspecific gingival manifestation of a variety of systemic disturbances, some of which are better understood at present than others. A provisional classification can now be suggested based on etiologic considerations.

1. Dermatoses
   a. Lichen planus
   b. Mucous membrane pemphigoid
   c. Bullous pemphigoid
   d. Pemphigus
2. Endocrine Imbalance
   a. Estrogen deficiency in females following hysterectomy with oophorectomy or after menopause
   b. Testosterone deficiency in males
3. Aging (senile atrophic gingivitis)
4. Metabolic Disturbances
   a. Nutritional deficiency (gingivosis)
5. Abnormal Response to Irritation (modification of chronic marginal gingivitis)

6. Idiopathic
7. Chronic Infections
   a. Tuberculosis
   b. Chronic candidiasis
   c. Histoplasmosis
8. Drug Reactions
   a. Toxic—antimetabolites
   b. Allergic—barbiturates, antibiotics, etc.

The large majority of cases of so-called chronic desquamative gingivitis are now understood to represent either lichen planus or mucous membrane pemphigoid, and these and other systemic diseases affecting the gingiva will be discussed in some detail.

Prinz[12] first used the term *chronic diffuse desquamative gingivitis* in 1932, describing 12 patients with chronic diffuse inflammations of the marginal gingiva characterized by desquamation of the epithelium of the papillae and adjacent gingiva. The denuded connective tissue bled upon the slightest irritation. The condition had been described earlier under other names by Tomes and Tomes[23] and by Goadby,[6] who thought that the disease was associated with an anemia. Merritt[10] and Sorrin[21] offered further descriptions and Ziskin and Zegarelli[26] suggested that the condition resulted from a metabolic disorder such as estrogen deficiency or hypothyroidism, and they used estrogen ointment to treat the gingival erythema and desquamation. Ziskin and Zegarelli studied their cases histologically and found vesicle formation in almost half of them. Foss et al.[3] also suggested a disturbance of endocrine function and used topical cortisone to treat their patients. Glickman and Smulow[5] studied the histopathology of desquamative gingivitis and described two principal types— a bullous type characterized by edema and subepithelial vesiculation and a lichenoid type characterized by a dense subepithelial band of chronic inflammatory cells, primarily lymphocytes. Histochemical[2, 20] and ultrastructural studies[1, 11, 24] have not contributed significant information. The electron microscopic changes described are extremely variable and resemble many of the changes described in lichen planus[8, 13] or mucous membrane pemphigoid.[22] Marked multiplication of the basal lamina was noted, as well as interruptions of the basal lamina and its separation from the basal cells.[11] Similar basal lamina changes were described in mucous membrane pemphigoid, including thickening and irregularity.[22] Separation of the epithelium and connective tissue was seen to start with a separation of collagen fibrils and a decrease in the number of anchoring fibrils.

Changes in oral lichen planus were described as a disruption of the basement membrane and an increased irregularity of nuclear membranes of epithelial cells with increased tonofibril thickness.[8, 13]

It is apparent that *the microscopic changes described in so-called desquamative gingivitis are consistent with those of either lichen planus or mucous membrane pemphigoid*. All cases of mucous membrane pemphigoid[17] and those cases of bullous pemphigoid with oral involvement[19] present a desquamative or erosive gingivitis. *However, since mucous membrane pemphigoid is a relatively rare disease, it is probable that the majority of cases of so-called desquamative gingivitis are in fact lichen planus*. A desquamative gingivitis is a rare manifestation of lichen planus (10 to 20 per cent of cases),[16, 25] but lichen planus is a relatively common disease of the mouth, and the incidence of gingival lichen planus should be higher than that of mucous membrane pemphigoid. Careful examination of the mouth in these cases should reveal other manifestations of lichen planus, such as reticulate lesions of the buccal mucosa. However, some cases of lichen planus start with gingival involvement, and other lesions may appear as the disease progresses. Diagnosis may be possible by histologic studies. In mucous membrane pemphigoid, there may be conjunctival lesions as well as involvement of other mucous membrane sites, such as the nasal mucosa, vagina, rectum, and urethra. However, the involvement may be confined to the gingiva in the early stages of the disease, and other oral lesions may follow. Biopsy studies may reveal the characteristic clean separation of the epithelium from the underlying connective tissue. In some cases of desquamative gingivitis, a history of a severe nutritional deficiency may be elicited, as suggested by Schour and Massler's observations[15] on "gingivosis" in Italian children of the immediate post–World War II era.

CLINICAL FEATURES. The clinical features of so-called desquamative gingivitis vary in severity, and mild, moderate, and severe forms have been described by Glickman and Smulow.[4]

Mild Form. In its mildest form there is diffuse erythema of the marginal, interdental, and attached gingivae; the condition is usually painless and comes to the attention of the patient or dentist because of the overall discoloration. The mild form occurs most frequently in females between 17 and 23 years of age.

Moderate Form. This is a more advanced

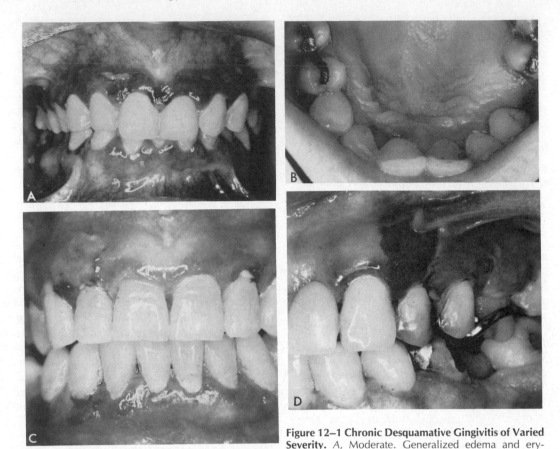

Figure 12–1 Chronic Desquamative Gingivitis of Varied Severity. *A,* Moderate. Generalized edema and erythema associated with inflammation and exposure of underlying connective tissue. *B,* Lingual view of patient shown in *A.* Aside from slight marginal erythema, there is little evidence of change in the gingiva and adjacent mucosa. *C,* Severe. Scattered, irregularly shaped, denuded areas produce a mosaic appearance. Note the ulceration between the right maxillary lateral and canine teeth. *D,* Severe. Complete denudation of the epithelium with exposure of underlying erythematous inflamed connective tissue.

form. It presents a patchy distribution of bright red and gray areas involving the marginal and attached gingivae (Fig. 12–1*A*). The surface is smooth and shiny, and the normally resilient gingiva becomes soft. There is slight pitting upon pressure, and the epithelium is not firmly adherent to the underlying tissues. Massaging the gingiva with the finger results in peeling of the epithelium and exposure of the underlying bleeding connective tissue surface.

The oral mucosa in the remainder of the mouth is extremely smooth and shiny. This condition is seen most frequently in persons between 30 and 40 years of age. Patients complain of a burning sensation and sensitivity to thermal changes. Inhalation of air is painful. The patient cannot tolerate condiments, and toothbrushing causes painful denudation of the gingival surface.

Severe Form. In this and other forms of desquamative gingivitis the lingual surface is usually less severely involved than the labial

(Fig. 12–1*B*) because the tongue and friction from food excursion reduce the accumulation of local irritants and limit the inflammation. This form is characterized by scattered, irregularly shaped areas in which the gingiva is denuded and strikingly red in appearance (Fig. 12–1*C*). Since the gingiva separating these areas is grayish blue, in overall appearance the gingiva seems speckled. The surface epithelium seems shredded and friable and can be peeled off in small patches (Fig. 12–1*D*).

There are occasionally surface vessels which rupture, releasing a thin, aqueous fluid and exposing an underlying surface that is red and raw. A blast of air directed at the gingiva causes elevation of the epithelium and the consequent formation of a bubble. The areas of involvement seem to shift to different locations on the gingiva. The mucous membrane other than the gingiva is smooth and shiny and may present a fissuring in the cheek adjacent to the line of occlusion.

The condition is extremely painful. The patient cannot tolerate coarse foods, condiments, or temperature changes. There is a constant dry, burning sensation throughout the oral cavity which is accentuated in the denuded gingival zones.

HISTOPATHOLOGY. Microscopically, so-called desquamative gingivitis often appears as one of two types: bullous lesions, resembling the histopathologic features of mucous membrane pemphigoid (Fig. 12–2), or lichenoid lesions, with features similar to those of lichen planus (Fig. 12–3). Occasionally there will be a thin, atrophic epithelium with little or no keratin at the surface and a dense, diffuse infiltration of chronic inflammatory cells in the underlying connective tissue. This tends to be the histopathologic picture in those rare cases of desquamative gingivitis due to menopausal alterations or the atrophic changes of aging.

THERAPY. The therapy for so-called desquamative gingivitis must be based, if possible, on an understanding of the basic disease process causing the gingival reaction.

A careful oral examination must be carried out so that other lesions may be discovered. In lichen planus the gingivae are rarely affected without other oral mucosal lesions being present.

A careful history should be taken to uncover possible coexistent extraoral disease. Conjunctivitis and symptoms of burning on urination or vaginal irritation may suggest multiple sites of mucosal disease and point to mucous membrane pemphigoid. The presence of papular skin lesions, particularly on sites such as wrists or ankles, would suggest lichen planus. Menopausal history or a history of hysterectomy would suggest a possible hormonal etiology.

Biopsy studies often point to the diagnosis of lichen planus or mucous membrane pemphigoid. They will also reveal those unusual cases in which a desquamative gingivitis represents a chronic bacterial infection such as tuberculosis or a mycotic infection such as candidiasis.

Local treatment is essential for all forms of desquamative gingivitis. The patient must be carefully instructed in plaque control using a soft toothbrush, since the gingival surface is easily abraded with a hard brush. Oxidizing mouthwashes (hydrogen peroxide USP 3 per cent diluted to one third peroxide:two thirds warm water) should be used twice daily. The reduction of marginal gingivitis results in some reduction of the inflammation and desquama-

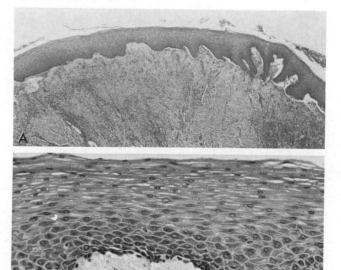

Figure 12–2 Chronic Desquamative Gingivitis—Bullous Type. *A,* There is massive replacement of the papillary and reticular connective tissue by inflammatory exudate, disruption of the epithelial–connective tissue junction, and formation of large subepithelial bullae. *B,* Detailed view showing blunting of epithelial rete pegs and inflammatory exudate of edema, fibrin, and leukocytes which have replaced the connective tissue.

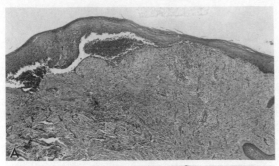

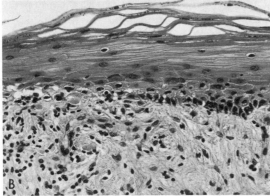

Figure 12–3 Chronic Desquamative Gingivitis–Lichenoid Type. *A,* The epithelium is atrophic, the connective tissue is inflamed, and the epithelium is separated from the connective tissue by a subepithelial vesicle. *B,* Detailed view showing atrophic parakeratotic epithelium with vacuolization of the basal cells and microvesicle formation at the epithelial-connective tissue junction.

tion of the attached gingiva. The use of topical corticosteroid ointments[7] and creams may be attempted, but their success has been limited. The gingival tissue is gently dried with a sterile sponge and an ointment or cream such as triamcinolone 0.1 per cent (Kenalog, Aristocort), fluocinonide 0.05 per cent (Lidex), or desonide 0.05 per cent (Tridesilon) is applied and gently rubbed into the gingiva several times daily.

Systemic therapy may be used in cases of severe gingival involvement. Systemic corticosteroid therapy is not to be considered lightly, since a variety of side effects are possible. The patient's general health should be discussed with his or her physician prior to the use of systemic corticosteroids. If a diagnosis of mucous membrane pemphigoid is entertained, moderate doses of corticosteroids are often helpful in alleviating discomfort and improving the tissue response. Prednisone can be used in a daily or every-other-day dose of 30 to 40 mg and gradually reduced to a daily maintenance dose of 5 to 10 mg or every-other-day maintenance dose of 10 to 20 mg. Other steroids in

comparable doses can be used. Systemic steroid therapy in lichen planus is helpful only in rare cases.

In a desquamative gingivitis due to a deficiency of estrogen or androgens, replacement therapy can be instituted, in consultation with the patient's physician. The estradiol or testosterone may stimulate growth of the atrophic gingival epithelium.

It must be emphasized that in many cases of desquamative gingivitis it may not be possible to determine the basic etiology. However, local therapy together with diligence and patience will eventually improve the condition, and the etiologic background may be discovered upon the eventual appearance of other lesions or symptoms. Particular care and patience are required in the atrophic gingivitis of aging, since there is no systemic therapy that has been found useful, other than nutritional supplements if the patient's nutritional status is deficient. Nutritional supplements[14] may be of value if the patient suffers from a true nutritional deficiency, such as vitamin B deficiency.

REFERENCES

1. Brusati, R., and Bracchetti, A.: Electron microscopic study of chronic desquamative gingivitis. J. Periodontol., *40*:388, 1969.
2. Engel, M., Ray, H. G., and Orban, B.: The pathogenesis of desquamative gingivitis. J. Dent. Res., *29*:410, 1950.
3. Foss, C. L., Grupe, H. E., and Orban, B.: Gingivosis. J. Periodontol., *24*:207, 1953.
4. Glickman, I., and Smulow, J. B.: Chronic desquamative gingivitis: its nature and treatment. J. Periodontol., *35*:397, 1964.
5. Glickman, I., and Smulow, J. B.: Histopathology and histochemistry of chronic desquamative gingivitis. Oral Surg., *21*:325, 1966.
6. Goadby, K.: Diseases of the gums and oral mucous membrane. London, Henry Froude and Hodder and Staughton, 1923, p. 22.
7. Goldman, H. M., and Ruben, M. P.: Desquamative gingivitis and its response to topical triamcinolone therapy. Oral Surg., *21*:579, 1966.
8. Hashimoto, K., Dibella, R., Shklar, G., and Lever, W.: Electron microscopic studies of oral lichen planus. G. Ital. Dermatol., *107*:765, 1966.
9. McCarthy, F. P., McCarthy, P. L., and Shklar, G.: Chronic desquamative gingivitis: a reconsideration. Oral Surg., *13*:1300, 1960.
10. Merritt, A. H.: Chronic desquamative gingivitis. J. Periodontol., *4*:30, 1933.
11. Nikai, H., Rose, G., and Cattoni, M.: Electron microscopic study of chronic desquamative gingivitis. J. Periodont. Res., *6*(Suppl.):1, 1971.
12. Prinz, H.: Chronic diffuse desquamative gingivitis. Dent. Cosmos, *74*:331, 1932.
13. Pullon, P. A.: Ultrastructure of oral lichen planus. Oral Surg., *28*:365, 1969.
14. Roth, H., and Ross, I. F.: The treatment of desquamative gingivitis. Oral Surg., *9*:391, 1956.
15. Schour, I., and Massler, M.: Gingival disease in postwar Italy: gingivosis in hospitalized children in Naples. Am. J. Orthod., *33*:756, 1947.

16. Shklar, G.: Lichen planus as an oral ulcerative disease. Oral Surg., *33*:376, 1972.
17. Shklar, G., and McCarthy, P. L.: Oral lesions of mucous membrane pemphigoid. A study of 85 cases. Arch. Otolaryngol., *93*:354, 1971.
18. Shklar, G., and Meyer, I.: The histopathology and histochemistry of dermatologic lesions in the mouth. Oral. Surg., *14*:1069, 1961.
19. Shklar, G., Meyer, I., and Zacarian, S.: Oral lesions in bullous pemphigoid. Arch. Dermatol., *99*:663, 1969.
20. Sognnaes, R. F., Weisberger, D., and Albright, J. T.: Pathologic desquamation of oral epithelium examined by electron microscopy and histochemistry. J. Natl. Cancer Inst., *17*:329, 1956.
21. Sorrin, S.: Chronic desquamative gingivitis. J. Am. Dent. Assoc., *27*:250, 1940.
22. Susi, F. R., and Shklar, G.: Histochemistry and fine structure of oral lesions of mucous membrane pemphigoid. Arch. Dermatol., *104*:244, 1971.
23. Tomes, J., and Tomes, C.: Dental Surgery. 4th ed. London, J. & A. Churchill, Ltd., 1894.
24. Whitten, J. B.: The fine structure of desquamative stomatitis. J. Periodontol., *39*:75, 1968.
25. Ziskin, D., and Silvers, H. F.: Report of a case of desquamative gingivitis and lichen planus. J. Periodontol., *16*:7, 1945.
26. Ziskin, D., and Zegarelli, E. V.: Chronic desquamative gingivitis. Am. J. Orthod., *33*:756, 1947.

DERMATOSES

Many dermatologic diseases may be accompanied by involvement of the oral mucous membrane, as well as of other mucosal sites. Although oral and skin lesions often occur together in dermatologic disease, changes in the oral cavity may mark the onset of the disease and precede the skin lesions by months or years. In many conditions, such as lichen planus, erythema multiforme, and pyostomatitis vegetans, oral lesions may constitute the only manifestation. Oral manifestations in the absence of skin involvement often result from drugs capable of causing dermatoses. Gingival involvement in dermatologic disorders and drug reactions presents a challenging diagnostic and therapeutic problem.

Lichen Planus

Lichen planus is an inflammatory disease of skin and mucous membranes characterized by the eruption of papules. The papules are violaceous and pointed on the skin, but tend to be white and flattened on the mucosa. When the disease is confined to the skin, it may be acute, subacute, or chronic; oral involvement is usually chronic. The etiology is generally considered to be psychosomatic.

ORAL LESIONS. Lichen planus may be confined to the skin or oral mucosa or may develop in both locations.[19, 25] However, it has become apparent that a *large percentage of cases remain confined to the oral cavity, and the lesions often present a diagnostic problem because of their variability in clinical appearance.*[1, 19]

Frictional factors play a role in determining the location of lesions of lichen planus, and the most common oral sites are the buccal mucosa in relation to the occlusal plane of the teeth, the lateral borders of the tongue, the labial and buccal surfaces of the attached gingiva, the hard palate, and the lower lip. The lesions are often symmetrical and tend to be dendritic and papular. The dendritic or reticulate lesions consist of grayish-white, linear, lace-like elevations composed of large numbers of small individual papules. Isolated papules of pin-head size may also be observed (Figs. 12–4 to 12–6). In addition to the raised dendritic lesions, there may also be raised plaque-like lesions and reddened areas of erosion and ulceration. Vesicles and bullae may also appear in lichen planus and will confuse the clinical picture by suggesting the possibility of a vesiculobullous dermatosis such as pemphigus or pemphigoid. The bullae eventually rupture, leaving areas of ulceration and erosion or desquamation. The great variability in the clinical appearance of the oral lesions of lichen planus depends upon the unique microscopic alterations and the severity of the degenerative changes in the basal layer of the epithelium.

The skin involvement of lichen planus usually results in a pruritus, but the oral lesions tend to be asymptomatic unless erosion or ulceration is present. These areas may be sensitive to hot, acid, or spicy foods, and extensive areas of ulceration may be painful. The disease tends to run a chronic or subacute course, with the duration varying from several months to many years. Periods of exacerbation of lesions tend to relate to episodes of emotional stress.

GINGIVAL LESIONS. The gingival tissue is often involved in oral lichen planus, and the pattern is extremely variable.[16, 35] Lesions may occur as one or more types of four distinctive patterns.

1. *Keratotic lesions*. These raised white lesions may present as groups of individual papules, as linear or reticulate lesions, or as plaque-like configurations (Fig. 12–4*B* to *E*).

2. *Erosive or ulcerative lesions*. These red areas may present as a patchy distribution among keratotic lesions or as extensive involvement. They may be hemorrhagic upon slight trauma, such as toothbrushing (Fig. 12–4*F* and *G*).

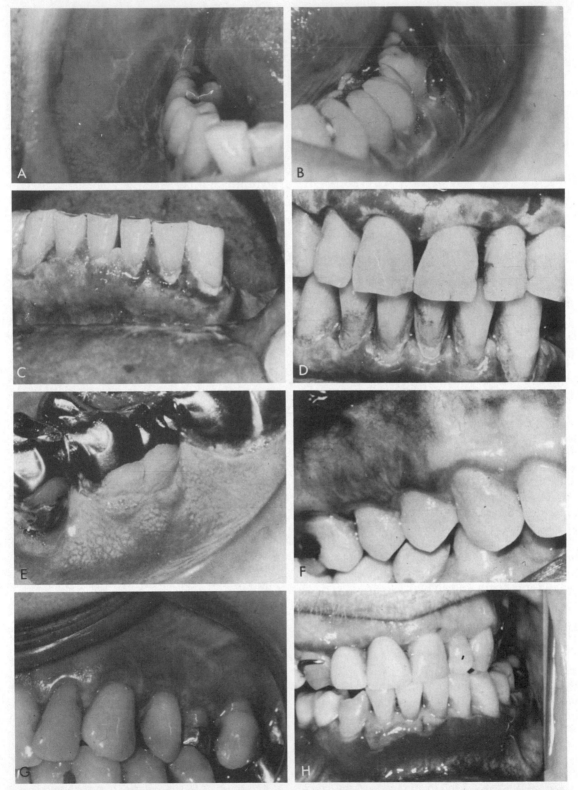

Figure 12–4 Different Clinical Patterns of Oral Lichen Planus. *A,* Reticulate lesions on buccal mucosa. *B,* Reticulate lesions on gingiva. *C,* Reticulate and plaque-like lesions on gingiva and labial mucosa. *D,* Plaque-like and erosive lesions on gingiva. *E,* Papular lesions on gingiva. *F,* Erosive and striated lesions on gingiva. *G,* Erosive and desquamative lesions on gingiva. *H,* Bullous involvement of mandibular gingiva. A large bulla has ruptured, leaving extensive ulceration.

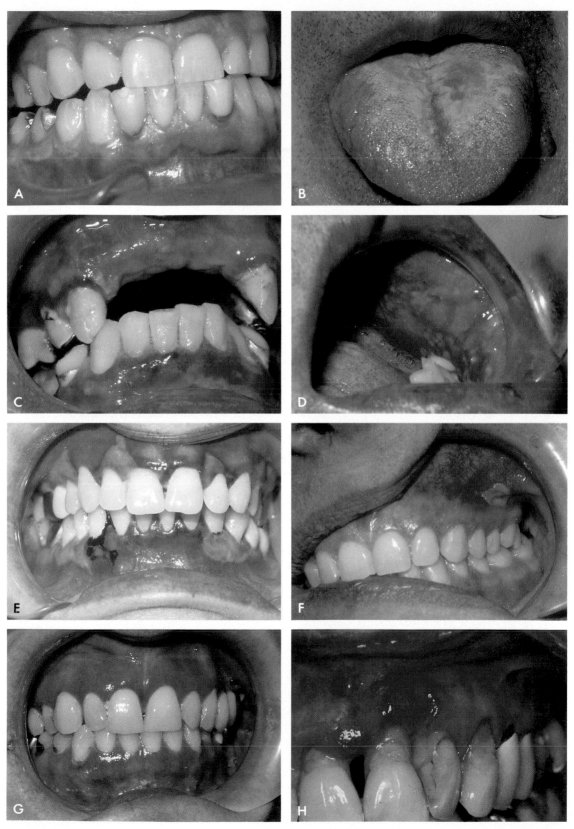

Plate III Desquamative Lesions

A, Lichen planus.   C, Lichen planus.   E, Pemphigus.   G, Mucous membrane pemphigoid.
B, Lichen planus.   D, Lichen planus.   F, Pemphigus.   H, Carcinoma.

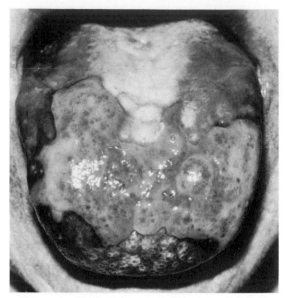

Figure 12–5 Bullous Lichen Planus of the Tongue. A ruptured bulla appears anteriorly and plaque-like lesions posteriorly.

3. *Vesicular or bullous involvement.* Raised fluid-filled lesions will rupture, leaving ulceration (Fig. 12–4*H*).

4. *Atrophic involvement.* Atrophic forms of lichen planus usually occur on the tongue or gingiva. Atrophic involvement of the dorsum of the tongue is characterized by the loss of filiform and fungiform dorsal surface. Atrophic involvement of the gingiva results in a thinning of the epithelium and a resulting erosive or desquamative gingivitis. Since lichen planus is a common disease of the oral mucosa, most cases of so-called desquamative gingivitis are in reality cases of erosive gingival lichen planus. If the mouth is carefully examined, lesions in sites other than the gingiva are usually found. In a small number of cases of oral lichen planus (less than 10 per cent), the involvement is confined to the gingiva, and the clinical pattern is one of erosion and desquamation.

HISTOPATHOLOGY. Microscopically, lichen planus is characterized by three main features—hyperkeratosis or parakeratosis, hydropic degeneration of the basal layer of the stratum germinativum, and a dense infiltration of lymphocytes as a broad band in the upper corium adjacent to the epithelium (Figs. 12–7 and 12–8). Occasionally, there may be extension of rete pegs in a saw-tooth pattern but this feature is more typical of lesions on the skin. The hydropic degeneration of the basal

layer of the epithelium may be sufficiently extensive that the epithelium becomes thin and atrophic or lifts off the underlying corium and produces either a subepithelial vesicle or an ulcer. The nature of the clinical lesion depends upon the microscopic pattern. The white papular or reticulate lesions demonstrate hyperkeratosis or parakeratosis and lymphocytic infiltration. Erosive or ulcerative lesions demonstrate extensive degeneration of the basal layer and patchy loss of epithelium. Vesicular lesions show degenerative and epithelial separation from underlying connective tissue. Atrophic lesions show a thin degenerating epithelium. A microscopic diagnosis can usually be made of oral lesions of lichen planus, but the characteristic pattern is found in the keratotic lesions, and biopsy specimens should be taken in these areas if possible. Oral lesions of lichen planus change in pattern, and occasionally a second or even third biopsy may be necessary before a definitive diagnosis can be made in certain unusual cases.

Electron microscopic studies indicate that lichen planus can be divided into three stages. The earliest stage is degeneration of the cytoplasm of the epithelial cells, with aggregation of particulate material. The intercellular spaces are enlarged, accompanied by lymphocytic infiltration. In the second stage there is loss of collagen fibers in the superficial lamina propria. The final stage shows degeneration and necrosis of the basal and lower spinous layers of the epithelium with the exception of the desmosomes, which are for the most part structurally unaltered. The superficial lamina

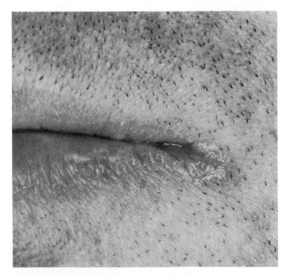

Figure 12–6 Lichen Planus at the labial commissure showing typical papules.

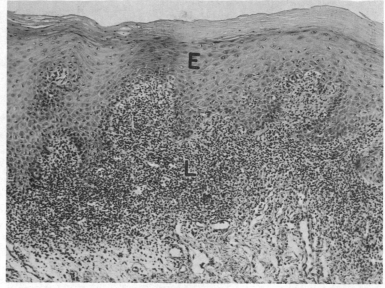

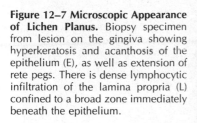

Figure 12–7 Microscopic Appearance of Lichen Planus. Biopsy specimen from lesion on the gingiva showing hyperkeratosis and acanthosis of the epithelium (E), as well as extension of rete pegs. There is dense lymphocytic infiltration of the lamina propria (L) confined to a broad zone immediately beneath the epithelium.

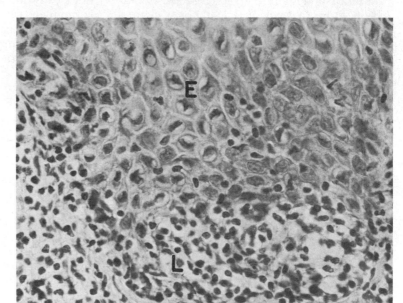

Figure 12–8 High-power view of Figure 12–7 showing hydropic degeneration in the basal layer of the epithelium (E) with lymphocytic infiltration of the lamina propria (L).

propria is also degenerated and necrotic, and the basement lamina is no longer visible. Secondary bacterial involvement of the necrotic tissue is often observed.[47] Separation of the basal lamina from the basal cell layer is an early manifestation of lichen planus.[40]

DIFFERENTIAL DIAGNOSIS. Among the conditions to be considered in the differential diagnosis of oral lichen planus are leukoplakia, white sponge nevus, chronic discoid lupus erythematosus, pemphigus, and mucous membrane pemphigoid.

Leukoplakia. Leukoplakia usually appears on the oral mucosa as raised plaques of varia-ble size (Fig. 12–9). Linear lesions of oral leukoplakia can resemble the reticulate lesions of lichen planus, and the more common discrete lesions of leukoplakia can resemble plaque-like configurations of lichen planus. However, in lichen planus lesions, the papular structure can usually be discerned grossly. Microscopic study will differentiate the two diseases. Leukoplakia usually occurs in heavy smokers.[30, 46]

White Sponge Nevus (White Folded Gingivostomatitis). This is a benign genetic disease, manifested at birth or during childhood by the development of white plaque-like areas on the

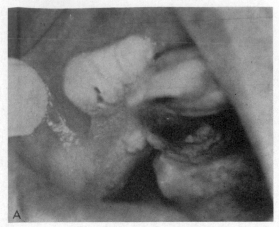
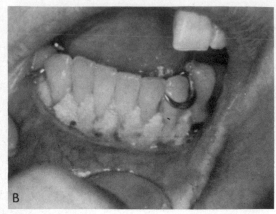

Figure 12–9 *A,* **Leukoplakia of Buccal Mucosa and** *B,* **Leukoplakia of Gingiva** in a 53-year-old female. Microscopic examination revealed evidence of dysplasia.

intercellular edema of the spongy layer of the skin.

oral mucosa (Fig. 12–10). Microscopic examination shows a thickened epithelium characterized by extensive spongiosis.

Chronic Discoid Lupus Erythematosus. Coexistent skin lesions on the face are present in almost all cases, so that the oral lesions, when present, do not present a significant diagnostic problem. They appear as slightly raised white plaques or white linear configurations and present a characteristic histopathologic pattern. Biopsy studies reveal parakeratosis or hyperkeratosis, hydropic degeneration of the basal layer, collagen degeneration, and a perivascular lymphocytic infiltrate.

Pemphigus. Pemphigus may resemble bullous or ulcerative lesions of oral lichen planus. However, the characteristic clinical white striations of lichen planus are usually evident even

in cases of bullous lichen planus. Diagnosis of pemphigus can be made by the microscopic findings of acantholysis and is usually confirmed by immunofluorescent antibody studies.

Mucous Membrane Pemphigoid. Mucous membrane pemphigoid may resemble oral lichen planus of the bullous type. In addition, pemphigoid invariably presents an erosive or desquamative gingivitis, and this type of gingival reaction may also appear in lichen planus. Microscopic evaluation of the oral lesions of pemphigoid reveals a subepithelial vesiculation without hydropic degeneration of the basal layer. In oral lichen planus of the bullous or ulcerative variety, the keratotic white striations can usually be found at the periphery of the ulcerated areas.

THERAPY. The most important aspect of the management of oral lichen planus is definitive

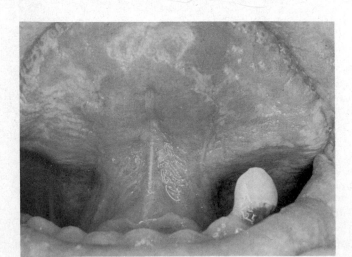

Figure 12–10 White Sponge Nevus (White Folded Gingivostomatitis) showing thickened epithelium with minute surface folds on the tongue and lips.

diagnosis, so that the patient can be given a specific diagnosis for the disease and reassured that the condition is neither infectious, contagious, nor precancerous. If the oral lesions are of the keratotic variety, no therapy is required. Skin lesions of lichen planus are often characterized by a pruritus, but oral keratotic lesions usually present no discomfort. If the oral lesions are erosive, bullous, or ulcerative, they may be painful and uncomfortable. Peroxide mouthwashes two or three times per day are recommended. If the ulcerative areas are well defined and reasonably localized, they may be dried with a sterile sponge and covered with a corticosteroid ointment or cream several times daily. The ointment can be rubbed gently into the lesions. Intralesional injections of corticosteroids are occasionally beneficial. For severe discomfort, topical anesthetics or a Kaopectate-Benadryl rinse can be used. In severe, widespread lesions, systemic corticosteroids may be helpful, such as 30 to 40 mg of prednisone every other day, reduced to a 10- to 20-mg maintenance dose after 2 weeks. This low maintenance dose, every other day, can be used for many months without evidence of steroid side effects.

Pemphigus

Pemphigus is a chronic vesiculobullous lesion involving the skin and mucous membranes. The oral mucosa is invariably affected, and oral lesions usually precede the extensive skin involvement. Early diagnosis of pemphigus is of considerable value, since therapy tends to be simplified if the disease is confined to the mouth. Systemic corticosteroid therapy at this point in the natural history of the disease may prevent the development of skin lesions, and a lower maintenance dose of steroids may be successfully utilized. Pemphigus has a distinctive microscopic appearance, and a definitive diagnosis can usually be made from an oral biopsy specimen.

The etiology of pemphigus is now considered to be autoimmune, and antibodies can be demonstrated by the use of immunofluorescent techniques.

ORAL LESIONS. Oral lesions of pemphigus range from small vesicles to large bullae (Fig. 12–11). The bullae rupture, leaving extensive areas of ulceration. Any region of the mouth can be involved, but lesions often develop at sites of irritation or trauma, such as the occlusal line of the buccal mucosa or edentulous alveolar ridges. An erosive or desquamative type of gingivitis is occasionally seen as a manifestation of oral pemphigus.

HISTOPATHOLOGY. Lesions of pemphigus demonstrate acantholysis, a separation of the epithelial cells of the lower stratum spinosum.[10, 22, 49] The upper layers of the epithelium separate from the basal layer, which remains attached to the underlying corium. The intraepithelial vesiculation begins as a microscopic alteration (Fig. 12–12) and gradually results in a grossly visible lesion as a fluid-filled bulla is formed. The separating cells of the stratum spinosum present degenerative changes—the cell outlines are round rather than polyhedral, the intercellular bridges are lost, and the nuclei are large and hyperchromatic. Many of these acantholytic cells are found within the clear fluid of the vesicle. The underlying connective tissue is densely infil-

[handwritten margin note: any disease of the skin accompanied by degeneration of the adhesive elements of the cells of the outer layer of the skin.]

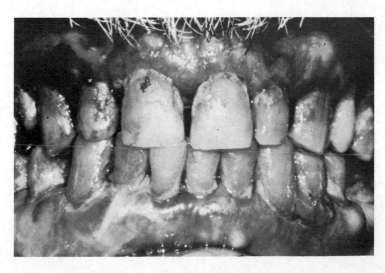

Figure 12–11 Pemphigus of the Gingiva. Note ruptured bulla.

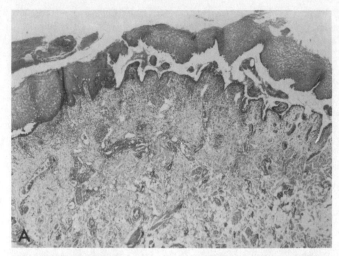

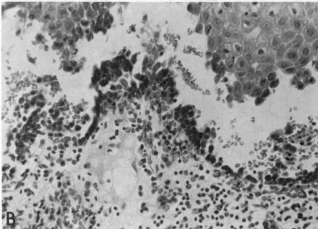

Figure 12–12 Pemphigus Vulgaris. *A,* Oral mucosa showing acantholysis and intraepithelial vesicle. *B,* Detailed view of intraepithelial vesicle in pemphigus vulgaris.

trated with chronic inflammatory cells, and these may also enter the vesicular fluid. As the vesicle or bulla ruptures, the ulcerated lesion becomes infiltrated with polymorphonuclear leukocytes, and the surface may show suppuration.

CYTOLOGY. Cytologic smears of oral pemphigus lesions may be used as corroborating evidence for a definitive diagnosis. A positive smear will show large numbers of rounded acantholytic cells with serrated borders and large hyperchromatic nuclei.[6, 36]

ELECTRON MICROSCOPY. Electron microscopic studies indicate that breakdown of the epithelial intercellular cement substance is the first stage in the development of acantholysis.[14, 15] Others feel that the destruction starts in the tonofilaments[48] or the desmosomes[41] (Fig. 12–13).

IMMUNOFLUORESCENCE. The presence of antibodies can be demonstrated in the oral mucosa of patients with oral pemphigus by the use of immunofluorescent techniques.[5] In the direct fluorescent techniques, an oral biopsy specimen is incubated with fluorescein-labeled IgG from the patient's serum. An indirect technique can be used but is less sensitive than the direct technique. In the indirect technique, a piece of oral or esophageal mucosa from a laboratory animal such as a rhesus monkey is first incubated with the patient's serum to attach the serum antibodies to the mucosal tissue. The tissue is then incubated with fluorescein-labeled antihuman IgG serum. If the test is positive, the immunofluorescence is observed in the intercellular spaces of the stratified squamous epithelium of the mucosa.

VARIETIES OF PEMPHIGUS. The common form of pemphigus is referred to as *pemphigus vulgaris.* A variant, *pemphigus vegetans*, may be considered a subacute form of pemphigus vulgaris with comparable but somewhat less severe clinical features. This form of the disease may be confined to the oral cavity for several weeks or months before the skin is

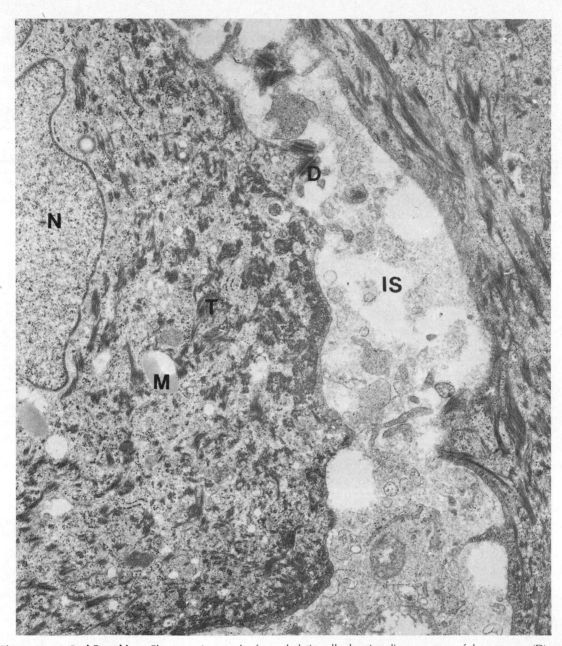

Figure 12–13 Oral Pemphigus. Electron micrograph of acantholytic cells showing disappearance of desmosomes (D) and separation of cells by widening of intercellular space (IS). Tonofibrils (T) show clumping. Mitochondria (M) are degenerating. Nucleus (N) demonstrates intact membrane.

involved. In the vegetative type of pemphigus, oral lesions dominate the picture, with crusted lesions of the skin being seen in intertriginous areas. However, the vegetating or hyperplastic lesions do not occur in the mouth. The oral lesions are of the common vesiculobullous and ulcerative form.

DIFFERENTIAL DIAGNOSIS. The oral lesions of erythema multiforme are frequently similar to those seen in pemphigus. In the former condition, however, there are recurrent active episodes of comparatively short duration followed by long intervals without skin or oral lesions. Erythema multiforme affects the lips with considerable severity. Biopsy studies can differentiate between oral lesions of pemphigus and erythema multiforme, since both have a characteristic histopathology. Mucous membrane pemphigoid may resemble pemphigus when the latter condition is confined to the mouth. Biopsy studies will demonstrate subepithelial vesiculation, with "lifting off" of the epithelium from the underlying corium, instead of the acantholysis characteristic of pemphigus.

Bullous lichen planus must also be considered in the differential diagnosis. The primary lesion of pemphigus may be of a bullous character, followed by erosion with associated pain and discomfort. In lichen planus, however, the characteristic dendritic lesions are invariably found associated with the bullae. Biopsy studies are usually sufficient to differentiate this condition from pemphigus, with its acantholytic changes.

THERAPY. Therapy for pemphigus involves the use of systemic corticosteroids, usually with a moderate to high dosage. If the patient responds well to the corticosteroid agent, the dosage can be gradually reduced, but a low maintenance level of the drug is usually necessary to prevent the recurrence of lesions. In some patients the steroid can be withdrawn completely. In patients who do not respond to corticosteroids or who gradually adapt to them, antimetabolite agents such as methotrexate or azathioprine are used. In general, oral lesions of pemphigus are more resistant to therapy than are skin lesions. The minimization of irritation in the mouth is essential in patients with oral pemphigus. Optimal oral hygiene is essential, since there is usually widespread involvement of the marginal and attached gingivae as well as other areas of the mouth, and the gingival disease represents an exaggerated response to local irritation. Periodontal care is an important part of the overall management of patients with pemphigus. Attention should be given to the fit and design of removable prosthetic appliances, since even slight irritation from these prostheses can result in severe inflammation with vesiculation and ulceration.

Local medication for oral pemphigus may include corticosteroid ointments or creams to reduce the painful symptomatology. Topical anesthetics, such as dyclonine hydrochloride (Dyclone) diluted 50 per cent with water, may be used as a mouth rinse several times daily. The anesthetic effect may last for 40 minutes or longer.[25]

Bullous Pemphigoid

Bullous pemphigoid is a chronic vesiculobullous dermatosis with oral involvement in a small percentage of cases.[47] The skin lesions resemble those of pemphigus clinically, but the microscopic picture is quite distinct from that of pemphigus. There is no evidence of acantholysis, and the developing vesicles are subepithelial rather than intraepithelial. The epithelium separates from the underlying connective tissue at the basement membrane zone. Electron microscopic studies show an actual horizontal splitting or replication of the basal lamina. The separating epithelium remains relatively intact, and the basal layer is present and appears regular.

Bullous pemphigoid is also considered to be an autoimmune disease. Antibodies can be demonstrated by immunofluorescent techniques, and they are seen in the basement membrane area.

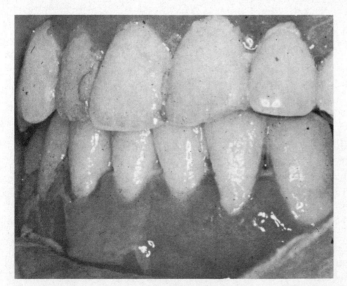

Figure 12–14 Benign Mucous Membrane Pemphigoid. Note remnant of ruptured bullous lesion in lower left area.

ORAL LESIONS. Oral lesions are seen in about 10 per cent of cases. There is an erosive or desquamative gingivitis and occasional vesicular or bullous lesions.[42]

THERAPY. Therapy involves the systemic use of corticosteroids in moderate dosage.

Mucous Membrane Pemphigoid (Benign Mucous Membrane Pemphigoid)

This is an unusual chronic vesiculobullous disease with involvement of the oral mucosa and other mucosal tissues. Skin is usually not affected. The oral mucous membrane is usually involved, and other sites of predilection are the conjunctiva, nasal mucosa, vaginal mucosa, rectal mucosa, and urethra. The ocular lesions can be severe and may result in scarring and eventual blindness.

ORAL LESIONS. The mouth is affected in almost all cases of mucous membrane pemphigoid. The most characteristic feature of the oral involvement is an erosive or desquamative gingivitis (Fig. 12–14), with notable erythema of the attached gingiva and areas of desquamation, ulceration, and often vesiculation.[37] Lesions may occur elsewhere in the mouth, and these are vesiculobullous in nature. The bullae tend to have a relatively thick roof (Fig. 12–15A), and they rupture in 2 to 3 days, leaving irregularly shaped areas of ulceration. Healing of the lesions may take up to 3 weeks.

HISTOPATHOLOGY. The microscopic appearance of the oral lesions, while not completely diagnostic for mucous membrane pemphigoid, is sufficiently distinctive so that a tentative diagnosis can be considered. There is a striking subepithelial vesiculation, with the epithelium lifting off from the underlying corium, leaving an intact basal layer (Fig. 12–16). The separation of the epithelium and the connective tissue is at the basement membrane zone, and electron microscopic studies have shown a split in the basal lamina.

Varying amounts of chronic inflammatory infiltration are found in the connective tissue. The epithelium remains intact until the bulla ruptures and then degenerates. The desquamative or erosive gingivitis presents a thin epithelium with some evidence of degeneration and occasional ulceration. Inflammatory infiltration may be notable.

IMMUNOFLUORESCENCE. Positive immunofluorescence localized to the basement membrane area has been reported in occasional cases of mucous membrane pemphigoid.[11]

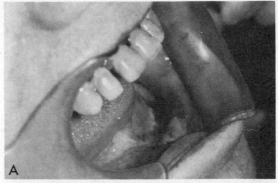

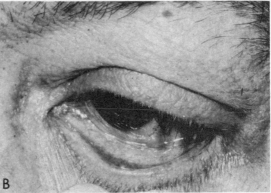

Figure 12–15 *A*, **Bullae on Floor of Mouth** and edentulous mucosa in mucous membrane pemphigoid. *B*, **Conjunctivitis** with symblepharon in mucous membrane pemphigoid.

OCULAR LESIONS. The eyes are affected in many cases of mucous membrane pemphigoid. There is conjunctivitis with the development of fibrous adhesions between the palpebral and bulbar conjunctivae (Fig. 12–15B). There may be adhesions of eyelid to eyeball (symblepharon). Adhesions at the edges of the eyelids (ankyloblepharon) may result in narrowing of the palpebral fissure. Small vesicular lesions may develop on the conjunctiva. Eventually the conjunctival involvement may lead to scarring, corneal damage, and blindness.

DIFFERENTIAL DIAGNOSIS. In the differential diagnosis one must consider the vesiculobullous diseases, such as pemphigus, erythema multiforme, and bullous lichen planus. Pemphigus may be confined to the oral cavity in its early stage, and the vesicular and ulcerative lesions may resemble those of mucous membrane pemphigoid. An erosive or desquamative gingivitis may also be seen in pemphigus as a rare manifestation. Biopsy studies can quickly rule out pemphigus by noting the absence of acantholytic changes. In erythema multiforme there are obvious vesiculobullous lesions, but the onset is usually acute rather than chronic, the labial involvement is severe,

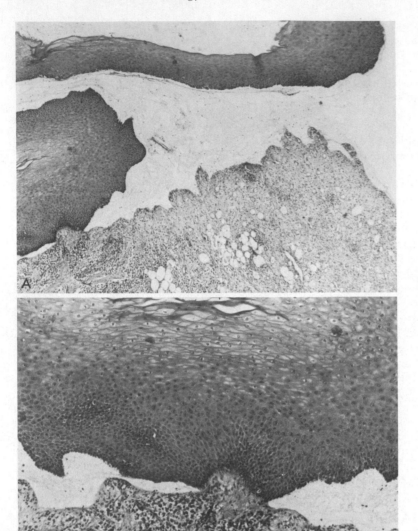

Figure 12–16 Biopsy specimen from oral lesion of **Mucous Membrane Pemphigoid.** *A*, Low-power view shows clean separation of epithelium from underlying connective tissue. *B*, High-power view shows intact basal layer as the epithelium separates from connective tissue at the basement membrane zone. Inflammatory infiltration is noted.

and the gingivae are usually not affected. A desquamative gingivitis is not seen in erythema multiforme, although occasional vesicular lesions may develop. A biopsy study of an oral lesion will reveal an unusual degeneration of the upper stratum spinosum, characteristically seen in oral erythema multiforme lesions.

THERAPY. Mucous membrane pemphigoid can be treated with systemic corticosteroids, using moderate daily or every-other-day doses and gradually lowering this to a very small maintenance dose (5 to 10 mg of prednisone or comparable doses of other corticosteroids). Topical corticosteroids have limited value, but occasionally applications of corticosteroid ointment may ameliorate severe desquamative gingivitis and help to promote healing. Optimal oral hygiene is essential, since local irritants on the tooth surface will result in an exaggerated gingival inflammatory response. A soft toothbrush and oxidizing mouthwashes are helpful in maintaining good oral hygiene. If the disease is not severe and the symptomatology is mild, systemic corticosteroids may be omitted. If ocular involvement exists, systemic corticosteroids are indicated.

Erythema Multiforme

Erythema multiforme is an acute inflammatory eruptive disease involving the skin and oral cavity. More than 80 per cent of the patients with skin involvement present oral lesions,[25] and in rare instances erythema multiforme may be confined to the mouth.[23] *The pathognomonic skin lesions are of a target or iris variety, with a central vesicle* or *bulla* surrounded by an *urticarial zone.*

Erythema multiforme is usually a *recurrent disease.* It may be ushered in with fever preceded by a chill, and the duration of the average episode is from 10 days to several weeks. The frequency of involvement varies from three or more attacks per year to a single attack every few years.

Erythema multiforme is probably not an etiologic entity, but a symptom complex or reaction pattern representing many possible causative factors, such as drugs, emotional stress, systemic disease, and so forth.

ORAL LESIONS. The oral lesions consist of *purplish-red macules* or *papules* with interspersed *bullous lesions.* The *tongue* often presents *severe involvement,* with erosion of the bullae followed by ulceration. The lesions are so painful that chewing and swallowing are impaired.

The lips are invariably involved, usually with considerable severity, so that extensive bullous and ulcerative lesions are present on the mucosal surface and secondary crusting occurs on the dry skin surface. The extensive labial lesions are often helpful in arriving at a clinical diagnosis.

HISTOPATHOLOGY. Microscopically, there is liquefaction degeneration of the upper epithelium and the development of intraepithelial vesicles, but without the acantholysis which occurs in pemphigus. Degenerative changes also occur in the basement membrane.[34]

TREATMENT. There is no specific treatment. Systemic steroid therapy suppresses the symptoms while the disease runs its course.

Stevens-Johnson Syndrome

The Stevens-Johnson syndrome is a rare form of erythema multiforme,[44] characterized by *erythematous, hemorrhagic,* and *bullous lesions.* The oral cavity, conjunctivae, and genitals are involved, as well as other areas of the skin (Fig. 12–17). This hemorrhagic type of erythema multiforme is associated with high fever and prostration, and it may be fatal in a small percentage of cases. The oral lesions appear as purpuric vesicles or bullae. Suppurating superficial and deep erosions of the gingiva are also seen. Steroid therapy is the treatment of choice.

Lupus Erythematosus

Lupus erythematosus used to be considered one of the so-called collagen diseases[12] but is now interpreted as an autoimmune disease.[38] It is classified into two forms, a chronic discoid type and an acute systemic type. The incidence of oral involvement in lupus erythematosus varies, depending upon the acuteness of the disease. Although not more than 10 per cent of patients with the chronic discoid type present oral lesions, as many as 75 per cent of patients with the acute systemic type have some oral manifestation before death. The *characteristic "butterfly" distribution* of the lesions *on the face* is a diagnostic aid in this disease (Fig. 12–18). Lupus erythematosus may occur on the oral mucous membrane

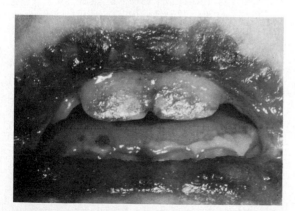

Figure 12–17 Stevens-Johnson Syndrome. Note the crusting of the lips and vesicular eruption on the tongue.

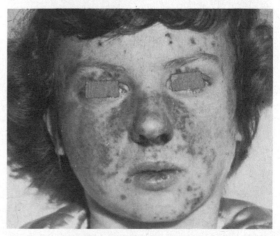

Figure 12–18 Lupus Erythematosus showing "butterfly" distribution of lesions on the face and crusting of the lips.

without skin lesions in extremely rare instances.

CHRONIC DISCOID TYPE. In the oral cavity the disease appears as *well-defined, slightly elevated,* and *infiltrated white lesions* with an erythematous periphery. The lesions are usually localized and are seen most often on the buccal mucosa (Fig. 12–19).[3] At the border of the lesion there may be numerous dilated blood vessels having a radial arrangement extending into the surrounding tissue, coupled with whitish pinhead papules. In the early stages, the center of the lesion is slightly depressed and eroded and is covered with a bluish-red epithelial surface showing scarring. In older lesions, the erythematous border becomes less elevated and is transformed into a whitish or bluish-white peripheral zone of thickened epithelium. The dilated vessels are replaced by white lines having the same diverging radial arrangement. On the tongue the disease occurs as circumscribed, smooth, reddened areas in which the papillae are lost or as patches with a whitish sheen resembling leukoplakia.

On the lip, the lesions are somewhat similar to those in the mouth, and, in most cases, the lip is involved by direct extension from perioral skin lesions. Localized patches may be present, or the entire lip may be involved. Early in the disease, the lip is swollen, bluish red, and often everted. The lip lesions may be covered with adherent scales and crusts, which remain localized and are rarely diffuse (Fig. 12–18). At the margins of the patches, dilated capillaries or fine branching radial lines may be seen. The lip is tender and sensitive, and, on removal

of the adherent scales, bleeding from the raw surface is noted. Depressed scars may follow healing of the deeper lesions.

Microscopically, the epithelial changes in the chronic discoid type consist of keratinization, keratotic plugging, acanthosis, atrophy, pseudocarcinomatous hyperplasia, and liquefaction degeneration of the basal cell layer.[2]
The histopathology of the oral lesions is characteristic and consists of hyperkeratosis or parakeratosis, hydropic degeneration of the basal layer of the epithelium, collagen degeneration in the corium, and a perivascular infiltration of lymphocytes.[39] **The collagen degeneration shows up clearly with a periodic acid–Schiff stain for mucopolysaccharides.**

Periods of activity and quiescence occur. The lesions enlarge by peripheral extension, accompanied by the occurrence of fresh erosions and superficial ulcerations, followed by atrophic changes. Some burning sensation occurs in the erosions and deeper ulcerations.

ACUTE SYSTEMIC TYPE. In the systemic variety, the oral lesions are more *acute,* and *greater destruction* occurs. The lesions are characterized by soft, irregular, superficial, or moderately deep erosions, usually covered with a necrotic, grayish pseudomembrane.

DIFFERENTIAL DIAGNOSIS. Diagnosis usually depends upon the identification of the accompanying skin lesions. The diagnosis of discoid lupus erythematosus confined to the oral cavity is very difficult to make, but microscopic studies usually reveal the characteristic histopathology.[2] The acute systemic variety may present a variety of oral lesions that are essentially nonspecific and erosive in nature. *Erythema multiforme* and *pemphigus* may sometimes look quite similar. Biopsy studies will aid in differentiating between lupus erythematosus and other erosive diseases.

TREATMENT. The treatment of lupus erythematosus is nonspecific. Systemic bismuth and gold have been used in the past. Corticotropin (ACTH) and corticosteroids are used currently for the systemic varieties of the disease. The antimalarial drugs are very successful in controlling the chronic discoid variety, but in systemic lupus erythematosus these drugs have no effect.

Scleroderma

Scleroderma is characterized by a primary induration and edema of the skin in localized

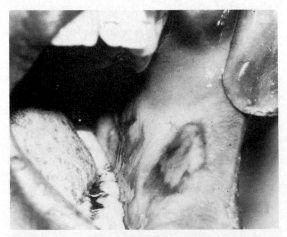

Figure 12–19 Lesions of Discoid Lupus Erythematosus on Buccal Mucosa. Note bulla and radiating striations.

patches or diffuse areas and later atrophy and pigmentation. There are three distinct forms: diffuse scleroderma, acrosclerosis, and circumscribed scleroderma (morphea).[28, 32] The etiology is obscure, although scleroderma is considered by many investigators to be of autoimmune origin. In all types of the disease the first sign is usually a moderate induration of the skin, gradually followed by the atrophic stage, which results in permanent disfiguration. Ulceration can occur, but it is rare and is seen only in advanced cases. Hemiatrophy is fairly common in cases of facial involvement, sometimes being accompanied by false ankylosis of the temporomandibular joint.

ORAL LESIONS. The diffuse and acrosclerotic types frequently involve the oral cavity.[32] Although the entire mucous membrane may be involved, it is the tongue that is most commonly observed to show pathologic changes, followed in frequency by the buccal mucosa and the gingiva. There may be painful induration of the tongue and gingiva.[45] The usual symptom is a minor speech defect due to impaired mobility of the tongue. The progress of scleroderma of the mucous membrane is chronic, but it is reportedly more rapid than that of the skin lesions.

In the acrosclerotic variety, the lips become thin and rigid, and their movements are greatly restricted. The opening of the oral cavity is usually materially reduced. Difficulty in eating and talking may follow. Obliterative endarter-

itis may result in avascularity, with increased susceptibility to infection.[17]

In acrosclerosis and diffuse scleroderma, Stafne and Austin[43] have described a characteristic roentgenographic picture consisting of an increase in the width of the periodontal space. This widening was found in 8 of 127 cases of acrosclerosis and in one case of diffuse scleroderma, with the findings much less marked in the latter condition. The authors noted that the amount of widening in acrosclerosis varies. All of the teeth may not be affected, and the posterior teeth are involved more often than the anterior teeth. Radiographically, the periodontal space in relation to the entire root is widened to an almost uniform thickness.[40] The increase in width of the periodontal spaces occurs at the expense of the alveolar bone. The lamina dura is obliterated. Clinically the teeth are firm.

Microscopically, the continuity of the periodontal fibers from the cementum to the alveolar bone is broken near the cementum.

TREATMENT. There is no effective treatment; however, use of an immunosuppressive agent (azathioprine) has been described.[17]

Pyostomatitis Vegetans

This rare disease may be confined to the oral cavity or associated with skin lesions.

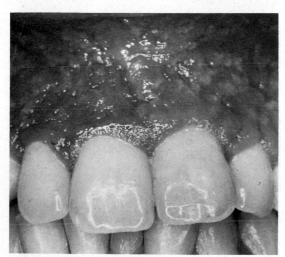

Fig. 12–20

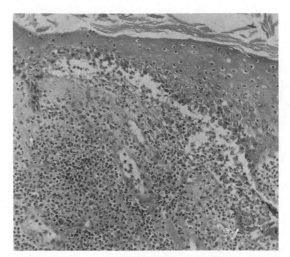

Fig. 12–21

Figure 12–20 Pyostomatitis Vegetans. Multiple small abscesses create granular appearance of the gingiva and adjacent mucosa.
Figure 12–21 Pyostomatitis Vegetans. Section showing hyperkeratosis of the epithelium and granulomatous inflammation in the connective tissue.

ORAL LESIONS. In the oral cavity the primary lesions appear as *multiple small pustules* with a *yellowish tip* and a *reddened base*[24] (Fig. 12–20). The process spreads within a very few weeks to involve the entire oral cavity and creates a diffuse granular surface. As the oral lesions become chronic, the buccal mucosa proliferates to form folds, and miliary abscesses are found on the summits of the rugae and in the deep invaginations. Oral involvement is accompanied by a mild degree of pain.

HISTOPATHOLOGY. Microscopically, there is pronounced hyperkeratosis and acanthosis, with broadening and elongation of the rete pegs (Fig. 12–21). The connective tissue presents a granulomatous inflammatory process with unruptured miliary abscesses. Degeneration of the epithelium and focal areas of surface necrosis are also seen.

TREATMENT. The disease tends to be chronic and resistant to therapy. Because it is frequently associated with an ulcerative colitis, both of these conditions must be treated simultaneously. Iron, liver, and vitamins are of value, but no specific therapy has been discovered to date.

CHRONIC INFECTIONS

Syphilis

Syphilis is a chronic, specific infection of the body by the spirochete *Treponema pallidum*, which results in many cutaneous and mucous membrane manifestations. Oral lesions can occur in any of the three stages of the disease.[26]

PRIMARY STAGE. This stage is marked by the appearance of the chancre and ends with its disappearance. The chancre or primary lesion of syphilis develops at the point of inoculation, usually in a period of 2 to 6 weeks after the entrance of the spirochete.

From 5 to 10 per cent of chancres are found in places other than on the genitalia, and about 70 per cent of these extragenital lesions are found on the lips or within the oral cavity. The lips are more frequently involved, and multiple primary lesions may occur.

Lip and intraoral chancres *vary from small, slightly indurated lesions to deep, indolent ulcerations*. Chancres of the oral cavity may be divided into two general types: erosive and ulcerative. Lymph node enlargement is noted in the cervical region, and, if the lesion is on or near the median line, the cervical adenop-

athy may be bilateral. The ulcerative type of mucous membrane chancre may vary from a relatively small ulcer the size of a fingernail to a large, ulcerating nodule. The base and border of the lesion are markedly indurated, and there may be evidence of secondary pyogenic infection.

These lesions tend to have an adherent crust when present on the lip, but within the oral cavity they show a broad, ulcerating, granulating surface. **As a rule, the primary lesion is relatively painless, but those with associated secondary infection may be very tender and painful.**

On the *tongue* the chancre is more often located near the tip, and it is usually markedly indurated and shows early ulceration. Chancre of the gingiva is comparatively rare. It appears as an indurated ulcer, which may be covered with a pseudomembrane (Fig. 12–22). Recession of the gingival tissue, exposing the tooth root, occurs if the lesions begin at the gingival

Fig. 12–22

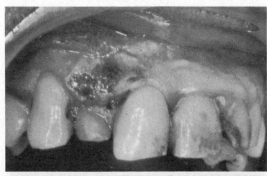

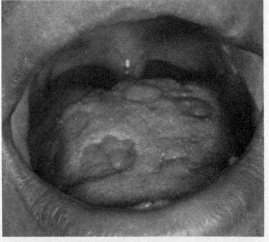

Fig. 12–23

Figure 12–22 Primary Stage of Syphilis. Chancre of the gingiva.

Figure 12–23 Secondary Stage of Syphilis. Patchy denudation of the tongue.

margin. Chancres of the gingiva may also be of the nodular type, with superficial erosions varying in size from that of a split pea to larger lesions that involve the gingiva in relation to several teeth.

Chancre of the gingiva tends to grow rapidly and is apt to be more painful than the slower growing tubercular lesions.

SECONDARY STAGE. The secondary stage is characterized by *cutaneous eruption* and *mucous patches* in the oral cavity. The mucous patch is the most *contagious lesion of syphilis,* as its surface is covered with an abundance of spirochetes. Mucous patches are slightly elevated, well-demarcated, grayish-white lesions with a smooth, glistening surface surrounded by an erythematous margin.

There is a *macular type of syphilid,* involving the oral cavity early in the secondary stage, which represents a manifestation of the generalized skin eruption.[36] The tongue and palate are most commonly involved, but the *tongue shows the more classic picture of this type of lesion* (Fig. 12–23). These lesions appear on the tongue as *reddish, round, multiple, symmetrical, nonindurated plaques.* Slow denudation of the normal coating of the tongue occurs, with shedding of the filiform papillae. The lesions are usually smooth and nonerosive early in their development and may assume a grayish color and either disappear or develop into a true mucous patch.

A papular type of syphilid is a rare form seen on the dorsum of the tongue or the external commissures of the labial orifice. These lesions are about the size of a split pea, and at the angles of the mouth they show a split arrangement, with one half of the papule on the upper lip and the other half on the lower lip. Such lesions must be differentiated from the common intertrigo labialis or maceration due to other causes.

TERTIARY STAGE. The tertiary stage of syphilis includes visceral, cutaneous, and oral lesions. The two types of tertiary luetic infection in the oral cavity are gummatous and interstitial. Both conditions tend to leave secondary changes, namely, perforations of the hard and soft palates and atrophic interstitial glossitis, respectively.

The Gummatous Reaction. The *tongue* is a common site of a single or multiple gummatous process. **The gumma is characterized by a growth of epithelioid (granulomatous) tissue in which the spirochetes are absent. It usually develops slowly as a relatively painless nodule that may grow to a rather large mass.** It tends to ulcerate, producing a thick, sanguineous

secretion. Healing of the gumma results in the formation of cicatricial tissue, resulting in a lobulated appearance of the tongue known as *lingua lobulata.* Other locations of gummata are the *hard and soft palates.*

The Interstitial Reaction. More commonly, the tongue is involved in a *sclerosing process,* with the development of the atrophic glossitis of tertiary syphilis referred to as "bald tongue." **The tongue is smooth, red, and glistening in its entirety or may present isolated patches of normal papillae.** The tongue may be shriveled, owing to replacement of the musculature by connective tissue (Fig. 12–24).

The production of this lesion may be explained by a sequence of related pathologic changes. The tongue, a mobile organ subject to mild trauma, receives a large dose of spirochetes in the secondary stage, and if the disease is untreated or inadequately treated, **endarteritis of the smaller vessels results. Later, owing to the interstitial sclerosing process, together with the resulting decrease in the blood supply, the papillae undergo atrophy, with the production of patchy smooth bald areas on the surface.** *Leukoplakia* is a common secondary feature, usually as the result of irritation from the products of combustion and heat from smoking. Because the leukoplakic lesions may undergo malignant change, the incidence of carcinoma of the tongue in patients with syphilitic glossitis is high.

HISTOPATHOLOGY. Lesions of the primary and secondary stages present ulceration and necrosis of the surface epithelium, with a

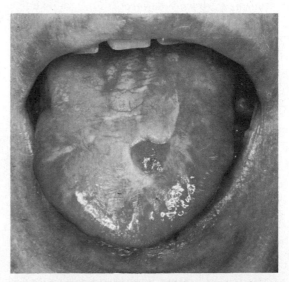

Figure 12–24 Tertiary Stage of Syphilis. Atrophic glossitis and leukoplakia of the tongue.

dense inflammatory infiltration of the underlying connective tissue. The deeper corium presents a characteristic pattern of endarteritis and a perivascular localization of lymphocytes.[26]

The gumma appears microscopically as a granulomatous process with epithelioid tissue (histiocytes), multinucleate giant cells, and areas of coagulation necrosis. *T. pallidum* is not demonstrable in the lesion. The diagnosis is confirmed by serologic tests.[31]

Biopsy studies of syphilitic interstitial glossitis reveal a wide subepithelial zone in which there is disorganization of the musculature caused by an interstitial proliferation of connective tissue. Marked narrowing of the lumina of the efferent arteries is also noted. Atrophy of the epithelial surface and filiform papillae is pronounced in the smooth areas noted clinically on the surface of the tongue. A perivascular lymphocytic infiltration is found in the deeper corium.

Tuberculosis

Tuberculous involvement of the oral cavity is relatively rare. The lesions may involve any area of the mouth, including the gingiva, but the usual site of involvement is the tongue, and the typical lesion is a *chronic ulcer.*[33]

Two types of tuberculous ulcers are seen in the oral cavity, primary and secondary. The **primary type of lesion** occurs in nontuberculous individuals, principally children, and involves the lip or tongue. The lesion resembles the primary lesion of syphilis, beginning as an *indurated, sharply defined lesion,* followed by ulceration with lymph node involvement. The diagnosis is made by a biopsy study showing a typical granulomatous process, with the demonstration of tubercle bacilli in the tissues.

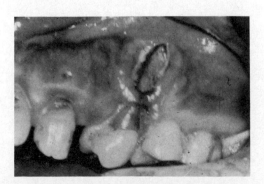

Figure 12–25 Ulcerative Tuberculous Lesion on the Gingiva. (Courtesy of Dr. Irving Meyer.)

The **secondary type** of tuberculous ulcer is seen more frequently. It occurs in individuals with tuberculosis and may be subdivided into *nodular, ulcerative,* and *verrucous types* (Fig. 12–25). The nodular type is most often found at the tip of the tongue, although it may occur elsewhere in the oral cavity. It is characterized by a slowly developing, relatively painless nodule, which may enlarge to a considerable size without showing any appreciable evidence of ulceration. This lesion resembles a syphilitic gumma, especially if it is located on the tongue. Considering the number of cases of pulmonary tuberculosis, this type of lesion is rare.

The verrucous type of tuberculous lesion in the oral cavity is the rarest of this group. Its usual location is on the dorsum of the tongue in the region of the circumvallate papillae or on the lips. The lesion may simulate the verrucous type of epidermoid carcinoma.

HISTOPATHOLOGY. The tuberculous ulcer is characterized microscopically by tubercle formation. Caseation necrosis is usually seen in addition to the granulomatous reaction of histiocytes and Langhans' giant cells. Tubercle bacilli can occasionally be demonstrated within the Langhans' giant cells, using special stains.

DRUG ERUPTIONS

An increase in the incidence of skin and oral manifestations of hypersensitivity to drugs has been noted since the advent of the sulfonamides, barbiturates, and various antibiotics. The eruptive skin and oral lesions are attributed to the fact that the drug acts as an *allergen,* either alone or in combination, *sensitizing* the tissues and then causing the allergic reaction.

Eruptions in the oral cavity resulting from sensitivity to drugs that have been taken by mouth or parenterally are termed **stomatitis medicamentosa.** *The local reaction from the use of a medicament in the oral cavity, such as a so-called aspirin burn and the stomatitis resulting from topical penicillin, is referred to as* **stomatitis venenata** *or* **contact stomatitis.**

Such changes may result either from the irritating local action of the drug or from drug sensitivity. In many cases skin eruptions may accompany the oral lesions.

In general, drug eruptions in the oral cavity are *multiform. Vesicular* and *bullous lesions* occur most commonly, but *pigmented* or *non-*

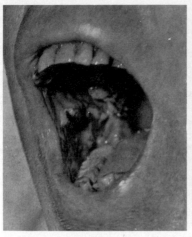
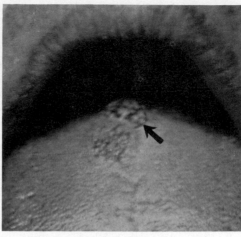

Fig. 12–26   Fig. 12–27

Figure 12–26 Stomatitis Medicamentosa resulting from bismuth salicylate showing necrosis of the buccal mucosa with pigmentation.
Figure 12–27 Fixed Eruption Due to Phenolphthalein. Note the bullous lesion on dorsum of tongue (*arrow*).

pigmented macular lesions are also frequently observed. Erosions, often followed by deep ulceration with purpuric lesions, may also occur. The lesions are seen in different areas of the oral cavity, with the gingiva frequently being affected.

There are hundreds of drugs capable of producing skin eruptions with or without mouth lesions. Constitutional symptoms may be severe or entirely absent. Only a few of the important and most commonly used drugs that may be associated with skin and oral eruptions will be considered here.

Agranulocytosis characterized by *necrotic oral lesions, sore throat,* and *leukopenia* may follow the use of gold salts, arsphenamine, aminopyrine, phenacetin, sulfonamides, and antibiotics. The barbiturates[20] and salicylates[8] (Fig. 12–26) occasionally produce vesicular or bullous lesions, followed by erosions in the oral cavity. Phenolphthalein, found in many proprietary laxatives, may produce bullous lesions, followed by erosions (usually confined to a single lesion) on the skin and in the oral cavity (Fig. 12–27).

Iodides and bromides may give rise to bullous and hemorrhagic eruptions in the oral cavity and, on the skin, to acne, urticaria, or suppurating and vegetating lesions. The sulfonamides are responsible for a variety of skin and oral lesions, including vesicles, bullae, and ulcerations. Sulfonamide ointment has been a factor in producing sensitization in a large percentage of cases.[45] A so-called fixed eruption of mucous membrane and skin caused by

sulfadiazine[9] has been reported. Atabrine (quinacrine hydrochloride), used in the prevention and treatment of malaria in World War II, produced a skin eruption called atypical lichenoid dermatitis that was characterized by lesions resembling lichen planus on the skin and oral mucosa.

Skin and oral eruptions and acute monilial infection have been associated with the widespread use of antibiotics (Fig. 12–28).

Cancer chemotherapeutic agents are currently responsible for a significant number of cases of oral ulcerative lesions.[7, 13]

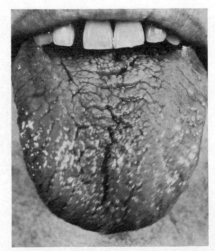

Figure 12–28. Prominent Papillae and Discoloration of the Tongue Associated with the Local Use of Penicillin.

FUNGUS DISEASES OF THE ORAL CAVITY

Although fungus disease of the oral cavity is relatively uncommon, the following conditions are occasionally seen.

Acute Candidiasis (Moniliasis, Thrush)

Acute candidiasis is the most common mycotic infection of the oral mucosa. It is seen in three types of individuals—the debilitated or immunosuppressed adult, the infant, and the adult who has been on antibiotic therapy for some time. The causative organism is *Candida albicans,* a common inhabitant of the mouth that is normally nonpathogenic. In the severely debilitated adult, with significantly lowered tissue resistance, the organism may become invasive and destructive, penetrating the oral mucosa and producing necrosis of the epithelium. Candidiasis is seen in immunosuppressed patients and is becoming increasingly frequent in cancer patients who have been treated with high dosages of radiation or chemotherapeutic drugs. The infant is born with a sterile mouth, and the normal oral bacterial-mycotic flora gradually develops. During this early stage, while the flora is becoming established, the candidal organisms may proliferate and produce disease. *C. albicans* may proliferate and invade the oral tissues if the normal bacterial components of the oral flora are removed by the use of antibiotics. However, the development of candidiasis as a complication of antibiotic therapy has been overemphasized. It usually requires the use of several different antibiotics over a period of several weeks or months, and these patients also tend to be debilitated by the conditions requiring the antibacterial therapy. An increased incidence of candidiasis is also seen in certain metabolic disorders such as diabetes and the hypothyroid–adrenocortical insufficiency syndrome. Women developing oral candidiasis may also develop vaginal candidiasis, since the organism is also a common inhabitant of the vaginal tract. Pregnancy and the use of contraceptive steroids tend to predispose the female to the development of both oral and vaginal candidiasis.

Microscopic examination of oral lesions of candidiasis reveals the invading mycelia of the organisms within epithelium that is undergoing necrosis. Biopsy studies are not necessary for diagnostic purposes, since a smear can adequately demonstrate the organisms. Culture of the organisms is unnecessary and misleading, since *C. albicans* is usually present in normal mouths as part of the bacterial-mycotic flora. This disease is not contagious, since the organisms are normally present, and some predisposing loss of tissue resistance or depression of the immune response is required.

ORAL LESIONS. The oral lesions may appear anywhere on the mucosal surface as a simple patch, but usually the lesions are multiple. *The characteristic lesions are creamy white, resembling coagulated milk, adherent, and, when forcibly removed, give rise to bleeding points* (Figs. 12–29 and 12–30). Intertriginous maceration at the labial commissures in both children and adults may reveal *C. albicans.*

DIAGNOSIS. The diagnosis is based upon the history, the clinical appearance of the lesions, and microscopic study of smears of scrapings from them. The smears are stained with gentian violet or methylene blue and will show spores and mycelia of *C. albicans* (Fig. 12–31).

Clinically, thrush may simulate *diphtheria, macerated epithelium* of the buccal mucosa

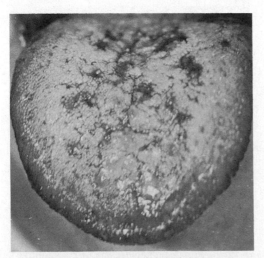

Figure 12–29 Acute Moniliasis of the Tongue.

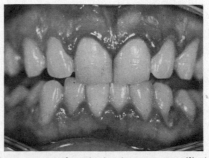

Figure 12–30 The Gingiva in Acute Moniliasis.

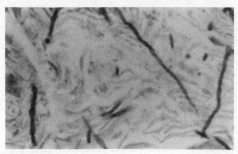

Figure 12–31 Smear from Lesion of Candidiasis Showing Proliferating Mycelia of *Candida albicans*.

from chronic irritation (biting habit), *leukoplakia,* and possibly *lichen planus.* These conditions are readily ruled out by smears of the necrotic white lesions.

TREATMENT. Current treatment of acute oral candidiasis favors the use of the antimycotic agent nystatin in a suspension or as a troche. A spoonful of the suspension (100,000 units/ml) is gently moved around in the mouth for about 1 minute and then swallowed. This is repeated four times daily for 7 to 10 days. Troches are more effective and are kept in the mouth until dissolved. This is repeated four times daily for 7 to 10 days. If oral troches or tablets are not available, vaginal tablets (100,000 units) are used as oral troches. Painting the lesions with 1 per cent gentian violet is an older but effective treatment if the clinician can paint all lesions every day for 7 days.

Chronic Candidiasis

This is a rare type of *C. albicans* infection resulting in a *granulomatous lesion* that begins

in infancy or early childhood and may persist for several years.[21] The oral lesions are often accompanied by involvement of the nails and skin (Figs. 12–32 to 12–34). In contrast to the mild, superficial acute forms of monilial infection, monilial granuloma[12] manifests itself by a deep inflammatory reaction with the production of granulation tissue. Ultimate involvement of the lungs with multiple abscesses, often associated with kidney lesions, results in death in many cases.

DIAGNOSIS. The diagnosis is confirmed by laboratory studies, as for acute candidiasis.

TREATMENT. In chronic or systemic candidiasis, the treatment involves the systemic use of amphotericin B, a potent but relatively toxic antimycotic agent. Newer antimycotic agents for systemic use are currently being tested.

Actinomycosis

Actinomycosis, caused by *Actinomyces (A. bovis* and *A. israelii),* is a disease that involves many parts of the body and is most frequently seen about the oral cavity. The actinomyces are classified as an intermediate group between the fungi and the bacteria and may be considered as bacteria-like fungi. Actinomyces are common normal inhabitants of the oral cavity.

Approximately 90 per cent of the cases of actinomycosis are of the cervicofacial type, and a large percentage of these follow extraction of teeth. One of the characteristics of actinomycosis is the lack of immediate tissue reaction following the invasion by the actinomyces. Clinically, the cervicofacial type of actinomycosis presents the following features: **dark-red discoloration of the skin, slate-blue elevated lesions, multiple nodules with formation of ridges and furrows in the creases of the skin**

Figure 12–32 Chronic Candidiasis involving gingiva in 18-year-old female.

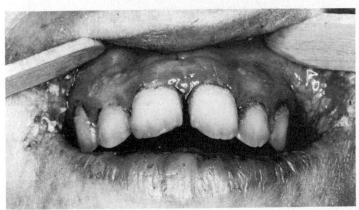

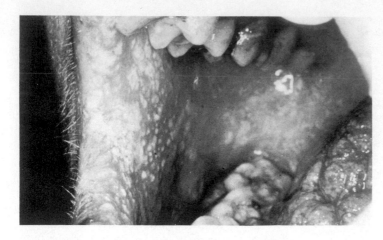

Figure 12–33 Lesions of **Chronic Candidiasis** on buccal mucosa.

and neck, distinct board-like induration, and multiple sinuses with both macroscopic and microscopic granules in the purulent discharge. Pain is usually mild and sometimes absent.

The *tongue* or *buccal mucosa* is occasionally the primary site of the disease. It starts as a *deep-seated, painless nodule* that grows slowly and eventually breaks through the mucosa, discharging a *yellowish purulent material*. On the *gingiva*, the picture is somewhat similar. It takes about 4 to 6 weeks for an actinomycotic nodule to soften and discharge its contents.

DIAGNOSIS. The purulent exudate from the lesions is collected from the draining sinuses and examined grossly for the yellow sulfur granules.

Microscopically, the granules appear as lobulated bodies composed of delicate branching, intertwined filaments. The organism can be grown anaerobically in thioglycolate medium.

TREATMENT. Surgical drainage of the lesion is effective; filtered x-irradiation, systemic penicillin, amphotericin B, and other antibiotics and sulfa drugs are also used.

Histoplasmosis

Histoplasmosis, one of the rare fungus diseases of man, shows cutaneous or mucomembranous lesions in half of the cases reported to date.[29]

Oral lesions occurred in 28 of 88 cases compiled by Miller et al.[27] The lesions may occur anywhere in the oral cavity, including the gingiva, but the *tongue* is the most common site. The most common form is a *very indurated ulcer*, although *nodular lesions* are almost as common as ulcers. The lesion also presents as verrucous or granular masses.[4] Purpuric, macular areas may accompany the ulcerations.

The skin lesions may be multiform in character and include papules, ulcerations, purpuric lesions, impetiginous eruptions, and generalized scaling dermatoses. The disease

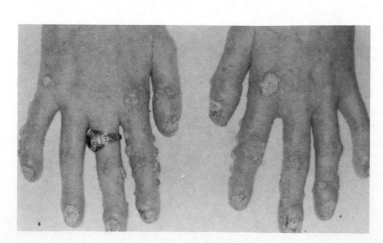

Figure 12–34 Lesions of **Chronic Candidiasis** on skin of hands and on fingernails.

presents systemic manifestations as well as cutaneous and oral lesions. The symptoms include elevated temperature, anemia, and leukopenia. Lymph node and pulmonary involvement resembling that of both lymphoblastoma and pulmonary tuberculosis occurs in many cases.

HISTOPATHOLOGY. Microscopically, histoplasmosis is classified among the chronic infectious granulomas and cannot be definitely differentiated on the basis of cellular changes from other members of this group. Multinucleated macrophages containing the yeast-like fungus *Histoplasma capsulatum* are diagnostic. Lymphocytic and plasma cell infiltration may be associated with focal areas of necrosis. Epithelial hyperplasia and fibrosis occur around the necrotic areas, and typical Langhans' giant cells are often present.

REFERENCES

1. Andreasen, J. O.: Oral lichen planus. A clinical evaluation of 115 cases. Oral Surg., 25:31, 1968.
2. Andreasen, J. O., and Poulsen, H. E.: Oral manifestations in discoid and systemic lupus erythematosus. Histologic investigation. Acta Odontol. Scand., 22:389, 1964.
3. Archard, H. O., Roebuck, N. F., and Stanley, H. R.: Oral manifestations of chronic discoid lupus erythematosus. Oral Surg., 16:696, 1963.
4. Bennett, D. E.: Histoplasmosis of the oral cavity and larynx. Arch. Intern. Med., 120:417, 1967.
5. Beutner, E. H., et al.: The immunopathology of pemphigus and bullous pemphigoid. J. Invest. Dermatol., 51:63, 1968.
6. Blank, H., and Burgoon, C. F.: Abnormal cytology of epithelial cells in pemphigus vulgaris: a diagnostic aid. J. Invest. Dermatol., 18:213, 1952.
7. Bottomley, W. K., Perlin, E., and Ross, G. R.: Antineoplastic agents and their oral manifestations. Oral Surg., 44:527, 1977.
8. Claman, H. N.: Mouth ulcers associated with prolonged chewing of gum containing aspirin. J.A.M.A., 202:651, 1967.
9. Cole, L. W.: Fixed eruption of mucous membrane and skin caused by sulfadiazine. Arch. Derm. Syph., 54:675, 1946.
10. Combes, F. L., and Canizares, O.: Pemphigus vulgaris, a clinico-pathological study of one hundred cases. Arch. Derm. Syph., 62:786, 1950.
11. Dabelsteen, E., et al.: Demonstration of basement membrane autoantibodies in patients with benign mucous membrane pemphigoid. Acta Derm. Venereol. (Stockh.), 54:189, 1974.
12. Gahan, E.: Lupus erythematosus. Clinical observations in 443 cases. Arch. Derm. Syph., 45:685, 1942.
13. Guggenheimer, J., et al.: Clinicopathological effects of cancer chemotherapeutic agents on human buccal mucosa. Oral Surg., 44:58, 1977.
14. Hashimoto, K.: Electron microscopy and histochemistry of pemphigus and pemphigoid. Oral Surg., 33:206, 1972.
15. Hashimoto, K., and Lever, W.: An electron microscopic study of pemphigus vulgaris of the mouth and skin with special reference to the intercellular cement. J. Invest. Dermatol., 48:540, 1967.
16. Jandinski, J., and Shklar, G.: Lichen planus of the gingiva. J. Periodontol., 47:724, 1976.
17. Jansen, G. T., et al.: Generalized scleroderma. Treatment with immunosuppressive agents. Arch. Dermatol., 97:690, 1968.
18. Komori, A., Welton, N. A., and Kelln, E. E.: The behavior of the basement membrane of skin and oral lesions in patients with lichen planus, erythema multiforme, lupus erythematosus, pemphigus vulgaris, pemphigoid and epidermolysis bullosa. Oral Surg., 22:752, 1966.
19. Laufer, J., and Kuffer, R.: Le Lichen Plan Buccal. Paris, Masson et Cie, 1970.
20. Lawson, B. F.: Severe stomatitis associated with barbiturate ingestion. J. Oral Med., 24:13, 1969.
21. Lehner, T.: Chronic candidiasis. Br. Dent. J., 116:539, 1964.
22. Lever, W. F.: Pemphigus. Medicine, 32:1, 1953.
23. Lozada, F., and Silverman, S.: Erythema multiforme: clinical characteristics and natural history in fifty patients. Oral Surg., 46:628, 1978.
24. McCarthy, F. P.: Pyostomatitis vegetans. Arch. Derm. Syph., 60:750, 1949.
25. McCarthy, P. L., and Shklar, G.: Diseases of the Oral Mucosa. 2nd ed. Philadelphia, Lea & Febiger, 1980.
26. Meyer, I., and Shklar, G.: The oral manifestations of acquired syphilis. Oral Surg., 23:45, 1967.
27. Miller, H. E., et al.: Histoplasmosis, cutaneous and mucomembranous lesions. Arch. Derm. Syph., 56:715, 1947.
28. O'Leary, P. A., and Nomland, R.: A clinical study of one hundred and three cases of scleroderma. Am. J. Med. Sci., 180:85, 1930.
29. Parsons, R. G., and Zarofonetis, C. J. D.: Histoplasmosis in man. Arch. Intern. Med., 75:1, 1945.
30. Pindborg, J. J., Roed-Peterson, B., and Renstrup, G.: Role of smoking in floor of the mouth leukoplakias. J. Oral Pathol., 1:22, 1972.
31. Schroeter, A. L., et al.: Treatment for early syphilis and reactivity of serologic tests. J.A.M.A., 211:471, 1972.
32. Scopp, I. W., and Schlagel, E.: Scleroderma: its orofacial manifestations. Oral Surg., 15:1510, 1962.
33. Shengold, M. A., and Sheingold, H.: Oral tuberculosis. Oral Surg., 20:29, 1951.
34. Shklar, G.: Oral lesions of erythema multiforme: histologic and histochemical observations. Arch. Dermatol., 92:495, 1965.
35. Shklar, G.: Lichen planus as an oral ulcerative disease. Oral Surg., 33:376, 1972.
36. Shklar, G., and Cataldo, E.: Histopathology and cytology of oral pemphigus vulgaris. Arch. Dermatol., 101:36, 1970.
37. Shklar, G., and McCarthy, P. L.: The oral lesions of mucous membrane pemphigoid. A study of 85 cases. Arch. Otolaryngol., 93:354, 1971.
38. Shklar, G., and McCarthy, P. L.: The Oral Manifestations of Systemic Disease. Boston, Butterworth, 1976.
39. Shklar, G., and McCarthy, P. L.: Histopathology of oral lesions of chronic discoid lupus erythematosus. Arch. Dermatol., 114:1031, 1978.
40. Shklar, G., Flynn, E., and Szabo, G.: Basement membrane changes in oral lichen planus. J. Invest. Dermatol., 70:45, 1978.
41. Shklar, G., Frim, S., and Flynn, E.: Gingival lesions of pemphigus. J. Periodontol., 49:428, 1978.
42. Shklar, G., Meyer, I., and Zacarian, S.: Oral lesions in bullous pemphigoid. Arch. Dermatol., 99:663, 1969.
43. Stafne, E. C., and Austin, L. T.: A characteristic dental finding in acrosclerosis and diffuse scleroderma. Am. J. Orthod. Oral Surg., 30:25, 1944.
44. Stevens, A. M., and Johnson, F. C.: Eruptive fever with stomatitis and ophthalmia. Am. J. Dis. Child., 24:526, 1922.
45. Sulzberger, M. B., Kanof, A., Baer, R. L., and Lowenberg, C.: Sensitization by topical application of sulfonamides. J. Allergy, 18:92, 1947.
46. Waldron, C. A., and Shafer, W. G.: Leukoplakia revisited: a clinico-pathologic study of 3,256 oral leukoplakias. Cancer. 36:1386, 1975.
47. Whitten, J. B.: Intraoral lichen planus simplex: an ultrastructural study. J. Periodontol., 41:261, 1970.
48. Wilgram, G. F., Caulfield, J. B., and Lever, W. F.: An electron microscopic study of acantholysis in pemphigus vulgaris. J. Invest. Dermatol., 36:373, 1961.
49. Zegarelli, D. J., and Zegarelli, E. V.: Intraoral pemphigus vulgaris. Oral Surg., 44:384, 1977.

Part II

Periodontal Disease

chapter thirteen

Classification of Periodontal Disease

The term *chronic destructive periodontal disease* describes all forms of periodontal disease caused primarily by local factors (bacterial plaque and trauma from occlusion). As useful background information, some of the more relevant classifications proposed for the clinical management of periodontal disease are presented in Table 13–1.

CLASSIFICATION

The following classification includes all forms of chronic destructive periodontal disease and attempts to provide a useful tool for the analysis and diagnosis of clinical cases: Chronic destructive periodontal disease
    I. Periodontitis
      A. Simple periodontitis
      B. Compound periodontitis
      C. Juvenile form of periodontitis
        1. Generalized form
        2. Localized form
    II. Trauma from occlusion*
    III. Periodontal atrophy*
      A. Presenile atrophy
      B. Disuse atrophy

---

*Both trauma from occlusion and periodontal atrophy, in their pure forms, are accommodation phenomena to changes in the environment. They are included under *diseases* for the sake of completeness and convenience for the clinician.

PERIODONTITIS

Periodontitis† is the most common type of periodontal disease and results from the extension of the inflammatory process initiated in the gingiva to the supporting periodontal tissues (see Chapters 14 to 16).

Periodontitis can be classified as *simple* or *marginal* periodontitis, in which the destruction of periodontal tissues is associated with inflammation alone; *compound* periodontitis, in which the tissue destruction resulting from inflammation is modified by trauma from occlusion; and *juvenile forms,* which constitute a special group of advanced lesions in children and adolescents.

Simple Periodontitis

CLINICAL FEATURES. Chronic inflammation of the gingiva, pocket formation, and bone loss usually accompany simple periodontitis. Tooth mobility and pathologic migration appear in advanced cases. This disease may be localized to a single tooth or group of teeth or generalized throughout the mouth, depending

---

†Synonyms not in current usage include: schmutz pyorrhea (Gottlieb), paradentitis (Weski-Becks), periodontoclasia, pericementitis, alveolar pyorrhea, alveoloclasia, Riggs' disease, and chronic suppurative periodontitis.

TABLE 13–1 REPRESENTATIVE CLASSIFICATIONS OF PERIODONTAL DISEASE

Weski, 1937[18]

Pardentitis (Gingivitis)
Hypertrophic
Simple
Ulcerative
Pardentosis
Partial atrophic (true form of paradentosis)
Total atrophic (alveolar atrophy)
Pardentoma
Localized form
Epulis
Generalized form
Elephantiasis gingivae

Gottlieb, 1928[6]

Inflammatory
Schmutz pyorrhea (poor oral hygiene)
Degenerative or atrophic
Diffuse alveolar atrophy (systemic or metabolic causes)
Paradental pyorrhea

Häupl and Lang, 1927[8]

Paradentitis
Marginal paradentitis
Etiology includes mechanical, thermal, chemical, and infectious factors, as well as functional disturbarces, tooth malformation, systemic disturbances, general resistance, etc.
Superficial marginal paradentitis
Epithelial changes
Regressive
Progressive
Formation of the pocket
Connective tissue changes
Subepithelial
Supra-alveolar
Changes in paradental bone
Marginal paradentitis profunda
Apical paradentitis

Carranza and Carranza, 1959[3]

Inflammatory periodontal syndrome { Superficial / Deep
Traumatic periodontal syndrome { Compensated / Uncompensated
Combined periodontal syndrome { Compensated / Uncompensated

McPhee and Cowley, 1969[11]

Gingivitis
Acute gingivitis
Acute specific
Ulceromembranous gingivitis
Herpetic gingivitis
Coccal gingivitis
Acute nonspecific
Acute gingivitis which does not present the features characteristic of ulceromembranous, herpetic, or coccal gingivitis
Chronic gingivitis
Chronic nonspecific
Chronic edematous gingivitis
Chronic hyperplastic gingivitis
Chronic atrophic gingivitis
Periodontitis
Acute nonspecific
Periodontal abscess
Chronic nonspecific
Periodontitis simplex
Periodontitis complex

Bernier, 1957[1]

Inflammation
Gingivitis
Periodontitis
Primary (simplex)
Secondary (complex)
Dystrophy
Occlusal traumatism
Periodontal disuse atrophy
Gingivosis
Periodontosis

Thoma and Goldman, 1937[17]

Inflammatory conditions
Gingivitis (may be of local or systemic origin)
Marginal, Hypertrophic, Ulcerative
Marginal paradentitis (poor oral hygiene)
Degenerative conditions
Paradontosis (bone resorption, in turn affecting other periodontal structures)
Atrophy
Gingival recession (faulty toothbrushing)
Presenile atrophy (normal physiologic process, recession of gingivae, and resorption of alveolar crest)
Disuse atrophy
Decreased dental function or lack of function of jaws
Atrophy due to abnormal occlusal trauma
Syndrome of paradontitis and paradontosis

Grant, Stern, and Everett, 1979[7]

Inflammatory
Gingivitis
Periodontitis
Juvenile periodontitis
Traumatic/degenerative
Periodontal trauma
Gingival recession
Alveolar atrophy
Systemic/genetic/immunologic
Hereditary gingival fibromatosis
Chédiak-Higashi syndrome
Down's syndrome
Hypophosphatasia
Cyclic neutropenia
Lazy leukocyte syndrome
Diabetes mellitus
Juvenile periodontitis
Hyperkeratosis palmaris et plantaris

Orban, 1949[12]

Inflammatory conditions
Gingivitis
Acute or chronic according to duration
Ulcerative, purulent, etc., according to symptoms
Local or systemic according to etiology
Local (extrinsic)
Infectious
Physical
Chemical
Systemic (intrinsic)
Dietary deficiency
Endocrine disturbance
Periodontitis
Simplex—following gingivitis
Complex—following periodontosis
Degenerative conditions
Gingivosis—systemic etiology
Degeneration of connective tissue
Periodontosis
Early—no inflammation
Late—deep pockets with periodontitis
Atrophic conditions
Periodontal atrophy—bone recession
Periodontal traumatism
Primary—overstress, bruxism, etc.
Secondary—loss of supporting tissue
Gingival hyperplasia
Infectious—pyogenic granuloma
Endocrine dysfunction—pregnancy
Drugs—Dilantin
Idiopathic

Goldman and Cohen, 1972[5]

I. Inflammation
  A. Gingivitis—with or without gingival enlargement (acute and chronic)
  B. Periodontitis
    1. Secondary to long-standing gingivitis
    2. Initial lesion
    3. May occur in conjunction with occlusal traumatism
    4. Secondary to periodontosis
II. Dystrophy
  A. Occlusal traumatism
  B. Degenerative disease of attachment apparatus: periodontosis

McCall and Box, 1925[10] and Box, 1940[2]

Gingivitis
Acute
Chronic
Periodontitis
Acute
Chronic
Periodontitis simplex (exogenous factors)
Periodontitis complex or rarefying pericementitis fibrosa (endogenous factors)

Fish, 1944[4]

Gingivitis
Acute ulcerative
Subacute marginal
Chronic marginal
Traumatic
Pyorrhea
Pyorrhea simplex
Pyorrhea profunda
Senile alveolar resorption
Neoplasia
Odontoclasma
Cementoma
Fibrous epulis

Table continued on following page

TABLE 13–1 REPRESENTATIVE CLASSIFICATIONS OF PERIODONTAL DISEASE *(Continued)*

Held and Chaput, 1960[9]	Prichard, 1972[14]	Ramfjord and Ash, 1979[15]	Schluger, Yuodelis and Page, 1977[16]
Parodontopathies	Diseases affecting the surface or gingiva	Gingivitis	Gingivitis
Superficial	Inflammation without surface destruction	Simplex	Plaque-associated gingivitis
Inflammatory—gingivitis	Marginal gingivitis	Complex	Acute ulcerative necrotizing gingivitis
Degenerative—gingivosis	Generalized diffuse gingivitis	Gingival hyperplasia	Hormonal gingivitis
Deep	Gingival enlargement	Necrotizing lesions	Drug-induced gingivitis
Inflammatory—parodontitis } parodontolysis	Inflammation with surface destruction	Traumatic	Marginal periodontitis
Degenerative—parodontosis	Necrotizing ulcerative gingivitis	Gingival atrophy or recession	Adult type
Superficial and deep	Herpetic gingivostomatitis	Systemic factors	Juvenile type
Neoplastic—parodontoma	Desquamative gingivitis	Local causes	
Reticular—parodontoreticulosis	Oral ulcers	Trauma from occlusion	
	Diseases that affect the deeper structures	Periodontitis	
Page and Schroeder, 1982[13]	Chronic destructive periodontal disease or periodontitis	Simple	
Prepubertal	Periodontal abscess	Complex	
Generalized	Periodontal traumatism	Juvenile, etc.	
Localized	Primary traumatism		
Juvenile	Secondary traumatism		
Rapidly Progressing Periodontitis			
"Adult" Type Periodontitis			

REFERENCES TO TABLE 13–1

1. Bernier, J. L.: Report of the committee on classification and nomenclature. J. Periodontol., 28:56, 1957.
2. Box, H. K.: Periodontal studies. D. Items Int., 62:915, 1940.
3. Carranza, F. A., Sr., and Carranza, F. A., Jr.: A suggested classification of common periodontal disease. J. Periodontol., 30:140, 1959.
4. Fish, E. W.: Paradontal Disease. London, Eyre and Spottiswoode, 1944, p. 52.
5. Goldman, H. M., and Cohen, D. W.: Periodontal Therapy. 5th ed. St. Louis, C. V. Mosby Company, 1972.
6. Gottlieb, B.: Parodontal pyorrhea and alveolar atrophy. J. Am. Dent. Assoc. 15:2196, 1928.
7. Grant, D. A., Stern, J., and Everett, F.: Periodontics. 5th ed. St. Louis, C. V. Mosby Company, 1979.
8. Häupl, K., and Lang, F. J.: Marginal Paradentitis. Berlin, H. Meusser, 1927.
9. Held, A.-J., and Chaput, A.: Les Parodontologes. Paris, Julien Prélat, 1960.
10. McCall, J. O., and Box, H. K.: Chronic periodontitis. J. Am. Dent. Assoc., 12:1300, 1925.
11. McPhee, T., and Cowley, G.: Essentials of Periodontology and Periodontitis. London, Blackwell Scientific Publications, 1969.
12. Orban, B.: Classification of periodontal disease. Paradentologie, 3:159, 1949.
13. Page, R. C., and Schroeder, H. E.: Periodontitis in Man and Other Animals. Basel, S. Karger, 1982.
14. Prichard, J. F.: Advanced Periodontal Disease. 2nd ed. Philadelphia, W. B. Saunders Company, 1972.
15. Ramfjord, S. P., and Ash, M. M.: Periodontology and Periodontics. Philadelphia, W. B. Saunders Company, 1979.
16. Schluger, S., Yuodelis, R., and Page, R.: Periodontal Disease. Philadelphia, Lea & Febiger, 1977.
17. Thoma, K. H., and Goldman, H. M.: Classification and histopathology of parodontal disease. J. Am. Dent. Assoc., 24:1915, 1937.
18. Weski, O.: Paradentopathia and paradentosis. Paradentium, 8:169, 1937.

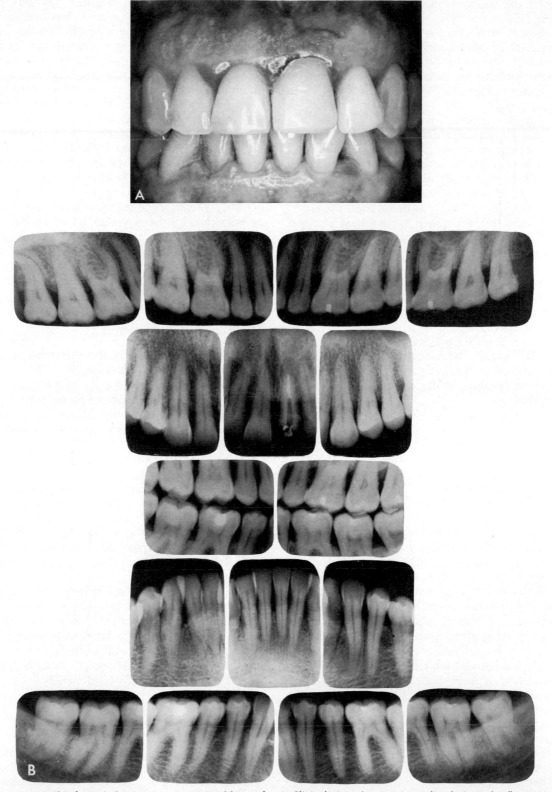

Figure 13–1 Simple Periodontitis in a 47-Year-Old Female. *A,* Clinical view showing generalized gingival inflammation and periodontal pocket formation. *B,* Radiographs showing generalized horizontal bone loss which varies in severity in different areas.

upon the distribution of the etiologic factors (Fig. 13–1).

Simple periodontitis progresses at a varied rate; its advanced stages are usually seen in the fifth and sixth decades of life. This contrasts with the juvenile form, which reaches its advanced stages in the late teens and early adulthood.

Simple periodontitis is usually painless, but it may be accompanied by such symptoms as (1) sensitivity to thermal changes, food, and tactile stimulation, associated with denudation of the roots; (2) dull, deep, radiating pain during and after chewing, caused by the forceful wedging of food into periodontal pockets; (3) acute symptoms such as throbbing pain and sensitivity to percussion, caused by periodontal abscess formation or superimposed acute necrotizing ulcerative gingivitis; and (4) pulpal symptoms such as sensitivity to sweets, thermal changes, or throbbing pain, which result from pulpitis associated with carious destruction of the root surfaces.

ETIOLOGY. Simple periodontitis is caused by dental plaque. The accumulation of plaque can be favored by a large variety of local irritants such as calculus, faulty restorations, and food impaction.

Compound Periodontitis*

CLINICAL FEATURES. The clinical features are the same as those of simple periodontitis, with the following exceptions: there is a higher incidence of infrabony pockets and angular rather than horizontal bone loss[2] (Fig. 13–2), widening of the periodontal ligament space is a more common finding, and tooth mobility tends to occur earlier and to be more severe.

ETIOLOGY. Compound periodontitis is caused by the combined effect of bacterial plaque and the resultant inflammation and trauma from occlusion.

On the basis of the rate of tissue destruction and some clinical features, simple and compound periodontitis can be subclassified into two groups. One is a *slowly progressing lesion* associated with abundant plaque and calculus deposits. Obvious signs of gingival inflammation are found (changes in color, surface texture, abundant exudate, and so forth). (See Chapter 9.)

The other type is a more *rapidly progressing lesion,* associated with scantier amounts of plaque and calculus. Page et al.[4] have recently described this condition as a distinct clinical entity with the following characteristics: seen most commonly in young adults in their twenties, but can occur up to the age of 35; extreme inflammation; hemorrhage; proliferation of the marginal gingiva; exudation; rapid bone loss (extreme loss within a few weeks or months). It may subside and become quiescent or progress to tooth loss. Most patients have serum antibodies for various species of Bacteroides, Actinobacillus, or both and show defects in either neutrophil or monocyte chemotaxis.

Clinical features of the slow and rapid types of periodontitis have yet to be more clearly defined, and differential diagnosis may therefore be difficult, except by determining the rate of progression of periodontal destruction and the response to treatment.

Juvenile Form of Periodontitis

This form includes advanced destructive lesions in children and adolescents.* The distribution of lesions is the basis for its classification into generalized and localized forms. The generalized form involves the whole dentition, whereas the localized form attacks first molars and incisors.

GENERALIZED FORM. These are the diseases associated with systemic conditions such as Papillon-Lefèvre syndrome, hypophosphatasia, agranulocytosis, Down's syndrome, and others. They have different characteristics depending on the systemic condition and are dealt with in Chapter 22. Patients without underlying systemic predisposing factors have also been described.

LOCALIZED FORM. This includes the disease we now call "idiopathic juvenile periodontitis" (Fig. 13–3) and that in the past received the name "periodontosis."[1, 3] It is characterized by deep angular lesions localized in the first molars and incisors and occurs in otherwise healthy adolescents (see Chapter 22).

TRAUMA FROM OCCLUSION

Because gingival inflammation is so common, trauma from occlusion seldom occurs without it. When it is the sole pathologic

---

*Other terms used for this condition include occlusal periodontitis and traumatic periodontitis.

*The terms precocious advanced alveolar atrophy, juvenile atrophy, paradentose juvenile, and juvenile parodontopathia have been used to describe this condition.

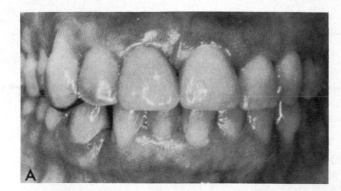

Figure 13–2 Compound Periodontitis in a 44-Year-Old Female. *A,* Generalized gingival inflammation with periodontal pocket formation. *B,* Generalized bone loss with angular destruction of the interdental septa caused by the combination of inflammation and trauma from occlusion.

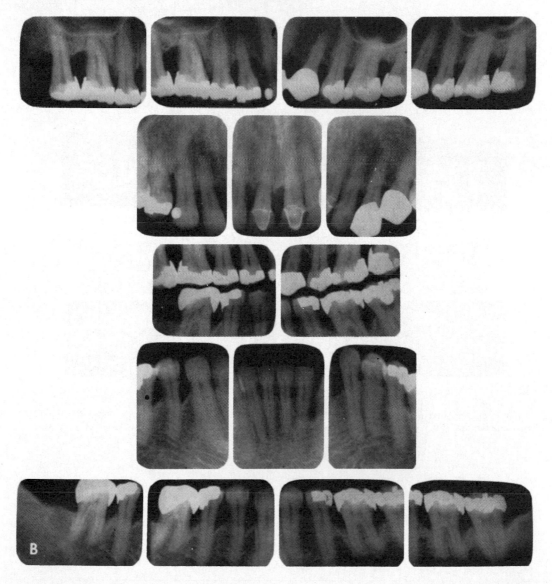

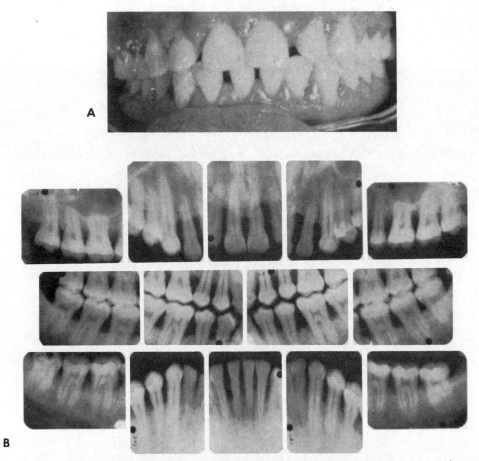

Figure 13–3 Idiopathic Juvenile Periodontitis in a 24-Year-Old Male. *A,* Pathologic migration of the maxillary and mandibular anterior teeth. *B,* Generalized bone loss accentuated in the maxillary and mandibular anterior areas.

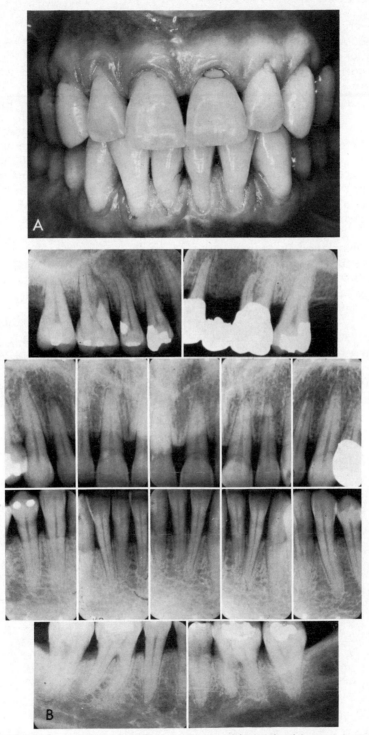

Figure 13–4 Presenile Atrophy in a 38-Year-Old Male. *A,* Reduction in the height of the periodontium and recession with slight gingival inflammation. *B,* Premature generalized bone loss.

process trauma from occlusion presents the following clinical features: tooth mobility, pronounced widening of the periodontal space in the gingival region of the root (with an associated angular destruction of bone), and thickening of the periodontal ligament at the apex. Isolated teeth and their antagonists are affected. It does not produce gingival inflammation or the formation of periodontal pockets.

PERIODONTAL ATROPHY

Atrophy is a decrease in the size of the tissue or organ or of its cellular elements after it has attained its normal mature size. Generalized reduction in the height of the alveolar bone, accompanied by recession of the gingiva without overt inflammation or trauma from occlusion, occurs with increasing age and has been termed physiologic or senile atrophy. It is due not to aging but to the cumulative effect of repeated injuries to the periodontium.

Presenile Atrophy

Presenile atrophy is premature reduction in the height of the periodontium that is uniform throughout the mouth and without apparent local cause (Fig. 13–4).

Disuse Atrophy

Disuse atrophy results when the functional stimulation required for the maintenance of the periodontal tissues is markedly diminished or absent. Disuse atrophy is characterized by thinning of the periodontal ligament, thinning and reduction in the number of periodontal fibers and disruption of the fiber bundle arrangement, thickened cementum, reduction in the height of the alveolar bone, and osteoporosis, which appears as a reduction in the number and thickness of the bony trabeculae.

REFERENCES

1. Baer, P. N.: The case of periodontosis as a clinical entity. J. Periodontol., *42*:516, 1971.
2. Erausquin, R., and Carranza, F. A.: Primeros hallazgos paradentosicos. Rev. Odontol. (Buenos Aires), *27*:485, 1939.
3. Gottlieb, B.: Die diffuse Atrophy des Alveolarknochens. Z. Stomatol., *21*:195, 1923.
4. Page, R. C., et al.: Rapidly progressive periodontitis. A distinct clinical condition. J. Periodontol., *54*:197, 1983.

The Periodontal Pocket

A periodontal pocket is a pathologically deepened gingival sulcus; it is one of the important clinical features of periodontal disease. Progressive pocket formation leads to destruction of the supporting periodontal tissues and loosening and exfoliation of the teeth.

SIGNS AND SYMPTOMS

The only reliable method of locating periodontal pockets and determining their extent is careful probing of the gingival margin along each tooth surface (see Chapter 32).

The following clinical signs may suggest the presence of periodontal pockets:

1. Enlarged, bluish-red marginal gingiva with a "rolled" edge separated from the tooth surface (Fig. 14–1).

2. A reddish-blue vertical zone extending from the gingival margin to the attached gingiva and sometimes into the alveolar mucosa (Fig. 14–2).

3. A break in the faciolingual continuity of the interdental gingiva.

4. Shiny, discolored, and puffy gingiva associated with exposed root surfaces (Fig. 14–3).

5. Gingival bleeding.

6. Purulent exudate of the gingival margin (Fig. 14–4) or its appearance in response to digital pressure on the lateral aspect of the gingival margin (Fig. 14–5).

7. Looseness, extrusion, and migration of teeth.

8. The development of diastemata where none had existed (Fig. 14–6).

Periodontal pockets are generally painless but may give rise to the following symptoms: localized pain or a sensation of pressure after eating, which gradually diminishes; a foul taste in localized areas; a tendency to suck material from the interproximal spaces; radiating pain "deep in the bone"; a "gnawing" feeling or feeling of itchiness in the gums; the urge to dig a pointed instrument into the gums with relief obtained from the resultant bleeding; complaints that food "sticks between the teeth" or that the teeth "feel loose" or a preference to "eat on the other side"; sensitivity to heat and cold; and toothache in the absence of caries.

CLASSIFICATION

Periodontal pockets are classified according to morphology and their relationship to adjacent structures as follows:

Gingival Pocket (Relative or False)

A gingival pocket is formed by gingival enlargement without destruction of the underlying periodontal tissues. The sulcus is deepened because of the increased bulk of the gingiva (Fig. 14–7). Gingival pockets are dealt with in Chapter 10.

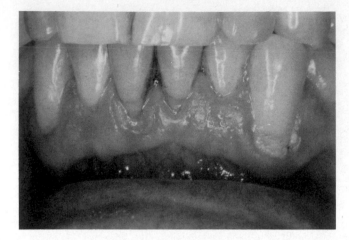

Figure 14–1 Periodontal Pockets around the central incisors and left canine, showing rolled margins and separation from the tooth surfaces. Note the materia alba on the canine.

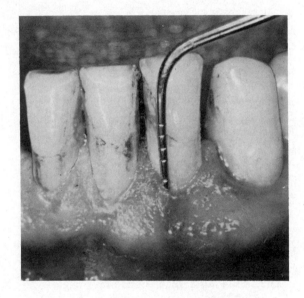

Figure 14–2 Periodontal Pocket with vertical discolored zone extending to the alveolar mucosa.

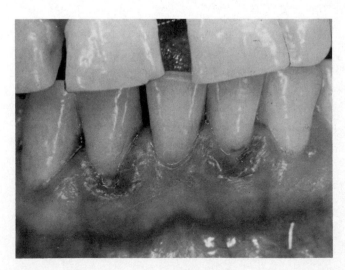

Figure 14–3 Periodontal Pockets with puffy, discolored gingiva and exposed root surfaces.

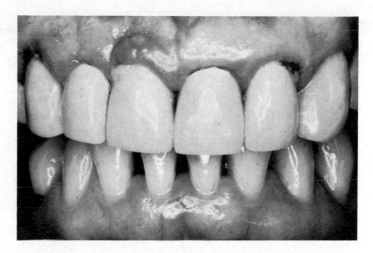

Figure 14–4 Purulent Exudate from periodontal pocket on the maxillary left central incisor.

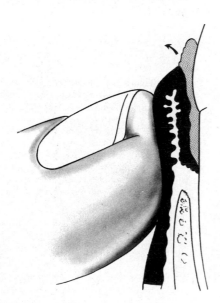

Figure 14–5 Purulent Exudate Expressed from Periodontal Pocket by Digital Pressure.

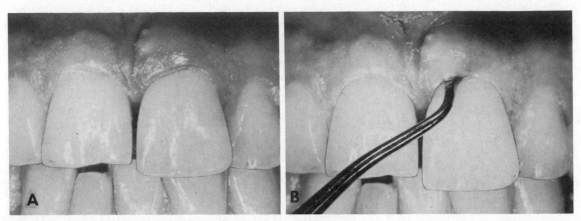

Figure 14–6 *A,* **Extrusion of Maxillary Left Incisor** and diastema associated with periodontal pocket. *B,* Entire length of periodontal probe inserted to the base of periodontal pocket on central incisor.

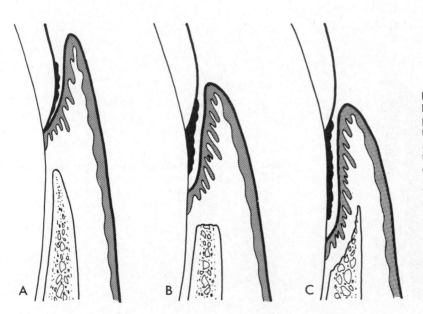

Figure 14–7 Different Types of Periodontal Pockets. *A,* Gingival pocket. There is no destruction of the supporting periodontal tissues. *B,* Suprabony pocket. The base of the pocket is coronal to the level of the underlying bone. Bone loss is horizontal. *C,* Infrabony pocket. The base of the pocket is apical to the level of the adjacent bone. Bone loss is vertical

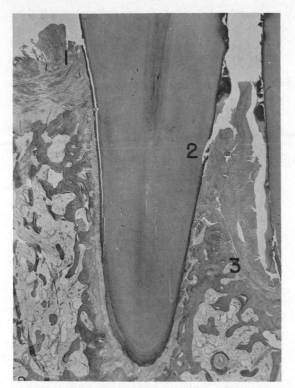

Figure 14–8 Suprabony Pockets of different depths on the distal (1) and mesial (2) surfaces of second premolar. Interdental space with suprabony pocket (2) and **Infrabony Pocket** (3) on the approximating tooth surfaces.

Periodontal Pocket (Absolute or True)

This is the type of pocket that occurs with destruction of the supporting periodontal tissues (Fig. 14–7). The remainder of this chapter refers to this type of pocket.

Absolute pockets are of two types: (1) **suprabony** (supracrestal), in which the bottom of the pocket is coronal to the underlying alveolar bone; and (2) **infrabony** (intrabony, subcrestal, or intra-alveolar), in which the bottom of the

pocket is apical to the level of the adjacent alveolar bone. In this second type the lateral pocket wall lies between the tooth surface and the alveolar bone (Fig. 14–7).

Pockets of different depths and types may occur on different surfaces of the same tooth and on approximating surfaces of the same interdental space (Fig. 14–8).

Pockets can also be classified according to the number of surfaces involved as follows:

SIMPLE. One tooth surface (Fig. 14–9).

COMPOUND. Two or more tooth surfaces. The base of the pockets is in direct communication with the gingival margin along each of the involved surfaces (Fig. 14–9).

COMPLEX. This is a spiral-type pocket that originates on one tooth surface and twists around the tooth to involve one or more additional surfaces (Figs. 14–9 and 14–10). The only communication with the gingival margin is at the surface where the pocket originates. To avoid missing the compound or complex types, all pockets should be probed laterally as well as vertically. These types of pockets are most common in furcation areas.

PATHOGENESIS

Periodontal pockets are caused by microorganisms and their products, which produce pathologic tissue changes and deepening of the gingival sulcus. On the basis of depth alone, it is sometimes difficult to differentiate between a deep normal sulcus and a shallow periodontal pocket. In such borderline cases pathologic changes in the gingiva differentiate the two conditions.

Deepening of the gingival sulcus may occur by (1) movement of the gingival margin in the direction of the crown (this produces a gingival rather than a periodontal pocket; sulcus depth

Figure 14–9 Classification of Pockets According to Involved Tooth Surfaces. *A*, Simple pocket. *B*, Compound pocket. *C*, Complex pocket.

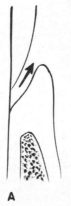

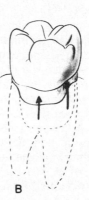

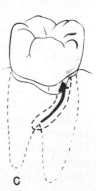

A   B   C

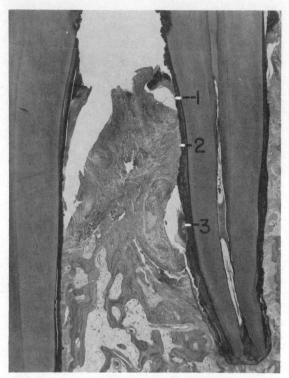

Figure 14–10 Complex Pocket. The base of the pocket is shown at 3. The pocket then spirals around onto another surface of the tooth and communicates with the oral cavity at 1. In the area marked 2, the periodontal ligament is attached to the tooth.

is increased by enlargement of the gingiva without destruction of supporting tissues); (2) migration of the junctional epithelium apically and its separation from the tooth surface; or (3) what is usually the case, a combination of both processes (Fig. 14–11).

Changes involved in the transition from the normal gingival sulcus to the pathologic periodontal pocket are associated with different proportions of bacterial cells in dental plaque. Healthy gingiva contains few microorganisms, mostly coccoid cells and straight rods. Diseased gingiva shows increased numbers of spirochetes and motile rods.[28, 30]

Pocket formation starts as an inflammatory change in the connective tissue wall of the gingival sulcus caused by bacterial plaque. The cellular and fluid inflammatory exudate causes degeneration of the surrounding connective tissue, including the gingival fibers.

Several zones have been described in the process of destruction of connective tissue attachment.[14, 47] Just apical to the junctional epithelium is an area of destroyed collagen fibers, which becomes occupied by inflamma-

tory cells and edema. Immediately apical to this is a zone of partial destruction, then an area of normal attachment. Two hypotheses have been advanced regarding the mechanism of collagen loss: (1) collagenases and other lysosomal enzymes from polymorphonuclear leukocytes[57] and macrophages[39] become extracellular and destroy collagen, and (2) fibroblasts phagocytize collagen fibers by extending cytoplasmic processes to the ligament-cementum interface and resorbing the inserted collagen fibrils and the fibrils of the cementum matrix.[14, 15]

In association with the inflammation, the junctional epithelium proliferates along the root in the form of finger-like projections two or three cells in thickness. The coronal portion of the junctional epithelium detaches from the root as the apical portion migrates.

The coronal portion of the junctional epithelium is subject, as a result of inflammation, to increased invasion by polymorphonuclear leukocytes, which are not joined to each other or to the remaining epithelial cells by desmosomes. When the relative volume of polymorphonuclear leukocytes reaches approximately 60 per cent or more of the junctional epithelium tissue, this tissue detaches from the tooth surface. Thus, the sulcus bottom shifts apically, and the oral sulcular epithelium occupies a gradually increasing portion of the sulcular lining.[48]

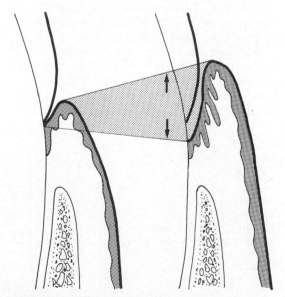

Figure 14–11 Diagrammatic Representation of Pocket Formation indicating expansion in two directions (*arrows*) from the normal gingival sulcus (*left*) to the periodontal pocket (*right*).

The degree of leukocyte infiltration of the junctional epithelium is independent of the volume of inflamed connective tissue, so this process may occur in gingiva with only slight signs of clinical inflammation.[47]

With continued inflammation, the gingiva increases in bulk, and the crest of the gingival margin extends toward the crown. The junctional epithelium continues to migrate along the root and separate from it. The epithelium of the lateral wall of the pocket proliferates to form bulbous and cord-like extensions into the inflamed connective tissue. Leukocytes and edema from the inflamed connective tissue infiltrate the epithelium lining the pocket, resulting in varying degrees of degeneration and necrosis.

The transformation of a gingival sulcus into a periodontal pocket creates an area where plaque removal becomes impossible, and the following feedback mechanism is established:

Plaque → gingival inflammation → pocket formation → more plaque formation.

The rationale for pocket reduction is based on the need to eliminate areas of plaque accumulation.

PERIODONTAL DISEASE ACTIVITY

For many years the loss of attachment produced by periodontal disease was thought to be a slow but continuously progressive phenomenon. In recent years and as a consequence of studies on the specificity of plaque bacteria (see Chapter 25), the concept of periodontal disease activity has evolved.

According to this concept, periodontal pockets go through periods of quiescence and exacerbation. **Periods of quiescence** are characterized by a reduced inflammatory response and little or no loss of bone and connective tissue attachment. A build-up of unattached plaque, with its gram-negative, motile, and anaerobic bacteria (see Chapter 25), starts a **period of exacerbation** in which bone and connective tissue attachments are lost and the pocket deepens. This period may last for days, weeks, or months and is eventually followed by a period of remission or quiescence in which gram-positive bacteria proliferate and a more stable condition is established. Based on a study of ^{125}I absorptiometry, McHenry et al. have reported that bone loss in untreated periodontal disease occurs in an episodic manner.[34]

These periods of quiescence and exacerbation are also known as *periods of activity and inactivity*. Clinically active periods show bleeding, either spontaneously or upon probing, and greater amounts of gingival exudate. Histologically, thinned or ulcerated pocket epithelium and an infiltrate composed predominantly of plasma cells[13] and/or polymorphonuclear leukocytes[39] are seen, whereas bacterial samples from the pocket lumen, analyzed with darkfield microscopy, show high proportions of motile organisms and spirochetes.[30] Over a period of time, loss of bone should be detected radiographically.

Methods to detect periods of activity or inactivity are being investigated at present (see Chapter 32).

TABLE 14–1   CORRELATION OF CLINICAL AND HISTOPATHOLOGIC FEATURES OF THE PERIODONTAL POCKET

Clinical Features	Histopathologic Features
1. The gingival wall of the periodontal pocket presents varying degrees of bluish-red discoloration, flaccidity, a smooth, shiny surface, and pitting on pressure.	1. The discoloration is caused by circulatory stagnation; the flaccidity, by destruction of the gingival fibers and surrounding tissues; the smooth, shiny surface, by the atrophy of the epithelium and edema; the pitting on pressure, by edema and degeneration.
2. Less frequently the gingival wall may be pink and firm.	2. In such cases fibrotic changes predominate over exudation and degeneration, particularly in relation to the outer surface of the pocket wall. However, despite the external appearance of health, the inner wall of the pocket invariably presents some degeneration and is often ulcerated (Fig. 14–21).
3. Bleeding is elicited by gently probing the soft tissue wall of the pocket.	3. Ease of bleeding results from increased vascularity, thinning and degeneration of the epithelium, and the proximity of the engorged vessels to the inner surface.
4. When explored with a probe the inner aspect of the periodontal pocket is generally painful.	4. Pain upon tactile stimulation is due to ulceration of the inner aspect of the pocket wall.
5. In many cases pus may be expressed by applying digital pressure.	5. This occurs in pockets with suppurative inflammation of the inner wall.

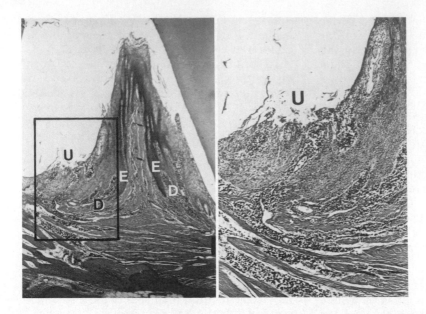

Figure 14–12 *Left,* **Interdental Papilla with Suprabony Pockets on Proximal Tooth Surfaces.** D, Densely inflamed connective tissue; E, proliferating pocket epithelium; U, ulcerated pocket epithelium. *Right,* Higher magnification of rectangle in Figure 14–12A. Note the ulcerated area (U) and the infiltrate between the collagen fibers.

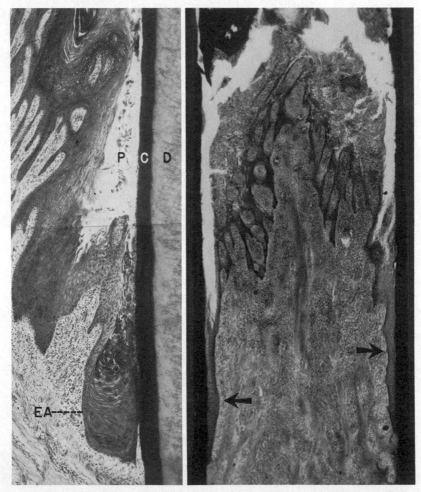

Figure 14–13 Varied Conformations of Junctional Epithelium. *Left,* Hyperkeratotic nodular junctional epithelium (EA) at the base of pocket (P), cementum (C), dentin (D). *Right,* Interdental papilla showing lengthy junctional epithelium (*arrows*) in two proximal pockets.

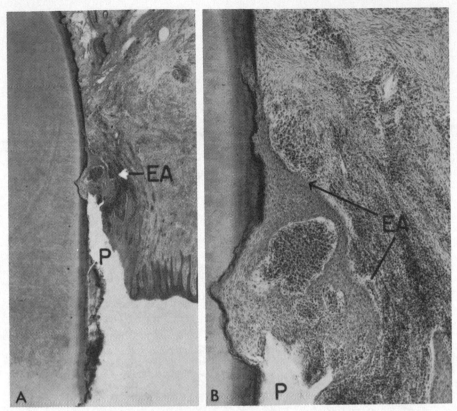

Figure 14–14 *A*, **Low-Power Section of Periodontal Pocket** (P). The location of the junctional epithelium is indicated by the arrow (EA). The lateral epithelial wall is ulcerated, *B*, **Detailed Study of Junctional Epithelium** (EA) at the base of the pocket (P). Note extension of well-formed epithelial cells (*arrow*) along the resorbed root surface. There is a dense accumulation of leukocytes enclosed within the epithelium.

HISTOPATHOLOGY

Changes occurring in the initial stages of pocket formation are presented in Chapter 8. Once the pocket is formed, the following microscopic features are present:

The Soft Tissue Wall

The connective tissue is edematous and densely infiltrated with plasma cells (approximately 80 per cent[64]) and lymphocytes and a scattering of polymorphonuclear leukocytes. The blood vessels are increased in number, dilated, and engorged. The connective tissue presents varying degrees of degeneration. Single or multiple necrotic foci are occasionally present.[38] In addition to exudative and degenerative changes, the connective tissue presents proliferation of the endothelial cells, with newly formed capillaries, fibroblasts, and collagen fibers (Fig. 14–12).

The junctional epithelium at the base of the pocket varies as to length, width, and condition of the epithelial cells. **The variations range from the extremes of a long, narrow band to a comparatively short, wide clump of cells (Fig. 14–13). The cells may be well formed and in good condition or present slight to marked degeneration (Fig. 14–14).**

Special note should be made of the fact that extension of the junctional epithelium along the root requires the presence of *healthy epithelial cells*. Degeneration of the junctional epithelium would retard rather than accelerate pocket formation. Degenerative changes are seen in the junctional epithelium at the base of periodontal pockets, but they are usually less severe than those in the epithelium of the lateral pocket wall. Since migration of the junctional epithelium requires healthy, viable cells, it is reasonable to assume that the degenerative changes seen in this area occurred after the junctional epithelium reached its position on the cementum.

The most severe degenerative changes in the periodontal pocket occur along the lateral wall (Fig. 14–15). The epithelium of the lateral wall

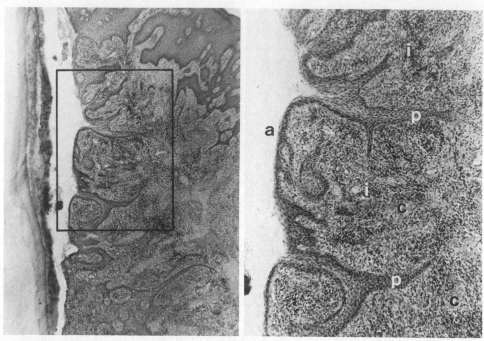

Figure 14–15 *A,* Low-power view of the lateral wall of a periodontal pocket. Note the dense inflammatory infiltrate and the proliferating epithelium. *B,* High-power view of rectangle in Figure 14–15*A.* Note the areas of atrophic epithelium (a) and areas of epithelial proliferation (p). The connective tissue is densely infiltrated (i); some remnants of collagen fibers (c) can be seen.

of the pocket presents striking proliferative and degenerative changes. **Epithelial buds or interlacing cords of epithelial cells project from the lateral wall into the adjacent inflamed connective tissue and frequently extend farther apically than the junctional epithelium. These epithelial projections, as well as the remainder of the lateral epithelium, are densely infiltrated by leukocytes and edema from the inflamed connective tissue. The cells undergo vacuolar degeneration and rupture to form vesicles. Progressive degeneration and necrosis of the epithelium lead to ulceration of the lateral wall, exposure of the underlying markedly inflamed connective tissue, and suppuration. In some cases acute inflammation is superimposed upon the underlying chronic changes.**

A detailed electron microscopic description of the pocket epithelium in experimentally induced pockets in dogs has been done by Müller-Glauser and Schroeder.[36]

It has recently been shown that **bacterial invasion of the apical and lateral areas of the pocket wall** may occur in human chronic periodontitis. Filaments, rods, and coccoid organisms with predominant gram-negative cell walls have been reported to appear in intercellular spaces of the epithelium.[16, 17] Bacteria invade

the intercellular space initially under exfoliating epithelial cells, but they are also found between deeper epithelial cells and accumulating on the basement lamina.[46] Some bacteria traverse the basement lamina and invade the subepithelial connective tissue[46] (Fig. 14–16).

The severity of the degenerative changes is not necessarily related to pocket depth. Ulceration of the lateral wall may occur in shallow pockets, and deep pockets are occasionally observed in which the lateral epithelium is intact and presents only slight degeneration (Fig. 14–17).

The epithelium at the crest of the periodontal pocket is generally intact and thickened, with prominent rete pegs. When acute inflammation occurs on the surface of the periodontal pocket, however, the crest of the gingiva undergoes degeneration and necrosis.

Microtopography of the Gingival Wall of the Pocket[45]

Scanning electron microscopy has permitted the description of several areas in the soft tissue wall of the pocket where different types of activity take place. These areas are irreg-

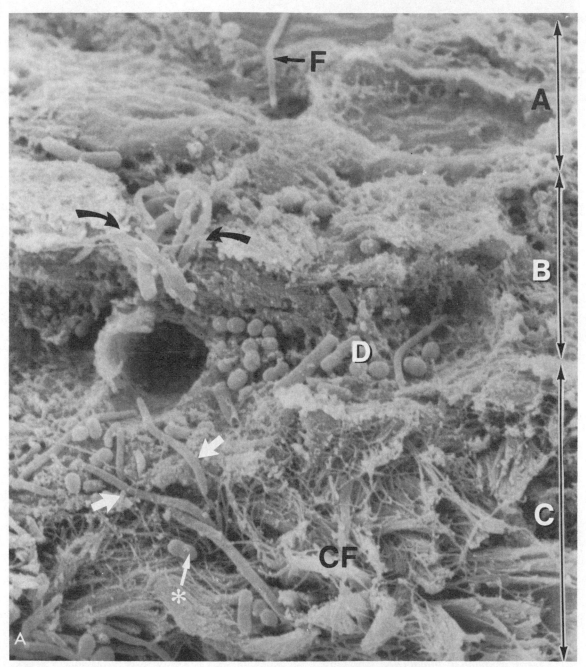

Figure 14–16 Electron Micrograph of Section of Pocket Wall in Advanced Periodontitis in a Human Specimen, Showing Bacterial Penetration into the Epithelium and Connective Tissue. *A,* **Scanning Electron Microscope** view of surface of pocket wall (A), sectioned epithelium (B), and sectioned connective tissue (C). Curved arrows point to areas of bacterial penetration into the epithelium. Thick white arrows point to bacterial penetration into the connective tissue through a break in the continuity of the basal lamina. F, filamentous organism on surface of epithelium; D, accumulation of bacteria (rods, cocci, filaments) on basal lamina; CF, connective tissue fibers. Asterisk points to coccobacillus in connective tissue.

Illustration continued on following page

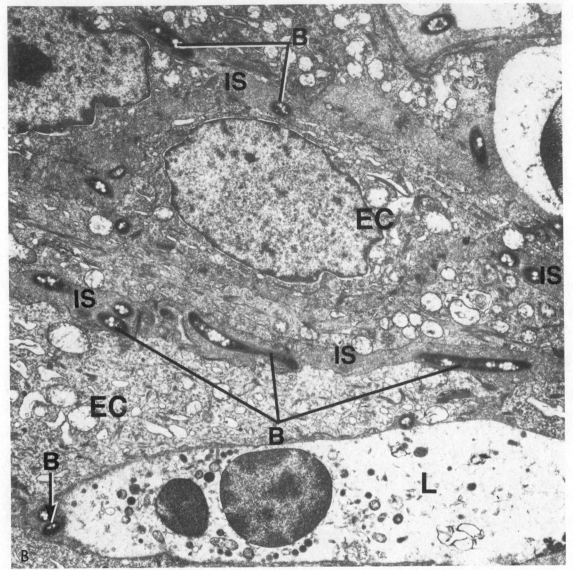

Figure 14–16 *Continued B,* **Transmission Electron Microscope** view of epithelium in periodontal pocket wall showing bacteria in intercellular spaces. EC, epithelial cell; IS, intercellular space; B, bacteria; L, leukocyte about to engulf bacteria. X 8000.

ularly oval or elongated, adjacent to one another, and measure about 50 to 200 microns. These findings suggest that the pocket wall is constantly changing as a result of the interaction between the host and the bacteria.

1. *Areas of relative quiescence,* showing a relatively flat surface with minor depressions and mounds and occasional shedding of cells (Fig. 14–18,A).

2. *Areas of bacterial accumulation,* which appear as depressions on the epithelial surface, with abundant debris and bacterial clumps penetrating into the enlarged intercellular

spaces. These bacteria are mainly cocci, rods, and filaments, with a few spirochetes (Fig. 14–18,B).

3. *Areas of emergence of leukocytes,* where leukocytes appear in the pocket wall through holes located in the intercellular spaces (Figs. 14–18 and 14–19).

4. *Areas of leukocyte-bacterial interaction,* where numerous leukocytes are present and covered with bacteria in an apparent process of phagocytosis. Bacterial plaque associated with the epithelium is seen either as an organized matrix covered by a fibrin-like material

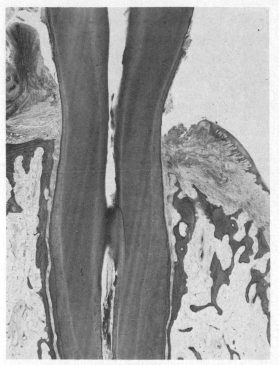

Figure 14–17 Shallow Ulcerated Pocket in Relation to One Surface of a Tooth (right) in contrast with intact deeper pocket in relation to other tooth surface (left).

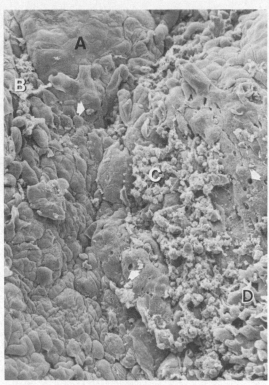

Figure 14–18 Scanning electron microscopic frontal view of periodontal pocket wall. Different areas can be seen in the pocket wall surface. A, area of quiescence; B, bacterial accumulation; C, bacterial-leukocyte interaction; D, intense cellular desquamation. Arrows point to emerging leukocytes and holes left by them in the pocket wall. × 800.

Figure 14–19 Scanning electron micrograph of periodontal pocket wall, frontal view, in a case of advanced periodontitis in a human. Note the desquamating epithelial cells and leukocytes (white arrows) emerging onto the pocket space. Scattered bacteria can also be seen (black arrow). × 150.

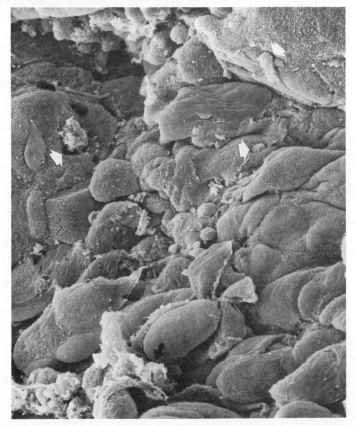

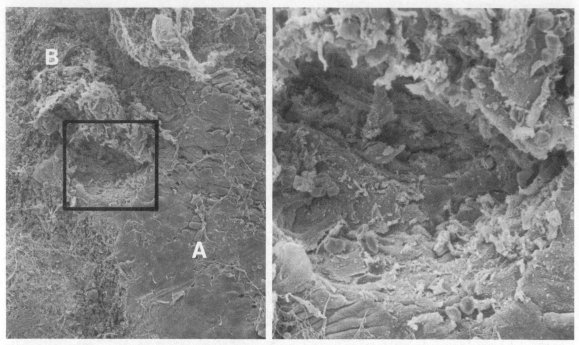

Figure 14–20 *Left,* Area of ulceration in lateral wall of deep periodontal pocket in human specimen. A, surface of pocket epithelium in a quiescent state; B, area of hemorrhage. × 800. *Right,* Higher magnification of square in Figure 14–20*A.* Connective tissue fibers and cells can be seen in bottom of ulcer. Scanning electron microscopy. × 3000.

in contact with the surface of cells or as bacteria penetrating into the intercellular spaces (Fig. 14–18,C).

5. *Areas of intense epithelial desquamation,* which consist of semiattached and folded epithelial squames, sometimes partially covered with bacteria (Fig. 14–18,D).

6. *Areas of ulceration,* with exposed connective tissue (Fig. 14–20).

7. *Areas of hemorrhage,* with numerous erythrocytes.

The transition from one area to another could be postulated as follows: bacteria accumulate in previously quiescent areas, triggering the emergence of leukocytes and the leukocyte-bacterial interaction. This would lead to intense epithelial desquamation and, finally, to ulceration and hemorrhage.

Periodontal Pockets Are Healing Lesions

Periodontal pockets are chronic inflammatory lesions and as such are constantly undergoing repair.

The condition of the soft tissue wall of the periodontal pocket results from a balance between destructive and constructive tissue changes. The destructive changes are charac- terized by the fluid and cellular inflammatory exudate and the associated degenerative changes stimulated by the local irritation. The constructive changes consist of the formation of blood vessels in an effort to repair the tissue damage caused by inflammation.

Complete healing does not occur because of the persistence of local irritants. These irritants continue to stimulate fluid and cellular exudate, which in turn causes degeneration of the new tissue elements formed in the continuous effort at repair.

The balance between exudative and constructive changes determines the color, consistency, and surface texture of the pocket wall. If the inflammatory fluid and cellular exudate predominate, the pocket wall is bluish red, soft, spongy, and friable, with a smooth, shiny surface. If there is a relative predominance of newly formed connective tissue cells and fibers, the pocket wall is firm and pink. At the clinical level the former condition is generally referred to as an edematous pocket, the latter as a fibrotic pocket (see Chapter 32).

Edematous and fibrotic pockets represent opposite extremes of the same pathologic process rather than different disease entities. They are subject to constant modification, depend-

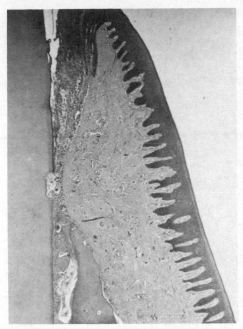

Figure 14–21 Periodontal Pocket Wall. The inner half is inflamed and ulcerated, the outer half is densely collagenous.

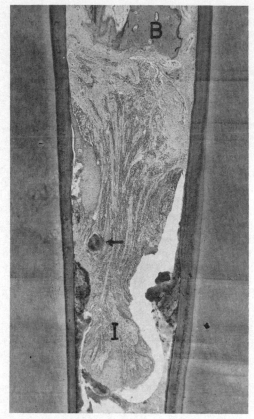

Figure 14–22 Interdental Papilla (I) with ulcerated suprabony periodontal pockets on its mesial and distal aspects. Calculus is present on the approximal tooth surfaces and within the gingiva *(arrow)*. The bone is shown at B.

ing upon the relative predominance of exudative and constructive changes.

The outer appearance of a periodontal pocket may be misleading because it is not necessarily a true indication of what is taking place throughout the pocket wall. The most severe degenerative changes in periodontal pockets occur along the inner aspect. In some cases inflammation and ulceration on the inside of the pocket are walled off by fibrous tissue on the outer aspect (Fig. 14–21). Outwardly the pocket appears pink and fibrotic, despite the degeneration taking place within.

The Contents

Periodontal pockets contain debris consisting principally of microorganisms and their products (enzymes, endotoxins, and other metabolic products), dental plaque, gingival fluid, food remnants, salivary mucin, desquamated epithelial cells, and leukocytes. Plaque-covered calculus usually projects from the tooth surface (Fig. 14–22). If a purulent exudate is present, it consists of living, degenerated, and necrotic leukocytes (predominantly polymorphonuclear), living and dead bacteria, serum, and a scant amount of fibrin.[35] The contents of periodontal pockets filtered free of organ-

isms and debris have been demonstrated to be toxic when injected subcutaneously into experimental animals.[24]

The Significance of Pus Formation

There is a tendency to overemphasize the importance of the purulent exudate and to equate it with severity of periodontal disease. Because it is a dramatic clinical finding, early observers assumed that it was responsible for the loosening and exfoliation of the teeth. *Pus is a common feature of periodontal disease, but it is only a secondary sign.* The presence of pus or the ease with which it can be expressed from the pocket merely reflects the nature of the inflammatory changes in the pocket wall. It is no indication of the depth of the pocket or the severity of the destruction of the supporting tissues. Extensive pus formation may occur in shallow pockets, whereas deep pockets may present little or no pus.

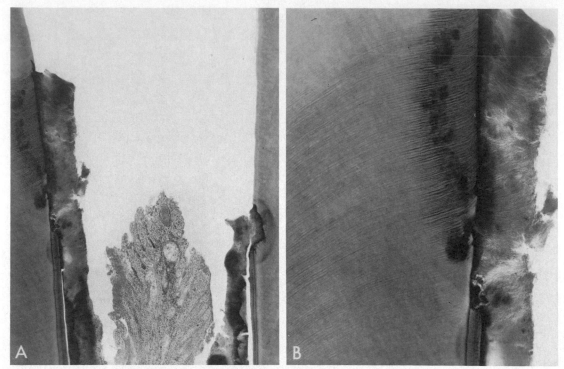

Figure 14–23 Caries on Root Surfaces Exposed by Periodontal Disease. *A,* Interdental space, showing inflamed gingiva and caries on proximal tooth surfaces. *B,* Caries of cementum and dentin, showing bacterial invasion of dentinal tubules. Note the filamentous structure of the dental plaque and darker staining of calculus adherent to the root.

The Root Surface Wall

The root surface wall of periodontal pockets often undergoes changes that are significant because they may *perpetuate the periodontal infection, cause pain,* and *complicate periodontal treatment.* Changes in cementum can be classified according to structural, chemical, and cytotoxic features.

STRUCTURAL CHANGES. (1) **Presence of pathologic granules,**[7] which have been observed with optical and electron microscopy[4] and may represent areas of collagen degeneration or areas where collagen fibrils had not been fully mineralized initially.

(2) **Areas of increased mineralization,**[52] probably due to an exchange, upon exposure to the oral cavity, of minerals and organic components at the cementum-saliva interface. The hypermineralized zone is detectable by electron microscopy. Selvig[52] studied these hypermineralized zones in detail and found that the increased mineral content was associated with increased perfection of the crystal structure and organic changes suggestive of a subsurface cuticle.

These zones have also been seen in microradiographic studies[54] as a layer 10 to 20 microns thick, with areas as thick as 50 microns. No decrease in mineralization was found in deeper areas, indicating that increased mineralization does not come from adjacent areas.

A loss or a reduction in the cross-banding of collagen near the cementum surface[18, 19] and a subsurface condensation of organic material of exogenous origin[52] have also been reported.

(3) **Areas of demineralization,** probably related to **root caries.** Exposure to oral fluid and bacterial plaque results in proteolysis of the embedded remnants of Sharpey's fibers; the cementum may be softened and undergo fragmentation and cavitation.[26]

Involvement of the cementum is followed by bacterial penetration of the dentinal tubules, resulting in destruction of the dentin (Fig. 14–23). In severe cases, large sections of necrotic cementum become detached from the tooth and separated from it by masses of bacteria (Fig. 14–24).

The tooth may not be painful, but exploration of the root surface reveals the presence of a defect; penetration of the involved area with a probe causes pain.

A prevalence rate study of root caries in 20- to 64-year-old individuals revealed that 42 per

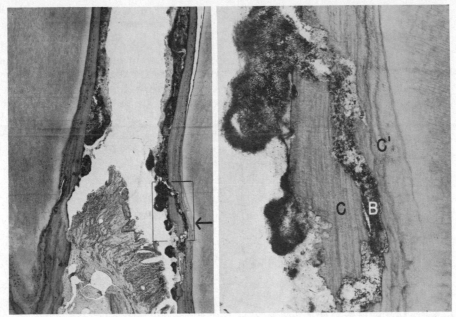

Figure 14–24 *Left,* Mesiodistal section through an interdental space in a patient with extensive periodontal destruction. An area of **Cementum Necrosis** is enclosed within the rectangle designated by the arrow.

Right, Detailed section of area enclosed in the rectangle showing **Necrotic Fragment of Cementum** (C) separated from lamellated cementum (C') by clumps of bacteria (B).

cent had one or more root caries lesions and that they tend to increase with age.[27a]

Caries of the root may lead to *pulpitis,* sensitivity to sweets and thermal changes, or severe pain. Pathologic exposure of the pulp occurs in severe cases. **It is well to bear in mind that root caries may be the cause of toothache in patients with periodontal disease without evidence of coronal decay.**

Caries of the cementum requires special attention when the pocket is treated. The necrotic cementum must be removed by scaling and root planing until firm tooth surface is reached, even if this entails extension into the dentin.

Areas of *cellular resorption* of cementum and dentin are common in roots uninvolved with periodontal disease.[55] These are of no particular significance because they are symptom-free, and so long as the root is covered by the periodontal ligament, they are apt to undergo repair. However, if the root is exposed by progressive pocket formation before repair of such areas occurs, they appear as isolated cavitations that penetrate into the dentin. These areas can be differentiated from caries of the cementum by their clear-cut outline and hard surface. Once exposed to the oral cavity, they may be sources of considerable pain and require restoration.

CHEMICAL CHANGES. The mineral content of exposed cementum is increased.[51] The following minerals are increased in diseased root surfaces; calcium,[54] magnesium,[37, 54] phosphorus,[37] and fluoride.[37] Microhardness, however, remains unchanged.[42, 63]

Exposed cementum may absorb calcium, phosphorus, and fluoride from its local environment, making possible the development of a highly calcified layer, resistant to decay.[1] This ability of cementum to absorb substances from its environment may be harmful if the absorbed materials are toxic.

CYTOTOXIC CHANGES. Bacterial penetration into the cementum can be found as deep as the cemento-dentinal junction.[12, 65] In addition, bacterial products such as endotoxins[2, 3] have also been detected in the cementum wall of periodontal pockets.

When root fragments from teeth with periodontal disease are placed in tissue culture, they induce irreversible morphologic changes in the cells of the culture. Such changes are not produced by normal roots.[25] Diseased root fragments also prevent the in vitro attachment of human gingival fibroblasts, whereas normal root surfaces allow the cells to attack freely.[2, 3] When reimplanted in the oral mucosa of the patient, diseased root fragments induce an inflammatory response even if autoclaved.[31]

The surface morphology of the tooth wall of a periodontal pocket has been studied by sev-

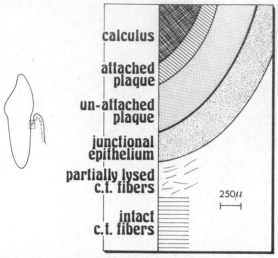

Figure 14–25 Diagrammatic Representation of the Area of the Bottom of a Pocket.

eral authors[6, 9, 27, 43, 44, 60] *The following zones can be found in the bottom of a periodontal pocket* (Fig. 14–25):

1. Cementum covered by calculus, where all the changes described in the preceding paragraphs can be found.

2. Attached plaque, which covers calculus and extends apically from it to a variable degree, probably 100 to 500 microns.

3. In extracted teeth a plaque-free zone between the most apical level of attached plaque and the coronal border of the periodontal ligament fibers has been described; it has been suggested that this area corresponds to the junctional epithelium. However, attached plaque is surrounded by unattached plaque[29] which extends apically; this unattached plaque is washed away in extracted teeth. It probably makes up most of this so-called plaque-free region. The plaque-free area would therefore be composed as follows: (a) a coronal portion of unattached plaque and (b) the area covered by the junctional epithelium. The total width of the plaque-free zone varies according to the type of tooth (it is wider in molars than in incisors) and the depth of the pocket (it is narrower in deeper pockets).[43]

Pulp Changes Associated with Periodontal Pockets

The spread of infection from periodontal pockets may cause pathologic changes in the pulp. *Such changes may give rise to painful*

symptoms or adversely affect the response of the pulp to restorative procedures.

Involvement of the pulp in periodontal disease occurs through either the apical foramen or the lateral canals in the root after infection spreads from the pocket through the periodontal ligament. Atrophy or hypertrophy of the odontoblastic layer, hyperemia, leukocytic infiltration, interstitial calcification, and fibrosis are the types of pulpal changes that occur in such cases.

The pulpal changes are correlated with the severity of periodontal involvement,[66] but not in all cases.[33]

Gingival Recession and Pocket Depth

Pocket formation causes recession of the gingiva and denudation of the root surface. The severity of recession is generally, but not always, correlated with the depth of the pocket. This is because the *degree of recession depends upon the location of the base of the pocket on the root surface, whereas the depth is the distance between the base of the pocket and the crest of the gingiva.* Pockets of the same depth may be associated with different degrees of recession (Fig. 14–26), and pockets of different depths may be associated with the same amount of recession (Fig. 14–27).

Exposure of the roots after pockets are eliminated depends upon the amount of recession before treatment is instituted. A realistic appraisal of the recession associated with periodontal pockets will prevent the erroneous impression that it is caused by the treatment.

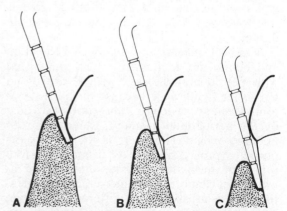

Figure 14–26 Same Pocket Depth—Different Amounts of Recession. *A,* Gingival pocket—no recession. *B,* Periodontal pocket of similar depth as *A,* but with some degree of recession. *C,* Pocket depth same as in *A* and *B* but still more recession.

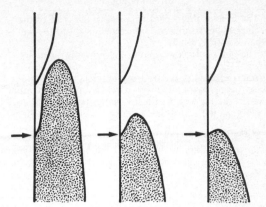

Figure 14–27 Different Pocket Depths with the Same Amount of Recession. Arrows point to bottom of pocket. Distance between arrow and cemento-enamel junctions remains the same in spite of different pocket depths.

THE RELATIONSHIP OF THE PERIODONTAL POCKET TO BONE

In **infrabony pockets,** the base is apical to the level of the alveolar bone, and the pocket wall lies between the tooth and bone. Infrabony pockets most often occur interproximally but may be located on the facial and lingual tooth surfaces. Most often the pocket spreads from the surface on which it originated to one or more contiguous surfaces. The **suprabony pocket** has its base coronal to the crest of the bone.

The inflammatory, proliferative, and degenerative changes in infrabony and suprabony pockets are the same, and both lead to destruction of the supporting periodontal tissues.

Relation of Pocket Depth to Alveolar Bone Destruction

Severity of bone loss may generally be correlated with pocket depth—but not always. Extensive bone loss may be associated with shallow pockets and slight loss with deep pockets. Destruction of alveolar bone may occur in the absence of periodontal pockets, in association with trauma from occlusion and in cases of marked recession.

The Area Between the Base of the Pocket and the Alveolar Bone

Normally, the distance between the junctional epithelium and the alveolar bone is relatively constant. Stanley[56] used histometric measurements to determine the distance between the bottom of the calculus and the alveolar crest in human periodontal pocket specimens and found it to be most constant, having a mean length of 1.97 mm ± 33.16 per cent. This was confirmed by Wade.[59]

Waerhaug measured the distance from attached plaque to bone and found it to be never less than 0.5 mm and never more than 2.7 mm.[61, 62] These findings suggest that the bone-resorbing activity induced by the bacteria is exerted within these distances. However, the recent finding of isolated bacteria and/or clumps of bacteria in the connective tissue[46] and on the bone surface[17] may modify these considerations.

Differences Between Infrabony and Suprabony Pockets

The principal differences between infrabony and suprabony pockets are the relationship of the soft tissue wall of the pocket to the alveolar bone, the pattern of bone destruction, and the direction of the transseptal fibers of the periodontal ligament[11] (Figs. 14–28 to 14–33).

In a suprabony pocket the alveolar crest and the fibrous apparatus attached to it gradually attain a more apical position in relation to the tooth but retain their general morphology and architecture, whereas in infrabony pockets the morphology of the alveolar crest changes completely. This may have an effect on the function of the area.[10]

The distinguishing features of suprabony and infrabony pockets are summarized in Table 14–2. The morphologic features of the infrabony pocket are important because they necessitate modification in treatment techniques (see Chapter 54).

Classification of Infrabony Pockets

See Chapter 16.

The Etiology of the Angular Bone Loss

Infrabony pockets are caused by the same local irritants as suprabony pockets. Trauma from occlusion may add to the effect of the inflammation by causing bone resorption lat-

TABLE 14–2 DISTINGUISHING FEATURES OF SUPRABONY AND INFRABONY POCKETS

Suprabony Pocket	Infrabony Pocket
1. The base of the pocket is coronal to the level of the alveolar bone.	1. The base of the pocket is apical to the crest of the alveolar bone, so that the bone is adjacent to the soft tissue wall (Fig. 14–7).
2. The pattern of destruction of the underlying bone is horizontal.	2. The bone destructive pattern is vertically angular (Fig. 14–29).
3. Interproximally, the transseptal fibers that are restored during progressive periodontal disease are arranged horizontally in the space between the base of the pocket and the alveolar bone (Fig. 14–30).	3. Interproximally, the transseptal fibers are oblique rather than horizontal. They extend from the cementum beneath the base of the pocket along the bone, and over the crest to the cementum of the adjacent tooth (Fig. 14–31).
4. On the facial and lingual surfaces, the periodontal ligament fibers beneath the pocket follow their normal horizontal-oblique course between the tooth and the bone.	4. On the facial and lingual surfaces, the periodontal ligament fibers follow the angular pattern of the adjacent bone. They extend from the cementum beneath the base of the pocket along the bone and over the crest to join with the outer periosteum.

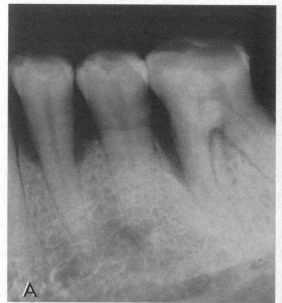

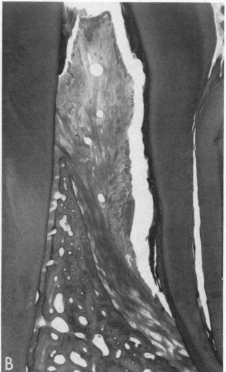

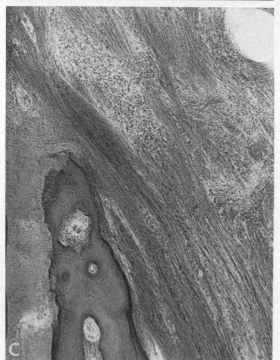

Figure 14–28 Infrabony Pocket on Mesial Surface of Molar. *A,* Radiograph showing deep angular defect on the mesial surface of the first molar. The bifurcation is also involved. Note the calculus on the mesial surface of the molar. *B,* Interdental space between the second premolar with a suprabony pocket *(left)* and the first molar with an infrabony pocket. Note the following: the transseptal fibers which extend from the base of the infrabony pocket along the bone to the root of the premolar; the relationship of the epithelial lining of the pocket to the transseptal fibers; the calculus on the root. *C,* Transseptal fibers extending from the distal surface of the premolar over the crest of the bone into the infrabony pocket. Note the leukocytic infiltration of the transseptal fibers.

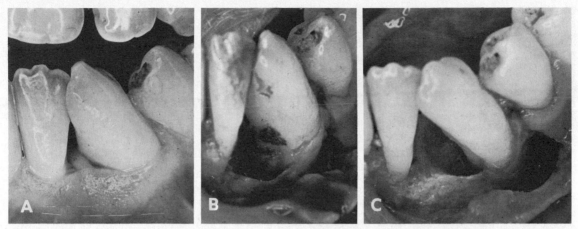

Figure 14–29 Infrabony Pocket on the Mesial Surface of the Mandibular Canine. *A,* Rolled gingival margin and space between gingiva and canine suggest presence of periodontal pocket. *B,* Flap reflected to show calculus on root and three wall bone defect. *C,* Bone defect, calculus removed.

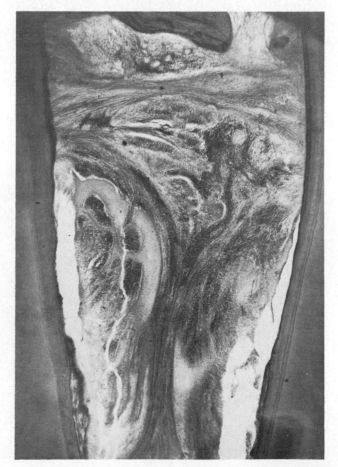

Figure 14–30 Two Suprabony Pockets in an Interdental Space between the maxillary cuspid and lateral incisor. Note the normal horizontal arrangement of the transseptal fibers.

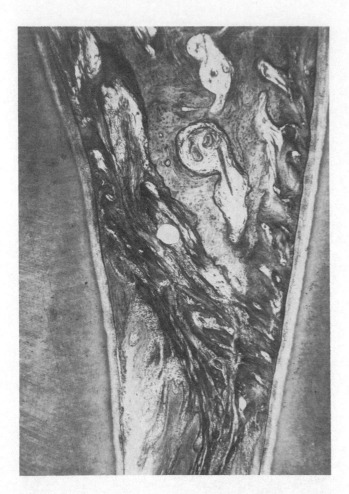

Figure 14–31 Vertical bone loss and suprabony pocket in maxillary incisor *(left)*. Note the oblique arrangement of the transseptal fibers.

Figure 14–32 Shallow, Broad Infrabony Pocket. Cementicles in the pocket wall (C′) represent an infrequent complication which may occur in any type of periodontal pocket. The epithelium at the base of the pocket is attached to a cementicle (C) which is adherent to the tooth (D).

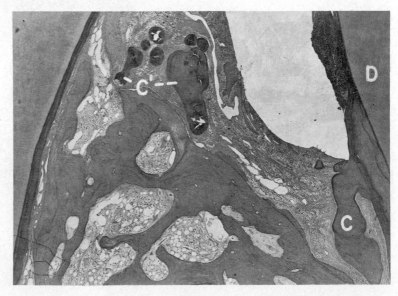

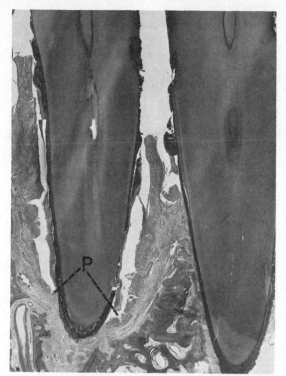

Figure 14–33 Deep Narrow Infrabony Pocket (P) on the mesial surface of the mandibular lateral incisor *(left)*. Deep wide infrabony pocket (P) on the distal surface *(right)*.

eral to the periodontal ligament, worsening the bone loss caused by inflammation alone and leading to the creation of the osseous defect as associated with infrabony pockets.*

Trauma may also add to the effect of inflammation in the following ways[20, 21]: (1) By altering the alignment of the transseptal periodontal fibers, it diverts the inflammation directly into the periodontal ligament space rather than into the interdental septum. (2) By injuring the periodontal ligament fibers, trauma may aggravate the destruction produced by inflammation. This further reduces the obstruction to the proliferating pocket epithelium. Instead of remaining coronal to the bone, the epithelium extends between the root and the bone (Fig. 14–34), creating an infrabony pocket.

There are other opinions regarding the etiology of infrabony pockets.[41, 61, 62] The causative role of inflammation combined with trauma from occlusion has been studied extensively, but other etiologic factors may also play a role. Anatomic characteristics of the area, such as wide bone margins, may favor the production of angular lesions and infrabony

---

*This subject is discussed in detail in Chapter 19.

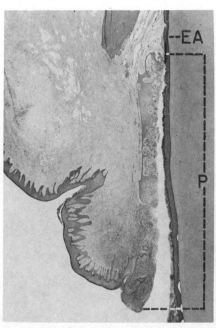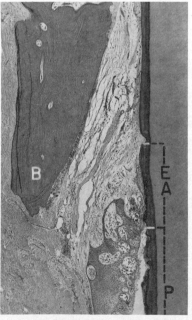

Figure 14–34 Transition from Suprabony Pocket to Infrabony Pocket. *Left,* Deep pocket (P) on the facial surface of a maxillary tooth. The junctional epithelium is shown at EA. *Right,* Base of the pocket. The junctional epithelium (EA) has migrated beyond the crest of the bone (B) and started to change the suprabony pocket to an infrabony pocket. At this early stage, the base of the pocket (P) is still coronal to the bone.

pockets. Food impaction and infrabony pockets often occur together,[40] but it has not been established whether the food impaction produces the pockets or aggravates infrabony pockets caused by other factors.

COMMENT REGARDING POCKET FORMATION

The following facts regarding pocket formation are worthy of special note:

Local irritation is required for the initiation and progression of pocket formation.

Proliferation of the junctional epithelium along the root and degeneration of the underlying gingival fibers are primary changes in pocket formation.

Proliferation of the junctional epithelium is stimulated by local irritation. Inflammation caused by local irritation produces degeneration of the gingival fibers, making it easier for the epithelium to move along the root.

Systemic disorders do not initiate pocket formation, but they may affect pocket depth by causing degeneration of the gingival and periodontal fibers.

REFERENCES

1. Aleo, J. J., and Vandersall, D. C.: Cementum. Recent concepts related to periodontal disease therapy. Dent. Clin. North Am., 24:627, 1980.
2. Aleo, J. J., DeRenzis, F. A., and Farber, P. A.: In vitro attachment of human gingival fibroblasts to root surfaces. J. Periodontol., 46:639, 1975.
3. Aleo, J. J., DeRenzis, F. A., Farber, P. A., and Varboncoeur, A. P.: The presence and biologic activity of cementum bound endotoxin. J. Periodontol., 45:672, 1974.
4. Armitage, G. C., and Christie, T. M.: Structural changes in exposed cementum. I. Light microscopic observations. J. Periodont. Res., 8:343, 1973. II. Electron-microscopic observations. J. Periodont. Res., 8:356, 1973.
5. Arnim, S. S., and Holt, R. T.: The defense mechanism of the gingiva. J. Periodontol., 26:79, 1955.
6. Bass, C. C.: A demonstrable line on extracted teeth indicating the location of the outer border of the epithelial attachment. J. Dent. Res., 25:401, 1946.
7. Bass, C. C.: A previously undescribed demonstrable pathologic condition in exposed cementum and the underlying dentine. Oral Surg., 4:641, 1951.
8. Benson, L. A.: A study of a pathologic condition in exposed cementum. Oral Surg., 16:1137, 1963.
9. Brady, J. M.: A plaque-free zone on human teeth—scanning and transmission electron microscopy. J. Periodontol., 44:416, 1973.
10. Carranza, F. A., and Carranza, F. A., Jr.: The management of alveolar bone in the treatment of the periodontal pocket. J. Periodontol., 27:29, 1956.
11. Carranza, F. A., Jr., and Glickman, I.: Some observations on the microscopic features of the infrabony pockets. J. Periodontol., 28:33, 1957.
12. Daly, C. G., Seymour, G. J., Kieser, J. B., and Corbet, E. F.: Histological assessment of periodontally involved cementum. J. Clin. Periodontol., 9:266, 1982.
13. Davenport, R. H., Jr., Simpson, D. M., and Hassell, T. M.: Histometric comparison of active and inactive lesions of advanced periodontitis. J. Periodontol., 53:285, 1982.
14. Deporter, D. A., and Brown, D. J.: Fine structural observations on the mechanisms of loss of attachment during experimental periodontal disease in the rat. J. Periodont. Res., 15:304, 1980.
15. Deporter, D. A., and Ten Cate, A. R.: Collagen resorption by periodontal ligament fibroblasts at the hard tissues–ligament interfaces of the mouse molar periodontium. J. Periodontol., 51:429, 1980.
16. Frank, R. M.: Bacterial penetration in the apical wall of advanced human periodontitis. J. Periodont. Res., 15:563, 1980.
17. Frank, R. M., and Volgel, R. C.: Bacterial bone resorption in advanced cases of human periodontitis. J. Periodont. Res., 13:251, 1978.
18. Furseth, R.: Further observations on the fine structure of orally exposed carious human dental cementum. Arch. Oral Biol., 16:71, 1971.
19. Furseth, R., and Johanson, E.: The mineral phase of sound and carious human dental cementum studies by electron microscopy. Acta Odontol. Scand., 28:305, 1970.
20. Glickman, L., and Smulow, J. B.: Alterations in the pathway of gingival inflammation into the underlying tissues induced by excessive occlusal forces. J. Periodontol., 33:7, 1962.
21. Glickman, I., and Smulow, J. B.: The combined effects of inflammation and trauma from occlusion in periodontitis. Int. Dent. J., 19:393, 1969.
22. Goldman, H. M.: The relationship of the epithelial attachment to the adjacent fibers of the periodontal membrane. J. Dent. Res., 23:177, 1944.
23. Gottlieb, B., and Orban, B.: Biology and Pathology of the Tooth. (Trans. M. Diamond.) New York, Macmillan Company, 1938, p. 64.
24. Graham, J. W.: Toxicity of sterile filtrate from parodontal pockets. Proc. R. Soc. Med., 30:1165, 1937.
25. Hatfield, C. G., and Baumhammers, A.: Cytotoxic effects of periodontally involved surfaces of human teeth. Arch. Oral Biol., 16:465, 1971.
26. Herting, H. C.: Electron microscope studies of the cementum surface structures of periodontally healthy and diseased teeth. J. Dent. Res., 46(Suppl.):1247, 1967.
27. Hoffman, I. D., and Gold, W.: Distances between plaque and remnants of attached periodontal tissues on extracted teeth. J. Periodontol., 42:29, 1971.
27a. Katz, R. V., Hazen, S. P., Chilton, N. W., and Mumma, R. D., Jr.: Prevalence and intraoral distribution of root caries in an adult population. Caries Res., 16:265, 1982.
28. Lindhe, J., Liljenberg, B., and Listgarten, M. A.: Some microbiological and histopathological features of periodontal disease in man. J. Periodontol., 52:264, 1980.
29. Listgarten, M. A.: Structure of the microbial flora associated with periodontal health and disease in man. J. Periodontol., 47:1, 1976.
30. Listgarten, M. A., and Hellden, L.: Relative distributions of bacteria at clinically healthy and periodontally diseased sites in humans. J. Clin. Periodontol., 5:665, 1978.
31. Lopez, N. J., Belvederessi, M., and de la Sotta, R.: Inflammatory effects of periodontally diseased cementum studied by autogenous dental root implants in humans. J. Periodontol., 51:582, 1980.
32. Masi, P. L., and Benini, A.: Richerche su la microdurezza del dente umano parodontosico. Riv. Ital. Stomatol., 18:293, 1963.
33. Mazur, B., and Massler, M.: Influences of periodontal disease on the dental pulp. Oral Surg., 17:592, 1964.
34. McHenry, K. R., Hausman, E., Genco, R. J., and Slots, J.: ^{125}I absorptiometry: alveolar bone mass measurements in untreated periodontal disease. J. Dent. Res., 60(Suppl. A):387, 1981 (abstract).
35. McMillan, L., Burrill, D. Y., and Fosdick, L. S.: An electron microscope study of particulates in periodontal exudate. Abstract. Dent. Res., 37:51, 1958.
36. Müller-Glauser, W., and Schroeder, H. E.: The pocket epithelium: a light and electronmicroscopic study. J. Periodontol., 53:133, 1982.

37. Nakata, T., Stepnick, R., and Zipkin, I.: Chemistry of human dental cementum. The effect of age and exposure on the concentration of F, Ca, P and Mg. J. Periodontol., *43*:115, 1972.
38. Orban, B., and Ray, A. G.: Deep necrotic foci in the gingiva. J. Periodontol., *19*:91, 1948.
39. Page, R. C., and Schroeder, H. H.: Structure and pathogenesis. *In* Schluger, S., Youdelis, R., and Page, R.: Periodontal Disease. Philadelphia, Lea & Febiger, 1977.
40. Prichard, J.: A technique for treating infrabony pockets based on alveolar process morphology. Dent. Clin. North Am., March 1960, p. 85.
41. Proceedings, World Workshop in Periodontics. The University of Michigan, 1966, p. 272.
42. Rautiola, C. A., and Craig, R. G.: The micro hardness of cementum and underlying dentin of normal teeth and teeth exposed to periodontal disease. J. Periodontol., *32*:113, 1961.
43. Saglie, R., Johansen, J. R., and Flotra, L.: The zone of completely and partially destroyed periodontal fibers in pathologic pockets. J. Clin. Periodontol., *2*:198, 1975.
44. Saglie, R., Johansen, J. R., and Tollefsen, T.: Plaque-free zones on human teeth in periodontitis. J. Clin. Periodontol., *2*:190, 1975.
45. Saglie, R., Carranza, F. A., Jr., Newman, M. G., and Pattison, G. L.: Scanning electron microscopy of the gingival wall of deep periodontal pockets in humans. J. Peridont. Res., *17*:284, 1982.
46. Saglie, R., Newman, M. G., Carranza, F. A., Jr., and Pattison, G. L.: Bacterial invasion of gingiva in advanced periodontitis in humans. J. Periodontol., *53*:217, 1982.
47. Schroeder, H. E.: Quantitative parameters of early human gingival inflammation. Arch. Oral Biol., *15*:383, 1970.
48. Schroeder, H. E., and Listgarten, M. A.: Fine Structure of the Developing Epithelial Attachment of Human Teeth. Monographs in Developmental Biology. Vol. 2. Basel, S. Karger, 1971
49. Seltzer, S., Bender, I. B., and Ziontz, M.: The interrelationship of pulp and periodontal disease. Oral Surg., *16*:1474, 1963.
50. Seltzer, S., Bender, I., Nazimov, H., and Sinai, I.: Pulpitis-induced interradicular periodontal changes in experimental animals. J. Periodontol., *38*:124, 1967.
51. Selvig, K. A.: Ultrastructural changes in cementum and adjacent connective tissue in periodontal disease. Acta Odontol. Scand., *24*:459, 1966.
52. Selvig, K. A.: Biological changes at the tooth-saliva interface in periodontal disease. J. Dent. Res., *48*(Suppl.):846, 1969.
53. Selvig, K. A., and Hals, E.: Periodontally diseased cementum studied by correlated microradiography, electron probe analysis and electron microscopy. J. Periodont. Res., *12*:419, 1977.
54. Selvig, K. A., and Zander, H. A.: Chemical analysis and microradiography of cementum and dentin from periodontally diseased human teeth. J. Periodontol., *33*:303, 1962.
55. Sottosanti, J. S.: A possible relationship between occlusion, root resorption, and the progression of periodontal disease. J. Western Soc. Periodontol., *25*:69, 1977.
56. Stanley, H. R.: The cyclic phenomenon of periodontitis. Oral Surg., *8*:598, 1955.
57. Taichman, N.: Potential mechanisms of tissue destruction in periodontal disease. J. Dent. Res., *47*:928, 1968.
58. Thilander, H.: Some structural changes in periodontal disease. Dent. Pract., *11*:191, 1961.
59. Wade, A. B.: The relation between the pocket base, the epithelial attachment and the alveolar process. In "Les Parodontopathies," 16th A.R.P.A. Congress, Vienna, 1960.
60. Waerhaug, J.: The gingival pocket. Odont. Tidsk., *60*(Suppl. 1), 1952.
61. Waerhaug, J.: The angular bone defect and its relationship to trauma from occlusion and downgrowth of subgingival plaque. J. Clin. Periodontol., *6*:61, 1979.
62. Waerhaug, J.: The infrabony pocket and its relationship to trauma from occlusion and subgingival plaque. J. Periodontol., *50*:355, 1979.
63. Warren, E. B., Hanse, N. M., Swartz, M. L., and Phillips, R. W.: Effects of periodontal disease and of calculus solvents on microhardness of cementum. J. Periodontol., *35*:505, 1964.
64. Wittwer, J. W., Dickler, E. H., and Toto, P. D.: Comparative frequencies of plasma cells and lymphocytes in gingivitis. J. Periodontol., *40*:274, 1969.
65. Zander, H. A.: The attachment of calculus to root surfaces. J. Periodontol., *24*:16, 1953.
66. Zilkens, K.: Some observations regarding the pulp in periodontal disease. Fortschr. Zahnheilk., *3*:289, 1927.

chapter fifteen

Extension of Inflammation from the Gingiva to the Supporting Periodontal Tissues

The extension of inflammation from the marginal gingiva into the supporting periodontal tissues marks the transition from *gingivitis* to *periodontitis*. **Periodontitis is always preceded by gingivitis, but not all gingivitis proceeds to periodontitis.** Some cases will apparently never become periodontitis, and others will go through their "gingivitis phase" in a brief period of time. The factor or factors that are responsible for the extension of inflammation to the supporting structures and bring about the conversion of gingivitis to periodontitis are not known.

The transition from gingivitis to periodontitis is associated with changes in the composition of bacterial plaque. In advanced stages of disease the number of motile organisms and spirochetes increases, whereas the number of coccoid rods and straight rods decreases.[11] Table 15–1 shows these variations in the bacterial composition of plaque with advancing disease.

The cellular composition of the infiltrated connective tissue also changes with increased severity of the lesion (see Chapter 8). Fibroblasts and lymphocytes predominate in Stage I gingivitis, whereas plasma cells and blast cells increase gradually in more severe disease. Seymour et al.[18, 19] postulate a stage of "contained" gingivitis in which T-lymphocytes predominate and believe that this becomes a progressively destructive lesion, which the authors consider to be a B-lymphocyte lesion.

In experimental animals, Heijl et al.[9] were able to convert a confined, naturally occurring chronic gingivitis into a progressive periodontitis by placing a silk ligature into the sulcus, tying it around the neck of the tooth. This induced ulceration of the sulcular epithelium,

a shift in the connective tissue population from predominantly plasma cells to predominantly polymorphonuclear leukocytes, and osteoclastic resorption of the alveolar crest. Recurring episodes of acute destruction over a period of time may be one mechanism leading to progressive bone loss in marginal periodontitis.

The extension of the inflammation to the supporting structures of a tooth may be modified by the pathogenic potential of plaque or by resistance factors of the host. The latter include immunologic factors, which are described in Chapter 24, and other tissue factors such as the degree of fibrosis of the gingiva, probably the width of the attached gingiva, and the reactive fibrogenesis and osteogenesis that occur peripheral to the inflammatory lesion. Recently, a fibrin-fibrinolytic system has been mentioned as "walling off" the advancing lesion.[17]

THE PATHWAYS OF GINGIVAL INFLAMMATION

For many years opinion differed regarding the pathway of gingival inflammation into the supporting tissues. Some considered it to be by way of the lymphatics of the periodontal ligament[2, 7, 21]; some felt that the inflammation extended along the fibers of the periodontal ligament or the outer periosteum of the alveolar bone[5, 11]; and others maintained that the inflammation spread from the gingiva into the alveolar bone and that it rarely, if ever, extended directly into the periodontal ligament.[3, 10, 22] The findings of Weinmann[23] led to a general acceptance of the last concept,

TABLE 15–1   PERCENTAGE DISTRIBUTION (MEAN AND STANDARD ERROR IN PERCENT) OF BACTERIA IN SUBGINGIVAL SAMPLES FROM SITES WHICH CLINICALLY WERE CHARACTERIZED AS "HEALTHY," "ESTABLISHED GINGIVITIS," AND "ADVANCED DISEASE"*

Microorganisms	Sites		
	Healthy	Established Gingivitis	Advanced Disease
	$\bar{X}$ SE	$\bar{X}$ SE	$\bar{X}$ SE
1. Coccoid cells + straight rods	76 ± 8.9	40.1 ± 6.9	16.4 ± 2.3
2. Filaments + fusiforms	19.2 ± 4.1	42.9 ± 12.4	10.8 ± 1.3
3. Curved + motile rods	2.9 ± 0.9	7.9 ± 1.5	15.3 ± 3.6
4. Spirochetes	21 ± 0.6	8.1 ± 9.8	57.2 ± 8.6

Significant difference:
"Healthy"   1 vs. 2, 3, 4, $P < 0.001$
                    2 vs. 3, 4, $P < 0.001$
"Established gingivitis"   1 vs. 2, NS
                    1, 2 vs. 3, 4, $P < 0.001$
"Advanced disease"   4 vs. 1, 2, 3, $P < 0.001$
                    1 vs. 2, 3, NS
Between sites: 1; relatively healthy > established gingiv. > adv. disease.
                    4; relatively healthy < established gingiv. < adv. disease.

*From Lindhe, J., Liljenberg, B., and Listgarten, M. A.: J. Periodontol., *51*:264; 1980.

namely, that gingival inflammation follows the course of the blood vessels through the loosely arranged tissues around them into the alveolar bone. *The pathway of the spread of inflammation is critical, because it affects the pattern of bone destruction in periodontal disease.*

Bacterial plaque causes inflammation in the marginal gingiva and interdental papillae. The inflammation penetrates and destroys the gingival fibers, usually at a short distance from their attachment to the cementum (Figs. 15–1 and 15–2). It then spreads into the supporting tissues along the following pathways (Fig. 15–3):

INTERPROXIMAL PATHWAYS. Interproximally, inflammation spreads in the loose connective tissue around the blood vessels, through the transseptal fibers, and then into the bone through vessel channels which perforate the crest of the interdental septum. *The location at which the inflammation enters the bone depends upon the location of the vessel channels.* It may enter the interdental septum at the center of the crest (Fig. 15–4), toward

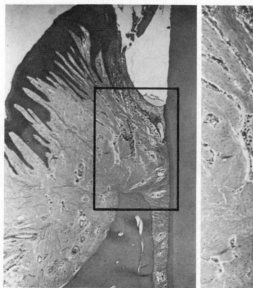
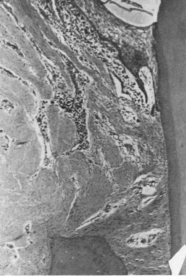

Figure 15–1 *A,* Area of inflammation extending from the gingiva into the suprabony area. *B,* Detailed view of rectangle in Figure 15–1*A,* showing extension of inflammation along blood vessels in between collagen bundles.

A   B

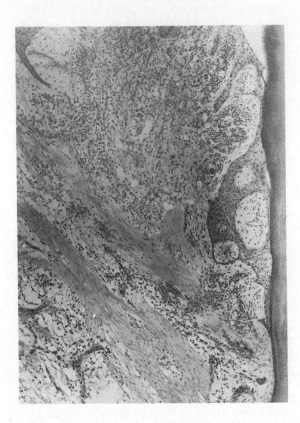

Figure 15–2 Destruction of Gingival Fibers associated with the extension of inflammation from the gingiva into the supporting periodontal tissues.

Figure 15–3 Pathways of Inflammation from the Gingiva into the Supporting Periodontal Tissues in Periodontitis. *A*, **Interproximally**. (1) From the gingiva into the bone, (2) from the bone into the periodontal ligament, (3) from the gingiva into the periodontal ligament. *B*, **Facially and Lingually**. (1) from the gingiva along the outer periosteum, (2) from the periosteum into the bone, (3) from the gingiva into the periodontal ligament.

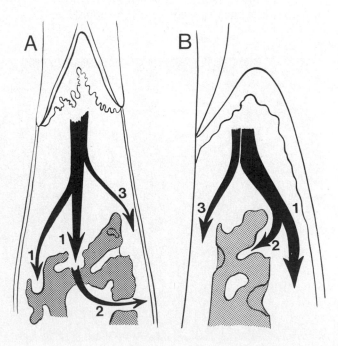

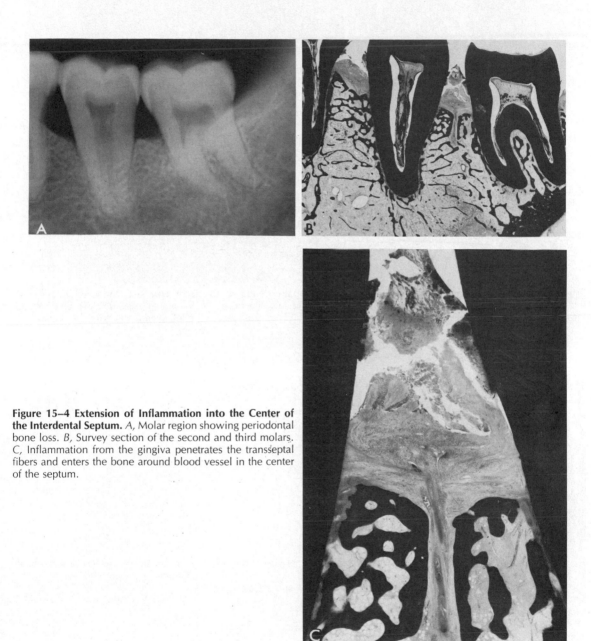

Figure 15–4 Extension of Inflammation into the Center of the Interdental Septum. *A,* Molar region showing periodontal bone loss. *B,* Survey section of the second and third molars. *C,* Inflammation from the gingiva penetrates the transseptal fibers and enters the bone around blood vessel in the center of the septum.

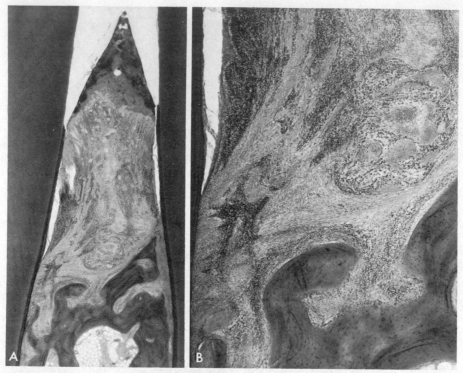

Figure 15–5 Inflammation Enters the Interdental Septum at the Center of the Crest and Near the Crestal Angle. *A,* Interdental periodontal pockets with inflammation extending into the bone. *B,* Inflammation enters the crest of the interdental bone at two areas. Note the granular necrosis of the collagen fibers in the inflamed area above the bone.

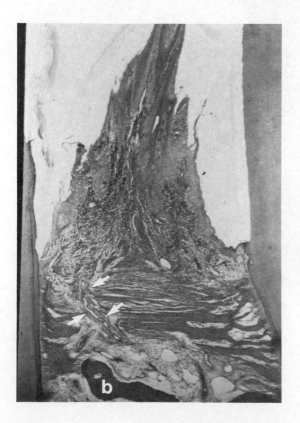

Figure 15–6 Interruption and/or destruction of transseptal fibers *(arrows)* as inflammation extends to the bone (b) around blood vessels.

the side of the crest (Fig. 15–5), or at the angle of the septum (Fig. 15–6), and it may enter the bone through more than one channel (Fig. 15–6). After reaching the marrow spaces, the inflammation may return from the bone into the periodontal ligament (see Fig. 15–3). Less frequently, the inflammation spreads from the gingiva directly into the periodontal ligament and from there into the interdental septum (see Fig. 15–3).[1]

FACIAL AND LINGUAL PATHWAYS. Facially and lingually, inflammation from the gingiva spreads **along the outer periosteal surface of the bone** (see Fig. 15–3) and penetrates into

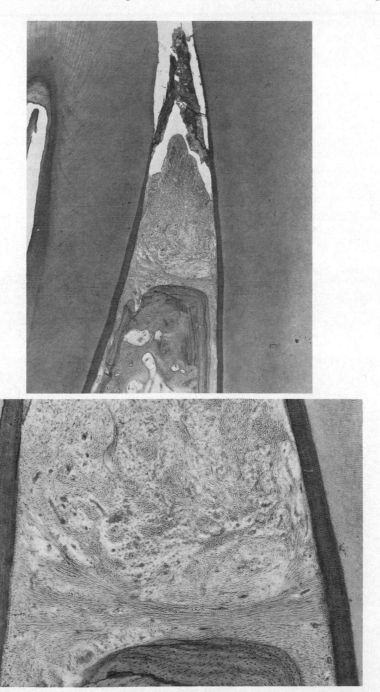

Figure 15–7 Re-formation of the Transseptal Fibers in Periodontal Disease. *Top,* Mesiodistal section through the interdental septum showing gingival inflammation with pocket formation and bone loss. *Bottom,* Bone margin showing recreated transseptal fibers of the periodontal ligament just above the bone. Note pronounced degeneration of the connective tissue above the transseptal fibers.

the marrow spaces through **vessel channels in the outer cortex.**

REESTABLISHMENT OF TRANSSEPTAL FIBERS. Along its course from the gingiva to the bone, the inflammation destroys the transseptal fibers and reduces them to disorganized granular fragments interspersed among the inflammatory cells and edema (Fig. 15–6; see also Fig. 15–5*B*).[15] However, there is a continuous tendency to recreate transseptal fibers across the crest of the interdental septum farther along the root as the bone destruction progresses. As a result, transseptal fibers are present even in cases of extreme periodontal bone loss (Fig. 15–7).

The dense transseptal fibers are of clinical significance when surgical procedures are employed for the eradication of periodontal pockets. They form a firm covering over the bone, which is encountered after the superficial granulation tissue is removed.

THE EFFECT OF TRAUMA FROM OCCLUSION. Considerable controversy has existed with reference to the possible changes in the pathway of gingival inflammation under the influence of trauma from occlusion. Excessive pressure affects the alignment of the transseptal fibers so that they become angular instead of horizontal; it also causes compression, degeneration, and realignment of periodontal ligament fibers so that they are more parallel than perpendicular to the tooth and bone. Glickman and Smulow[8] have stated that, instead of following its usual course into the interdental bone, the inflammatory exudate is channeled between the transseptal fibers directly into the periodontal ligament (Fig. 15–8). Other authors[5, 20] have been unable to arrive at similar conclusions. This change in the pathway of inflammation under the influence of trauma from occlusion would lead to vertical bone losses and infrabony pocket formation. Other mechanisms for this trauma-inflammation interaction have been suggested (see Chapter 19).

Excessive tension has also been described as affecting the pathway of inflammation.[12] Tension causes stretching and unraveling of the

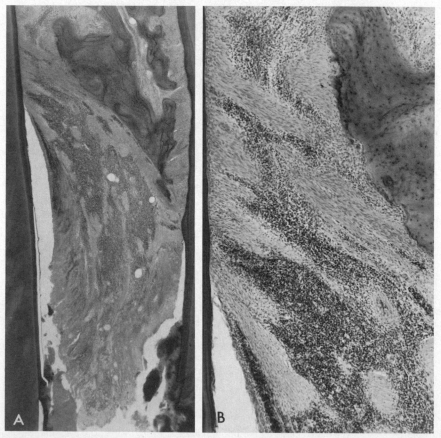

Figure 15–8 Inflammation Extends Directly into the Periodontal Ligament. *A,* Infrabony pocket on the mesial surface of maxillary premolar *(left). B,* Inflammation at the base of infrabony pocket extends directly into the periodontal ligament. Note the funnel-shaped widening of the periodontal ligament space and the osteoclastic resorption along the bone surface.

principal fiber bundles of the periodontal ligament, reducing the barrier provided by the intact bundles and permitting the inflammation direct access to the periodontal ligament.

CLINICAL ASPECTS OF INFLAMMATION IN THE PERIODONTAL LIGAMENT

Regardless of whether it extends directly from the gingiva or indirectly through the alveolar bone, inflammation is often present in the periodontal ligament in periodontal disease and contributes to tooth mobility and pain.

TOOTH MOBILITY. Inflammation in the periodontal ligament is one of the factors responsible for pathologic tooth mobility, along with loss of alveolar bone and trauma from occlusion. The inflammatory exudate reduces tooth support by causing degeneration and destruction of the principal fibers and a break in the continuity between the root and the bone. The extent to which inflammation in the periodontal ligament contributes to tooth mobility is dramatically demonstrated when the inflammation is eliminated by treatment and the tooth becomes firm.

PAIN. Inflammation in the periodontal ligament is usually chronic and asymptomatic. However, superimposed acute inflammation is frequently the cause of considerable pain. With the influx of the acute exudate, the tooth becomes elevated in its socket and there is a desire on the part of the patient to "grind" on it. Repeated contact with the opposing teeth causes the tooth to become sensitive to percussion. The condition may develop into an acute periodontal abscess unless the irritating agents are removed.

REFERENCES

1. Akiyoshi, M., and Mori, K.: Marginal periodontitis: a histological study of the incipient stage. J. Periodontol., *38*:45, 1967.
2. Black, G. V.: Operative Dentistry. Chicago, Medical-Dental Publishing Company, 1936, p. 165.
3. Box, H. K.: Twelve Periodontal Studies. Toronto, University of Toronto Press, 1940.
4. Carranza, F. A., Jr., Simes, R. J., Mayo, J., and Cabrini, R. L.: Histometric evaluation of periodontal bone loss in rats. J. Periodont. Res., *6*:65, 1971.
5. Comar, M. D., Kollar, J. D., and Gargiulo, A. W.: Local irritation and occlusal trauma as cofactors in the periodontal disease process. J. Periodontol., *40*:193, 1969.
6. Coolidge, E. D.: Inflammatory changes in the gingival tissue due to local irritation. J. Am. Dent. Assoc., *18*:2255, 1931.
7. Fish, E. W.: Bone infection. J. Am. Dent. Assoc., *26*:691, 1939.
8. Glickman, I., and Smulow, J. B.: Alterations in the pathway of gingival inflammation into the underlying tissues induced by excessive occlusal forces. J. Periodontol., *33*:7, 1962.
9. Heijl, L., Rifkin, B. R., and Zander, H. A.: Conversion of chronic gingivitis to periodontitis in squirrel monkeys. J. Periodontol., *47*:710, 1976.
10. Kronfeld, R.: Histopathology of the Teeth and Their Surrounding Structures. Philadelphia, Lea & Febiger, 1939, p. 315.
11. Lindhe, J., Liljenberg, B., and Listgarten, M. A.: Some microbiological and histopathological features of periodontal disease in man. J. Periodontol., *51*:264, 1980.
12. Macapanpan, L. C., and Weinmann, J. P.: The influence of injury to the periodontal membrane on the spread of gingival inflammation. J. Dent. Res., *33*:263, 1954.
13. Melcher, A. H.: Some histological and histochemical observations on the connective tissue of chronically inflamed human gingiva. J. Periodont. Res., *2*:127, 1967.
14. Noyes, F. B.: A review of the work on the lymphatics of dental origin. J. Am. Dent. Assoc., *14*:714, 1927.
15. Ooya, K., and Yamamoto, H.: A scanning electron microscopic study of the destruction of human alveolar crest in periodontal disease. J. Periodont. Res., *13*:498, 1978.
16. Ramirez, J. M., and Hunt, W. C.: Bone remodelling in periodontal lesions. J. Periodontol., *48*:74, 1977.
17. Ruben, M., and Cooper, S. J.: Tissue factors modifying the spread of periodontal inflammation: a perspective. Cont. Ed. Dent., *2*:387, 1981.
18. Seymour, G. J., Dockrell, H. M., and Greenspan, J. S.: Enzyme differentiation of lymphocyte subpopulations in sections of human lymph nodes, tonsils, and periodontal disease. Clin. Exp. Immunol., *32*:169, 1978.
19. Seymour, G. J., Powell, R. N., and Davies, W. J. R.: Conversion of a stable T cell lesion to a progressive B cell lesion in the pathogenesis of chronic inflammatory periodontal disease: a hypothesis. J. Clin. Periodontol., *6*:267, 1979.
20. Stahl, S. S.: The response of the periodontium to combined gingival inflammation and occluso-functional stresses in four surgical specimens. Periodontics, *6*:14, 1968.
21. Talbot, E. S.: Interstitial Gingivitis. Philadelphia, S. S. White Manufacturing Company, 1899.
22. Thoma, K. H., and Goldman, H. M.: The classification and histopathology of parodontal disease. J. Am. Dent. Assoc., *24*:1915, 1937.
23. Weinmann, J. P.: Progress of gingival inflammation into the supporting structures of the teeth. J. Periodontol., *12*:71, 1941.

chapter sixteen

Bone Loss and Patterns of Bone Destruction in Periodontal Disease

The crux of the problem of chronic destructive periodontal disease lies in the changes that occur in the bone. Changes in the other tissues of the periodontium are important, but in the final analysis it is the destruction of bone that is responsible for the loss of teeth.

PHYSIOLOGIC ALVEOLAR BONE EQUILIBRIUM

The height of the alveolar bone is normally maintained by an equilibrium, regulated by local and systemic influences,[7, 9] between bone formation and bone resorption[1] (Fig. 16–1). When resorption exceeds formation, bone height is reduced. It has been claimed that a reduction in the height of the alveolar bone, termed *physiologic* or *senile atrophy*, occurs with age.[14] This concept has not been proved (see Chapter 6).

In bone destruction in periodontal disease the equilibrium is altered so that resorption exceeds formation. Any factor or combination of factors that changes the physiologic bone equilibrium so that resorption exceeds formation results in loss of alveolar bone.

Bone loss in periodontal disease may result from any of the following changes (Fig. 16–1):

1. Increased resorption in the presence of normal or increased formation.

2. Decreased formation in the presence of normal resorption.

3. Increased resorption combined with decreased formation.

BONE DESTRUCTION IN PERIODONTAL DISEASE

Bone destruction in periodontal disease is caused principally by local factors. It may also be caused by systemic factors, but their role has not been defined. Local factors responsible for bone destruction in periodontal disease fall into two groups: *those that cause gingival inflammation* and *those that cause trauma from occlusion.* Acting singly or together, inflammation and trauma from occlusion are responsible for the locally caused bone destruction in periodontal disease and determine its severity and pattern.

Bone loss caused by extension of gingival inflammation is responsible for reduction in height of the alveolar bone, whereas trauma from occlusion causes bone loss lateral to the root surface.

Bone destruction in periodontal disease is not a process of bone necrosis. It involves the activity of living cells along viable bone. When tissue necrosis and pus are present in periodontal disease, they occur in the soft tissue

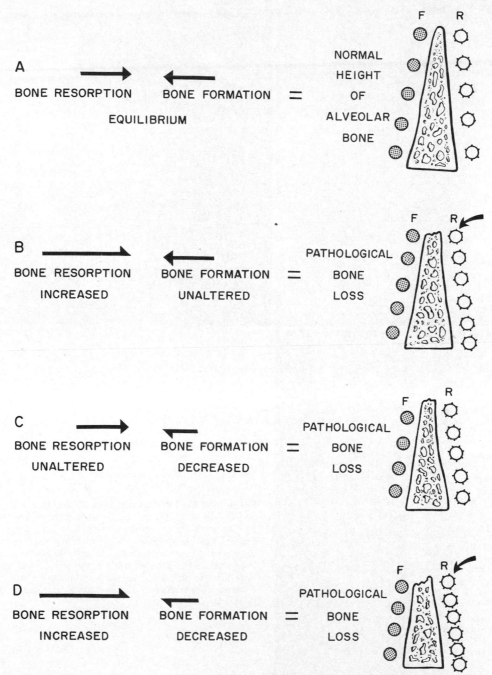

Figure 16–1 Diagrammatic Representation of Bone Formative–Bone Resorptive Relationships in Periodontal Health and Disease. *A,* Physiologic equilibrium between bone resorption (R) and bone formation (F) responsible for the maintenance of normal alveolar bone height. *B,* Pathologic bone loss produced when bone resorption is increased *(arrow). C,* Pathologic bone loss produced when bone formation is decreased. *D,* Pathologic bone loss produced when bone resorption is increased *(arrow)* and bone formation decreased.

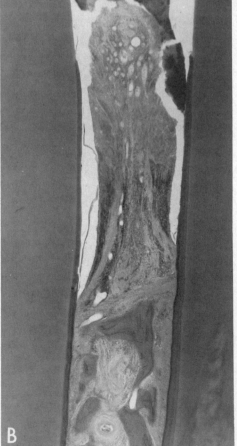

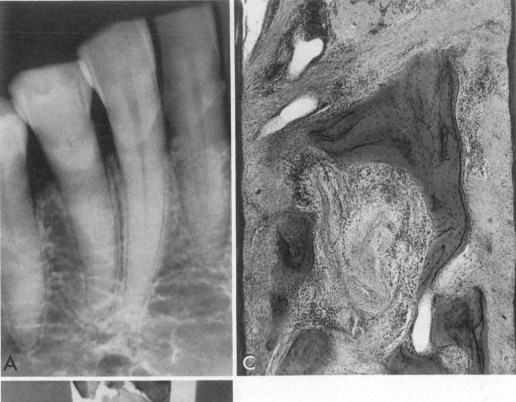

Figure 16–2 Early Periodontal Bone Destruction. *A*, Early periodontal bone loss in the canine and premolar areas. *B*, Interdental space between the canine and first premolar, showing calculus and periodontal pockets. *C*, Interdental septum beneath the periodontal pockets. The inflammation has invaded the marrow space, and there is lacunar resorption of the surrounding bone surface. Note the inflammation in the periodontal ligament on the right side.

walls of periodontal pockets, not along the resorbing margin of the underlying bone. The level of bone is the consequence of past pathologic experiences, whereas changes in the soft tissue of the pocket wall reflect the present inflammatory condition. Therefore, the degree of bone loss is not necessarily correlated with the depth of periodontal pockets, the severity of ulceration of the pocket wall, or the presence or absence of pus.

Bone Destruction Caused by Chronic Inflammation

Chronic inflammation is the most common cause of bone destruction in periodontal disease.

The *rate of bone loss* has been found to average about 0.2 mm a year for facial surfaces and about 0.3 mm a year for interproximal surfaces when periodontal disease is allowed to progress untreated.[26]

HISTOPATHOLOGY. **Inflammation reaches the bone by extension from the gingiva (see Chapter 15). It spreads into the marrow spaces and replaces the marrow with a leukocytic and fluid exudate, new blood vessels, and proliferating fibroblasts (Fig. 16–2). Multinuclear osteoclasts and mononuclear phagocytes are increased in number, and the bone surfaces are lined with cove-like resorption lacunae (Fig. 16–3).**

A recent hypothesis has assumed that two cell types are involved in bone resorption: the *osteoclast,* which removes the mineral portion of the bone, and the *mononuclear cell,* which plays a role in organic matrix degradation.[17] Both kinds of cells have been found in resorbing bone surfaces in experimental periodontitis in animals.

In the marrow spaces resorption proceeds from within, causing first a thinning of the surrounding bony trabeculae and enlargement of the marrow spaces, followed by destruction of the bone and reduction in bone height.

A histometric study of human autopsy material has shown that the amount of inflammatory infiltrate correlates significantly with the degree of bone loss, but not with the number of osteoclasts. However, the distance from the apical border of the inflammatory infiltrate to the alveolar bone crest correlates significantly with both the number of osteoclasts on the alveolar crest and the total number of osteoclasts.[37] Similar findings have been seen in studies of experimentally induced periodontitis in animals.[24]

Schroeder and Lindhe[39] concluded in a study of experimental periodontitis in dogs that the onset and maintenance of the lesion depend on the subgingival ulceration of the junctional epithelium; rapid destruction of the alveolar bone is the consequence of acute inflammation. Bone degradation and root resorption

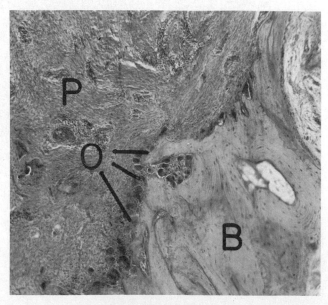

Figure 16–3 Pronounced Osteoclastic Activity. Osteoclasts (O) along the bone (B) surface adjacent to inflammation in a periodontal pocket (P).

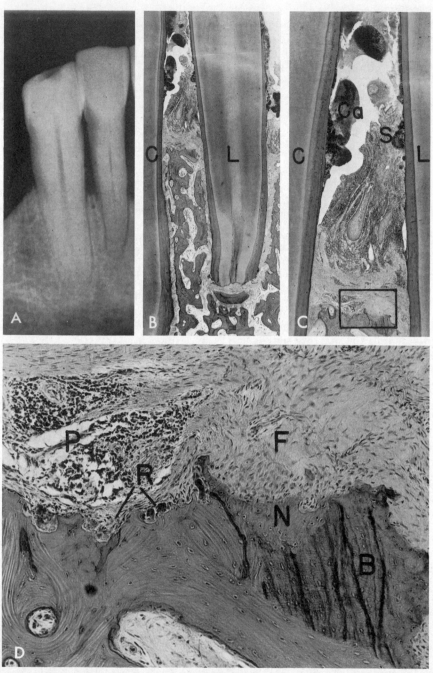

Figure 16–4 Bone Resorption and Formation in Active Periodontal Disease. *A,* Lateral incisor and canine with bone loss. *B,* Survey section of lateral incisor (L) and canine (C). *C,* Interdental space between lateral incisor (L) and canine (C), showing calculus (Ca) and periodontal pockets with suppuration (S). A detailed view of the bone margin within the rectangle is shown in *D. D,* Bone margin beneath the periodontal pockets. Note the following: osteoclastic resorption (R) beneath the inflammation (P) and newly formed bone (N) with a thin surface layer of osteoid and osteoblasts adjacent to the resorption. The new bone is separated from the lamellated bone (B) by an irregular resorption line. An area of fibrosis is shown at F.

are the results of osteoclastic activity, with fibroblasts degrading collagenous remnants.

The inflammation also stimulates bone formation immediately adjacent to active bone resorption (Fig. 16–4) and along trabecular surfaces at a distance from the inflammation in an apparent effort to reinforce the remaining bone (buttressing bone formation) (Fig. 16–5). This osteogenic response is clear in experimental periodontitis in animals.[4] In humans it is less obvious but is nevertheless confirmed by histometric[2] and histologic studies.[8] Normally fatty bone marrow is partially or totally replaced by a fibrous type of marrow in the vicinity of the resorption.

Mechanisms by Which Inflammation and/or Plaque-Derived Products Destroy Bone in Periodontal Disease

Many investigations have been conducted and many explanations considered, but the mechanism or mechanisms of bone destruction in inflammatory periodontal disease have not yet been determined.

Inflammation in periodontal disease is accompanied by an increase in osteoclasts and mononuclear phagocytes, both of which resorb bone by removing the mineral crystals and digesting the exposed collagen. The increased vascularity associated with inflammation may also cause bone resorption by stimulating an increase in osteoclasts and by elevating the local oxygen tension.

The possible pathways by which plaque products could cause alveolar bone loss in periodontal disease have been listed by Hausmann[15]:

1. Direct action of plaque products on bone progenitor cells induces their differentiation into osteoclasts.

2. Plaque products act directly on bone, destroying it through a noncellular mechanism.

3. Plaque products stimulate gingival cells, causing them to release mediators which in turn induce bone progenitor cells to differentiate into osteoclasts.

4. Plaque products cause gingival cells to release agents that can act as cofactors in bone resorption.

5. Plaque products cause gingival cells to

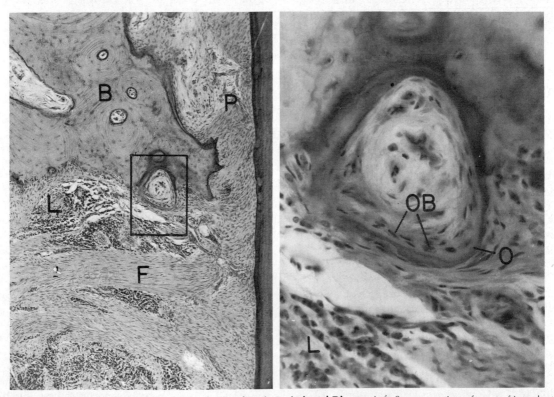

Figure 16–5 Central Buttressing Bone Formation in Chronic Periodontal Disease. *Left,* Survey section of crest of interdental bone (B) beneath inflamed connective tissue (L). The periodontal ligament is shown at P, the transseptal fibers at F. *Right,* High-power study of area in rectangle showing osteoblasts (OB) and layer of osteoid buttressing thinned remnant of resorbed bone (O). Leukocytic infiltration is shown at L.

release agents that destroy bone by direct chemical action, without osteoclasts.

The presence of bacteria on the bone surface has been described in advanced cases of periodontitis[5] and in juvenile periodontitis.[3] This information, as well as the exact role and frequency of bacteria on bone, awaits further study.

Pharmacologic Agents and Bone Resorption

Several local agents that are capable of inducing bone resorption in vitro can play a role in periodontal disease (for a review see references 10 and 11). These include prostaglandins and their precursors and osteoclast-activating factor, all of which are present in inflamed gingiva, and endotoxins produced by plaque bacteria. Endotoxin from *Bacteroides melaninogenicus* stimulates osteoclastic bone resorption[16, 36]; lipoteichoic acid acts in a similar way.[15]

Prostaglandins are a group of naturally occurring lipids that participate in the inflammatory process and have hormone-like effects.[13] When injected intradermally, they induce the vascular changes seen in inflammation. When injected over a bone surface, they induce bone resorption[20] in the absence of inflammatory cells and with few multinucleated osteoclasts.[13] Complement may enhance the synthesis of prostaglandins by the bone and therefore induce bone resorption.[34]

Bone resorption can also be induced by supernatants of leukocyte cultures stimulated by antigens from dental plaque.[18] Horton et al. hypothesized that lymphocytes produce an **osteoclast-activating factor** which induces osteoclast formation and activity.[18]

Proteolytic enzymes produced in the periodontal tissue or by plaque bacteria may also participate in bone resorption.[19] Collagenase is present in the normal periodontium and increased in inflamed gingiva; it is also produced by oral bacteria. Collagenolytic activity is produced in resorbing bone in vitro, but the collagen content is not correlated with the severity of bone loss.[6] By breaking down the bone matrix ground substance, hyaluronidase produced by oral bacteria may influence the resorptive process.

In an experiment with gnotobiotic rats monoinfected with *Actinomyces naeslundii, Actinomyces viscosus,* or *Streptococcus mutans,* and in another experiment with conventional rats superinfected with *A. naeslundii,* Irving found that bone loss was not accompanied by osteoclasts and seemed to be more a result of gradual cessation of bone formation than of active resorption.[19]

Bone Formation in Periodontal Disease

It is significant that the response of alveolar bone to inflammation includes bone formation as well as resorption. This means that *bone loss in periodontal disease is not simply a destructive process, but results from the predominance of resorption over formation.* New bone formation retards the rate of bone loss, compensating in some degree for the bone destroyed by inflammation. Newly formed osteoid is more resistant to resorption than mature bone. Because of the interaction between bone resorption and bone formation, *bone loss in periodontal disease is not necessarily continuous. It is a progressive process, but its rate cannot be predicted.*

Autopsy specimens from patients with untreated disease occasionally show areas where bone resorption had ceased and new bone was being formed on the previously eroded bone margin. **This finding indicates that bone resorption in periodontal disease may occur as an intermittent process, with periods of remission and exacerbation.** This is consistent with the varied rates of progression observed clinically in untreated periodontal disease.

These periods of remission and exacerbation, also known as periods of activity and inactivity, appear to coincide with the quiescence or exacerbation of gingival inflammation, manifested by changes in the bleeding index, in the amount of exudate, and in the composition of bacterial plaque (see Chapters 14 and 15).

The microscopic bone formation in response to inflammation varies in amount and distribution. It is governed by the severity and distribution of the inflammation and by systemic influences. In this way systemic factors which affect the metabolic processes involved in bone formation influence the bone loss in periodontal disease.[2]

The presence of bone formation in response to inflammation even in active periodontal disease has a bearing on the outcome of treatment. Elimination of inflammation to remove the stimulus for bone resorption and the establishment of conditions conducive to healing are basic aims in periodontal treatment. Healing of the periodontium following treatment depends upon the body's reparative processes, one of which is the formation of new bone. An active tendency toward bone formation in untreated disease could benefit healing if it were carried over into the posttreatment period.

The radiograph is extremely useful in diagnosis, but it does not detect microscopic resorptive and formative activities. Sometimes endosteal bone formation in periodontal disease produces increased radiodensity (condensing osteitis) adjacent to eroded bone margins. However, there may be bone formation in periodontal disease without any radiographic suggestion of its presence (Fig. 16–6).

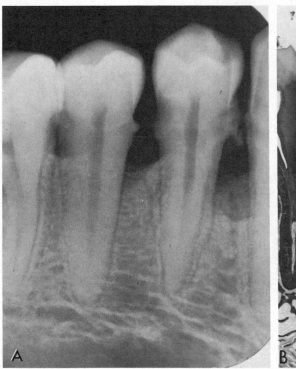

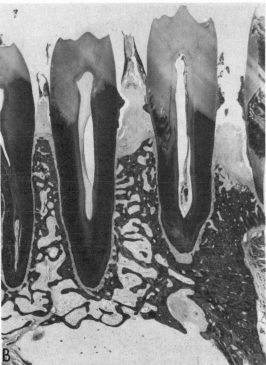

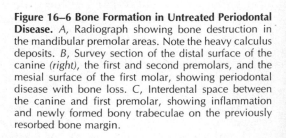

Figure 16–6 Bone Formation in Untreated Periodontal Disease. *A,* Radiograph showing bone destruction in the mandibular premolar areas. Note the heavy calculus deposits. *B,* Survey section of the distal surface of the canine *(right),* the first and second premolars, and the mesial surface of the first molar, showing periodontal disease with bone loss. *C,* Interdental space between the canine and first premolar, showing inflammation and newly formed bony trabeculae on the previously resorbed bone margin.

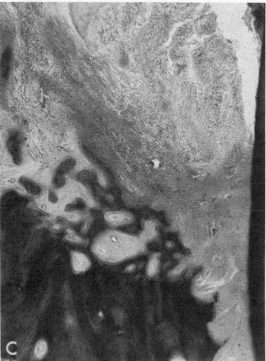

Bone Destruction Caused by Trauma from Occlusion

Inflammation is the more common cause of periodontal destruction; the other is trauma from occlusion. Trauma from occlusion can produce bone destruction in the absence of inflammation or combined with it.

TRAUMA IN THE ABSENCE OF INFLAMMATION. In the absence of inflammation, the changes caused by trauma from occlusion vary from increased compression and tension of the periodontal ligament and increased osteoclasis of alveolar bone[27] to necrosis of the periodontal ligament and bone and resorption of bone and tooth structure. These changes are reversible in that they are repaired if the offending forces are removed. However, persistent trauma from occlusion causes funnel-shaped widening of the crestal portion of the periodontal ligament, with resorption of the adjacent bone.[25] These changes, which may result in an angular shape of the bony crest, represent adaptation of the periodontal tissues in order to "cushion" increased occlusal force, but they produce defects in the bone which weaken tooth support and cause tooth mobility.

TRAUMA COMBINED WITH INFLAMMATION. When combined with inflammation, trauma from occlusion acts as a co-destructive factor in periodontal disease. It aggravates the bone destruction caused by the inflammation[25] and causes bizarre bone patterns.

Bone Destruction Caused by Systemic Disorders

Local and systemic factors regulate the physiologic equilibrium of bone.[7] When there is a generalized tendency toward bone resorption, bone loss initiated by local inflammatory processes may be magnified. This systemic influence upon the response of alveolar bone loss has been termed the **bone factor** in periodontal disease.[7]

The bone factor concept, developed by Irving Glickman,[7] envisions a systemic component in all cases of periodontal disease.

In addition to the amount and virulence of plaque bacteria, it is the nature of the systemic component, not its presence or absence, that influences the severity of periodontal destruction.

Periodontal bone loss may also occur in generalized skeletal disturbances, such as hyperparathyroidism, leukemia, Hand-Schüller-Christian disease, and so forth, by mechanisms which may be totally unrelated to the usual periodontal problem.

BONE LOSS AND TOOTH MOBILITY

Loss of alveolar bone in periodontal disease is an important cause of tooth mobility, but other factors are also involved. As a result, the degree of tooth mobility in periodontal disease is not necessarily correlated with the amount of bone loss (see Chapter 20).

FACTORS DETERMINING BONE MORPHOLOGY IN PERIODONTAL DISEASE

Normal Variation in the Morphology of Alveolar Bone

There is considerable normal variation in the morphology of alveolar bone (see Chapter 4), and it affects the osseous contours produced by periodontal disease. The bone features that significantly affect the bone destructive pattern in periodontal disease are the *thickness, width, and crestal angulation of the interdental septa, the thickness of the facial and lingual alveolar plates, the presence of fenestrations and dehiscences on the root surfaces, thickening of the alveolar bone margins to accommodate functional demands,* and *the alignment of the teeth.*

For example, angular osseous defects cannot form in thin facial or lingual alveolar plates, which have little or no cancellous bone between the outer and inner cortical layers. In such instances, the entire crest of the plate is destroyed and the height of the bone is reduced.

Exostoses

Exostoses are outgrowths of bone of varied size and shape. They occur more often on the facial surface than on the lingual and apparently serve no useful purpose. The cervical margin of the alveolar bone is often thickened in response to increased functional demands, so it is sometimes difficult to differentiate between linear exostoses and functional adaptation.

The Pathway of Inflammation

Because chronic inflammation is an important cause of bone destruction, its pathway in the supporting tissues is a significant determinant of the bone morphology produced by periodontal disease.

Trauma from Occlusion

Trauma from occlusion is a critical factor in determining the dimension and shape of bone deformities. It may cause a change in the morphology of the bone (angular defects, buttressing bone—see below) upon which inflammatory changes will later be superimposed. Also, trauma from occlusion may be a co-destructive factor that changes the bone destructive pattern of inflammation.

Buttressing Bone Formation (Lipping)

Bone formation sometimes occurs in an attempt to buttress bony trabeculae weakened by resorption. When it occurs within the jaw, it is termed *central buttressing bone formation.*[8] When it occurs on the external surface, it is referred to as *peripheral buttressing bone.* The latter may cause bulging of the bone contour, termed *lipping*, which sometimes accompanies the formation of osseous craters and infrabony defects (Fig. 16–7).

Food Impaction

Interdental bone defects often occur where the proximal contact is abnormal or absent. Pressure and irritation from food impaction contribute to the inverted bone architecture.

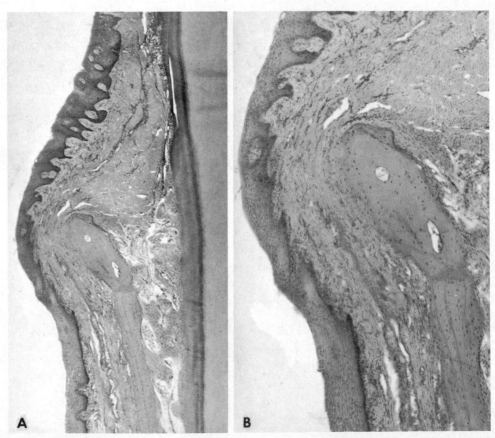

Figure 16–7 Lipping of Facial Bone. *A,* Peripheral buttressing bone formation along the external surface of the facial bony plate and at the crest. Note the deformity in the bone produced by the buttressing bone formation and the bulging of the mucosa. *B,* Detailed view showing lipping and deformity produced by buttressing bone formation.

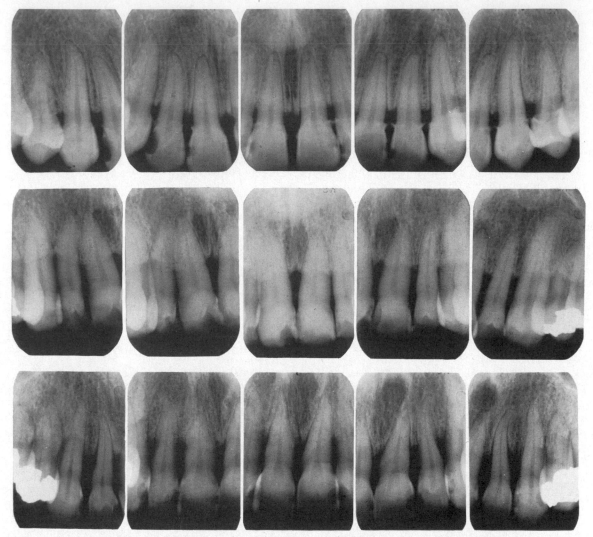

Figure 16–8 Horizontal Bone Loss. Radiographs of three patients with different degrees of destruction in the anterior maxilla.

In some instances the poor proximal relationship may be the result of a shift in tooth position because of extensive bone destruction that preceded food impaction. In such cases food impaction is a complicating factor, rather than the cause of the bone defect.

Localized Juvenile Periodontitis

Vertical or angular destruction of alveolar bone is found in juvenile periodontitis. The cause of the bone destructive pattern in this type of periodontal disease is unknown.

BONE DESTRUCTIVE PATTERNS IN PERIODONTAL DISEASE

In addition to reducing bone height, periodontal disease alters the morphology of the bone. An understanding of the nature and pathogenesis of these alterations is essential for effective diagnosis and treatment.

Horizontal Bone Loss

This is the most common pattern of bone loss in periodontal disease. The bone is re-

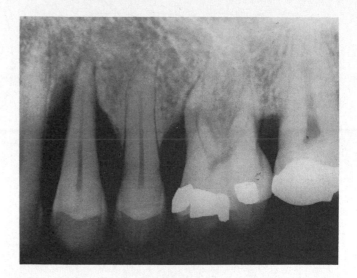

Figure 16–9 Angular (Vertical) Defects of different depths.

duced in height, and the bone margin is roughly perpendicular to the tooth surface. The interdental septa and the facial and lingual plates are affected, but not necessarily to an equal degree around the same tooth (Fig. 16–8).

Bone Deformities (Osseous Defects)

The following are types of bone deformities produced by periodontal disease. They usually occur in adults but have been reported in human skulls with deciduous dentitions.[23] Their presence may be suggested by radiographs, but **careful probing and surgical exposure of the areas are required to determine their conformation and dimensions.**

VERTICAL OR ANGULAR DEFECTS. Vertical or angular defects are those that occur in an oblique direction, leaving a hollowed-out trough in the bone alongside the root; the base of the defect is located apical to the surrounding bone (Figs. 16–9 and 16–10). In most instances angular defects have accompanying infrabony pockets; infrabony pockets always have an underlying angular defect.

Infrabony pockets are classified on the basis of the *number of walls*[12] *and the depth and width of their underlying osseous defect* since these are important features which may influence the selection of a treatment technique. Angular defects may have one wall, two walls, or three walls (Figs. 16–11 to 16–13). The number of walls in the apical portion of the defect may be greater than that in its occlusal portion; in these cases the term combined

osseous defect is used (Fig. 16–14). Angular defects can be shallow and narrow, shallow and wide; deep and narrow, or deep and wide; they generally occur in forms which represent gradients of these types.

Vertical defects occurring interdentally can generally be seen in the radiograph, although sometimes thick bony plates may obscure them. Angular defects can also appear in facial and lingual or palatal surfaces, but these defects are not seen in the radiographs. Surgical exposure is the only sure way to determine the presence and configuration of vertical osseous defects.

Vertical defects increase with age.[32] Approx-

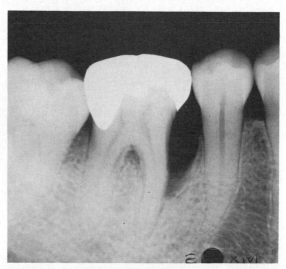

Figure 16–10 Angular Defect on the Mesial Surface of the First Molar. Note also the furcation involvement.

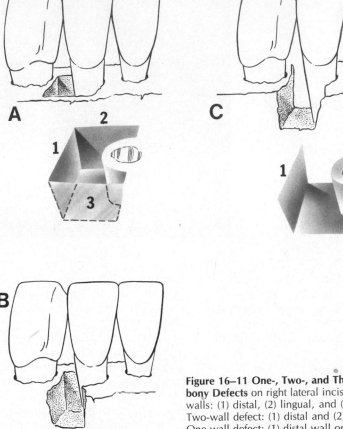

Figure 16–11 One-, Two-, and Three-Walled Infra-bony Defects on right lateral incisor. *A,* Three bony walls: (1) distal, (2) lingual, and (3) facial walls. *B,* Two-wall defect: (1) distal and (2) lingual walls. *C,* One-wall defect: (1) distal wall only.

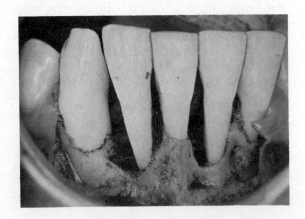

Figure 16–12 One-Wall Infrabony Defect on the mesial surface of the left lateral incisor and 1½-wall defect (distal wall and half of the labial wall) on the distal surface of the right lateral incisor.

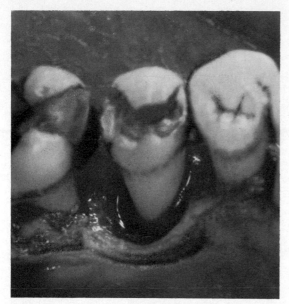

Figure 16–13 Circumferential vertical defect viewed from the lingual surface, consisting of facial, lingual, mesial, and distal walls in relation to the second premolar. The facial bony wall is obscured by the tooth. This type of defect has also been classified as a "four-wall vertical defect."

imately 60 per cent of individuals with interdental angular defects have only a single defect.[32] The most common location of vertical defects, as viewed radiographically, is on distal surfaces of molar teeth.[32]

The three-wall vertical defect has also been called an *intrabony defect.* These appear most frequently on the mesial aspects of second and third maxillary and mandibular molars. The one-wall vertical defect is also called a *hemiseptum.*

OSSEOUS CRATERS. Osseous craters are concavities in the crest of the interdental bone confined within the facial and lingual walls (Fig. 16–15). Craters have been found to make up about one third of all defects (35.2 per cent) and about two thirds (62.0 per cent) of all mandibular defects. They are twice as common in posterior segments as in anterior segments.[28, 29]

The heights of the facial and lingual crests of a crater have been found to be identical in 85 per cent of cases, with the remaining 15 per cent being nearly equally divided between higher facial and higher lingual crests.[38] The following reasons for the high frequency of interdental craters have been suggested: the interdental area collects plaque and is difficult to clean, the normal flat or even concave faciolingual shape of the interdental septum in lower molars may favor crater formation, and vascular patterns from the gingiva to the center of the crest may provide a pathway for inflammation.[28, 29, 38]

BULBOUS BONE CONTOURS. These are bony enlargements caused by exostoses, adaptation to function, or buttressing bone formation (Fig. 16–16). They are found more frequently in the maxilla than in the mandible.

INCONSISTENT MARGINS. These are angular or U-shaped defects produced by resorption of the facial or lingual alveolar plate or abrupt differences between the height of the facial or lingual margins and the height of the interdental septa (Fig. 16–17). These defects have also

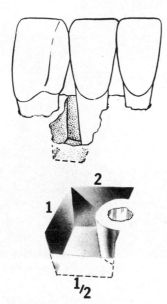

Figure 16–14 Combined Type of Osseous Defect. Because the facial wall is half the height of the distal (1) and lingual (2) walls, this is an osseous defect with three walls in its apical half and two walls in the occlusal half.

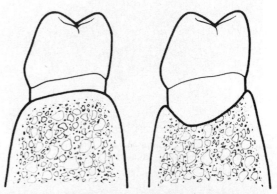

Figure 16–15 Diagrammatic Representation of an Osseous Crater in a Faciolingual Section Between Two Lower Molars. *Left,* Normal bone contour. *Right,* Osseous crater.

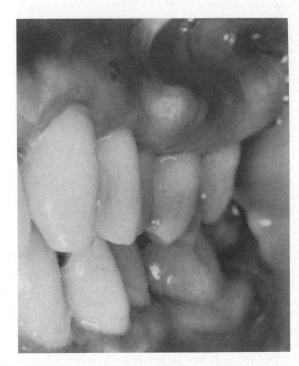

Figure 16–16 Exostoses.

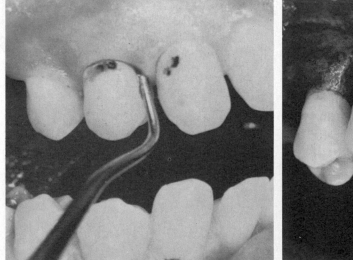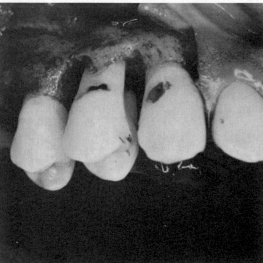

Figure 16–17 Irregular Bone Margin. *Left,* Probe in deep infrabony pocket on the mesial surface of maxillary premolar. *Right,* Elevated flap shows irregular bone margin with notching of interdental bone.

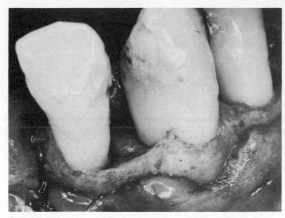

Figure 16–18 Labial Ledge produced by interproximal resorption.

been termed *reversed architecture.* They are more frequent in the maxilla.[28]

LEDGES. Ledges are plateau-like bone margins caused by resorption of thickened bony plates (Fig. 16–18).

REFERENCES

1. Carranza, F. A., Jr.: Histometric evaluation of periodontal pathology. A review of recent studies. J. Periodontol., *38*:741, 1967.
2. Carranza, F. A., Jr., and Cabrini, R. L.: Histometric studies of periodontal tissues. Periodontics, *5*:308, 1967.
3. Carranza, F. A., Jr., Saglie, R., and Newman, M. G.: Scanning and transmission electron microscopy study of tissue invading microorganisms in juvenile periodontitis. J. Periodontol., in press.
4. Carranza, F. A., Jr., Simes, R. J., Mayo, J., and Cabrini, R. L.: Histometric evaluation of periodontal bone loss in rats. J. Periodont. Res., *6*:65, 1971.
5. Frank, R. M., and Voegel, J. C.: Bacterial bone resorption in advanced cases of human periodontitis. J. Periodont. Res., *13*:251, 1978.
6. Fullmer, H. M., et al.: Collagenase and gingival disease. Proceedings, First Pan-Pacific Congress of Dental Research, 1970, p. 167.
7. Glickman, I.: The experimental basis for the "bone factor" concept in periodontal disease. J. Periodontol., *20*:7, 1951.
8. Glickman, I., and Smulow, J.: Buttressing bone formation in the periodontium. J. Periodontol., *36*:365, 1965.
9. Glickman, I., and Wood, H.: Bone histology in periodontal disease. J. Dent. Res., *21*:35, 1942.
10. Goldhaber, P., and Rabadjija, L.: Influence of pharmacological agents on bone resorption. In Genco, R., and Mergenhagen, S. E. (eds.): Host-Parasite Interactions in Periodontal Diseases. Washington, D.C., American Society for Microbiology, 1982, p. 363.
11. Goldhaber, P., Rabadjija, L., Beyer, W. R., and Kornhauser, A.: Bone resorption in tissue culture and its relevance to periodontal disease. J. Am. Dent. Assoc., *87*:1027, 1973.
12. Goldman, H. M., and Cohen, D. W.: The intrabony pocket: classification and treatment. J. Periodontol., *29*:272, 1958.
13. Goodson, J. M., McClatchy, K., and Revell, C.: Prostaglandin-induced resorption of the adult calvarium. J. Dent. Res., *53*:670, 1974.
14. Gottlieb, B., and Orban, B. J.: Biology and Pathology of the Tooth and Its Supporting Mechanism. New York, Macmillan, Inc., 1938.
15. Hausmann, E.: Potential pathways for bone resorption in human periodontal disease. J. Periodontol., *45*:338, 1974.
16. Hausmann, E., Raisz, L. G., and Miller, W. A.: Endotoxin: stimulation of bone resorption in tissue culture. Science, *168*:862, 1970.
17. Heersche, J. N. M.: Mechanism of osteoclastic bone resorption: a new hypothesis. Calcif. Tissue Res., *26*:81, 1978.
18. Horton, J. E., Raisz, L. G., Simmons, H. A., Oppenheim, J. J., and Mergenhagen, S. E.: Bone resorbing activity in supernatant fluid from cultured human peripheral blood leukocytes. Science, *177*:793, 1972.
19. Irving, J. T.: Factors concerning bone loss associated with periodontal disease. J. Dent. Res., *49*:262, 1970.
20. Klein, D. C., and Raisz, L. G.: Prostaglandins: stimulation of bone resorption in tissue culture. Endocrinology, *86*:1436, 1970.
21. Kronfeld, R.: Condition of alveolar bone underlying periodontal pockets. J. Periodontol., *6*:22, 1935.
22. Larato, D. C.: Intrabony defects in the dry human skull. J. Periodontol., *41*:496, 1970.
23. Larato, D. C.: Periodontal bone defects in the juvenile skull. J. Periodontol., *41*:473, 1970.
24. Lindhe, J., and Ericsson, I.: Effect of ligature placement and dental plaque on periodontal tissue breakdown in the dog. J. Periodontol., *49*:343, 1978.
25. Lindhe, J., and Svanberg, G.: Influence of trauma from occlusion on progression of experimental periodontitis in beagle dogs. J. Clin. Periodontol., *1*:3, 1974.
26. Löe, H., Anerud, A., Boysen, H., and Smith, M.: The natural history of periodontal disease in man. The rate of periodontal destruction before 40 years of age. J. Periodontol., *49*:607, 1978.
27. Lopez-Otero, R., et al.: Histologic and histometric study of bone resorption after tooth movement in rats. J. Periodont. Res., *8*:327, 1973.
28. Manson, J. D.: Bone morphology and bone loss in periodontal disease. J. Clin. Periodontol., *3*:14, 1976.
29. Manson, J. D., and Nicholson, K.: The distribution of bone defects in chronic periodontitis. J. Periodontol., *45*:88, 1974.
30. Melcher, A. H., and Eastoe, J. E.: Biology of the Periodontium. New York, Academic Press, 1969, p. 315.
31. Newman, M. G.: The role of *Bacteroides melaninogenicus* and other anaerobes in periodontal infections. Rev. Infect. Dis., *1*:313, 1979.
32. Nielsen, J. I., Glavind, L., and Karring, T.: Interproximal periodontal intrabony defects. Prevalence, localization and etiological factors. J. Clin. Periodontol., *7*:187, 1980.
33. Prichard, J. F.: Periodontal Surgery, Practical Dental Monographs. Chicago, Year Book Medical Publishers, 1961, p. 16.
34. Raisz, L. G., Sandberg, A. L., Goodson, J. M., Simmons, H. A., and Mergenhagen, S. E.: Complement-dependent stimulation of prostaglandin synthesis and bone resorption. Science, *185*:789, 1974.
35. Rifkin, B. R., and Heijl, L.: The occurrence of mononuclear cells at sites of osteoclastic bone resorption in experimental periodontitis. J. Periodontol., *50*:636, 1979.
36. Rizzo, A. A., and Mergenhagen, S. E.: Histopathologic effects of endotoxin injected into rabbit oral mucosa. Arch. Oral Biol., *9*:659, 1964.
37. Rowe, D. J., and Bradley, L. S.: Quantitative analyses of osteoclasts, bone loss and inflammation in human periodontal disease. J. Periodont. Res., *16*:13, 1981.
38. Saari, J. T., Hurt, W. C., and Briggs, N. L.: Periodontal bony defects on the dry skull. J. Periodontol., *39*:278, 1968.
39. Schroeder, H. E., and Lindhe, J.: Conditions and pathological features of rapidly destructive experimental periodontitis in dogs. J. Periodontol., *51*:6, 1980.

Furcation Involvement

The term *furcation involvement* refers to commonly occurring conditions in which the bifurcation and trifurcation of multirooted teeth are denuded by periodontal disease.[4] The mandibular first molars are the most common sites and the maxillary premolars the least common; the number of furcation involvements increases with age.[8]

CLINICAL FEATURES

The denuded bifurcation or trifurcation may be visible or obscured by the inflamed wall of a periodontal pocket. The extent of involvement is determined by exploration with a blunt probe, with a simultaneous blast of warm air to facilitate visualization. The tooth may or may not be mobile and is usually symptom-free, but there may be painful complications. These include **sensitivity to thermal changes,** caused by caries or lacunar resorption of the root in the furcation area; **recurrent or constant throbbing pain,** caused by pulp changes; and **sensitivity to percussion,** caused by acute inflammatory involvement of the periodontal ligament. Furcation involvement may result in acute periodontal or periapical abscess formation, with all the symptoms that accompany such lesions (Figs. 17–1 and 17–2).

MICROSCOPIC FEATURES

Microscopically, furcation involvement presents no unique pathologic features. It is simply a phase in the rootward extension of the periodontal pocket. In its early stages, it presents a widening of the periodontal space, with cellular and fluid inflammatory exudation (Fig. 17–3), followed by epithelial proliferation into the bifurcation area from an adjoining periodontal pocket (Fig. 17–4). Extension of the inflammation into the bone leads to resorption and reduction in bone height (Fig. 17–5). Bone formation is often present adjacent to areas of resorption and along adjoining medullary spaces (Fig. 17–6). The bone destructive pattern may be horizontal or may produce angular osseous defects associated with infrabony pockets (Fig. 17–7). Plaque, calculus, and bacterial debris occupy the denuded furcation space. Findings that complicate furcation involvement and account for painful symptoms include caries of the cementum and dentin, with involvement of the dentinal tubules (Fig. 17–8); idiopathic tooth resorption, in which cementum is absent and the dentin present a clear-cut, irregular margin with hollowed-out lacunae (Fig. 17–4); and abscess formation in the furcation area.

ETIOLOGY

Bifurcation and trifurcation involvement are stages of progressive periodontal disease and have the same etiology. The difficulty, and sometimes impossibility,[1, 2] of controlling plaque in furcations is responsible for extensive lesions in this area[10] (see Chapter 33).

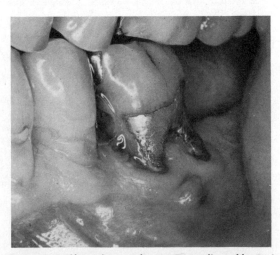

Figure 17–1 Bifurcation Involvement Complicated by Periodontal Abscess.

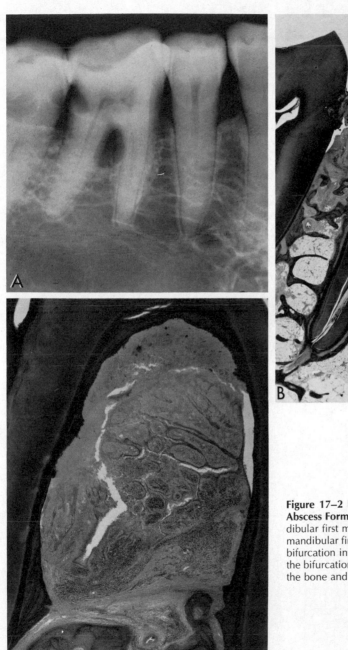

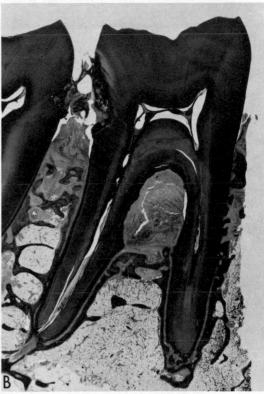

Figure 17–2 Bifurcation Involvement Complicated by Abscess Formation. *A*, Bifurcation involvement of mandibular first molar. Also note caries. *B*, Section through mandibular first molar showing periodontal disease with bifurcation involvement. Note the caries. *C*, Abscess in the bifurcation. Note extension of the inflammation into the bone and thickened blood vessel.

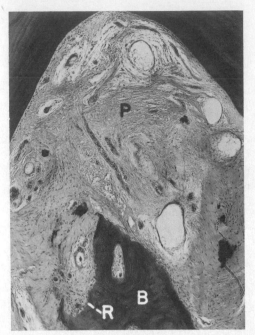

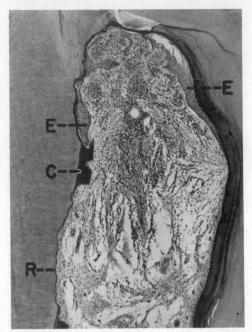

Fig. 17–3   Fig. 17–4

Figure 17–3 Bifurcation Area in a Mandibular Molar. The periodontal space is widened. There is edema, degeneration, and slight leukocytic infiltration of the periodontal ligament and an area of resorption (R) at the margin of the bone (B).
Figure 17–4 Bifurcation Area showing proliferation of epithelium (E), edema and degeneration of connective tissue, bone loss, and destruction of cementum (C) and dentin with irregularly hollowed-out lacunae along the dentinal surface (R).

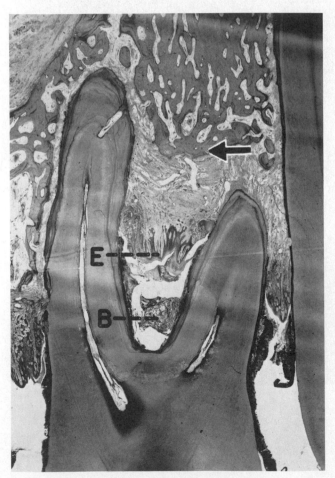

Figure 17–5 Trifurcation Involvement. Maxillary first molar showing pronounced bone loss, inflammation, and epithelial proliferation (E). Bacterial debris is shown at B. Note different height of bone between the mesial surface *(left)* and the furcation area *(arrow)*.

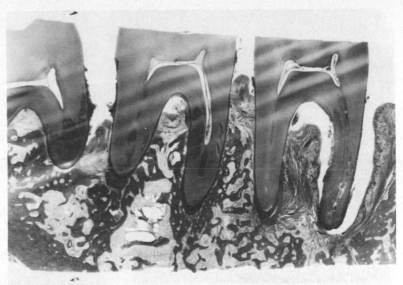

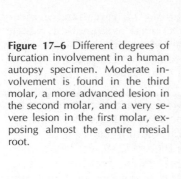

Figure 17–6 Different degrees of furcation involvement in a human autopsy specimen. Moderate involvement is found in the third molar, a more advanced lesion in the second molar, and a very severe lesion in the first molar, exposing almost the entire mesial root.

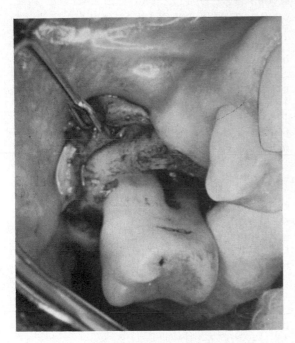

Figure 17–7 Crater-like Osseous Defect in Trifurcation of Molar.

Figure 17–8 Trifurcation Showing Destruction of Cementum (C) and Caries of Dentin (D).

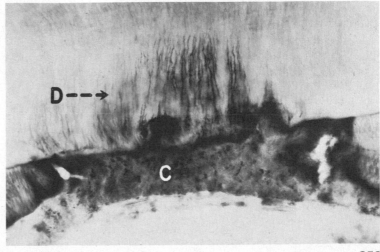

253

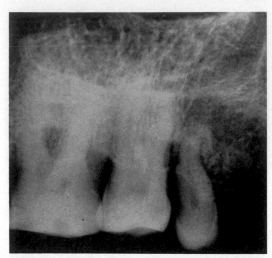

Figure 17–9 Radiograph Showing Trifurcation Involvement of the Maxillary First Molar. Compare with Figures 17–10 and 17–11.

RADIOGRAPHIC FEATURES

Definitive diagnosis of furcation involvement is made by clinical examination, which includes careful probing with one of the specially designed probes (Nabers probe). Radiographs are helpful but show artefacts which make it possible for furcation involvement to be present without detectable radiographic changes. As a general rule, bone loss is always greater than the radiograph shows.

For example, in Figure 17–9, the trifurcation of the maxillary first molar appears involved, whereas that of the second molar does not. Microscopic sections of the autopsied jaw indicate that both the first (Fig. 17–10) and second (Fig. 17–11) molars are involved. The opaque palatal root of the second molar hides the bone loss in the trifurcation.

Variations in radiographic technique may obscure the presence and extent of furcation involvement. A tooth may present marked bifurcation involvement in one film (Fig. 17–12A) but appear uninvolved in another (Fig. 17–12b). Radiographs should be taken at different angles to reduce the risk of missing furcation involvement.

Aids in Radiographic Interpretation. The recognition of large, clearly defined radiolucency in the furcation area presents no problem (Fig. 17–12A), but less clearly defined radiographic changes produced by furcation involvement are often overlooked. To assist in the radiographic detection of furcation involvement, the following diagnostic criteria are suggested:

1. The slightest radiographic change in the furcation area should be investigated clinically, especially if there is bone loss on adjacent roots (Fig. 17–13).

2. Diminished radiodensity in the furcation area in which outlines of bony trabeculae are visible (Fig. 17–14) suggests furcation involvement.

3. Whenever there is marked bone loss in relation to a single molar root, it may be assumed that the furcation is also involved (Figs. 17–15 and 17–16). This is an extremely important rule. Treatment limited to the root with extensive bone loss may seal the infected bifurcation or trifurcation, prevent drainage, and lead to the formation of a periodontal abscess.

References follow on page 258

The role of trauma from occlusion in the etiology of furcation lesions is controversial. Some assign a key role to trauma, considering that furcation areas are most sensitive to injury from excessive occlusal forces.[5] Others deny the initiating effect of trauma and consider that inflammation and edema caused by plaque in the furcation area will tend to extrude the tooth, which then will become traumatized and sensitive.[10]

Trauma from occlusion should be particularly suspect as a contributing etiologic factor in cases of furcation involvement with crater-like or angular deformities in the bone and, especially, when bone destruction is localized to one of the roots.

Other factors that may play a role are the presence of enamel projections into the furca,[9] which occur in about 13 per cent of multirooted teeth, and the proximity of the furcation to the cemento-enamel junction, which occurs in about 75 per cent of the cases.[8] The presence of accessory pulpal canals in the furcation area may extend pulpal inflammation to the furca[6]; this possibility should be carefully explored, particularly when mesial and distal bone retain their normal height. Frequently, the sequence of therapy in endodontic-periodontal cases depends on the sequence of etiologic factors involved.

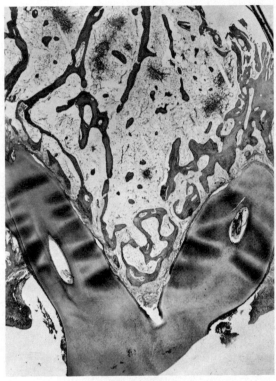

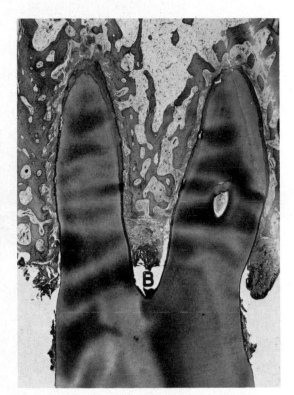

Fig. 17–10   **Fig. 17–11**

Figure 17–10 Buccopalatal section through the **Maxillary First Molar** shown in Figure 17–9. The trifurcation is involved, and there are periodontal pockets on the buccal *(left)* and palatal roots *(right)*.

Figure 17–11 Buccopalatal section through the **Maxillary Second Molar** shown in Figure 17–9. There is involvement of the trifurcation at B, which is clearly detectable in the radiograph.

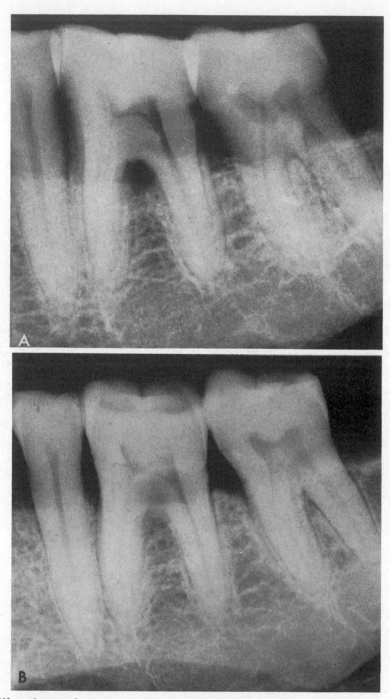

Figure 17–12 *A,* **Bifurcation Involvement** indicated by triangular radiolucence in bifurcation area of mandibular first molar. The second molar presents only a slight thickening of the periodontal space in the bifurcation area. *B,* Same area, different angulation. The triangular radiolucence in the bifurcation of the first molar is obliterated, and involvement of the second molar bifurcation is apparent.

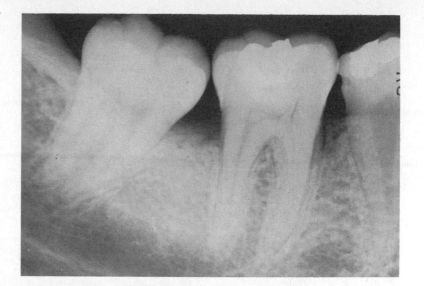

Figure 17–13 Early Furcation Involvement suggested by fuzziness in the bifurcation of the mandibular first molar, particularly when associated with bone loss on the roots.

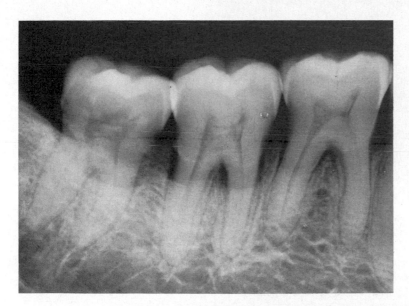

Figure 17–14 Bifurcation Involvement of Mandibular First and Second Molars Indicated by Thickening of Periodontal Space in Bifurcation Area. The bifurcation of the third molar is also involved, but the thickening of the periodontal space is partially obscured by the external oblique line.

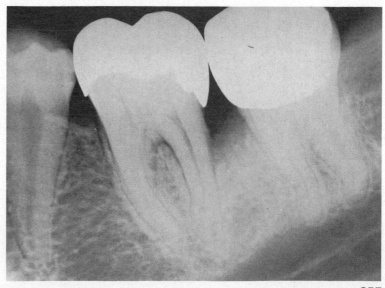

Figure 17–15 Bifurcation Involvement of first molar, associated with bone loss on the distal root.

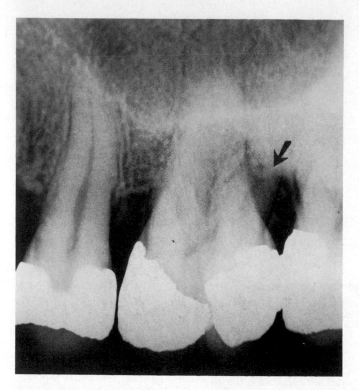

Figure 17–16 Trifurcation Involvement of the First Molar Partially Obscured by the Radiopaque Lingual Root. The horizontal line across the distobuccal root demarcates the apical portion *(arrow)*, which is covered by bone, from the remainder of the root, where the bone has been destroyed.

REFERENCES

1. Bower, R. C.: Furcation morphology relative to periodontal treatment. Furcation entrance architecture. J. Periodontol., *50*:23, 1979.
2. Bower, R. C.: Furcation morphology relative to periodontal treatment. Furcation root surface anatomy. J. Periodontol., *50*:366, 1979.
3. Easley, J. R., and Drennan, G. A.: Morphological classification of the furca. J. Can. Dent. Assoc., *35*:104, 1969.
4. Glickman, I.: Bifurcation involvement in periodontal disease. J. Am. Dent. Assoc, *40*:528, 1950.
5. Glickman, I., Stein, R. S., and Smulow, J. B.: The effects of increased functional forces upon the periodontium of splinted and non-splinted teeth. J. Periodontol., *32*:290, 1961.
6. Gutman, J. L.: Prevalence, location and patency of accessory canals in the furcation region of permanent molars. J. Periodontol., *49*:21, 1978.
7. Larato, D. C.: Furcation involvements: incidence of distribution. J. Periodontol., *41*:499, 1970.
8. Larato, D. C.: Some anatomical factors related to furcation involvements. J. Periodontol., *46*:608, 1975.
9. Masters, D. H., and Hoskins, S. W.: Projection of cervical enamel into molar furcations. J. Periodontol., *35*:49, 1963.
10. Waerhaug, J.: The furcation problem. Etiology, pathogenesis, diagnosis, therapy and prognosis. J. Clin. Periodontol., *7*:73, 1980.

The Periodontal Abscess

A periodontal abscess is a localized purulent inflammation in the periodontal tissues. It is also known as a *lateral* or *parietal abscess.* Periodontal abscess formation may occur as follows:

1. Deep extension of infection from a periodontal pocket into the supporting periodontal tissues and localization of the suppurative inflammatory process along the lateral aspect of the root.

2. Lateral extension of inflammation from the inner surface of a periodontal pocket into the connective tissue of the pocket wall. Localization of the abscess results when drainage into the pocket space is impaired (Fig. 18–1).

3. In a pocket that describes a tortuous course around the root (complex pocket), a periodontal abscess may form in the cul-de-sac, the deep end of which is shut off from the surface.

4. Incomplete removal of calculus during treatment of a periodontal pocket. In this instance, the gingival wall shrinks, occluding the pocket orifice, and a periodontal abscess occurs in the sealed-off portion of the pocket.

5. A periodontal abscess may occur in the absence of periodontal disease, following trauma to the tooth or perforation of the lateral wall of the root in endodontic therapy.

CLASSIFICATION

Periodontal abscesses are classified according to location as follows:

1. *Abscess in the supporting periodontal tissues* along the lateral aspect of the root. In this condition, there is generally a sinus in the bone, which extends laterally from the abscess to the external surface (Fig. 18–2).

2. *Abscess in the soft tissue wall of a deep periodontal pocket* (Figs. 18–3 and 18–4).

CLINICAL FEATURES

Periodontal abscesses may be *acute* or *chronic.* Acute lesions often subside but persist in the chronic state, whereas chronic lesions may exist without having been acute. Chronic lesions frequently undergo acute exacerbations.

Acute Abscess. The acute periodontal abscess is accompanied by symptoms such as *throbbing, radiating pain, exquisite tenderness of the gingiva to palpation, sensitivity of the tooth to percussion, tooth mobility, lymphadenitis, and systemic effects such as fever, leukocytosis, and malaise.*

The acute periodontal abscess appears as an ovoid elevation of the gingiva along the lateral aspect of the root (Figs. 18–5 and 18–6). The gingiva is edematous and red, with a smooth, shiny surface. The shape and consistency of the elevated area vary. It may be dome-like and relatively firm or pointed and soft. In most instances, pus may be expressed from the gingival margin by gentle digital pressure. Occasionally, the patient may present symptoms of an acute periodontal abscess *without any notable clinical lesion or radiographic changes.* Microorganisms which colonize the periodontal abscess are primarily gram-negative anaerobic rods.[3]

Chronic Abscess. The chronic periodontal abscess usually presents a sinus that opens onto the gingival mucosa somewhere along the length of the root. There may be a history of intermittent exudation (Fig. 18–7). The orifice of the sinus may appear as a difficult-to-detect pinpoint opening, which when probed reveals a sinus tract deep in the periodontium (Fig. 18–8). The sinus may be covered by a small, pink, bead-like mass of granulation tissue (Fig. 18–9).

The chronic periodontal abscess is usually asymptomatic. However, the patient may re-

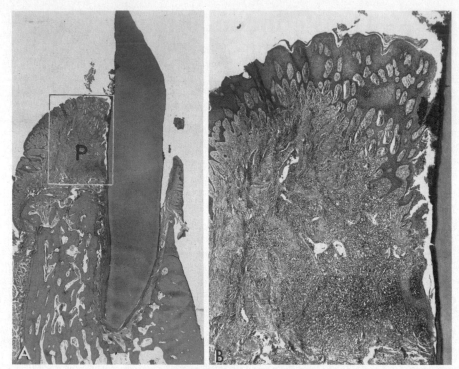

Figure 18–1 *A*, **Periodontal Abscess (P) on the Lingual Surface of Mandibular Incisor** (abscess enclosed in rectangle). *B*, Detailed view of periodontal abscess showing dense leukocytic infiltration and suppuration.

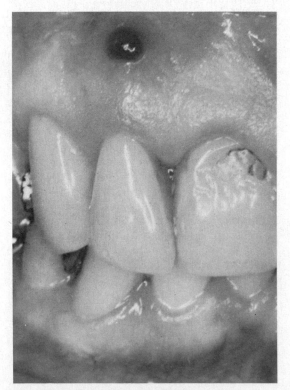

Figure 18–2 Periodontal Abscess deep in the periodontium showing hemorrhagic tissue at the sinus orifice.

port episodes of *dull, gnawing pain, slight elevation of the tooth, and a desire to bite down on and grind the tooth.* The chronic periodontal abscess often undergoes acute exacerbations, with all the associated symptoms.

RADIOGRAPHIC APPEARANCE

The typical radiographic appearance of the periodontal abscess is of a discrete area of radiolucence along the lateral aspect of the root (Figs. 18–10 and 18–11). *However, the radiographic picture is often not typical* (Fig. 18–12) because of many variables, such as:

1. The stage of the lesion. In the early stages the acute periodontal abscess is extremely painful but presents no radiographic changes.

2. The extent of bone destruction and the morphology of the bone.

3. The location of the abscess.

Lesions in the soft tissue wall of a periodontal pocket are less likely to produce radiographic changes than those deep in the supporting tissues.

Abscesses on the facial or lingual surface are obscured by the radiopacity of the root;

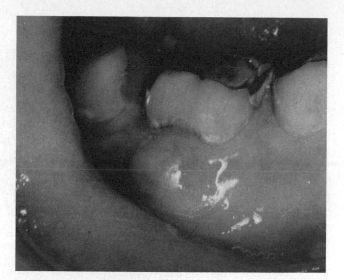

Figure 18–3 Chronic Periodontal Abscess in the Wall of a Deep Pocket.

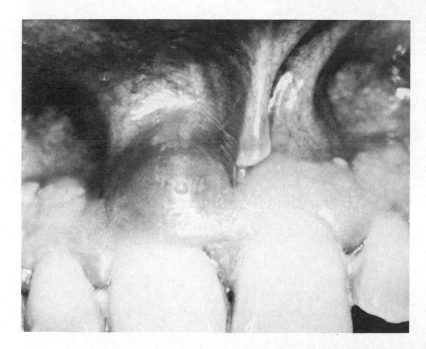

Figure 18–4 Periodontal Abscess on Upper Central Incisor.

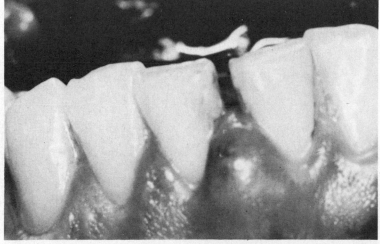

Figure 18–5 Acute Periodontal Abscess Between Lower Central Incisors.

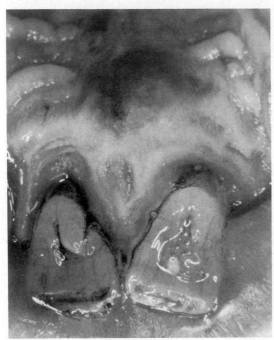

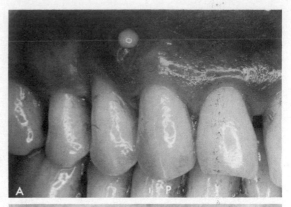

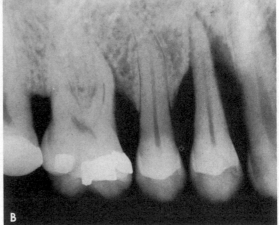

Figure 18–6 Acute Periodontal Abscess on the Lingual Surface. The fibrotic tissue obscures some of the "typical" features of the abscess.

Figure 18–7 Suppuration from a Chronic Periodontal Abscess. *A,* Suppurative draining sinus between the canine and first premolar. *B,* Radiograph showing extensive bone destruction in the area of the draining sinus.

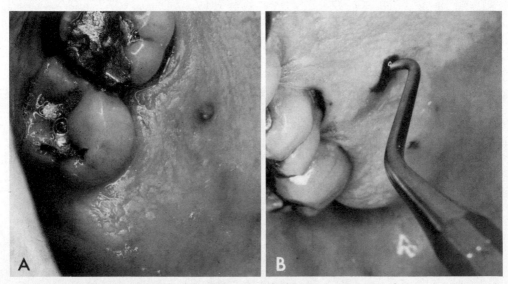

Figure 18–8 Pinpoint Orifice of Sinus from Palatal Periodontal Abscess. *A,* Pinpoint orifice on the palate indicative of sinus from periodontal abscess. *B,* Probe extends into abscess deep in the periodontium.

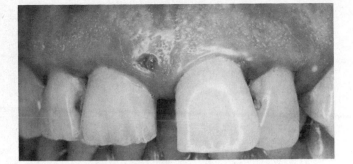

Figure 18–9 Granulation Tissue at the orifice of sinus from periodontal abscess.

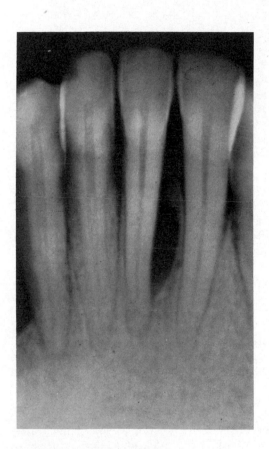

Figure 18–10 Radiolucent Area on the lateral aspect of root with chronic periodontal abscess.

Figure 18–11 Typical Radiographic Appearance of Periodontal Abscess on Right Central Incisor.

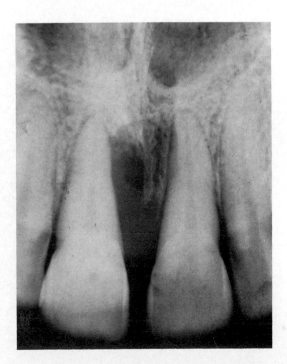

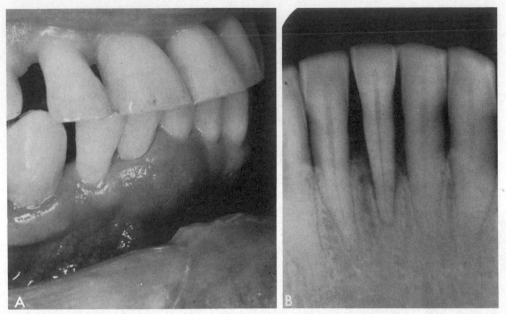

Figure 18–12 Chronic Periodontal Abscess. *A,* Periodontal abscess in the right central and lateral incisor area. *B,* Extensive bone destruction and thickening of the periodontal ligament space around the right central incisor.

interproximal lesions are more likely to be visualized radiographically.

The radiograph alone cannot be relied upon for the diagnosis of a periodontal abscess.

DIAGNOSIS

Diagnosis of the periodontal abscess requires correlation of the history and clinical and radiographic findings. *Continuity of the lesion with the gingival margin is clinical evidence of a periodontal abscess.* The suspected area should be probed carefully along the gingival margin in relation to each tooth surface to detect a channel from the marginal area to the deeper periodontal tissues. *The abscess is not necessarily located on the same surface of the root as the pocket from which it is formed.* A pocket on the facial or lingual surface may give rise to a periodontal abscess interproximally. It is common for a periodontal abscess to be localized on a root surface other than that along which the pocket originated, because impairment of drainage is more likely to occur when a pocket follows a tortuous course.

DIFFERENTIAL DIAGNOSIS BETWEEN A PERIODONTAL AND A PERIAPICAL ABSCESS

The following are useful guides in the differential diagnosis between a *periodontal* and a *periapical* abscess:

If the tooth is nonvital, the lesion is most likely periapical. In severe cases a periodontal abscess may extend to the apex and cause pulpal involvement and necrosis. Except in such cases, however, periodontal abscesses do not cause devitalization of teeth.

An apical abscess may spread along the lateral aspect of the root to the gingival margin, but when the apex and lateral surface of a root are involved by a single lesion that can be probed directly from the gingival margin, it is more likely to have originated as a periodontal abscess.

Radiographic findings are helpful in differentiating between a periodontal and a periapical lesion, but their usefulness is limited. Early acute periodontal and periapical abscesses present no radiographic changes. Ordinarily an area of radiolucence along the lateral surface of the root suggests the presence of a periodontal abscess, whereas apical rarefaction suggests a periapical abscess. *However, acute periodontal abscesses that show no radiographic changes frequently cause symptoms in teeth with long-standing, radiographically detectable periapical lesions that are not contributing to the patient's complaint.* Clinical findings, such as the presence of extensive caries, pocket formation, tooth vitality, and the existence of continuity between the gingival margin and the abscess area, often prove to be of greater diagnostic value than radiographs.

A draining sinus on the lateral aspect of the root suggests periodontal rather than apical involvement; a sinus from a periapical lesion is more likely to be located farther apically. However, sinus location is not conclusive. In many instances, particularly in children, the sinus from a periapical lesion drains on the side of the root rather than at the apex (see also Chapter 55).

THE PERIODONTAL ABSCESS AND THE GINGIVAL ABSCESS

The principal differences between the periodontal abscess and the gingival abscess are location and history (see Chapter 10). The gingival abscess is confined to the marginal gingiva, and it often occurs in previously disease-free areas. It is usually an acute inflammatory response to foreign material forced into the gingiva. In rare instances it results from infection of an epithelium-lined gingival cyst.[4] The periodontal abscess involves the supporting periodontal tissues and generally occurs in the course of chronic destructive periodontal disease.

THE PERIODONTAL CYST

This is an uncommon lesion which produces localized destruction of the periodontal tissues along a lateral root surface, most often in the mandibular canine-premolar area.[2] The following possible etiologies have been suggested:

1. Odontogenic cyst caused by proliferation of the epithelial rests of Malassez; the stimulus initiating the cellular activity is not known.

2. Lateral dentigerous cyst retained in the jaw after tooth eruption.

3. Primordial cyst of supernumerary tooth germ.

4. Stimulation of epithelial rests of the periodontal ligament by infection from a periodontal abscess or from the pulp through an accessory root canal.

A periodontal cyst is usually asymptomatic and without grossly detectable changes, but it may present as a localized tender swelling. *Radiographically,* when located interproximally the periodontal cyst appears on the side of the root as a radiolucent area bordered by a radiopaque line. Its radiographic appearance cannot be differentiated from that of a periodontal abscess.

Microscopically, the cystic lining may be (1) a loosely arranged, nonkeratinized, thickened, proliferating epithelium; (2) a thin, nonkeratinized epithelium; or (3) an odontogenic keratocyst.[2]

REFERENCES

1. Cross, W. G.: Lateral peridontal cyst: report of a case. J. Periodontol., *25*:287, 1954.
2. Fantasia, J. E.: Lateral periodontal cyst. An analysis of 46 cases. Oral Surg., *48*:237, 1979.
3. Newman, M. G., and Sims, T. N.: The predominant cultivable microbiota of the periodontal abscess. J. Periodontol., *50*:350, 1979.
4. Ritchey, B., and Orban, B.: Cysts of the gingiva. Oral Surg., *6*:765, 1952.
5. Standish, S. N., and Shafer, W. G.: The lateral periodontal cyst. J. Periodontol., *29*:27, 1958.

chapter nineteen

Trauma from Occlusion

THE FUNCTIONAL COMPONENT IN PERIODONTAL HEALTH

Periodontal health depends upon a balance between an internal, systemically controlled milieu that governs tissue metabolism and the external environment of the tooth, of which occlusion is an important component. To remain structurally and metabolically sound, the periodontal ligament and alveolar bone require the mechanical stimulation of occlusal forces.

The relationship of occlusion to periodontal health starts with the development of the tooth. When the crown of the tooth is completed, it is contained within a bony crypt in the jaw, protected from external environmental factors. As the tooth erupts into the oral cavity, it is confronted with an entirely new world. Pressure from the lips and the tongue, the cheeks, the child's fingers, the pacifier, and food is thrust upon it. To enable the crown to withstand such forces, the root is built as the tooth erupts, and the periodontium develops around the root to hold it in the jaw. **The periodontium is custom-built to meet the functional demands of the tooth; support of the tooth is the only reason for its existence.**

Just as the tooth depends upon the periodontal tissues to keep it in the jaw, so do the periodontal tissues depend upon the functional activity of the tooth to remain healthy. When there is insufficient functional stimulation, the periodontal tissues atrophy; when the tooth is extracted, the periodontium disappears. *Occlusion is the life line of the periodontium.* In periodontal health, it provides the mechanical stimulation which marshals the complex bio-logic mechanisms responsible for the well-being of the periodontium.

PHYSIOLOGIC ADAPTIVE CAPACITY OF THE PERIODONTIUM TO OCCLUSAL FORCES

When there is an increased functional demand upon it, the periodontium tries to accommodate that demand. The adaptive capacity varies in different persons and in the same person at different times. The effect of occlusal forces upon the periodontium is influenced by their **magnitude, direction, duration,** and **frequency.**

When the **magnitude of occlusal forces** is increased, the periodontium responds with a thickening of the periodontal ligament, an increase in the number and width of periodontal ligament fibers, and an increase in the density of alveolar bone.

Changing the **direction of occlusal forces** causes a reorientation of the stresses and strains within the periodontium.[32] The principal fibers of the periodontal ligament are arranged so that they can best accommodate occlusal forces in the long axis of the tooth. When *axial forces* are increased, there is viscoelastic distortion of the periodontal ligament and ultimate compression of the periodontal fibers and resorption of bone in the apical areas. The fibers in relation to the remainder of the root are placed under tension, and new bone is formed.[65] **In designing dental restorations and prostheses, every effort is made to direct occlusal forces axially in order to make** use of the greater tolerance of the periodontium to forces in this direction.[39]

Lateral or *horizontal forces* are ordinarily accommodated by bone resorption in areas of pressure and bone formation in areas of tension (Fig. 19–1). The most advantageous point of application of a lateral force is near the cervical line. As the point of application is moved coronally, the distance from the center of rotation is lengthened and the force upon the periodontal ligament increases.[78]

Torques or *rotational forces* cause both tension and pressure; this force, under physiologic conditions, results in bone formation and bone resorption.[64] Torques are the type of force most likely to injure the periodontium.

The **duration** and **frequency of occlusal forces** affect the response of alveolar bone. Constant pressure on the bone causes resorption, whereas intermittent force favors bone formation. The time lapse between pressure applications apparently influences the bone response. Recurrent forces over short intervals of time have essentially the same resorbing effect as constant pressure.

An inherent "margin of safety" common to all tissues permits some variation in occlusion without the periodontium being adversely affected. However, when occlusal forces exceed the adaptive capacity of the tissues, tissue injury results.[5, 7, 15, 26, 36, 50, 52] The injury is called trauma from occlusion.

TRAUMA FROM OCCLUSION

Periodontal tissue injury caused by occlusal forces is called trauma from occlusion.* **Trauma from occlusion is the tissue injury— not the occlusal force.** An occlusion which produces such injury is called a traumatic occlusion.[3] Excessive occlusal forces may also disrupt the function of the masticatory musculature and *cause painful spasms, injure the temporomandibular joints,* or *produce excessive tooth wear,* but the term "trauma from occlusion" is generally used in connection with injury in the periodontium.

Trauma from occlusion may be *acute* or *chronic.* **Acute trauma from occlusion** results from an abrupt change in occlusal force such as that produced by restorations or prosthetic appliances which interfere with or alter the

direction of occlusal forces on the teeth. The results are tooth pain, sensitivity to percussion, and increased mobility. If the force is dissipated by a shift in the position of the tooth or by wearing away or correction of the restoration, the injury heals and the symptoms subside. Otherwise, periodontal injury may worsen and develop into necrosis, with periodontal abscess formation, or it may persist as a symptom-free chronic condition. Acute trauma can also produce cemental tears (see Chapter 3).

Chronic trauma from occlusion is more common than the acute form and is of greater clinical significance. It most often develops from gradual changes in the occlusion produced by tooth wear, drifting, and extrusion of teeth, combined with parafunctional habits such as bruxism and clenching, rather than as a sequel to acute periodontal trauma. The features of chronic trauma from occlusion and their significance are discussed below.

The criterion which determines whether an occlusion is traumatic is whether it produces injury, rather than how the teeth occlude. Any occlusion which produces periodontal injury is traumatic. Malocclusion is not necessary to produce trauma; it may occur when the occlusion appears normal.[47] The dentition may be anatomically and esthetically acceptable, but functionally injurious. Conversely, not all malocclusions are necessarily injurious to the periodontium. Occlusal relationships which are traumatic are referred to by such terms as "occlusal disharmony," "functional imbalance," and "occlusal dystrophy." This is because of their effect upon the periodontium, not because of the position of the teeth. Since trauma from occlusion refers to the tissue injury rather than to the occlusion, an increased occlusal force is not traumatic if the periodontium can accommodate it.

The Causes of Trauma from Occlusion

Trauma from occlusion may be caused by (1) alterations in occlusal forces, (2) reduced capacity of the periodontium to withstand occlusal forces, or (3) a combination of both. When trauma from occlusion is the result of alterations in the occlusal forces, it is called primary trauma from occlusion. When it results from reduced ability of the tissues to resist the occlusal forces, it is known as secondary trauma from occlusion.

PRIMARY TRAUMA FROM OCCLUSION.

---

*This term is used throughout the text to designate periodontal tissue injury produced by occlusal forces. It is also known as "traumatism" and "occlusal trauma."

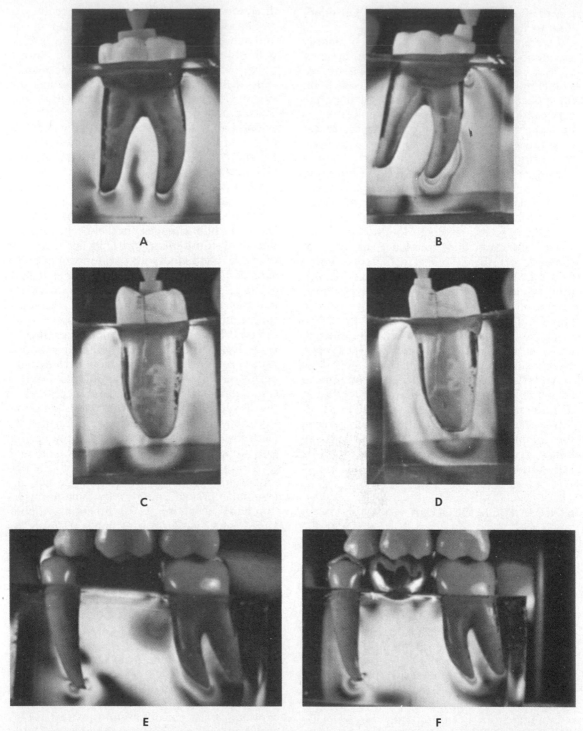

Figure 19–1 Stress Patterns Around the Roots Changed by Shifting the Direction of Occlusal Forces (Experimental Model Using Photoelastic Analysis). *A*, Buccal view of ivorine molar subjected to an **Axial Force.** The shaded fringes indicate that the internal stresses are at the root apices. *B*, Buccal view of ivorine molar subjected to a **Mesial Tilting Force.** The shaded fringes indicate that the internal stresses are along the mesial surface and at the apex of the mesial root. *C*, Ivorine molar subjected to **Axial Force** viewed from the mesial proximal surface. The shaded fringes indicate that the stresses are concentrated at the apex. *D*, Ivorine molar subjected to **Lingual Tilting Force** viewed from the mesial proximal surface. The shaded fringes indicate that the internal stresses are along the lingual surface and at the apex. *E*, **Stress Patterns Around the Roots of Teeth Adjacent to an Edentulous Space.** Note particularly the stress fringes in the mesial cervical region of the molar. *F*, **Changes in Stress Patterns Produced by Inserting a Fixed Bridge.** Note the disappearance of the fringes in the cervical region of the molar (compare with *E*). (From Glickman, I., et al.: J. Periodontol., *41*:30, 1970.)

Trauma from occlusion may be considered the primary etiologic factor in periodontal destruction if the only local alteration to which a tooth is subjected is one of occlusion. Examples are periodontal injury produced around teeth with a *previously healthy periodontium* following: (1) insertion of a "high filling," (2) insertion of a prosthetic replacement which creates excessive forces on abutment and antagonistic teeth, (3) the drifting or extrusion of teeth into spaces created by unreplaced missing teeth, and (4) the orthodontic movement of teeth into functionally unacceptable positions. Most of the studies made on experimental animals of the effect of trauma from occlusion have been on this primary type of trauma. These changes do not alter the level of connective tissue attachment and do not initiate pocket formation. This is probably because the supracrestal gingival fibers are not affected and therefore prevent the apical migration of the junctional epithelium.[55]

SECONDARY TRAUMA FROM OCCLUSION. Trauma from occlusion is considered a secondary cause of periodontal destruction when the adaptive capacity of the tissues to withstand occlusal forces is impaired. The periodontium becomes vulnerable to injury, and previously well-tolerated occlusal forces become traumatic.

Bone loss and systemic factors impair the capability of the periodontium to withstand occlusal forces. Bone loss due to marginal inflammation reduces the periodontal attachment area. This increases the burden upon the remaining tissues, because there is less tissue to support the forces and because the leverage upon the remaining tissues is altered. Alveolar bone loss is the most common cause of secondary trauma and may be very difficult to remedy. Systemic disorders may inhibit anabolic activity or induce degenerative changes in the periodontium,[30, 71] causing previously tolerable forces to become excessive.

Three Stages of Trauma from Occlusion

Trauma from occlusion occurs in three stages.[10, 17] The first is injury, the second is repair, and the third is adaptive remodeling of the periodontium. Tissue injury is produced by excessive occlusal forces. Nature attempts to repair the injury and restore the periodontium. This can occur if the forces are diminished or if the tooth drifts away from them. If, however, the offending force is chronic, the periodontium is remodeled in order to cushion its impact. The ligament is widened at the expense of the bone, angular bone defects occur without periodontal pockets, and the tooth becomes loose.

STAGE I: INJURY. The severity, location, and pattern of the tissue damage depend upon the severity, frequency, and direction of the injurious forces. *Slightly excessive pressure* stimulates resorption of the alveolar bone, with a resultant widening of the periodontal ligament space. *Slightly excessive tension* causes elongation of the periodontal ligament fibers and apposition of alveolar bone. In areas of increased pressure the blood vessels are numerous and reduced in size; in areas of increased tension they are enlarged.[83]

Greater pressure produces a gradation of changes in the periodontal ligament, starting with compression of the fibers, which produces areas of hyalinization.[61, 62] Subsequent injury to the fibroblasts and other connective tissue cells leads to necrosis of areas of the ligament.[59, 63] Vascular changes are also produced: within 30 minutes, retardation and stasis of blood flow occur; at 2 to 3 hours, blood vessels appear packed with erythrocytes, which start to fragment; and between 1 and 7 days, there is disintegration of the blood vessel walls and release of the contents into the surrounding tissue.[60] Also, excessive resorption of alveolar bone and resorption of tooth surface may occur[36, 41] (Figs. 19–2 and 19–3).

Severe tension causes widening of the periodontal ligament, thrombosis, hemorrhage, tearing of the periodontal ligament, and resorption of alveolar bone.

Pressure severe enough to force the root against bone causes **necrosis of the periodontal ligament and bone. The bone is resorbed from viable periodontal ligament adjacent to necrotic areas and from marrow spaces, a process called "undermining resorption."[34, 50]**

The bifurcation and trifurcation are the areas of the periodontium most susceptible to injury from excessive occlusal forces.[31]

With injury to the periodontium there is a temporary depression in mitotic activity and in the rate of proliferation and differentiation of fibroblasts,[72] collagen, and bone formation.[36, 67, 72] These return to normal following dissipation of the forces.

STAGE II: REPAIR. Repair is constantly occurring in the normal periodontium. During trauma from occlusion the injured tissues stimulate increased reparative activity. **The damaged tissues are removed, and new connective**

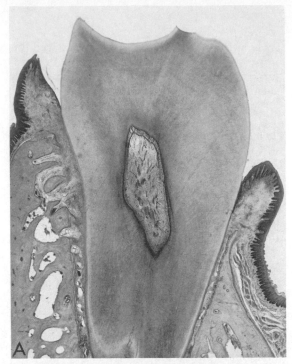

Figure 19–2 Periodontal Accommodation to Lateral Forces. *A,* Mandibular premolar. *B,* Lingual surface, showing new bone formation in response to tension on the periodontal ligament. Note the pale-staining osteoid bordered by osteoblasts and the incremental lines indicative of previous additions to the bone. *C,* Facial surface shows compression of the periodontal ligament and osteoclastic resorption of the bony plate. Note the new bone formed on the external surface. This is **Peripheral Buttressing Bone,** which reinforces the resorbing facial plate. Note, too, that the buttressing bone has produced a bulge in the bony contour.

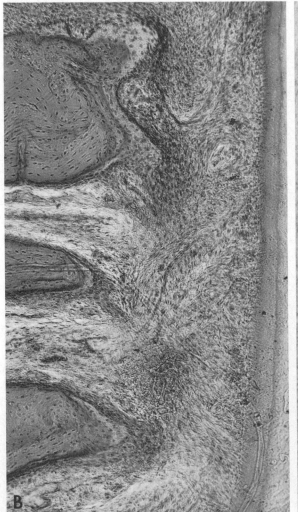

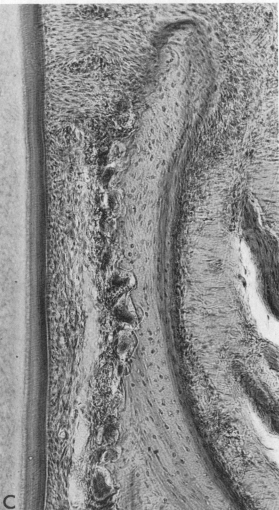

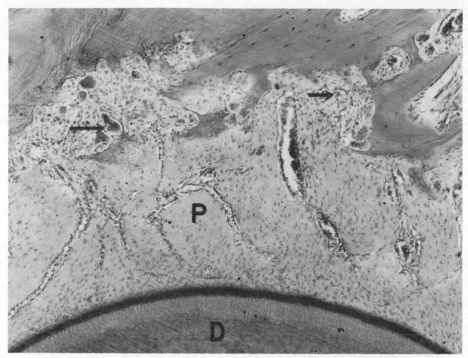

Figure 19–3 Trauma from Occlusion at Root Apex. Note bone resorption with prominent osteoclasts (*arrows*). The periodontal ligament (P) is widened as the result of bone resorption, and the blood vessels are engorged. The root is shown at D.

tissue cells and fibers, bone, and cementum are formed in an attempt to restore the injured periodontium (Figs. 19–4 and 19–5). Forces remain traumatic only so long as the damage produced exceeds the reparative capacity of the tissues. Cartilage-like material sometimes develops in the periodontal ligament spaces as an aftermath of the trauma.[21] Formation of crystals from erythrocytes has also been shown.[64]

Buttressing Bone Formation. When bone is resorbed by excessive occlusal forces, nature attempts to reinforce the thinned bony trabeculae with new bone (Fig. 19–6). This attempt to compensate for lost bone is called buttressing bone formation and is an important feature of the reparative process associated with trauma from occlusion.[27] It also occurs when bone is destroyed by inflammation or osteolytic tumors.

Buttressing bone formation occurs within the jaw (central buttressing) and on the bone surface (peripheral buttressing). In central buttressing the endosteal cells deposit new bone, which restores the bony trabeculae and reduces the size of the marrow spaces (Fig. 19–6). Peripheral buttressing occurs on the facial and lingual surfaces of the alveolar plate. Depending upon its severity, it may produce a shelf-like thickening of the alveolar margin, referred to as lipping (Fig. 19–7; see also Fig. 19–2), or a pronounced bulge in the contour of the facial and lingual bone[17, 25] (see Chapter 16).

STAGE III: ADAPTIVE REMODELING OF THE PERIODONTIUM. If the repair cannot keep pace with the destruction caused by the occlusion, the periodontium is remodeled in an effort to create a structural relationship in which the forces are no longer injurious to the tissues. **To cushion the impact of the offending forces, the periodontal ligament is widened and the adjacent bone loss is absorbed.[27] The involved teeth become loose.[82] The results are a thickened periodontal ligament, funnel-shaped at the crest, and angular defects in the bone, with no pocket formation. An increased vascularization has also been reported.[18]**

The three stages in the evolution of traumatic lesions have been differentiated histometrically by means of the relative amounts of periodontal bone surface undergoing resorption or formation[11, 17] (Fig. 19–8). The injury phase shows an increase in areas of resorption and a decrease in bone formation, whereas the repair phase demonstrates increased formation and decreased resorption. After adaptive remodeling of the periodontium, resorption and formation return to normal (Fig. 19–8).

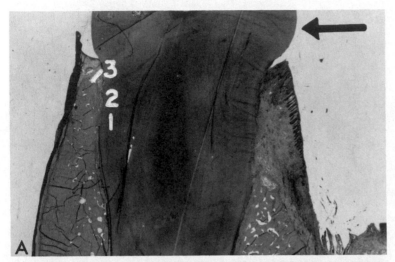

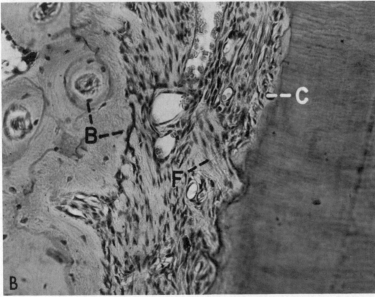

Figure 19–4 *A*, Faciolingual survey section of mandibular tooth of dog, subjected to **Excessive Lateral Force** *(arrow)* that injured periodontium in area marked 1,2,3. *B*, **Reversibility of Trauma from Occlusion.** Healing in area marked 1,2,3, 1 month after cessation of force. There is new bone formation (B) in relation to the periodontal ligament and endosteal bone margins. Cementum (C) is being deposited along the eroded dentinal surface. Note the fibroblasts with collagen fibers (F) being embedded in the cementum and extending into the newly formed bone.

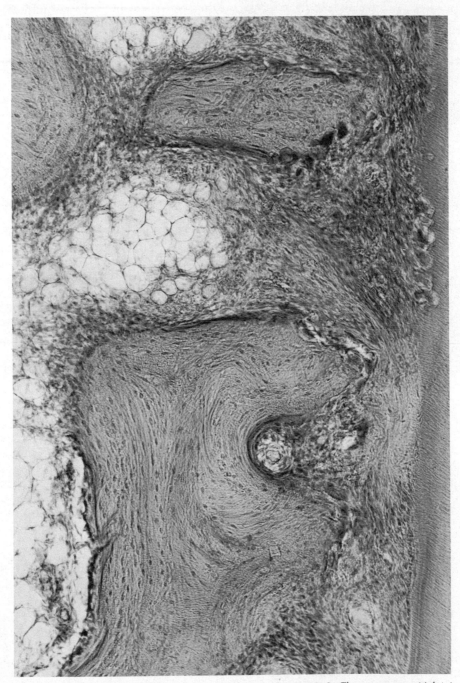

Figure 19–5 Trauma from Occlusion. Injury more severe than in Figure 19–3. The cementum *(right)* is undergoing resorption, the periodontal ligament is compressed and necrotic, and the bone is undergoing resorption. Note the osteoblasts and new bone (central buttressing bone formation) on the trabecular margins adjacent to the marrow.

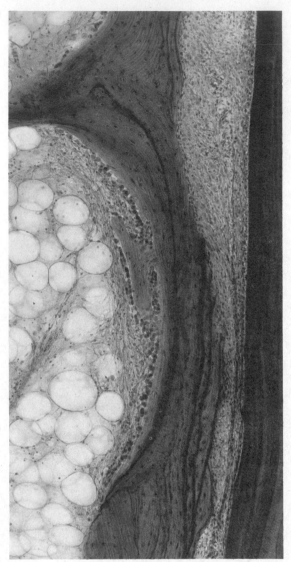

Figure 19–6 Central Buttressing Bone. New bone formation on the marrow side of alveolar bone which is undergoing resorption on the side of the periodontal ligament.

Effects of Insufficient Occlusal Force

Insufficient occlusal force may also be injurious to the supporting periodontal tissues.[13, 43] Insufficient stimulation causes degeneration of the periodontium, manifested by thinning of the periodontal ligament, atrophy of the fibers, osteoporosis of the alveolar bone, and reduction in bone height. Hypofunction results from an open bite relationship, absence of functional antagonists, or unilateral chewing habits that neglect one side of the mouth.

Trauma from Occlusion Is Reversible

Trauma from occlusion is reversible. When trauma is artificially induced in experimental animals, the teeth move away or are intruded into the jaw. The impact of the artificially created force is relieved, and the tissues undergo repair. The fact that trauma from occlusion is reversible under such conditions does not mean that it always corrects itself and is therefore temporary and of limited clinical significance. The injurious force must be relieved in order for repair to occur.[31, 56] If conditions in humans do not permit the teeth to escape from or adapt to excessive occlusal force, periodontal damage persists[15] until the excessive forces are corrected by the clinician.

Traumatic forces that affect the teeth in balancing positions, i.e., nonaxial, are often such that severe lesions result because there is a tendency for teeth to be maintained in the position dictated by axial forces, i.e., in intercuspal position. Axial forces are most important in determining tooth position.

The presence in the periodontium of inflammation due to plaque accumulation may impair the reversibility of traumatic lesions.[37, 56]

The Effects of Excessive Occlusal Forces on the Dental Pulp

The effects of excessive occlusal forces upon the dental pulp have not been established. Some clinicians report the disappearance of pulpal symptoms following correction of occlusal forces. Pulpal reactions have been noted in animals subjected to increased occlusal forces,[16, 42] but not when the forces were light and occurred over short periods.[42]

THE INFLUENCE OF TRAUMA FROM OCCLUSION ON THE PROGRESSION OF MARGINAL PERIODONTITIS

The role of trauma from occlusion in gingivitis and periodontitis is best understood if the periodontium is considered as consisting of two zones (Figs. 19–9 and 19–10); the *zone of irritation* and the *zone of co-destruction.*

The Zone of Irritation

The zone of irritation consists of the marginal and interdental gingivae; its boundary is

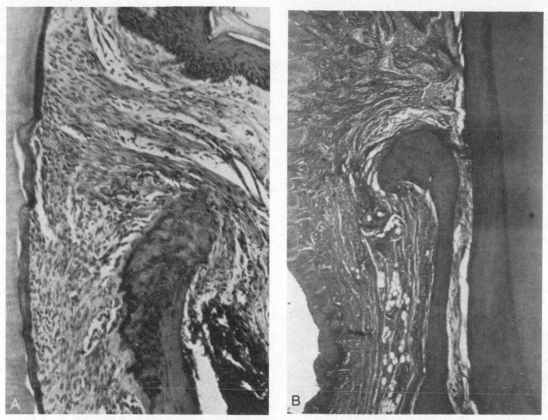

Figure 19–7 *A,* Widening of periodontal ligament space in cervical area and change in shape of marginal alveolar bone as a result of chronic prolonged trauma from occlusion in rats. *B,* Comparable change in shape of marginal bone found in a human autopsy case.

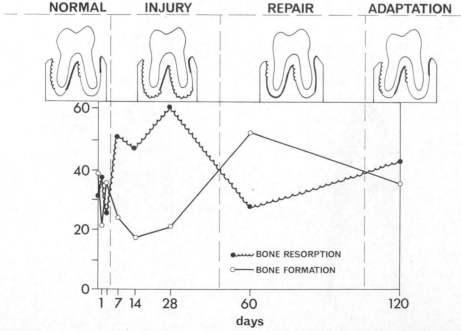

Figure 19–8 Evolution of traumatic lesions as depicted experimentally in rats by variations in relative amounts of areas of bone formation and bone resorption in periodontal bone surfaces. Horizontal axis: days after initiation of traumatic interference. Vertical axis: percentage of bone surface undergoing resorption or formation. The stages in the evolution of the lesions are represented in the top drawings, which show the average amount of bone activity for each group. See reference 17.

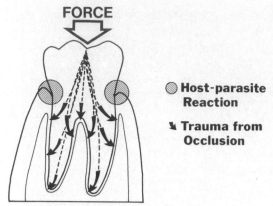

Figure 19–9 The reaction between dental plaque and the host takes place in the gingival sulcus region. Trauma from occlusion appears in the supporting tissues of the tooth.

formed by the gingival fibers (Fig. 19–10). This is where gingivitis and periodontal pockets start. They are caused by local irritation from bacteria. With few exceptions,[6, 76] researchers agree that trauma from occlusion does not cause gingivitis or periodontal pockets.[3, 29, 36, 57, 80, 82, 84]

The local irritants which initiate gingivitis and periodontal pockets affect the marginal gingiva, but trauma from occlusion occurs in the supporting tissues and does not affect the gingiva. The marginal gingiva is unaffected by

trauma from occlusion because its blood supply is sufficient to maintain it even when the vessels of the periodontal ligament are obliterated by excessive occlusal forces.[33]

As long as inflammation is confined to the gingiva, the inflammatory process is not affected by occlusal forces.[40] When it extends from the gingiva into the supporting periodontal tissues (i.e., when gingivitis becomes periodontitis), plaque-induced inflammation enters the zone of co-destruction.

The Zone of Co-destruction

The zone of co-destruction begins with the transseptal fibers interproximally and with the alveolar crest fibers facially and lingually (Fig. 19–10). It consists of the supporting periodontal tissues, the periodontal ligament, the alveolar bone, and the cementum. When inflammation reaches the supporting periodontal tissues, the destruction it causes comes under the influence of the occlusion.

Investigations conducted in monkeys[48, 53] and in dogs[38, 45] have found that trauma from occlusion, in association with marginal periodontitis, **increases the amount of alveolar bone loss and changes the shape of the alveolar crest.** The change in shape consists of a widening of the marginal periodontal ligament

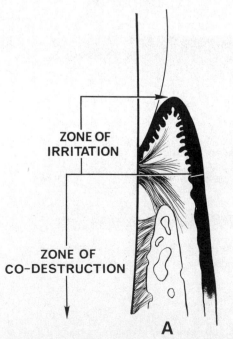
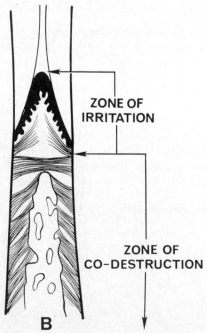

Figure 19–10 Zones of Irritation and Co-destruction in Periodontal Disease. *A,* Facial or lingual surface. *B,* Interproximal area.

space and a narrowing of the interproximal alveolar bone.[45, 48] Only in isolated cases was a loss of connective tissue attachment found.

When trauma from occlusion is eliminated, a significant reversibility of bone loss occurs, except in the presence of periodontitis. This indicates that inflammation inhibits the potential for bone regeneration.[37, 55, 56] These studies point out the importance of eliminating the marginal inflammatory component of trauma from occlusion, since the presence or absence of inflammation will affect bone regeneration after the removal of the traumatizing contacts.[37] It has also been shown in experimental animals that trauma from occlusion will not induce progressive destruction of the periodontal tissues in tooth regions kept healthy after the elimination of pre-existent periodontitis.[20]

Trauma from occlusion does not alter the inflammatory process but changes the tissue environment and the architecture of the area around the inflamed site.[17, 45] For this reason, in the absence of inflammation the response to trauma from occlusion is limited to adaptation to the increased forces. However, in the presence of inflammation the changes in the shape of the alveolar crest may be conducive to angular bone loss and infrabony pockets in some cases. Other theories that have been proposed to explain the interaction of trauma and inflammation include:

1. Trauma from occlusion may alter the pathway of the extension of gingival inflammation to the underlying tissues. Inflammation then may proceed to the periodontal ligament rather than to the bone. As a consequence, bone loss would be angular and pockets could become infrabony.[2, 23, 24, 26, 46]

2. Trauma-induced areas of root resorption uncovered by apical migration of the inflamed gingival attachment may offer a favorable environment for the formation and attachment of plaque and calculus and may therefore be responsible for deeper lesions.[68]

The existence of a co-destructive relationship between inflammation and trauma from occlusion does not rule out the possibility that both may be present without producing infrabony pockets and angular defects. The inflammation or the trauma may not be severe enough, or the anatomy of the tooth or bone may not be conducive to their formation. For example, if the facial or lingual bone is very thin, it may undergo resorption before an angular defect can develop. For these reasons, the absence of infrabony pockets and osseous defects does not rule out the presence of trauma from occlusion. Such periodontal lesions may be produced by etiologic factors other than the combination of inflammation and trauma from occlusion. *In summary, not every infrabony pocket develops because of a combination of trauma and inflammation, but this combination apparently increases the likelihood of a periodontal pocket becoming infrabony.*

Changes Produced by Trauma from Occlusion Alone

In the absence of local irritants severe enough to produce periodontal pockets, trauma from occlusion may cause excessive loosening of teeth, widening of the periodontal ligament, and angular (vertical) defects in the alveolar bone without pockets.[17, 44]

The most common sign of trauma to the periodontium is *increased tooth mobility*. Tooth mobility produced by trauma occurs in two phases. The *initial phase* is the result of alveolar bone resorption increasing the width of the periodontal ligament and reducing the number of periodontal fibers. The *second phase* occurs after repair of the traumatic lesion and adaptation to the increased forces, which results in permanent widening of the periodontal ligament space. See Chapter 20 for a more detailed description of tooth mobility.

Radiographic Signs of Trauma from Occlusion

The radiographic signs of trauma from occlusion are shown in Figures 19–11 and 19–12. They include (1) widening of the periodontal space, often with thickening of the lamina dura along the lateral aspect of the root, in the apical region, and in bifurcation areas; (2) "vertical" rather than "horizontal" destruction of the interdental septum, with the formation of infrabony defects; (3) radiolucence and condensation of the alveolar bone; and (4) root resorption.

It should be understood that widening of the periodontal space and thickening of the lamina dura do not necessarily indicate destructive changes. They may result from thickening and strengthening of the periodontal ligament and alveolar bone, which constitute a favorable response to increased occlusal forces (Fig. 19–13) (see Chapter 32).

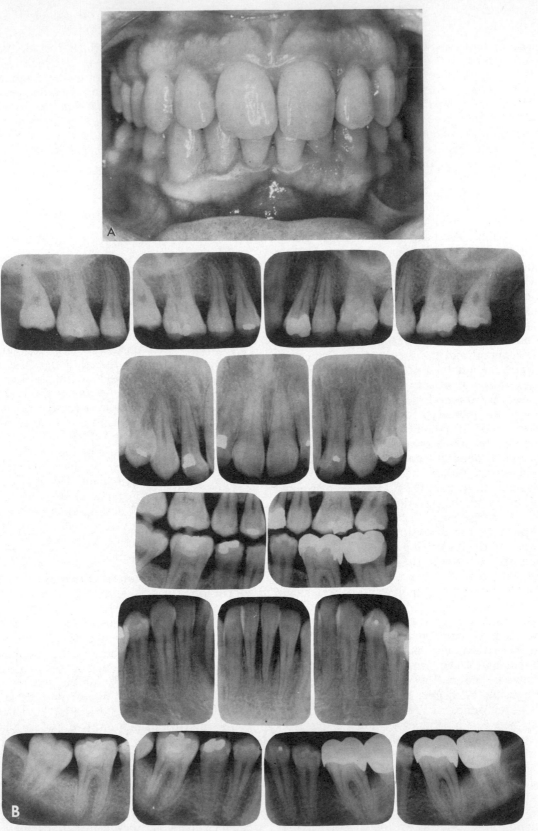

Figure 19–11 Radiographic Signs of Trauma from Occlusion. *A*, Twenty-seven-year-old female with only slight clinical evidence of periodontal disease. Little suggestion of the bone destruction shown radiographically. *B*, Radiographs show typical signs of trauma from occlusion: widening of the periodontal space in the mandibular anterior region, early angular bone destruction, and furcation involvement in the molar areas.

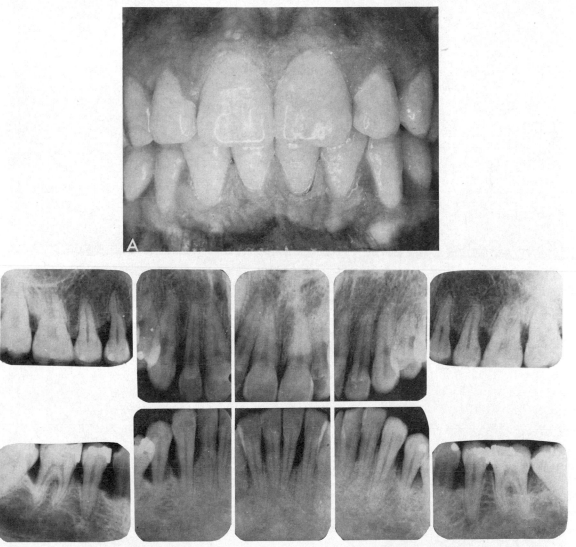

Figure 19–12 Radiographic Signs of Trauma from Occlusion. *A,* Thirty-year-old female with slight gingival disease. *B,* Radiographs show typical signs of trauma from occlusion: thickening of lamina dura, varied degrees of angular bone destruction, and furcation involvement.

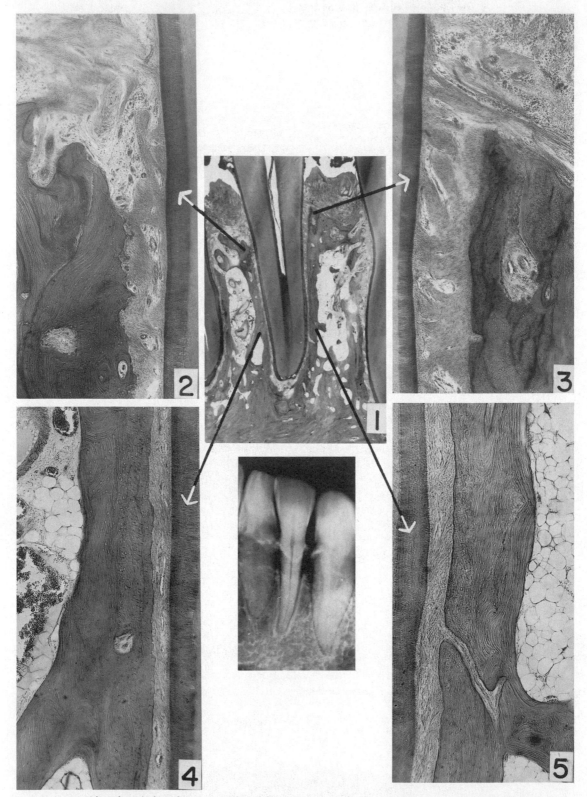

Figure 19–13 Widened Periodontal Space Produced by Two Types of Tissue Response to Increased Occlusal Forces.
Radiograph shows thickening of periodontal space and lamina dura around the lateral incisor. *1,* Survey microscopic section of lateral incisor. *2,* Mesial surface widening of the periodontal space has resulted from resorption of alveolar bone associated with pressure. *3,* Distal surface widening of the periodontal space has resulted from thickening of the periodontal ligament, which is a favorable response to increased tension. *4* and *5,* Thinned periodontal ligament at axis of rotation, one-third the distance from the apex.

Other Clinical Changes Attributed to Trauma from Occlusion

A wide variety of clinical changes have been attributed to trauma from occlusion, *based upon clinical impressions rather than substantiated evidence.*[47, 49, 73, 75] These are listed as a matter of interest: food impaction, abnormal habits, obscure facial pain, erosion, recession, gingival bleeding, cheek biting, sensitivity of the occlusal and incisal surfaces, chronic necrotizing ulcerative gingivitis, hyperplasia of the gingiva, pericementitis, bruxism, unilateral mastication, limited excursion of the mandible (insufficient wear), unlimited excursion of the mandible (excessive wear), interproximal caries, formation of subgingival calculus and gingivitis, tendency toward epulis formation, blanching of the gingiva upon the application of occlusal force, pulpal hyperemia resulting in hypersensitivity to cold, pulpitis, pulpal necrosis, and pulp stones.

Box[4] and Stillman[74] considered trauma to be the causative factor for the following signs of incipient periodontal disease:

Traumatic crescent, a crescent-shaped, bluish-red zone of gingiva confined to about one sixth of the circumference of the root.

Congestion, ischemia, or hyperemia of the marginal gingiva.

Recession of the gingiva, which may be asymmetrical, associated with resorption of the alveolar crest.

Stillman's clefts, indentations in the gingival margin, generally on one side of the tooth. Two clefts frequently occur on the same tooth. Intermittent compressions of the periodontal ligament followed by abnormal flushing of the gingival capillaries and enlargement and engorgement of the gingival vessels were considered to be the mechanism responsible for the clefting.

McCall's festoons, discrete semilunar enlargement of the marginal gingiva.

Absence of stippling, interpreted as evidence of edema secondary to trauma.

Injection of the blood vessels in the marginal gingiva.

Sharply demarcated linear depressions in the alveolar mucosa, parallel to the long axis of the root and overlying the septal bone.

Distended veins in the oral mucosa.

It must be emphasized that none of these changes has been shown conclusively to be associated with trauma to the periodontium.

SUMMARY

Trauma from occlusion is an important factor in periodontal disease, an integral part of the destructive process. It does not initiate gingivitis or periodontal pockets, but it affects the progress and severity of periodontal pockets started by local irritation. Understanding the effect of trauma from occlusion on the periodontium is useful in the clinical management of periodontal problems.

REFERENCES

1. Akiyoshi, M., and Mori, K.: Marginal periodontitis: a histologic study of the incipient stage. J. Periodontol., 38:45, 1967.
2. Balbe, R., Carranza, F. A., and Erausquin, R.: Los paradencios del caso ocho. Rev. Odont. (Buenos Aires), 26:606, 1938.
3. Bhaskar, S. N., and Orban, B.: Experimental occlusal trauma. J. Periodontol., 26:270, 1955.
4. Box, H. K.: Signs of incipient periodontal disease. J. Am. Dent. Assoc., 12:1150, 1925.
5. Box, H. K.: Traumatic occlusion and traumatogenic occlusion. Oral Health, 20:642, 1930.
6. Box, H. K.: Experimental traumatogenic occlusion in sheep. Oral Health, 25:9, 1935.
7. Box, H. K.: Twelve Periodontal Studies, Toronto, University of Toronto Press, 1940, p. 55.
8. Breitner, C.: Tissue changes caused by so-called bite-raising acting on the front teeth. Z. Stomatol., 30:1185, 1932.
9. Budtz-Jorgensen, E.: Bruxism and trauma from occlusion. J. Clin. Periodontol., 7:149, 1980.
10. Carranza, F. A., Jr.: Histometric evaluation of periodontal pathology. J. Periodontol., 38:741, 1970.
11. Carranza, F. A., Jr., and Cabrini, R. L.: Histometric studies of periodontal tissues. Periodontics, 5:308, 1967.
12. Carranza, F. A., Jr., and Glickman, I.: Some observations on the microscopic features of the infrabony pocket. J. Periodontol., 28:33, 1957.
13. Cohn, S. A.: Disuse atrophy of the periodontium in molar teeth of mice. J. Dent. Res., 40:707, 1961.
14. Comar, M. D., Kollar, J. A., and Gargiulo, A. W.: Local irritation and occlusal trauma as co-factors in the periodontal disease process. J. Periodontol., 40:193, 1969.
15. Coolidge, E. D.: Traumatic and functional injuries occurring in the supporting tissues on human teeth. J. Am. Dent. Assoc., 25:343, 1938.
16. Cooper, M. B., Landay, M. A., and Seltzer, S.: The effects of excessive occlusal forces on the pulp. II. Heavier and longer term forces. J. Periodontol., 42:353, 1971.
17. Dotto, C. A., Carranza, F. A., Jr., and Itoiz, M. E.: Efectos mediatos del trauma experimental en ratas. Rev. Asoc. Odontol. Argent., 54:48, 1966.
18. Dotto, C. A., Carranza, F. A., Jr., Cabrini, R. L., and Itoiz, M. E.: Vascular changes in experimental trauma from occlusion. J. Periodontol., 38:183, 1967.
19. Erausquin, R., and Carranza, F. A.: Primeros hallazgos paradentosicos. Rev. Odont. (Buenos Aires), 27:486, 1939.
20. Ericsson, I., and Lindhe, J.: Lack of effect of trauma from occlusion on the recurrence of experimental periodontitis. J. Clin. Periodontol., 4:115, 1977.
21. Everett, F. G., and Bruckner, R. J.: Cartilage in the periodontal ligament space. J. Periodontol., 41:165, 1970.
22. Ewen, S. J., and Stahl, S. S.: The response of the periodontium to chronic gingival irritation and long term tilting forces in adult dogs. Oral Surg., 15:1426, 1962.
23. Glickman, I.: Occlusion and the periodontium. J. Dent. Res., 46(Suppl. 53), 1967.
24. Glickman, I., and Smulow, J. B.: Alterations in the pathway of gingival inflammation into the underlying tissues induced by excessive occlusal forces. J. Periodontol., 33:7, 1962.
25. Glickman, I., and Smulow, J. B.: Buttressing bone formation in the periodontium. J. Periodontol., 36:365, 1965.
26. Glickman, I., and Smulow, J. B.: Effect of excessive occlusal forces upon the pathway of gingival inflammation in humans. J. Periodontol., 36:141, 1965.
27. Glickman, I., and Smulow, J. B.: Adaptive alterations in the periodontium of the Rhesus monkey in chronic trauma from occlusion. J. Periodontol., 39:101, 1968.
28. Glickman, I., and Smulow, J. B.: The combined effects of inflammation and trauma from occlusion to periodontitis. Int. Dent. J., 19:393, 1969.

29. Glickman, I., and Weiss, L.: Role of trauma from occlusion in initiation of periodontal pocket formation in experimental animals. J. Periodontol., *26*:14, 1955.
30. Glickman, I., Smulow, J. B., and Moreau, J.: Effect of alloxan diabetes upon the periodontal response to excessive occlusal forces. J. Periodontol., *37*:146, 1966.
31. Glickman, I., Stein, R. S., and Smulow, J. B.: The effects of increased functional forces upon the periodontium of splinted and non-splinted teeth. J. Periodontol., *32*:290, 1961.
32. Glickman, I., Roeber, F., Brion, M., and Pameijer, J.: Photoelastic analysis of internal stresses in the periodontium created by occlusal forces. J. Periodontol., *41*:30, 1970.
33. Goldman, H.: Gingival vascular supply in induced occlusal traumatism. Oral Surg., *9*:939, 1956.
34. Gottlieb, B., and Orban, B.: Changes in the Tissue Due to Excessive Force Upon the Teeth. Leipzig, G. Thieme, 1931.
35. Gottlieb, B., and Orban, B.: Tissue changes in experimental traumatic occlusion with special reference to age and constitution. J. Dent. Res., *11*:505, 1931.
36. Itoiz, M. E., Carranza, F. A., Jr., and Cabrini, R. L.: Histologic and histometric study of experimental occlusal trauma in rats. J. Periodontol., *34*:305, 1963.
37. Kantor, M., Polson, A. N., and Zander, H. A.: Alveolar bone regeneration after removal of inflammatory and traumatic factors. J. Periodontol., *46*:687, 1976.
38. Kaufman, H., Carranza, F. A., Jr., Enders, B., Murphy, N. C., and Newman, M. G.: Effect of occlusal trauma on periodontal pocket bacterial flora. J. Dent. Res., *61*:350, 1982 (abstract).
39. Kemper, W. W., Johnson, J. F., and Van Huysen, G.: Periodontal tissue changes in response to high artificial crowns. J. Prosthet. Dent., *20*:160, 1968.
40. Kenney, E. B.: A histopathologic study of incisal dysfunction and gingival inflammation in the Rhesus monkey. J. Periodontol., *42*:3, 1971.
41. Kvam, E.: Scanning electron microscopy of tissue changes on the pressure surface of human premolars following tooth movement. Scand. J. Dent. Res., *80*:357, 1972.
42. Landay, M. A., Nazimov, H., and Seltzer, S.: The effects of excessive occlusal forces on the pulp. J. Periodontol., *41*:3, 1970.
43. Levy, G., and Mailland, M. L.: Etude quantitative des effets de l'hypofonction occlusale sur la largeur desmodontale et la resorption osteoclastique alveolaire chez le rat. J. Biol. Buccale, *8*:17, 1980.
44. Lindhe, J., and Ericsson, I.: The influence of trauma from occlusion on reduced but healthy periodontal tissues in dogs. J. Clin. Periodontol., *3*:110, 1976.
45. Lindhe, J., and Svanberg, G.: Influence of trauma from occlusion on progression of experimental periodontitis in the beagle dog. J. Clin. Periodontol., *1*:3, 1974.
46. Macapanpan, L. C., and Weinmann, J. P.: The influence of injury to the periodontal membrane on the spread of gingival inflammation. J. Dent. Res., *33*:263, 1954.
47. McCall, J. O.: Traumatic occlusion. J. Am. Dent. Assoc., *26*:519, 1939.
48. Meitner, S.: Co-destructive factors of marginal periodontitis and repetitive mechanical injury. J. Dent. Res., *54*:C78, 1975.
49. Miller, S. C.: Textbook of Periodontia. 3rd ed. Philadelphia, Blakiston Company, 1950, p. 350.
50. Orban, B.: Tissue changes in traumatic occlusion. J. Am. Dent. Assoc., *15*:2090, 1928.
51. Orban, B.: Classification of periodontal diseases. Paradentologie, *3*:159, 1949.
52. Orban, B., and Weinmann, J.: Signs of traumatic occlusion in average human jaws. J. Dent. Res., *13*:216, 1933.
53. Polson, A. M.: Trauma and progression of marginal periodontitis in squirrel monkeys. II. Co-destructive factors of periodontitis and mechanically-produced injury. J. Periodont. Res., *9*:108, 1974.
54. Polson, A. M., Kennedy, J. E., and Zander, H. A.: Trauma and progression of marginal periodontitis in squirrel monkeys. I. Co-destructive factors of periodontitis and thermally-produced injury. J. Periodont. Res., *9*:100, 1974.
55. Polson, A. M., Meitner, S. W., and Zander, H. A.: Trauma and progression of marginal periodontitis in squirrel monkeys. III. Adaption of interproximal alveolar bone to repetitive injury. J. Periodont. Res. *11*:279, 1976.
56. Polson, A. M., Meitner, S. W., and Zander, H. A.: Trauma and progression of marginal periodontitis in squirrel monkeys. IV. Reversibility of bone loss due to trauma alone and trauma superimposed upon periodontitis. J. Periodont. Res., *11*:290, 1976.
57. Ramfjord, S. P., and Kohler, C. A.: Periodontal reaction to functional occlusal stress. J. Periodontol., *30*:95, 1959.
58. Rothblatt, J. M., and Waldo, C. M.: Tissue response to tooth movement in normal and abnormal metabolic states. J. Dent. Res., *32*:678, 1953.
59. Rygh, P.: Ultrastructural cellular reactions in pressure zones of rat molar periodontium incident to orthodontic movement. Acta Odontol. Scand., *30*:575, 1972.
60. Rygh, P.: Ultrastructural vascular changes in pressure zones of rat molar periodontium incident to orthodontic movement. Scand. J. Dent. Res., *80*:307, 1972.
61. Rygh, P.: Ultrastructural changes in pressure zones of human periodontium incident to orthodontic tooth movement. Acta Odontol. Scand., *31*:109, 1973.
62. Rygh, P.: Ultrastructural changes of the periodontal fibers and their attachment in rat molar periodontium incident to orthodontic tooth movement. Scand. J. Dent. Res., *81*:467, 1973.
63. Rygh, P.: Elimination of hyalinized periodontal tissues associated with orthodontic tooth movement. Scand. J. Dent. Res., *82*:57, 1974.
64. Rygh, P., and Selvig, K. A.: Erythrocytic crystallization in rat molar periodontium incident to tooth movement. Scand. J. Dent. Res., *81*:62, 1973.
65. Schwarz, A. M.: Movement of teeth under traumatic stress. D. Items Intern., *52*:96, 1930.
66. Skillen, W. C., and Reitan, K.: Tissue changes following rotation of teeth in the dog. Angle Orthod., *10*:140, 1940.
67. Solt, C. W., and Glickman, I.: A histologic and radioautographic study of healing following wedging interdental injury in mice. J. Periodontol., *39*:249, 1968.
68. Sottosanti, J. S.: A possible relationship between occlusion, root resorption and the progression of periodontal disease. J. Western Soc. Periodontol., *25*:69, 1977.
69. Stahl, S. S.: The responses of the periodontium to combined gingival inflammation and occluso-functional stresses in four human surgical specimens. Periodontics, *6*:14, 1968.
70. Stahl, S. S.: Accommodation of the periodontium to occlusal trauma and inflammatory periodontal disease. Dent. Clin. North Am., *19*:531, 1975.
71. Stahl, S. S., Miller, S. C., and Goldsmith, E. D.: The effects of vertical occlusal trauma on the periodontium of protein deprived young adult rats. J. Periodontol., *28*:87, 1957.
72. Stallard, R. E.: The effect of occlusal alterations on collagen formation within the periodontium. Periodontics, *2*:49, 1964.
73. Stillman, P. R.: Early clinical evidences of disease in the gingiva and periodontium. J. Dent. Res., *3*:25, 1921.
74. Stillman, P. R.: Differential diagnosis of early periodontal lesions. Bull. Ont. Dent. Assoc., 1925.
75. Stillman, P. R., and McCall, J. O.: Textbook of Clinical Periodontia. New York, Macmillan, Inc., 1937, p. 116.
76. Stones, H. H.: An experimental investigation into the association of traumatic occlusion with paradontal disease. Proc. Soc. Med., *31*:479, 1938.
77. Svanberg, G., and Lindhe, J.: Vascular reactions to the periodontal ligament incident to trauma from occlusion. J. Clin. Periodontol., *1*:58, 1974.
78. Thurow, R. C.: The periodontal membrane in function. Angle Orthod., *15*:8, 1945.
79. Ubios, A. M.: Estudio Autorradiografico de la Reabsorcion Osea en los Movimientos Ortodoncicos de los Molares de Rata. Thesis, University of Buenos Aires, 1972.
80. Waerhaug, J.: Pathogenesis of pocket formation in traumatic occlusion. J. Periodontol., *26*:107, 1955.
81. Waerhaug, J., and Hansen, E. R.: Periodontal changes incidental to prolonged occlusal overload in monkeys. Acta Odontol. Scand., *24*:91, 1966.
82. Wentz, F. M., Jarabak, J., and Orban, B.: Experimental occlusal trauma imitating cuspal interferences. J. Periodontol., *29*:117, 1958.
83. Zaki, A. E., and Van Huysen, G.: Histology of the periodontium following tooth movement. J. Dent. Res., *42*:1373, 1963.
84. Zander, H. A., and Muhlemann, H. R.: The effect of stresses on the periodontal structures. Oral Surg., *9*:380, 1956.

chapter twenty

Tooth Mobility and Pathologic Migration

TOOTH MOBILITY

Normal Mobility

Teeth normally have a certain range of mobility. Single-rooted teeth have more mobility than multirooted teeth, and the incisors have the most. The mobility is principally in a horizontal direction; it also occurs axially, but to a much lesser degree.[7] The range of physiologic tooth mobility varies among individuals and from hour to hour in individual teeth in the same person. It is highest upon arising, possibly because of slight extrusion in the absence of function during the night, and diminishes during the day, possibly owing to intrusion caused by pressure from chewing and swallowing. The 24-hour variations in tooth mobility are less in persons with a healthy periodontium than in persons with periodontal disease or occlusal habits such as bruxism and clenching.

Tooth mobility occurs in two stages: (1) The **initial or intrasocket stage,** in which the tooth moves within the confines of the periodontal ligament. This is associated with viscoelastic distortion of the ligament and redistribution of the periodontal fluids, interbundle content, and fibers.[3] (2) The **secondary stage,** which occurs gradually and entails elastic deformation of the alveolar bone in response to increased horizontal forces.[5] The tooth itself is also deformed by the impact of a force applied to the crown, but not to a clinically significant degree.

When a force such as that normally applied to teeth in occlusion is discontinued, the teeth return to their original positions in two stages: the first is an **immediate, spring-like elastic recoil;** the second is a **slow, asymptomatic recovery movement.** The recovery movement is pulsating and is apparently associated with the normal pulsation of the periodontal vessels, which occurs in synchrony with the cardiac cycle.[4]

Abnormal (Pathologic) Mobility

Mobility beyond the physiologic range is termed abnormal or pathologic. It is pathologic in the sense that it exceeds the limits of normal mobility values, rather than that the periodontium is necessarily diseased at the time of examination. Pathologic mobility is caused by one or more of the following factors:

1. **Loss of tooth support (bone loss).** The amount of mobility depends upon the severity and distribution of the tissue loss on individual root surfaces, the length and shape of the roots, and the root size compared to that of the crown.[8] A tooth with short, tapered roots is more likely to loosen than one with normal-sized or bulbous roots with the same amount of bone loss. Because bone loss is not the sole cause of tooth mobility and tooth mobility usually results from a combination of factors, the severity of tooth mobility does not necessarily correspond to the amount of bone loss.

2. **Trauma from occlusion.** Injury produced by excessive occlusal forces or incurred because of abnormal occlusal habits such as bruxism and clenching, which are aggravated by emotional stress, is a common cause of tooth mobility. Mobility is also increased by hypofunction. Mobility produced by trauma from occlusion occurs initially as a result of resorption of the cortical layer of bone and later as an adaptation phenomenon resulting in a widened periodontal space.

3. **The extension of inflammation from the gingiva into the periodontal ligament results in degenerative changes which increase mobility.** The changes usually occur in periodontal disease which has advanced beyond the early stages, but tooth mobility is sometimes observed in severe gingivitis. The spread of inflammation from an acute periapical abscess produces a temporary increase in tooth mobility in the absence of periodontal disease.

Mobility is also temporarily increased for a short period after periodontal surgery.

4. **Tooth mobility is increased in pregnancy and is sometimes associated with the menstrual cycle or the use of hormonal contraceptives.** It occurs in patients with or without periodontal disease, presumably because of physicochemical changes in the periodontal tissues.

Mobility can also result from jaw processes that destroy the alveolar bone and/or the roots of the teeth. Osteomyelitis and tumors of the jaws belong in this category.

PATHOLOGIC MIGRATION

Pathologic migration refers to tooth displacement that results when the balance among the *factors which maintain physiologic tooth position is disturbed by periodontal disease.* Pathologic migration is relatively common and may be an early sign of disease, or it may occur in association with gingival inflammation and pocket formation as the disease progresses.

Pathologic migration occurs most frequently in the anterior region, but posterior teeth may also be affected. The teeth may move in any direction, and the migration is usually accompanied by mobility and rotation. Pathologic migration in the occlusal or incisal direction is termed extrusion or elongation, the former term being preferred. All degrees of pathologic migration are encountered, and one or more teeth may be affected (Fig. 20–1). It is important to detect it in its early stages (Fig. 20–2) and to prevent more serious involvement by eliminating the causative factors. Even in the early stage, some degree of bone loss has occurred.

Pathogenesis

Two major factors play a role in maintaining the normal position of the teeth: (1) the health

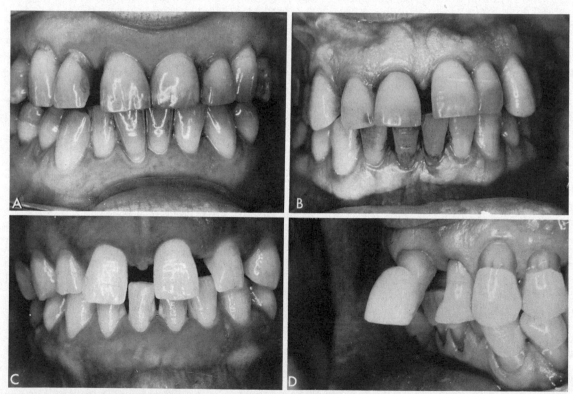

Figure 20–1 Stages in Pathologic Migration. *A,* Migration of right maxillary lateral incisor. *B,* Labial migration of maxillary central incisors and left canine and mesial migration of right lateral incisor. *C,* Migration and extrusion of maxillary and mandibular incisors. *D,* Severe migration of maxillary central incisor.

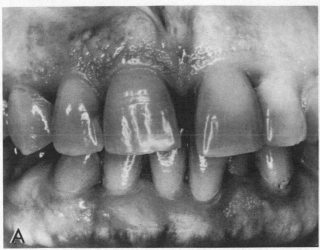
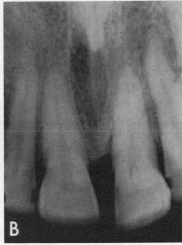

Figure 20–2 *A,* **Pathologic Migration and Early Extrusion** of maxillary central incisor. *B,* Radiograph showing bone loss on extruded central incisor.

and normal height of the periodontium and (2) the forces exerted upon the teeth. The latter can be the forces of occlusion or pressure from the lips, cheeks, and tongue. With relation to the forces of occlusion, the following factors are important: tooth morphology and cuspal inclination; the presence of a full complement of teeth; a physiologic tendency toward mesial migration; the nature and location of contact-point relationships; proximal, incisal, and occlusal attrition; and the axial inclination of the teeth.

Alterations in any of these factors start an interrelated sequence of changes in the environment of a single tooth or a group of teeth that results in pathologic migration.

Pathologic migration, therefore, occurs under conditions that weaken the periodontal support and/or increase or modify the forces exerted upon the teeth.

WEAKENED PERIODONTAL SUPPORT. The inflammatory destruction of the periodontium in *periodontitis* creates an imbalance between the tooth and the occlusal and muscular forces it is ordinarily called upon to bear. The weakened tooth is unable to maintain its normal position in the arch and moves away from the force, unless it is restrained by proximal contact. The force that moves the weakened tooth may be created by factors such as occlusal contacts or pressure from the tongue.

It is important to understand that **the abnormality in pathologic migration rests with the weakened periodontium.** The force itself need not be abnormal. Forces that are acceptable to the intact periodontium become injurious when periodontal support is reduced. An

example of this is the tooth with abnormal proximal contacts. Abnormally located proximal contacts convert the normal anterior component of force to a wedging force, which moves the tooth occlusally or incisally. The wedging force, which is withstood by the intact periodontium, causes the tooth to extrude when the periodontal support is weakened by disease. **As its position changes, the tooth is subjected to abnormal occlusal forces which aggravate the destruction and the migration** (Fig. 20–3).

Pathologic migration may continue after a tooth no longer contacts its antagonist (Fig. 20–4). Pressure from the tongue, from the food bolus in mastication, and from proliferating granulation tissue provides the force.

Pathologic migration is also an early sign of *localized juvenile periodontitis.* The teeth are weakened by loss of periodontal support. The maxillary and mandibular anterior incisors drift labially, rotate and extrude, and create diastemata between the teeth (Fig. 20–5).

CHANGES IN THE FORCES EXERTED UPON THE TEETH. Changes in magnitude, direction, or frequency of the forces exerted upon the teeth can induce pathologic migration of a tooth or a group of teeth. These forces need not be abnormal if the periodontium is sufficiently weakened. Changes in the forces may occur in the following conditions:

Unreplaced Missing Teeth. **Drifting of teeth** into the spaces created by unreplaced missing teeth often occurs. **Drifting differs from pathologic migration in that it does not result from destruction of the periodontal tissues.** However, drifting usually creates conditions that

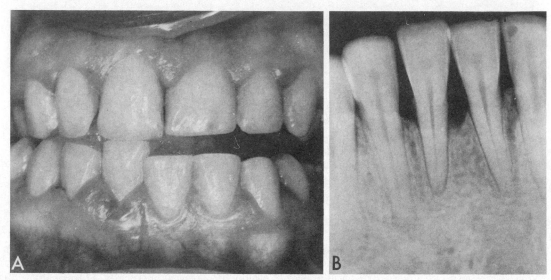

Figure 20–3 Pathologic Migration Aggravated by Excessive Occlusal Force. *A,* Mandibular central incisor extruded beyond the line of occlusion. Note that the maxillary central incisor is also extruded. *B,* Thickening of the periodontal ligament space around the central incisor and angular bone destruction pattern typical of injury produced by excessive occlusal forces.

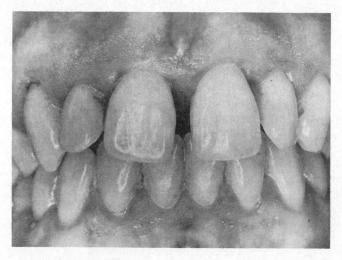

Figure 20–4 Pathologic Migration continues despite absence of contact between mandibular and maxillary incisors.

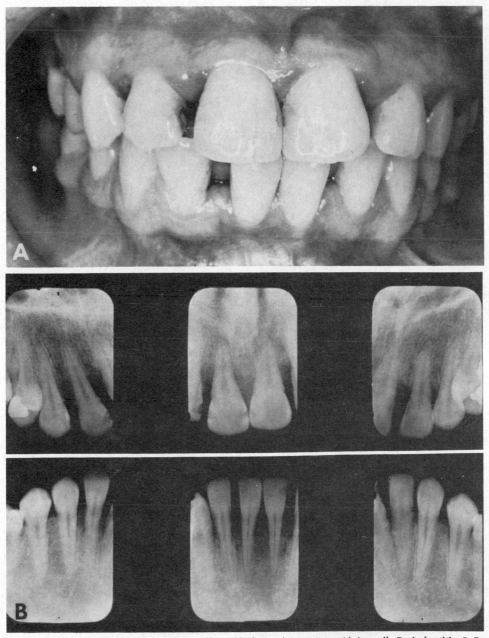

Figure 20–5 *A,* **Pathologic Migration** of maxillary and mandibular teeth in patient with **Juvenile Periodontitis.** *B,* Radiographs showing bone loss around the anterior teeth.

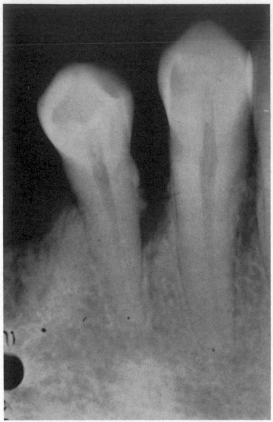

Figure 20–6 Calculus and Bone Loss on mesial surface of canine that has drifted distally.

lead to periodontal disease, so that the initial tooth movement is aggravated by loss of periodontal support (Fig. 20–6).

Drifting generally occurs in a mesial direction, combined with tilting or extrusion beyond the occlusal plane. The premolars frequently drift distally (Figs. 20–7 and 20–8). Although drifting is a common sequel when missing teeth are not replaced, it does not always occur (Fig. 20–9).

Failure to Replace First Molars. The pattern of changes that may follow failure to replace missing first molars is characteristic. In extreme cases it consists of the following:

1. The second and third molars tilt, resulting in a decrease in vertical dimension (Fig. 20–10).

2. The premolars move distally, and the mandibular incisors tilt or drift lingually. The mandibular premolars, while drifting distally, lose their intercuspating relationship with the maxillary teeth and may tilt distally.

3. Anterior overbite is increased. The mandibular incisors strike the maxillary incisors near the gingiva or traumatize the gingiva.

4. The maxillary incisors are pushed labially and laterally (Fig. 20–11).

5. The anterior teeth extrude because the incisal apposition has largely disappeared.

6. Diastemata are created by the separation of the anterior teeth (see Fig. 20–10).

The disturbed proximal contact relationships lead to food impaction, gingival inflammation, and pocket formation, followed by bone loss and tooth mobility. Occlusal disharmonies created by the altered tooth positions traumatize the supporting tissues of the periodontium and aggravate the destruction caused by the inflammation. Reduction in periodontal support leads to further migration of the teeth and mutilation of the occlusion.

Other Causes. **Trauma from occlusion** may cause a shift in tooth position either by itself

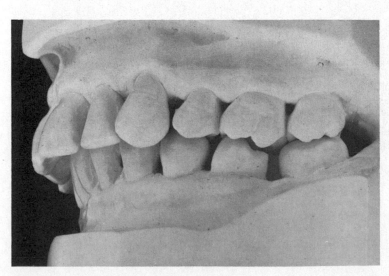

Figure 20–7 Maxillary First Molar Tilted and Extruded into space created by missing mandibular tooth.

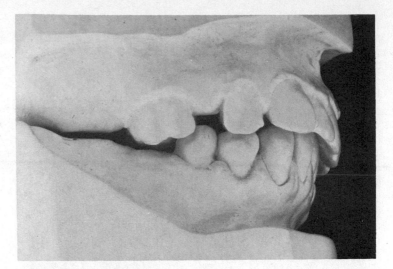

Figure 20–8 Distal Drifting of Maxillary and Mandibular Premolars. The maxillary molar is extruded and tilted.

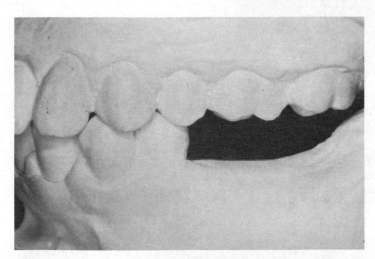

Figure 20–9 No Drifting or Extrusion despite 4 years' absence of mandibular teeth.

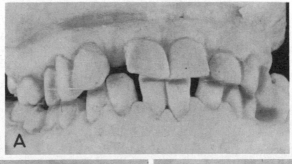

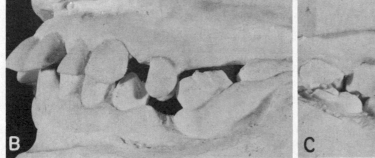
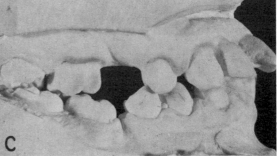

Figure 20–10 Mutilation of Occlusion Associated with Unreplaced Missing Teeth. Note pronounced pathologic migration, disturbed proximal contacts, and functional relationships with "closing of the bite."

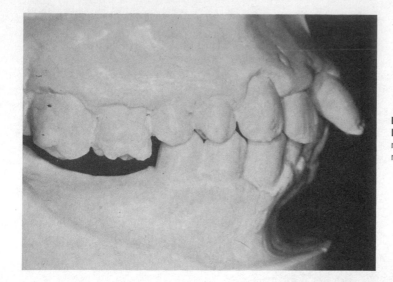

Figure 20–11 Maxillary Incisors Pushed Labially in Patient with bilateral unreplaced mandibular molars. Note extrusion of the maxillary molars.

Figure 20–12 Pathologic Migration associated with tongue pressure.

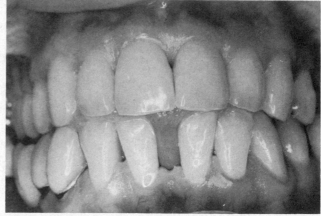

or in combination with inflammatory periodontal disease. The direction of movement depends upon the occlusal force.

Pressure from the tongue may cause drifting of the teeth in the absence of periodontal disease or contribute to pathologic migration of teeth with reduced periodontal support (Fig. 20–12).

In teeth weakened by periodontal destruction, **pressure from the granulation tissue of periodontal pockets** has been mentioned as contributing to pathologic migration. The teeth may return to their original positions after the pockets are eliminated, but, if there has been more destruction on one side of a tooth than on the other, the healing tissues tend to pull in the direction of the lesser destruction.

Gottlieb[1] considered pathologic migration to be caused by a **disturbance in the balance between active and passive eruption.** It is produced when the teeth do not erupt at an even rate and when some are more worn down by attrition than others. Teeth with least attrition must bear the entire biting force and are most susceptible to pathologic migration.

REFERENCES

1. Gottlieb, B.: Formation of the pocket: diffuse atrophy of alveolar bone. J. Am. Dent. Assoc., *15*:462, 1928.
2. Hirschfeld, I.: The dynamic relationship betwen pathologically migrating teeth and inflammatory tissue in periodontal pockets: a clinical study. J. Periodontol., *4*:35, 1933.
3. Kurashima, K.: Viscoelastic properties of periodontal tissue. Bull. Tokyo Med. Dent. Univ., *12*:240, 1965.
4. Mühlemann, H. R.: Tooth mobility: a review of clinical aspects and research findings. J. Periodontol., *38*:686, 1967.
5. Mühlemann, H. R., Savdir, S., and Rateitschak, K. H.: Tooth mobility—its causes and significance. J. Periodontol., *36*:148, 1965.
6. O'Leary, T. J.: Tooth mobility. Dent. Clin. North Am., *13*:567, 1969.
7. Parfitt, G. J.: Measurement of the physiologic mobility of individual teeth in an axial direction. J. Dent. Res., *39*:608, 1960.
8. Perlitsch, M. J.: A systematic approach to the interpretation of tooth mobility and clinical implications. Dent. Clin. North Am., *24*:177, 1980.

Gingival Disease in Childhood

The effects of periodontal disease observed in adults have their inception earlier in life. The gingival disease of childhood may progress to jeopardize the periodontium of the adult. The increasing awareness of the prevalence of gingival and periodontal disease in children,[26] coupled with the need for more information regarding the early stages of periodontal disease, has focused attention upon the periodontium in childhood.[4, 5, 26]

The developing dentition and certain systemic metabolic patterns are peculiar to childhood. There are also gingival and periodontal disturbances that occur more frequently in childhood and are, therefore, identified with this period. Consequently, some degree of coherence is provided by grouping the facts regarding gingival and periodontal problems in childhood in separate chapters (this chapter and Chapter 22).

THE PERIODONTIUM OF THE DECIDUOUS DENTITION

The *gingiva* of the deciduous dentition is pale pink, firm, and either smooth or stippled (the latter in 35 per cent of children from 5 to 13 years old[24]) (Fig. 21–1). The interdental gingiva is broad faciolingually and tends to be relatively narrow mesiodistally, in conformity with the contour of the approximal tooth surfaces. It is comparable to that of the adult in that it consists of a facial and lingual papilla with an intervening depression or *col*. The mean gingival sulcus depth for the primary dentition is 2.1 mm $\pm$ 0.2 mm.[23]

Microscopically, the stratified squamous epithelium of the gingiva presents well-differen- tiated rete pegs with a parakeratinized (Fig. 21–2) or keratinized surface, the latter correlated with stippling. The connective tissue is predominantly fibrillar and is differentiated into papillary and reticular layers. The well-differentiated collagen bundles seen in the adult are not present in childhood.

The epithelium initially covering the col is a few cells thick and nonkeratinized. The *periodontal ligament* of the deciduous teeth is wider than that of the permanent dentition. During eruption the principal fibers are parallel to the long axis of the teeth; the bundle arrangement seen in the adult dentition occurs when the teeth encounter their functional antagonists.

The *alveolar bone* in relation to the deciduous dentition shows a prominent lamina dura radiographically, both in the crypt stage and during eruption. The trabeculae of the alveolar bone are fewer but thicker and the marrow spaces tend to be larger than in the adult. The crests of the interdental septa are flat.[5]

In beagle dogs, the juvenile gingiva shows a thicker keratinized layer of the oral epithelium than does the gingiva of the adult. Also, the juvenile junctional epithelium structurally resembles the oral epithelium, and there is a cuticular structure at the surface of the junctional epithelium.[16] These differences might explain the reduced inflammatory response to plaque accumulation in juvenile dogs.

PHYSIOLOGIC GINGIVAL CHANGES ASSOCIATED WITH TOOTH ERUPTION

During the transitional period in the development of the dentition, changes associated

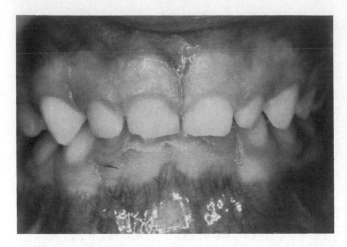

Figure 21–1 Deciduous Dentition with Stippled Gingiva.

with eruption of the permanent teeth occur in the gingiva. It is important to recognize these physiologic changes and to differentiate them from the gingival disease that often accompanies tooth eruption. The following are physiologic changes in the gingiva associated with tooth eruption:

PRE-ERUPTION BULGE. Before the crown appears in the oral cavity, the gingiva presents a bulge which is firm, may be slightly blanched, and conforms to the contour of the underlying crown.

FORMATION OF THE GINGIVAL MARGIN. The marginal gingiva and sulcus develop as the crown penetrates the oral mucosa. In the course of eruption the gingival margin is usually edematous, rounded, and slightly reddened (Fig. 21–3).

NORMAL PROMINENCE OF THE GINGIVAL MARGIN. During the period of the mixed dentition it is normal for the marginal gingiva around the permanent teeth to be quite prominent, particularly in the maxillary anterior region. At this stage in tooth eruption the

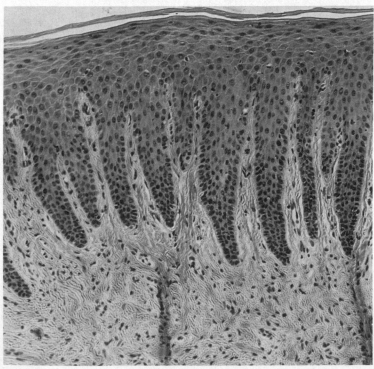

Figure 21–2 Normal Gingiva in a 4-Year-Old Patient Showing Stratified Squamous Epithelium with Rete Pegs and Surface Keratinization. The papillary arrangement of the underlying connective tissue can also be seen.

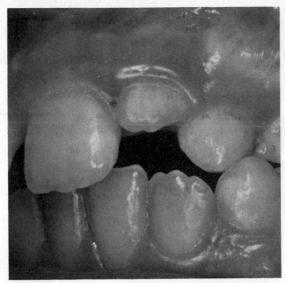

Figure 21–3 Gingivitis Associated with Tooth Eruption. Prominent rolled gingival margin which is slightly inflamed and edematous around erupting maxillary lateral incisor.

gingiva is still attached to the crown, and it appears prominent when superimposed upon the bulk of the underlying enamel (Fig. 21–4).

GINGIVAL DISEASE

Chronic Marginal Gingivitis

This is the most prevalent type of gingival change in childhood. The gingiva presents all the changes in color, size, consistency, and surface texture characteristic of chronic inflammation. A fiery red surface discoloration is often superimposed upon underlying chronic changes.

ETIOLOGY. In children, as in adults, the most common cause of gingivitis is local irritation, as well as local conditions which lead to the accumulation of bacterial plaque. In studies in preschool children the gingival response to bacterial plaque was found to be reduced.[14, 15] Gingivitis in children is caused by dental plaque; materia alba and poor oral hygiene favor the accumulation of plaque (Fig. 21–5). Dental plaque appears to form more rapidly in children (aged 8 to 12) than in adults.

Calculus. Calculus is uncommon in infants; it occurs in approximately 9 per cent of children between the ages of 4 and 6, 18 per cent between 7 and 9, and 33 to 43 per cent between 10 and 15.[6] In children with *cystic fibrosis,* calculus formation is more common (77 per cent at ages 7 to 9, 90 per cent at ages 10 to 15) and more severe; it is probably related to increased concentrations of phosphate, calcium, and protein in the saliva.[18]

Gingivitis Associated with Tooth Eruption. The frequency with which gingivitis occurs around erupting teeth has given rise to the term *eruption gingivitis.* However, *tooth eruption per se does not cause gingivitis.* The inflammation results from plaque accumulation around erupting teeth. The initiation of gingivitis appears to be related to plaque accumulation rather than to tissue remodeling associated with eruption.[8] Plaque retention around deciduous teeth facilitates plaque formation around juxtaposed permanent teeth.[8] The inflammatory changes accentuate the normal prominence of the gingival margin and create the impression of a marked gingival enlargement (Fig. 21–6).

Loose and Carious Teeth. Partially exfoliated, loose deciduous teeth frequently cause gingivitis. The eroded margin of partially re-

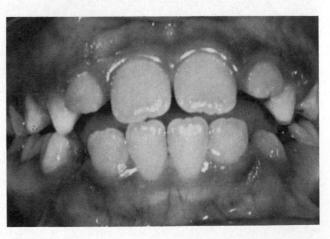

Figure 21–4 Prominent Marginal Gingiva on the cervical third of partially erupted maxillary anterior teeth.

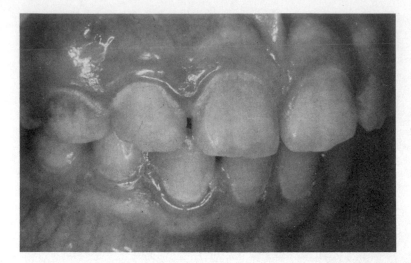

Figure 21–5 Chronic Marginal Gingivitis associated with plaque and materia alba.

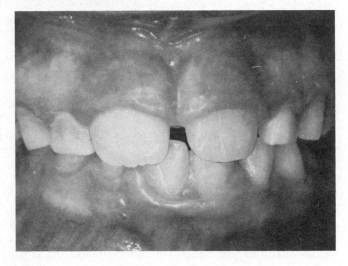

Figure 21–6 Developmental Gingival Enlargement caused by inflammation superimposed upon the normal prominence of the gingiva at this stage of tooth eruption.

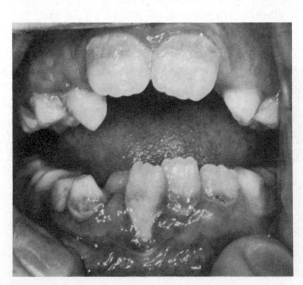

Figure 21–7 Severe Gingivitis associated with accumulation of plaque around malposed teeth.

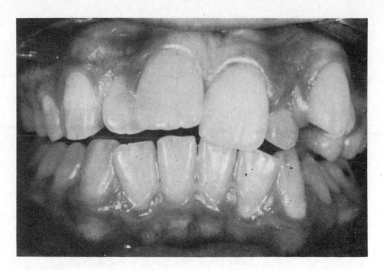

Figure 21–8 Gingival Enlargement in relation to malposed maxillary lateral and canine teeth (*left*). (Courtesy of Dr. Coenraad F. Moorrees.)

sorbed teeth favors plaque accumulation that causes gingival changes varying from slight discoloration and edema to abscess formation with suppuration. Other factors favoring plaque build-up are food impaction and materia alba accumulation around teeth partially destroyed by caries. Children frequently develop *unilateral chewing habits* to avoid loose or carious teeth, aggravating the accumulation of plaque on the nonchewing side.

Malposed Teeth and Malocclusion. Gingivitis occurs more frequently and with greater severity around malposed teeth because of their increased tendency to accumulate plaque and materia alba. Severe changes include gingival enlargement, bluish-red discoloration, ulceration (Fig. 21–7), and the formation of deep pockets from which pus can be expressed. Gingival health and contour are restored by correction of the malposition (Figs. 21–8 and

21–9), elimination of local irritants, and, when necessary, surgical removal of the enlarged gingiva.

Gingivitis is increased in children with *excessive overbite* and *overjet*, with *nasal obstruction*, and with *mouth breathing*.

Mucogingival Problems. According to Maynard and Wilson,[17] mucogingival problems start in the primary dentition as a consequence of developmental aberrations in eruption and deficiencies in the thickness of the periodontium. If there is also inadequate plaque control or excessive toothbrushing trauma, a mucogingival problem develops. However, the width of the attached gingiva increases with age, and these problems may resolve.

HISTOPATHOLOGY. Chronic gingivitis in children[12, 13] is characterized by loss of collagen in the area around the junctional epithe-

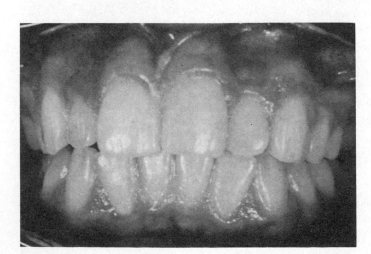

Figure 21–9 Disappearance of gingival enlargement shown in Figure 21–8 following orthodontic correction of the malposed teeth. (Courtesy of Dr. Coenraad F. Moorrees.)

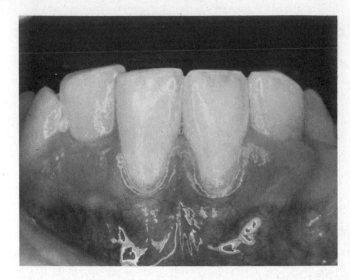

Figure 21–10 Gingival Recession on labially positioned mandibular central incisors.

lium, an important vascular component, and an infiltrate consisting mostly of lymphocytes and small numbers of polymorphonuclear leukocytes, plasma cells, monocytes, mast cells, fibroblasts, and endothelial cells.

This description corresponds to that of a Stage II gingivitis (the "initial lesion" of Page and Schroeder), rather than the Stage III gingivitis (Page and Schroeder's "established lesion") that is usually seen in adults.

Localized Gingival Recession

Gingival recession around individual teeth or groups of teeth is a common source of concern. The gingiva may be inflamed or free of disease, depending upon the presence or absence of local irritants. There are many causes of gingival recession (see Chapter 9), but in children the *position of the tooth in the arch* is the most important.[21] Gingival recession occurs on teeth in labial version (Fig. 21–10) or on those which are tilted or rotated so that the roots project labially. The recession may be a transitional phase in tooth eruption and may correct itself when the teeth attain proper alignment, or it may be necessary to realign the teeth orthodontically.

Acute Gingival Infections

ACUTE HERPETIC GINGIVOSTOMATITIS. This is the most common type of acute gingival infection in childhood. It often occurs as a sequel to upper respiratory tract infection. (For a full discussion, see Chapter 11.)

CANDIDIASIS. This is a mycotic infection of the oral cavity caused by the fungus *Candida albicans*. It is most often *acute* (Fig. 21–11) but may be *chronic*. (For a full discussion, see Chapter 12.)

ACUTE NECROTIZING ULCERATIVE GINGIVITIS. The incidence of acute necrotizing ulcerative gingivitis in childhood is low. (For a full discussion, see Chapter 11.) In children living in areas of chronic malnutrition and in children with Down's syndrome, the incidence and severity of acute necrotizing ulcerative gingivitis seem to increase.[10, 22] Acute herpetic gingivostomatitis, which is more common in childhood, is occasionally erroneously diagnosed as acute necrotizing ulcerative gingivitis.

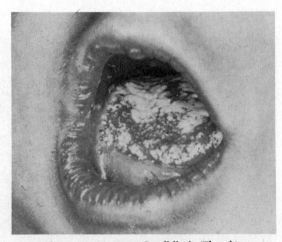

Figure 21–11 Acute Candidiasis (Thrush).

TRAUMATIC CHANGES IN THE PERIODONTIUM

Traumatic changes may occur in the periodontal tissues of deciduous teeth under several conditions. In shedding deciduous teeth, resorption of teeth and bone weakens the periodontal support so that the existing functional forces are injurious to the remaining supporting tissues.[2] Excessive occlusal forces may be produced by malalignment, mutilation, loss, or extractions of teeth or by dental restorations. In the mixed dentition, the periodontium of the permanent teeth may be traumatized because they bear an increased occlusal load when the adjacent deciduous teeth are shed. The periodontal ligament of an erupting permanent tooth may be injured by occlusal forces transmitted through the deciduous tooth it is replacing.[7]

Microscopically,[11, 19, 20] the least severe traumatic changes involve compression, ischemia, and hyalinization of the periodontal ligament. With severe injury there is crushing and necrosis of the periodontal ligament (see Chapter 19).

In most instances the injuries are repaired and tooth loss does not result. However, such traumatized teeth may be sore or loose. Repair may result in *ankylosis* of the tooth to the bone, fixing the tooth in situ. When the permanent dentition erupts, ankylosed deciduous teeth appear to be *submerged.*

THE ORAL MUCOUS MEMBRANE IN CHILDHOOD DISEASES

Certain childhood diseases present specific alterations in the oral cavity.[3, 9] Among these are the communicable diseases.

CHICKENPOX (VARICELLA). Successive papillary eruptions and vesicles appear on the buccal mucosa as well as on the face and the rest of the cutaneous body surface (Fig. 21–12). On the buccal mucosa the vesicles break down to become small, ulcerated craters with surrounding erythemas; they resemble the lesions of acute herpetic stomatitis. Comparable but more extensive oral lesions are seen in *smallpox* (variola).

MEASLES (RUBEOLA). Koplik's spots are pathognomonic of measles and are found in 97 per cent of patients. They are seen 2 to 3 days before the rash appears. They most often occur on the buccal mucosa opposite the first molars or on the inner aspect of the lower lip and appear as bluish-white specks–pinpoint in size–surrounded by a bright red areola. They are best seen in daylight. At first only a few are present, but later they become numerous and coalesce. In addition to these specific lesions, measles may also be accompanied by erythema and edema of the gingiva and the remainder

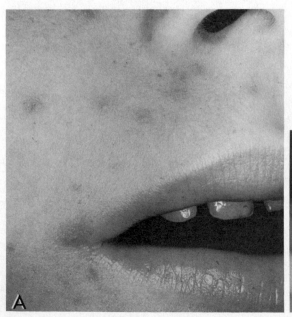
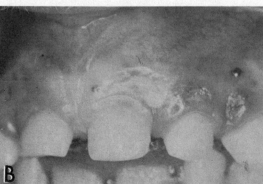

Figure 21–12 Chickenpox (Varicella). *A,* Skin lesions. *B,* Vesicles on gingiva.

of the oral mucosa and by discrete, bluish-red discolored areas on the soft palate.

SCARLET FEVER (SCARLATINA). Diffuse, fiery red discoloration of the oral mucosa occurs in scarlet fever. Characteristic tongue changes include (1) "raspberry tongue," a bright red, shiny discoloration with prominent papillae; and (2) "strawberry tongue," a coated surface covering an underlying bright red discoloration with prominent papillae.

DIPHTHERIA. Diphtheria is characterized by pseudomembrane formation in the oropharynx that appears as a gray, friable, curtain-like extension in the area of the anterior faucial pillars. Diffuse erythema of the oral mucous membrane with vesicle formation is also commonly seen in this condition.

REFERENCES

1. Baer, P. N., and Benjamin, S. D.: Periodontal Disease in Children and Adolescents. Philadelphia, J. B. Lippincott Company, 1974.
2. Bernick, S., and Freedman, N.: Microscopic studies of the periodontium of the primary dentitions of monkeys. II. Posterior teeth during the mixed dentitional period. Oral Surg., 7:322, 1954.
3. Blackstone, C. H.: A clinical and roentgenographic study of periodontic problems in children with systemic disease. J. Am. Dent. Assoc., 29:1664, 1942.
4. Bradley, R. F.: Periodontal lesions of children–their recognition and treatment. Dent. Clin. North Am., 5:671, 1961.
5. Brauer, J. C., Highley, L. B., Massler, M., and Schour, I.: Dentistry for Children. 2nd ed. Philadelphia, Blakiston Company, 1947.
6. Everett, F. G., Tuchler, H., and Lu, K. H.: Occurrence of calculus in grade school children in Portland, Oregon. J. Periodontol., 34:54, 1963.
7. Grimmer, E. A.: Trauma in an erupting premolar. J. Dent. Res., 18:267, 1939.
8. Hock, J.: A clinical study of gingivitis of deciduous and succedaneous permanent teeth in dogs. J. Periodont. Res., 13:68, 1978.
9. Jacobs, M. H.: Oral lesions in childhood. Oral Surg., 9:871, 1956.
10. Jimenez, M., Ramos, J., Garrington, G., and Baer, P. N.: The familial occurrence of acute necrotizing gingivitis in Colombia. J. Periodontol., 40:414, 1969.
11. Kronfeld, R., and Weinmann, J.: Traumatic changes in the periodontal tissues of deciduous teeth. J. Dent. Res., 19:441, 1940.
12. Longhurst, P., Gillett, R., and Johnson, N. W.: Electron microscope quantitation of inflammatory infiltrates in childhood gingivitis. J. Periodont. Res., 15:255, 1980.
13. Longhurst, P., Johnson, N. W., and Hopps, R. M.: Differences in lymphocyte and plasma cell densities in inflamed gingiva from adults and young children. J. Periodontol., 48:705, 1977.
14. Mackler, S. B., and Crawford, J. J.: Plaque development in the primary dentition. J. Periodontol., 44:18, 1973.
15. Mattson, L.: Development of gingivitis in preschool children and young adults. A comparative experimental study. J. Clin. Periodontol., 5:24, 1978.
16. Mattson, L., and Attstrom, R.: Histologic characteristics of experimental gingivitis in the juvenile and adult beagle dog. J. Clin. Periodontol., 6:334, 1979.
17. Maynard, J. G., and Wilson, R. D.: Diagnosis and management of mucogingival problems in children. Dent. Clin. North Am., 24:683, 1980.
18. Notman, S., Mandel, I. D., and Mercadante, J.: Calculus in normal children and children with cystic fibrosis. Intern. Assoc. for Dent. Res. Program and Abstracts, 48th General Meeting, 1970, p. 64.
19. Oppenheim, A.: Histologische Befunde beim Zahnwechsel. Z. Stomatol., 20:543, 1922.
20. Orban, B., and Weinmann, J.: Signs of traumatic occlusion in average human jaws. J. Dent. Res., 13:216, 1933.
21. Parfitt, G. J., and Mjor, I. A.: A clinical evaluation of local gingival recession in children. J. Dent. Child., 31:257, 1964.
22. Pindborg, J. J., Bhat, M., Devanath, K. R., Narayana, H. R., and Ramachandra, S.: Occurrence of acute necrotizing gingivitis in South India children. J. Periodontol., 37:14, 1966.
23. Rosenblum, F. N.: Clinical study of the depth of the gingival sulcus in the primary dentition. J. Dent. Child., 5:289, 1966.
24. Soni, N. N., Silberkweit, M., and Hayes, R. L.: Histological characteristics of stippling in children. J. Periodontol., 34:31, 1963.
25. Standish, S. M., and Shafer, W. G.: Gingival reparative granulomas in children. J. Oral Surg., 19:367, 1961.
26. Thomas, B. O. A.: The child patient as a future periodontal problem. J. Am. Dent. Assoc., 35:763, 1947.

chapter twenty-two

Juvenile Periodontitis

Generalized Form	Localized Form
Papillon-Lefèvre Syndrome	Historical Background
Down's Syndrome (Mongolism, Trisomy 21)	Prevalence
Neutropenias	Age and Sex Distribution
Hypophosphatasia	Distribution of Lesions
Eosinophilic Granuloma and Related Syndromes	Clinical Findings
Congenital Heart Disease	Radiographic Findings
Diabetes	Clinical Course
Cerebral Palsy	Heredity
Beta-Thalassemia (Erythroblastic Anemia, Cooley's Anemia)	Histopathology
	Bacteriology
Acute and Subacute Leukemia	Immunology

There are cases of severe rapid periodontal destruction and premature tooth loss in children and teenagers, the etiology of which is not well understood. These cases occur infrequently; they are referred to as "juvenile periodontitis"* and can be classified as those occurring in otherwise healthy individuals and those associated with a variety of diseases of other systems. The term "localized" is used with reference to the first group, although some cases may show generalized involvement. Cases of the second kind are termed "generalized juvenile periodontitis," since the whole dentition is usually involved.

GENERALIZED FORM

This type of juvenile periodontitis attacks the whole dentition or a large part of it and is associated with systemic disturbances. Generalized juvenile periodontitis appears in the following diseases:

PAPILLON-LEFÈVRE SYNDROME. This is a syndrome characterized by hyperkeratotic skin lesions, severe destruction of the periodontium, and, in some cases, calcification of the dura.[2, 11, 21, 28, 38, 45] The skin and periodontal changes usually appear together before the age of 4 years. The skin lesions consist of hyperkeratosis and ichthyosis of localized areas in the palms, soles, knees, and elbows (Figs. 22–1 and 22–2).

Periodontal lesions consist of early inflammatory involvement leading to bone loss and exfoliation of teeth. Primary teeth are lost by 5 or 6 years of age. The permanent dentition then erupts normally, but within a few years the teeth are exfoliated owing to destructive periodontal disease. By the age of 15, patients are usually edentulous except for the third molars. These, too, are lost a few years after they erupt.

The microscopic changes observed in one case[38] included marked chronic inflammation of the lateral wall of the pocket, with considerable osteoclastic activity and an apparent lack of osteoblastic activity; in the tooth studied, the cementum was very thin or almost nonexistent except in the apical area, where a comparatively wide area of cellular cementum was seen.

Bacterial studies of plaque in a case of Papillon-Lefèvre syndrome revealed a flora similar to that of "adult" type periodontitis, not to that of juvenile periodontitis.[42] Spirochete-rich zones in the apical portion of the pockets, as well as spirochete adherence to the cementum and microcolony formation of mycoplasmas, have been reported in Papillon-Lefèvre syndrome.[31]

The syndrome is inherited and appears to follow an autosomal recessive pattern.[23] Parents are not affected, and both must carry the autosomal genes for the syndrome to appear in the offspring. It may occur in siblings; males and females are equally affected. The estimated frequency is one to four cases per million.[25]

---

*The term "periodontosis" has been used to designate this condition. At present the term "juvenile periodontitis" is preferred.

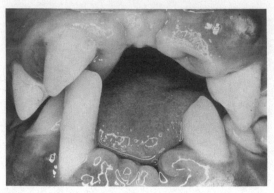

Figure 22–1 Dentition of a 17-year-old male patient with **Papillon-Lefèvre Syndrome.** The missing teeth were exfoliated.

Patients with skin lesions similar to those of Papillon-Lefèvre syndrome but without periodontal destruction are diagnosed as having Meleda disease.

DOWN'S SYNDROME (Mongolism, Trisomy 21). This is a congenital disease caused by a chromosomal abnormality and characterized by mental deficiency and growth retardation. The prevalence of periodontal disease in Down's syndrome is high, and although plaque, calculus, and periodontal pockets are present, the severity of periodontal destruction exceeds that explainable by local factors alone.[17, 30, 56]

Periodontal disease in Down's syndrome is characterized by formation of deep periodontal pockets associated with a high plaque score and moderate gingivitis (Fig. 22–3). These findings are usually generalized, although they tend to be more severe in the lower anterior region; marked recession is also sometimes seen in this region, apparently associated with high frenum attachment. Acute necrotizing lesions are a frequent finding.

No satisfactory explanation has been offered for the increased prevalence and severity of periodontal destruction in children with Down's syndrome. The following factors have been mentioned: general physical deterioration of these patients at an early age[4]; reduced resistance to infections because of poor circulation, especially in areas of terminal vascularization such as the gingival tissues[19]; and neurodystrophic processes.[17] Increased numbers of *Bacteroides melaninogenicus* have been reported in these children's mouths.[36]

NEUTROPENIAS. See Chapter 30.

HYPOPHOSPHATASIA. This is a rare familial skeletal disease which in some cases results in loss of primary teeth, particularly the incisors. An association with abnormal alkaline phosphatase activity has been suggested but not proven.[3]

EOSINOPHILIC GRANULOMA AND RELATED SYNDROMES. This is a group of diseases char-

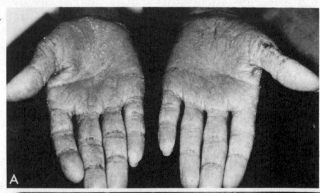

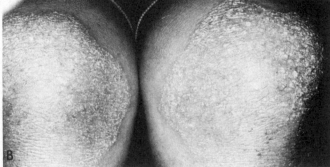

Figure 22–2 *A,* Palms and *(B)* knees of the patient in Figure 22–1. Note the hyperkeratotic scaly lesions.

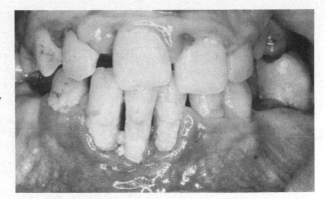

Figure 22–3 Down's syndrome patient, 14 years old, with severe periodontal destruction.

acterized by proliferation of eosinophils and mononuclear cells that infiltrate the bone marrow and other tissues. Three disease entities are usually included in this group: (1) **Eosinophilic granuloma,** which is the most benign and presents unifocal bone lesions[10, 53]; (2) **Hand-Schüller-Christian disease,** which shows multifocal bone lesions and occurs mostly in young children; and (3) **Letterer-Siwe disease,** which is widespread to all major organs and occurs in babies and young children.

One of the initial manifestations, particularly of Hand-Schüller-Christian disease but also of the others, may be *radiolucent lesions in the jaws and severe gingival inflammation, with loss of bone leading to looseness and exfoliation of teeth.*[9, 10, 52]

CONGENITAL HEART DISEASE. Gingival disease and other oral symptoms may occur in children with congenital heart disease.[6, 32] In cases of **tetralogy of Fallot,** which is characterized by pulmonary stenosis, right ventricular enlargement, a defect in the interventricular septum, and malposition of the aorta to the right, the oral changes include a purplish-red discoloration of the lips and severe marginal gingivitis and periodontal destruction (Figs.

22–4 and 22–5). The tongue is coated, fissured, and edematous, and there is extreme reddening of the fungiform and filiform papillae. There are an increased number of subepithelial capillaries, which return nearly to normal following cardiac surgery.[20]

In cases of **tetralogy of Eisenmenger** there is pulmonary insufficiency and a diastolic murmur; the lips, cheeks, and buccal mucous membranes are cyanotic, but less markedly so than in tetralogy of Fallot. Severe generalized marginal gingivitis is a common finding. In cases in which there is **transposition of the aorta and superior vena cava,** cyanotic discoloration and marginal gingivitis of a lesser degree are noted. In **coarctation of the aorta** there is a narrowing of the vessel in the region where it is joined by the ductus arteriosus. These patients show marked inflammation of the gingiva in the anterior part of the mouth.

DIABETES. In childhood, uncontrolled diabetes may be accompanied by marked destruction of alveolar bone. Although gingival inflammation is a frequent finding in such cases, the extent of alveolar bone loss is in excess of that generally seen in children with comparable gingival involvement (see Chapter 29).

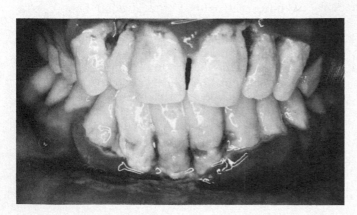

Figure 22–4 Extensive marginal inflammation with ulceronecrotic lesions and periodontal destruction in an adolescent with tetralogy of Fallot.

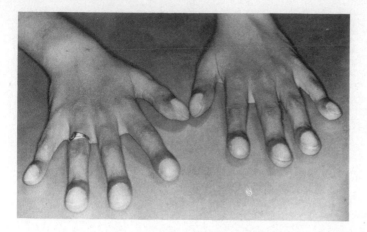

Figure 22–5 Characteristic clubbing of the fingers in the patient shown in Figure 22–4.

CEREBRAL PALSY. Hypoplasia, attrition, malocclusion, and temporomandibular dysfunction are increased in cerebral palsy.[55] Because oral hygiene is a problem for individuals with cerebral palsy, the incidence of periodontal disorders and caries may be high.

BETA-THALASSEMIA (Erythroblastic Anemia, Cooley's Anemia). This is an inherited disorder characterized by a hemolytic anemia, splenomegaly, nucleated red blood cells in the peripheral blood, and generalized skeletal lesions.[16] Skeletal changes are absent or minimal during the first year of life. The osteoporosis characteristic of the disease occurs during early childhood and is followed by sclerosis. The most characteristic bony changes are noted in the metacarpals and femora. Pneumatization of the paranasal sinuses is retarded.

Oral changes[16] include pallor and cyanosis of the mucous membrane and marked malocclusion due to the overgrowth of the alveolar ridge of the maxilla (Fig. 22–6). There is an associated spreading of the teeth, with creation of large interproximal spaces. Radiographic examination reveals generalized rarefaction of the bones of the jaw, with an alteration in the trabecular pattern characterized by an irregularly arranged heterogeneous lattice. The lam-

ina dura is obliterated in some areas (Fig. 22–7).

ACUTE AND SUBACUTE LEUKEMIA. These diseases in children are accompanied by gingival changes (see Chapter 30).

PREPUBERTAL PERIODONTITIS, GENERALIZED FORM. Children with advanced periodontal destruction and no systemic disease have also been described.[44] These cases are very rare, and they start during or immediately following eruption of the primary teeth. An extremely acute inflammation and proliferation of the gingival tissues, with very rapid destruction of bone, are found. Defects in peripheral blood neutrophils and monocytes have been found in these patients; they also have frequent respiratory infections and sometimes otitis media. All primary teeth are affected, but the permanent dentition may or may not be affected.[43a]

LOCALIZED FORM

HISTORICAL BACKGROUND. The localized form of juvenile periodontitis was first described by Gottlieb[26] in 1923, under the name "diffuse atrophy of the alveolar bone," in a patient with a fatal case of epidemic influenza. He described it as different from marginal atrophy and as consisting of a loss of collagen fibers in the periodontal ligament and their replacement by loose connective tissue and extensive bone resorption, resulting in a widened periodontal ligament space. The gingiva was apparently not involved. In 1928 Gottlieb attributed this condition to the inhibition of continuous cementum formation, which he considered essential for maintenance of the periodontal ligament fibers; he then termed it "deep cementopathia." Expanding his theory,

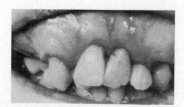

Figure 22–6 Patient with Erythroblastic Anemia. Note the prominence of the maxilla and pallor of the gingival mucosa. (Courtesy of Dr. M. M. Cohen and Dr. J. M. Baty.)

Gottlieb hypothesized that deep cementopathia was a "disease of eruption." Senescent cementum could act like a foreign body in an attempt by the host to exfoliate the tooth, resulting in bone resorption and pocket formation.[27] In 1938 Wannenmacher[59] described the incisor–first molar location of the disease, which he called "parodontitis marginalis progressiva." Contrary to others at that time, Wannenmacher considered this disease an inflammatory process.

In 1940 Thoma and Goldman[57] used the term "paradontosis" to refer to this disease; the initial abnormality was located in the alveolar bone rather than in the cementum and consisted of vascular resorption and halisteresis rather than "lacunar resorption." In 1947, Goldman[24] again described vascular resorption and halisteresis in a spider monkey as being due to a degenerative noninflammatory disease of the supporting structures.

In 1942 Orban and Weinmann[43] introduced the term "periodontosis" and, on the basis of one autopsy case studied in detail, described three stages in the development of the disease.

Stage 1 involves the degeneration and desmolysis of the principal fibers of the periodontal ligament and the probable cessation of cementum formation; there is simultaneous resorption of the alveolar bone due to lack of functional stimulation from the tooth and increased tissue pressure caused by edema and capillary proliferation. In this stage, tooth migration is the earliest clinical sign, and it occurs without detectable inflammatory involvement.

Stage 2 is characterized by the rapid proliferation of the junctional epithelium along the root and sometimes by proliferation of the epithelial rests of Malassez. In this stage, the earliest signs of inflammation appear. Clinically, both the first and second stages are of short duration; they cannot be differentiated from each other.

Stage 3 is characterized by progressive in-

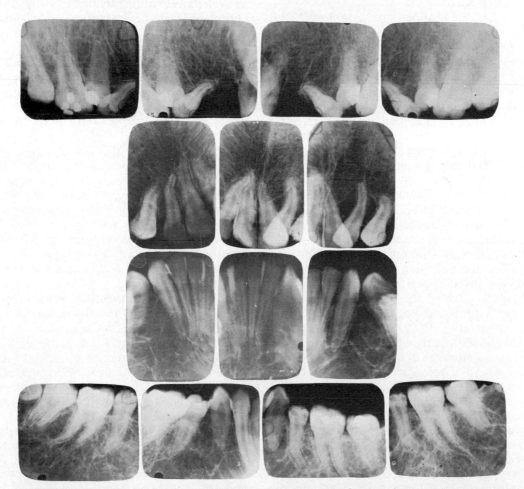

Figure 22–7 Radiographs of Patient with Erythroblastic Anemia. There is generalized rarefaction of the bone and enlarged irregularly arranged medullary spaces. (Courtesy of Drs. M. M. Cohen and J. M. Baty.)

flammation and the development of deep periodontal pockets of the infrabony type. This is the stage most frequently seen.

All of the above-mentioned studies consider "periodontosis" a degenerative disease caused by unknown systemic factors. Glickman in 1952[23] felt that the conditions described in these studies did not represent a different type of periodontal disease but, rather, extreme variants of destructive processes common to all periodontal disease.

Other authors have denied the existence of a degenerative type of periodontal disease and have attributed the changes observed to trauma from occlusion.[8, 39, 46] In 1966, the World Workshop in Periodontics[60] opined that the conventional concept of "periodontosis" as a degenerative entity was unsubstantiated and that the term should be eliminated from periodontal nomenclature. The committee did recognize that a clinical entity different from "adult" periodontitis may occur in adolescents and young adults.

Baer in 1971[2] defined "periodontosis" as a "disease of the periodontium occurring in an otherwise healthy adolescent which is characterized by a rapid loss of alveolar bone about more than one tooth of the permanent dentition. There are two basic forms in which it occurs. In one form, the teeth affected are the incisors and the first molars, in the other, more generalized form, most of the dentition can be affected. The amount of destruction manifested is not commensurate with the amounts of local irritants present."

The term "juvenile periodontitis" was introduced by Chaput et al. in 1967 in the French literature and by Butler[7] in 1969 in the English literature.

PREVALENCE. Differences of opinion with regard to the definition of and diagnostic criteria for juvenile periodontitis make it very difficult to establish the real prevalence of the disease in different populations. Saxen, in a study population of 8096 16-year-olds from a geographically restricted area of Finland, using the above-mentioned criteria delineated by Baer, found a prevalence of 0.1 per cent.[49] Earlier studies do not offer clear evidence of sound criteria for differentiating juvenile periodontitis from other forms of the disease.

AGE AND SEX DISTRIBUTION. Juvenile periodontitis affects both males and females and is seen most frequently in the period between puberty and the age of 25. There is a predilection for female patients, particularly in the youngest age groups.[29]

DISTRIBUTION OF LESIONS. The distribution of lesions in the mouth is characteristic and as yet unexplained. *The classic distribution is in the first molars and incisors, with the least destruction in the cuspid-premolar area* (Fig. 22–8). Recently three types of bone loss localization have been defined[29]: (1) first molars and/or incisors; (2) first molars, incisors, and some additional teeth (total < 14 teeth); and (3) generalized involvement. There is an increase in the number of affected teeth with advancing age.

Frequently bilateral symmetrical patterns of bone loss occur.[12] Manson and Lehner[37] have classified the typical pattern of bone loss (first molar–incisor) according to symmetrical and asymmetrical distribution; in their series of 28 patients they found 15 symmetrical and 13 asymmetrical cases.

CLINICAL FINDINGS. The onset of osseous destruction is insidious, especially during the circumpubertal period from 11 to 13 years of age. The most striking feature of early juvenile periodontitis is the *lack of clinical inflammation*. Late in the incipient stages there is the beginning of deep pocket formation in the periodontium around affected teeth, and, clinically, the *most common presenting symptoms are mobility and migration of the incisors and first molars*.

As the disease progresses, however, other symptoms may arise. Denuded root surfaces become sensitive to thermal changes, foods, and tactile stimuli such as toothbrush bristles or curette blades. Deep, dull, radiating pain may be present upon mastication and is probably due to irritation of the supporting structures by mobile teeth and impacted food. Periodontal abscesses may form at this stage. Manson and Lehner[37] have reported a high incidence of regional lymph node enlargement in affected individuals.

RADIOGRAPHIC FINDINGS. *Vertical loss of alveolar bone around the first molars and incisors in otherwise healthy individuals* is taken to be a diagnostic sign of classic juvenile periodontitis. Roentgenographic findings include "an arc-shaped loss of alveolar bone extending from the distal surface of the second premolar to the mesial surface of the second molar."[40] Evidence indicates that the bone loss is not the result of any developmental or congenital absence or defect. Alveolar bone in patients in this age group develops normally with tooth eruption, and only subsequently does it undergo resorptive changes. *Classically, one sees a distolabial migration of the maxillary*

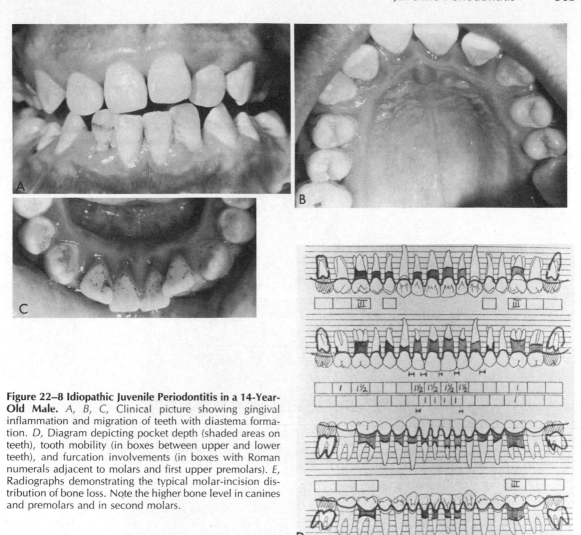

Figure 22–8 Idiopathic Juvenile Periodontitis in a 14-Year-Old Male. *A, B, C,* Clinical picture showing gingival inflammation and migration of teeth with diastema formation. *D,* Diagram depicting pocket depth (shaded areas on teeth), tooth mobility (in boxes between upper and lower teeth), and furcation involvements (in boxes with Roman numerals adjacent to molars and first upper premolars). *E,* Radiographs demonstrating the typical molar-incision distribution of bone loss. Note the higher bone level in canines and premolars and in second molars.

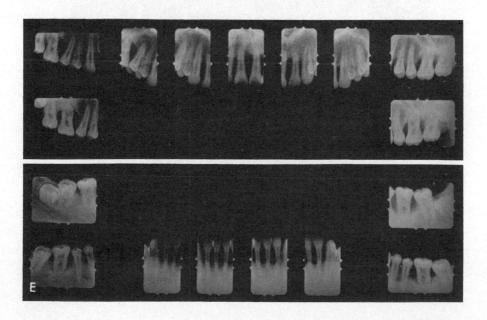

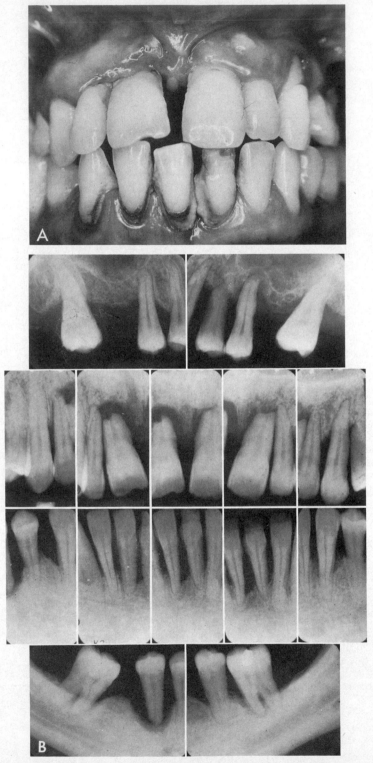

Figure 22–9 Advanced Juvenile Periodontitis in a 28-Year-Old Female. *A,* Gingival inflammation, heavy calculus deposits, anterior open bite with diastema formation associated with tongue-thrusting habit. *B,* Severe generalized bone destruction obscures the limitation of bone loss to the anterior and molar regions seen in early periodontosis.

incisors, with diastema formation. The lower incisors seem to have less of a propensity to migrate than do the upper ones. Occlusal patterns and tongue pressure can vary the amount and type of migration noted. Along with anterior tooth migration, an apparent increase in the size of the clinical crown, accumulation of plaque and calculus, and clinical inflammation appear.

CLINICAL COURSE. Juvenile periodontitis progresses rapidly. Evidence indicates that the *rate of bone loss is about three to four times faster* than in typical periodontitis.[2, 3] In affected persons, bone resorption progresses until the teeth are either treated, exfoliated, or extracted. There is no consistent or reliable evidence to indicate that the disease process per se spreads to unaffected areas. However, it has been reported that, in later stages of the disease, other teeth are involved with a form of periodontitis accompanied by the usual inflammatory changes (Fig. 22–9).

HEREDITY. Several authors have described a familial pattern of alveolar bone loss and have implicated (without substantial evidence) a genetic factor in localized juvenile periodontitis.[7, 14] Benjamin and Baer,[5] in the most comprehensive study on familial patterns, described the disease in identical twins, siblings, and first cousins, as well as in parents and offspring. Newman and Socransky[41] have also described a familial pattern and have suggested the possibility of a transmissible microbiologic component in the pathogenesis of the disease.

Several investigators have concluded that juvenile periodontitis is inherited as an autosomal recessive trait. Others have considered it to be transmitted as an X-linked dominant disease.

HISTOPATHOLOGY. A thin, frequently ulcerated pocket epithelium, infiltrated by numerous leukocytes, covers large areas of inflammatory cell accumulation composed mainly of plasma cells and blast cells, with lymphocytes and macrophages present in small numbers.[35] Collagen and other tissue components constitute only a small proportion of the diseased site as compared with adult-type periodontitis.[35]

Electron microscopy has revealed **bacterial invasion of connective tissue** in cases of juvenile periodontitis,[22] reaching the bone surface.[8a] The invading flora has been described as morphologically mixed but composed mainly of gram-negative bacteria including cocci, rods, filaments, and spirochetes.[22] Using different methods, including immunocyto-chemistry and electronmicroscopy, Saglie et al.[47] have identified the following tissue-invading microorganisms in localized juvenile periodontitis: *Actinobacillus actinomycetemcomitans, Capnocytophaga sputigena, Mycoplasma,* and spirochetes.

Subgingival plaque in juvenile periodontitis remains relatively thin (20 to 200 microns) and does not tend to mineralize.[58] A scanning electron microscopic study of the root surface in a tooth with juvenile periodontitis showed scattered clumps of rods, cocci, and filaments, with the apical 400 microns occupied by large numbers of rods of uniform morphology on the cemental and soft tissue surfaces.[1]

BACTERIOLOGY. In recent years the relationship of lesions of localized juvenile periodontitis to a bacterial flora different from that of adult periodontitis has been described.[44] This flora consists mainly of gram-negative anaerobic rods, along with a minimal amount of attached plaque with a larger unattached component. The two bacteria that have been considered pathogens in juvenile periodontitis are *Actinobacillus actinomycetemcomitans*[54, 54a] and *Capnocytophaga.*[41] For further details, see Chapter 25.

IMMUNOLOGY. Some immune defects have been implicated in the pathogenesis of localized and generalized juvenile periodontitis. Impaired neutrophil chemotaxis and inhibition of macrophage migration[12, 13, 34] have been reported, although proofs are still lacking (see Chapter 24).

TREATMENT. See Chapter 45.

REFERENCES

1. Allen, A. L., and Brady, J. M.: Periodontosis: a case report with SEM observations. J. Periodontol., *49*:415, 1978.
2. Baer, P. N.: The case for periodontosis as a clinical entity. J. Periodontol., *42*:516, 1971.
3. Baer, P. N., and Benjamin, S. D.: Periodontal Disease in Children and Adolescents. Philadelphia, J. B. Lippincott Company, 1974.
4. Benda, C. E.: Mongolismo y Cretinismo. 2nd ed. Barcelona, Científica Médica, 1954.
5. Benjamin, S. D., and Baer, P. N.: Familial patterns of advanced alveolar bone loss in adolescence (periodontosis). Periodontics, *5*:82, 1967.
6. Blitzer, B., Sznajder, N., and Carranza, F. A., Jr.: Hallazgos clínicos periodontales en niños con cardiopatias congénitas. Rev. Asoc. Odontol., Argent., *63*:169, 1975.
7. Butler, J. H.: A familial pattern of juvenile periodontitis (periodontosis). J. Periodontol., *40*:115, 1969.
8. Carranza, F. A., Sr., and Carranza, F. A., Jr.: A suggested classification of common periodontal disease. J. Periodontol., *30*:140, 1959.
8a. Carranza, F. A., Jr., Saglie, R., and Newman, M. G.: Scanning and transmission electron microscopy study of tissue invading microorganisms in localized juvenile periodontitis. J. Periodontol., in press.
9. Carraro, J. J., Sereday, M., and Sznajder, N.: Oral manifestations of histiocytosis X. J. Periodontol., *38*:521, 1967.

10. Carraro, J. J., Sznajder, N., Barros, R., and Martinez Lalis, R.: Periodontal involvement in eosinophilic granuloma. J. Periodontol., *43*:427, 1972.

11. Carvel, R. I.: Palmar-plantar hyperkeratosis and premature periodontal destruction. J. Oral Med., *24*:73, 1969.

11a. Christersson, L. A., Albini, B., Zambon, J., Slots, J., and Genco, R. J.: Demonstration of *Actinobacillus actinomycetemcomitans* in gingiva in localized juvenile periodontitis in humans. J. Dent. Res., *62*:255, 1983 (abstract).

12. Cianciola, R. J., et al.: Defective polymorphonuclear leukocyte function in a human periodontal disease. Nature, *265*:445, 1977.

13. Clark, R. A., Page, R. C., and Wilde, G.: Defective neutrophil chemotaxis in juvenile periodontitis. Infect. Immun., *18*:694, 1977.

14. Cohen, D. W., and Goldman, H. M.: Clinical observations on the modification of human oral tissue metabolism by local intraoral factors. Ann. N.Y. Acad. Sci., *85*:68, 1960.

15. Cohen, D. W., and Goldman, H. M.: Periodontal disease in children. P. D. M., July, 1962, p. 3.

16. Cohen, M. M., and Baty, J. M.: Oral manifestations of erythroblastic anemia. J. Am. Dent. Assoc., *32*:1396, 1945.

17. Cohen, M. M., Winer, R. A., Schwartz, S., and Shklar, G.: Oral aspects of mongolism. Part I. Periodontal disease in mongolism. Oral Surg., *14*:92, 1961.

18. Cooley, T. B., Witwer, E. R., and Lee, P.: Anemia in children with splenomegaly and peculiar changes in bones. Am. J. Dis. Child., *34*:347, 1927.

19. Dow, R. S.: Preliminary study of periodontoclasia in mongolian children at Polk State School. Am. J. Ment. Defic., *55*:535, 1951.

20. Forsslund, G.: Occurrence of subepithelial gingival blood vessels in patients with morbus caeruleus (tetralogy of Fallot). Acta Odontol. Scand., *20*:301, 1962.

21. Galanter, D. R., and Bradford, S.: Hyperkeratosis palmoplantaris and periodontosis: the Papillon-Lefèvre syndrome. J. Periodontol., *40*:40, 1969.

22. Gillett, R., and Johnson, N. W.: Bacterial invasion of the periodontium in a case of juvenile periodontitis. J. Clin. Periodontol., *9*:93, 1982.

23. Glickman, I.: Periodontosis: a critical evaluation. J. Am. Dent. Assoc., *44*:706, 1952.

24. Goldman, H. M.: Similar condition to periodontosis in two spider monkeys. Am. J. Orthod., *33*:749, 1947.

25. Gorlin, R. J., Sedano, H., and Anderson, V. E.: The syndrome of palmar-plantar hyperkeratosis and premature periodontal destruction of the teeth. J. Pediatr., *65*:895, 1964.

26. Gottlieb, B.: Die diffuse Atrophy des Alveolarknochens. Z. Stomatol., *21*:195, 1923.

27. Gottlieb, B.: The formation of the pocket: diffuse atrophy of alveolar bone. J. Am. Dent. Assoc., *15*:462, 1928.

28. Haneke, E.: The Papillon-Lefèvre syndrome; keratosis palmoplantaris with periodontopathy. Hum. Genet., *51*:1, 1979.

29. Hormand, J., and Frandsen, A.: Juvenile periodontitis. Localization of bone loss in relation to age, sex, and teeth. J. Clin. Periodontol., *6*:407, 1979.

30. Johnson, N. P., and Young, M. A.: Periodontal disease in Mongols. J. Periodontol., *34*:41, 1963.

31. Jung, J. R., Carranza, F. A., Jr., and Newman, M. G.: Scanning electronmicroscopy of plaque in Papillon-Lefèvre syndrome. J. Periodontol., *52*:442, 1981.

32. Kaner, A., Losch, P., and Green, M.: Oral manifestations of congenital heart disease. J. Pediatr., *29*:269, 1946.

33. Kaslick, R. S., and Chasens, A. I.: Periodontosis with periodontitis: a study involving young adult males. Oral Surg., *25*:327, 1968.

34. Lavine, W. S., et. al.: Impaired neutrophil chemotaxis in patients with juvenile and rapidly progressing periodontitis. J. Periodont. Res., *14*:10, 1979.

35. Liljenberg, B., and Lindhe, J.: Juvenile periodontitis. Some microbiological, histopathological and clinical characteristics. J. Clin. Periodontol., *7*:48, 1980.

36. Loesche, W. J., Hockett, R. N., and Syed, S. A.: The predominant cultivable flora of tooth surface plaque removed from institutionalized subjects. Arch. Oral Biol., *17*:1311, 1972.

37. Manson, J. D., and Lehner, T.: Clinical features of juvenile periodontitis (periodontosis). J. Periodontol., *45*:636, 1974.

38. Martinez Lalis, R. R., Lopez Otero, R., and Carranza, F. A., Jr.: A case of Papillon-Lefèvre syndrome. Periodontics, *3*:292, 1965.

39. Mezl, Z.: Contribution a l'histologie pathologique du paradentium. Paradentologie, *2*:60, 1948.

40. Miller, S. C.: Precocious advanced alveolar atrophy. J. Periodontol., *19*:146, 1948.

41. Newman, M. G., and Socransky, S. S.: Predominant cultivable microbiota in periodontosis. J. Periodont. Res., *12*:120, 1977.

42. Newman, M. G., Angel, I., Karge, H., Weiner, M., Grinenko, V., and Schusterman, L.: Bacterial studies of the Papillon-Lefèvre syndrome. J. Dent. Res., *56*:545, 1977.

43. Orban, B., and Weinmann, J. P.: Diffuse atrophy of alveolar bone. J. Periodontol., *21*:31, 1942.

44. Page, R. C., and Schroeder, H. E.: Periodontitis in Man and Other Animals. Basel, S. Karger, 1982.

45. Papillon, M. M., and Lefèvre, P.: Deux cas de keratodermie palmaire et plantaire symetrique familiale (maladie de Meleda) chez le frere et la soeur. Coexistance dans les deux cas d'alterations dentaires graves. Soc. Franc. Derm. Syph., *31*:82, 1924.

46. Ramfjord, S. P.: Effect of acute febrile diseases on the periodontium of Rhesus monkeys with reference to poliomyelitis. J. Dent. Res., *30*:615, 1951.

47. Saglie, F. R., Carranza, F. A., Jr., Newman, M. G., Cheng, L., and Lewin, K.: Identification of tissue invading bacteria in juvenile periodontitis. J. Periodont. Res., *17*:452, 1982.

48. Saxen, L.: Juvenile periodontitis. J. Clin. Periodontol., *7*:1, 1980.

49. Saxen, L.: Prevalence of juvenile periodontitis in Finland. J. Clin. Periodontol., *7*:177, 1980.

50. Saxen, L.: Heredity of juvenile periodontitis. J. Clin. Periodontol., *7*:276, 1980.

51. Saxen, L., Aula, S., and Westermarck, T.: Periodontal disease associated with Down's syndrome: an orthopantomographic evaluation. J. Periodontol., *48*:337, 1977.

52. Sedano, H., Cernea, P., Hosxe, G., and Gorlin, R. J.: Histiocytosis X. Oral Surg., *27*:760, 1969.

53. Shklar, G., Taylor, R., and Schwartz, S.: Oral lesions of eosinophilic granuloma. Oral Surg., *19*:613, 1965.

54. Slots, J., Reynolds, H. S., and Genco, R. J.: *Actinobacillus actinomycetemcomitans* in human periodontal disease: a cross-sectional microbiological investigation. Infect. Immun., *29*:1013, 1980.

54a. Slots, J., Zambon, J. J., Rosling, B. C., Reynolds, H. S., Christersson, L. A., and Genco, R. J.: *Actinobacillus actinomycetemcomitans* in human periodontal disease. Association, serology, leukotoxicity, and treatment. J. Periodont. Res., *17*:447, 1982.

55. Sznajder, N.: Oral diseases in cerebral palsy children. Rev. Assoc. Odontol. Argent., *52*:96, 1964.

56. Sznajder, N., Carraro, J. J., Otero, E., and Carranza, F. A., Jr.: Clinical periodontal finding in trisomy 21 (mongolism). J. Periodont. Res., *3*:1, 1968.

57. Thoma, K. H., and Goldman, H. M.: Wandering and elongation of the teeth and pocket formation in paradontosis. J. Am. Dent. Assoc., *27*:335, 1940.

58. Waerhaug, J.: Subgingival plaque and loss of attachment in periodontosis as well as observed in autopsy material. J. Periodontol., *47*:636, 1976.

59. Wannenmacher, E.: Ursachen auf dem Gebiet der Paradentopathien. Zbl. Gesant. Zahn-, Mund-, Kieferheilk., *3*:81, 1938.

60. World Workshop in Periodontics. Ramfjord, S. P., Ash, M. M., and Kerr, D. A. (eds.). Ann Arbor, University of Michigan, 1966.

chapter twenty-three

The Epidemiology of Gingival and Periodontal Disease

Epidemiologic surveys conducted throughout the world point to the universal distribution of gingival and periodontal disease.[140, 142] From the earliest times, diseases of the supporting structures of the teeth have been recognized in almost every culture. Paleontologic studies indicate that periodontal disease existed in early man as far back as 2000 B.C.[134, 180]

Progress in the study of the periodontal diseases has been retarded because of several important factors that do not exist in the study of dental caries. The pathology of dental caries involves hard calcified tissues, whereas periodontal disease involves soft and hard tissues. Unlike dental caries, which has its greatest attack rate from the time the permanent teeth erupt in the mouth through the middle twenties, the greatest incidence and prevalence* of destructive periodontal disease do not occur until approximately 35 years of age. Finally, periodontal disease does not lend itself easily to objective measurement because the signs of periodontal pathology involve color changes in the soft tissues; swelling, bleeding, and bone changes that are reflected in crevice depth changes or pathologic pockets; and loss of tooth function because of mobility. Hence, examining the teeth for the signs of dental caries is far easier than is evaluating the pathologic parameters used to define periodontal diseases.[35]

Dental epidemiology, by simple definition, is the study of the **pattern (distribution)** and **dynamics** of dental diseases in a human population. **Pattern** implies that certain people are selected for attack by a disease and that the association between a disease and a people can be described by variables such as age, sex, racial-ethnic group, occupation, social characteristics, place of residence, susceptibility, and exposure to specific agents, to name only a few. The term **dynamics** refers to a temporal pattern (distribution) and is concerned with trends, cyclic patterns, and the time that elapses between the exposure to inciting factors and the onset of the specific disease.[151] Russell's definition of dental epidemiology may provide a better overview: "It is not so

---

Incidence is defined as the rate of occurrence of new disease in a population during a given period of time. *Prevalence* is the proportion of persons affected by a disease at a specific point in time, such as a cross-sectional survey.

much the study of disease as a process as it is a study of the condition of the people in whom the disease occurs."[144]

The **purpose or objective** of epidemiology is to increase understanding of the disease process, thereby leading to methods of control and prevention. In addition, epidemiology attempts to discover populations at high and low risk and to define the specific problem under investigation. The design, conduct, and interpretation of clinical trials of preventive and curative measures are also within its purview.[151] One of the most valuable techniques employed in dental epidemiology is the epidemiologic index.

Epidemiologic indices are attempts to quantitate clinical conditions on a graduated scale, thereby facilitating comparison among populations examined by the same criteria and methods. Unlike the absolute or definitive diagnosis that can be made for a solitary patient, an epidemiologic index (i.e., a numerical value) will estimate only the **relative** prevalence or occurrence of the clinical condition. In general, indices are actually **underestimates** of the true clinical condition. The **criteria** of a good epidemiologic index are that it must be easy to use, permit the examination of many people in a short period of time, define clinical conditions objectively, be highly reproducible in assessing a clinical condition when used by one or more examiners, be amenable to statistical analysis, and be strongly related numerically to the clinical stages of the specific disease under investigation. Calibration or standardization of the examiner(s) in reference to the use of an index's criteria is imperative to ensure the reliability of the data.[144]

In general, there are two types of dental indices. The first type of index measures the **number or proportion** of people in a population with or without a specific condition at a specific point in time or interval of time. The second type of dental index measures the **number** of people affected **and the severity** of the specific condition at a specific time or interval of time.[144] More explicitly, the second type of index will not only help to identify the person in the population affected with a specific condition, but it will also assess the condition under study on a graduated scale. Most of the indices described in this chapter will be of the latter type.

INDICES USED TO STUDY PERIODONTAL PROBLEMS

Although there are many indices for recording and quantitating the entities that make up

periodontal disease, space limitations permit the inclusion only of indices that historically contributed to our understanding of periodontal diseases or that are currently in frequent use. An excellent comprehensive review of indices not covered in this chapter is available in two symposium publications.[24, 27]

The indices that will be discussed in this chapter can, for the purposes of convenience and reason, be divided into those that evaluate:

A. The degree of inflammation of the gingival tissues
B. The degree of periodontal destruction
C. The amount of plaque accumulated
D. The amount of calculus present

A. Indices Used to Assess Gingival Inflammation

Papillary-Marginal-Attachment Index (Schour and Massler[155])

Originally the Papillary-Marginal-Attachment (PMA) Index was used to count the number of gingival units affected with gingivitis.[154, 155] This approach was predicated on the belief that the number of units affected correlated with the degree or severity of gingival inflammation. The facial surface of the gingiva around a tooth was divided into three gingival scoring units: the mesial dental papilla (P), the gingival margin (M), and the attached gingiva (A). The presence or absence of inflammation on each gingival unit was recorded as 1 or 0, respectively. The P, M, and A numerical values were totaled separately, added together, and expressed numerically as the PMA Index *score per person*. Although all of the facial tissues surrounding all of the teeth could be assessed in this manner, usually only the maxillary and mandibular incisors, canines, and premolars were examined. The developers of this index eventually added a severity component for assessing gingivitis; then, the papillary units (P) were scored on a scale of 0 to 5 and the marginal (M) and attached (A) gingivae were scored on a scale of 0 to 3.[91] The value of this index lies in its broad application to epidemiologic surveys and clinical trials and in its capacity for use on individual patients. The criteria for and approach to assessing gingival inflammation developed by Schour and Massler[155] have served as the basis for many of the indices to be discussed.

Examples of indices that are based on modifications of the PMA Index are those developed by Mühlemann and Mazor,[107] Lobene,[73] and Suomi and Barbano.[169] Mühlemann and Mazor[107] assessed the prevalence and severity of gingivitis only on the gingival and papillary units surrounding each tooth. The areas were scored on a scale of 0 to 4, and light probing was used to determine the extent of bleeding.

Examining only the papilla and the gingival margin of the facial and lingual surfaces surrounding each tooth (i.e., six scoring units per tooth), Lobene[73] assessed the presence of gingivitis on a scale of 0 to 3.

Suomi and Barbano[169] assessed the presence and severity of gingivitis on each papilla and the gingival margin of all of the teeth on a scale of 0 to 2. When this criterion was applied to the entire facial and lingual surfaces of eight selected teeth only (teeth numbered 3, 8, 12, 14, 19, 24, 28, and 30), it became known as the Dental Health Center Index (DHCI),[166] after the place where it was developed.

Periodontal Index (Russell[136])

The Periodontal Index (PI) was intended to estimate deeper periodontal disease than the PMA Index by measuring the presence or absence of gingival inflammation and its severity, pocket formation, and masticatory function. The criteria appearing in Table 23–1 are used to assess all of the gingival tissue circumscribing each tooth (i.e., all of the tissue circumscribing a tooth is considered a scoring or gingival unit). Because the PI measures both reversible and irreversible aspects of periodontal disease, it is an epidemiologic index with a true biologic gradient.[144] A PI *score per individual* is determined by adding all of the tooth scores and dividing by the number of teeth examined.

Since only a mouth mirror, and no calibrated probe or radiographs, is used when performing the PI examination, the results tend to under-

TABLE 23–1 THE PERIODONTAL INDEX (RUSSELL[136])

Score	Criteria and Scoring for Field Studies	Additional X-ray Criteria Followed in the Clinical Test
0	NEGATIVE. There is neither overt inflammation in the investing tissues nor loss of function due to destruction of supporting tissues.	Radiographic appearance is essentially normal.
1	MILD GINGIVITIS. There is an overt area of inflammation in the free gingivae, but this area does not circumscribe the tooth.	
2	GINGIVITIS. Inflammation completely circumscribes the tooth, but there is no apparent break in the epithelial attachment.	
4	(Used when radiographs are available.)	There is early, notchlike resorption of the alveolar crest.
6	GINGIVITIS WITH POCKET FORMATION. The epithelial attachment has been broken and there is a pocket (not merely a deepened gingival crevice due to swelling in free gingivae). There is no interference with normal masticatory function, the tooth is firm and has not drifted.	There is horizontal bone loss involving the entire alveolar crest, up to half of the length of the tooth root.
8	ADVANCED DESTRUCTION WITH LOSS OF MASTICATORY FUNCTION. The tooth may be loose; may have drifted; may sound dull on percussion with a metallic instrument; may be depressible in its socket.	There is advanced bone loss, involving more than one-half of the length of the tooth root, or a definite infrabony pocket with widening of the periodontal ligament. There may be root resorption, or rarefaction at the apex.

RULE: When in doubt, assign the lesser scores.

$$\text{Periodontal Index Score per Person} = \frac{\text{Sum of individual scores}}{\text{Number of teeth present}}$$

Clinical Condition	Group PI Scores*	Stage of Disease
Clinically normal supportive tissues	0 to 0.2	
Simple gingivitis	0.3 to 0.9	
Beginning destructive periodontal disease	0.7 to 1.9	Reversible
Established destructive periodontal disease	1.6 to 5.0	Irreversible
Terminal disease	3.8 to 8.0	

*From reference 132.

TABLE 23–2 CRITERIA FOR SEVERAL COMPONENTS OF THE
PERIODONTAL DISEASE INDEX (RAMFJORD[130])

Gingival Status (Gingivitis Index)
0 = Absence of signs of inflammation.
1 = Mild to moderate inflammatory gingival changes, not extending around the tooth.
2 = Mild to moderately severe gingivitis extending all around the tooth.
3 = Severe gingivitis characterized by marked redness, swelling, tendency to bleed, and ulceration.[131]

Crevicular Measurements
A. If the gingival margin is on the enamel, measure from the gum margin to the cemento-enamel junction and
record the measurement. If the epithelial attachment is on the crown and the cemento-enamel junction
cannot be felt by the probe, record the depth of the gingival sulcus on the crown. Then record the distance
from the gingival margin to the bottom of the pocket if the probe can be moved apically to the cemento-
enamel junction without resistance or pain. The distance from the cemento-enamel junction to the bottom of
the pocket can then be found by subtracting the first from the second measurement.
B. If the gingival margin is on the cementum, record the distance from the cemento-enamel junction to the
gingival margin as a minus value. Then record the distance from the cemento-enamel junction to the bottom
of the gingival sulcus as a plus value. Both loss of attachment and actual sulcus depth can easily be assessed
from the scores.[131]

Periodontal Disease Index (PDI) Criteria for Surveys
If the gingival sulcus in none of the measured areas extended apically to the cemento-enamel junction, the
recorded score for gingivitis is the PDI score for that tooth. If the gingival sulcus in any of the two measured
areas extended apically to the cemento-enamel junction but not more than 3 mm (including 3 mm in any area),
the tooth is assigned a PDI score of 4. The score for gingivitis is then disregarded in the PDI score for that
tooth. If the gingival sulcus in either of the two recorded areas of the tooth extends apically to from 3 to 6 mm
(including 6 mm) in relation to the cemento-enamel junction, the tooth is assigned a PDI score of 5 (again, the
gingivitis score is disregarded). Whenever the gingival sulcus extends more than 6 mm apically to the cemento-
enamel junction in any of the measured areas of the tooth, the score of 6 is assigned as the PDI score for that
tooth (again disregarding the gingivitis score).[131]

Shick-Ash Modification[164] of Plaque Criteria
0 = Absence of dental plaque.
1 = Dental plaque in the interproximal or at the gingival margin covering less than one third of the gingival
half of the facial or lingual surface of the tooth.
2 = Dental plaque covering more than one third but less than two thirds of the gingival half of the facial or
lingual surface of the tooth.
3 = Dental plaque covering two thirds or more of the gingival half of the facial or gingival surface of the tooth.

Calculus Criteria
0 = Absence of calculus.
1 = Supragingival calculus extending only slightly below the free gingival margin (not more than 1 mm).
2 = Moderate amount of supra- and subgingival calculus or subgingival calculus alone.
3 = An abundance of supra- and subgingival calculus.[131]

estimate the true level of periodontal disease, especially early bone loss, in a population.[163] The index was developed for use in epidemiologic surveys, but with care it may be used in clinical trials. The abstractness of the numerical score, an often-stated criticism of epidemiologic indices, is minimized in the PI because group scores may be associated with the clinical conditions of periodontal disease (Table 23–1).[143]

The significance of the PI lies in the fact that more data have been assembled using it than any other index of periodontal disease. Thus, much of what we know about the distribution of periodontal disease in the United States and throughout the world resulted from using this index. The PI also is used in the National Health Survey (NHS),[62] the largest ongoing health survey in the United States.

Several years ago, the World Health Organization (WHO) discontinued the PI and the Simplified Oral Hygiene Index (OHI-S) as its recommended procedures for assessing periodontal status in surveys in favor of the Periodontal Status Index (PSI).[181] The PSI assesses oral hygiene, gingivitis, calculus, and periodontal health. Its advantages over the PI and OHI-S are that it simplifies the examination and recording of oral conditions and assesses treatment requirements in terms of the time needed to complete them. In a study that compared the PSI with the PI and OHI-S, Cutress et al.[30] found that the PSI lacked quantitation and was difficult to use in diagnosing severe gingivitis, as well as localized and general conditions. The PI and OHI-S are clearly more objective, sensitive, and quantitative than the PSI. The advocation by the

WHO of the PSI in preference to the PI and the OHI-S at this point in its development seems to be premature.[30]

Gingivitis Component of the Periodontal Disease Index (Ramfjord[130])

The Periodontal Disease Index (PDI) is similar to the PI in that both are used to measure the presence and severity of periodontal disease. The PDI does so by combining the assessments of gingivitis and gingival sulcus depth on six selected teeth (numbered 3, 9, 12, 19, 25, and 28). Calculus and plaque are also examined to assist in formulating a comprehensive assessment of periodontal status. Only gingivitis will be discussed here. Other components of the PDI will be described in later sections of this chapter.

The tissue circumscribing each of six selected teeth is assessed using the criteria described in Table 23–2. The criteria combine elements of the PMA Index and the PI. The six index teeth have been tested as reliable indicators for the various regions of the mouth. A numerical score for the *gingival status component* of the PDI (i.e., the Gingivitis Index score per person) is obtained by adding all of the gingival units and dividing by the number of teeth present.[131] The PDI has been used in epidemiologic surveys, longitudinal studies of periodontal disease, and clinical trials of therapeutic or preventive procedures. It is considered the gingival index of choice in longitudinal studies of periodontal disease.[47]

Gingival Index (Löe and Silness[75])

The Gingival Index (GI) was developed solely for the purpose of assessing the severity of gingivitis and its location in four possible areas. The tissues surrounding each tooth are divided into four gingival scoring units: distal-facial papilla, facial margin, mesial-facial papilla, and the entire lingual gingival margin. Unlike the facial surface, the lingual surface is not subdivided in an effort to minimize examiner variability in scoring, since it will most likely be viewed indirectly with a mouth mirror. A blunt instrument, such as a periodontal pocket probe, is used to assess the bleeding potential of the tissues. Each of the four gingival units is assessed according to the criteria appearing in Table 23–3.

Totaling the scores around each tooth yields the GI score for the *area*. If the scores around each tooth are totaled and divided by four, the GI score for the *tooth* is obtained. Totaling all of the scores per tooth and dividing by the number of teeth examined provides the GI *score per person*. The GI may be used to evaluate a segment of the mouth or a group of teeth in the same way.[74]

Except for the consideration of bleeding, the criteria used in the GI are similar to those used by Lobene.[73] The numerical scores of the GI may be associated with varying degrees of clinical gingivitis as follows:

Gingival Scores	Condition
0.1–1.0	Mild gingivitis
1.1–2.0	Moderate gingivitis
2.1–3.0	Severe gingivitis

The index can be used to determine the prevalence and severity of gingivitis in epidemiologic surveys, as well as in the individual dentition. This latter attribute has contributed to making the GI the index of choice in controlled clinical trials of preventive or therapeutic agents.[47]

TABLE 23–3 CRITERIA FOR THE GINGIVAL INDEX (LÖE AND SILNESS[75]) AND THE PLAQUE INDEX (SILNESS AND LÖE[165])

Gingival Index (GI)
0 = Normal gingiva.
1 = Mild inflammation, slight change in color, slight edema; *no bleeding on palpation.*
2 = Moderate inflammation, redness, edema, and glazing; *bleeding on palpation.*
3 = Severe inflammation, marked redness and edema; ulcerations; *tendency to spontaneous bleeding.*[74]

Plaque Index (PlI)
0 = No plaque in the gingival area.
1 = A film of plaque adhering to the free gingival margin and adjacent area of the tooth. The plaque may be recognized only by running a probe across the tooth surface.
2 = Moderate accumulation of soft deposits within the gingival pocket and on the gingival margin and/or adjacent tooth surface, which can be seen by the naked eye.
3 = Abundance of soft matter within the gingival pocket and/or on the gingival margin and adjacent tooth surface.[74]

Indices of Gingival Bleeding

So far, two indices that combine the clinical parameters of inflammation and bleeding have been described. The Sulcus Bleeding Index (SBI) of Mühlemann and Mazor[107] uses bleeding upon gentle probing as the first criterion for indicating gingival inflammation. In 1971, Mühlemann and Son[108] added an additional category to the original criteria, resulting in a 0 to 5 scale for assessing inflammation or sulcular bleeding. Both of Mühlemann's indices are predicated on an understanding of sulcular bleeding as a precursor of gingival inflammation and as the first sign of inflammation. The GI of Löe and Silness,[75] on the other hand, uses the presence of a slight color change and the absence of bleeding when a blunt instrument is used to palpate the soft tissue wall at the gingival margin to indicate initial gingival inflammation. Although the correlation between the two parameters (inflammation and bleeding) is not perfect, the histologic evidence for associating inflammation with the GI criteria is stronger than is that for an association between gingival fluid flow and the SBI. From the epidemiologic viewpoint, it is better to measure single parameters than to combine several into one measure. As it happens, the criteria for the GI can easily be separated into an index of gingival inflammation and an index of gingival bleeding without destroying the integrity of the scoring system.

Several other indices are worthy of mention. The Bleeding Points Index (Lenox and Kopczyk[72]) was developed to assess a patient's oral hygiene performance. It assesses the presence or absence of gingival bleeding interproximally and on the facial and lingual surfaces of each tooth. A periodontal probe is drawn horizontally through the gingival crevice of a quadrant, and the gingiva is examined for bleeding after 30 seconds. The Gingival Bleeding Index of Carter and Barnes[23] also assesses the presence or absence of gingival bleeding, but only at the interproximal spaces, using unwaxed dental floss. The floss is thought to assess a larger area more quickly than a periodontal probe, and it can be used by both the professional and the patient when the latter is instructed to perform self-evaluation in a control program. The Gingival Bleeding Index (GBI) of Ainamo and Bay[1] was developed as an easy and suitable technique for the practitioner to assess a patient's progress in plaque control. The presence or absence of gingival bleeding is determined by gentle probing of the gingival crevice with a periodontal probe.

The appearance of bleeding within 10 seconds indicates a positive score that is expressed as a percentage of the total number of gingival margins examined.

In conclusion, the use of gingival bleeding indices is desirable because bleeding is a more objective indicator than early gingival color changes and because it provides evidence of recent plaque exposure.[72] *In general, the indices that utilize palpation or dental floss are more suitable for diagnosis and assessing a patient's progress in plaque control than are indices that utilize probing of the gingival sulcus. The latter indices, however, are more suitable for assessing the effects of subgingival periodontal therapy.*

Gingival Periodontal Index (O'Leary et al.[119])

The Gingival Periodontal Index (GPI) is a modification of the PDI of Ramfjord for the purpose of screening individuals to determine who needs periodontal treatment. The GPI assesses three components of periodontal disease: gingival status; periodontal status (crevice depth); and, collectively, materia alba, calculus, and overhanging restorations. The latter triad is independently called the **Irritation Index.** Only the criteria for the gingival status component will be described in this section.

The maxillary and mandibular arches are each divided into three segments: the six anterior teeth, the left posterior teeth, and the right posterior teeth. The primary objective in using the index is to determine the tooth, or its surrounding tissues, with the severest condition within each segment. Hence, each segment is assessed for each of the three components of periodontal disease described above. The specific criteria for the gingival status component of the GPI are as follows:

0 = Tissue tightly adapted to the teeth, firm consistency with physiologic architecture.
1 = Slight to moderate inflammation, as indicated by changes in color and consistency, involving one or more teeth in the same segment but not completely surrounding any one tooth.
2 = The above changes either singularly or combined completely encircle one or more teeth in a segment.
3 = Marked inflammation, as indicated by loss of surface continuity (ulceration), spontaneous hemorrhage, loss of faciolingual continuity or any interdental papilla,

marked deviation from normal contour, such as gross thickening or enlargement covering more than one third of the anatomic crown, recession, and clefts.

The area with the highest score counts as the gingival score for the entire segment, and the *gingival status* for the mouth is obtained by dividing the sum of the gingival scores by the number of segments.

The GPI has been used extensively in military populations. Unlike the traditional indices used in epidemiology (which attempt primarily to assess the status of a specific disease condition, with only the crudest suggestion of determining treatment needs), the GPI was developed for the specific purpose of detecting periodontal disease early so that treatment may be instituted promptly.[115]

Another index, the Periodontal Treatment Need System (PTNS), has been used in Oslo with interesting results.[47] It attempts to place individuals into one of four classes based on treatment procedures relative to time requirements. It considers the presence or absence of gingivitis and plaque and the presence of pockets of 5 mm or deeper in each quadrant of the mouth, as shown in Table 23–4.

B. Indices Used to Measure Periodontal Destruction

In 1973 Ramfjord summarized the state of the art in measuring periodontal destruction by saying "categorically . . . none of the present periodontal indices provide data with adequate details for studies and clinical trials involving loss or gain of periodontium."[132] Although little has changed since this statement was made, it is possible and necessary to make the most of what is known and to describe the epidemiologic indices and techniques that have made it possible to quantitate the irreversible loss of alveolar bone. At a workshop on quantitative evaluation of periodontal diseases, the majority of participants agreed that the destruction of bone is still the most important criterion for assessing the severity of periodontal disease.[128] Some of the approaches to measuring bone loss that will be discussed in this section are gingival crevice measurements, radiographic evaluations of bone loss, and assessments of gingival recession and tooth mobility.

Gingival Sulcus Measurement Component of the Periodontal Disease Index (Ramfjord[131])

The technique developed by Ramfjord for measuring gingival sulcus depth with a calibrated periodontal probe is the most quantitative method currently available for assessing periodontal support. It involves measuring the distance from the cemento-enamel junction to the free gingival margin and the distance from the free gingival margin to the bottom of the gingival sulcus or pocket. The difference between the two measurements yields the gingival *sulcus depth,* which translates into epithelial attachment level. This is considered the most important clinical measurement in determining the status of the periodontium. Ramfjord's technique is considered useful in epidemiologic surveys, longitudinal studies of periodontal disease, and clinical trials of preventive and therapeutic agents.[132]

The first measurement in this two-step process may be used in assessing **gingival loss (recession) or gain.** It is considered more accurate and reliable in clinical trials than the Gingival Recession Index used in epidemiologic surveys.[132]

The probe used for the sulcus depth measurements is graduated in 3-mm increments. All measurements are rounded to the nearest millimeter. Anything close to 0.5 mm is rounded to the lower whole number. This "underscoring" has increased the reproducibility of measurements using the above crite-

TABLE 23–4 CRITERIA FOR THE PERIODONTAL TREATMENT NEED SYSTEM (PTNS) CLASSIFICATION*

PTNS classification	Unit	Plaque	Calculus and/or overhangs	Inflammation	Pocket depth
Class 0	mouth	no	no	no	not considered
Class A	mouth	yes	no	yes	≤ 5 mm.
Class B	quadrant	yes	yes	yes	< 5 mm.
Class C	quadrant	yes	yes	yes	> 5 mm.

*Adapted from Bellini, H. T.: A System to Determine the Periodontal Therapeutic Needs of a Population. Oslo, Universitetsforlagets Trykningssentral, 1973.

ria. The placement of the periodontal probe in a standardized position relative to the tooth and the gingival crevice is also crucial. Measurements are made on the facial surface, equidistant between the mesial and distal surfaces; the mesial-facial line angle at the interproximal contact area; the lingual surface, equidistant between the mesial and distal surfaces; and the distal-lingual line angle at the interproximal contact area. In making the facial-mesial and distal-lingual measurements, the probe is in contact with the adjacent tooth.[131] Measurements at the distal-lingual line angle are considered optional because their omission does not significantly decrease the accuracy of the Periodontal Disease Index (PDI) score.[132] The criteria developed by Ramfjord for making sulcular determinations appear in Table 23–2.

When the measurements are rounded to the nearest millimeter, as described above, the Ramfjord criteria are most applicable to longitudinal studies of periodontal disease and clinical trials of preventive or therapeutic agents. Either the six teeth (teeth numbered 3, 9, 12, 19, 25, and 28) used by Ramfjord or whatever teeth are appropriate to the objective of the study may be assessed.

In an epidemiologic survey (i.e., cross-sectional survey), when the purpose is to determine the prevalence of total periodontal disease, only the six index teeth should be used. The set of criteria for a cross-sectional survey is called the **Periodontal Disease Index (PDI)** for surveys and appears in Table 23–2. The PDI score for the *individual* is obtained by totaling the scores of the teeth and dividing by the number of teeth examined (a maximum of six).[131]

Radiographic Approaches to Measuring Bone Loss

In general, the use of radiographs in the study of the epidemiology of periodontal disease would appear to overcome some of the criticisms of the more subjective clinical measurements. Radiographs present a permanent objective record of interdental bone levels; in longitudinal studies they may present less variability than poorly standardized dental examiners; and they offer the only method available for making crown and root measurements. Their disadvantages are that they are not useful in the buccal or lingual assessment of bone level; they do not provide adequate information on soft tissue attachment; and their value may be lost if improper angulation is used[40] (see Chapter 32).

There are only a few indices that have been specifically designed to evaluate the radiographic assessment of periodontal disease, but other more precise techniques for making reasonably accurate measurements from radiographs have been developed.

GINGIVAL-BONE COUNT INDEX (DUNNING AND LEACH[36]). The Gingival-Bone (GB) Count Index records the gingival condition and the level of the crest of the alveolar bone. The bone level is assessed by clinical examination, but radiographs are recommended for greater accuracy. The GB Count Index is scored as shown in Table 23–5. The average gingival (G) score per person is added to the average bone (B) score per person to yield the *GB count per person.*

Sheiham and Striffler[163] developed an index similar to the bone count component of the

---

TABLE 23–5 THE GINGIVAL-BONE (GB) COUNT (DUNNING AND LEACH[36])

Gingival score (One score is assigned to each tooth studied. A mean is then computed for the whole mouth.)

Negative	0
Mild gingivitis involving the free gingiva (margin, papilla, or both)	1
Moderate gingivitis involving both free and attached gingivae	2
Severe gingivitis with enlargement and easy hemorrhage	3

Bone score (One score is assigned to each tooth studied. A mean is then computed for the whole mouth.)

No bone loss	0
Incipient bone loss or notching of the alveolar crest	1
Bone loss approximating one fourth of root length or pocket formation one side not over one half root length	2
Bone loss approximating one half of root length or pocket formation one side not over three fourths root length; mobility slight*	3
Bone loss approximating three fourths of root length or pocket formation one side to apex; mobility moderate*	4
Bone loss complete; mobility marked*	5
Maximum possible GB count per person	8

*If mobility or impairment of masticatory function varies considerably from that to be expected with bone loss seen, the score may be altered up or down one point.

GB Count Index. The criteria for evaluating radiographs are as follows:

0 = Normal.
4 = Lack of continuity of cortical plate at the crest of the interdental bone, with possible widening of the periodontal ligament.
5 = Up to one third of supporting bone lost.
6 = More than one third and up to two thirds of supporting bone lost.
7 = More than two thirds of supporting bone lost.[40]

The strength of each of the above indices is in epidemiologic surveys in which evaluation time is limited because of large study populations.

TECHNIQUES USED TO OBTAIN MORE ACCURATE MEASUREMENTS OF RADIOGRAPHS. Miller and Seidler[101, 102] used a scale of 0 to 5 to assess tooth–to–marginal bone level ratios from radiographs. A percentage value was used as the index of periodontal disease. Schei et al.[153] introduced a graded scale to estimate bone loss using the cemento-enamel junction as a point of reference. Bjorn et al.[14, 15] developed a method involving the projection of radiographs at a fixed distance onto a screen with a graded scale of 20 divisions. The number of divisions between the most coronal level of bone and the apical base of the bone was counted.

One additional technique that offers great practicality is the use of wire grids (with 1-mm squares) embedded in thin plastic that are attached to the radiograph before exposure.[44, 170] Either direct observation or projection of the radiograph permits measurements relative to the cemento-enamel junction rounded to the nearest 0.5 mm.

The time constraints of epidemiologic surveys limit the use of radiographic assessment of periodontal support to longitudinal studies of periodontal disease, whether descriptive or experimental.

Techniques Used to Measure Horizontal Tooth Mobility*

The most subjective method used to assess horizontal tooth mobility was described by Miller[100] and involves assessing the mobility of a tooth when held between two instruments on a scale of 0 to 3. The numerical values correspond to movement in 1-mm increments. Although this approach is useful in clinical diagnosis and treatment planning, it is of little value in longitudinal or clinical studies.

Parfitt[121, 123] used an electronic instrument to measure tooth movement with an accuracy of 0.001 mm $\pm$ 7 per cent. Picton[125, 126] developed a method that used resistance-wire strain gauges to measure any movement relative to the adjacent tooth. A system using electronic transducers was developed by Körber and Körber.[68-70] All of these devices are complex, and the time required to use them is prohibitive for epidemiologic surveys or large clinical trials.

Mühlemann[104, 105] has developed two instruments for measuring tooth mobility: the macroperiodontometer and microperiodontometer. Although many studies have been completed using the first device, its value is limited to specific areas of the mouth.[106] The latter device is more difficult to master, and its results are less reproducible.[116]

The Periodontometer (United States Air Force School of Aerospace Medicine) developed by O'Leary and Rudd[117] has been used more extensively than any other device to measure tooth mobility. It measures the facial or palatal deflection of tooth mobility in increments of 0.0001 inch when 500 grams of force are applied. It requires two investigators, extensive training in its use, and a minimum of 8 to 10 minutes per quadrant. Therefore, its use can be considered only in clinical trials.[116]

C. Indices Used to Measure Plaque Accumulation

In general, most of the indices used to measure plaque accumulation utilize a numerical scale to measure the extent of the surface area of a tooth covered by plaque. For our purposes, *plaque* will be defined as a nonmineralized soft tooth deposit that includes debris and materia alba. No attempt will be made to present the various indices according to the subtle differences that exist in their definitions of plaque, debris, and materia alba (i.e., the terms *plaque* and *debris* will be used interchangeably unless otherwise stated) (see Chapters 25 and 26).

Plaque Component of the Periodontal Disease Index (Ramfjord[131])

The first index that attempted to use a numerical scale to assess the extent of plaque

---

*The reader is referred to an excellent review of this subject by Timothy O'Leary.[116]

covering the surface area of a tooth was developed by Ramfjord. The plaque component of the Periodontal Disease Index (PDI) is used on the six teeth selected by Ramfjord (teeth numbered 3, 9, 12, 19, 25, and 28) after staining with Bismarck brown solution. The criteria measure the presence and extent of plaque on a scale of 0 to 3, looking specifically in all interproximal facial and lingual surfaces of the index teeth. The criteria are suitable for longitudinal studies of periodontal disease.[131] Even though the plaque component is not a part of the PDI score, it is helpful in a total assessment of periodontal status.

Shick and Ash[164] modified the original criteria of Ramfjord by excluding consideration of the interproximal areas of the teeth and "restricting the scoring of plaque to the gingival half"[132] of the facial and lingual surfaces of the index teeth. The criteria for the Shick-Ash modification of the Ramfjord plaque criteria appear in Table 23–2.

The plaque *score per person* is obtained by totaling all of the individual tooth scores and dividing by the number of teeth examined. These modified plaque criteria are suitable for clinical trials of preventive or therapeutic agents.

Simplified Oral Hygiene Index (Green and Vermillion[54])

In the early development of the indices used to measure gingivitis and periodontal disease, it became apparent that the data lacked meaning or significance unless the level of oral hygiene or cleanliness was evaluated as a separate component. The lack of a simple, objective set of criteria that minimized examiner variability prompted Green and Vermillion to develop the Oral Hygiene Index (OHI).[53] Their goal was to develop a measuring technique that could be used in "studying the epidemiology of periodontal disease and oral calculus, when assessing toothbrushing efficiency, and when evaluating the dental health practices of a community and the immediate as well as the long-term effects of dental health education" programs.[52] Realizing that it was neither necessary nor practical to assess all of the teeth to determine a person's level of oral cleanliness, Green and Vermillion selected six index tooth surfaces that were representative of all anterior and posterior segments of the mouth based on whole-mouth examinations. This modification of the OHI was called the Simplified Oral Hygiene Index (OHI-S).[54] The

OHI-S measures the surface area of the tooth covered by debris and calculus. The imprecise term *debris* was used because it was not practical to observe the soft deposits microscopically and make the subtle distinctions between plaque, debris, and materia alba. In addition, the practicality of determining the weight and thickness of the soft deposits prompted the assumption that the dirtier the mouth, the greater the tooth surface area covered by debris. This assumption also implied a time factor, because the longer oral hygiene practices are neglected, the greater is the likelihood that the surface area of the tooth will be covered by debris.

The OHI-S consists of two components: a Simplified Debris Index (DI-S) and a Simplified Calculus Index (CI-S). Each component is assessed on a scale of 0 to 3. Only a mouth mirror and a shepherd's crook or sickle-type dental explorer, and no disclosing agent, are used for the examination. The six tooth surfaces examined in the OHI-S are the facial surfaces of the teeth numbered 3, 8, 14, and 24 and the lingual surfaces of the teeth numbered 19 and 30. Each tooth surface is divided horizontally into gingival, middle, and incisal thirds.

For the DI-S a dental explorer is placed on the incisal third of the tooth and moved toward the gingival third according to the criteria illustrated in Figure 23–1. The DI-S *score per person* is obtained by totaling the debris score per tooth surface and dividing by the number of the surfaces examined.

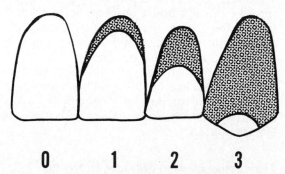

Figure 23–1 Criteria for Scoring Oral Debris (DI-S) Component of the Simplified Oral Hygiene Index (OHI-S). (From Greene, J. C., and Vermillion, J. R.: J. Am. Dent. Assoc., 68:7, 1964.)
0—No debris or stain present.
1—Soft debris covering not more than one third of the tooth surface, or the presence of extrinsic stains without other debris regardless of surface area covered.
2—Soft debris covering more than one third but not more than two thirds of the exposed tooth surface.
3—Soft debris covering more than two thirds of the exposed tooth surface.

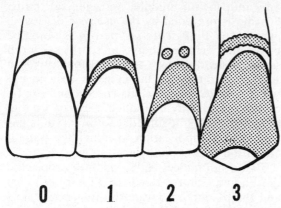

Figure 23–2 Criteria for Scoring Calculus (CI-S) Component of the Simplified Oral Hygiene Index (OHI-S). (From Greene, J. C., and Vermillion, J. R.: J. Am. Dent. Assoc., 68:7, 1964.)

0—No calculus present.

1—Supragingival calculus covering not more than one third of the exposed tooth surface.

2—Supragingival calculus covering more than one third but not more than two thirds of the exposed tooth surface or the presence of individual flecks of subgingival calculus around the cervical portion of the tooth or both.

3—Supragingival calculus covering more than two thirds of the exposed tooth surface or a continuous heavy band of subgingival calculus around the cervical portion of the tooth or both.

The CI-S assessment is performed by gently placing a dental explorer into the distal gingival crevice and drawing it subgingivally from the distal contact area to the mesial contact area (one half of a tooth's circumference is considered a scoring unit). The criteria for scoring the calculus component of the OHI-S appear in Figure 23–2. The CI-S *score per person* is obtained by totaling the calculus scores per tooth surface and dividing by the number of surfaces examined. The OHI-S *score per person* is the total of the DI-S and CI-S scores per person.

The clinical levels of oral cleanliness for debris that can be associated with group DI-S scores are as follows[52]:

Good	0.0–0.6
Fair	0.7–1.8
Poor	1.9–3.0

The clinical levels of oral hygiene that can be associated with group OHI-S scores are as follows[52]:

Good	0.0–1.2
Fair	1.3–3.0
Poor	3.1–6.0

The significance of the OHI-S is that, like the Periodontal Index (PI) of Russell,[136] it has been used extensively throughout the world and has contributed greatly to our understanding of periodontal disease. It is also used in the National Health Survey (NHS).[63] The high degree of correlation ($r = 0.82$)[157] between the OHI-S and the PI makes it possible, knowing one of the two scores, to calculate the other score using regression analysis.[51] The major strength of the OHI-S is its use in epidemiologic surveys[82] and in evaluating dental health education programs (longitudinal). It can also be used to evaluate an individual's level of oral cleanliness and, to a more limited extent, in clinical trials. The index is easy to use because the criteria are objective, the examination may be performed quickly, and a high level of reproducibility is possible with a minimum of training sessions.[52]

Turesky-Gilmore-Glickman Modification[175] of the Quigley-Hein[129] Plaque Index

In 1962, Quigley and Hein[129] presented the results of a plaque index that focused attention on the gingival third of the tooth surface. They examined only the facial surfaces of the anterior teeth, after utilizing a basic fuchsin mouthwash as a disclosing agent, using a numerical scoring system of 0 to 5.

Turesky et al.[175] strengthened the objectivity of the Quigley-Hein criteria by redefining the scores of the gingival third area. The Turesky-Gilmore-Glickman modification of the Quigley-Hein criteria appears in Table 23–6. They assessed plaque on the facial and lingual surfaces of all of the teeth after using a disclosing agent. A plaque *score per person* was obtained by totaling all of the plaque scores and dividing by the number of surfaces examined. This system of scoring plaque is relatively easy to use because of the objective definitions of each

TABLE 23–6 TURESKY-GILMORE-GLICKMAN MODIFICATION[175] OF THE QUIGLEY-HEIN PLAQUE INDEX[129]

0 =	No plaque.
1 =	Separate flecks of plaque at the cervical margin of the tooth.
2 =	A thin, continuous band of plaque (up to 1 mm) at the cervical margin.
3 =	A band of plaque wider than 1 mm but covering less than one third of the crown.
4 =	Plaque covering at least one third but less than two thirds of the crown.
5 =	Plaque covering two thirds or more of the crown[80]

numerical score. The strength of this plaque index is its application to longitudinal studies and clinical trials of preventive and therapeutic agents. Mandel has suggested that, if the Turesky-Gilmore-Glickman modification of the Quigley-Hein criteria were applied to the distal, middle, and mesial thirds of the facial and lingual surfaces of the teeth, it would be the plaque index of choice in clinical trials.[80, 81]

Glass Criteria for Scoring Debris[48]

The only other index that assesses the presence and extent of debris accumulation is a system developed by Glass[48] for evaluating toothbrushing efficacy. All of the teeth are scored, and the facial and lingual surfaces are scored as a unit. In addition to assessing debris, Glass also developed criteria for measuring gingival changes, tooth stain, and calculus accumulation. Only the debris criteria will be described here. The criteria for scoring debris according to the Glass criteria are as follows:

0 = No visible debris.
1 = Debris visible at gingival margin—but discontinuous—less than 1 mm in height.
2 = Debris continuous at gingival margin—greater than 1 mm in height.
3 = Debris involving entire gingival third of tooth.
4 = Debris generally scattered over tooth surface.

The debris index *score per person* is obtained by totaling all of the debris scores per tooth and dividing by the number of teeth examined. Because it places more emphasis on the gingival third of the tooth than does the OHI-S, the strength of this index is in clinical trials of preventive or therapeutic agents.[80]

Patient Hygiene Performance Index (Podshadley and Haley[127])

The Patient Hygiene Performance (PHP) Index[127] was the first index developed for the sole purpose of assessing an individual's performance in removing debris after toothbrushing instruction (i.e., after patient education). It assesses the presence or absence of debris as a 1 or a 0, respectively, using the six OHI-S teeth (six surfaces). The PHP Index is relatively more sensitive than the OHI-S because it divides each tooth surface into five areas: three longitudinal thirds—distal, middle, and mesial; the middle third is subdivided horizon-

tally into incisal, middle, and gingival thirds. Scoring is preceded by the use of a disclosing agent. The PHP *score per person* is obtained by totaling the five subdivision scores per tooth surface and dividing by the number of tooth surfaces examined. This index is easy to use because of its dichotomous criteria and can be performed quickly. Although it can be used in group studies of health education, its value lies chiefly in its application to individual patient education (i.e., as an education aid).

Two other indices with a similar purpose are the Plaque Control Record (O'Leary et al.[118]) and the plaque portion of the Bleeding Points Index (Lenox and Kopczyk[72]).

Plaque Index (Silness and Löe[165])

The Plaque Index (PlI) is unique among the indices described so far because it ignores the coronal extent of plaque on the tooth surface area and assesses only the **thickness** of plaque at the gingival area of the tooth. Since it was developed as a component to parallel the Gingival Index (GI) of Löe and Silness,[75] it examines the same scoring units of the teeth: distal-facial, facial, mesial-facial, and lingual surfaces. A mouth mirror, dental explorer, and air drying of the teeth are used to assess plaque in the PlI. Unlike most indices, it does not exclude or substitute for teeth with gingival restorations or crowns. Either all or only selected teeth may be used in the PlI. The criteria for the PlI of Silness and Löe appear in Table 23–3.

The PlI score for the **area** is obtained by totaling the four plaque scores per tooth. If the sum of the PlI scores per tooth is divided by four, the PlI score for the *tooth* is obtained. The PlI *score per person* is obtained by adding the PlI scores per tooth and dividing by the number of teeth examined. The PlI may be obtained for a segment of the mouth or a group of teeth in a similar manner.

The strength of the PlI is in its application to longitudinal studies and clinical trials. In spite of the studies that have been conducted to ensure the reliability of the PlI data, the assessment of plaque thickness is so subjective that it requires highly trained and experienced examiners to ensure valid data.[80]

Modified Navy Plaque Index[39]

This index was developed for the purpose of evaluating oral hygiene performance (health education) in Navy personnel. It records the presence or absence of plaque, by a score of 1 or 0, respectively, on nine areas of each tooth surface of the six index teeth used by Ramfjord. Each tooth surface is divided horizontally into a gingival, middle, and incisal third. The gingival third is further divided horizontally, following the scalloped shape of the gingiva, into two halves. The lower half is immediately adjacent to the gingiva and does not exceed 1 mm in width. Both of the gingival halves are divided longitudinally into distal, middle, and mesial thirds. The middle third (horizontally) of the tooth surface is divided into a distal and mesial half, and the incisal third is coronal to the contact area and is not subdivided. This approach emphasizes the gingival two thirds of the tooth, with the gingival third weighted twice as heavily (i.e., the plaque in closest proximity to the gingival tissues is weighted more heavily because of its importance). A Modified Navy Plaque Index *score per person* is obtained by totaling all nine of the subdivision scores per tooth surface and dividing by the number of tooth surfaces examined. Like the PHP Index of Podshadley and Haley, the Modified Navy Plaque Index is of value in assessing health education programs and the ability of individuals to perform oral hygiene practices.

Other Plaque Indices

Plaque is one of the two factors measured in the Irritants Index,[115, 119] which is a component of the Gingival Periodontal Index (GPI) of O'Leary et al. The presence and coronal extent of plaque are scored on a scale of 0 to 3. Other factors that contribute to the Irritants Index are supra- and subgingival calculus and subgingival irritants, such as overhanging or deficient restorations.

Bjorby and Löe[13] developed a Retention Index that not only examined supra- and subgingival calculus, but also grossly assessed dental caries and the quality of the margins of restorations. Collectively, all of these parameters were scored on a numerical scale of 0 to 3.[74]

D. Indices Used to Measure Calculus

In general, the indices used to assess calculus may be conveniently divided into those that are most appropriate to epidemiologic surveys; those that are appropriate to longitudinal studies, with an examination every 3 to 6 months;

and those that are used in short-term clinical studies, usually no longer than 6 weeks.

Calculus Component of the Simplified Oral Hygiene Index (Greene and Vermillion[54])

The Simplified Calculus Index (CI-S) component of the Simplified Oral Hygiene Index (OHI-S) was presented in detail under "Indices Used to Measure Plaque Accumulation" because it is less separable from its scoring system than any of the other indices that combine several component measures. The value of the CI-S component is its application to epidemiologic surveys and longitudinal studies of periodontal disease.[52] Figure 23–2 presents the specific criteria of the OHI-S used to assess calculus.

Calculus Component of the Periodontal Disease Index (Ramfjord[130])

The calculus component of the Periodontal Disease Index (PDI) assesses the presence and extent of calculus on six index teeth (i.e., the facial and lingual surfaces of teeth numbered 3, 9, 12, 19, 25, and 28) on a numerical scale of 0 to 3. A mouth mirror and a dental explorer and/or a periodontal probe are used in the examination. The criteria for assigning a score to each tooth surface for the calculus component of the PDI appear in Table 23–2.

The calculus scores per tooth are totaled and then divided by the number of teeth examined to yield the calculus *score per person*. Like the CI-S of the OHI-S, the calculus component of the PDI has a high degree of examiner reproducibility, can be performed quickly, and has its best application in epidemiologic surveys and longitudinal studies.[131]

Probe Method of Calculus Assessment (Volpe et al.[177])

The Probe Method of Calculus Assessment was developed to assess the quantity of supragingival calculus formed in longitudinal studies. A periodontal probe graduated in millimeter divisions is used to measure the deposits of calculus on the lingual surfaces of the six mandibular anterior teeth. The smallest unit used to record the presence of calculus is 0.5 mm. A mouth mirror is used to visualize and air is used to dry the teeth prior to examination. Measurements are made in three planes: gingival, distal, and mesial. The gingival measurement is made with the probe held parallel to the long axis of the tooth and equidistant from the mesial and distal surfaces. The probe should be simultaneously in contact with the calculus and the incisal edge of the tooth. The distal measurement is made by holding the probe diagonally so that the tip is in contact with the distal aspect of the tooth and the opposite end (i.e., the portion toward the shank of the probe) is bisecting the mesial-incisal line angle of the tooth. The opposite is true for the mesial measurement. The measurement may be calculated and expressed in three different ways: per measurement score, per tooth score, and per subject score. The *measurement score* is simply the total of all of the scores divided by the number of measurements made. The *tooth score* is the total of all of the scores divided by the number of teeth scored. The *subject score* is simply the total of all of the scores (subjects with fewer than six teeth are excluded).[176]

The Probe Method of Calculus Assessment has been shown to possess a high degree of inter- and intraexaminer reproducibility. However, extensive training under an experienced investigator is required to master it.

Calculus Surface Index (Ennever et al.[43])

The Calculus Surface Index (CSI) is one of two indices that are used in short-term (i.e., less than 6 weeks) clinical trials of calculus inhibitory agents. The objective of this type of study is to determine rapidly whether a specific agent has any effect on reducing or preventing supra- or subgingival calculus. The CSI assesses the presence or absence of supra- and/or subgingival calculus on the four mandibular incisors. The index has also been applied to the six mandibular anterior teeth. The presence or absence of calculus is determined by visual examination or by tactile examination using a mouth mirror and a sickle-type dental explorer. Each incisor is divided into four scoring units. The facial (or labial) surface is considered one unit, and the lingual surface is divided longitudinally into three subsections: the distal-lingual third, the lingual third, and mesial-lingual third. The total number of surfaces with calculus is considered the CSI score per person. The index has been shown to have good intraexaminer reproducibility, and the examination can be performed in a relatively short period of time. Hence, using a 1 to indicate the presence of calculus (and a 0 the absence of calculus), the maximum number of surfaces (scoring mandibular incisors) per person that could have calculus is 16.[176]

A companion index to the CSI is the Calculus Surface Severity Index (CSSI).[43] The CSSI measures the quantity of calculus present on a scale of 0 to 3 on each of the surfaces examined for the CSI. The criteria for the CSSI are as follows[28]:

0 = No calculus present.
1 = Calculus observable, but less than 0.5 mm in width and/or thickness.
2 = Calculus not exceeding 1.0 mm in width and/or thickness.
3 = Calculus exceeding 1.0 mm in width and/or thickness.

Marginal Line Calculus Index (Mühlemann and Villa[109])

The second index that is frequently used in short-term (i.e., less than 6 weeks) clinical trials of anticalculus agents is the Marginal Line Calculus Index (MLCI). This index was developed to assess the accumulation of supragingival calculus on the gingival third of the tooth or, more specifically, supragingival calculus along the margin of the gingiva.

Using a mouth mirror to examine and air to dry the tooth surfaces, only the cervical areas on the lingual surfaces of the four mandibular incisors are examined. The cervical third of each lingual surface is divided into a distal half and a mesial half. Each half is examined for the extent of calculus covering the surface, and a score on a scale of percentages is assigned as follows: 0, 12.5, 25, 50, 75, and 100 per cent. The MLCI *score per tooth* is determined by averaging the two units for each tooth. The MLCI *score per person* is determined by totaling the scores per tooth and dividing by the number of teeth examined. Like the CSI, the MLCI has shown good reproducibility.[176]

RELIABILITY OF DENTAL INDICES*

In the context of epidemiologic indices, the term *reliability* means the ability of a dental index to measure a condition in the same subject repeatedly and obtain the same score results each time. The definition† implies that reliability is a matter of degree, since all measurements are subject to error (method and

---

*The reader is referred to an excellent discussion of this subject by Clemmer and Barbano.[26]

†Term *reliability* is considered a more general term than *reproducibility* or *repeatability*, the latter of which is usually restricted to repeat examination data.[135]

observer) or variability. Replicate (repeat) examinations by one examiner will assess intraexaminer variability, whereas duplicate examinations by two or more examiners will assess interexaminer variability. The most obvious implications of unreliable measures are that prevalence estimates (from surveys) become questionable in making comparisons between groups and that measurements from longitudinal studies may no longer reveal the likelihood of differences between treatment and control groups.

The literature describing the reliability of the indices used in measuring periodontal disease and oral hygiene status, in contrast to similar literature about dental caries, is sparse. Clemmer and Barbano[26] have described several statistical techniques used in assessing intra- and interexaminer reproducibility of periodontal scores. They discussed the proportion of agreement (similarity or "alikeness" on each unit scored), the paired *t* test, the analysis of variance (ANOVA), and the correlation coefficient. The last three tests measure the alikeness of the average score per person. The kappa statistic* was applied to quantitative and qualitative data on categorical scales by Fleiss et al.[45]

Davies et al.[33] tested the intraexaminer variability of the Periodontal Index (PI) using the statistic of percentage discrepancy (the discrepancy between scores of two examinations, with the repeat examination score expressed as a percentage of the first). Among individual examiners the greatest differences (discrepancies) occurred at the lowest clinical ranges (no gingivitis to mild gingivitis). These discrepancies ranged from 0 to 264 per cent. The fewest discrepancies occurred between the categories of moderate gingivitis and loss of tooth function, scores of 2 and 8, respectively. The range of discrepancies for pocket formation was from 0 to 60 per cent. The range of percentages for the consistency ratio (the number of times the condition is recorded at both examinations divided by the total number of times the condition is recorded as present at least once) was also greatest for gingivitis, from 19 to 76.

Davies et al.[32] examined the intra- and interexaminer variability of the PI and the Simplified Oral Hygiene Index (OHI-S) and determined that the examiners were applying the criteria for groups reliably and reproducibly. The comparison of the mean index scores for

interexaminer variability showed slight but insignificant differences. In addition, two other studies found the intraexaminer variability (percentage agreements) for the OHI-S to be quite acceptable (80 per cent and 84 per cent for assessing debris, 95 per cent and 93 per cent for supragingival calculus, and 81 per cent and 76 per cent for subgingival calculus).[52, 166]

Crowley[29] was one of the first to show that examiners were able to reproduce their own scores (intraexaminer variability) 79 per cent of the time when evaluating gingival inflammation. Using the Dental Health Center Index (DHCI), Smith et al.[166] showed that, over a 3-day period, intraexaminer agreement (percentage agreement) for gingival inflammation improved from 59.3 per cent on the first day of duplicate examinations to 86.9 per cent by the third day (agreement averaged 80.4 per cent over the 3-day period). Over a 16-week period, Suomi et al.[170] found the reversal rate (the number of units described as inflamed on the first examination and noninflamed on the second, or vice versa) for DHCI scores (scale of 0 to 2) between two consecutive examinations to range from 14 to 25 per cent.

Elliott and Clemmer[38] studied intra- and interexaminer variability of a gingival index (scale of 0 to 2), pocket scores (scale of 0 to 3), and plaque scores using the Modified Navy Plaque Index. Using the statistic of proportion of agreement in scores, they found intraexaminer agreement to be 0.76 to 0.81 for gingivitis, 0.74 to 0.78 for gingival depth, and 0.46 to 0.49 for plaque. The interexaminer proportion of agreement for these three conditions was 0.64 for gingivitis, 0.69 for gingival depth, and 0.44 for plaque.

In a study of intra- and interexaminer agreement in scoring gingivitis with the Papillary-Marginal-Attachment (PMA) Index and the Gingival Index (GI), Alexander et al.[2] found that they were able to achieve a nonsignificant difference in duplicate examinations for interexaminer reliability only after three extensive training periods. Four extensive training periods were needed before there was a nonsignificant difference in intraexaminer variability in training three different examiners. In a study of the diagnostic reproducibility of the GI and the Plaque Index (PlI), Shaw and Murray[159] found simple correlation coefficients to range from 0.81 to 0.84 for intraexaminer reproducibility using the GI; interexaminer reproducibility was 0.79. The intraexaminer reproducibility for the PlI ranged from 0.83 to 0.84, and the interexaminer reproducibility was 0.70. Löe et al.[77] used

---

*The kappa statistic "corrects the observed proportion of agreement for the proportion of agreement to be expected by chance alone."[45]

the statistic of percentage agreement to examine intraexaminer reproducibility on duplicate examinations. The percentage agreement ranged from 69 to 87 for the Gingival Index, 58 to 79 for the Loss of Attachment Index, 60 to 95 for the Plaque Index, and 65 to 99 for the Calculus Index.

In conclusion, our understanding of the reliability of periodontal indices dictates that all studies should incorporate some system to measure reliability, describe it in publications, and report the results. Since there is no common agreement as to the best statistical method for describing reliability, a combination of methods should be used and presented rather than limiting the topic to a single statistic.

DESCRIPTIVE EPIDEMIOLOGY OF GINGIVAL AND PERIODONTAL DISEASE

Prevalence of Gingivitis

Gingivitis has been observed in children younger than 5 years of age.[95, 173] In general, the prevalence and severity of gingivitis increase with age, beginning at approximately 5 years of age, reaching their highest point in puberty, and then very gradually decreasing but remaining relatively high throughout life (Fig. 23–3).[60] The rapid increase in the incidence of gingivitis prior to 10 years of age is associated with the eruption of the permanent dentition.[94] Surveys of the prevalence and severity of gingivitis are summarized in Table 23–7. Data from the National Health Survey (NHS) (Fig. 23–4) show that for children 6 to 11 years of age[61] the prevalence of gingivitis (i.e., periodontal disease with no pockets) is approximately 38 per cent; for adolescents 12 to 17 years of age[149] it is 62 per cent, and for young adults 18 to 24 years of age[62] it is 57 per cent. Thereafter, the prevalence of gingivitis continues to decrease gradually with increasing age. Hence, **the highest prevalence of gingivitis occurs during puberty**. More recent data from the first Health and Nutrition Examination Survey (HANES I) suggest that there has been a dramatic decrease in the prevalence of gingivitis over the past decade (for adults 18 to 74 years, a decrease from 48.7 to 24.3 per cent).[60] A concomitant decrease in oral hygiene scores over this period, in conjunction with an increase in preventive services, provides some basis for believing that a decrease in the prevalence of gingivitis has in fact occurred. The magnitude of the decreases (48 per cent for 6- to 11-year-olds, no change for 12- to 17-year-olds, and 35 per cent for 18- to 74-year-olds), however, may be partially attributable to interexaminer variability in applying the Periodontal Index (PI) criteria, especially in the lower end of the PI scale that classifies the presence or absence of gingivitis or its severity. Therefore, a small decrease in gingivitis prevalence is reasonable, but not one of the magnitude reported in the HANES I study.

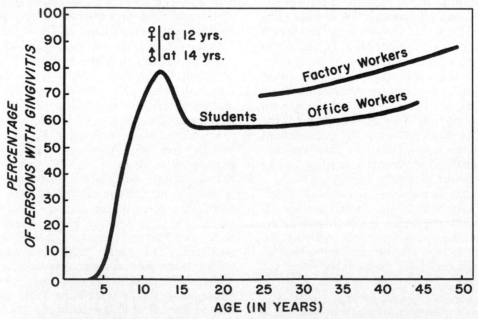

Figure 23–3 Incidence of Gingivitis in 10,000 Persons. (Courtesy of Dr. Maury Massler.)

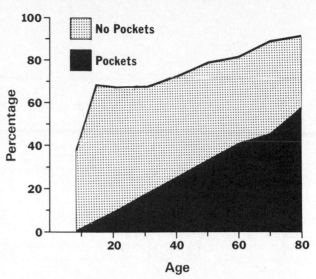

Figure 23–4 Prevalence of Periodontal Disease by Age. Data are from the National Health Survey and cover the following periods: 1963 to 1965 (children, aged 6 to 11 years), 1966 to 1970 (youths, aged 12 to 17 years), and 1960 to 1962 (adults, aged 18 to 79 years). The percent distribution is by mild to moderate gingivitis (no pockets) and periodontal disease with one or more pockets; it is based on Periodontal Index (PI) scores. Data for males and females were combined. (Adapted from Kelly, J. E., and Sanchez, M. J.: Periodontal Disease and Oral Hygiene Among Children, United States. Washington, D.C., U.S. Department of Health, Education, and Welfare, 1972; Sanchez, M. J.: Periodontal Disease Among Youths 12–17 Years, United States. Washington, D.C., U.S. Department of Health, Education, and Welfare, 1974; and Kelly, J. E., and Van Kirk, L. E.: Periodontal Disease in Adults, United States 1960–1962. Washington, D.C., U.S. Department of Health, Education, and Welfare, 1966.)

Prevalence of Periodontal Disease

On a worldwide basis, the United States ranks relatively low in the magnitude and prevalence of periodontal disease. Table 23–8 shows mean PI scores by various population groups throughout the world. Compared with that in South America and the Asian countries, the severity of periodontal disease in groups in the United States is relatively low.[142]

Although there is no precise method of determining the absolute magnitude of periodontal disease in the United States, sufficient data do exist to allow a relatively accurate estimate of its prevalence. In adults 18 to 79 years of age in the 1960 to 1962 cycle of the NHS, for example, three of four (73.9 per cent) had some form of periodontal disease, and one of four (25.4 per cent) had destructive periodontal disease.[62] Data from the HANES I survey (1971 to 1974) suggest that two of four adults (49.7 per cent) have some form of periodontal disease, and one of four (25.4 per cent) has destructive periodontal disease.[60] Hence, the decrease in periodontal disease is attributable to a decrease in gingivitis, whereas the prevalence of destructive disease has remained almost constant. Again, the prevalence of 74 per cent shown in the NHS data may be high, but the lower prevalence of 50 per cent in the HANES I survey is lower than expected, based on the discussion of gingivitis prevalence. Of the 14.7 per cent of the adult population that is completely edentulous,[55] it is reasonable to assume a substantial number of people lost their teeth owing to periodontal disease. Also, adults who have teeth in only one arch have more severe periodontal disease

than people with some teeth in both arches.[62] All adults will at some point during their lifetime experience some deterioration of their periodontal structures. Collectively, all of these observations lead to the conclusion that periodontal disease has a graver effect on dental health than the percentage values indicate. *As more people retain their teeth throughout their lifetime, and as the proportion of older people increases, more teeth will be at risk for periodontal disease. Hence, the prevalence of destructive periodontal disease will likely increase in the future.*

Prevalence of Juvenile Periodontitis

It is difficult to arrive at a statement of prevalence for juvenile periodontitis because few studies have been specifically designed to determine the extent of this degenerative disease. The lack of uniform criteria for recognizing and classifying juvenile periodontitis and the small sample size of the study groups have contributed to the problem. A review of the literature will reveal a range of prevalence values from 0.1 to 17.6 per cent.[8, 90, 98, 113, 120, 133, 139, 146, 152] The age group that appears to be most affected by juvenile periodontitis is that between puberty and approximately 30 years of age.[90, 98, 146] Most investigators agree on this generalization. An examination of the percent-age distribution of periodontal disease for persons in the United States (Fig. 23–4) shows that the prevalence of destructive periodontal disease (i.e., disease with pockets) is 5.8 per cent for adolescents 12 to 17 years of age,[149] 10 per cent for young

TABLE 23–7 PREVALENCE OF GINGIVITIS IN CHILDREN AND YOUNG ADULTS

Investigators	Year	Group Studied	No. Children in Group	Age Group	Percentage of Persons Affected with Gingivitis
McCall[95]	1933	New York	4600	1–14 yrs	98.0
Messner et al.[97]	1938	Children in 26 states of United States	1,438,318	6–14 yrs	3.5–8.6
Marshall-Day and Tandan[89]	1940	Middle-class children in Lahore, India	756	approx. 13 yrs	68.0
Marshall-Day[82]	1940	Fluoride endemic area in northern India	203	5–18 yrs	59.6
King[65]	1940	Isle of Lewis	2280	6–15 yrs	90.0
Campbell and Cook[22]	1942	Dundee Hospital in Scotland	1924		2.2
Marshall-Day[83]	1944	Boys in Kangra district of India (poor nutrition)	200	approx. 13 yrs	81.0
Marshall-Day and Shourie[85]	1944	Low-middle-class school children	613	5–15 yrs	80.0
King et al.[67]	1944	English boys	403	11–14 yrs Group A Group B	77.4 87.6
	1944	Gibraltar evacuees in England	135	10–14 yrs	85.2
King[66]	1945	Primary school children in Dundee, Scotland	103	12–14 yrs	90.0
	1945	Harpenden Institution, England	170	11–14 yrs	Groups vary 56.4–97.5
Marshall-Day and Shourie[86]	1947	Low- to middle-class male school children in Lahore, India	1054	9–17 yrs	99.4
Marshall-Day and Shourie[86]	1947	Girls of high socioeconomic level in Lahore, India	179	9–17 yrs	73.3
Schour and Massler[154]	1947	Four communities in Italy suffering from malnutrition	682 721	6–10 yrs 11–20 yrs	40.3 55.3
Marshall-Day and Shourie[88]	1948	Puerto Rico	1648	6–18 yrs	60.0–79.0
Massler et al.[94]	1950	Suburban Chicago school children	804	5–14 yrs	64.3
Marshall-Day and Shourie[88]	1950	Virgin Islands (91% black population)	823 860	6–18 yrs 5–13 yrs	57.0 26.9
Stahl and Goldman[167]	1953	School children in Massachusetts	1300	13–17 yrs	29.0
Russel[139]	1957	Urban United States	White { 6682 15,922 4031	5–9 yrs 10–14 yrs 15–19 yrs	10.8 25.5 37.3
			Black { 37 494	5–9 yrs 10–19 yrs	8.1 28.7

Table continued on opposite page

TABLE 23–7 PREVALENCE OF GINGIVITIS IN CHILDREN AND YOUNG ADULTS (*Continued*)

Investigators	Year	Group Studied	No. Children in Group	Age Group	Percentage of Persons Affected with Gingivitis
Greene[50]	1960	School boys in low socioeconomic area of India	1613	11–17 yrs	96.9
		School boys in low socioeconomic area of Atlanta, Georgia	577	11–17 yrs	92.0
Zimmerman and Baker[182]	1960	White children from Maryland	529	6–12 yrs	35.0
		Black children from Texas	442	6–12 yrs	67.0
		White children from Texas	435	6–12 yrs	79.0
Jamison[57]	1963	Tecumseh, Michigan (deciduous teeth only)	159	5–14 yrs	99.4
McHugh et al.[96]	1964	Dundee, Scotland, boys and girls	2905	13 yrs	99.4
Dutta[37]	1965	Calcutta, India, boys and girls	1424	6–12 yrs	89.8
Wade[178]	1966	Iraq	200	13–15 yrs	97.0
		London	222	13–15 yrs	
Sheiham[161]	1968	Nigeria	1620	10 yrs and older	99+
Sheiham[162]	1969	Surrey	756	11–17 yrs	99.7
Murray[110]	1969	West Hartlepool, 1.5–2.0 ppm fluoride			
		Boys	211	15 yrs	94.8
		Girls	175	15 yrs	86.3
		York, 0.2 ppm fluoride			
		Boys	202	15 yrs	95.5
		Girls	179	15 yrs	85.5
Downer[34]	1970	Secondary school children in London, England	373	11–14 yrs	79.0
Murray[111]	1972	West Hartlepool, 1.5–2.0 ppm fluoride			
		Boys	141	15–19 yrs	90.1
		Girls	449	15–19 yrs	88.4
		York, 0.2 ppm fluoride			
		Boys	61	15–19 yrs	86.9
		Girls	102	15–19 yrs	84.3
Jorkjend and Birkeland[59]	1973	Primary school children in Porsgrunn, Norway	154	11–13 yrs	99.0
Bowden et al.[18]	1973	Cheshire, England	622	15 yrs	81.2
Murray[112]	1974	West Hartlepool, 1.5–2.0 ppm fluoride			
		Boys	1470	8–18 yrs	92.9
		Girls	1406	8–18 yrs	91.1

TABLE 23–8 AVERAGE PERIODONTAL INDEX SCORES IN CIVILIANS (BOTH SEXES), AGED 40–49 YEARS, SURVEYED BY EXAMINERS OF THE NATIONAL INSTITUTE OF DENTAL RESEARCH, UNITED STATES*

Population Group	Average Periodontal Index Score
Baltimore, Maryland (white)	1.03
Colorado Springs, Colorado	1.04†
Alaska; primitive Eskimos	1.17‡
Ecuador	1.85
Ethiopia	1.86
Baltimore, Maryland (black)	1.99
Uganda	2.50§
Vietnam; Vietnamese	2.18
Colombia	2.21
Alaska; urban Eskimos	2.31‡
Chile	2.74
Lebanon; Lebanese	2.98
Thailand	3.30
Lebanon; Palestinian refugees	3.52
Burma	3.58
Jordan; Jordanian civilians	3.96
Vietnam; hill tribesmen	3.97
Trinidad	4.21
Jordan; Palestinian refugees	4.41

*Modified from Russell, A. L.: J. Periodontol., *38*:585, 1967.

†Ages 40–44 only.
‡Males only.
§Age over 40.

adults 18 to 24 years of age, and approximately 17 per cent for adults 30 to 34 years of age.[62] Assuming that approximately half of these individuals had juvenile periodontitis, it would be reasonable to expect that the true prevalence of juvenile periodontitis would be somewhat less than 8 per cent, and even this may be a high estimate. Some investigators[8, 133] believe that females are affected more frequently than males, but this has not been clearly established.[113] Intraorally, the teeth that are most severely affected are the maxillary and mandibular incisors and the first molars; the least affected teeth are the mandibular premolars.[8, 99] When greater agreement among investigators is reached relative to the parameters used to describe juvenile periodontitis, a more accurate estimate of its prevalence will be possible.

FACTORS AFFECTING THE PREVALENCE AND SEVERITY OF GINGIVITIS AND PERIODONTAL DISEASE

AGE. *The prevalence of periodontal disease increases directly with increasing age.*[142] Figure 23–4 shows the distribution of periodontal disease, with and without pockets.[61, 62, 149] The prevalence of periodontal disease is approximately 45 per cent at 10 years of age, 67 per cent at 20 years, 70 per cent at 35 years, and 80 per cent at 50 years. Although these prevalences may be high, the lower values suggested by the HANES I survey are lower than expected: approximately 15 per cent at 10 years of age, 38 per cent at 20 years, 46 per cent at 35 years, and 54 per cent at 50 years.[60] *This gradual increase in the prevalence of periodontal disease supports the statement that virtually no one escapes the ravages of this disease.* The distribution of periodontal disease with pockets is approximately 1 per cent at 10 years of age, 10 per cent at 20 years, 20 per cent at 35 years, 30 per cent at 50 years. There is a dramatic ninefold increase in the prevalence of destructive disease with pockets between 20 and 70 years of age. The HANES I data (1971 to 1974)[60] coincide almost perfectly with the NHS data presented in Figure 23–4 (1960 to 1962). This pattern of disease with pockets closely parallels that of the reduction in bone height that occurs with increasing age.[87] Although destructive periodontal disease is primarily a disease of adults, its onset during puberty has been observed with greater frequency in countries[138] other than the United States.[149]

The severity of periodontal disease, as indicated by mean Periodontal Index (PI) scores, *increases directly with age* (Fig. 23–5). Between 35 and 40 years of age, the average adult enters the beginning phase of destructive periodontal disease. It then takes approximately 20 more years before the average adult (55 to 60 years of age) enters the advanced phase of destructive periodontal disease.[62] This is consistent with the newest data available.[60]

SEX. *In general, males consistently have a higher prevalence and severity of periodontal disease than females* (Fig. 23–6). Before 20 years of age the difference between males and females are very slight.[61, 149] At 20 years of age males have only a 30 per cent higher PI score (0.14 PI unit) than females.[58, 62] Between 18 and 74 years of age, males have almost 45 per cent more severe periodontal disease than females. As a group, males enter the beginning phase of destructive periodontal disease at approximately 35 years of age, and females enter the beginning phase at approximately 45 years of age. Males enter the advanced stage of periodontal disease at approximately 55 years of age, whereas females enter the advanced stage at approximately 75 years of age.

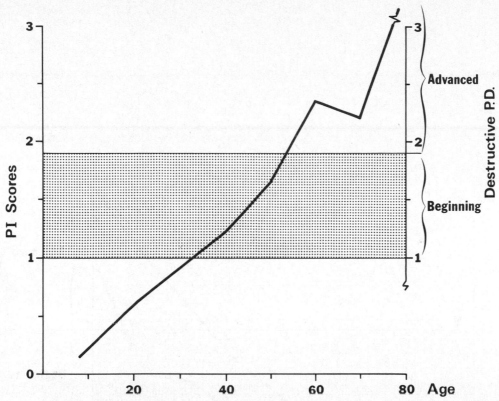

Figure 23–5 Distribution of Periodontal Disease Severity by Age. Data are from the National Health Survey and are combined for whites and blacks. Severity is indicated by mean Periodontal Index (PI) scores. The subdivisions of destructive periodontal disease approximate the group PI scores that correspond to the various clinical conditions (see Table 23–1). (Adapted from Kelly, J. E., and Sanchez, M. J.: Periodontal Disease and Oral Hygiene Among Children, United States. Washington, D.C., U.S. Department of Health, Education, and Welfare, 1972; Sanchez, M. J.: Periodontal Disease Among Youths 12–17 Years, United States. Washington, D.C., U.S. Department of Health, Education, and Welfare, 1974; and Kelly, J. E., and Van Kirk, L. E.: Periodontal Disease in Adults, United States 1960–1962. Washington, D.C., U.S. Department of Health, Education, and Welfare, 1966.)

However, newer data suggest that women enter the advanced stage at closer to 65 years of age than 75 years.[60]

RACE. Figure 23–7 compares the severity of periodontal disease by racial-ethnic group for the National Health Survey (NHS)[61, 62, 149] and the Ten-State Nutrition Survey (10-SNS or National Nutrition Survey).[173] When whites and blacks from the NHS are compared, blacks appear consistently to have more severe periodontal disease than whites.[62] After 20 years of age, blacks average 50 per cent more severe periodontal disease than whites. Even though the differences that exist between whites and blacks are not as great in the data from the 10-SNS, the same general trend still holds (i.e., blacks have more periodontal disease than whites). The severity of periodontal disease among Spanish-Americans appear to be higher than that among both whites and blacks, but disproportionate differences in the number of persons being compared make any definitive statement on the severity of periodontal disease among Spanish-Americans invalid.

EDUCATION. Figure 23–8 illustrates two important associations relative to periodontal disease.[62] First, *periodontal disease is inversely related to increasing levels of education.*[55a, 138] In whites the decrease in periodontal disease severity is 63 per cent (three fifths), and in blacks the decrease is 47 per cent (one half). Second, *the differences that were observed between whites and blacks with periodontal disease* (see Fig. 23–7) *may be explained by differences in education, since no significant differences exist between whites and blacks of similar education.* It is not surprising that occupation, which is so closely tied to education in the United States, shows a relationship to periodontal disease that is similar to that of education. For example, the prevalence and severity of periodontal disease are lower in

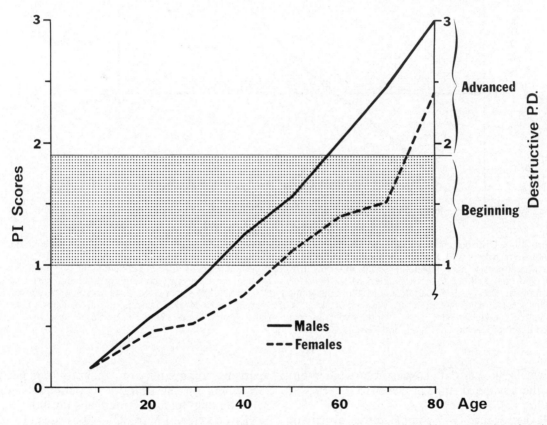

Figure 23–6 Severity of Periodontal Disease by Sex and Age. Data are from the National Health Survey and are for whites only. (Adapted from Kelly, J. E., and Sanchez, M. J.: Periodontal Disease and Oral Hygiene Among Children, United States. Washington, D.C., U.S. Department of Health, Education, and Welfare, 1972; Sanchez, M. J.: Periodontal Disease Among Youths 12–17 Years, United States. Washington, D.C., U.S. Department of Health, Education, and Welfare, 1974; Kelly, J. E., and Van Kirk, L. E.: Periodontal Disease in Adults, United States 1960–1962. Washington, D.C., U.S. Department of Health, Education, and Welfare, 1966.)

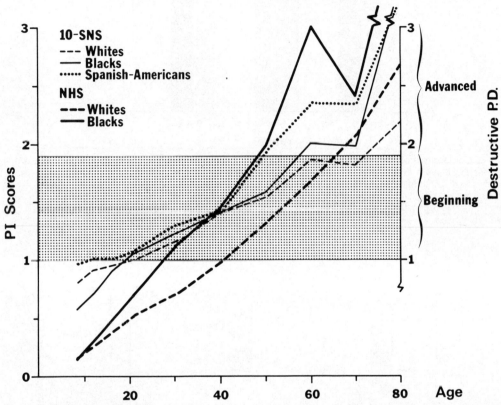

Figure 23–7 Severity of Periodontal Disease by Racial-Ethnic Group and Age. Data are from the National Health Survey and the Ten-State Nutrition Survey (10–SNS) (1968 to 1970), high income ratio states. (Adapted from Kelly, J. E., and Sanchez, M. J.: Periodontal Disease and Oral Hygiene Among Children, United States. Washington, D.C., U.S. Department of Health, Education, and Welfare, 1972; Sanchez, M. J.: Periodontal Disease Among Youths 12–17 Years, United States. Washington, D.C., U.S. Department of Health, Education, and Welfare, 1974; Kelly, J. E., and Van Kirk, L. E.: Periodontal Disease in Adults, United States 1960–1962. Washington, D.C., U.S. Department of Health, Education, and Welfare, 1966; and Ten-State Nutrition Survey 1968–1970. Atlanta, Centers for Disease Control, 1972.)

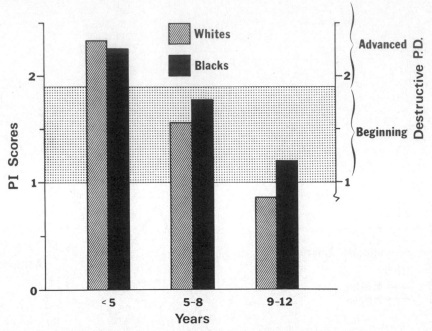

Figure 23–8 Comparison of Periodontal Disease Severity by Education and Racial-Ethnic Group. Data are from the National Health Survey and are for adults according to the number of years or the highest grade of elementary or high school completed. (Adapted from Kelly, J. E., and Van Kirk, L. E.: Periodontal Disease in Adults, United States 1960–1962. Washington, D.C., U.S. Department of Health, Education, and Welfare, 1966.)

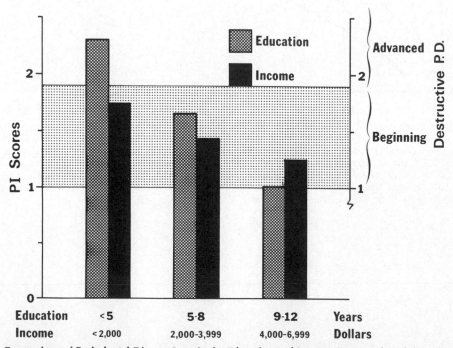

Figure 23–9 Comparison of Periodontal Disease Severity by Education and Income. Data are for adults, whites and blacks combined, from the National Health Survey. (Adapted from Kelly, J. E., and Van Kirk, L. E.: Periodontal Disease in Adults, United States 1960–1962. Washington, D.C., U.S. Department of Health, Education, and Welfare, 1966.)

office personnel than in factory workers, and they are generally lower among persons in occupations that require more educational background.[6, 92]

INCOME. The association between periodontal disease and income is similar to that observed between periodontal disease and education. *Periodontal disease is inversely related to increasing levels of income.* Data from the NHS show that the decrease in the severity of periodontal disease that occurs with increasing income is 38 per cent for whites and 20 per cent for blacks.[62] The differences that were observed between whites and blacks in Figure 23–7 are not influenced as strongly by income as they are by education.

The stronger influence of education than of income relative to periodontal disease is vividly illustrated in Figure 23–9.[62] When the PI scores of whites and blacks are combined according to education and income, the decrease due to education is 55 per cent, whereas the decrease due to income is only 28 per cent.

PLACE OF RESIDENCE. In general, the prevalence and severity of periodontal disease are slightly higher in rural areas than in urban areas.[11, 62]

GEOGRAPHIC AREA. Within the United States, some investigators have shown geographic differences in the prevalence and severity of periodontal disease,[93, 182] but no significant differences were observed for adults (6672 persons, 18 to 79 years of age) in the NHS[62] and adults (13,645 persons, 18 to 74 years of age) in the HANES I Survey.[60] Children (7109; 6 to 11 years)[61] and youths (6,768; 12 to 17 years)[149] living in the South, however, did have slightly higher PI scores than their counterparts living in the Midwest and West.

ETIOLOGIC FACTORS OF GINGIVAL AND PERIODONTAL DISEASE

ORAL HYGIENE. The strong positive association that exists between poor oral hygiene and gingival and periodontal disease[50, 51, 54, 63, 78, 162, 172] makes poor hygiene the primary etiologic agent. On the basis of observations of periodontal disease in the United States and throughout the world, Russell states that "active (gingival and periodontal) disease is rarely found in the absence of oral debris (plaque) or calculus."[145] One vivid example that puts in perspective the importance of oral hygiene relative to the other demographic variables, detailed under the descriptive epidemiology of periodontal disease, is a multiple correlation analysis of the combined effects of age, sex, and oral hygiene (Simplified Oral Hygiene Index [OHI-S] scores) to Periodontal Index (PI) scores in 752 South Vietnamese over 15 years of age.[148] The coefficient of multiple correlation was $r = 0.82$, which, under the above conditions, means that statistically 67 per cent (two thirds) of the variance was attributed to oral hygiene and approximately 31 per cent was attributed to age. In the National Health Survey (NHS), a comparison of the partial correlation coefficients of oral hygiene (OHI-S), age, education of the head of the household, and family income to PI scores showed that oral hygiene was the best predictor of the prevalence and severity of periodontal disease.[149, 150] Hence, **statistically as well as clinically, plaque is a primary etiologic factor of periodontal disease**.

NUTRITION. The nutrients that have been specifically associated with the periodontal tissues are vitamins A, B complex, C, and D and the elements calcium and phosphorus (see Chapter 28). Deficiencies in each of these nutrients and their effects on the periodontium have been clearly demonstrated in appropriately designed animal studies. The evidence for deficiencies in these nutrients being associated with periodontal disease in humans, however, has been less than convincing.[158] In a series of nutrition surveys (conducted under the auspices of the Interdepartmental Committee on Nutrition for National Defense [ICNND]),[141] designed specifically to determine associations between nutrient levels and disease, the strongest residual associations between periodontal disease and nutritional deficiencies were expressed in partial correlations (holding the effects of age, debris, and calculus constant) of -0.11 for vitamin A and -0.19 for hematocrit levels.[142] The partial correlation coefficient (-0.11) for the vitamin A deficiency accounts for approximately 1 per cent of the variance in the PI scores; the strongest partial correlation coefficient (-0.19) accounts for less than 4 per cent of the variance in the PI scores. Little or no effect could be attributed to serum ascorbic acid, serum carotene, total serum protein, urinary thiamine, riboflavin, and N'methylnicotinamide, and hemoglobin. A vitamin A deficiency and a subnormal hematocrit level were found in a South Vietnamese population, but neither of these deficiencies was found to be associated with periodontal disease in subsequent ICNND surverys. In the Ten-State Nutrition Survey

(10-SNS),[173] the simple correlation coefficient (-0.03) for PI scores and plasma vitamin A deficiency accounted for 0.1 per cent of the variance in PI scores. All of these correlation coefficients are at best weak associations. The ICNND nutrition surveys found no consistent correlation between nutrition and periodontal disease. They concluded, however, that "despite the independence of the nutritive state of the individual adult and his periodontal condition, there is a trend towards a higher prevalence and severity of periodontal disease in adults in areas[65] where protein calorie malnutrition and vitamin A deficiency are common in children."[137]

Nutrition is, therefore, a secondary factor in the etiology of periodontal disease.

FLUORIDES. No definitive statement can be made concerning the prevalence and severity of gingival or periodontal disease in cities with optimal or high levels of fluoride in the drinking water. Some investigators have reported that optimal levels of fluoride do not have any effect on the gingival tissues,[41, 56, 103, 110] but others have reported a lower prevalence and severity of gingivitis and periodontal disease in optimally fluoridated areas.[7, 42, 137]

ADVERSE HABITS. Tobacco smoking[5, 6, 168] and betel nut chewing[9] have been associated with increased periodontal disease.[31] Although this association is not unequivocal, it seems reasonable that any habit that increases irritation of the gingival tissues or lowers their resistance would be a predisposing or secondary factor in initiating periodontal disease (see Chapter 26).

PROFESSIONAL DENTAL CARE

The incidence and severity of periodontal disorders are lower in individuals under regular dental care.[19, 79, 147, 172, 179] The prevalence and severity of disease increase with neglect (see Chapter 59).

DISTRIBUTION OF DISEASE IN DIFFERENT AREAS OF THE MOUTH

The strong association that was previously described between plaque and calculus and periodontal disease may in its initial stages be explained by the dynamics of plaque and gingivitis formation over time. Figure 23–10 shows the rate of plaque and gingivitis formation that Löe et al.[76] observed in their classic study of experimental gingivitis. It shows that, when brushing is omitted from oral hygiene cleansing procedures, the formation of plaque and gingivitis closely parallels each other. In the study, both increased with time, reaching a maximum between 15 and 21 days, when all subjects experienced a maximum of gingivitis. Reinstituting toothbrushing not only demonstrated the reversible nature of gingival inflammation, but also showed a concomitant decrease in the plaque and gingivitis formation.

Dividing the mouth into interproximal, buccal, and lingual areas by upper and lower arches (Table 23–9), Löe et al. showed that the interproximal area was most severely affected by gingivitis, followed by the buccal and lingual surfaces. Dividing each of the areas into upper and lower arches revealed that gingivitis was more severe in the upper arch than in the lower arch for the interproximal and buccal areas, and in the lingual area it was more severe in the lower arch than in the upper arch.[76] Suomi and Barbano[169] examined the severity of gingivitis by facial and lingual surfaces for three areas of the mouth (Fig. 23–11) and found the same general pattern observed by Löe et al. For facial surfaces, the areas most severely affected by gingivitis, in descending order, were the upper first and second molars, lower anteriors, upper anteriors, upper premolars, lower first and second molars, and lower premolars. For lingual surfaces, the areas most severely affected by gingivitis, in descending order, were the lower first and second molars, lower premolars, lower anteriors, upper first and second molars, upper premolars, and upper anteriors. This intraoral pattern of gingivitis was similar to that observed by Marshall-Day,[84] with the exception of the facial surfaces of the upper anteriors, which he found to be the most severely affected by gingivitis. Several investigators[12, 169] have observed a slightly higher tendency to gingivitis on the right half of the arch than on the left half. This may be

TABLE 23–9 SEVERITY OF GINGIVITIS FOR THREE DIFFERENT AREAS BY ARCH*

Area	Arch	Mean Gingival Index Score
Interproximal	Upper > lower	1.44 > 1.20
Buccal	Upper > lower	1.23 > 1.13
Lingual	Lower > upper	0.89 > 0.46

*Adapted from Löe, H., Theilade, E., and Jensen, S. B.: J. Periodontol., 36:177, 1965.

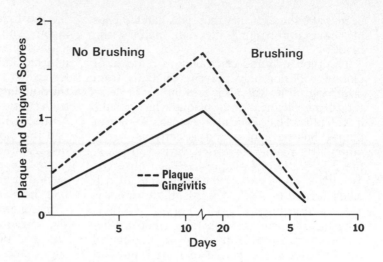

Figure 23–10 Rate of Plaque and Gingivitis Formation. Data are for 12 young Scandinavian adults, averaging 23 years of age. The Gingival Index (GI) and the Plaque Index (PII) were used for the clinical assessments. (Adapted from Löe, H., Theilade, E., and Jensen, S. B.: J. Periodontol., 36:177, 1965.)

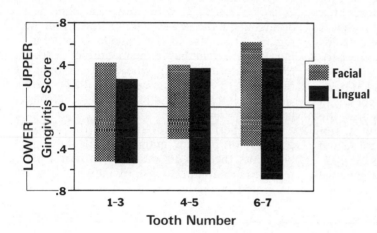

Figure 23–11 Intraoral Distribution of Gingivitis Severity by Tooth Surface and Area of Mouth. Data are for 400 males 15 to 34 years of age. The Dental Health Center Index (DHCI) was used to assess gingivitis by marginal and papillary units for all teeth. Tooth numbers are defined as follows: 1 = central incisor, 2 = lateral incisor, 3 = canine, 4 = first premolar, 5 = second premolar, 6 = first molar, 7 = second molar. (Adapted from Suomi, J. D., and Barbano, J. P.: J. Periodontol., 39:71, 1968.)

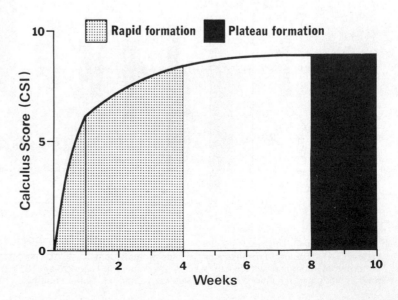

Figure 23–12 Rate of Calculus Formation. Data are for 39 subjects who were heavy calculus formers. The Calculus Surface Index (CSI) was used to assess calculus on the four mandibular incisors. (Adapted from Conroy, C. W., and Sturzenberger, O. P.: J. Periodontol., 39:142, 1968.)

because of the difficulty that right-handed people have in brushing the right half of the mouth.

The thorough and conscientious removal of plaque will not only prevent gingivitis from occurring, but will also prevent or at least retard the calcification of plaque which results in calculus. Histologically, the calcification of plaque has been observed as early as 4 to 8 hours after plaque formation starts. Clinically, the calcification of plaque has been observed as early as 48 hours.[174] The dynamics of calculus formation in heavy calculus formers is illustrated in Figure 23–12.[28] Following a thorough prophylaxis, calculus was clinically detected in measurable quantities by the end of the first week, the period of most rapid formation. The rapid formation of calculus continued until the fourth week, and then the rate started to diminish, reaching a plateau at 8 weeks. The significance of this study is that it suggests an upper limit on the rate of calculus formation that may be expected in some people.

The intraoral pattern of supra- and subgingival calculus by individual teeth appears in Figure 23–13.[156] For supragingival calculus, the upper first molars had the most calculus, followed by the lower centrals and laterals, and the upper anteriors (centrals, laterals, and canines) had the least calculus. For subgingival calculus, the lower centrals and laterals had the most calculus, followed by the upper first molars; the upper anteriors (centrals, laterals, and canines) and upper second molars had intermediate percentages of calculus; and the lower first and second premolars and the lower third molars had the least calculus. Combining both supra- and subgingival calculus, the lower centrals and laterals and the upper first molars had the most calculus; the upper second premolars and the upper second molars had intermediate percentages of calculus; and the lower second premolars and the lower third molars had the least calculus.[122, 156]

In general, the severity of bone loss follows the intraoral pattern of subgingival calculus and the intraoral pattern of calculus when supra- and subgingival calculus are combined. The incisor and molar areas are more severely involved than are the canine and premolar areas,[46, 87, 102, 153, 172a] with the least bone loss occurring in the lower canine and premolar region. Bone loss in the maxilla is generally more severe than that in the mandible,[10] except for the anterior region, where the situation is reversed.[87, 179] Also, the severity of bone loss is greater interproximally than it is facially and lingually.

The upper and lower limits of the various patterns of plaque, gingivitis, calculus, and bone loss together produce the intraoral pattern of periodontal disease by individual teeth presented in Figure 23–14.[17] The result of all

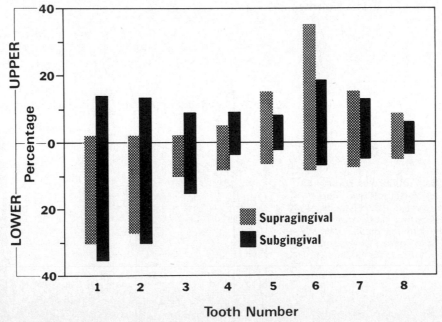

Figure 23–13 Intraoral Prevalence of Calculus by Individual Teeth. The percentage of supra- and subgingival calculus is presented by tooth and arch. Tooth numbers are defined in Figure 23–11. 8 = third molar. (Adapted from Schroeder, H. E.: Formation and Inhibition of Dental Calculus. Vienna, H. Huber Publishers, 1969.)

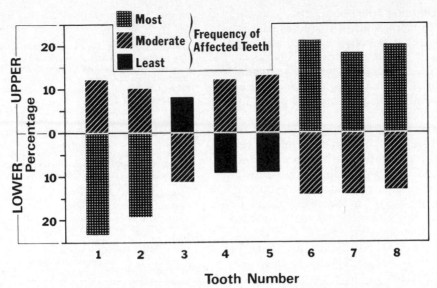

Figure 23–14 Intraoral Prevalence of Periodontal Disease by Individual Teeth. The percentages of teeth affected by periodontal disease are classified as most, moderate, and least. Data are for industrial workers 40 to 44 years of age, with males and females combined. Tooth numbers are defined in Figures 23–11 and 23–13. (Adapted from Bossert, W. A., and Marks, H. H.: J. Am. Dent. Assoc., *52*:429, 1956.)

of the above parameters shows that the *teeth that are most severely affected* by periodontal disease are the lower centrals and laterals and upper molars (first, second, and third). The teeth that are moderately affected by periodontal disease are the lower first molars (first, second, and third), the upper centrals, laterals, and premolars (first and second), and the lower canines. Finally, the *teeth that are least affected* by periodontal disease are the lower premolars (first and second) and the upper canines.

THE RELATIONSHIP BETWEEN PERIODONTAL DISEASE AND DENTAL CARIES

Even though numerous investigators have attempted to determine the relationship between the occurrence of periodontal disease and dental caries, no clear-cut positive or negative relationship has been established.[25, 49, 64, 71] Some investigators consider these antagonistic processes, with the presence

Figure 23–15 Tooth Extractions Due to Dental Caries and Periodontal Disease. A comparison of the percentage of teeth indicated for extraction due to caries and periodontal disease by age was determined from almost 225,000 dental records of the U.S. Public Health Service facilities from 1948 through 1952. (Adapted from Pelton, W. J., Pennell, E. H., and Druzina, A.: J. Am. Dent. Assoc., *49*:439, 1954.)

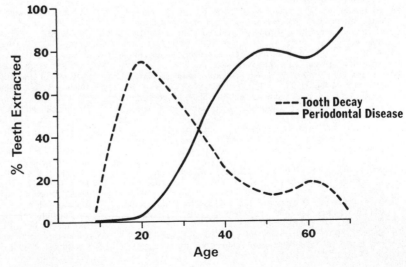

of one precluding the occurrence of the other.[20, 49, 64] Several statistical studies suggest a positive correlation between caries and gingival disease,[16, 160] but this has not been substantiated.[66, 83, 179] Although both have dental plaque as their chief etiologic factor, caries and periodontal disease appear to be two independent processes.[101, 179]

The final result of either dental caries or periodontal disease is the loss of teeth. Hence, comparing the percentages of teeth extracted owing to caries and to periodontal disease will provide a common denominator for describing the relationship between the two processes. Figure 23–15 shows that the ravages of caries start shortly after the teeth erupt in the mouth, reach their greatest prevalence at approximately 20 years of age, and gradually decrease in a skewed pattern.[124] The greatest incidence of tooth extraction due to periodontal disease occurs between 20 and 50 years of age, and **after 35 years of age more teeth are lost owing to periodontal disease than to dental caries.**[3, 4] Even when there had been an absence of dental caries early in life (before 20 years of age), the need for tooth extraction is high before 40 years of age in those with moderate to advanced periodontal disease.[77]

It has been shown that periodontal disease is responsible for approximately 50 per cent of the total tooth loss after age 15 and caries for approximately 38 per cent. The remainder of the teeth are lost owing to other causes, such as accidents and impactions, or are removed for orthodontic or prosthetic reasons.[124]

REFERENCES

1. Ainamo, J., and Bay, I.: Problems and proposals for recording gingivitis and plaque. Int. Dent. J., *25*:229, 1975.
2. Alexander, A. G., Leon, A. R., Ribbons, J. W., and Morganstein, S. I.: An assessment of the inter- and intraexaminer agreement in scoring gingivitis clinically. J. Periodont. Res., *6*:146, 1971.
3. Allen, E. F.: Statistical study of the primary causes of extraction. J. Dent. Res., *23*:453, 1944.
4. Andrews, G., and Krogh, H. W.: Permanent tooth mortality. D. Progress, *1*:130, 1961.
5. Arno, A., Schei, O., Lovdal, A., and Waerhaug, J.: Alveolar bone loss as a function of tobacco consumption. Acta Odontol. Scand., *17*:3, 1959.
6. Arno, A., Waerhaug, J., Lovdal, A., and Schei, O.: Incidence of gingivitis as related to sex, occupation, tobacco consumption, toothbrushing and age. Oral Surg., *11*, 587, 1958.
7. Ast, D. B., and Schlesinger, E. R.: The conclusion of a tenyear study of fluoridation. Am. J. Public Health, *46*:265, 1956.
8. Baer, P. N, and Benjamin, S. D.: Periodontal Disease in Children and Adolescents. Philadelphia, J. B. Lippincott Company, 1974, pp. 139–181.
9. Balendra, W.: The effect of betel chewing on the dental and oral tissues and its possible relationship to buccal carcinoma. Br. Dent. J., *87*:83, 1949.
10. Beagrie, G. S., and James, G. A.: The association of posterior tooth irregularity and periodontal disease. Br. Dent. J., *113*:239, 1962.
10a. Bellini, H. T.: A System to Determine the Periodontal Therapeutic Needs of a Population. Oslo, Universitetsforlagets Trykningssentral, 1973.
11. Benjamin, E. M., Russell, A. L., and Smiley, R. D.: Periodontal disease in rural children of 25 Indian countries. J. Periodontol., *28*:294, 1957.
12. Beube, F. E., Schwartz, M., and Thompson, R. H.: A comparison of effectiveness in plaque removal of an electric toothbrush and a conventional hand toothbrush. Periodontics, *2*:71, 1964.
13. Bjorby, A., and Löe, H.: The relative significance of different local factors in the initiation and development of periodontal inflammation. J. Periodont. Res., *2*:76, 1967 (abstract).
14. Bjorn, H., and Holmberg, K.: Radiographic determination of periodontal bone destruction in epidemiological research. Odontol. Revy, *17*:232, 1966.
15. Bjorn, H., Halling, A., and Thyberg, H.: Radiographic assessment of marginal bone loss. Odontol. Revy, *20*:165, 1969.
16. Black, G. V.: Something of the etiology and early pathology of the diseases of the periodontal membrane with suggestions as to treatment Dent. Cosmos, *55*:1219, 1913.
17. Bossert, W. A., and Marks, H. H.: Prevalence and characteristics of periodontal disease of 12,800 persons under periodic dental observation. J. Am. Dent. Assoc., *52*:429, 1956.
18. Bowden, D. E. J., Davies, R. M., Holloway, P. J., Lennon, M. A., and Rugg-Gunn, A. J.: A treatment need survey of a 15-yeard-old population. Br. Dent. J., *134*:375, 1973.
19. Brandtzaeg, P., and Jamison, H. C.: The effect of controlled cleansing of the teeth on periodontal health and oral hygiene in Norwegian army recruits. J. Periodontol., *35*:308, 1964.
20. Broderick, F. W.: Angagonism between dental caries and pyorrhea. Am. D. Surg., *49*:103, 1929.
21. Burnham, C. E.: Edentulous Persons, United States 1971. Washington, D.C., U.S.P.H.S., U.S. Department of Health, Education, and Welfare, National Center for Health Statistics, Publication No. (HRA) 74–1516, Series 10, No. 89, 1974.
22. Campbell, H. G., and Cook, R. P.: Incidence of Gingivitis at Dundee Dental Hospital. Year Book of Dentistry. Chicago, Year Book Publishers, 1942.
23. Carter, H. G., and Barnes, G. P.: The Gingival Bleeding Index. J. Periodontol., *45*:801, 1974.
24. Chilton, N. W. (ed.): International Conference on Clinical Trials of Agents Used in the Prevention/Treatment of Periodontal Diseases. J. Periodont. Res., *9*(Suppl. 14):7–211, 1974.
25. Citron, J.: About the question of the internal etiology of paradentosis. Zahnärztl. Rdsch., *37*:1319, 1928.
26. Clemmer, B. A., and Barbano, J. P.: Reproducibility of periodontal score in clinical trials. J. Periodont. Res., *9*(Suppl. 14):118, 1974.
27. Cohen, D. W., and Ship., I. I. (eds.): Clinical Methods in Periodontal Diseases Based on a Conference Held on May 20–23, 1967. J. Periodontol., *38*:580–795, 1967.
28. Conroy, C. W., and Strurzenberger, O. P.: The rate of calculus formation in adults. J. Peridontol., *39*:142, 1968.
29. Crowley, R. E.: A method for evaluating consistency in diagnosis of gingivitis. Oral Surg., *8*:1128, 1955.
30. Cutress, T. W., Hunter, P. B. V., Beck, D. J., and deSouza, P.: A comparison of WHO Periodontal Status Index with the Periodontal and Oral Hygiene Indices. Community Dent. Oral Epidemiol., *6*:245, 1978.
31. Davies, G. N.: Social customs and habits and their effect on oral disease. J. Dent. Res., *42*:209, 1963.
32. Davies, G. N., Horowitz, H. S., and Wada, W.: The assessment of periodontal disease for public health purposes. J. Periodont. Res., *9*:62, 1974.
33. Davies, G. N., Kruger, B. J., and Homan, B. T.: An epidemiological training course. Aust. Dent. J., *12*:17, 1967.
34. Downer, M. C.: Dental caries and periodontal disease in girls of different ethnic groups: a comparison in a London secondary school. Br. Dent. J., *128*:379, 1970.
35. Dunning, J. M.: Principles of Dental Public Health, 3rd ed. Cambridge, Mass., Harvard University Press, 1979, pp. 68–69, 161–162.

36. Dunning, J. M., and Leach, L. B.: Gingival-bone count: a method for epidemiological study of periodontal disease. J. Dent. Res., *39*:506, 1960.

37. Dutta, A.: A study on prevalence of periodontal disease and dental caries amongst the school-going children in Calcutta. J. All India Dent. Assoc., *37*:367, 1965.

38. Elliott, J. R., and Clemmer, B. A.: On the reproducibility of periodontal indices. U.S. Navy Med., *59*:41, 1972.

39. Elliott, J. R., Bowers, G. M., Clemmen, B. A., and Rovelstad, G. H.: Evaluation of an oral physiotherapy center in the reduction of bacterial plaque and periodontal disease. J. Periodontol., *43*:221, 1972.

40. Emslie, R. D.: Formal discussion. *In* Ramfjord, S. P.: Design of studies or clinical trials to evaluate the effectiveness of agents or procedures for the prevention, or treatment, of loss of the periodontium. J. Periodont. Res., *9*:(Suppl. 14):78, 1974.

41. Englander, H. R., and White, C. L.: Periodontal and oral hygiene status of teenagers in optimum and fluoride-deficient cities. J. Am. Dent. Assoc., *68*:173, 1964.

42. Englander, H. R., Kesel, R. G., and Gupta, O. P.: Effect of natural fluoride on the periodontal health of adults. Am. J. Public Health, *53*:1233, 1963.

43. Ennever, J., Sturzenberger, C. P., and Radike, A. W.: Calculus Surface Index for scoring clinical calculus studies. J. Periodontol., *32*:54, 1961.

44. Everett, F. G., and Fixott, H. C.: Use of an incorporated grid in the diagnosis of oral roentgenograms. Oral Surg., *16*:1061, 1963.

45. Fleiss, J. L., Fischman, S. L., Chilton, N. W., and Park, M. H.: Reliability of discrete measurements in caries trials. Caries Res., *13*:23, 1979.

46. Fleming, W. C.: Localization of pyorrhea involvement. Dent. Cosmos, *54*:538, 1926.

47. Gjermo, P.: Formal discussion. *In* Hazen, S. P.: Indices for the measurement of gingival inflammation in clinical studies of oral hygiene and periodontal disease. J. Periodont. Res., *9*(Suppl. 14):61, 1974.

48. Glass, R. L.: Hand and electric toothbrushing. J. Periodontol., *36*:323, 1965.

49. Gottlieb, B.: Zur Atiologie und Therapie der Alveolarpyorrhoe. Z. Stomatol., *18*:59, 1920.

50. Greene, J. C.: Periodontal disease in India: report of an epidemiological study. J. Dent. Res., *39*:302, 1960.

51. Greene, J. C.: Oral hygiene and periodontal disease. Am. J. Public Health, *53*:913, 1963.

52. Greene, J. C.: The Oral Hygiene Index—development and uses. J. Periodontol., *38*:625, 1967.

53. Greene, J. C., and Vermillion, J. R.: Oral Hygiene Index: a method for classifying oral hygiene status. J. Am. Dent. Assoc., *61*:172, 1960.

54. Greene, J. C., and Vermillion, J. R.: The Simplified Oral Hygiene Index. J. Am. Dent. Assoc., *68*:7, 1964.

55. Harvey, C., and Kelly, J. E.: Decayed, Missing, and Filled Teeth Among Persons 1–74 Years, United States. Hyattsville, Md., U.S.P.H.S., U.S. Department of Health and Human Services, National Center for Health Statistics, DHHS Publication No. (PHS) 81–1673, Series 11, No. 223, 1981.

55a. Horton, J. E., and Sumnicht, R. W.: Relationships of educational levels to periodontal disease and oral hygiene with variables of age and geographic regions. J. Periodontol., *38*:335, 1967.

56. James, P. M. C., et al.; Gingival health and dental cleanliness in English school children. Arch. Oral Biol., *3*:57, 1960.

57. Jamison, H. C.: Prevalence of periodontal disease of the deciduous teeth. J. Am. Dent. Assoc., *66*:207, 1963.

58. Johnson, E. S., Kelly, J. E., and Vankirk, L. E.: Selected Dental Findings in Adults by Age, Race and Sex, United States 1960–1962. Washington, D.C., U.S. Department of Health, Education, and Welfare, National Center for Health Statistics, Publication No. 1000, Series 11, No. 7, 1965.

59. Jorkjend, L., and Birkeland, J. M.: Plaque and gingivitis among Norwegian children participating in a dental health program. Community Dent. Oral Epidemiol., *1*:41, 1973.

60. Kelly, J. E., and Harvey, C. R.: Basic Dental Examination Findings of Persons 1–74 Years, United States 1971–1974. Hyattsville, Md., U.S.P.H.S., U.S. Department of Health, Education, and Welfare, National Center for Health Statistics, DHEW Publication No. (PHS) 79–1662, Series 11, No. 214, 1979.

61. Kelly, J. E., and Sanchez, M. J.: Periodontal Disease and Oral Hygiene Among Children, United States. Washington, D.C., U.S.P.H.S., U.S. Department of Health, Education, and Welfare, National Center for Health Statistics, Publication No. (HSM) 72–1060, Series 11, No. 117, 1972.

62. Kelly, J. E., and Van Kirk, L. E.: Periodontal Disease in Adults, United States 1960 1962. Washington, D.C., U.S.P.H.S., U.S. Department of Health, Education, and Welfare, National Center for Health Statistics, Publication No. 1000, Series 11, No. 12, 1966.

63. Kelly, J. E., Van Kirk, L. E., and Garst, C. C.: Oral Hygiene in Adults, United States 1960–1962. Washington, D.C., U.S.P.H.S., U.S. Department of Health, Education, and Welfare, National Center for Health Statistics, Publication No. 1000, Series 11, No. 16, 1966.

64. Kesel, R. G.: Are dental caries and periodontal disease incompatible? J. Periodontol., *21*:30, 1950.

65. King, J. D.: Dental Disease in the Isle of Lewis. Medical Research Council, Special Report Series, No. 241. London, His Majesty's Stationery Office, 1940.

66. King, J. D.: Gingival disease in Dundee. D. Record, *65*:9, 32, 55, 1945.

67. King, J. D., Franklyn, A. B., and Allen, I.: Gingival disease in Gibraltar evacuee children. Lancet, *1*:495, 1944.

68. Körber, K. H.: Periodontal pulsation. J. Periodontol., *41*:382, 1970.

69. Körber, K. H.: Electronic registration of tooth movements. Int. Dent. J., *21*:466, 1971.

70. Körber, K. H., and Körber, E.: Untersuchungen zur Biophysik des Parodontiums. Dtsch. Zahnärztl. Z., *17*:1585, 1962.

71. Landgraph, E., and Banhigyi, S.: Untersuchungen über den Cholesterin-, Bilirubin- und Reservealkaligehalte des Blutes bei Paradentosekranken. Z. Stomatol., *29*:11, 1931.

72. Lenox, J. A., and Kopczyk, R. A.: A clinical system for scoring a patient's oral hygiene performance. J. Am. Dent. Assoc., *86*:849, 1973.

73. Lobene, R. R.: The effect of an automatic toothbrush on gingival health. J. Periodontol., *35*:137, 1964.

74. Löe, H.: The Gingival Index, the Plaque Index and the Retention Index systems. J. Periodontol. *38*:610, 1967.

75. Löe, H., and Silness, J.: Periodontal disease in pregnancy. Acta Odontol. Scand., *21*:533, 1963.

76. Löe, H., Theilade, E., and Jensen, S. B.: Experimental gingivitis in man. J. Periodontol. *36*:177, 1965.

77. Löe, H., Anerud, A., Boysen, H., and Smith, M.: The natural history of periodontal disease in man—study design and baseline data. J. Periodont. Res., *13*:550, 1978.

78. Lovdal, A., Arno, A., and Waerhaug, J.: Incidence of clinical manifestations of periodontal disease in light of oral hygiene and calculus formation. J. Am. Dent. Assoc., *56*:21, 1958.

79. Lovdal, A., Arno, A., Schei, O., and Waehaug, J.: Combined effect of subginival scaling and controlled oral hygiene on the incidence of gingivitis. Acta Odontol. Scand., *19*:537, 1961.

80. Mandel, I. D.: Indices for measurement of soft accumualtions in clinical studics of oral hygiene and periodontal disease. J. Periodont. Res., *9*(Suppl. 14):7, 1974.

81. Mandel, I. D.: Indices for measurement of soft accumulations in clinical studies of oral hygiene and periodontal disease (continued). J. Periodont. Res., *9*(Suppl. 14):106, 1974.

82. Marshall-Day, C. D.: Chronic endemic fluorosis in Northern India. Br. Dent. J., *68*:409, 1940.

83. Marshall-Day, C. D.: Nutritional deficiencies and dental caries in northern India. Br. Dent. J., *76*:115, 143, 1944.

84. Marshall-Day, C. D.: The epidemiology of periodontal disease. J. Periodontol., *22*:13, 1951.

85. Marshall-Day, C. D., and Shourie, K. L.: The incidence of periodontal disease in the Punjab. Indian J. Med. Res., *32*:47, 1944.

86. Marshall-Day, C. D., and Shourie, K. L.: Hypertrophic gingivitis in Indian children and adolescents. Indian J. Med. Res., *35*(4):261, 1947.

87. Marshall-Day, C. D., and Shourie, K. L.: A roentgenographic study of periodontal disease in India. J. Am. Dent. Assoc., *39*:572, 1949.

88. Marshall-Day, C. D., and Shourie, K. L.: Gingival disease in the Virgin Islands. J. Am. Dent. Assoc., *40*:175, 1950.

89. Marshall-Day, C. D., and Tandan, G. C.: The incidence of dental caries in the Punjab. Br. Dent. J., *69*:389, 1940.

90. Marshall-Day, C. D., Stephens, R. G.,. and Quigley, L. F.: Periodontal disease: prevalence and incidence. J. Periodontol., *26*:185, 1955.

91. Massler, M.: The P-M-A Index for the assessment of gingivitis. J. Periodontol., *38*:592, 1967.

92. Massler, M., and Schour, I.: The P-M-A Index of Gingivitis. J. Dent. Res., *28*:634, 1949 (abstract).

93. Massler, M., Cohen, A., and Schour, I.: Epidemiology of gingivitis in children. J. Am. Dent. Assoc., *45*:319, 1952.

94. Massler, M., Schour, I., and Chopra, B.: Occurrence of gingivitis in suburban Chicago school children. J. Periodontol., *21*:146, 1950.

95. McCall, J. O.: The periodontist looks at children's dentistry. J. Am. Dent. Assoc., *20*:1518, 1933.

96. McHugh, W. D., McEven, J. D., and Hitchin, A. D.: Dental disease and related factors in 13-year-old children in Dundee. Br. Dent. J., *117*:246, 1964.

97. Messner, C. T., Gafaver, W. M., Cady, F. C., and Dean, H. T.: Dental Survey of School Children Ages 6 to 14 Years Made in 1933–1934 in 26 States. Public Health Bulletin 226. Washington, D.C., U.S. Government Printing Office, 1938.

98. Miglani, D. C.: Incidence of acute necrotizing ulcerative gingivitis and periodontosis among cases seen at the Government Hospital, Madras. J. All India Dent. Assoc., *37*:183, 1965.

99. Miller, S. C.: Precocious advanced alveolar atrophy. J. Periodontol., *19*:146, 1948.

100. Miller, S. C.: Textbook of Periodontia. 3rd ed. Philadelphia, Blakiston, 1950.

101. Miller, S. C., and Seidler, B. B.: A correlation between periodontal disease caries. J. Dent. Res., *19*:549, 1940.

102. Miller, S. C., and Seidler, B. B.: Relative alveoloclastic experience of the various teeth. J. Dent. Res., *21*:365, 1942.

103. Moore, R. M., Muhler, J. C., and McDonald, R. E.: A study of the effect of water fluoride content and socioeconomic status on the occurrence of gingivitis in school children. J. Dent. Res., *43*:782, 1964.

104. Mühlemann, H. R.: Periodontometry, a method for measuring tooth mobility. Oral Surg., *4*:1220, 1951.

105. Mühlemann, H. R.: Tooth mobility. I. The measuring method—initial and secondary tooth mobility. J. Periodontol., *25*:125, 1954.

106. Mühlemann, H. R.: Ten years of tooth-mobility measurements. J. Periodontol., *31*:110, 1960.

107. Mühlemann, H. R., and Mazor, Z. S.: Gingivitis in Zurich school children. Helv. Odontol. Acta, *2*:3, 1958.

108. Mühlemann, H. R., and Son, S.: Gingival sulcus bleeding—a leading symptom in initial gingivitis. Helv. Odontol. Acta, *15*:107, 1971.

109. Mühlemann, H. R., and Villa, P.: The Marginal Line Calculus Index. Helv. Odontol. Acta, *11*:175, 1967.

110. Murray, J. J.: Gingivitis in 15-year-old children from high fluoride and low fluoride areas. Arch. Oral Biol., *14*:951, 1969.

111. Murray, J. J.: Gingivitis and gingival recession in adults from high-fluoride and low-fluoride areas. Arch. Oral Biol., *17*:1269, 1972.

112. Murray, J. J.: The prevalence of gingivitis in children continuously resident in a high fluoride area. J. Dent. Child., *41*:133, 1974.

113. Newman, M. G.: Periodontosis. J. Western Soc. Periodontol./Periodont. Abs., *24*:5, 1976.

114. Nizel, A. E.: The Science of Nutrition and Its Application in Clinical Denistry. 2nd ed., Philadelphia, W. B. Saunders Company 1966, pp. 408–420.

115. O'Leary, T. J.: The periodontal screening examination. J. Periodontol., *38*:617, 1967.

116. O'Leary, T. J.: Indices for measurement of tooth mobility in clinical studies. J. Periodont. Res., *9*(Suppl. 14):94, 1974.

117. O'Leary, T. J., and Rudd, K. D.: An instrument for measuring horizontal tooth mobility. Periodontics, *1*:249, 1963.

118. O'Leary, T. J., Drake, R. B., and Naylor, J. E.: The plaque control record. J. Periodontol., *43*:38, 1972.

119. O'Leary, T. J., Gibson, W. A., Shannon, I. L., Schuessler, C. F., and Nabers, C. L.: A screening examination for detection of gingival and periodontal breakdown and local irritants. Periodontics, *1*:167, 1963.

120. Orban, B.: Classification of periodontal disease. Parodontologie, *4*:159, 1949.

121. Parfitt, G. J.: Development of an instrument to measure tooth mobility. J. Dent. Res., *37*:64, 1958 (abstract).

122. Parfitt, G. J.: A survey of the oral health of Navajo Indian children. Arch. Oral Biol., *1*:193, 1959.

123. Parfitt, G. J.: Measurement of the physiological mobility of individual teeth in an axial direction. J. Dent. Res., *39*:608, 1960.

124. Pelton, W. J., Pennell, E. H., and Druzina, A.: Tooth morbidity experience of adults. J. Am. Dent. Assoc., *49*:439, 1954.

125. Picton, D. C. A.: A method of measuring physiological tooth movements in man. J. Dent. Res., *36*:814, 1957.

126. Picton, D. C. A.: A study of normal tooth mobility and the changes with periodontal disease. Dent. Practit., *12*:167, 1962.

127. Podshadley, A. G., and Haley, J. V.: A method for evaluating patient hygiene performance by observation of selected tooth surfaces. Public Health Rep., *83*:259, 1968.

128. Proceedings of the Workshop on Quantitative Evaluation of Periodontal Diseases by Physical Measurement Techniques. J. Dent. Res., *58*:547, 1979.

129. Quigley, G., and Hein, J.: Comparative cleansing efficiency of manual and power brushing. J. Am. Dent. Assoc., *65*:26, 1962.

130. Ramfjord, S. P.: Indices for prevalence and incidence of periodontal disease. J. Periodontol., *30*:51, 1959.

131. Ramfjord, S. P.: The Periodontal Index (PDI). J. Periodontol., *38*:602, 1967.

132. Ramfjord, S. P.: Design of studies or clinical trials to evaluate the effectiveness of agents or procedures for the prevention, or treatment, of loss of the periodontium. J. Periodont. Res., *9*(Suppl. 14):78, 1974.

133. Rao, S. S., and Tewani, S. V.: Prevalence of periodontosis among Indians. J. Periodontol., *37*:27, 1968.

134. Ruffer, M. A.: Studies in the Palaeopathology of Ancient Eygpt. Chicago, University of Chicago Press, 1921.

135. Rgug-Gunn, A. J., and Holloway, P. J.: Methods of measuring the realiability of caries prevalence and incremental data. Community Dent. Oral Epidemicol., *2*:287, 1974.

136. Russell, A. L.: A system of classification and scoring for prevalence surveys of periodontal disease. J. Dent. Res., *35*:350, 1956.

137. Russell, A. L.: Fluoride, domestic water and periodontal disease. Am. J. Public Health, *47*:688, 1957.

138. Russell, A. L.: A social factor associated with the severity of periodontal disease. J. Dent. Res., *36*:922, 1957.

139. Russell, A. L.: Some epidemiological characteristics of periodontal disease in a series of urban populations. J. Periodontol., *28*:286, 1957.

140. Russell, A. L.: The Geographical Distribution and Epidemiology of Periodontal Disease. World Health Organization Expert Committee on Dental Health (Periodontal Disease). WHO/DH/34. Geneva, 1960.

141. Russell, A. L.: International nutrition surveys: a summary of preliminary dental findings. J. Dent. Res., *42*:233, 1963.

142. Russell, A. L.: Epidemiology of periodontal disease. Int. Dent. J., *17*:282, 1967.

143. Russell, A. L.: The Periodontal Index. J. Periodontol., *38*:585, 1967.

144. Russell, A. L.: Epidemiology and the rational bases of dental public health and dental practice. In Young, W. O., and Striffler, D. F. (eds.): The Dentist, His Practice, and His Community, 2nd ed. Philadelphia, W. B. Saunders Company, 1969, pp. 35–57.

145. Russell, A. L.: The epidemiology of dental caries and periodontal diseases. In Young, W. O., and Striffler, D. F. (eds.): The Dentist, His Practice, and His Community. 2nd ed. Philadelphia, W. B. Saunders Company, 1969, pp. 73–86.

146. Russell, A. L.: The prevalence of periodontal disease in different populations during the circumpubertal period. J. Periodontol. *42*:508, 1971.

147. Russell, A. L., and Ayers, P.: Periodontal disease and socioeconomic status in Birmingham, Ala. Am. J. Public Health., *50*:206, 1960.

148. Russell, A. L., Leatherwood, E. C., Consolazio, C. F., and Van Reen, R.: Periodontal disease and nutrition in South Vietnam. J. Dent. Res., *44*:775, 1965.

149. Sanchez, M. J.: Periodontal Disease Among Youth 12–17 Years, United States. Washington, D. C., U.S.P.H.S., U.S. Department of Health, Education, and Welfare, National Center for Health Statistics, Publication No. (HRA) 74–1623, Series 11, No. 141, 1974.

150. Sanchez, M. J.: Oral Hygiene Among Youths 12–17 Years, United States. Washington, D.C., U.S.P.H.S., U.S. Department of Health, Education, and Welfare, National Center for Health Statistics, Publication No. (HRA) 76–1633, Series 11, No. 151, 1975.

151. Sartwell, P. E. (ed.): Maxcy-Rosenau Preventive Medicine and Public Health. 10th ed. New York, Appleton-Century-Crofts, 1973, pp. 1–58.

152. Saxen, L.: Juvenile periodontics. J. Clin. Periodontol., *7*:1, 1980.

153. Schei, O., Waerhaug, J., Lovdal, A., and Arno, A.: Alveolar bone loss as related to oral hygiene and age. J. Periodontol., *30*:7, 1959.

154. Schour, I., and Massler, M.: Gingival disease in postwar Italy (1945). I. Prevalence of gingivitis in various age groups. J. Am. Dent. Assoc., *35*:475, 1947.

155. Schour, I., and Massler, M.: Survey of gingival disease using the PMA Index. J. Dent. Res., *27*:733, 1948.

156. Schroeder, H. E.: Formation and Inhibition of Dental Calculus. Berne, Stuttgart, Vienna, H. Huber Publishers, 1969, pp. 66–68.

157. Shapiro, S., Pollack, B. R., and Gallant, D.: A special population available for periodontal research. Part II. A correlation and association analysis between oral hygiene and periodontal disease. J. Periodontol., *42*:161, 1971.

158. Shaw, J. H., and Sweeney, E. A.: Nutrition in relation to dental medicine. *In* Goodhart, R. S., and Shils, M. E. (eds.): Modern Nutrition in Health and Disease. Philadelphia, Lea & Febiger, 1973, p. 756.

159. Shaw, L., and Murray, J. J.: Diagnostic reproducibility of periodontal indices. J. Periodont. Res., *12*:141, 1977.

160. Shay, H., and Smart, G. A.: The association of local factors with gingivitis. Br. Dent. J., *78*:135, 1945.

161. Sheiham, A.: The epidemiology of chronic periodontal disease in western Nigerian children. J. Periodont. Res., *3*:257, 1968.

162. Sheiham, A.: The prevalence and severity of periodontal disease in Surrey school chidlren. Dent. Practit., *19*:232, 1969.

163. Sheiham, A., and Striffler, D. F.: A comparison of four epidemiological methods of assessing periodontal disease. J. Periodont. Res., *5*:155, 1970.

164. Shick, R. A., and Ash, M. M.: Evaluation of the vertical method of toothbrushing. J. Periodontol., *32*:346, 1961.

165. Silness, P., and Löe, H.: Periodontal disease in pregnancy. Acta Odontol. Scand., *22*:121, 1964.

166. Smith, L. W., Suomi, J. D., Green, J. C., and Barbano, J. P.: A study of intraexaminer variation in scoring oral hygiene

status, gingival inflammation and epithelial attachment level. J. Periodontol., *41*:671, 1970.

167. Stahl, D. G., and Goldman, H. M.: Incidence of gingivitis among a sample of Massachusetts school children. Oral Surg., *6*:707, 1953.

168. Summers, C., and Oberman, A.: Association of oral disease with twelve selected variables. I. Periodontal disease. J. Dent. Res., *47*:457, 1968.

169. Suomi, J. D., and Barbano, J. P.: Patterns of gingivitis. J. Periodontol., *39*:71, 1968.

170. Suomi, J. D., Plumbo, J., and Barbano, J. P.: A comparative study of radiographs and pocket measurements in periodontal disease evaluation. J. Periodontol., *39*:311, 1968.

171. Suomi, J. D., Smith, L. W., and McClendon, B. J.: Marginal gingivitis during a sixteen week period. J. Periodontol., *42*:268, 1971.

172. Suomi, J. D., Greene, J. C., Vermillion, J. R., Doyle, J., Chang, J. J., and Leatherwood, E. C.: The effect of controlled oral hygiene procedures on the progression of periodontal disease in adults: results after third and final year. J. Periodontol., *42*:152, 1971.

172a. Tenenbaum, B., Karshan, M., Ziskin, D., and Nahoun, K. I.: Clinical and microscopic study of the gingivae in periodontosis. J. Am. Dent. Assoc., *40*:302, 1950.

173. Ten-State Nutrition Survey 1968–1970, by Health Services and Mental Health Administration, U. S. Department of Health, Education, and Welfare. Atlanta Center for Disease Control. Atlanta, Publication No. (HSM) 72–8131, 1972, Vol. 3, pp. 111, 126–131.

174. Tibbetts, L. S., and Kashiwa, H. K.: A histochemical study of early plaque mineralization, *In* I.A.D.R. Program and Abstracts of Papers, Abstract No. 616, 1970, p. 202.

175. Turesky, S., Gilmore, N. D., and Glickman, I.: Reduced plaque formation by the chloromethyl analogue of Victamine C. J. Periodontol., *41*:41, 1970.

176. Volpe, A. R.: Indices for the measurement of hard deposits in clinical studies of oral hygiene and periodontal disease. J. Periodont. Res., *9*(Suppl. 14):31, 1974.

177. Volpe, A. R., Manhold, J. H., and Hazen, S. P.: *In vivo* calculus assessment: a method and its reproducibility. J. Periodontol., *36*:292, 1965.

178. Wade, A. B.: Validity of anterior segment gingival scores in epidemiologic studies. J. Periodontol., *37*:55, 1966.

179. White, C. L., and Russell, A. L.: Some relations between dental caries experience and active periodontal disease in two thousand adults. N.Y. J. Dent., *32*:211, 1962.

180. Wilkinson, F. C., Adamson, K. T., and Knight, F.: A study of the incidence of dental disease in the aborigines, from the examination of 65 in the collection found in the Melbourne University. Aust. J. Dent., *33*:109, 1929.

181. World Health Organization: Oral Health Surveys: Basic Methods. 2nd ed. Geneva, WHO, 1977.

182. Zimmerman, E. R., and Baker, W. A.: Effect of geographic location and race on gingival disease in children. J. Am. Dent. Assoc., *61*:542, 1960.

Part III

Etiology of Periodontal Disease

Etiologic factors of periodontal disease have customarily been classified into local and systemic factors, although their effects are interrelated. *Local factors* are those in the immediate environment of the periodontium, whereas *systemic factors* result from the general condition of the patient.

Local factors cause inflammation, which is the principal pathologic process in periodontal disease; systemic factors monitor the tissue response to local factors, so that the effect of local irritants may be dramatically aggravated by unfavorable systemic conditions. The following diagram, modified from that developed by Bahn, shows in schematic form the role of the different factors:

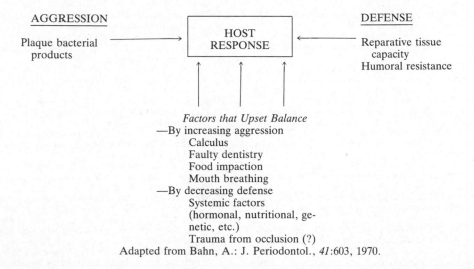

Adapted from Bahn, A.: J. Periodontol., *41*:603, 1970.

Plaque is necessary to initiate the disease. A small but variable amount of plaque can, however, be controlled by the body defense mechanisms, resulting in an equilibrium between aggression and defense. This equilibrium can be broken either by increasing the amount and/or the virulence of the bacteria or by reducing the defensive capacity of the tissues. The following factors favor the accumulation of plaque: calculus, faulty dentistry (inadequate restorations), food impaction, and mouth breathing.

Factors that reduce the defensive capacity of the tissues include all the systemic conditions that may disturb the tissue response to irritation. Their exact mechanism of action is in most cases obscure.

It should also be clearly understood that diseases besides periodontal disease can attack the periodontal tissues. These other diseases may result from a variety of causes, by direct extension from the oral mucosa or the jaw bones or owing to a systemic involvement. Within this group of diseases, which we shall term "periodontal manifestations of other diseases," the following can be found: herpetic gingivostomatitis; tuberculous, syphilitic, and other bacterial infections; different dermatoses; blood diseases; and various benign and malignant tumors.

Systemic factors can therefore act either by reducing tissue resistance to plaque or by producing changes per se. In the former case, the resulting disease will be periodontal disease; in the latter, it will be a periodontal manifestation of the systemic disease.

The Host Response in Periodontal Disease

It is now recognized that host responses play a role in most forms of periodontal disease. *In gingivitis, periodontitis, and juvenile periodontitis, the development of the disease depends upon the interaction between the resident microbiota and the host response. In other types of periodontal disease, such as desquamative gingivitis, the lesions frequently result from a host response.*

Emphasis in periodontal disease research has been focused on understanding the immunopathologic mechanisms which may operate in the development and maintenance of periodontal inflammatory changes. This chapter will briefly review the basis of the immunologic and inflammatory responses as they may relate to the etiology and pathogenesis of periodontal diseases. Responses occurring in gingivitis and periodontitis will be emphasized.

Previous investigators considered periodontal disease to be one disease process, in which the nature and severity differed according to the individual host's resistance and the specific etiologic and predisposing factors present. Evidence now suggests that the term *periodontal disease* may in fact represent different diseases of the periodontium, each demonstrating unique clinical, bacterial, pathologic,

biochemical, and immunologic patterns.[122, 136] In most individuals, the host response mechanisms depend on the presence of specific microorganisms and their particular toxic and/or antigenic products.[13, 94, 109] The nature and severity of periodontal pathology are now thought to be dependent on specific microorganisms and modified by factors such as white blood cell defects,[19] mechanical and traumatic forces, drug ingestion, nutritional deficiencies, systemic disease, and age.

The histopathology of gingivitis and periodontitis suggests that an immunologic response occurs in the pathogenesis of these diseases (Fig. 24–1). Inflammation in the periodontal tissues is triggered to some extent by the host response to the continuous bacterial antigenic exposure and the direct nonimmunologic effects of bacterial products from the dental plaque microorganisms. In disease, the gingival tissues are infiltrated with all the elements necessary to elicit immune responses: **plasma cells,** which produce immunoglobulins that can participate in immediate hypersensitivity and immune complex disease; **lymphocytes,** including T-cells actively responsible for cell-mediated immunity and B-cells responsible for antibody-mediated reactions; **mast cells; poly-**

343

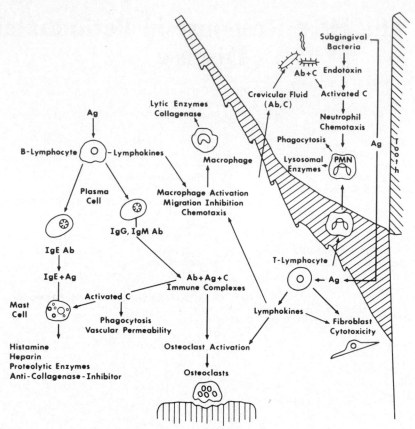

Figure 24–1 Immunologic Responses in Gingivitis and Periodontitis. Potential immunopathologic processes which may occur in the course of human gingivitis and periodontitis. (From Nisengard, R. J.: J. Periodontol., *48*:505, 1977.)

morphonuclear leukocytes; and **macrophages.** *Although inflammation is a host defense mechanism to localize and destroy foreign materials, the host's own tissues may also be destroyed in the process.*[122] *Thus, inflammation may account for part of the soft tissue destruction and alveolar bone loss seen in the course of human periodontal disease.*

INITIAL HOST RESPONSE

Following the accumulation of bacteria or their products in the gingival sulcus, there is a host response. This includes the migration of polymorphonuclear leukocytes into the gingival crevice and a vascular response. The vascular response consists of increased blood flow and permeability of the small vessels of the gingiva.[31, 32] Serum components, fibrin, erythrocytes, and granulocytes accumulate and form an inflammatory exudate. Clinically, this type of response can occur within 2 to 4 days of plaque accumulation and is characterized as **acute gingivitis.**[109] The events which take place as a result of the host response may be protective or destructive.

The nature and character of the host response determine whether the initial lesion resolves rapidly, with the tissue restored to normal, or evolves into a chronic inflammatory lesion. If the latter occurs, an infiltrate of macrophages and lymphoid cells appears in a few days.[109]

The acute inflammatory exudate and the changes in the microcirculation are induced biochemically by substances released in the gingiva. Increased vascular permeability results from released histamine, 5-hydroxytryptamine, kinins, complement components, and prostaglandins. Histamine has many sources, including mast cells, platelets, and endothelial cells. Mast cell degranulation results from direct bacterial effects, endotoxins, IgE-mediated immediate hypersensitivity, immune complexes, complement components, mechanical trauma, basic peptides, and proteolytic enzymes.[62, 122]

The increased permeability which occurs in the gingival microvasculature increases the number of cells and chemical constituents which have the potential for causing tissue damage. The resulting edema, together with the increased permeability of the junctional epithelium, allows the flow of gingival fluid into the gingival sulcus or pocket. Because of its cellular and chemical constituents, the gingival fluid could serve to neutralize bacteria and their products and/or to furnish essential nutrients to potentially pathogenic organisms located deep in periodontal pockets.[93] The presence of the protein-rich gingival fluid and reduced oxygen tension are very important ecologic factors favoring the accumulation and growth of the protein- and amino acid–requiring gram-negative rods and spirochetes. These organisms increase in number during the development of gingivitis and in periodontitis (see Chapter 25).

INFLAMMATORY CELL RESPONSE

In response to specific biochemical stimuli, inflammatory cells chemotactically migrate and concentrate in localized areas where they phagocytize bacteria or their components (Fig. 24–1). Some of these, such as T- and B-lymphocytes, divide and increase in number by blastogenesis. Others release vasoactive products, and still others may produce substances that cause the lysis of other host cells or the destruction of alveolar bone.[122] The cells involved are mast cells, polymorphonuclear leukocytes (neutrophils), macrophages, and lymphocytes.

Mast Cells

Mast cells may play a role in the pathogenesis of gingivitis and periodontitis, since their numbers are inversely related to the degree of gingival inflammation.[16, 27, 129, 152] Normal gingiva contains more mast cells than does moderately inflamed tissue. Severely inflamed gingiva contains the fewest mast cells.[16] This suggests that degranulation occurs during the development of periodontal disease. Mast cell counts decrease during periodontitis and in-

crease following successful periodontal therapy.[94] During periods when mast cell numbers are found to be reduced, mast cell granules are seen in tissue spaces.[6]

Mast cells are important because their cytoplasmic granules contain histamine, slow-reacting substance of anaphylaxis (SRS-A), and bradykinin, which are released into the gingival tissues.[8] Degranulation of mast cells occurs during immediate hypersensitivity when antigens react with surface-bound IgE antibody. The reactions form the basis of anaphylaxis. In addition, a mast cell "factor" has been shown to enhance collagenase activity,[142] and heparin (contained in other granules)[78] may enhance bone resorption[46] by potentiating the effect of parathyroid hormone (Fig. 24–1).

Neutrophils

Neutrophils (polymorphonuclear leukocytes) are important in the host defense against injury and infection. These cells are found in all inflammatory lesions, particularly more acute lesions, where they concentrate at sites of injury and engulf, kill, and digest microorganisms and neutralize other noxious substances (Fig. 24–1). In **periodontal diseases**, systemic neutrophils apparently play both a protective and a destructive role.[2, 94, 109, 122] When these cells are depressed in number, as in cyclic neutropenia, or have impaired function, as in localized juvenile periodontitis,[10] host defenses are inadequate and periodontal destruction is more severe. Experimental neutropenia alters the initial appearance of gingivitis.[3] Rather than collagen being destroyed, gingival collagen fibers are displaced. Also, it appears that reduced numbers of neutrophilic granulocytes are associated with a more rapid apical proliferation of subgingival plaque.

In patients with localized **juvenile periodontitis,**[19, 69] there is a reduction in phagocytosis and a decreased response of neutrophils to chemotactic stimuli. In the majority of these patients, the chemotactic dysfunction is due to an intrinsic cellular defect.[69] Healthy siblings of patients with this disease also have a chemotactic defect. Approximately half the adults with rapidly progressing, generalized loss of periodontal attachment have a chemotactic defect. In these cases, dysfunction commonly results from leukocyte cellular defects. These alterations may impair host defenses against implicated gram-negative bacteria. Recent findings suggest that some of the gram-negative bacteria, such as strains of *Actinobacillus acti-nomycetemcomitans,* also produce a leukotoxin which can kill neutrophils, including those in the gingival crevice.[4, 139] A similar severe alveolar bone loss occurs in other disorders in which there is neutrophil dysfunction: cyclic neutropenia, agranulocytosis,[7] Chédiak-Higashi syndrome, and diabetes.[42, 68, 143] Neutrophil defects have been described in patients with chronic infections[150] and chronic candidiasis[51] and are thought to be responsible for the increased incidence of bacterial infections in cirrhosis[83] and rheumatoid arthritis.[89]

In rapidly progressive and juvenile periodontitis, neutrophils from the periodontal pockets also demonstrated reduced phagocytic capacity.[91] This appears to be at least partly a local phenomenon, since neutrophils from nondiseased sites did not display this reduced capacity.

Neutrophils may also cause tissue destruction. Their granules contain substances capable of killing, digesting, and neutralizing microorganisms and/or their products, and they also contain a specific collagenase.[37, 49, 56, 140, 141] It is important to note that the localized tissue damage seen in the Arthus reaction (see below) depends upon the presence of neutrophils.

The subgingival bacteria associated with inflammatory periodontal disease appear to influence neutrophils in two ways. Bacteria, including *Treponema denticola, Actinomyces viscosus, Bacteroides gingivalis,* and *Capnocytophaga ochraceus,* contain factors chemotactic for neutrophil granulocytes.[76] Once the neutrophils are attracted to the site of bacteria, some bacteria, such as *Capnocytophaga, Bacteroides melaninogenicus, Leptotrichia buccalis,* and, to a lesser extent, *Actinobacillus actinomycetemcomitans,* can induce the lysosomal release from the neutrophils.[144]

Macrophages

Macrophages play a direct, important function in cell-mediated immunity (discussed below). These large, highly phagocytic cells are part of the scavenger reticuloendothelial system.[26] They participate with T-lymphocytes in aiding the response of B-lymphocytes to many immunogens.[33] Recognition of this helper function stems from observations which demonstrate that trace amounts of antigen bound to the macrophage surface are far more potent immunogenically than the same amount of free, unbound antigen.[85] It is thought that the macrophage "processes" the antigen for the B-lymphocyte. In inflammatory lesions, macrophages are formed by differentiation of monocytes carried to the lesion by the blood. These cells act nonspecifically with antigens, which provide them with the capability of destroying a diverse, antigenically unrelated group of bacteria.[137]

Macrophages and monocytes are not the most common cell types found in periodontal lesions, but they may play an important role in the pathogenesis of these lesions.[110] In chronic periodontitis, activated macrophages can be identified in the gingival epithelium, lamina propria, perivascular tissues, and blood vessels.[17] Mononuclear cells are attracted to sites of inflammation by lymphokines (substances released by lymphocytes) and complement factors. Once present, they are retained at these sites by other lymphokines (Fig. 24–1). The ability of the macrophages to ingest, kill, and digest microorganisms is dependent upon interaction with other leukocytes, the immune system in general, and complement. The efficiency of bacterial phagocytosis by the macrophages is enhanced by the reaction of antibody with the antigen and subsequent complement activation.

Macrophages are also important because they produce prostaglandins,[88] cyclic adenosine monophosphate (cyclic AMP), and collagenase[39, 70, 111, 145] in response to stimulation by bacterial endotoxin, immune complexes, or lymphokines. Macrophage collagenase may play a significant role in collagen destruction in the diseased periodontal tissues.

ANTIBODY

The host can respond to the presence of oral bacteria and their products by the production of antibodies, primarily by mature plasma cells. The possible role of antibodies in periodontal and gingival disease is summarized in Table 24–1.

These proteins, derived from the blood and functioning as antibodies, are the effectors of humoral immunity.[26] They are referred to as **immunoglobulins.** All immunoglobulins have a similar structural organization, but they differ according to their antigenic properties, carbohydrate content, weight, and amino acid sequences. Every antibody molecule has a specific group of antigens with which it can react at the "antibody-combining site" because of its specific amino acid sequence and tertiary structure.

TABLE 24–1 POSSIBLE ROLE OF ANTIBODIES IN PERIODONTAL AND GINGIVAL DISEASE*

Reaction or Process‡	Effects
Activation of C′ by Ag-Ab complexes	Protective early changes in inflammation
Phagocytosis of Ag-Ab complexes by PMN's with release of lysosomes	Destructive
Enhanced lymphocyte stimulation by Ag-Ab complexes	Release of lymphokines with protective and destructive effects
Blocking of lymphocytes by free antibody or by Ag-Ab complexes	Suppression of cell-mediated immune reactions
Neutralization of bacterial allergins, toxins, or histolytic enzymes	Protective
Enhanced opsonization or bacteriolysis of plaque bacteria	Protective

*Adapted from Genco, R., et al.: J. Periodontol., *45*:336, 1974.
‡PMN's = polymorphonuclear leukocytes. Ag-Ab complexes = antigen-antibody complexes.

Human immunoglobulin is divided into five classes on the basis of structural differences. These differences are responsible for different biologic effects subsequent to antigen binding (Table 24–2). The five classes are IgG, IgM, IgA, IgE, and IgD. Four subclasses of IgG have been identified (IgG$_1$, IgG$_2$, IgG$_3$, and IgG$_4$), as have two subclasses of IgA (IgA$_1$ and IgA$_2$) and two subclasses of IgM (IgM$_1$ and IgM$_2$). Immunoglobulin molecules are made up of one of two types of light (small) and one of five types of heavy (large) polypeptide chains. The class is determined by the type of heavy chain. Each of the five classes of immunoglobulins has similar sets of light chains but antigenically distinct sets of heavy chains. Any particular immunoglobulin molecule has identical heavy chains and identical light chains.[26]

A variety of studies have suggested that IgG molecules are Y-shaped. The tail of the Y is made up of part of a set of heavy chains, the end of which is referred to as the Fc fragment. It is in this region that the complement binding takes place. The V area of the Y-shaped molecule is made up of the rest of the set of heavy chains and light chains. This is the Fab or antibody-binding site. The number of these binding sites is called the valence of the molecule.

Biologic Properties of Immunoglobulins

IgG. IgG is the most abundant of the serum immunoglobulins and is distributed equally between the blood and the extravascular fluids. Its major role is to neutralize bacterial toxins by binding to organisms, thereby enhancing their phagocytosis. Although IgG concentration in serum is very high, its concentration in secretions is low. IgG constitutes 80 per cent of the total serum immunoglobulin, passes the placental barrier, and provides newborns with the humoral immunity of the mother.[26]

IgM. Antibodies of the IgM class are the first to be formed after challenge with most antigens, but they are usually present in much lower concentrations than IgG. The levels of IgM during the later stages of an infection become negligible in comparison with those of IgG. This early synthesis suggests an important role for IgM in the early stages of infection. IgM is also the most efficient activator of the complement system. IgM molecules are composed of five basic immunoglobulin structural units, each unit similar to the IgG molecule, with a corresponding larger number of sites for interaction with antigen.

IgE. IgE (reaginic antibody) is present in human serum at about 1/125,000 the level of IgG. Despite the low concentration, this class

TABLE 24–2 PROPERTIES OF IMMUNOGLOBULINS*

	IgG				IgA	IgM	IgD	IgE
	1	*2*	*3*	*4*				
Serum concentration (mg./ml.)	total IgG: 12				2	1.2	0.03	0.00004
Complement fixation								
Classic pathway	+	±	+	−	−	+	−	−
Alternate pathway	+	+	+	?	+	+	−	+
Placental transfer	+	+	+	+	−	−	−	−
Reaginic activity	−	−	−	−	−	−	−	+
Antibacterial lysis	+	+	+	+	+	+	?	?

*From Nisengard, R. J.: J. Periodontol., *48*:505, 1977.

of antibody is responsible for severe acute allergic reactions and may be important in some phases of periodontal disease. The cells that produce IgE are abundant in the mucosa of the respiratory and intestinal tracts. Because of this, IgE is also found in exocrine secretions. Higher concentrations of these antibodies are found in patients with asthma, hay fever, and drug and food allergies. This class of antibodies has an affinity for cell surfaces which is mediated by an attachment site on their Fc fragment. In man, IgE is homocytotropic or attaches to mast cells and basophilic leukocytes. Thus, when antigens bind to two IgE antibodies that are already attached to mast cells, the antigen-antibody reaction causes histamine and other pharmacologically active substances to be released.

IgD. IgD is an immunoglobulin which is found at extremely low levels in serum. Although its role in the immune system is not clear, evidence suggests that it is the antigen receptor on the surface of lymphocytes. It may play an important role in triggering lymphocyte stimulation by antigen, thus initiating the immune response.

IgA. IgA occurs in a variety of polymeric forms of the basic IgG molecule, from monomer to trimer and even higher forms. IgA is the principal immunoglobulin in exocrine secretions (saliva, milk, respiratory secretions, intestinal mucin, and tears). It is present at one fifth the concentration of IgG in human serum. The cells that produce IgA are concentrated in the subepithelial tissue of the exocrine glands and apparently respond to antigens that are present locally. Serum IgA is mostly monomer, whereas secretory IgA is a dimer. Gingival tissue and crevicular fluid contain serum IgA rather than secretory IgA.

Properties of secretory IgA antibodies make them unique and influence the way in which they function on mucosal surfaces. Secretory IgA is more resistant to digestion by proteolytic enzymes than are other immunoglobulins. It has been suggested that the secretory component of a polypeptide chain which is attached to the Fc portion of secretory IgA stabilizes this portion of the molecule, facilitating its transport across the glandular epithelium. It is also possible that the J chain, the fourth type of polypeptide chain associated with secretory IgA, may function in making secretory IgA more resistant to proteolysis. The valence of the secretory IgA molecules generally found in saliva is 4.[85]

There has been wide interest in the protective effects of secretory antibodies against bac-terial and viral diseases on mucosal surfaces. IgA, unlike IgG and IgM, does not activate complement by the classical pathway, which begins with fixation of complement to the Fc portion of the immunoglobulin molecule. An alternate pathway of complement activation has been described which involves the later complement components, C3 through C9, but not C1, C4, or C2 (see section on "Complement"). This alternate pathway can be activated by aggregated immunoglobulin, including IgA.

Adhesion of bacteria to tissue surfaces may be prevented or reduced by secretory antibodies.[44] This mechanism of protection is thought to be active in bacterial diseases such as cholera and dental caries and possibly in the early phase of periodontal disease, in which bacterial adhesion and colonization of mucosal or dental tissues are necessary steps in the pathogenesis[87] (see Chapter 25). An antibacterial role of secretory IgA in established periodontal lesions is doubtful, since saliva probably does not penetrate into the depths of the lesion.

Antibody and Periodontal Disease

The presence of IgG, IgM, IgE, and (serum-derived) IgA in the gingival tissue of clinically healthy individuals suggests that these immunoglobulins gain access to the gingival sulcus.[123] Some of these immunoglobulins are detected in higher concentrations in the sulcular fluid of individuals with periodontal disease.[41, 94, 97, 117] IgG synthesis and IgA synthesis, but not IgM synthesis, have been identified in chronically inflamed gingival tissue.[67] The local synthesis of these antibodies and the demonstration of immunoglobulin-coated bacteria in subgingival plaque indicate that some of these immunoglobulins are specific for oral microorganisms.[9, 52]

The in vivo coating of subgingival bacteria with immunoglobulins and complement may directly influence the numbers and types of subgingival bacteria.[96, 126] Reactions with gram-negative bacteria could promote lysis, and reactions with gram-positive bacteria could promote phagocytosis. In vivo coating could also affect the growth characteristics of the bacteria by limiting their numbers.[14, 48]

Antibody titers to oral bacteria may also have a protective effect. Frequently, but not always, titers increase with increased severity of disease.[34, 45] In a few cases, higher titers are seen in healthy control subjects or in patients with gingivitis than in patients with periodontitis.[28, 45] Localized antibody production also occurs in gingival tissues.[94] Antibodies to bacilli,[86] spirochetes,[100, 138] cocci, and filamentous bacteria,[45] and specifically to *Fusobacterium, Leptotrichia,*[86] *Veillonella, Bacteroides,*[84] and *Actinobacillus,*[29] have been identified. These antibodies could aid in phagocytosis and in the removal of bacterial products from the tissues through complement activation by immune complexes.

The reaction of antibodies and bacterial antigens within the gingival tissues creates the potential for adverse tissue responses. The host, in the process of attempting to destroy or remove the foreign antigens, may exhibit an inflammatory response excessive for elimination of the antigens. Such responses occur in immediate hypersensitivity and in immune complex or Arthus reactions. Repetitive, experimentally induced immediate hypersensitivity and Arthus reactions in the gingiva can result in a chronic inflammatory infiltrate. In addition, Arthus reactions also cause osteoclastic alveolar bone loss.[1, 101]

Serum antibody and complement titers to plaque flora and to organisms isolated in lesions of idiopathic juvenile periodontitis have been assayed.[99] Significantly elevated titers occurred in association with *Bacteroides* species. For some of the other juvenile periodontitis–associated organisms, titers were significantly greater in patients with the disease than in older healthy subjects, adults with periodontitis, and siblings of patients with idiopathic juvenile periodontitis. In patients with juvenile periodontitis, serum concentrations of IgG, IgA, and IgM are elevated compared with those of normal subjects.[63, 73, 147] However, no significant changes occurred in IgG subclass levels. Plasma cells in lesions contain only K or λ chains, but no heavy chain, suggesting an immunologic defect.[148] Compared with patients with periodontitis and control subjects, there is also a marked increase in C3 deposits within the tissue.[60] Patients with juvenile periodontitis have elevated serum and gingival fluid antibody titers to *A. actinomycetemcomitans.*[90] Antibody responses in serum to the leukotoxin of *Actinobacillus* were also elevated in patients with juvenile periodontitis, compared with those of edentulous patients and patients with acute necrotizing ulcerative gingivitis and adult periodontitis.[30]

The general concept that develops from studies of antibody titers to oral bacteria is that most humans with clinically healthy periodontal tissues have a spectrum of antibodies to plaque organisms. In periodontitis, antibody titers vary in concentration depending on the specific organism to which antibodies have been detected. Further work must be done to elucidate the significance of these antibody responses in the pathogenesis of periodontal diseases. Some gram-negative bacteria indirectly influence antibody production because they possess potent polyclonal B-cell activators.[15] These B-cell activators can induce B-lymphocytes to produce antibody.

COMPLEMENT

An important and potentially harmful biologic consequence of antigen-antibody interaction is the activation of complement (Fig. 24–2). Complement consists of at least 11 proteins that make up approximately 10 per cent of the proteins in the normal sera of man and other vertebrates.[26] These proteins are not immunoglobulins, and they do not increase in concentration after immunization. These substances are synthesized in the liver, small intestine, macrophages, and other mononuclear cells.[122] They react with a wide variety of antibody-antigen complexes when the antibodies are of the IgG and IgM classes and exert their primary biologic effects on cell membranes, causing lysis and functional alteration that can promote phagocytosis. Of primary importance is their effect on mast cells. In these cells, degranulation by complement causes the release of histamine and other biologically active substances which increase the permeability of small blood vessels. Migration of polymorphonuclear leukocytes, increased phagocytic activity by leukocytes and macrophages, hemolysis, and bacteriolysis also take place. Red blood cell lysis (hemolysis) as a consequence of complement activation when antibody has reacted with the red blood cell has been analyzed in greatest detail because it is simple to measure. This provides the basis for the complement fixation assay, an important laboratory procedure for detecting and measuring many different kinds of antigens and antibodies and their effect on the complement system.

The reaction sequence in the activation of the complement system has a cascading-type pathway similar to that of the blood coagulation system (Fig. 24–2). After one component of the complement system is bound by the Fc portion of the antibody in the antibody-antigen complex, the other components of the complement system react in an ordered sequence. In general, each activated complement compo-

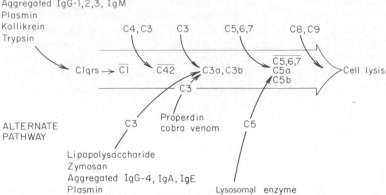

Figure 24–2 Schematic diagram of the complement sequence. Direct (classical) and alternate pathways in the activation of complement components. (From Page, R.: *In* Schluger, S., Yuodelis, R. A., and Page, R. C.: Periodontal Disease. Philadelphia, Lea & Febiger, 1977.)

nent cleaves the next reacting member of the series into fragments, until the cascade has been completed. Some of the smaller fragments formed during cleavage have phlogistic activity; that is, they cause inflammatory tissue changes[85] (Table 24–3). These include increased vascular permeability and the attraction of polymorphonuclear leukocytes. Other biologic activities of complement fixation are shown in Table 24–3. The classical pathway is activated by antigen reacting with IgG or IgM antibodies and by aggregated immunoglobulins. The sequence is C1, C4, C2, C3, C5, C6, C7, C8, C9. C3 is cleaved by the complex C42 into C3b, which binds to the cell membrane, and C3a, which has biologic activity (Fig. 24–2).

An alternate pathway for complement activation also exists. Aggregated antibodies of the IgG, IgA, and IgE classes, as well as endotoxin, can initiate the complement se-

quence by the direct activation of the third component of complement (C3) without triggering the beginning of the cascade starting with C1. The alternate pathway begins with cleavage of C3 after the conversion of C3 proactivator. The sequence after C3 activation is identical with that of the classical pathway: C5, C6, C7, C8, C9.

Studies have demonstrated that *the alternate pathway of complement activation occurs in most periodontal pockets* and that the classical pathway is activated only occasionally.[94, 122] Bacterial antigens such as endotoxins and polysaccharides such as dextran are also activators of the alternate pathway.[132] Dental plaque and pure cultures of oral bacteria can also activate complement by the alternate pathway in the absence of antibody.[105] Upon activation of complement by endotoxin, biologically active fragmentation products are released. Complement components that are present in the gingival sulcular fluid have been shown to be activated by some plaque bacteria and bacterial proteases.[125, 130] Complement activation by these various pathways could result in mechanisms which destroy the periodontal tissues.[118]

Although most attention has focused on cell lysis as a result of complement activation, the main physiologic effects are the cellular and tissue changes associated with inflammation. When C3 and C5 components are activated to C3a and C5a, they cause the degranulation of mast cells with the liberation of histamine, leading to a marked increase in capillary permeability. Injection of C3a into human skin elicits a wheal caused by increased capillary permeability. This effect can be specifically blocked by antihistamine drugs.

Chemotaxis of polymorphonuclear leukocytes is brought about by the activation of C5

TABLE 24–3 BIOLOGIC EFFECTS OF COMPLEMENT*

Activity	Complement Components
Cytolytic and cytotoxic damage to cells	C1–9
Chemotactic activity for leukocytes	C3a, C5a, C567
Histamine release from mast cells	C3a, C5a
Increased vascular permeability	C3a, C5a
Kinin activity	C2, C3a
Lysosomal enzyme release from leukocytes	C5a
Promotion of phagocytosis	C3, C5
Enhancement of blood clotting	C6
Promotion of clot lysis	C3, C4
Inactivation of bacterial lipopolysaccharides from endotoxin	C5, C6

*From Nisengard, R. J.: J. Periodontol., *48*:505, 1977.

to the C5a component of the complement system.[133-135] There is some speculation that the C3a component is also involved in this activity. Chemotaxis is neither stimulated by histamine nor blocked by antihistamine drugs and therefore does not appear to be related to the effects of C3 and C5 on histamine release.

In addition to complement chemotactic factors, certain species of bacteria produce peptides of low molecular weight that are also directly chemotactic and do not require complement.[122] These products could contribute to the accumulation of inflammatory cells in the periodontal lesion.

An important effect of complement occurs when antibodies react with invading gram-negative bacteria, leading to complement activation. These bacteria can by lysed by complement acting through the same reaction sequence as occurs in the lysis of red blood cells. It appears that gram-positive bacteria are not susceptible to this lytic action of complement but are phagocytosed more rapidly after complement activation. The overall effect of complement activation in the course of periodontal disease may be increased permeability of the gingival tissues, allowing a greater penetration of bacteria and/or toxic products from plaque. This initiates a vicious circle in the destruction of the periodontal tissues (see Fig. 24–1).

The prerequisites for complement activation via either pathway or by direct enzymatic cleavage are all present in the periodontal lesion. Endotoxin from gram-negative bacteria can activate the alternate pathway, immune complexes can activate the classical pathway, and bacterial and host tissue proteases can cleave complement components directly.

Several complement components (C3, C4, and factor B) have been identified in sulcular fluid and in the gingival connective tissue of normal individuals, as well as in those with clinical symptoms of periodontal disease.[122] Immunofluorescent staining for C3 demonstrates a more intense fluorescent pattern in inflamed gingiva than in nondiseased tissue. As indicated earlier, the finding of a conversion product of C3 and reduced C4 levels in sulcular fluid from inflamed gingiva strongly suggests local complement activation.[125, 126]

Extracts of inflamed human gingival tissue, but not of clinically healthy attached gingiva, are chemotactic for human mononuclear cells.[121] Because chemotaxis could be suppressed by anti-C5, C5 activation is thought to be a major factor in the chemotaxis of mononuclear cells in periodontal disease. The C5 activation in the inflamed gingival tissue occurs as a result of complement activation by both the classical and the alternate pathways.[104] It is thought that there are three possible activators for the complement-derived chemotactic activity in inflamed gingiva: immune complexes, endotoxins, and tissue enzymes.

Complement studies of sulcular fluid from patients with localized juvenile periodontitis suggest that complement is activated by the alternate pathway.[147] This activation may be induced by endotoxins from the predominantly gram-negative flora in this type of periodontal lesion.

IMMUNE MECHANISMS

Immune mechanisms are usually protective responses of the host to the presence of foreign substances such as bacteria and viruses, but they may, at the same time, also cause local tissue destruction by triggering several types of overreaction or *hypersensitivity*. Tissue damage (immunopathology) may occur in a sensitized host upon subsequent exposure to the sensitizing antigen. Four types of hypersensitivity reactions are described by Gell and Coombs[11, 38]; they are designated as Type I, II, III, and IV (Fig. 24–3).

There are three *antibody*-mediated responses potentially of importance to periodontal disease which are classified as **hypersensitivity reactions.**[121] They are anaphylaxis or immediate hypersensitivity (Type I), cytotoxic reactions (Type II), and immune complex or Arthus reactions (Type III). In addition, reactions to transfused blood are involved with immediate hypersensitivity reactions. Another type of hypersensitivity, which depends upon the interaction of immunocompetent *cells,* is the delayed hypersensitivity or cell-mediated reaction (Type IV).

Anaphylaxis (Type I)

Two variations in anaphylactic hypersensitivity occur, depending on the route of administration of the antigen. If the antigen is injected locally into the skin, the reaction is called *cutaneous anaphylaxis.* If the antigen is injected intravenously, it is called *systemic* or *generalized anaphylaxis.* The basic mechanisms in both types of immediate hypersensitivity are the same.

Both IgG and IgE are involved in anaphylaxis; however, only IgE is capable of sensitizing the skin. This sensitizing capability is re-

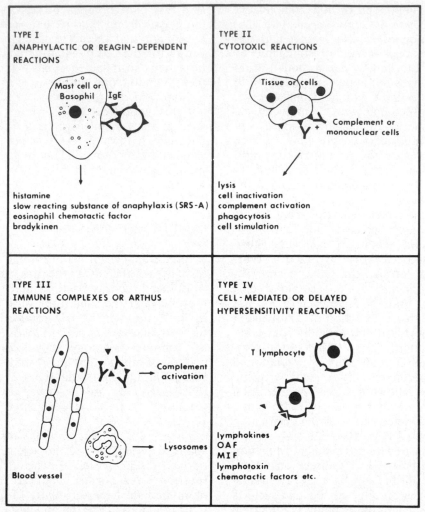

Figure 24–3 Immunologic Mechanisms of Tissue Damage. The four types of hypersensitivity reactions described by Gell and Coombs and depicted by Nisengard. (From Nisengard, R. J.: J. Periodontol., *48*:505, 1977.)

ferred to as *reaginic* and the IgE antibody as *reagin*. IgG antibody combines with antigen and prevents sensitization. These IgG antibodies are referred to as *blocking* antibodies. There are several major features which distinguish these blocking antibodies from reaginic or sensitizing antibodies.

IgE antibodies involved in anaphylactic reactions attach strongly at the Fc portion of the antibody to receptors found on mast cells and basophilic leukocytes, primarily in the skin and other connective tissues such as the gingiva. Experimentally, this binding lasts for several days. These sensitizing IgE antibodies are called *homocytotropic antibodies* because they normally bind in vivo to specific host cells, in this case both mast cells and basophilic leukocytes. In contrast, IgG blocking antibodies bind to mast cells of other phylogenetically distinct species and are termed *heterocytotropic*

antibodies. Experimentally, this binding usually lasts for only a few hours. A very important component in anaphylactic hypersensitivity is the fact that IgE antibodies normally do not fix (activate) complement.

Since plasma cells are known to produce immunoglobulins, the finding of IgE-containing cells in the periodontal and other tissues is thought to represent localized synthesis of IgE antibodies.[94, 97] These IgE-containing cells are found primarily in the respiratory and gastrointestinal mucosa and in regional lymph nodes. It has been suggested that IgE formed locally in tissue may then participate in local disease processes.

MECHANISMS OF ANAPHYLACTIC HYPERSENSITIVITY. Anaphylaxis occurs when two IgE antibodies that are fixed to a mast cell or basophil react with the sensitizing antigen through the Fab portion of the antibodies (Fig.

TABLE 24–4 PHARMACOLOGICALLY ACTIVE MEDIATORS RELEASED BY HUMAN MAST CELLS*

Mediator	Pharmacologic Action
Histamine	Increased capillary permeability
	Smooth muscle contraction
	Stimulation of exocrine glands
	Dilation and increased venule permeability
	Skin response: wheal and erythema
	Bone resorption?
SRS-A	Smooth muscle contraction
	Increased vascular permeability
Bradykinin	Smooth muscle contraction
	Vasodilation
	Increased capillary permeability
	Migration of leukocytes
	Stimulation of pain fibers
Alpha$_2$-macroglobulin	Collagenase activation

*Adapted from Nisengard, R. J.: J. Periodontol., *45*:345, 1972.

24–3). This antibody-antigen reaction causes the release of pharmacologically active substances from the sensitized cells (Table 24–4). It is these substances that cause the response and have the potential to induce tissue damage in periodontal disease.[95, 116]

Of the several active pharmacologic substances released during anaphylaxis, histamine pre-exists in the cells and is promptly released by antibody-antigen complexes. Other pharmacologically active substances, such as the kinins and slow-reacting substance of anaphylaxis (SRS-A), are produced only *after* the antigen-antibody complexes are formed.

An alpha$_2$-macroglobulin which blocks the normally found inhibitor for collagenase is also released from challenged sensitized cells, as are prostaglandins and an eosinophil chemotactic factor.

Histamine has been the most extensively studied chemical mediator of immediate hypersensitivity. As mentioned previously, it is widely found in mammalian tissues. Mast cells, platelets, and basophilic leukocytes contain this substance. Histamine levels in chronically inflamed gingiva are significantly higher than levels in normal gingiva. Some pharmacologic actions of histamine include increased capillary permeability, smooth muscle contraction, stimulation of the exocrine glands, and increased venule dilatation and permeability. The biologic effects of histamine can be blocked with antihistamine drugs, but no apparent change in the course of periodontal disease has been demonstrated with these drugs.

Slow-reacting substances of anaphylaxis (SRS-A) are acidic lipids which cause a sus-tained slow contraction of guinea pig ileum. This contraction is not inhibited by antihistamines and occurs even when histamine has been added to the point at which it can no longer cause ileum contraction. In addition to causing contraction of smooth muscle, SRS-A has some permeability-enhancing activity.

Bradykinin, a peptide formed by the enzymatic action of kallikrein on an alpha$_2$-globulin of plasma, has a number of pharmacologic activities and is considered to be a major pharmacologic mediator of anaphylactic hypersensitivity. These biologic activities include smooth muscle contraction, vasodilatation, increased capillary permeability, migration of leukocytes, and the stimulation of pain fibers. The action of bradykinin is not inhibited by antihistamine drugs.

Anaphylactic-type reactions to oral bacteria have been demonstrated to correlate with severity of periodontal disease in humans.[59, 94, 98] Skin test reagents prepared from an extract of *Actinomyces* and other oral bacteria have provided an in vivo test demonstrating that humans have immediate (anaphylactic) and delayed reactions to these oral filamentous bacteria.[96] A statistically significant correlation was found between the incidence of immediate hypersensitivity and the severity of periodontal disease. The greatest incidence of hypersensitivity was found in patients with periodontitis. In patients with generalized gingivitis, the incidence of immediate hypersensitivity was significantly depressed compared with that in patients with normal gingiva, localized gingivitis, and periodontitis.[94]

Cytotoxic Reactions (Type II)

In these Type II reactions (Fig. 24–3), antibodies react directly with antigens tightly bound to cells. These antigens may be natural surface components of the cell, such as the cell membrane polysaccharide antigens of red blood cells. A cytotoxic reaction in which these cells are involved may result in hemolysis. Cytotoxic antibodies may also react with antigens associated with tissue cells. These cell-associated antigens include normal cell surface antigens or those derived from bacteria, drugs, or altered tissue components.

Cytotoxic antibodies are of the IgG or IgM class. These antibodies have the ability to fix complement, although complement fixation is not required for all types of cytotoxic antibody reactions. In addition to inducing cell lysis, cytotoxic antibodies may cause tissue damage by increasing the synthesis and release of lysosomal enzymes by cells (polymorphonuclear leukocytes) coated with antigen. The tissues in the neighborhood of these enzymes may then be damaged. Hemolytic transfusion reactions, hemolytic disease of the newborn, and autoallergic hemolytic anemia are examples of cytotoxic reactions induced by these antibody-antigen reactions.[26] Cytotoxic reactions are seen in autoimmune disease in which antibodies react with a patient's own tissue components. This occurs, for example, in pemphigus, in which antibodies react with cell membranes, and in pemphigoid, in which antibodies react with the epithelial basement membrane.[10, 94] To date there is no evidence which suggests an important role for cytotoxic reactions in gingivitis and periodontitis.

Arthus Reactions (Type III)

When high levels of antigen to which the host has been sensitized are present, antigen-antibody (IgG and IgM) complexes precipitate in and around small blood vessels and, with complement activation, cause tissue damage at the site of the local reaction[20, 75] (Fig. 24–3). Inflammation, hemorrhage, and necrosis may occur. Tissue damage appears to be due to the release of lysosomal enzymes from polymorphonuclear leukocytes. This reaction is referred to as an Arthus reaction and is usually mediated by IgM- or IgG-type antibodies. These antibodies have the ability to fix complement, which is partially responsible for the chemotactic attraction of the polymorphonuclear leukocytes crucial to the Arthus reaction (see Fig. 24–1).

The presence of antibodies to many oral bacteria, together with the recognition of continual antigen penetration of the gingiva, provides the basis for an immune complex or Arthus reaction.[22, 23] Experimental gingival Arthus reactions have a histopathology similar to those of human gingivitis and periodontitis, including osteoclastic bone loss.[101, 119–121, 123] It has also been suggested that immune complex–induced complement activation may participate in the initiation of gingival inflammation.[61] Topical application of plaque to plaque-immunized animals leads to neutrophil chemotaxis and increased vascular permeability. In immunized, decomplemented dogs, neutrophil migration and vascular exudation upon topical plaque application are less than in immunized and nonimmunized normal dogs. In vitro studies have also demonstrated that immune

complexes with complement activation induce osteoclastic activity,[38, 94] possibly by prostaglandin E synthesis.[118]

A reduction in antibodies, which are necessary for immune complex disease, has little or no effect on gingivitis or periodontitis. Gingivitis can be seen in hypogammaglobulinemia.[94] Immunosuppression with azathioprine in combination with prednisone or Imuran and prednisone may also influence periodontal disease.[108, 127] When these drugs are employed after organ (usually kidney) transplants, the usual and expected correlation between the severity of periodontal disease and plaque accumulation has not been demonstrated. Whether this lack of relationship results from suppressed humoral immunity, cell-mediated immunity, a direct effect of the prednisone on inflammation by stabilization of lysosomal membranes, or nonimmune mechanisms such as the direct toxic effects of bacterial products is not known.[94, 108] It is also possible that these drugs may affect the plaque bacteria directly.

Cell-Mediated Immunity—Delayed Hypersensitivity (Type IV)

The phenomenon of delayed hypersensitivity belongs to the class of immune responses known as cell-mediated immunity. These reactions are referred to as Type IV reactions (Fig. 24–4).

Cellular immunity does not involve circulating antibodies but is based on the interaction of antigens with the surface of lymphocytes. There are actually two populations of lymphocytes (Fig. 24–4). Lymphocytes that can develop into plasma cells which produce antibodies are designated as B-cells because they were found to proliferate in the bursa of Fabricius in birds and the bone marrow of mammals. These cells circulate from the blood or thoracic duct to the lymphatic tissues, the cortical germinal centers of lymph nodes, and the red pulp of the spleen, where they differentiate into plasma cells.[85] These differentiated cells can then produce antibodies. B-lymphocytes have been shown to produce biologically active lymphokines[82, 146] (see below).

In contrast, the T-cells migrate from the bone marrow to the thymus, where they divide and become immunocompetent (Fig. 24–4). From the thymus they migrate to the pericortical areas of lymph nodes and the white pulp of the spleen.[85] The relationship between T- and B-lymphocytes and cellular and humoral immunity is not as simple as was previously

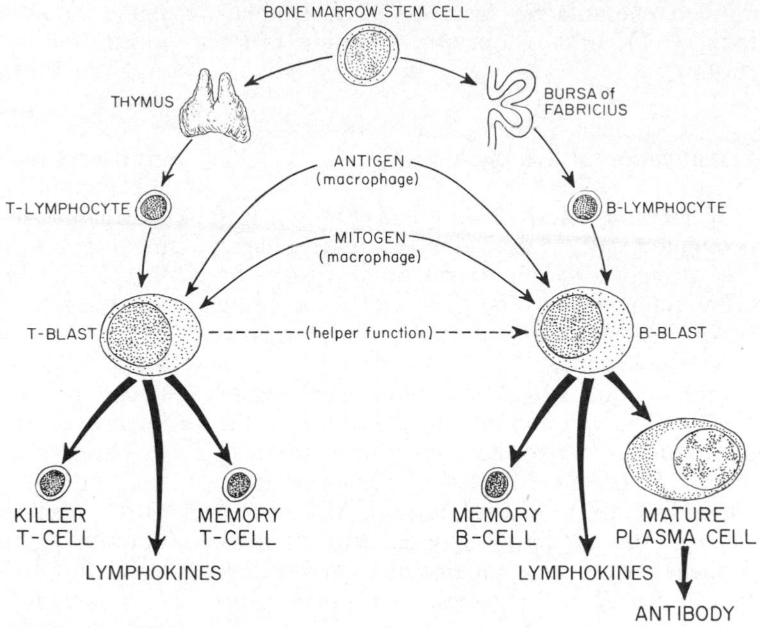

Figure 24–4 Schematic diagram illustrating the derivation and response of B- and T-lymphocytes. Antigen- and mitogen-induced responses result from the presence of macrophages. (From Page, R.: *In* Schluger, S., Yuodelis, R. A., and Page, R. C.: Periodontal Disease. Philadelphia, Lea & Febiger, 1977.)

thought, since interactions frequently occur between these cells.[94]

T-lymphocytes or B-lymphocytes sensitized to an immunizing antigen can be stimulated to undergo blastogenesis or transformation in vitro and presumably in vivo. This consists of morphologic enlargement and synthesis of proteins, RNA, and DNA and results, ultimately, in mitotic division. This increases the number of immunocompetent lymphoid cells which are specific for a particular antigen. Some oral bacteria, including *Actinomyces* and some strains of *Streptococcus,* produce extracellular substances that inhibit blast transformation of normal peripheral lymphocytes.[50] Similar substances from some bacteria also inhibit fibroblast growth.

LYMPHOKINES

In the process of blastogenesis, a variety of soluble, biologically active substances (mediators) are made by the cultured T-lymphocytes. These mediators, called lymphokines, appear in the supernatant of lymphocyte cultures.[24] B-lymphocytes can presumably produce lymphokines without prior blastogenesis. The accumulation of plasma cells and lymphocytes in the periodontal tissues suggests that lymphokines participate in periodontal pathology. Since the number of currently identified lymphokines is extensive[122] (Table 24–5), only the major ones will be discussed. These are macrophage-activating factor (MAF), macrophage migration inhibitory factor (MIF), leukocyte-

TABLE 24–5 LYMPHOKINES: BIOLOGIC ACTIVITY OF MEDIATORS OF CELL-MEDIATED IMMUNITY

Biologic Activity	Lymphokine (or Mediator)
Effects on Macrophages	
Chemotaxis	Leukocyte-derived chemotactic factor (CTX)
Inhibition of migration	Macrophage migration inhibitory factor (MIF)
Activation	Macrophage activating factor (MAF)
Effects on Other Cells	
Inhibition of leukocyte migration	Inhibition factors
Chemotaxis of neutrophils, basophils, and eosinophils	Chemotactic factors
Blast formation of lymphocytes	Eosinophil chemotactic factor (ECF)
Cytotoxicity (fibroblasts and other cells)	Mitogenic factor
Activation of osteoclasts	Lymphotoxin (LT)
	Osteoclast activating factor (OAF)
Other Effects	
Transfer of cell-mediated immunity	Transfer factors
Inhibition of virus replication	Interferon
Inhibition of yeast (in vitro)	Antifungal factors

derived chemotactic factor (CTX), lymphotoxin (LT), and osteoclast activating factor (OAF).

Classification of Lymphokines

Macrophage Activating Factor (MAF). It is postulated that, in periodontitis, macrophages are attracted to the periodontal tissues by CTX, retained there by MIF, and activated by MAF.[92] MAF stimulates the macrophages to secrete collagenase.

Macrophage Migration Inhibitory Factor (MIF). The lymphokine responsible for the inhibition of macrophage migration from an area in which the lymphokines have been released by activated lymphocytes is MIF.[8, 66, 128] In vivo, this mediator may concentrate macrophages at the local inflammatory site, where they function to phagocytize and digest antigen.

Leukocyte-Derived Chemotactic Factor (CTX). The inflammatory lesion in periodontal disease is characterized by polymorphonuclear and mononuclear leukocytes. It is suggested that this is due to the production of chemotactic factors.[150] These chemotactic factors may be from the complement system, plaque bacteria, or host lymphocytes, which produce CTX. T- or B-lymphocytes can be stimulated in vitro by endotoxins and other antigens to produce this lymphokine.

Lymphotoxin (LT). In vitro experiments have demonstrated that LT may be cytotoxic for cultures of human gingival fibroblasts.[65, 124] A correlation exists between the degree of periodontal disease of the lymphocyte donor and the amount of LT elaborated by the cells in response to plaque antigens. Thus, there may be some in vivo correlation with the in vitro experiments.

Cytotoxicity of tissue cells may also be affected by a direct lymphocyte interaction with target cells containing a specific stimulating antigen on their surface.[85] Although antigen recognition by sensitized lymphocytes is generally quite specific, the cytotoxic effect produced by lymphocyte host cell interaction is generally nonspecific. These lymphocyte interactions suggest that the persistent deposition of plaque antigens into the gingival tissue could favor the generation of LT-producing cells and/or direct lymphocytotoxicity, resulting in the tissue damage seen in periodontal diseases.[94]

Lymphocytes sensitized to plaque antigens undergo morphologic and functional transformation (in vitro), which results in a chronic infiltration with lymphocytes and macrophages and the formation of biologically active substances.

Another important type of reaction is the graft-versus-host reaction, which is seen when the lymphocytes are transferred from an immunologically competent donor to an allogenic incompetent recipient. These reactions have increasing clinical importance because of therapeutic attempts to transfer normal thymus or bone marrow cells to immunodeficient humans. These transplantation techniques are becoming increasingly common; they have been used in patients with genetic defects and in patients with leukemia treated with cytotoxic drugs and whole-body irradiation.[127] Often such patients have concomitant periodontal manifestations of their primary systemic disease (see Chapter 29).

Osteoclast Activating Factor (OAF). OAF induces osteoclastic resorption of bone in organ cultures.[53, 54] Histologically, the resorption is characteristically associated with the appearance of increased numbers of osteoclasts and the loss of the bony matrix. OAF can be distinguished from other bone-resorbing substances such as parathormone, active metabolites of vitamin D, and prostaglandins.

Assays

The assays for lymphocyte transformation are performed in vitro. Small lymphocytes harvested from either peripheral blood or lymphoid organs can be transformed (induced) to larger lymphocytes by blastogenesis. During the process of transformation, the cells synthesize DNA, RNA, and proteins. By labeling or incorporating radioactive precursors of the DNA, such as tritiated thymidine, the transformation reaction can be quantitated.[26, 107] The degree of transformation is compared with that of control substances capable of stimulating the majority of lymphocytes. These stimulants are nonspecific and are called *mitogens*. Mitogens include phytohemagglutinin, antilymphocyte serum, and mercuric chloride.[12, 35, 43]

CELLULAR IMMUNITY IN PERIODONTAL DISEASE

Delayed hypersensitivity reactions, as measured by lymphocyte transformation, may play an important role in the pathogenesis of periodontal disease[46, 57, 58, 72, 74] (see Fig. 24–1). Peripheral blood lymphocytes from patients with moderate periodontal disease react to a greater degree than those from patients with mild or no periodontal disease. In some studies, patients with more severe or extensive periodontal destruction manifested a diminished reaction to the particular stimulant. This phenomenon may occur because patients with extensive periodontal destruction have blocking factors which could limit the disease process in severe periodontal destruction. This assumption is made if one considers that this immunopathologic reaction actually occurs in vivo.

The experimental gingivitis model permits examination of cell-mediated immune responses in gingival health and through the early stages of gingival inflammation.[74, 112, 131] After plaque is allowed to accumulate, the blastogenic response to many bacteria increases. Later in the experimental gingivitis period, variable blastogenic responses have been reported, ranging from a biphasic response[74] to an increasing response[112] to a reduced response.[131] After the resumption of oral hygiene, there is a reduced blastogenic response.

A similar correlation of cell-mediated immunity and periodontal disease has been observed with sonicated plaque antigens.[39, 41] Lower concentrations of autogenous supragingival plaque are necessary for stimulating a maximal lymphoproliferative response in patients with more severe periodontitis.[18] A diminished response to plaque, however, was not observed in severe periodontitis. Cell-mediated immunity to other microorganisms, including *Actinomyces israelii, Actinomyces naeslundii, Arachnia propionica, Propionibacterium acnes, Leptotrichia buccalis,* and an anaerobic gram-negative rod from a lesion of idiopathic juvenile periodontitis[55, 93] also correlated with disease status.[66] When the cell-mediated immune responses to a battery of oral microorganisms were evaluated, three general patterns of responses could be identified.[36, 113] Regardless of periodontal disease status, *Actinomyces* species and *Rothia dentocariosa* stimulated lymphocyte blastogenesis in most subjects, whereas *Streptococcus sanguis, Campylobacter,* and *Eikenella corrodens* stimulated blastogenesis in few subjects. The third response occurred to several gram-negative anaerobic bacteria, including *Bacteroides asaccharolyticus* and *Treponema denticola,* which elicited a greater response in subjects with destructive periodontitis than in patients with gingivitis.

Cell-mediated immunity to some bacteria is frequently long lasting. Patients edentulous for at least 5 years respond as well to *Actinomyces viscosus, Actinomyces naeslundii,* and homologous dental plaque as do patients with gingivitis and periodontitis.[43, 102, 114, 151] This suggests that lymphocyte stimulation may occur or be maintained from sources other than the periodontium. These edentulous subjects, however, did not respond to *Veillonella alcalescens, Leptotrichia buccalis,* or *Bacteroides melaninogenicus.* Thus, cell-mediated immunity to gram-negative bacteria may relate more directly to periodontitis.

It has been recognized that the gingival inflammatory response to plaque is more severe during pregnancy. In the second trimester, there is a suppression or depression in the cell-mediated immune response to plaque bacteria, which resolves after parturition.[76, 106] This suppression may play a role in the altered response to plaque.

Cell-mediated immune responses in idiopathic juvenile periodontitis are dependent on the type of antigen. No statistically significant response was observed to *Veillonella, Bacteroides, Fusobacterium, Actinomyces,* or plaque,[73] whereas gram-negative bacteria isolated from lesions of patients with this disease did elicit a significant response.[5]

Clinical periodontal therapy consisting of scaling and root planing in patients with advanced periodontitis does not result in reduced cell-mediated immunity to *A. viscosus* or *A. naeslundii.*

REFERENCES

1. Asaro, J., Nisengard, R., Beutner, E. H., and Neider, M.: Experimental periodontal disease: immediate hypersensitivity. J. Periodontol., *54*:23, 1983.
2. Attström, R.: Studies on neutrophil polymorphonuclear leukocytes at the dento-gingival junction in gingival health and disease. J. Periodont. Res., *8*(Suppl):1, 1971.
3. Attström, R., and Schroeder, H. E.: Effect of experimental neutropenia on initial gingivitis in dogs. Scand. J. Dent. Res., *87*:7, 1979.
4. Baehni, P., Tsai, C., McArthur, W. C., Hammond, B. T., and Taichman, N. S.: Interaction of inflammatory cells and microorganisms. VII. Detection of leukotoxic activity of a plaque-derived gram-negative microorganism. Infect. Immun., *24*:233, 1979.
5. Baker, J. J., Chan, S. P., Socransky, S. S., Oppenheim, J. J., and Mergenhagen, S. E.: Importance of *Actinomyces* and certain gram-negative anaerobic organisms in the transformation of lymphocytes from patients with periodontal disease. Infect. Immun., *13*:1363, 1976. ·
6. Barnett, M. L.: The fine structure of human connective tissue mast cells in periodontal disease. J. Periodont. Res., *9*:84, 1974.
7. Bauer, W. H.: The supporting tissues of the tooth in acute secondary agranulocytosis (arsphenamin neutropenia). J. Dent. Res., *25*:501, 1946.
8. Benditt, E. P., and Lagunoff, D.: The mast cell: its structure and function. Prog. Allergy, *8*:195, 1964.

9. Berglund, S. E.: Immunoglobulins in human gingiva with specificity for oral bacteria. J. Periodontol., *42*:546, 1971.

10. Beutner, E. H., Chorzelski, T. P., and Jordan, R. E.: Autosensitization in pemphigus and bullous pemphigoid. Springfield, Ill., Charles C Thomas, 1970.

11. Bickley, H. C.: A concept of allergy with reference to oral disease. J. Periodontol., *41*:302, 1970.

12. Bourne, H. R., Epstein, L. B., and Melmon, L. L.: Lymphocyte cyclic adenosine monophosphate (AMP) synthesis and inhibition of phytohemagglutinin-induced transformation. J. Clin. Invest., *50*:10a, 1971.

13. Brandtzaeg, P.: Immunology of inflammatory periodontal lesions. Int. Dent. J., *23*:438, 1973.

14. Brandtzaeg, P., Fjellanger, I., and Gjeruldsen, S. T.: Adsorption of immunoglobulin A onto oral bacteria in vivo. J. Bacteriol., *96*:242, 1968.

15. Carpenter, A. B., Beck, P. H., Moore, W. E. C., and Tew, J. G.: Polyclonal B cell activation by gram negative bacteria frequently isolated from periodontitis. J. Dent. Res., *60A*:326, 1981.

16. Carranza, F. A., Jr., and Cabrini, R. L.: Mast cells in human gingiva. Oral Surg., *8*:1093, 1955.

17. Charon, J., Toto, P. D., and Gargiulo, A. W.: Activated macrophages in human periodontitis. J. Periodontol., *52*:328, 1981.

18. Church, H., and Dolby, A. E.: The relationship between the dose of dentogingival plaque and the in vitro lymphoproliferative response in subjects with periodontal disease. J. Oral Pathol. 7:318, 1978.

19. Cianciola, L. J., Genco, R. J., Patters, M. R., McKenna, J., and van Oss, C. J.: Defective polymorphonuclear leukocyte functions in a human periodontal disease. Nature, *265*:445, 1977.

20. Cochrane, C. G.: Mechanisms involved in the deposition of immune complexes in tissues. J. Exp. Med., *134*:75, 1971.

21. Cohen, S., and Winkler, S.: Cellular immunity and the inflammatory response. J. Periodontol., *45*:348, 1974.

22. Colbe, H. M.: Transitory bacteremia. Oral Surg., 7:609, 1954.

23. Corner, H. D., Hamberman, S., Collings, C. K., and Winford, T. E.: Bacteremias following periodontal scaling in patients with healthy appearing gingiva. J. Periodontol., *38*:466, 1967.

24. David, J. R.: Delayed hypersensitivity in vitro: its mediation by cell-free substances formed by lymphoid cell-antigen interaction. Proc. Natl. Acad. Sci. U.S.A., *56*:72, 1966.

25. David, J. R.: Lymphocyte mediators and cellular hypersensitivity. N. Engl. J. Med., *288*:143, 1973.

26. Davis, B. D. et al.: Microbiology. 2nd ed. New York, Harper & Row, Inc., 1973.

27. Diensten, B., Ratcliff, P. A., and Williams, R. K.: Mast cell density and distribution in gingival biopsies: quantitative study. J. Periodontol., *38*:198, 1967.

28. Doty, S. L., Lopatin, D. E., and Smith, T. N.: Humoral immune response to oral microorganisms in periodontitis. J. Dent. Res., *60A*:497, 1981.

29. Ebersole, J. L., Frey, D. E., Taubman, M. A., and Smith, D. J.: An ELISA for measuring serum antibodies to *Actinobacillus actinomycetemcomitans*. J. Periodont. Res., *15*:621, 1980.

30. Ebersole, J. L., Frey, D. E., Taubman, M. A., Smith, D. J., Genco, R. J., and Hammond, B. T.: Antibody response to antigens from *A. actinomycetemcomitans* (44): relationship to localized juvenile periodontitis. J. Dent. Res., *59A*:331, 1980.

31. Egelberg, J.: Permeability of the dento-gingival blood vessels. II. Clinically healthy gingivae. J. Periodont. Res., *1*:276, 1966.

32. Egelberg, J.: Permeability of the dento-gingival blood vessels. III. Chronically inflamed gingivae. J. Periodont. Res., *1*:287, 1966.

33. Erb, P., and Feldman, M.: Role of macrophages in in vitro induction of T-helper cells. Nature, *254*:352, 1975.

34. Evans, R. T., Spaeth, S., and Mergenhagen, S. E.: Bactericidal antibody in mammalian serum to obligatorily anaerobic gram-negative bacteria. J. Immunol., *97*:112, 1966.

35. Ferraris, V. A., and DeRubertis, F. R.: Release of prostaglandin by mitogen and antigen-stimulated leukocytes in culture. J. Clin. Invest., *54*:378, 1974.

36. Fotos, P. G., Gerencser, V. F., and Gerencser, M. A.: Blastogenic response of human lymphocytes to antigens of *Rothia dentocariosa*. J. Dent. Res., *60A*:325, 1981.

37. Freedman, H. L., Taichman, N. S., and Keystone, J.: Inflammation and tissue injury. II. Local release of lysosomal enzymes during mixed bacterial infection in the skin of rabbits. Proc. Soc. Exp. Biol. Med., *125*:1209, 1967.

38. Gell, P. G. H., Coombs, R. R. A., and Lachman, P. J.: Clinical Aspects of Immunology. 3rd ed. Oxford, Blackwell Scientific Publications, 1975.

39. Gemsa, D., et al.: Release of cyclic AMP from macrophages by stimulation with prostaglandins. J. Immunol., *144*:1422, 1975.

40. Genco, R. J., and Cianciola, L. J.: Relationship of the neutrophil to host resistance in periodontal disease. Alpha Omegan, *10*:31, 1977.

41. Genco, R. J., and Krygier, G.: Localization of immunoglobulins, immune cells and complement in human gingiva. J. Periodont. Res., *10*(Suppl.):30, 1972.

42. Genco, R. J., Mashimo, P. A., Krygier, G., and Ellison, S. A.: Antibody-mediated effects on the periodontium. J. Periodontol., *45*:330, 1974.

43. Gery, I., and Waksman, B. H.: Potentiation of the T-lymphocyte response to mitogens. J. Exp. Med., *136*:143, 1972.

44. Gibbons, R. J., and Van Houte, J.: Selective bacterial adherence to oral epithelial surfaces and its role as an ecological determinant. Infect. Immun., *3*:567, 1971.

45. Gilmour, M. N., and Nisengard, R. J.: Interactions between serum titers to filamentous bacteria and their relationship to human periodontal disease. Arch. Oral Biol., *19*:959, 1974.

46. Goldhaber, P.: Heparin enhancement of factors stimulating bone resorption in tissue culture. Science, *147*:407, 1965.

47. Granger, G. A.: Lymphokines—the mediators of cellular immunity. Ser. Haematol., *4*:8, 1972.

48. Green, L. H., and Kass, E. H.: Quantitative determination of antibacterial activity of the rabbit gingival sulcus. Arch. Oral Biol., *15*:491, 1970.

49. Hawkins, D.: Neutrophilic leukocytes in immunologic reactions: evidence for the selective release of lysosomal constituents. J. Immunol., *108*:310, 1972.

50. Higerd, T. B., Vesole, D. H., and Goust, J.: Inhibitory effects of extracellular products from oral bacteria on human fibroblasts and stimulated lymphocytes. Infect. Immun., *21*:567, 1978.

51. Hill, H. R., Estensen, R. D., Hogan, N. A., and Quie, P. G.: Severe staphylococcal disease associated with allergic manifestations, hyperimmunoglobulinemia E, and defective neutrophil chemotaxis. J. Lab. Clin. Med., *88*:796, 1976.

52. Horton, J. E., Leiken, S., and Oppenheim, J. J.: Human lymphoproliferative reaction to saliva and dental plaque deposits: an *in vitro* correlation with periodontal disease. J. Periodontol., *43*:522, 1972.

53. Horton, J. E., Oppenheim, J. J., and Mergenhagen, S. E.: A role for cell mediated immunity in the pathogenesis of periodontal disease. J. Periodontol., *45*:351, 1974.

54. Horton, J. E., Raisz, L. G., Simmons, H. A., Oppenheim, J. J., and Mergenhagen, S. E.: Bone resorbing activity in supernatant fluid from cultured human peripheral blood leukocytes. Science, *177*:793, 1972.

55. Irving, J. T., Newman, M. G., Socransky, S. S., and Heeley, J. O.: Histologic changes in experimental periodontal disease in rats monoinfected with a gram-negative organism. Arch. Oral Biol., *20*:219, 1975.

56. Ishikawa, I., Cimasoni, G., and Ahmad-Zadeh, C.: Possible role of lysosomal enzymes in the pathogenesis of periodontitis. A study on cathepsin D in human gingival fluid. Arch. Oral Biol., *17*:111, 1972.

57. Ivanyi, L., and Lehner, T.: Stimulation of lymphocyte transformation by bacterial antigens in patients with periodontal disease. Arch. Oral Biol., *15*:1089, 1970.

58. Ivanyi, L., Wilton, J. M. A., and Lehner, T.: Cell-mediated immunity in periodontal disease; cytotoxicity, migration inhibition and lymphocyte transformation studies. Immunology, *22*:141, 1972.

59. Jayawardine, A., and Goldner, M.: Reagin-like activity of serum in human periodontal disease. Infect. Immun., *15*:665, 1977.

60. Johnson, R. J., Matthews, J. L., Stone, M. J., Hurt, W. C.,

and Newman, J. T.: Immunopathology of periodontal disease. I. Immunologic profiles in periodontitis and juvenile periodontitis. J. Periodontol., *51*:705, 1980.

61. Kahnberg, K. E., Lindhe, J., and Attström, R.: The effect of decomplementation by carragheenin on experimental initial gingivitis in hyperimmune dogs. J. Periodont. Res., *12*:479, 1977.

62. Kaliner, M., and Austen, K. F.: Immunologic release of chemical mediators from human tissues. *In* Elliott, H. W., George, R., and Okum, R. (eds.), Annual Review of Pharmacology. Palo Alto, Calif., Annual Review, Inc., 1975, pp. 177–189.

63. Kaslick, R. S., West, T. L., Singh, S., and Chasens, H. I.: Serum immunoglobulins in periodontosis patients. J. Periodontol., *51*:343, 1980.

64. Kiger, R. D., Wright, W. H., and Creamer, H. R.: The significance of lymphocyte transformation responses to various microbial stimulants. J. Periodontol., *45*:780, 1974.

65. Kolb, W. P., and Granger, G. A.: Lymphocyte in vitro cytotoxicity: characterization of human lymphotoxin. Proc. Natl. Acad. Sci. U.S.A., *61*:1250, 1968.

66. Koopman, W., Gillis, M. H., and David, J. R.: Prevention of MIF activity by agents known to increase cellular cyclic AMP. J. Immunol., *110*:1609, 1973.

67. Lally, E. T., Boehni, P. C., and McArthur, W. P.: Local immunoglobulin synthesis in periodontal disease. J. Periodont. Res., *15*:159, 1980.

68. Lavine, W. S., Page, R. C., and Padgett, G. A.: Host response in chronic periodontal disease. V. The dental and periodontal status of mink and mice affected by Chédiak-Higashi Syndrome. J. Periodontol., *47*:621, 1976.

69. Lavine, W. S., Maderazo, E. G., Stolman, J., Ward, P. A., Cogen, R. B., Greenblatt, J., and Robertson, P. B.: Impaired neutrophil chemotaxis in patients with juvenile and rapidly progressing periodontitis. J. Periodont. Res., *14*:10, 1979.

70. Lazarus, G. S., et al.: Human granulocyte collagenase. Science, *159*:1483, 1968.

71. Lehner, T.: Cell-mediated immune responses in oral disease: a review. J. Oral Pathol., *1*:39, 1972.

72. Lehner, T., Challacombe, S. J., Wilton, J. M. A., and Ivanyi, L.: Immunopotentiation by dental microbial plaque and its relationship to oral disease in man. Arch Oral Biol., *21*:749, 1976.

73. Lehner, T., Wilton, J. M. A., Ivanyi, L., and Manson, J. B.: Immunologic aspects of juvenile periodontitis (periodontosis). J. Periodont. Res., *9*:261, 1974.

74. Lehner, T., et al.: Sequential cell-mediated immunoresponse in experimental gingivitis in man. Clin. Exp. Immunol., *16*:481, 1974.

75. Lerner, C.: Arthus reaction in the oral cavity of laboratory animals. J. Periodontol., *3*:18, 1965.

76. Lindhe, J., and Socransky, S. S.: Chemotaxis and vascular permeability produced by human periodontopathic bacteria. J. Periodont. Res., *14*:138, 1979.

77. Lopatin, D. E., Kornman, K. S., and Loesche, W. J.: Modulation of immunoreactivity to periodontal disease–associated microorganisms during pregnancy. Infect. Immun. *28*:713, 1980.

78. Lucas, O. N., and Wright, W. H.: Heparin in normal and inflamed gingival tissue. J. Dent. Res., Suppl. 55, Abstr. No. 793, 1976.

79. Mackaness, G. B.: The immunological basis of acquired cellular resistance. J. Exp. Med., *120*:105, 1964.

80. Mackaness, G. B.: The relationship of delayed hypersensitivity to acquired cellular resistance. Br. Med. Bull., *23*:52, 1967.

81. Mackler, B. F., Frostad, K. B., Robertson, P. B., and Levy, B. M.: Immunoglobulin bearing lymphocytes and plasma cells in human periodontal disease. J. Periodont. Res., *12*:37, 1977.

82. Mackler, B. F., et al.: Blastogenesis and lymphokine synthesis by T and B lymphocytes from patients with periodontal disease. Infect. Immun., *10*:844, 1974.

83. Maderazo, E. G., Ward, P. A., and Quintiliani, R.: Defective regulation of chemotaxis in cirrhosis. J. Lab. Clin. Med., *85*:621, 1975.

84. Mansheim, B. J., Stenstrom, M. L., and Clark, W. B.: Measurement of serum and salivary antibodies to the oral pathogen *Bacteroides asaccharolyticus* in human subjects. Arch. Oral Biol., *25*:553, 1980.

85. Mergenhagen, S. E., and Scherp, H. W. (eds.): Comparative Immunology of the Oral Cavity. DHEW Publ. No. 73–438, 1973.

86. Mergenhagen, S. E., DeAraujo, W. C., and Varah, E.: Antibody to *Leptotrichia buccalis* in human sera. Arch. Oral Biol., *10*:29, 1965.

87. Michalek, S. M., et al.: Ingestion of *Streptococcus mutans* induces secretory immunoglobulin A and caries immunity. Science, *192*:1238, 1976.

88. Morley, H.: Prostaglandins and lymphokines in arthritis. Prostaglandins, *8*:315, 1974.

89. Mowat, A. G., and Baum, J.: Chemotaxis of polymorphonuclear leukocytes from patients with rheumatoid arthritis. J. Clin. Invest., *50*:2541, 1971.

90. Murray, P. A., and Genco, R. J.: Serum and gingival fluid antibodies to *Actinobacillus actinomycetemcomitans* in localized juvenile periodontitis. J. Dent. Res., *59A*:329, 1980.

91. Murray, P. A., and Patters, M. R.: Gingival crevice neutrophil function in periodontal disease. J. Periodont. Res., *15*:463, 1980.

92. Nath, I., Poulter, L. W., and Turk, J. L.: Effect of lymphocyte mediators on macrophages in vitro. A correlation of morphological and cytochemical changes. Clin. Exp. Immunol., *13*:455, 1973.

93. Newman, M. G., Socransky, S., Savitt, E. D., Propas, E. D., and Crawford, A.: Studies of the microbiology of periodontosis. J. Periodontol., *47*:373, 1976

94. Nisengard, R. J.: The role of immunology in periodontal disease. J. Periodontol., *48*:505, 1977.

95. Nisengard, R. J., and Beutner, E. H.: Relation of immediate hypersensitivity to periodontitis in animals and man. J. Periodontol., *41*:223, 1970.

96. Nisengard, R. J., and Jarrett, C.: Coating of subgingival bacteria with immunoglobulin and complement. J. Periodontol., *47*:518, 1976.

97. Nisengard, R. J., Beutner, E. H., and Gauto, M. S.: Immunofluorescent studies of IgE in periodontal disease. Ann. N.Y. Acad. Sci., *177*:39, 1971.

98. Nisengard, R. J., Beutner, E. H., and Hazen, S. P.: Immunologic studies of periodontal disease. III. Bacterial hypersensitivity and periodontal disease. J. Periodontol., *39*:329, 1968.

99. Nisengard, R. J., Myers, D., and Newman, M. G.: Human antibody titers to periodontosis—associated microbiota. IADR Abstract, p. A23, 1977.

100. Nisengard, R. J., Myers, D., Fischman, S., and Socransky, S.: Immunologic studies of acute necrotizing ulcerative gingivitis. IADR Abstract, p. B206, 1976.

101. Nisengard, R. J., Beutner, E. H., Neugeboren, N., Neiders, M., and Asaro, J.: Experimental induction of periodontal disease with Arthus-type reactions. Clin. Immunol. Immunopathol., *8*:97, 1977.

102. Nobreus, N., Attström, R., and Egelberg, J.: Effect of antithymocyte serum on chronic gingival inflammation in dogs. J. Periodont. Res., *9*:236, 1974.

103. Okada, H., and Silverman, M. S.: Chemotactic activity in periodontal disease. I. The role of complement in monocyte chemotaxis. J. Periodont. Res., *14*:20, 1979.

104. Okada, H., and Silverman, M. S.: Chemotactic activity in periodontal disease. II. The generation of complement-derived chemotactic factors. J. Periodont. Res., *14*:147, 1979.

105. Okuda, K., and Takazoe, I.: Activation of complement by dental plaque. J. Periodont. Res., *15*:232, 1980.

106. O'Neil, T. C. A.: Maternal T-lymphocyte response and gingivitis in pregnancy. J. Periodontol., *50*:178, 1979.

107. Oppenheim, J. J.: Relationships of in vitro lymphocyte transformation to delayed hypersensitivity in guinea pig and man. Fed. Proc., *27*:21, 1968.

108. Oshrain, H. I., Mender, S., and Mandel, I. D.: Periodontal status of patients with reduced immunocapacity. J. Periodontol., *50*:185, 1979.

109. Page, R. C.: Pathogenic mechanisms. *In* Schluger, S., Yudalis, R., and Page, R. C. (eds.): Periodontal Disease: Basic Phenomena, Clinical Management and Restorative Interrelationships. Philadelphia, Lea & Febiger, 1977.

110. Page, R. C., Davies, P., and Allison, A. C.: Effects of dental

plaque on the production and release of lysosomal hydrolases by macrophages in culture. Arch. Oral Biol., *18*:1481, 1973.

111. Parakkal, P. F.: Involvement of macrophages in collagen resorption. J. Cell Biol., *41*:345, 1969.

112. Patters, M. R., Sedransk, N., and Genco, R. J.: The lymphoproliferative response during human experimental gingivitis. J. Periodont. Res., *14*:269, 1979.

113. Patters, M. R., Chen, P., McKenna, J., and Genco, R. J.: Lymphoproliferative responses to oral bacteria in humans with varying severities of periodontal disease. Infect. Immun., *28*:777, 1980.

114. Patters, M. R., Genco, R. J., Reed, M. J., and Mashimo, P. A.: Blastogenic response of human lymphocytes to oral bacterial antigens: comparison of individuals with periodontal disease to normal and edentulous subjects. Infect. Immun., *14*:1213, 1976.

115. Pick, E., and Turk, J. L.: The biological activities of soluble lymphocyte products. Clin. Exp. Immunol., *10*:1, 1972.

116. Piper, P. J., and Vane, J. R.: Release of additional factors in anaphylaxis and its antagonism by anti-inflammatory drugs. Nature, *223*:29, 1971.

117. Platt, D., Crosby, R. G., and Dalbow, N. H.: Evidence for the presence of immunoglobulins and antibodies in inflamed periodontal tissues. J. Periodontol., *41*:215, 1970.

118. Raisz, L. G., et al.: Complement-dependent stimulation of prostaglandin synthesis and bone resorption. Science, *185*:789, 1974.

119. Ranney, R. R., and Zander, H. A.: Allergic periodontal disease in sensitized squirrel monkeys. J. Periodontol., *41*:12, 1970.

120. Rizzo, A. A.: Histologic and immunologic evaluation of antigen penetration into oral tissues after topical application. J. Periodontol., *41*:210, 1970.

121. Rizzo, A. A., and Mergenhagen, S. E.: Studies on the significance of local hypersensitivity in periodontal disease. Periodontics, *3*:271, 1965.

122. Rizzo, A. A., and Mergenhagen, S. E.: Host responses in periodontal disease. Proceedings of the International Conference on Research on the Biology of Periodontal Disease. Chicago, 1977.

123. Rizzo, A. A., and Mitchell, C. T.: Chronic allergic inflammation induced by repeated deposition of antigen in rabbit gingival pockets. Periodontics, *4*:5, 1966.

124. Russell, S. W., et al.: Purification of human lymphotoxin. J. Immunol., *109*:784, 1972.

125. Schenkein, H. A., and Genco, R. J.: Gingival fluid and serum in periodontal diseases. I. Quantitative study of immunoglobulins, complement and other plasma proteins. J. Periodontol., *48*:772, 1977.

126. Schenkein, H. A., and Genco, R. J.: Gingival fluid and serum in periodontal diseases. II. Evidence for cleavage of complement components C3, C3 proactivator (factor B) and C4 in gingival fluid. J. Periodontol., *48*:778, 1977.

127. Schuller, P. D., Freedman, H. L., and Lewis, D. W.: Periodontal status of renal transplant patients receiving immunosuppressive therapy. J. Periodontol., *44*:167, 1973.

128. Seravalli, E., and Taranta, A.: Release of macrophage migration inhibitory factor(s) from lymphocytes stimulated by streptococcal preparations. Cell. Immunol., *8*:40, 1973.

129. Shelton, L. E., and Hall, W. B.: Human gingival mast cells. Effects of chronic inflammation. J. Periodont. Res. *3*:214, 1968.

130. Shillitoe, E. J., and Lehner, T.: Immunoglobulins and complement in crevicular fluid, serum and saliva in man. Arch. Oral Biol., *17*:241, 1972.

131. Smith, F. N., Lang, N. P., and Löe, H.: Cell-mediated immune responses to plaque antigens during experimental gingivitis in man. J. Periodont. Res., *13*:232, 1978.

132. Snyderman, R.: Role for endotoxin and complement in periodontal tissue destruction. J. Dent. Res., *51*(Suppl. 2):356, 1972.

133. Snyderman, R., Phillips, J. K., and Mergenhagen, S. E.: Biological activity of complement in vivo: role of C5 in the accumulation of polymorphonuclear leukocytes in inflammatory exudates. J. Exp. Med., *134*:1131, 1971.

134. Snyderman, R., Shin, H. S., and Dannenberg, A. M.: Macrophage proteinase and inflammation. Production of chemotactic activity from the fifth component of complement by macrophage proteinase. J. Immunol., *109*:896, 1972.

135. Snyderman, R., Shin, H. S., and Hausmann, M. H.: A chemotactic factor from mononuclear phagocytes. Proc. Soc. Exp. Biol. Med., *138*:378, 1971.

136. Socransky, S. S.: Microbiology of periodontal disease. Present status and future considerations. J. Periodontol., *48*:497, 1977.

137. Spector, W. G.: The macrophage in inflammation. Scr. Haematol., *3*:132, 1970.

138. Steinberg, A. I., and Gershoff, S.: Quantitative differences in spirochetal antibody observed in periodontal disease. J. Periodontol., *39*:286, 1968.

139. Taichman, N. S., and Wilton, J. M. A.: Cytotoxicity of *Actinobacillus actinomycetemcomitans* (Y4) leukotoxin for gingival crevice PMNs. J. Dent. Res., *59A*:323, 1980.

140. Taichman, N. S., Freedman, H. L., and Uriuhara, T.: Inflammation and tissue injury. I. The response to intradermal injections of human dentogingival plaque in normal and leukopenic rabbits. Arch. Oral Biol., *11*:1385, 1966.

141. Taichman, N. S., Pruzanski, W., and Ranadive, N. S.: Release of intracellular constituents from rabbit polymorphonuclear leukocytes exposed to soluble and insoluble immune complexes. Int. Arch. Allergy Appl. Immunol., *43*:182, 1972.

142. Taylor, A. C.: Collagenolysis in cultured tissue. II. Role of mast cells. J. Dent. Res., *50*:1301, 1971.

143. Temple, T. R., Kimball, H. R., Kakehashi, S., and Amen, C. R.: Host factors in periodontal disease: periodontal manifestations of Chédiak-Higashi Syndrome. J. Periodont. Res. *10*(Suppl.):26, 1973.

144. Tsai, C. C., Hammond, T. F., Baehni, P., McArthur, W. P., and Taichman, N. S.: Interaction of inflammatory cells and oral microorganisms. J. Periodont. Res., *13*:504, 1978.

145. Wahl, L. M., et al.: Collagenase production by lymphokine-activated macrophages. Science, *187*:261, 1975.

146. Wahl, S. M., Iverson, G. M., and Oppenheim, J. J.: Induction of guinea pig B-cell lymphokine synthesis by mitogenic and nonmitogenic signals to Fe, Ig and C3 receptors. J. Exp. Med., *140*:1631, 1974.

147. Waldrop, T. C., Mackler, B. T., and Schur, P.: IgG and IgG subclasses in human periodontosis (juvenile periodontitis): serum concentrations. J. Periodontol., *52*:96, 1981.

148. Waldrop, T. C., Mackler, B. T., Schur, P., and Kelloy, W.: Immunologic study of human periodontosis (juvenile periodontitis). J. Periodontol., *52*:8, 1981.

149. Ward, P. A., and Schlegel, R. J.: Impaired leukotactic responsiveness in a child with recurrent infections. Lancet, *2*:344, 1969.

150. Ward, P. A., Remold, H. G., and David, J. R.: Leukotactic factor produced by sensitized lymphocytes. Science, *163*:1079, 1967.

151. Wright, W. E., Oppenheim, J. J., Baker, J. J., and Chan, S. P.: Effect of clinical therapy on lymphocyte transformation in severe periodontitis. JADR Abstract, p. B206, 1976.

152. Zachrisson, B. U.: Mast cells of the human gingiva. J. Periodont. Res., *2*:87, 1967.

chapter twenty-five

The Role of Microorganisms in Periodontal Disease

Numerous investigations have documented the fact that bacterial plaque is the etiologic agent in most forms of periodontal disease. However, the exact nature of the microbiota associated with periodontal health and disease has not yet been determined.[9, 30, 35, 36, 61, 71, 86, 110–112, 125, 126]

Earlier theories regarding the role of dental plaque suggested that plaque consisted of a complex and homogeneous bacterial mass which would lead to disease where allowed to overgrow. It was later found that the bacterial composition of plaque associated with healthy sites is different from that of the plaque associated with disease. Even more important was the fact that a characteristic microbial flora may be associated with clinically different periodontal diseases. These findings opened a new era in periodontal bacteriology.

Widespread application of sophisticated technologies—such as computer-assisted bacterial and statistical analyses and immunoelectron microscopy, as well as electron microscopic studies of human plaque in situ—has permitted expansive growth and improved knowledge of the role of microorganisms in the etiology, treatment, and prevention of periodontal disease.

The clinical characteristics of periodontal disease present several problems in the search for its etiology (Table 25–1). One of the most important considerations is the chronic nature of periodontal disease. For many years it was not clear whether periodontal destruction occurred at a slow, steady rate or whether there were periods of exacerbation *(disease activity)* and remission which resulted in attachment loss. Recently the "episodic" nature of periodontal destruction has been documented. The rate of periodontal destruction or *periodontal disease activity* is difficult to assess. The correlation of microbiologic and clinical parameters with periodontal disease activity is at present one of the most important areas of periodontal research (Fig. 25–1). Any analysis of the microbiota associated with a particular periodontal lesion or healthy area must take into account the stage of disease activity in that location at the time, because certain bacteria appear to be associated with periods of destruction, whereas other groups of bacteria seem to be associated with remission or quiescent periods.[112]

Host resistance factors can influence conceptions regarding the role of microorganisms in periodontal diseases as well as the types of bacteria permitted to colonize a particular ecologic niche. The balance between host resistance and bacterial virulence will determine the state of periodontal health or disease.

TABLE 25–1 DIFFICULTIES IN STUDYING THE MICROBIOLOGY OF PERIODONTAL HEALTH AND DISEASE

Disease Characteristic	Problems Encountered
Disease activity	Periods of exacerbation and remission
Host resistance	Variable, difficult to measure
Animal models	Results not directly transferable
Response to treatment	Definition of criteria for success

361

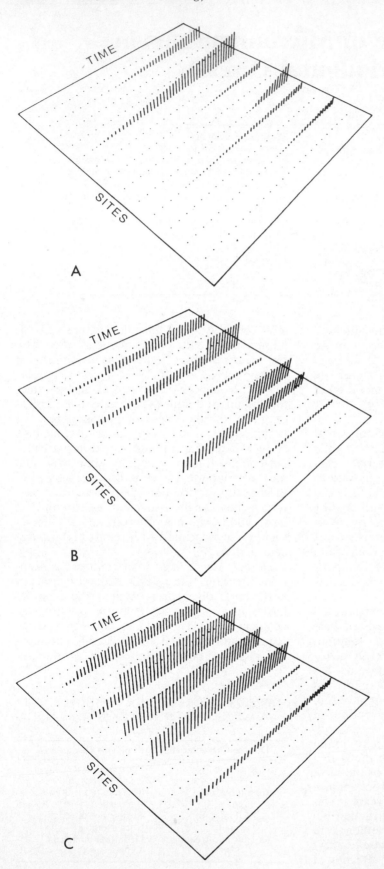

Figure 25–1 Diagrammatic representation of different possible modes of progression of chronic destructive periodontal disease. Sites on the x-axis are plotted against time on the y-axis, and activity is shown on the z-axis. *A*, some sites show progressive loss of attachment over time, whereas others show no destruction. The time of onset and the extent of destruction vary from site to site. *B*, "Random burst model." Activity occurs at random at any site. Some sites show no activity, whereas others show one or several bursts of activity. The cumulative extent of destruction varies from site to site. *C*, "Asynchronous multiple burst model." Several sites show bursts of activity over a finite period, followed by prolonged periods of inactivity. Occasional bursts may occur infrequently at certain sites at later periods. Other sites show no periodontal disease activity at any time. The difference from the model shown in part *b* is that here the majority of destructive disease activity takes place within a few years of the individual's life. (Courtesy of Drs. S. Socransky, A. Haffajee, M. Goodson, and J. Lindhe.)

Thus, it is important to consider the nature of the host's defensive (and potentially destructive) relationship with the bacteria colonizing the periodontal tissues. The complexity of the host response has been discussed in detail in Chapter 24.

COMPLEXITY OF PLAQUE BACTERIOLOGY

The bacteria which are associated with the periodontium exist in an extremely complex arrangement. There may be as many as 200 to 400 species of microorganisms in one individual. Earlier studies of the bacterial etiology of periodontal disease revealed problems in sampling the resident microorganisms, in cultivation, and in the description of the isolated bacteria (Table 25–2). In addition to the numerous variables among individual subjects, such as host factors and diet, the precise nature of the bacterial flora itself has been elusive. For example, the use of the pooled plaque samples described in earlier studies tended to obscure actual differences in bacterial distribution from site to site. Often bacteria from periodontally involved sites were mixed with bacteria from normal sites. Thus, any differences which may have existed could not be detected. The inability to adequately cultivate oxygen-sensitive microorganisms found in the gingival crevice led to further problems in completely characterizing the resident flora.

Examination of the microbiota associated with periodontal health and with different forms of disease revealed previously unsuspected differences in associated microbial composition. The once prevalent view that dental plaque composition was reasonably consistent from individual to individual and from site to site was found to be false. The idea that plaques were similar in composition was derived in part from studies of the microbial composition of pooled dental plaque and also from studies of the infectious potential of plaque by means of subcutaneous injection into experimental animals.[22, 26, 118, 120] Since supragingival plaque is usually more abundant (and more easily removed) than subgingival plaque, the samples often reflected the organisms dominant in the supragingival sites.

Different microbial complexes have been associated with different clinical forms of human periodontal disease. Clinical responses to the plaque bacteria are varied, with differences in the degree and nature of inflammation, the shape of the lesion and its location in the oral cavity, and the formation of pus, calculus, and so forth. Attempts to relate clinical symptomatology to the type of microorganisms present are under way, and limited progress has been made.

CRITERIA FOR DETERMINATION OF A MICROORGANISM AS A PERIODONTAL PATHOGEN

Classically, the criteria used to establish the bacterial etiology of human infectious disease are known as *Koch's postulates*. These postulates, formulated by Robert Koch in the late 1800s, provide a theoretical basis by which a specific bacterial agent may be defined as a causative agent.[30]

These criteria must be modified for the study of periodontal disease etiology because dental infections are associated with a complex array of factors which differ markedly from the diseases which concerned Koch. Recently Socransky has suggested an alternative to Koch's postulates that reflects the current understanding of the relationship of microorganisms to periodontal diseases:

1. The number of the etiologic organisms in the pathologic site must be increased, and, conversely, the organisms must be reduced or absent in healthy sites or sites with other forms of disease.

2. If the etiologic organism is eliminated or suppressed, the disease should stop; if it does not, either the wrong organism was eliminated or organisms which remain in high numbers in the site are sufficient by themselves for destruction to take place. This criterion for the deter-

---

TABLE 25–2   MAJOR CONCEPTUAL AND TECHNICAL PROBLEMS IN THE BACTERIAL ETIOLOGY OF PERIODONTAL DISEASE

Conceptual problems
  Anaerobic and capnophilic nature of flora
  Bacterial specificity
  Architectural arrangement of plaque
    Epithelium-associated plaque
    Bacterial invasion of gingiva
    Regional areas of pocket epithelium
  Unique bacterial types
  Host-bacterial interaction

Technical problems
  Anaerobic techniques
  Sampling methods
  Plaque dispersion
  Anatomic and immunologic methods
  Computer-aided analyses
  Development of taxonomy schemes

mination of a periodontopathogen has fostered the use of the term *"recolonization."* Currently, recolonization studies are being used in research as a measure of the effectiveness of a particular mode of therapy.

3. The response of the host may provide an important guide to the role of certain organisms in dental disease. An increased or decreased cellular and/or humoral immune response to a given species in a specific form of periodontal disease suggests a role for that organism in the disease process. The host response may also be influenced by the resident bacteria.

4. A relatively finite spectrum of organisms have been shown to initiate caries or some forms of periodontal disease in experimental animals. In each instance the organism tested was isolated in a pure culture. Uncultivable organisms or organisms which fail to implant in the oral cavity of experimental animals cannot be tested. Recently many anaerobic bacteria (see below) have been implicated in the etiology and/or progression of periodontal diseases, but these organisms are extremely difficult to implant in experimental animals. In spite of the many reservations regarding the applicability of animal pathogenicity to human disease processes, such testing should remain part of the effort to determine the possible etiologic role of different bacterial species.

5. *Bacterial virulence* is another criterion which could contribute to the determination of potential oral pathogens. For example, a potent mechanism of demineralization would be an essential prerequisite for organisms involved in the etiology of dental caries. Many bacterially mediated mechanisms can be considered in the etiology of destructive periodontal diseases and will be discussed below.

PLAQUE

Many types of deposits exist on the tooth surface above and below the gingival margin. In the past these were designated by a variety of terms; often the same term was applied to different aggregations.

The term *"plaque"* is used universally to describe the association of bacteria to the tooth surface.[9] Based on its relationship to the gingival margin, plaque is differentiated primarily into two categories: *supragingival* and *subgingival*. Some authors have described the plaque near the gingival margin as *marginal plaque*. Recently the presence of bacteria within the gingival tissues has been confirmed.[2, 25, 31, 97] These bacteria appear in the tissues either as isolated organisms or as bacterial aggregates. The applicability of the term "plaque" to these bacteria awaits further analysis.

Supragingival Plaque

Small amounts of supragingival plaque are not clinically visible unless they are disclosed by pigments from within the oral cavity or stained by disclosing solutions or wafers (Plate IV). As plaque develops and accumulates, it becomes a visible globular mass with a pinpoint nodular surface that varies in color from gray to yellowish-gray to yellow. Supragingival plaque develops mostly on the gingival third of the teeth, with a predilection for surface cracks, defects, rough areas, and overhanging margins of dental restorations.

Supragingival plaque formation begins with the adhesion of bacteria on the acquired pellicle or tooth surface, whether enamel, cementum, or dentin (Fig. 25–2).[10, 90] Plaque mass grows by (1) the addition of new bacteria,[19] (2) the multiplication of bacteria, and (3) the accumulation of bacterial and host products.

Measurable amounts of supragingival plaque may form within 1 hour after the teeth are thoroughly cleaned,[51] with maximum accumulation reached in 30 days or less. The rate of formation and the location vary among individuals, on different teeth in the same mouth, and on different areas of individual teeth.[62]

Irreversible bacterial colonization of the pellicle does not appear to take place until 2 to 4 hours after enamel has been exposed to the bacteria. Organisms *initially* colonize smooth surfaces and pits and grooves as single cells rather than as aggregates.[19] The earliest colonizers are mainly gram-positive cocci. Adhesion by means of polysaccharides produced by some of these bacteria is mediated by cell surface glycosyltransferase, the enzyme that governs the production of these polysaccharides. Although stagnation is the principal factor governing the retention of bacteria at periodontal disease–prone dental sites,[33] there is clear evidence that some organisms adhere more readily than others (Fig. 25–3).

The amount of plaque varies from individual to individual and is influenced by diet, age, salivary factors, oral hygiene, tooth alignment, systemic disease, and host factors.

Composition of Supragingival Dental Plaque

Supragingival plaque consists primarily of proliferating microorganisms (see below) and a scattering of epithelial cells, leukocytes, and

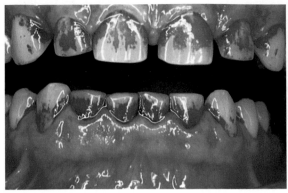

A

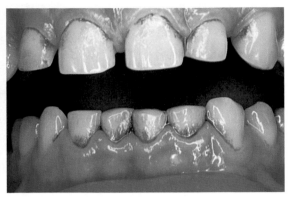

B

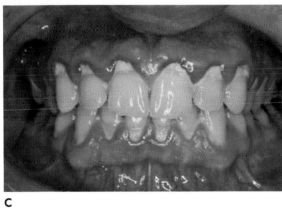

C

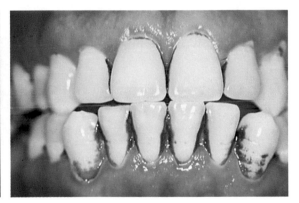

D

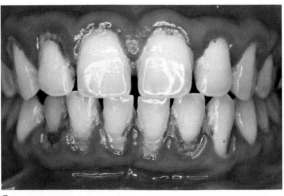

E

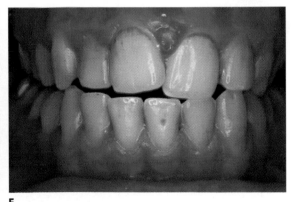

F

Plate IV

A, Disclosed supragingival plaque covering one half to two thirds of the clinical crowns. (Courtesy of Dr. S. Socransky.)

B, Supragingival plaque (same patient as in *A*) disclosed with an oxidation-reduction dye that indicates reduced (anaerobic) areas of plaque. The supragingival anaerobic areas (purple stain) are located interproximally and along the gingival margin. (Courtesy of Dr. S. Socransky.)

C, Materia alba generalized throughout the mouth, with heaviest accumulation near the gingiva. Note the gingivitis present.

D, Teeth stained by several weeks of mouth rinses with alexidine. This stain can be easily removed.

E, Supragingival calculus in a patient with gingival inflammation.

F, Green stain on anterior teeth. Note the inflamed, enlarged interdental papilla between the maxillary central incisors.

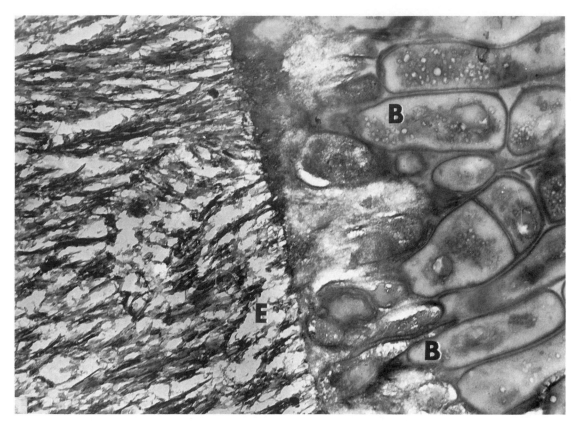

Figure 25–2 Plaque Formed Directly on Enamel Surface. Electronmicrograph of decalcified noncarious enamel surface showing remnants of enamel matrix (E) and bacteria (B) in attached plaque. (Courtesy of R. M. Frank and A. Brendel.)

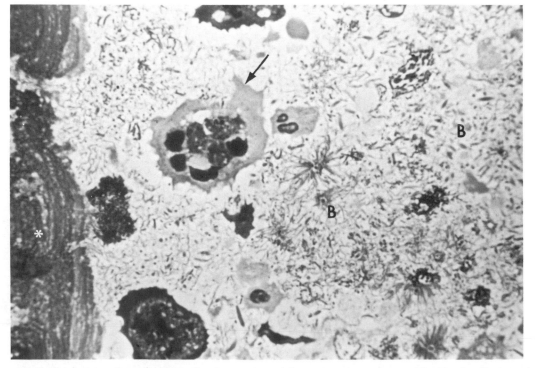

Figure 25–3 Histologic section of plaque showing nonbacterial components, such as white blood cells *(arrow)* and epithelial cells *(asterisk),* interspersed among bacteria (B). (Courtesy of Dr. Max Listgarten.)

macrophages in an adherent intercellular matrix.[10, 72] Organic and inorganic solids form about 20 per cent or more of the plaque; the remainder is water. Bacteria constitute approximately 70 to 80 per cent of the solid material, and the rest is intercellular matrix. Supragingival plaque stains positive with periodic acid–Schiff (PAS) stain, and it is orthochromatic with toluidine blue.

Supragingival Plaque Matrix

ORGANIC CONTENT. The organic matrix consists of a polysaccharide protein complex of which the principal components are carbohydrates and proteins (approximately 30 per cent each) and lipids (approximately 15 per cent), with the nature of the remainder unclear. These components represent extracellular products of plaque bacteria, their cytoplasmic and cell membrane remnants, ingested foodstuff, and derivatives of salivary glycoproteins. The carbohydrate present in greatest amounts in the matrix of supragingival plaque is *dextran,* a bacteria-produced polysaccharide which forms approximately 9.5 per cent of the total plaque (Table 25–3). Other matrix carbohydrates are levan, galactose, and methylpentose in the form of rhamnose. When *Streptococcus mutans* is present in the plaque, *mutan,* another type of extracellular carbohydrate, is found to contribute to the organic matrix. Bacterial remnants provide muramic acid, lipids, and some matrix protein, for which salivary glycoproteins are the principal source.

INORGANIC CONTENT. The principal inorganic components of the supragingival plaque matrix are calcium and phosphorus; there are small amounts of magnesium, potassium, and sodium. They are bound to the organic components in higher concentrations on the mandibular anterior teeth than in the remainder of the mouth, and they are also found in relatively high concentrations on lingual surfaces. The total inorganic content of early supragingival plaque is small; the greatest increase in inorganic content occurs in plaque which is transformed to calculus. Fluoride topically applied to the teeth and in drinking water, toothpaste, dental floss coated with fluoride, or mouthwash becomes incorporated in the plaque. This fluoride is thought to become incorporated ultimately on the tooth surface, whether on the enamel, cementum, or dentin. The fluoride may act to deter the metabolism of plaque bacteria, kill them directly,[133] or aid in remineralization of the tooth surface.

Diet and Supragingival Plaque Formation

Dental plaque is not a food residue. Supragingival plaque forms more rapidly during sleep, when no food is ingested, than following meals. This may be because the mechanical action of food and the increased salivary flow caused by mastication during the day may deter plaque formation. Patients who have dry mouths have increased amounts of supragingival plaque. Saliva and salivary flow are major ecologic influences on supragingival plaque. The consistency of the diet also affects the rate of plaque formation. Supragingival plaque forms rapidly in patients on soft diets, whereas hard, chewy foods retard formation (see Chapter 28) (Plate IV).

In man and in some laboratory animals, dietary supplements of sucrose increase supragingival plaque formation[17] and affect its bacterial composition. This effect is attributed to extracellular polysaccharides produced by bacteria; glucose supplements do not have a similar effect. Plaque formation occurs in patients on high-protein, low-fat diets and patients on carbohydrate-free diets, but in smaller amounts. These dietary alternatives not only alter the metabolism of existing plaque bacteria, but may also alter the environment and, subsequently, the plaque composition.

The relationship of supragingival plaque to the etiology of periodontal disease is still far from being completely understood, but it is quite clear that "marginal" plaque and subgingival plaque are directly responsible for the initiation and progression of periodontal diseases. It is probable that supragingival plaque strongly influences the growth, accumulation, and pathogenic potential of subgingival plaque, especially in the early stages of gingivitis and periodontitis. Once the disease has progressed and periodontal pocket formation has taken

TABLE 25–3 CARBOHYDRATE CONTENT OF PLAQUE MATRIX*

	Percentage of Lyophilized Matrix Weight	
	Mean	Range
Dextran (polymer of glucose)	9.5%	8–10%
Hexosamine	4%	3–6%
Methylpentose	3.1%	2–4%
Galactose	2.6%	1.7–4.4%
Levan (polymer of fructose)	0.4%	0.1–0.7%

*Modified from Mandel, I. D.

place, the influence of supragingival plaque on all but the most coronally located subgingival plaque is minimal.

Subgingival Plaque

Structure and Organization of Subgingival Plaque

The gingival sulcus and periodontal pocket harbor a diverse collection of bacteria. The nature of the organisms which colonize these retentive sites differs from that of organisms found in supragingival plaque. The morphology of the gingival sulcus and periodontal pocket makes them less subject to the cleansing activities of the mouth. Thus, these retentive areas form a relatively stagnant environment where organisms which cannot readily adhere to a tooth surface may have the oppor-

tunity to colonize. It is not surprising, therefore, to find that the majority of the motile bacteria in the mouth colonize these sites. These organisms may also adhere to other bacteria, to the tooth, and/or to the subgingival pocket epithelium.[85] In addition, organisms within these retentive sites have direct access to the nutrients and immunoglobulins[73] present in sulcular fluid. The oxidation-reduction potential (anaerobic nature) of the gingival sulcus and periodontal pocket has been demonstrated to be very low. Thus, organisms which can exist only in areas of low oxygen concentration can survive in the gingival sulcus area.

Light and electron microscopic observations of extracted teeth and adjacent tissues from humans have been of paramount importance in increasing our understanding of the colonization of microorganisms in subgingival sites.[8, 12, 55, 57, 65, 68–70, 97, 98] From these studies, subgingival plaque can be described as *tooth*

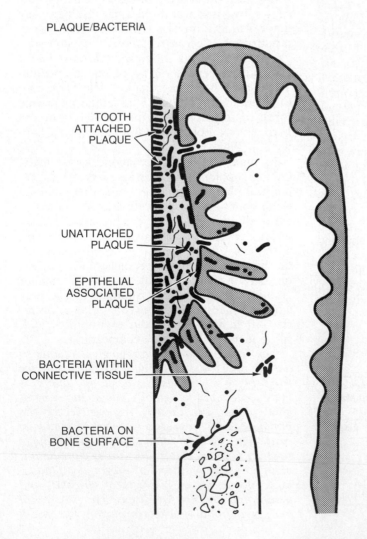

PLAQUE/BACTERIA

TOOTH ATTACHED PLAQUE

UNATTACHED PLAQUE

EPITHELIAL ASSOCIATED PLAQUE

BACTERIA WITHIN CONNECTIVE TISSUE

BACTERIA ON BONE SURFACE

Figure 25–4 Diagram depicting plaque/bacteria association with tooth surface and periodontal tissues.

associated, and epithelium associated. Bacteria and other microorganisms from the subgingival epithelium–associated plaque may penetrate, invade, and colonize the gingival connective tissue. These bacteria are referred to as *connective tissue associated* (Fig. 25–4).

TOOTH-ASSOCIATED (ATTACHED) SUBGINGIVAL PLAQUE. There are plaque bacteria attached to the tooth surface in the gingival sulcus and periodontal pocket. This can be observed after washing the tooth, staining it, and examining it for adherent plaque. The organisms are thought to be gram-positive rods and cocci, such as *Streptococcus mitis, S. sanguis, Eubacterium, Bifidobacterium, Actinomyces viscosus, A. naeslundii, Propionibacter-*

ium, Bacterionema matruchotii, and other species. In addition, some gram-negative cocci and rods can always be found in this attached subgingival plaque. The apical border of tooth-associated plaque is always found some distance away from the junctional epithelium. The surface morphology of the attached subgingival plaque appears to be granular at low magnification. At higher magnification the surface layer of this plaque appears to be composed of coccal or filamentous and fusiform microorganisms.

The tooth (attached) component of subgingival plaque is associated with the deposition of mineral salts, with the formation of calculus,[11] and with root caries and root resorption

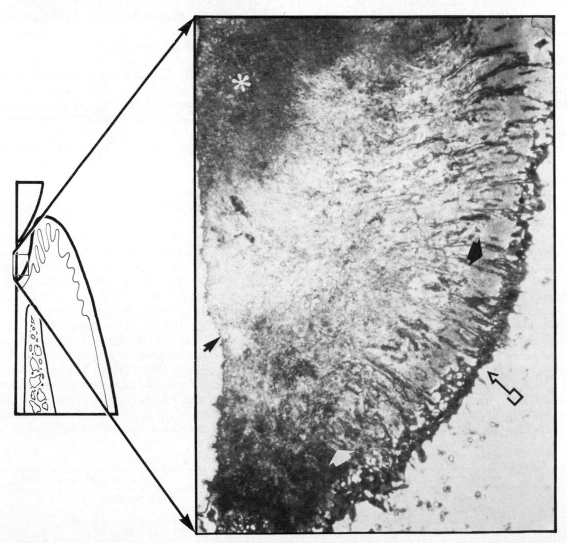

Figure 25–5 *Left,* Diagrammatic representation of the histologic structure of subgingival plaque. *Right,* Histologic section of subgingival plaque. *Arrow with box,* Sulcular epithelium. *White arrow,* Predominantly gram-negative unattached zone. *Black arrow,* Tooth surface. *Asterisk,* Predominantly gram-positive attached zone. (From Listgarten, M.: J. Periodontol., 46:10, 1975.)

areas. However, it is not clear whether this attached component develops before other bacteria are found in the gingival sulcus area.

EPITHELIUM-ASSOCIATED SUBGINGIVAL PLAQUE. A loosely adherent component of the subgingival plaque is in direct association with the subgingival epithelium and extends from the gingival margin to the junctional epithelium. In the past this zone has been called the zone of unattached subgingival plaque (Fig. 25–5). It contains one portion which is in contact with the epithelium and another which is loose in the pocket lumen. Conceptually, we now reserve the term "unattached" for the latter portion. However, little is known about differences between the unattached plaque and the epithelium-associated plaque, and therefore they will be dealt with together. Epithelium-associated plaque contains predominantly but not exclusively motile and gram-negative organisms (Table 25–4). Organisms within this zone are in direct contact with the epithelium of the gingival sulcus or periodontal pocket and with the surface of the tooth immediately coronal to the junctional epithelium (Fig. 25–6). Removal of teeth for study would disturb and eliminate the plaque loosely adherent to the tooth surface, leaving a zone immediately coronal to the junctional epithelium devoid of plaque bacteria. Use of a disclosing solution to stain this area would reveal no plaque since it is not adhering to the tooth. Therefore, some authors have called this the plaque-free zone even though loosely adherent plaque is present in vivo.

The relative proportions of the subgingival plaque zones appear to be related to the nature and activity of the disease which is present in a particular pocket. In rapidly advancing lesions, such as those of localized juvenile periodontitis (see below), the tooth-associated component of subgingival plaque appears to be minimal. Instead, the periodontal pocket contains predominantly loosely adherent gram-negative rods and spirochetes which make up the larger epithelium-associated subgingival plaque zone

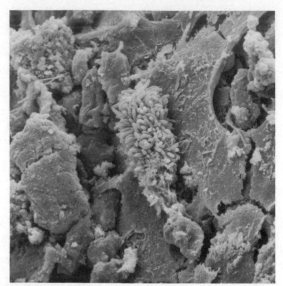

Figure 25–6 Scanning electron micrograph of bacteria between junctional epithelial cells. × 600

(see Fig. 25–4). A similar pattern of subgingival bacterial colonization has been demonstrated in patients with a rapidly progressing form of periodontitis. Several investigators have suggested that the plaque adjacent to the sulcular and junctional epithelia may be the "advancing front" of the periodontal lesion.

Further examination of the structure of subgingival plaque reveals characteristics of each component which are important for our understanding of the relationship of certain groups of microorganisms to disease. It is clear from clinical examination that calculus is attached to the tooth surface and not to the epithelium.[11] Thus, the tooth-associated subgingival plaque is most important in calculus formation. In addition, subgingival root caries undoubtedly results from a subgingival plaque, which is also in contact with the root surface (Fig. 25–7). Calculus is always covered by adherent plaque (Fig. 25–8). The plaque on the surface of calculus may gain entrance into the periodontal tissues because of the irritation and physical trauma to the thin inflamed pocket epithelium caused by the calculus.

TABLE 25–4   CHARACTERISTICS OF SUBGINGIVAL PLAQUE

Attached to Tooth	Unattached	Attached to Epithelium
Gram-positive bacteria predominate	Gram variable	Gram variable
Does not extend to junctional epithelium	Extends to junctional epithelium	Extends to junctional epithelium
May penetrate the cementum	—	May penetrate epithelium and connective tissue
Associated with calculus formation and root caries	Associated with gingivitis	Associated with gingivitis and periodontitis

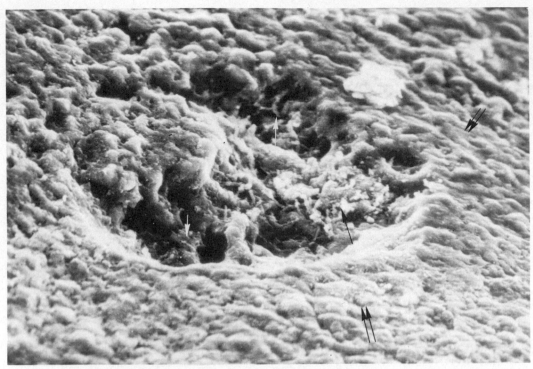

Figure 25–7 Minute lesion on surface of root (resorption concavity) previously covered by plaque. Note microorganisms *(single arrows)* within lesion. Cemental mounds can easily be identified *(double arrows)*. (Courtesy of Dr. J. Sottosanti.)

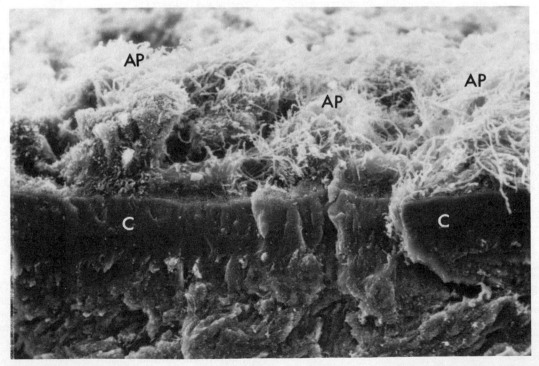

Figure 25–8 Scanning electron photomicrograph of cross section of cementum (C) with attached subgingival plaque (AP). Area shown is within a periodontal pocket. (Courtesy of Dr. J. Sottosanti.)

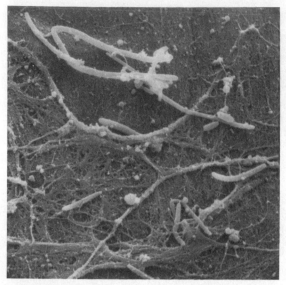

Figure 25–9 Scanning electron micrograph of cocci and filaments associated with surface of pocket epithelium in a case of marginal gingivitis. × 3000.

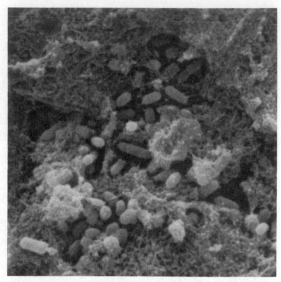

Figure 25–11 Scanning electron micrograph of frontal view of pocket wall showing short rods on epithelial surface. × 10,000.

RELATIONSHIP OF MICROORGANISMS TO THE POCKET EPITHELIAL SURFACE.

On examination of the surface of deep periodontal pockets, areas of bacterial accumulation are found on the epithelium. These areas trigger a host response consisting of the emergence of leukocytes and areas of leukocyte-bacterial interaction[94, 95] (see Chapters 8 and 14). The presence of microtopographically distinct areas

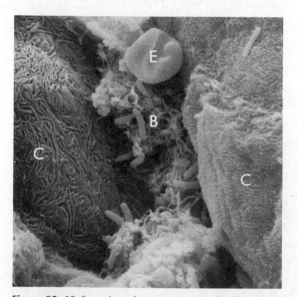

Figure 25–10 Scanning electron micrograph of epithelial intercellular spaces containing bacterial plaque (B) enmeshed in a fibrin-like material. C, epithelial cells; E, erythrocyte. The cell to the left show signs of necrosis. × 4000.

suggests that the pocket wall is constantly changing as a result of the interaction between the epithelium, the adjacent epithelium-associated bacteria, calculus, and host factors.[93]

Coccal bacteria and filaments are regularly seen on the pocket epithelial surface of gingivitis specimens; occasionally other morphologic forms are found as well (Fig. 25–9). The association of spirochetes, bacilli, and filaments on the epithelial surface is more frequently seen in the pocket epithelium in periodontitis. These bacteria are associated on the surface with extracellular bacterial products, fibrin, or other host-derived material (Figs. 25–10 and 25–11). The finding of a differential nature of bacterial colonization along the epithelial surface is most likely related to the adjacent subgingival plaque, the precise nature of the host response, or other factors. Microenvironments along the epithelial surface are important in permitting invasion, colonization, and growth of specific plaque bacteria.

BACTERIAL INVASION OF THE PERIODONTIUM

Direct invasion of the periodontal tissues has not generally been found in the past, except in the gingiva of patients with acute necrotizing ulcerative gingivitis (see Chapter 11). The presence of invading bacteria in gingivitis,[21] in the lateral wall of periodontal pock-

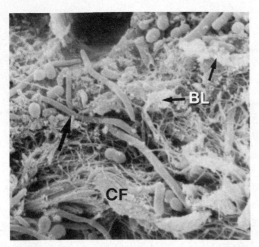

Figure 25–12 Scanning electron micrograph of connective tissue–epithelial junction in a deep periodontal pocket in a human. Note bacteria accumulated on basal lamina (BL) and penetrating the connective tissue through an interruption in the basal lamina (*arrow*). CF, collagen fiber. × 9000.

ets in advanced chronic periodontitis[25, 97] and juvenile periodontitis[12, 31] in humans, and in the gingival connective tissue of rats[2] has recently been demonstrated.

Invasion of the pocket epithelium by bacteria has been found in intercellular spaces of the stratum spinosum (Fig. 25–12). Widening of intercellular spaces and rupture of intercellular ridges are associated with abundant bacteria. Coccal forms, short rods, filaments, and spirochetes have been found occupying spaces between intercellular connections. Accumulations of bacteria are found on the epithelial side of the basal lamina. Bacteria appear in greater numbers in this area than in intercellular spaces, suggesting that they move toward the basal lamina. Bacteria that accumulate along the basement membrane penetrate into the connective tissue in areas where a perforation or interruption is found. Bacteria can also gain access to the epithelium through ulcerations in the pocket wall or through spaces on the surface created by emigrating polymorphonuclear leukocytes. This pattern of gingival epithelial invasion is similar to that of the invasion of other epithelial surfaces of man.

Gram-negative and gram-positive filamentous, rod-shaped, and coccoid bacteria have been found in the gingival connective tissue and in contact with the alveolar bone surface (Fig. 25–13). Spirochetes have been seen at the surface of alveolar bone, where they may attach. Table 25–5 summarizes findings on bacterial penetration of the periodontium.

Bacterial Invasion: Current Perspective

Bacterial penetration into the periodontium is an important factor in the pathogenesis of periodontal disease. Whether bacterial penetration represents a regular feature of the advanced stages of periodontitis, leading to exfoliation of the tooth or also occurs in less advanced stages remains to be determined. The clinical implications of bacterial invasion are also unknown.

MICROBIAL SPECIFICITY

In the past two decades there have been a number of changes in our concepts regarding the etiology of periodontal disease. In the 1960s the composition of plaque was thought to be relatively similar from patient to patient and from site to site within patients. Variability was recognized to exist, but the true extent of differences in bacterial composition was not appreciated. It was thought that the major event triggering destructive periodontal disease was an increase in the mass of bacterial plaque, possibly accompanied by a diminution in host resistance.

Certain observations, however, troubled clinicians and researchers. For example, the localized nature of destruction occurring in individual mouths was of considerable concern. If all plaques were alike and the host responded consistently to a constant challenge, why was destruction taking place adjacent to one tooth but not another? Another troublesome observation was the presence of large accumulations of plaque and severe gingivitis in some individuals for years without destruction of the supporting structures. In contrast, other individuals were observed with little detectable plaque or clinical inflammation but with dramatic loss of the periodontium.

An answer to some of these questions stemmed from the work of Socransky, Loesche, Slots, and others who developed the concept of specificity of periodontal lesions.

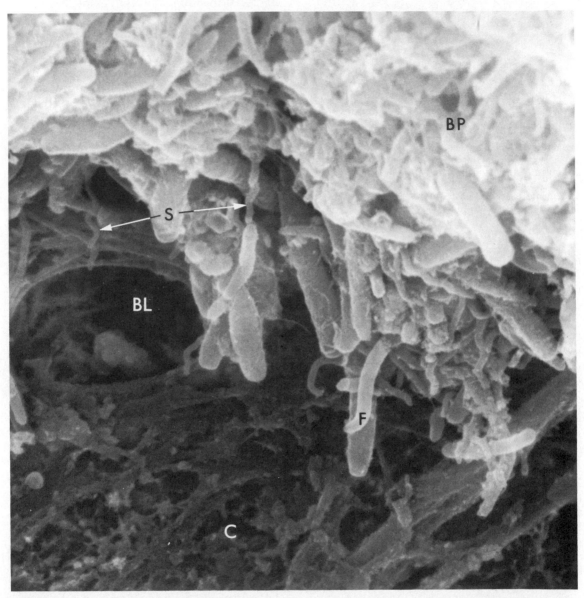

Figure 25–13 Scanning electron micrograph of bacterial plaque (BP) on bone surface in a case of juvenile periodontitis. S, spirochete; F, filament; BL, bone lacunae containing bacteria; C, bone collagen. × 10,000.

TABLE 25–5   INTRAGINGIVAL MICROORGANISMS IN HUMAN PERIODONTAL DISEASE

Penetration
    Through intercellular spaces of epithelium
    Through ulcers and clefts
Found in
    Pocket and junctional epithelium
        On surface
        In intercellular spaces
        On basal lamina
    Gingival connective tissue
    On bone surface
Diseases
    Acute necrotizing ulcerative gingivitis
    Advanced periodontitis
    Localized juvenile periodontitis
    Others (?)
Microorganisms identified
    Spirochetes (in acute necrotizing ulcerative gingivitis, advanced periodontitis, and
        localized gingival periodontitis)
    Mycoplasma (in advanced periodontitis and localized juvenile periodontitis)
    Actinobacillus actinomycetemcomitans (in localized juvenile periodontitis)
    Capnocytophaga sputigena (in localized juvenile periodontitis)

Concept of Specificity

The concept of bacterial specificity, formally discussed by Loesche as the *"specific plaque hypothesis"* in 1976, suggests that specific forms of periodontal disease have specific bacterial etiologies.[61]

Keyes and Jordan demonstrated bacterial specificity in animals,[45] but momentum with regard to bacterial specificity was achieved when Slots[107] and Newman, Socransky, and co-workers[74–77, 80, 83] isolated a characteristic bacterial flora from deep periodontal lesions in patients diagnosed as having localized juvenile periodontitis (see below).

The concept of bacterial specificity suggests that periodontal disease may be a group of diseases with different etiologies and clinical courses, but with similar symptomatologies. With the recognition of a diverse group of etiologic agents, more accurate clinical and laboratory diagnoses could be made.[112] Although this area of research is recent, it is beginning to improve our diagnostic acumen, as well as our basic understanding of periodontal disease pathogenesis. Accurate identification of specific etiologic agents is an absolute prerequisite to future advances.

Microbiologic Factors: Technical Considerations

The complexity of the flora is a major barrier to unraveling the answers to our questions regarding the periodontal microbiota. Comparison of information from various research laboratories indicates that different technical procedures used in deriving new data may influence the results obtained.[49, 92] Consideration of these technical differences is essential in analyzing current research.

SAMPLING. The analysis of the types of bacteria found in association with different anatomic sites or in patients with different diseases depends on the quality of the sample being analyzed.[66] The subgingival area presents conceptual, logistic, anatomic, and other technical problems, all of which can influence the quality of the microbial sample and, thus, the identification of the resident microorganisms. To date there is no best way to obtain samples from the subgingival area. Each method must be judged according to the results desired and achieved.

SAMPLE DISPERSION. Since some of the subgingival microbiota is a tightly adherent mass of bacteria, dispersion of the clumps of plaque will permit accurate identification of the various individual components that make it up.

ANAEROBIC ENVIRONMENT. The vast majority of subgingival isolates are anaerobic and require anaerobic methods of processing and characterization.

IDENTIFICATION OF MICROORGANISMS. There are hundreds of different types of bacteria that can colonize subgingival sites. Some have never been identified; thus, reference information may be unavailable or inaccurate. In order to compare data and communicate information, accurate identification of bacteria is an absolute prerequisite.[117] From accurate identification, diagnostic and therapeutic strategies can be developed.

STATISTICAL ANALYSIS. The generation of complex and voluminous data from clinical and cultural microbiology studies requires complex and voluminous statistical analysis. The frequency of occurrence of specific bacteria is usually not distributed in a normal manner and, thus, requires nonparametric statistical analysis or the use of transformed data. The complexity of the data calls for computer-assisted analysis, and this phase of periodontal microbiology research has assumed an important part in the overall quest to eliminate, control, or prevent periodontal diseases.

MECHANISMS OF BACTERIA-MEDIATED DESTRUCTION

Periodontal health is maintained as long as the balance between host resistance and bacterial virulence is in favor of the host. Periodontopathic microorganisms produce a variety of pathogenic and virulence factors which are undoubtedly involved in all stages of the disease process.

Bacteria can cause disease indirectly by (1) evading the host defense mechanisms, (2) minimizing or neutralizing the host defense mechanisms, and (3) triggering immunopathologic processes[64] (see Chapter 24).

Microbes that successfully infect the host resort to one or several strategies to counteract the defensive activities of the phagocyte. Mims lists the following strategies that may be used by bacteria: (1) killing the phagocyte by releasing soluble substances that are lethal to it, (2) inhibition of chemotaxis, (3) inhibition of adsorption of microorganisms to the surface of the phagocytic cell, (4) inhibition of phagocytosis, (5) inhibition of fusion of lysosomes with phagocytic vacuoles, (6) escape from the phagosome, and (7) resistance to killing and digestion in the phagolysosome, which may be followed by the growth of bacteria inside the phagocytic cell.[64]

Knowledge of these mechanisms is very sketchy, and much more basic information is required. No data are available with reference to these mechanisms in the gingival area. Further consideration of these possible actions is vital.

The bacteria which colonize the periodontal tissues may also cause tissue destruction by *direct* means. Considerable attention has been focused on characterizing the organisms which produce lytic enzymes or toxic products which could be responsible for destroying the periodontium. This attention is primarily due to the fact that, in earlier cultural studies, samples of pooled gingival bacteria from either healthy or diseased individuals suggested that specific groups of bacteria were not associated with clinical disease. It was therefore hypothesized that periodontitis was bacteriologically nonspecific and that certain bacterial metabolites such as lytic enzymes were probably responsible for the tissue destruction.[13, 14, 17, 29, 34, 37, 54, 84, 88, 89, 91, 100-104, 115, 116, 127, 132] Analysis of whole plaque demonstrated a variety of enzymes capable of destroying the major components of the gingival connective tissue.[17] Furthermore, specific gingival bacteria were also found to produce a variety of other substances.[36, 120, 121] In addition to lytic enzymes, there are a wide variety of other potentially toxic products elaborated by gingival bacteria. These factors can be divided into three major kinds (Table 25–6): (1) factors that affect the intercellular matrix, (2) direct

TABLE 25–6 BACTERIA-MEDIATED EFFECTS

	Bacteria	Substance Elaborated
Intercellular matrix	Staphylococci	Hyaluronidase-glucuronidase
	Streptococci	Hyaluronidase-glucuronidase
	Diphtheroids	Chondroitin sulfatase
	Bacteroides	Collagenase
Cytotoxic substances	Many plaque bacteria	Ammonia, proteases
	Many plaque bacteria	Hydrogen sulfide
	Many plaque bacteria	Indole, toxic amines
	Many plaque bacteria	Organic acids
	Actinobacillus	Leukotoxin
	Capnocytophaga	Cytotoxin
Inflammatory stimulants	Gram-negative organisms	Endotoxin
	Gram-positive organisms	Peptidoglycans

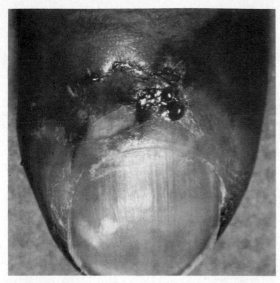

Figure 25–14 Infected finger from accidental puncture with periodontal curette. (Courtesy of Dr. R. Barbanell.)

cellular toxicity factors,[122] and (3) inflammatory stimulants.[22, 43, 48]

The pathogenic potential of organisms isolated in periodontal lesions has been demonstrated in other ways. For example, bacteria colonizing the mouth of humans can initiate dangerous infections in other parts of the body.[23, 24, 106] Infections initiated by oral organisms can occur accidentally, through skin punctures with dental probes (Fig. 25–14), or from human bite wounds.[26, 63] Organisms associated with periodontal disease have been found in infected surgical wounds and in pleuropulmonary abscesses as the result of aspiration,[23] and bacterial sepsis by *Capnocytophaga* of periodontal origin has been documented in patients with granulocytopenia.[24] Bacterial endocarditis due to bacteria associated with periodontal disease has also increased in occurrence.

Studies in Experimental Animals

The periodontopathic potential of organisms isolated from human periodontal disease can be demonstrated in experimental animals[7, 18, 27, 38–42, 47, 79] (Figs. 25–15 and 25–16). Ideally, animals in which such experiments are carried out should have conditions similar to those which occur in man. Unfortunately, a good animal model system which develops a periodontal pathology comparable with that of humans has not been found. Recently, however, great interest has been generated regard-

ing the beagle dog model system.[123, 124] These animals will develop gingivitis and a subsequent loss of supporting bone similar to that found in human disease if they are maintained on soft diets for long periods (Fig. 25–17). There are many similarities between the oral flora in the animals and that in humans, but it is quite clear that these dogs have a characteristic indigenous microbiota different from that of humans. Consequently, direct extrapolation of bacteriologic findings from animals to humans should be done with great caution.

MICROBIOLOGY OF PERIODONTAL HEALTH AND DISEASE

Oral Flora

The oral cavity is sterile at birth, but a simple, primarily facultative flora becomes established within 6 to 10 hours.[113] Anaerobes appear in some mouths within the first 10 days and are present in most by five months of age, before the teeth erupt, and in 100 per cent of mouths when the incisors appear. Anaerobes increase with age, but the facultative types remain numerically predominant. Microscopic counts in saliva range from 43 million to 5.5 billion organisms per milliliter, with an average of 750 million.[11] A representative census of the salivary bacterial population is shown in Table 25–7. Also present are fungi, including *Candida, Cryptococcus,* and *Saccharomyces,* and protozoa such as *Entamoeba gingivalis* and *Trichomonas tenax.*[11] Viruses and *Mycoplasma*[20, 78] can be found in the oral cavity. Bacteriophages are often found associated with the oral indigenous and pathogenic bacteria.

Most of the salivary bacteria are derived from the dorsum of the tongue, from which they are detached by mechanical action; lesser amounts come from the remainder of the oral mucous membrane. The number of microorganisms increases temporarily during sleep and decreases after eating and toothbrushing.

Supragingivally, bacteria associated with periodontal health are mainly gram-positive coccal and rod-shaped bacteria (Fig. 25–18).

These organisms initiate plaque growth by means of their ability to adhere to the tooth surface (pellicle) and then to proliferate in that particular ecologic niche. The colonization of the tooth surface by supragingival plaque bacteria appears to be quite specific and apparently depends upon the interaction of the bacterial surface with the salivary glycoprotein of

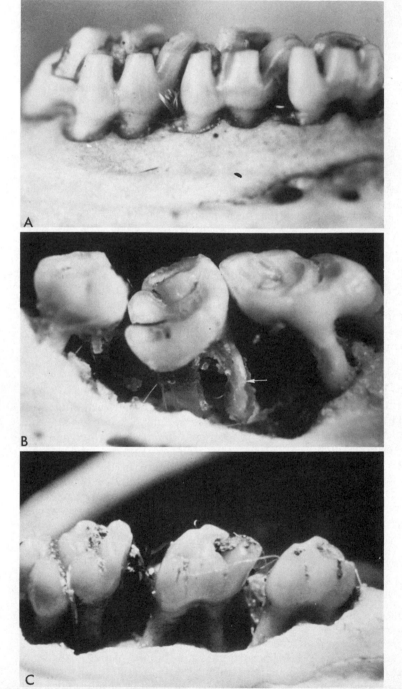

Figure 25–15 *A,* Jaw of noninfected control germ-free rat 90 days old. *B,* Massive alveolar bone destruction and root caries *(arrow)* caused by monoinfection with a periodontopathic strain of Actinomyces naeslundii in 90-day-old gnotobiotic rat. Organism isolated from a patient with periodontitis. *C,* Extreme alveolar bone loss caused by monoinfection with a periodontopathic strain of *Capnocytophaga* in 90-day-old gnotobiotic rat. Organism was isolated from lesion in patient with juvenile periodontitis (periodontosis). Note that these organisms did not cause root surface caries.

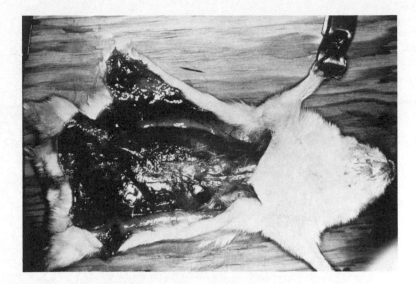

Figure 25–16 Transmissible mixed infection caused by bacteria isolated from human periodontal lesion. (Courtesy of Dr. S. Socransky.)

TABLE 25–7   INDIGENOUS FLORA OF HUMAN SALIVA*

Bacterial Group	Predominant Isolates of the Group	Percentage
Gram-positive facultative cocci	Streptococci represent 41 per cent of all isolates and are composed of *S. salivarius, S. mitis,* and small numbers of enterococci; the remainder are staphylococci	46.2
Gram-negative anaerobic cocci	*Veillonella*	15.9
Gram-positive anaerobic cocci	*Peptostreptococcus or Peptococcus*	13.0
Gram-positive facultative rods	Diphtheroids, *Actinomyces*	11.8
Gram-negative anaerobic rods	*Campylobacter sputorum, Bacteroides, Fusobacterium*	4.8
Gram-positive anaerobic rods	*Propionibacterium, Actinomyces*	4.8
Gram-negative facultative rods	Unidentified	2.3
Gram-negative facultative cocci	Unidentified	1.2

*Modified from Gordon, D. F., Jr., and Jong, B. B.: Appl. Microbiol., *16*:428, 1968.

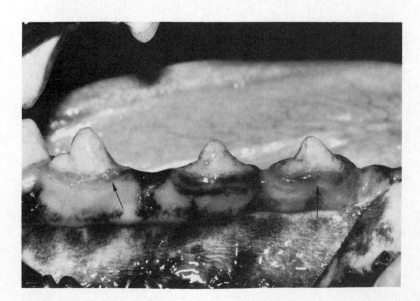

Figure 25–17 Mouth of beagle dog demonstrating classic signs of inflammatory periodontal disease. Note inflamed gingival margins *(arrows)* adjacent to plaque-laden teeth.

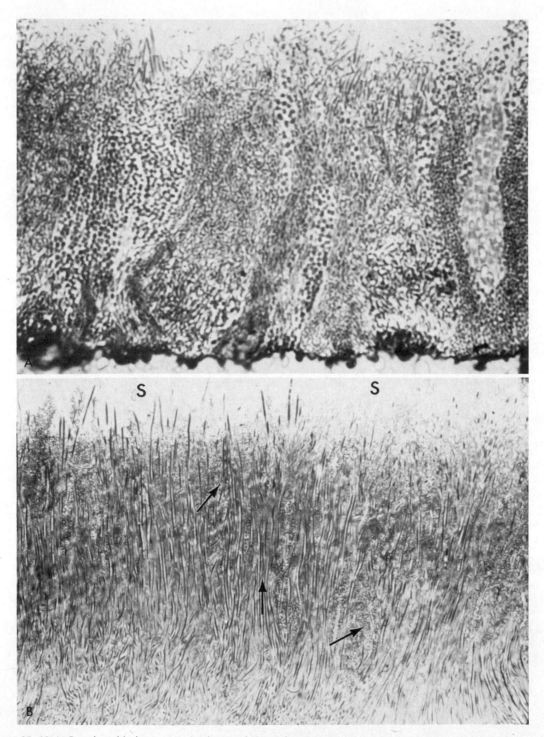

Figure 25–18 *A,* One-day-old plaque. Microcolonies of plaque bacteria extend perpendicularly away from tooth surfaces. (From Listgarten, M.: J. Periodontol., *46:*10, 1975.) *B,* Developed supragingival plaque showing overall filamentous nature and microcolonies *(arrows)* extending perpendicularly away from tooth surface. Saliva-plaque interface shown (S). (Courtesy of Dr. Max Listgarten.)

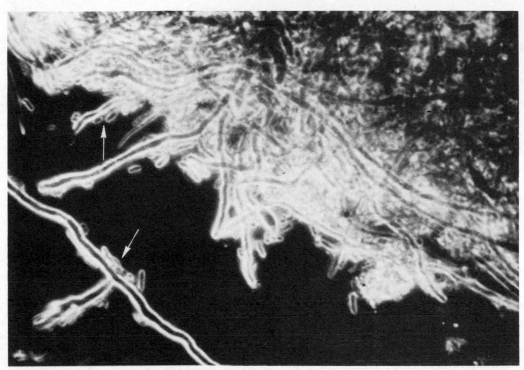

Figure 25–19 Darkfield photomicrograph demonstrates filamentous nature of plaque associated with gingivitis. Note attachment of smaller bacteria to filaments *(arrows)*

the pellicle. *Streptococcus sanguis* and gram-positive rods have been shown to be the major bacteria which initiate supragingival plaque.[30]

Once supragingival plaque is initiated, secondary growth and maturation take place. During this phase, bacterial population shifts occur *(bacterial succession)*. Filamentous organisms and gram-negative bacteria increase in proportion. In general, this plaque appears more compact (Fig. 25–19). Bacterial cohesive interactions are also more evident (Fig. 25–20) (Table 25–8).

The microorganisms commonly encountered in such sites in adults include *S. mitis, S. sanguis, Staphylococcus epidermidis, Rothia dentocariosa, Actinomyces viscosus, A. naeslundii,* and occasionally species of *Neisseria* and *Veillonella*.[80, 118, 128] This list is not meant to exclude other forms, which can frequently be detected, but to indicate the organisms most likely to be encountered.

Gingival Sulcus Bacteria and Periodontal Health

To date there have been few technically acceptable studies which have specifically documented the nature of the sulcular microbial flora associated with periodontal health. In general terms, the healthy periodontal tissues of humans appear to be associated with a minimal microbial flora, both supragingivally and subgingivally. Depending on the methods used for sampling and cultivating these flora, certain patterns have emerged.[81, 108, 119]

Subgingivally, the nature of the microbiota apparently conforms to the architectural arrangement previously described. Electron microscopic studies of in situ plaque located near the marginal gingiva and in the gingival crevice area at healthy sites have revealed a relatively thin layer (less than 60 microns) of predominantly gram-positive coccoid cells. Cultural studies have shown a predominance of streptococci (mainly *S. sanguis*); *A. viscosus, A. naeslundii,* and *A. israelii* are frequently present, sometimes in relatively high numbers. Gram-negative organisms such as *Capnocytophaga, Bacteroides* species, *Campylobacter,* and *Fusobacterium* can be isolated. *Mycoplasma* colonizes the gingival sulcus regularly.[20] Very few motile forms and spirochetes are present in this relatively scanty microflora. There appears to be no marked difference in bacterial composition between the supragingival and subgingival microflora associated with healthy sites.

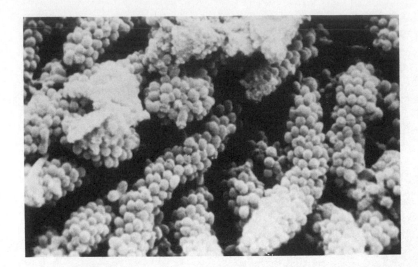

Figure 25–20 Long-standing supragingival plaque near the gingival margin demonstrates "corn cob" arrangement. Central gram-negative filamentous core (*Leptotrichia buccalis*). Coccal forms held in position by firm intercellular attachment (cohesion). (Courtesy of Dr. Z. Skobe.)

In the healthy host, bacteria colonize in a predictable sequence. As one group of bacteria colonizes, it alters the environment to allow new organisms to become established or to allow existing species to become dominant. Thus, supragingival plaque affects the establishment of the subgingival flora by lowering the oxidation reduction potential, providing essential growth factors, and altering the gingival tissues; these features in turn influence the numbers and types of subgingival microorganisms. In addition, the supragingival bacteria may provide sites of attachment for subgingival organisms.

Clinical studies indicate that supragingival plaque control in periodontally healthy persons appears to be sufficient to prevent the maturation of a simple, health-compatible plaque to a complex, disease-associated plaque.[4, 53] In patients with existing periodontal disease, the influence of supragingival microorganisms and plaque control (oral hygiene) procedures appears to be limited to approximately 4 mm into the pocket.

TABLE 25–8 COMMON MICROORGANISMS ISOLATED FROM THE HEALTHY AND THE DISEASED PERIODONTIUM

Health
  Streptococcus
  Actinomyces
  Capnocytophaga
  Veillonella

Gingivitis
  Actinomyces
  Bacteroides
  Fusobacterium
  Peptostreptococcus   } + Health
  Propionibacterium
  Streptococcus
  Veillonella
  Treponema

Pregnancy gingivitis
  Bacteroides melaninogenicus subspecies *intermedius*

Acute necrotizing ulcerative gingivitis
  Bacteroides melaninogenicus sp.
  Spirochetes

Periodontitis
  Eubacterium
  Eikenella
  Wolinella   } + Gingivitis
  Black-pigmented *Bacteroides*
  Selenomonas

Juvenile periodontitis
  Actinobacillus actinomycetemcomitans
  Capnocytophaga

Gingivitis

The initial development of gingivitis is thought to be a major consequence of the bacteria associated with an increase in supragingival plaque formation.[3, 58] The gram-positive filaments and rods, mainly *Actinomyces,* appear to be of major significance in this clinical condition. The sequence of development of supragingival plaque (discussed in an earlier section) is associated with an increase in absolute numbers and in percentages of *Actinomyces* species. The appearance of gram-negative forms, such as spirochetes, *Bacteroides, Fusobacterium,* vibrios, and other motile forms, in the late stages of the development of gingival redness (clinical inflammation) clearly indicates a sequential process in the development of gingivitis, since these organisms are associated with subgingival plaque. However, the initial insult to the periodontal structures in gingivitis may be associated with noxious elements of large masses of the gram-positive bacteria from supragingival plaque. In the early stages of gingivitis, edematous changes in the marginal gingiva may contribute to the successional acquisition of pathogenic subgingival species. This may be accomplished by an anatomic increase in the subgingival compartment (gingival swelling), providing mechanical retention and nutrients via the increase in gingival fluid.

It has been suggested by many investigators that repeated episodes of gingivitis can lead to periodontal bone loss (periodontitis). This fact is a generally accepted clinical observation (see Chapter 15). It stems from many epidemiologic studies which have demonstrated that the continued presence of bacterial plaque is associated with alveolar bone loss. *However, it is quite clear that some individuals may have recurrent episodes of gingivitis without developing periodontitis.* It is not clear whether the microbiota in these individuals is different from that in those who develop gingivitis and, subsequently, periodontitis. Gingivitis alone is reversible when plaque is removed.[3, 4, 58, 67]

Recently the epithelial invasion of gram-positive and gram-negative bacteria was reported in some cases of advanced gingivitis.[21] It is possible that this finding may have pinpointed the initiating event responsible for the progression of gingivitis to periodontitis.

PREGNANCY GINGIVITIS. The microbiota associated with pregnancy gingivitis has recently been described. Anaerobic *Bacteroides melaninogenicus subspecies intermedius* and *Capnocytophaga* were found in high concentrations. This proliferation may be due to a direct stimulating effect of increased hormone levels in saliva and sulcular fluid.[46]

ACUTE NECROTIZING ULCERATIVE GINGIVITIS. The microbiota associated with acute necrotizing ulcerative gingivitis has been described in Chapter 11.

Periodontitis

There are limited data which suggest that specific organisms, or groups of organisms, are associated with different forms of human periodontal diseases. This is especially evident when one considers the microbiota associated with periodontitis. There are important observations which demonstrate that trends or patterns of bacterial colonization in periodontal

pockets actually exist. The exact nature of this microbiota depends on the state of periodontal destruction, disease activity, and host resistance. Whether the lesion is associated with chronic disease or with a more rapid form of periodontal destruction is an important consideration.[109, 110, 130]

In the most common chronic forms of periodontitis, there is a large component of attached subgingival plaque. Filamentous organisms such as *Actinomyces israelii, A. naeslundii,* and *A. viscosus* are numerous[16] (Table 25–8). These organisms may constitute 30 to 40 per cent of the bacteria present. In almost all cases this attached plaque is associated with varying degrees of calculus formation.[105] *A. naeslundii* and *A. israelii* demonstrate a characteristic pathogenicity when implanted as monocontaminants in germ-free rats[36, 114] (see Fig. 25–15). These organisms form large accumulations of bacterial plaque and cause root caries. Alveolar bone loss appears to be associated with a suppression of osteoblasts.

The unattached component of the subgingival plaque in chronic periodontitis has not been adequately studied. However, electron microscopic observations suggest that this zone contains numerous gram-negative rods and spirochetes. Limited information from cultural studies also suggests that *B. melaninogenicus, Fusobacterium, Capnocytophaga, Campylobacter,* and *Selenomonas* species are present in various concentrations.

In rapidly destructive forms of periodontitis, the unattached component of the pocket flora predominates at the apical portion of the periodontal pocket[82] (Fig. 25–21). The microbiota associated with this rapidly progressing periodontitis is characterized by gram-negative microorganisms, including *Bacteroides gingivalis, B. melaninogenicus, Wolinella recta, Hemophilus,* and spirochetes. In addition, *Capnocytophaga* organisms and *Selenomonas sputigena* are found in periodontitis lesions.[15] When some organisms from this zone of the subgingival microbiota are implanted into germ-free animals as monocontaminants, they are extremely periodontopathic. However, the resultant destruction in these animals differs markedly from that observed when gram-positive organisms are established. Infection with these gram-negative organisms results in rapid alveolar bone destruction, a lack of large bacterial masses, no root caries, and a stimulation of osteoclastic activity.[30, 41, 42] Thus, it appears that the virulence of these organisms in experimental animals is of a higher order than that

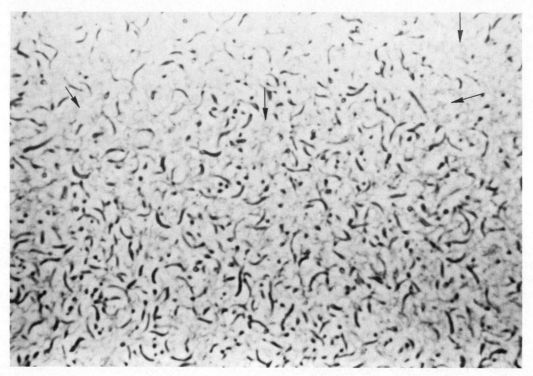

Figure 25–21 Histologic section of unattached plaque from a patient with a rapidly destructive form of periodontitis. Arrows indicate spirochetes forming a light-staining background. Vibrio and spiral-shaped organisms (*Selenomonas*) predominate. (From Listgarten, M., et al.: J. Periodontol., *47*:1, 1976.)

of the gram-positive organisms associated with the attached component of subgingival plaque from chronic periodontitis. It has been suggested that if infection with gram-negative organisms is superimposed upon that produced by gram-positive organisms, the rate of tissue destruction is accelerated.[28, 29] The findings of higher proportions of gram-negative anaerobic organisms in the depths of pockets in rapidly progressing periodontitis substantiate this suggestion. These organisms may accelerate the rate of destruction because of their elaboration of endotoxins and their ability to invade the adjacent gingival tissue.

Localized Juvenile Periodontitis

Since localized juvenile periodontitis (LJP) can be sharply defined, it may be considered a good model in which exacerbation and bone destruction can be accurately predicted and studied.[52, 129] (See Chapter 22 for a complete discussion of the clinical symptomatology of this type of periodontal disease.)

Although many details describing the microbiota of LJP lesions have not been clarified, a number of observations seem consistent (Table 25–9). The number of organisms in LJP lesions is less than in most forms of destructive periodontal disease, ranging from 10^5 to 10^6 bacteria per pocket. This may be one to three orders of magnitude lower than counts of organisms in adult periodontitis pockets of similar depth and with comparable bone loss.

The predominant cultivable microbiota of the LJP lesion is dominated by gram-negative rods.[74–77, 80, 83, 99, 107] Most of the isolates from such lesions have been saccharolytic and capnophilic, as well as anaerobic.

At present, three groups of organisms appear to be most frequently encountered in lesions of LJP patients. One group, which initially received considerable attention, con-

TABLE 25–9 MICROBIOLOGIC FEATURES ASSOCIATED WITH LOCALIZED JUVENILE PERIODONTITIS

Fewer bacteria (gram-negative rods)
Major proportion of subgingival plaque loosely adherent to tooth surface
Bacterial invasion demonstrated
Pathogenic potential in animal models
Immunologic response
Antibacterial treatment

sists of fusiform-shaped, capnophilic rods which have the ability to glide on agar surfaces. Members of this group had been called *Bacteroides ochraceus*, but now are designated by the genus name *Capnocytophaga*.[21, 25, 26] These organisms are not anaerobic (as originally described by Newman et al.[75, 80]) but require increased carbon dioxide tension for their growth; they are referred to as capnophilic ("carbon dioxide loving").

Some strains of *Capnocytophaga* produce a substance which inhibits the proliferation of human fibroblasts. In addition, these bacteria may cause distinctive abnormalities in host white blood cells.

A second group of capnophilic, gram-negative rods frequently isolated from LJP lesions includes the species *Actinobacillus actinomycetemcomitans*. Strains of this species produce a protein exotoxin capable of destroying polymorphonuclear leukocytes and gingival fibroblasts, and its endotoxin appears to be a potent stimulator of bone resorption, macrophage cytotoxicity, and platelet aggregation.[5] Both the exotoxin and the endotoxin may be associated with membrane vesicles shed during the growth of these organisms.

The exact role that *A. actinomycetemcomitans* plays in the pathogenesis of this disease is under intensive investigation and is one of the most exciting avenues of research concerning this disease entity. Serologic studies have demonstrated a significant host response to *Actinobacillus* in LJP patients.

A third group of organisms frequently encountered appear to fit descriptions of the species *Eubacterium saburreum*. This species is gram positive in very young cultures and gram negative in older preparations; cells are long, blunt-ended rods which often produce filaments.

The three groups of organisms briefly discussed above are by no means solely confined to LJP lesions. However, their frequency of isolation and their proportions when isolated are clearly much higher in these lesions than in lesions of adult destructive diseases or in healthy sites of adult patients or age-matched control subjects.

The pathogenic potential of *Capnocytophaga* and *Actinobacillus* isolated from juvenile periodontitis lesions has been demonstrated in germ-free rats[15, 41, 80, 112] (see Fig. 25–15). The destruction caused by monoinfection with individual organisms results in minimal plaque formation, no root caries, extensive loss of alveolar bone, and a marked osteoclastic response.

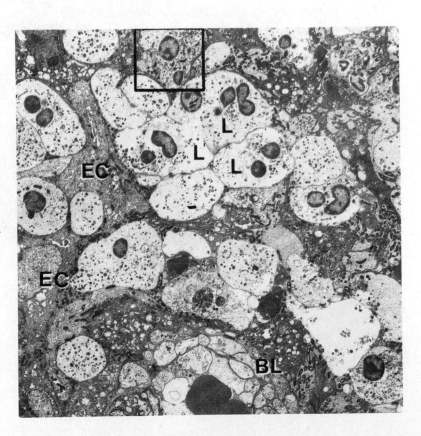

Figure 25–22 Interface between pocket epithelium and connective tissue separated by the basement lamina (BL). Abundant bacteria can be seen in the intercellular spaces. Numerous infiltrating polymorphonuclear leukocytes (L) are seen between epithelial cells (EC). Some of the leukocytes show engulfed bacteria. × 3908.

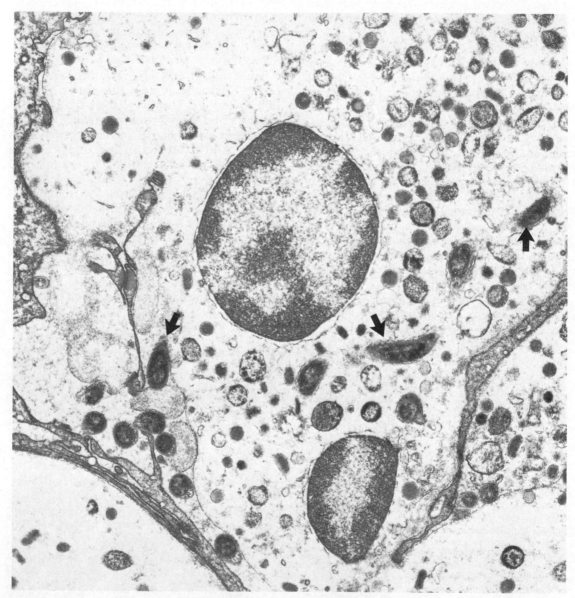

Figure 25–23 Higher magnification of a polymorphonuclear leukocyte in Figure 25–22 with engulfed bacteria *(arrows).* × 15,000.

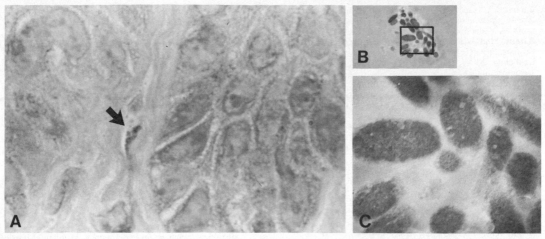

Figure 25–24 *A,* Gingival tissue of a patient with localized juvenile periodontitis showing granular positive (dark gray) staining, in the connective tissue, for *Actinobacillus actinomycetemcomitans (arrow).* Formalin paraffin section, peroxidase-antiperoxidase method, anti–*Actinobacillus actinomycetemcomitans,* counterstained with hematoxylin. × 1200. *B,* Electron micrograph of same paraffin section showing the area indicated by the arrow in part *A* which was re-embedded in plastic (modified "pop off" technique). × 40,000. *C,* Higher magnification of the rectangle in part *B* showing the short coccobacillary rod with approximately the size and shape of *A. actinomycetemcomitans.* × 80,000.

The bone destruction occurs rapidly and differs from that seen when gram-positive organisms are implanted as monocontaminants. Irving et al. described superficial penetration of *Capnocytophaga* in the lesions of monoinfected germ-free rats.[39–42]

Anatomic studies of the subgingival microbiota in LJP lesions by Listgarten et al. revealed that the majority of the subgingival bacteria are loosely adherent to the tooth surface.[56, 57] Electron microscopically, many of those microorganisms were shown to be gram negative (see Fig. 25–24). Allen and Brady found rod-shaped microorganisms which were continuously present along the entire cemental surface of extracted LJP-involved teeth.[1] Bacterial penetration of the gingival epithelium and connective tissue by several types of microorganisms has also been documented[12, 31] (Figs. 25–22 and 25–23), and the following organisms have been identified within the periodontal epithelium and connective tissues: spirochetes, gram-negative fusiform rods, *Mycoplasma,* and *A. actinomycetemcomitans*[12, 96] (Figs. 25–24 and 25–25).

The cultural and anatomic association of microorganisms with LJP lesions provide the basis for research which may clarify the exact role of these bacteria. Such observations are prerequisite to a more accurate assessment of the response (or failure to respond) of the host to potentially pathogenic bacteria and/or their products.

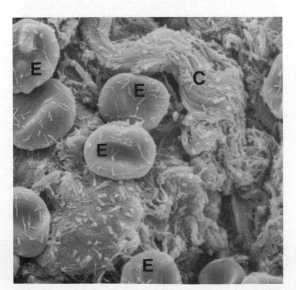

Figure 25–25 Invasive mycoplasma on top of extravascular erythrocytes (E). C, collagen fibers. × 8000.

REFERENCES

1. Allen, A. L., and Brady, J. M.: Periodontosis: a case report with scanning electron microscopic observations. J. Periodontol., *49*:415, 1978.
2. Allenspach-Petrzilka, G. E., and Guggenheim, B.: *Bacteroides melaninogenicus* subsp. *intermedius* invades rat gingival tissue. J. Dent. Res. *61*, I.A.D.R. Abstracts 728, 1982.
3. Arno, A., Waerhaug, J., Lovdahl, A., and Schei, O.: Incidence of gingivitis as related to sex, occupation, tobacco consumption, tooth-brushing and age. Oral Surg., *11*:587, 1958.
4. Axelsson, P., and Lindhe, J.: The effect of a preventive programme on dental plaque, gingivitis and caries in school children. Results after one and two years. J. Clin. Periodontol., *1*:126, 1974.

5. Baehni, P., Tsai, C. C., Taichman, N. S., and Mc Arthur, W.: Interaction of inflammatory cells and oral microorganisms. J. Periodont. Res., *13*:333, 1978.
6. Barrett, M. T.: Clinical report upon amoebic pyorrea. Dent. Cosmos, *56*:1345, 1914.
7. Behbehani, M. J., and Jordan, H. V.: Comparative colonization of human *Actinomyces* species in hamsters under different dietary conditions. J. Periodont. Res., *15*:395, 1980.
8. Berthold, P., Lai, C. H., and Listgarten, M. A.: Immunoelectron microscopic studies of *Actinomyces viscosus*. J. Periodont. Res., *17*:26, 1982.
9. Bowen, W.: Nature of plaque. Oral Sci. Rev., *9*:3, 1976.
10. Brecx, M., Ronstrom, A., Theilade, J., and Attstrom, R.: Early formation of dental plaque on plastic films. J. Periodont. Res., *16*:213, 1981.
11. Burnett, G. W., and Scherp, H. W.: Oral Microbiology and Infectious Diseases. Third ed. Baltimore, Williams & Wilkins Company, 1968.
12. Carranza, F. A., Jr., Saglie, R., Newman, M. G., and Valentin, P.: Scanning and transmission electron microscopic study of tissue-invading microorganisms in localized juvenile periodontitis. J. Periodontol., 1983, in press.
13. Courant, P. R., Paunio, I., and Gibbons, R. J.: Infectivity and hyaluronidase activity of debris from healthy and diseased gingiva. Arch. Oral Biol., *10*:119, 1965.
14. Cowley, G.: Effect of plaque on gingival epithelium. Oral Sci. Rev., *1*:103, 1972.
15. Crawford, A., Socransky, S. S., and Bratthall, G.: Predominant cultivable microbiota of advanced periodontitis. J. Dent. Res., *54*:209, 1975.
16. Darwish, S., Hyppa, T., and Socransky, S. S.: Studies of the predominant cultivable microbiota of early periodontitis. J. Periodont. Res., *13*:1, 1978.
17. Dewar, M. R.: Bacterial enzymes and periodontal disease. J. Dent. Res., *37*:100, 1958.
18. Dick, D. S., and Shaw, J. H.: The infectious and transmissible nature of the periodontal syndrome of the rice rat. Arch. Oral Biol., *11*:1095, 1966.
19. Ellen, R. P., and Balcerzak-Raczkowski, T. B.: Interbacterial aggregation of *Actinomyces naeslundii* and dental plaque streptococci. J. Periodont. Res., *12*:11, 1977.
20. Engee, M.: *Mycoplasma salivarium* in human gingival sulcus. J. Periodont. Res., *5*:163, 1970.
21. Fillery, E. D., and Pekovic, D. D.: Identification of microorganisms in immunopathological mechanisms on human gingivitis. J. Dent. Res., *61*:253, 1982.
22. Fine, D. H., Tabak, L., Oshrain, H., Salkind, A., and Siegel, K.: Studies in plaque pathogenicity. I. Plaque collection and limulus lysate screening of adherent and loosely adherent plaque. J. Periodont. Res., *13*:17, 1978.
23. Finegold, S.: Anaerobic Bacteria in Human Disease. New York, Academic Press, 1977.
24. Forlenza, S., Blachman, V., Newman, M. G.: *Capnocytophaga* sepsis in granulocytopenic patients. Lancet, March 15, 1980.
25. Frank, R. M.: Bacterial penetration in the apical pocket wall of advanced human periodontitis. J. Periodont. Res., *15*:563, 1980.
26. Fritzell, K. E.: Infections of hand due to human mouth organisms. Lancet, *60*:135, 1940.
27. Garant, P. R.: An electron microscopic study of the periodontal tissues of germ-free rats and rats monoinfected with *Actinomyces naeslundii*. J. Periodont. Res., *15*(Suppl.):1, 1976.
28. Gibbons, R. J.: Studies of the predominant cultivable microbiota of dental plaque. Arch. Oral Biol., *8*:281, 1963.
29. Gibbons, R. J., and Macdonald, J. B.: Degradation of collagenous substrates by *Bacteroides melaninogenicus*. J. Bacteriol., *81*:614, 1961.
30. Gibbons, R. J., and Van Houte, J.: Microbiology of periodontal disease. *In* Shaw, J. H., et al.: Textbook of Oral Biology. Philadelphia, W. B. Saunders Company, 1978.
31. Gillett, R., and Johnson, N. W.: Bacterial invasion of the periodontium in a case of juvenile periodontitis. J. Clin. Periodontol., *9*:93, 1982.
32. Gottlieb, D. S., and Miller, L. H.: Entamoeba gingivitis in periodontal disease. J. Periodontol., *42*:412, 1971.
33. Griffiths, G. S., and Addy, M.: Effects of malalignment of teeth in the anterior segments on plaque accumulation. J. Clin. Periodontol., *8*:481, 1981.
34. Hampp, E. G., Mergenhagen, S. E., and Omata, R. R.: Studies of mucopolysaccharase activity on oral spirochetes, J. Dent. Res., *38*:979, 1959.
35. Hardie, J.: Normal microbial flora of mouth. Soc. Appl. Bacteriol. Symp. Ser., *3*:47, 1974.
36. Van Palestein Halderman, W. H.: Microbial etiology of periodontal disease. J. Clin. Periodontol., *8*:261, 1981.
37. Horton, J. E., Oppenheim, J. J., and Mergenhagen, S. E.: Elaboration of lymphotoxin by cultured human peripheral blood leukocytes stimulated with dental plaque deposits. Clin. Exp. Immunol., *13*:383, 1973.
38. Hunter, N., Schwab, J. H., and Simpson, D. M.: Experimental periodontitis induced in rats by streptococcal cell wall fragments. J. Periodont. Res., *14*:453, 1979.
39. Irving, J. T., Socransky, S. S., and Heeley, J. D.: Histological changes in experimental periodontal disease in gnotobiotic rats and conventional hamsters. J. Periodont. Res., *9*:73, 1974.
40. Irving, J. T., Socransky, S. S., and Tanner, A. C. R.: Histological changes in experimental periodontal disease in rats monoinfected with gram-negative organisms. J. Periodont. Res., *13*:326, 1978.
41. Irving J. T., Newman, M. G., Socransky, S. S., and Heeley, J. D.: Histological changes in experimental periodontal disease in rats monoinfected with gram negative organism. Arch. Oral Biol., *20*:219, 1975.
42. Irving, J. T., Socransky, S. S., Newman, M. G., and Savitt, E.: Periodontal destruction induced by *Capnocytophaga* in gnotobiotic rats. J. Dent. Res., *55*:B257, 1976 (abstract).
43. Ivanyi, L., and Lehner, T.: Stimulation of lymphocyte transformation by bacterial antigen in patients with periodontal disease. Arch. Oral Biol., *15*:1089, 1970.
44. Kaplan, G. B., Ruben, M. P., and Pameijer, C. H.: Scanning electron microscopy of the epithelium of the periodontal pocket. Part II. J. Periodontol., *48*:634, 1977.
45. Keyes, P. H., and Jordan, H. V.: Periodontal lesions in the Syrian hamster. III. Findings related to an infectious and transmissible component. Arch. Oral Biol., *9*:377, 1964.
46. Kornman, K. S., and Loesche, W. J.: The subgingival microbial flora during pregnancy. J. Periodont. Res., *15*:111, 1980.
47. Kornman, K. S., Holt, S. C., and Robertson, P. B.: The microbiology of ligature induced periodontitis in the cytomolgus monkey. J. Periodont. Res., *16*:371, 1981.
48. Lang, N. P., and Smith, F. N.: Lymphocyte blastogenesis to plaque antigens in human periodontal disease. I. Populations of varying severity of disease. J. Periodont. Res., *12*:298, 1977.
49. Leadbetter, E. R., and Holt, S. A.: Influence of sonication on cultivable microbiota of dental plaque. J. Dent. Res., *53*:208, 1974.
50. Lehner, T., and Clarry, E. D.: Acute ulcerative gingivitis, an immunofluorescent investigation. Br. Dent. J., *120*:366, 1966.
51. Lie, T.: Early dental plaque morphogenesis, J. Periodont. Res., *12*:73, 1977.
52. Liljenberg, B., and Lindhe, J.: Juvenile periodontitis. J. Clin. Res., *7*:48, 1980.
53. Lindhe, J., and Nyman, S.: The effect of plaque control and surgical pocket elimination on the establishment and maintenance of periodontal health. A longitudinal study of periodontal therapy in cases of advanced periodontitis. J. Clin. Periodontol., *2*:67, 1975.
54. Lindhe, J., and Socransky, S. S.: Chemotaxis and vascular permeability produced by human periodontopathic bacteria. J. Periodont. Res., *4*:138, 1979.
55. Listgarten, M. A.: Structure of the microbial flora associated with periodontal disease and health in man. A light and electron microscopic study. J. Periodontol., *47*:1, 1976.
56. Listgarten, M. A.: Structure of surface coatings on teeth. A review. J. Periodontol., *47*:139, 1976.
57. Listgarten, M. A., Mayo, H. E., and Tremblay, R.: Development of dental plaque on epoxy resin crowns in man. A light and electron microscopic study. J. Periodontol., *46*:10, 1975.
58. Löe, H. E., Theilade, E., and Jensen, S. B.: Experimental gingivitis in man. J. Periodontol., *36*:177, 1965.

59. Löe, H. E., Theilade, E., Jensen, S. B., and Schiott, C.: Experimental gingivitis in man. III. The influence of antibiotics on gingival plaque development. J. Periodont. Res., 2:282, 1967.

60. Loesche, W.: Oxygen sensitivity of various anaerobic bacteria. Appl. Microbiol., 18:723, 1969.

61. Loesche, W.: Chemotherapy of dental plaque infections. Oral Sci. Rev., 9:65, 1976.

61a. Mandel, I. D.: Plaque and calculus. J. Med. Sci., 5:313, 1968.

62. Manganiello, A. D., Socransky, S. S., Smith, C., Propas, D., Oram, V., and Dogan, I. L.: Attempts to increase viable count recovery of human supragingival dental plaque. J. Periodont. Res., 12:107, 1977.

63. McMaster, P. E.: Human bite infection. Am. J. Surg., 45:60, 1939.

64. Mims, C.: The pathogenesis of infectious disease. 2nd ed. New York, Academic Press, 1982.

65. Mousquès, T., Listgarten, M. A., and Phillips, R. W.: Effect of scaling and root planing on the composition of the human subgingival microbial flora. J. Periodont. Res., 15:144, 1980.

66. Mousquès, T., Listgarten, M. A., and Stoller, N. H.: Effect of sampling on the composition of the human subgingival microbial flora. J. Periodont. Res., 15:137, 1980.

67. Nayak, R. P., and Wade, A. B.: The relative effectiveness of plaque removal by the Proxabrush and rubber cone stimulator. J. Clin. Periodontol., 4:128, 1977.

68. Newman, H. N.: The approximal apical border of plaque on children's teeth. I. Morphology, structure and cell content. J. Periodontol., 50:561, 1979.

69. Newman, H. N.: The approximal apical border of plaque on children's teeth. II. Adhesion, interbacterial connections and carbohydrate metabolism. J. Periodontol., 50:568, 1979.

70. Newman, H. N.: Neutrophils and IgG at the host-plaque interface on children's teeth. J. Periodontol., 51:642, 1980.

71. Newman, H. N.: Update on plaque and periodontal disease. J. Clin. Periodontol., 7:251, 1980.

72. Newman, H. N.: Calcium, matrix polymers and plaque formation. J. Periodontol., 53:101, 1982.

73. Newman, H. N., Seymour, G. J., and Challacombe, S. J.: Immunoglobulins in human dental plaque. J. Periodont. Res., 14:1, 1979.

74. Newman, M. G.: Periodontosis. J. West. Soc. Periodontol., 24:5, 1976.

75. Newman, M. G., and Socransky, S. S.: Predominant cultivable microbiota in periodontosis. J. Periodont. Res., 12:120, 1977.

76. Newman, M. G., Socransky, S. S., and Listgarten, M. A.: Relationship of microorganisms to the etiology of periodontosis. J. Dent. Res., 53:290, 1974.

77. Newman, M. G., Williams, R. C., and Crawford, A.: Predominant cultivable microbiota of periodontosis. III. J. Dent. Res., 54:211, 1975.

78. Newman, M. G., Saglie, R., Carranza, F. A., Jr., and Kaufman, A. K.: *Mycoplasma* in periodontal disease. J. Periodontol., in press.

79. Newman, M. G., Sandler, M., Ormerod, W., Angel, L., and Goldhaber, P.: The effect of dietary gantrisin supplements on the flora of periodontal pockets in four Beagle dogs. J. Periodont. Res., 12:129, 1977.

80. Newman, M. G., Socransky, S. S., Savitt, E. D., Propas, D. A., and Crawford, A.: Studies of the microbiology of periodontosis. J. Periodontol., 47:373, 1976.

81. Newman, M. G., Weiner, M. S., Angel, I., Grinenko, V., and Karge, H. J.: Predominant cultivable microbiota of the gingival crevice in "supernormal" patients. J. Dent. Res., 56:277, 1977.

82. Newman, M. G., Angel, I., Karge, H., Weiner, M., Grinenko, V., and Schusterman, L.: Bacterial studies of Papillon-Lefèvre syndrome. J. Dent. Res., 56:220, 1977.

83. Newman, M. G., Socransky, S. S., Savitt, E., Krichevsky, M., Listgarten, M., and Lai, W.: Characterization of bacteria isolated from periodontosis. J. Dent. Res., 53:325, 1974.

84. Okuda, K., and Takazoe, I.: Activation of complement by dental plaque. J. Periodont. Res., 15:23, 1980.

85. Osterberg, S. K. A., Sudo, S. Z., and Folke, L. E. A.: Microbial succession in subgingival plaque of man. J. Periodont. Res., 11:243, 1976.

86. Page, R. C.: Dental deposits. In Schluger, S., Youdelis, R., and Page, R. (eds.): Periodontal Disease. Philadelphia, Lea & Febiger, 1977.

87. Passo, S. A., Tsai, C. C., McArthur, W. P., Leifer, C., and Taichman, N. S.: Interaction of inflammatory cells and oral microorganisms. J. Periodont. Res., 15:470, 1980.

88. Patters, M. R., Landesburg, R. L., Johansson, L. A., Trummel, C. L., and Robertson, P. B.: *Bacteroides gingivalis* antigens and bone resorbing activity in root surface fractions of periodontally involved teeth. J. Periodont. Res., 17:122, 1982.

89. Ranney, R. R.: Immunofluorescent localization of soluble dental plaque components in human gingiva affected by periodontitis. J. Periodont. Res., 13:99, 1978.

90. Ritz, H. L.: Microbial population shifts in developing human dental plaque. Arch. Oral Biol., 12:1561, 1967.

91. Rizzo, A. A.: The possible role of hydrogen sulfide in human periodontal disease. I. Hydrogen sulfide production in periodontal pockets. Periodontics, 5:233, 1967.

92. Robrish, S. A., Grove, S. B., Bernstein, R., and Amdur, B.: Differential breakage plaque dispersion. J. Dent. Res., 54:236, 1975.

93. Saglie, R.: A scanning electron microscopic study of the relationship between the most apically localized subgingival plaque and the epithelial attachment. J. Periodontol., 42:105, 1977.

94. Saglie, R., Newman, M. G., and Carranza, F. A., Jr.: A scanning electron microscopic study of leukocytes and their interaction with bacteria in human periodontitis. J. Periodontol., 53:752, 1982.

95. Saglie, R., Carranza, F. A., Jr., Newman, M. G., and Pattison, G. A.: Scanning electron microscopy of the gingival wall of deep periodontal pockets in humans. J. Periodont. Res., 17:284, 1982.

96. Saglie, R., Carranza, F. A., Jr., Newman, M. G., and Pattison, G. A.: Immunochemical localization of *Actinobacillus actinomycetemcomitans* in sections of gingival tissue in localized juvenile periodontitis. In preparation.

97. Saglie, R., Newman, M. G., Carranza, F. A., Jr., and Pattison, G. A.: Bacterial invasion of gingiva in advanced periodontitis in humans. J. Periodontol., 53:217, 1982.

98. Saglie, R., Carranza, F. A., Jr., Newman, M. G., Cheng, L., and Lewin, K. J.: Identification of tissue-invading bacteria in human periodontal disease. J. Periodont. Res., 17:452, 1982.

99. Savitt, E. D., Socransky, S. S., Hammond, B. F., and Newman, M. G.: Characterization of fusiform organisms isolated from periodontosis. J. Dent. Res., 54:208, 1975.

100. Schultz-Haudt, S., and Scherp, H. W.: Lysis of collagen by human gingival bacteria. Proc. Soc. Exp. Biol. Med., 89:697, 1955.

101. Schultz-Haudt, S., and Scherp, H. W.: Production of chondrosulfatase by microorganisms isolated from human gingival crevices. J. Dent. Res., 35:299, 1956.

102. Schultz-Haudt, S., Bibby, B. G., and Bruce, M. A.: Tissue destructive products of gingival bacteria from non-specific gingivitis. J. Dent. Res., 33:624, 1954.

103 Schuster, G. S., Hayashi, J. A., and Bahn, A. N.: Toxic properties of the cell wall of gram positive bacteria. J. Bacteriol., 93:47, 1967.

104. Shapiro, L., et al.: Endotoxin determinations in gingival inflammation. J. Periodontol., 43:591, 1972.

105. Sidaway, D. A.: A microbiological study of dental calculus. J. Periodont. Res., 15:240, 1980.

106. Silver, J. G., Martin, A. W., and McBride, B. C.: Experimental transient bacteraemias in human subjects with varying degrees of plaque accumulation and gingival inflammation. J. Clin. Periodontol., 4:92, 1977.

107. Slots, J.: The predominant cultivable organisms in juvenile periodontitis. Scand. J. Dent. Res., 84:1, 1976.

108. Slots, J.: The microflora in the healthy gingival sulcus in man. Scand. J. Dent. Res., 85:247, 1977.

109. Slots, J.: The predominant cultivable microflora of advanced periodontitis. Scand. J. Dent. Res., 85:114, 1977.

110. Slots, J.: Subgingival microflora and periodontal disease. J. Clin. Periodontol., 6:351, 1979.

111. Socransky, S. S.: The relationship of bacteria to the etiology of periodontal disease. J. Dent. Res., 49:2, 203, 1970.

112. Socransky, S. S.: Microbiology of periodontal disease. Present status and future considerations. J. Periodontol., *48*:497, 1977.
113. Socransky, S. S., and Manganiello, A. D.: The oral microbiota of man from birth to senility. J. Periodontol., *42*:485, 1971.
114. Socransky, S. S., Hubersak, C., and Propas, D.: Induction of periodontal destruction in gnotobiotic rats by a human oral strain of *Actinomyces naeslundii.* Arch. Oral Biol., *15*:993, 1970.
115. Socransky, S. S., Hubersak, C., Propas, D., and Rozanis, J.: "Pathogenic potential" of human gram positive rods for oral tissues. I.A.D.R. Abstracts, No. 151, 1970.
116. Socransky, S. S., Loesche, W. J., Hubersak, C., and Macdonald, J. B.: Dependency of *Treponema microdentium* on other oral organisms for isobutyrate, polyamines, and a controlled oxidation-reduction potential. J. Bacteriol., *88*:200, 1964.
117. Socransky, S. S., Listgarten, M. A., Hubersak, C., Cotmore, J., and Clark, A.: Morphological and biochemical differentiation of three types of small oral spirochetes, J. Bacteriol., *98*:878, 1969.
118. Socransky, S. S., Manganiello, A. D., Propas, D., Oram, V., and Van Houte, J.: Bacteriological studies of developing supragingival dental plaque. Periodont. Res., *12*:90, 1977.
119. Socransky, S. S., Gibbons, R. J., Dale, A. C., Bortnick, L., Rosenthal, E., and Macdonald, J.: The microbiota of the gingival crevice area of man. I. Total microscopic and viable count of specific organisms. Arch. Oral Biol., *8*:275, 1963.
120. Spiegel, C. A., Hayduk, S. E., Minah, G. E., and Krywolap, G. N.: Black-pigmented *Bacteroides* from clinically characterized periodontal sites. J. Periodont. Res., *14*:376, 1979.
121. Steenbergen, T. J. M. V., Kastelein, P., Touw, J. J. A., and de Graaff J.: Virulence of black-pigmented *Bacteroides* strains from periodontal pockets and other sites in experimentally induced skin lesions in mice. J. Periodont. Res., *17*:41, 1982.
122. Sundquist, G., Bloom, G. D., Kjell, E., and Johansson, E.: Phagocytosis of *Bacteroides melaninogenicus* and *Bacteroides gingivalis in vitro* by human neutrophils. J. Periodont. Res., *17*:113, 1982.
123. Svanberg, G. K., Syed, S. A., and Scott, B. W., Jr.: Differences between gingivitis and periodontitis associated microbial flora in the beagle dog. J. Periodont. Res., *17*:1, 1982.
124. Syed, S. A., Svanberg, M., and Svanberg, G.: The predominant cultivable dental plaque flora of beagle dogs with periodontitis. J. Clin. Periodontol., *8*:45, 1981.
125. Tanzer, J.: Microbiology section summary. Proceedings of the International Workshop in the Biology of Periodontal Disease. Chicago, University of Chicago Press, 1977.
126. Theilade, E., and Theilade, J.: Role of plaque in the etiology of periodontal disease and caries. Oral Sci. Rev., *9*:23, 1976.
127. Tsai, C. C., Hammond, B. F., Baehni, P., McArthur, W. C., and Taichman, N. S.: Interaction of inflammatory cells and oral microorganisms. VI. Exocytosis of PMN lysosomes in response to gram-negative plaque bacteria. J. Periodont. Res., *13*:504, 1978.
128. Van Palestein-Halderman, W. H.: Total viable count and differential count of *Vibrio (Campylobacter) sputorum, Fusobacterium nucleatum, Selenomonas sputigena, Bacteroides ochraceous* and *Veillonella* in the inflamed and non-inflamed human gingival crevice. J. Periodont. Res., *10*:294, 1976.
129. Waerhaug, J.: Subgingival plaque and loss of attachment in periodontosis as evaluated on extracted teeth. J. Periodontol., *48*:125, 1977.
130. Waerhaug, J.: The infrabony pocket and its relationship to trauma from occlusion and subgingival plaque. J. Periodontol., *50*:355, 1979.
131. Watanabe, S.: Possible role of mycoplasmas in periodontal disease. Bull. Tokyo Med. Dent. Univ., *19*:93, 1972.
132. Wennstrom, J., Heijl, L., Lindhe, J., and Socransky, S. S.: Migration of gingival leukocytes mediated by plaque bacteria. J. Periodont. Res., *15*:363, 1980.
133. Yoon, N., and Newman, M. G.: Antimicrobial effect of fluorides on *Bacteroides melaninogenicus* subspecies and *Bacteroides asaccharolyticus.* J. Clin. Periodontol., *7*:489, 1980.

chapter twenty-six

Calculus, Faulty Dentistry, and Other Local Factors in the Etiology of Periodontal Disease

The cause of gingival inflammation is bacterial plaque (see Chapter 25). Several factors previously considered to be of direct etiologic significance in periodontal disease now are known to act only by favoring plaque accumulation. These include calculus, faulty restorations and partial removable prostheses, food impaction, and other factors presented in this chapter.

This chapter also considers other factors (habits, toothbrush trauma, chemical irritation, and radiation) that will produce gingival inflammation and/or periodontal destruction by different mechanisms. It should be understood that they do not produce periodontal pockets or, therefore, so-called periodontitis unless they become complicated by bacterial plaque.

CALCULUS

Although acquired bacterial coatings have been demonstrated to be the major etiologic factor in periodontal disease, the presence of calculus is of great concern to the clinician.

The primary effect of calculus is not, as was originally thought, due to mechanical irritation, but to the fact that it is always covered by bacteria (Figs. 26–1 to 26–5). Experiments with germ-free animals have proved this point very clearly (see Chapter 25). However, these calcified deposits play a major role in maintaining and accentuating periodontal disease by keeping plaque in close contact with the gingival tissue and creating areas where plaque removal is impossible. When calculus is present, the gingival tissues are inflamed; when it is present in deep subgingival lesions, the potential for repair and reattachment is virtually nonexistent. Therefore, the clinician must be extremely competent in his or her ability to remove calculus and the necrotic cementum to which it attaches.

Supragingival and Subgingival Calculus

Calculus is an adherent calcified or calcifying mass that forms on the surface of natural teeth and dental prostheses (Plate V). Ordinarily calculus consists of mineralized bacterial plaque. It is classified according to its relation to the gingival margin as follows:

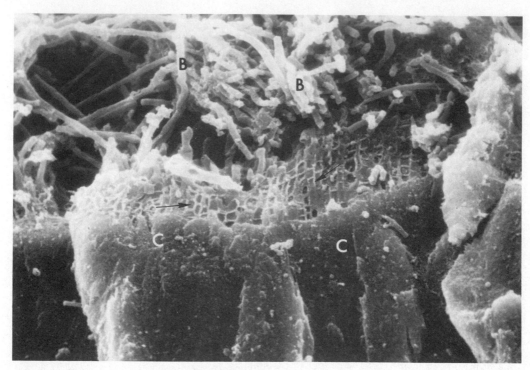

Figure 26–1 Attachment "spaces" (*arrows*) for subgingival bacteria (B) in pellicle-like substance on surface of cementum (C). (Courtesy of Dr. John Sottosanti.)

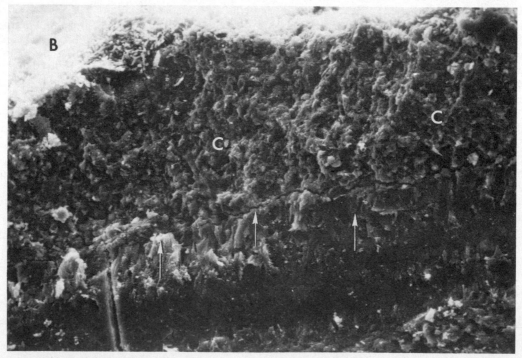

Figure 26–2 Subgingival calculus (C) attached to cementum surface (*arrows*). Adherent plaque bacteria on calculus surface (B). (Courtesy of Dr. John Sottosanti.)

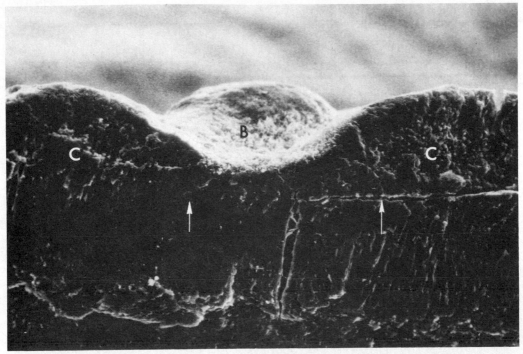

Figure 26–3 Subgingival calculus (C) attached to cementum surface (*arrows*). Adherent plaque bacteria (B) attached in depression on calculus surface. (Courtesy of Dr. John Sottosanti.)

Figure 26–4 Detailed Examination of Calculus showing an inner structure (C), filamentous organisms (F), other bacteria (B), and desquamated epithelial cells (E).

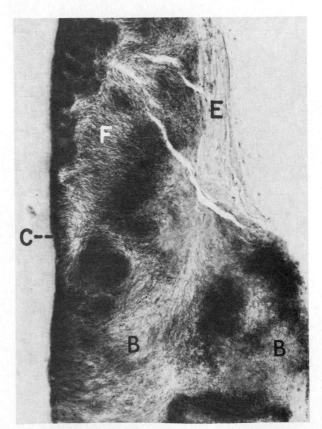

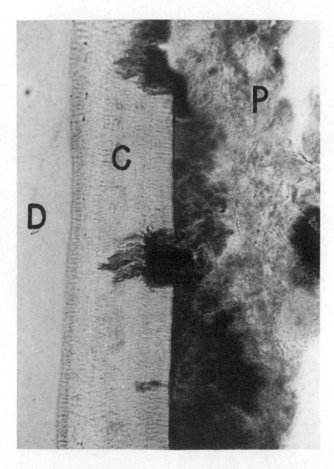

Figure 26–5 Calculus on Tooth Surface Embedded Within the Cementum (C). Note the early stage of penetration shown in the lower portion of the illustration. The dentin is at D. P, plaque attached to calculus.

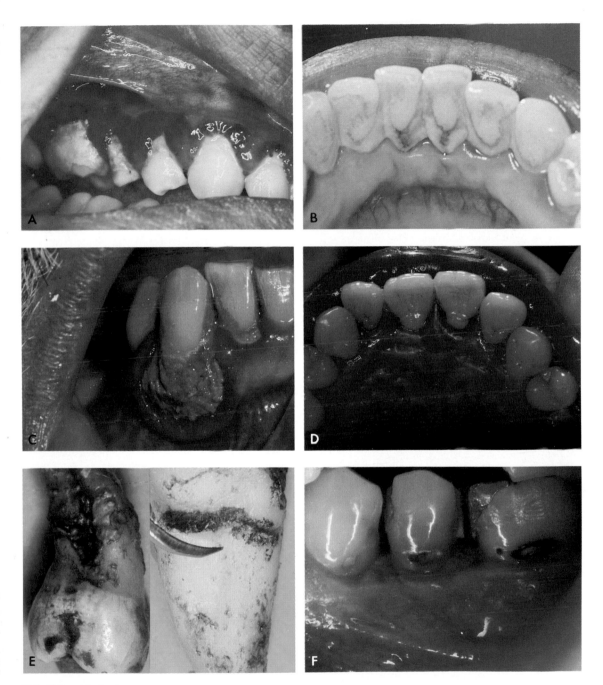

Plate V Local Irritants

A, Heavy calculus deposits on facial surfaces of upper first molar and second premolar. Note the severe gingival inflammation in the entire quadrant.

B, Calculus deposits on lingual surfaces of lower incisors forming a bridge over the interdental papillae. Gingival inflammation can also be seen.

C, Heavy calculus deposit on facial surface of lower cuspid with associated gingival recession.

D, Palatal view of upper anterior teeth with heavy calculus deposits, particularly in interdental spaces.

E, Different shapes of calculus on extracted teeth.

F, Overhanging margin of restoration and atrophied and inflamed gingival papilla.

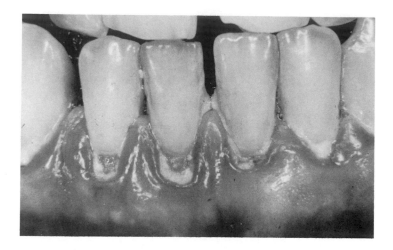

Figure 26–6 Supragingival Calculus.

Supragingival calculus (visible calculus) refers to calculus coronal to the crest of the gingival margin and visible in the oral cavity (Fig. 26–6). Supragingival calculus is usually white or whitish yellow, of hard, clay-like consistency, and easily detached from the tooth surface. Its recurrence after removal may be rapid, especially in the lingual area of the mandibular incisors. The color is affected by such factors as tobacco and food pigment. It may localize on a single tooth or a group of teeth or be generalized throughout the mouth. Supragingival calculus occurs most frequently and in greatest quantity on the buccal surfaces of the maxillary molars opposite Stensen's duct (Fig. 26–7) and on the lingual surfaces of the mandibular anterior teeth opposite Wharton's duct; it occurs more on the central incisors than on the lateral ones (Fig. 26–8). In extreme cases calculus may form a bridge-like structure along adjacent teeth (Fig. 26–9) or cover the occlusal surface of teeth without functional antagonists (Fig. 26–10).

Subgingival calculus refers to calculus below the crest of the marginal gingiva, usually in periodontal pockets, and is not visible upon usual oral examination. Determination of the location and extent of subgingival calculus requires careful examination with an explorer (Fig. 26–11). It is usually dense and hard, dark brown or greenish black, flint-like in consistency, and firmly attached to the tooth surface (Figs. 26–12 and 26–13). Supragingival calculus and subgingival calculus generally occur together, but one may be present without the other. Microscopic studies demonstrate that the deposits usually extend near but do not reach the base of periodontal pockets in chronic periodontal lesions.

Supragingival calculus has also been referred to as *salivary* and subgingival calculus as *serumal,* on the assumption that the former is derived from the saliva and the latter from the blood serum. This concept was overshadowed for a long time by the view that saliva was the sole source of all calculus. However, it is the current consensus that the minerals for the formation of supragingival calculus come from the saliva, whereas the gingival fluid, which resembles serum, is the main mineral source for subgingival calculus[23, 65]

When the gingival tissues recede, subgingival calculus becomes exposed and is classified as supragingival. Thus, supragingival calculus can be composed of both the supragingival and subgingival types.

Supragingival calculus and subgingival calculus usually appear in the early teens and increase with age.[19, 30, 49] The supragingival type is more common; subgingival calculus is uncommon in children, and supragingival calculus is uncommon up to the age of 9. The reported prevalence of both types of calculus at different ages varies considerably, according to the examination criteria of different investigators and in different population groups. In children between the ages of 9 and 15, supragingival calculus has been reported in from 37[14] to 70 per cent[28] of the individuals studied; in the 16 to 21 age group, it ranges from 44[56] to 88 per cent; and in those over 40, the figure is between 86 per cent[3] and 100 per cent. The prevalence of subgingival calculus is generally slightly lower than that of the supragingival type, but it appears in between 47 and 100 per cent of individuals after the age of 40.

Supragingival calculus and subgingival calculus are often seen in roentgenograms (see Chapter 32). Supragingivally, well-calcified deposits are readily detectable, forming irregular

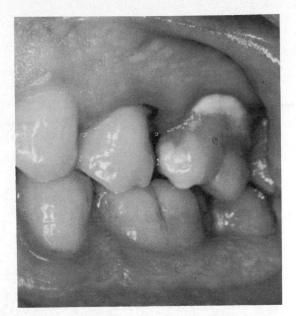

Figure 26–7 Calculus on Molar Opposite Stensen's Duct.

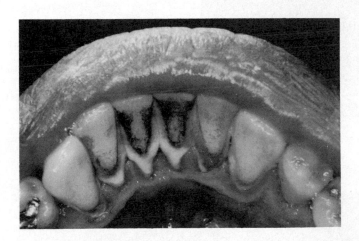

Figure 26–8 Calculus and Stain on lingual surface in relation to orifice of submaxillary and sublingual glands.

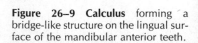

Figure 26–9 Calculus forming a bridge-like structure on the lingual surface of the mandibular anterior teeth.

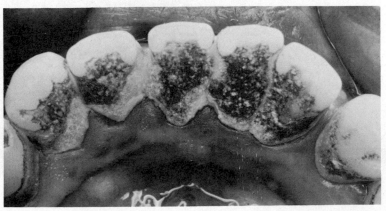

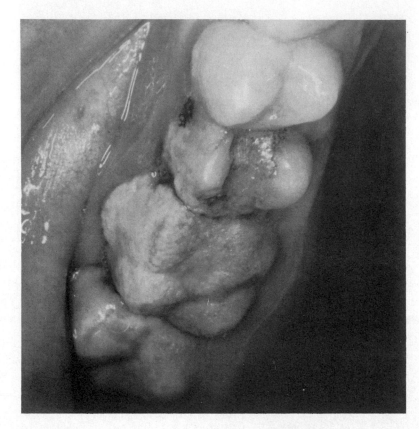

Figure 26–10 Calculus covering nonfunctioning maxillary molars and part of the second premolar. Compare with the first premolar, which has functional antagonists.

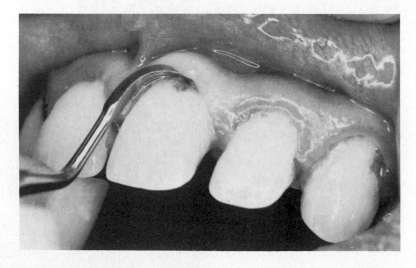

Figure 26–11 Subgingival Calculus revealed by deflecting the pocket wall. Note the inflammation of the marginal gingiva on adjacent lateral incisor and canine associated with supra- and subgingival calculus.

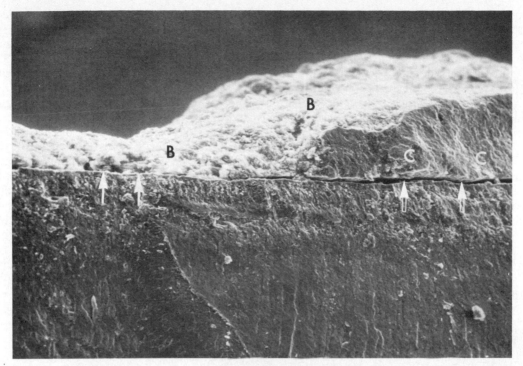

Figure 26–12 Cross-section of subgingival calculus (C) which is not firmly attached to the cemental surface (*arrows*). Note bacteria (B) attached to calculus and cemental surface. (Courtesy of Dr. John Sottosanti.)

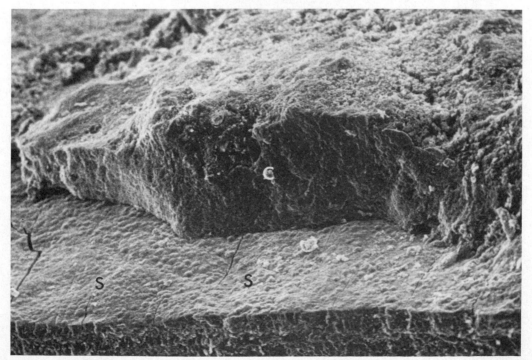

Figure 26–13 Cross-sectional view of subgingival calculus (C) attached to the cementum surface (S). (Courtesy of Dr. John Sottosanti.)

contours on the roentgenographic crown. Interproximal calculus, both supra- and subgingival, is even more easily detectable, since these deposits form irregularly shaped projections into the interdental space. Normally the location does not indicate the depth of the periodontal pocket, since the most apical plaque is not calcified enough to be roentgenographically visible.

Composition of Calculus

INORGANIC CONTENT. Supragingival calculus consists of inorganic (70 to 90 per cent[16]) and organic components. The inorganic portion consists of 75.9 per cent calcium phosphate, $Ca_3(PO_4)_2$; 3.1 per cent calcium carbonate, $CaCO_3$; and traces of magnesium phosphate, $Mg_3(PO_4)_2$, and other metals. The percentage of inorganic constituents of calculus is similar to that of other calcified tissues of the body. The principal inorganic components are calcium, 39 per cent; phosphorus, 19 per cent; carbon dioxide, 1.9 per cent; magnesium, 0.8 per cent; and trace amounts of sodium, zinc, strontium, bromine, copper, manganese, tungsten, gold, aluminum, silicon, iron, and fluorine.[44] At least two thirds of the inorganic component is crystalline in structure.[29] The four main crystal forms and their percentages are hydroxyapatite, $Ca_{10}(PO_4)_6(OH)_2$, approximately 58 per cent; magnesium whitlockite, $Ca_9(PO_4)_6$ X $PO_7 \cdot (X = Mg_{11} \cdot F_{11})$, and octacalcium phosphate, $Ca_4H(PO_4)_3 \cdot 2H_2O$, approximately 21 per cent each[52]; and brushite, $CaHOP_4 \cdot 2H_2O$, approximately 9 per cent. Generally two or more crystal forms occur in a calculus sample, with hydroxyapatite and octacalcium phosphate being the most com-

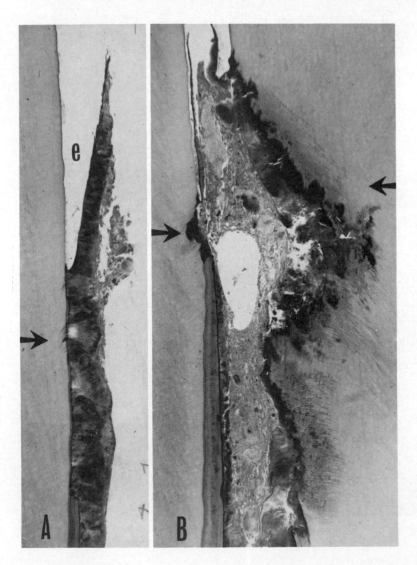

Figure 26–14 Calculus. *A*, Calculus attached to pellicle on enamel surface (e). The enamel was removed in preparation of the specimen. Also note calculus attached to dentin and associated penetration of dental tubules (*arrows*). *B*, Interproximal area with early and advanced root caries of adjacent teeth and with calculus attached to carious surfaces (*arrows*).

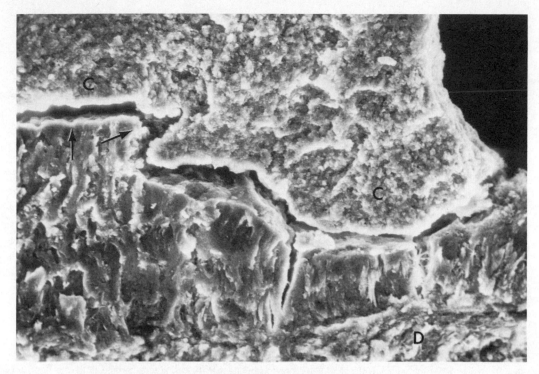

Figure 26–15 Subgingival calculus (C) embedded beneath the cementum surface (arrows) and penetrating to the dentin (D), making removal difficult. (Courtesy of Dr. John Sottosanti.)

mon (in 97 to 100 per cent of all supragingival calculus) and in the greatest amounts. Brushite is more common in the mandibular anterior region and magnesium whitlockite in the posterior areas. The incidence of the four crystal forms varies with the age of the deposit.[57]

ORGANIC CONTENT. The organic component of calculus consists of a mixture of protein-polysaccharide complexes, desquamated epithelial cells, leukocytes, and various types of microorganisms (see Fig. 26–6)[38]; 1.9 to 9.1 per cent of the organic component is carbohydrate, which consists of galactose, glucose, rhamnose, mannose, glucuronic acid, galactosamine, and sometimes arabinose, galacturonic acid, and glucosamine, all of which are present in salivary glycoprotein, except arabinose and rhamnose.[34, 63] Protein derived from the saliva accounts for 5.9 to 8.2 per cent of the organic component of calculus and includes most of the amino acids.[34, 36, 63] Lipids account for 0.2 per cent of the organic content in the form of neutral fats, free fatty acids, cholesterol, cholesterol esters, and phospholipids.[33]

The composition of subgingival calculus is similar to that of supragingival, with some differences. It has the same hydroxyapatite content,[66] more magnesium and whitlockite, and less brushite and octacalcium phosphate.[52] The ratio of calcium to phosphate is higher subgingivally, and the sodium content increases with the depth of periodontal pockets.[32] Salivary proteins present in supragingival calculus are not found subgingivally.[4] Dental calculus, salivary duct calculus, and calcified dental tissues are similar in inorganic composition.

Attachment of Calculus to the Tooth Surface

Differences in the manner in which calculus is attached to the tooth surface affect the relative ease or difficulty encountered in its removal. The various modes of attachment were first described by Zander.[77] Subsequent articles by others presented further information.[24, 39, 53, 58, 61]

The following modes of attachment have been described: attachment by means of an organic pellicle (Fig. 26–14); penetration of calculus bacteria into cementum (this mode of attachment is not accepted by some investigators[24]); mechanical locking into surface irregularities, such as resorption lacunae, caries, and so forth (Fig. 26–15); and close adaptation of calculus undersurface depressions to the gently sloping mounds of the unaltered cementum surface[64] (Fig. 26–16). Calculus embedded deeply in cementum may

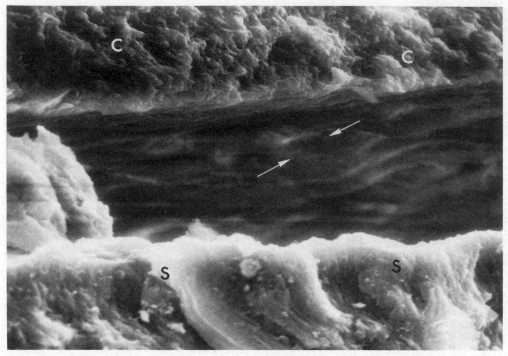

Figure 26–16 Undersurface of subgingival calculus (C) previously attached to cementum surface (S). Note impression of cementum mounds in calculus (*arrows*). (Courtesy of Dr. John Sottosanti.)

appear morphologically similar to cementum and has been termed "calculo-cementum."[58, 61]

Calculus Formation

Calculus is attached dental plaque which has undergone mineralization. The soft plaque is hardened by precipitation of mineral salts, which usually starts between the first and the fourteenth day of plaque formation; however, calcification has been reported as early as 4 to 8 hours.[67] Calcifying plaques may become 50 per cent mineralized in 2 days and 60 to 90 per cent mineralized in 12 days.[41, 54, 60]

All plaque does not necessarily undergo calcification. Early plaque contains a small amount of inorganic material, which increases as the plaque develops into calculus. Plaque which does not develop into calculus reaches a plateau of maximum mineral content by 2 days.[41, 55, 60] Microorganisms are not always essential in calculus formation, since it occurs readily in germ-free rodents.[15, 21]

Saliva is the mineral source for supragingival calculus, and the gingival fluid or exudate furnishes the minerals for subgingival calculus. Plaque has the ability to concentrate calcium at 2 to 20 times its level in saliva.[11] Early plaque of heavy calculus formers contains more calcium, three times more phosphorus, and less potassium than that of nonformers, suggesting that phosphorus may be more critical than calcium in plaque mineralization.[38]

Calcification entails the binding of calcium ions to the carbohydrate-protein complexes of the organic matrix[35] and the precipitation of crystalline calcium phosphate salts. Crystals form initially in the intercellular matrix and on the bacterial surfaces, and finally within the bacteria.[17, 78]

Calcification begins along the inner surface of the supragingival plaque (and in the attached component of subgingival plaque) adjacent to the tooth in separate foci that increase in size and coalesce to form solid masses of calculus (Fig. 26–17). It may be accompanied by alterations in the bacterial content and staining qualities of the plaque. With the occurrence of calcification, filamentous bacteria increase in number. In the calcification foci there is a change from basophilia to eosinophilia; the staining intensity of periodic acid-Schiff–positive groups and sulfhydryl and amino groups is reduced; and staining with toluidine blue, initially orthochromatic, becomes metachromatic and disappears.[72] Calculus is formed in layers, often separated by a thin cuticle which becomes embedded in it as calcification progresses.[40]

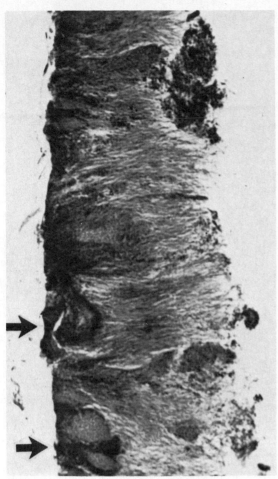

Figure 26–17 Five-Day Plaque, showing spherical calcification foci (*arrows*) and perpendicular alignment of filamentous organisms along the inner surface and colonies of cocci on the outer surface. (From Turesky, S., Renstrup, G., and Glickman. I.: J. Periodontol., 32:7, 1961.)

RATE OF FORMATION AND ACCUMULATION. *The starting time and rates of calcification and accumulation of calculus vary from person to person, in different teeth, and at different times in the same person.*[43, 68] Based on these differences, individuals may be classified as heavy, moderate, or slight calculus formers or as nonformers. The average daily increment in calculus formers is from 0.10 to 0.15 per cent of dry weight.[60, 68]

Calculus formation continues until it reaches a maximum, from which it may be reduced in amount. The time required to reach the maximum level has been reported as 10 weeks,[10] 18 weeks, and 6 months.[70] The decline from maximum accumulation (reversal phenomenon)[42, 70] may be explained by the vulnerability of bulky calculus to mechanical wear from food and from the cheeks, lips, and tongue.

THEORIES REGARDING THE MINERALIZATION OF CALCULUS. Theories regarding the mechanisms whereby plaque is mineralized to form calculus fit into two principal concepts:[44]

According to the first concept, mineral precipitation results from a local rise in the degree of saturation of calcium and phosphate ions, which may be brought about in several ways: (1) A rise in the pH of the saliva causes precipitation of calcium phosphate salts by lowering the precipitation constant. The pH may be elevated by the loss of carbon dioxide and by the formation of ammonia by dental plaque bacteria or by protein degradation during stagnation.[6, 22, 45] (2) Colloidal proteins in saliva bind calcium and phosphate ions and maintain a supersaturated solution with respect to calcium phosphate salts. With stagnation of saliva, colloids settle out; the supersaturated state is no longer maintained, leading to precipitation of calcium phosphate salts.[48] (3) Phosphatase liberated from dental plaque, desquamated epithelial cells, or bacteria is believed to play a role in the precipitation of calcium phosphate by hydrolyzing organic phosphates in saliva and thus increasing the concentration of free phosphate ions.[9, 75] Another enzyme, esterase, present in the cocci, filamentous organisms, leukocytes, macrophages, and desquamated epithelial cells of dental plaque may initiate calcification by hydrolyzing fatty esters into free fatty acids.[1] The fatty acids form soaps with calcium and magnesium that are later converted into the less soluble calcium phosphate salts.

According to the second concept, seeding agents induce small foci of calcification, which enlarge and coalesce to form a calcified mass.[46] This concept has been referred to as the "epitactic concept." The seeding agents in calculus formation are not known, but it is suspected that the intercellular matrix of plaque plays an active role.[39, 41, 78] The carbohydrate-protein complexes may initiate calcification by removing calcium from the saliva (chelation) and binding with it to form nuclei that induce subsequent deposition of minerals.[35, 71] Plaque bacteria have also been implicated as possible seeding agents (discussed in the following section).

ROLE OF MICROORGANISMS IN THE MINERALIZATION OF CALCULUS. Mineralization of plaque starts extracellularly around both gram-positive and gram-negative organisms[26]; it may also start intracellularly. Filamentous organisms, diphtheroids, and *Bacterionema* and *Veillonella* species have the ability to form intracellular apatite crystals. Calculus formation spreads until the matrix and bacteria are calcified.[17, 50, 78] Some feel that plaque bacteria actively participate in the mineralization of calculus by forming phosphatases, changing the plaque pH, or inducing mineralization,[13, 35] but the prevalent opinion is that these bacteria are only passively involved[17, 51, 74] and are simply calcified along with other plaque components. The occurrence of calculus-like deposits in germ-free animals supports this opinion.[15, 21] However, other experiments suggest that transmissible factors are involved in calculus formation and that penicillin in the diet of some of these animals reduces calculus formation.[2]

Etiologic Significance of Calculus

It is difficult to separate the effects of calculus and plaque upon the gingiva, because calculus is always covered with a nonmineralized layer of plaque.[55] There is a positive correlation between calculus and the prevalence of gingivitis,[49] but it is not as high as that between plaque and gingivitis.[18] In young individuals the periodontal condition is more closely related to plaque accumulation than to calculus, but the situation is reversed with age.[18, 30]

Calculus, gingivitis, and periodontal disease increase with age. It is extremely rare to find a periodontal pocket in adults without subgingival calculus, although in some cases the latter may be of microscopic proportion (Fig. 26–18).

The nonmineralized plaque on the calculus surface is the principal irritant, but the underlying calcified portion may be a significant contributing factor. **It does not irritate the gingiva directly, but it provides a fixed nidus for the continued accumulation of irritating surface plaque and holds the plaque against the gingiva.**

Subgingival calculus may be the product rather than the cause of periodontal pockets. Plaque initiates the gingival inflammation which starts pocket formation, and the pocket provides a sheltered area for plaque and bacterial accumulation. The increased flow of gingival fluid associated with gingival inflammation provides the minerals which convert the continually accumulating plaque into subgingival calculus.

Regardless of its primary or secondary relationship in pocket formation, and although the principal irritating feature of calculus is

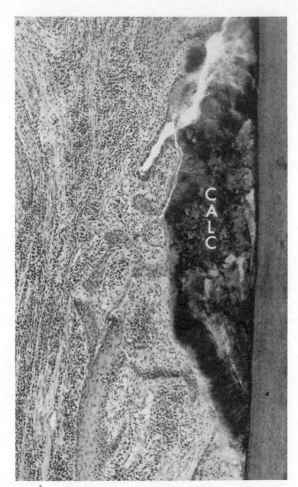

Figure 26–18 Suppurative Inflammation in periodontal pocket wall adjacent to uncalcified plaque on calculus surface (CALC).

surface plaque rather than its calcified interior, calculus is a significant pathogenic factor in periodontal disease.

MATERIA ALBA

Materia alba* is primarily an acquired bacterial coating which is a yellow or grayish-white, soft, sticky deposit somewhat less adherent than dental plaque.[56] Materia alba is clearly visible without the use of disclosing solutions and forms on tooth surfaces, restorations, calculus, and gingiva.[37, 41] It tends to accumulate on the gingival third of the teeth and on malposed teeth. It can form on previously cleaned teeth within a few hours and

---

*"Materia alba" is a traditional clinical term for a material which is essentially a heavy accumulation of plaque.

during periods when no food is ingested.[47] Materia alba can be flushed away with a water spray, but mechanical cleansing is required to ensure complete removal.

Long considered to consist of stagnant food debris, materia alba is now recognized to be *a concentration of microorganisms, desquamated epithelial cells, leukocytes, and a mixture of salivary proteins and lipids,*[37, 56, 76] *with few or no food particles.*[47] It lacks a regular internal pattern such as is observed in plaque. The irritating effect of materia alba upon the gingiva is most likely caused by bacteria and their products. Materia alba has also been demonstrated to be toxic when injected into experimental animals after the bacterial component has been destroyed by heat.[5]

FOOD DEBRIS

Most food debris is rapidly liquefied by bacterial enzymes and cleared from the oral cavity within 5 minutes after eating, but some remains on the teeth and mucosa.[7, 47] Salivary flow; mechanical action of the tongue, cheeks, and lips; and form and alignment of the teeth and jaws affect the rate of food clearance, which is accelerated by increased chewing and low viscosity of saliva.[25] Although it contains bacteria, food debris is different from the bacterial coatings (plaque and materia alba). *Dental plaque is not a derivative of food debris, nor is food debris an important cause of gingivitis.*[12] Food debris should be differentiated from fibrous strands trapped interproximally in areas of food impaction.

The rate of clearance from the oral cavity varies with the type of food and the individual. Liquids are cleared more readily than solids. For example, traces of sugar ingested in aqueous solution remain in the saliva for approximately 15 minutes, whereas sugar consumed in solid form is present for as long as 30 minutes after ingestion.[69] Sticky foods, such as figs, bread, toffee, and caramel, may adhere to tooth surfaces for over 1 hour, whereas coarse foods and raw carrots and apples are quickly cleared. Plain bread is cleared faster than bread with butter,[7, 20] brown rye bread faster than white,[25] and cold foods slightly faster than hot. The chewing of apples and other fibrous foods can effectively remove most of the food debris from the oral cavity, although it has no significant effect on the reduction of plaque.[8, 31]

REFERENCES

1. Baer, P. N., and Burstone, M. S.: Esterase activity associated with formation of deposits on teeth. Oral Surg., *12*:1147, 1959.
2. Baer, P. N., Keyes, P. H., and White, C. L.: Studies on experimental calculus formation in the rat. XII. On the transmissibility of factors affecting dental calculus. J. Periodontol., *39*:86, 1968.
3. Barros, L., and Witkop, C. P.: Oral and genetic study of Chileans, 1960. III. Periodontal disease and nutritional factors. Arch. Oral Biol., *8*:195, 1963.
4. Baumhammers, A., and Stallard, R. E.: A method for the labeling of certain constituents in the organic matrix of dental calculus. J. Dent. Res., *45*:1568, 1966.
5. Beckwith, T. B., and Williams, A.: Materia alba as toxic material. Am. Dent. Surg., *29*:73, 1929.
6. Bibby, B. G.: The formation of salivary calculus. Dent. Cosmos, *77*:668, 1935.
7. Bibby, B. G., Goldberg, H. J. V., and Chen, E.: Evaluation of caries-producing potentialities of various foodstuffs. J. Am. Dent. Assoc., *42*:491, 1951.
8. Birkeland, J., and Jorkjend, L.: The effect of chewing apples on dental plaque and food debris. Community Dent. Oral Epidemiol., *2*:161, 1974.
9. Citron, S.: The role of *Actinomyces israelii* in salivary calculus formation. J. Dent. Res., *24*:87, 1945.
10. Conroy, C., and Sturzenberger, O.: The rate of calculus formation in adults. J. Periodontol., *39*:142, 1968.
11. Dawes, C., and Jenkins, G. N.: Some inorganic constituents of dental plaque and their relationship to early calculus formation and caries. Arch. Oral Biol., *7*:161, 1962.
12. Egelberg, J.: Local effect of diet on plaque formation and development of gingivitis in dogs. III. Effect of frequency of meals and tube feeding. Odont. Revy, *16*:50, 1965.
13. Ennever, J.: Microbiologic mineralization: a calcifiable cell-free extract from a calcifiable microorganism. J. Dent. Res., *41*:1383, 1962.
14. Everett, F. G., Tuchler, H., and Lu, K. H.: Occurrence of calculus in grade school children in Portland, Oregon, J. Periodontol., *34*:54, 1963.
15. Glas, J. E., and Krasse, B.: Biophysical studies on dental calculus from germ free and conventional rats. Acta Odont Scand., *20*:127, 1962.
16. Glock, G. E., and Murray, M. M.: Chemical investigation of salivary calculus. J. Dent. Res., *17*:257, 1938.
17. Gonzales, F., and Sognnaes, R. F.: Electromicroscopy of dental calculus. Science, *131*:156, 1960.
18. Greene, J. C.: Oral hygiene and periodontal disease. Am. J. Public Health, *53*:913, 1963.
19. Greene, J. C., and Vermillion, J. R.: The Oral Hygiene Index. J. Am. Dent. Assoc., *68*:7, 1964.
20. Grenby, T.: The influence of sticky foods of high sugar content on dental caries in the rat. Arch. Oral Biol., *14*:1259, 1969.
21. Gustafsson, B. E., and Krasse, B.: Dental calculus in germ free rats. Acta Odontol. Scand., *20*:135, 1962.
22. Hodge, H. C., and Leung, S. W.: Calculus formation. J. Periodontol., *21*:211, 1950.
23. Jenkins, G. N.: The Physiology of the Mouth. Oxford, Blackwell Scientific Publications, 1966, p. 495.
24. Kupczyk, L., and Conroy, M.: The attachment of calculus to root planed surfaces. Periodontics, *6*:78, 1968.
25. Lanke, L. S.: Influence on salivary sugar of certain properties of foodstuffs and individual oral conditions. Acta Odontol. Scand., *15*(Suppl. 23):3, 1957.
26. Leach, S. A., and Saxton, C. A.: An electron microscopic study of the acquired pellicle and plaque formed on the enamel of human incisors. Arch. Oral Biol., *11*:1081, 1966.
27. Leung, S. W.: The uneven distribution of calculus in the mouth. J. Periodontol., *22*:7, 1951.
28. Leung, S. W.: Role of calculus deposits in periodontal disease. *In* A Symposium on Preventive Dentistry. St. Louis, C. V. Mosby Company, 1956, p. 206.
29. Leung, S. W., and Jensen, A. T.: Factors controlling the deposition of calculus. Int. Dent. J., *8*:613, 1958.
30. Lilienthal, B., Amerena, V., and Gregory, G.: An epidemiological study of chronic periodontal disease. Arch. Oral Biol., *10*:553, 1965.

31. Lindhe, J., and Wicen, P.: The effects on the gingivae of chewing fibrous foods. J. Periodont. Res., *4*:193, 1969.
32. Little, M. F., and Hazen, S. P.: Dental calculus composition. 2. Subgingival calculus: ash, calcium, phosphorus and sodium. J. Dent. Res., *43*:645, 1964.
33. Little, M. F., Bowman, L. M., and Dirksen, T. R.: The lipids of supragingival calculus. J. Dent. Res., *43*:836, 1964.
34. Little, M. F., Bowman, L., Casciani, C. A., and Rowley, J.: The composition of dental calculus. III. Supragingival calculus—the amino acid and saccharide component. Arch. Oral Biol., *11*:385, 1966.
35. Mandel, I. D.: Calculus formation. The role of bacteria and mucoprotein. Dent. Clin. North Am., *4*:731, 1960.
36. Mandel, I. D.: Histochemical and biochemical aspects of calculus formation. Periodontics, *1*:43, 1963.
37. Mandel, I. D.: Dental plaque: Nature, formation, and effects. J. Periodontol., *37*:357, 1966.
38. Mandel, I. D.: Biochemical aspects of calculus formation. J. Periodont. Res., *4*(Suppl. 4):7, 1969.
39. Mandel, I. D., Levy, B. M., and Wasserman, B. H.: Histochemistry of calculus formation. J. Periodontol., *28*:132, 1957.
40. Moskow, B. S.: Calculus attachment in cemental separations. J. Periodontol., *40*:125, 1969.
41. Mühlemann, H. R., and Schroeder, H.: Dynamics of supragingival calculus formation. Adv. Oral Biol., *1*:175, 1964.
42. Mühlemann, H. R., and Villa, P. R.: The Marginal Line Calculus Index. Helv. Odontol. Acta, *11*:175, 1967.
43. Muhler, J. C., and Ennever, J.: Occurence of calculus through several successive periods in a selected group of subjects. J. Periodontol., *33*:22, 1962.
44. Mukherjee, S.: Formation and prevention of supragingival calculus. J. Periodont. Res., *3*(Suppl. 2), 1968.
45. Naeslund, C.: A comparative study of the formation of concretions in the oral cavity and in the salivary glands and ducts. Dent. Cosmos, *68*:1137, 1926.
46. Neuman, W. F., and Neuman, M. W.: The Chemical Dynamics of Bone Mineral. Chicago, University of Chicago Press, 1958, p. 209.
47. Parfitt, G. J.: Summary of the problem of the prevention of periodontal disease. Ala. J. Med. Sci., *5*:305, 1968.
48. Prinz, H.: The origin of salivary calculus. Dent. Cosmos, *63*:231, 369, 503, 619, 1921.
49. Ramfjord, S. P.: The periodontal status of boys 11 to 17 years old in Bombay, India. J. Periodontol., *32*:237, 1961.
50. Rizzo, A. A., Scott, D. B., and Bladen, H. A.: Calcification of oral bacteria. Ann. N.Y. Acad. Sci., *109*:14, 1963.
51. Rizzo, A. A., Martin, G. R., Scott, D. B., and Mergenhagen, E. E.: Mineralization of bacteria. Science, *135*:439, 1962.
52. Rowles, S. L.: The inorganic composition of dental calculus. *In* Blackwood, H. J. J. (ed.): Bone and Tooth. Oxford, Pergamon Press, 1964, pp. 175–183.
53. Schoff, F. R.: Periodontia: an observation on the attachment of calculus. Oral Surg., *8*:154, 1955.
54. Schroeder, H. E.: Inorganic content and histology of early dental calculus in man. Helv. Odontol. Acta, 7:17, 1963.
55. Schroeder, H. E.: Crystal morphology and gross structures of mineralizing plaque and of calculus. Helv. Odontol. Acta, *9*:73, 1965.
56. Schroeder, H. E.: Formation and Inhibition of Dental Calculus. Berne, Stuttgart, and Vienna, Hans Huber Publ., 1969, pp. 12–15.
57. Schroeder, H. E., and Bambauer, H. U.: Stages of calcium phosphate crystallization during calculus formation. Arch. Oral Biol., *11*:1, 1966.
58. Selvig, J.: Attachment of plaque and calculus to tooth surfaces. J. Periodont. Res., *5*:8, 1970.
59. Selvig, K. A.: The formation of plaque and calculus on recently exposed tooth surfaces. J. Periodont. Res., *4*(Suppl. 4):10, 1969.
60. Sharawy, A., Sabharwal, K., Socransky, S., and Lobene, R.: A quantitative study of plaque and calculus formation in normal and periodontally involved mouths. J. Periodontol., *37*:495, 1966.
61. Sottosanti, J. S.: A possible relationship between occlusion, root resorption, and the progression of periodontal disease. J. Western Soc. Periodontol. *25*:69, 1977.
62. Sottosanti, J. S.: Relationship of calculus to root surfaces. Unpublished.
63. Standford, J. W.: Analysis of the organic portion of dental calculus. J. Dent. Res., *45*:128, 1966.
64. Stanton, G.: The relation of diet to salivary calculus formation. J. Periodontol., *40*:167, 1969.
65. Stewart, R. T., and Ratcliff, P. A.: The source of components of subgingival plaque and calculus. Periodont. Abstr., *14*:102, 1966.
66. Theilade, J., and Schroeder, H. E.: Recent results in dental calculus research. Int. Dent. J., *16*:205, 1966.
67. Tibbetts, L. S., and Kashiwa, H. K.: A histochemical study of early plaque mineralization. I.A.D.R. Abst. 1970, No. 616, p. 202.
68. Turesky, S., et al.: Effects of changing the salivary environment on progress of calculus formation. J. Periodontol., *33*:45, 1962.
69. Volker, J. F., and Pinkerton, D. M.: Acid production in saliva-carbohydrates. J. Dent. Res., *26*:229, 1947.
70. Volpe, A. R., Kupczak, L. J., King, W. J., Goldman, H., and Schulmann, S. M.: In vivo calculus assessment. Part IV. Parameters of human clinical studies. J. Periodontol., *40*:76, 1969.
71. Von der Fehr, F., and Brudevold, F.: In vitro calculus formation. J. Dent. Res., *39*:1041, 1960.
72. Waerhaug, J.: The source of mineral salts in subgingival calculus. J. Dent. Res., *34*:563, 1955.
73. Waerhaug, J.: Effect of rough surfaces upon gingival tissue. J. Dent. Res., *35*:323, 1956.
74. Wasserman, B. H., Mandel, J. D., and Levy, B. M.: In vitro calcification of calculus. J. Periodontol., *29*:145, 1958.
75. Wilkinson, F. C.: A patho-histological study of the tissue to tooth attachment. Dent. Record, *55*:105, 1935.
76. World Health Organization: Periodontal disease: report of an expert committee on dental health. Int. Dent. J., *11*:544, 1961.
77. Zander, H. A.: The attachment of calculus to root surfaces. J. Periodontol., *24*:16, 1953.
78. Zander, H. A., Hazen, S. P., and Scott, D. B.: Mineralization of dental calculus. Proc. Soc. Exp. Biol. Med., *103*:257, 1960.

FAULTY DENTISTRY

Faulty dental restorations and prostheses are common causes of gingival inflammation and periodontal destruction. Inadequate dental procedures may also injure the periodontal tissues. The following characteristics of restorations and partial dentures are of importance from a periodontal viewpoint; margins, contour, occlusion, materials, and design of removable partial dentures. They will be described in this chapter, as they play a role in the etiology of periodontal lesions; a more comprehensive review, with special emphasis on the recommended approach to restorative procedures, will be presented in Chapter 58.

MARGINS OF RESTORATIONS. Overhanging margins provide ideal locations for the accumulation of plaque and the multiplication of bacteria (Figs. 26–19 and 26–20). Removal of overhangs permits a more effective plaque control, resulting in the disappearance of gingival inflammation and increased alveolar bone support.[29, 33] A study has shown that 75 per cent of restorations show marginal defects and that 55 per cent of the defects equal or exceed 0.2 mm.[11] Other investigations have found 16.5 per cent[49] and 50 per cent[12, 28] of proximal

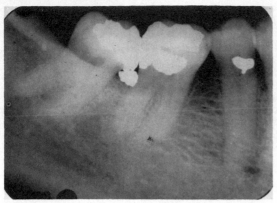

Figure 26–19 Amalgam Excess, which is source of irritation to the gingiva.

restorations defective. A highly significant statistical relationship was found between marginal defects and reduced bone height.[11, 33]

Silness[81] has described three different states of periodontal health related to differences in the position of the restoration margins. Larger amounts of plaque, more severe gingivitis, and deeper pockets are associated with subgingival location of margins; less severe conditions appear with margins at the level of the gingiva; and the degree of periodontal health associated with supragingival margins does not differ from that seen with intact control surfaces. Numerous studies[28, 37, 41, 69] have shown a positive correlation between subgingival margins and gingival inflammation. It has also been shown that even high quality restorations, if placed subgingivally, will increase plaque accumulation, gingival inflammation,[49, 70] and the rate of gingival fluid flow.[59]

Roughness in the subgingival area is considered the major cause of plaque build-up and the resultant inflammatory response.[79] The subgingival zone is made up of the crown and the margin of the restoration, the luting ma-

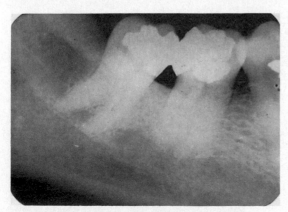

Figure 26–20 Amalgam Excess Removed.

terial, and the prepared tooth surface. Silness[81] has described the following sources of roughness: stripes and scratches in the surface of carefully polished acrylic resin, porcelain, or gold restorations (Fig. 26–21); separation of the cervical crown margin and the cervical margin of the finishing line by the luting material, exposing the rough surface of the prepared tooth (Fig. 26–22); dissolution and disintegration of the luting material, causing crater formation between the preparation and the restoration (Fig. 26–23); and inadequate marginal fit of the restoration.

The undersurface of pontics in fixed bridges should barely touch the mucosa. When this contact is excessive, it will prevent cleaning. Plaque will accumulate, causing inflammation and even pseudopocket formation (Fig. 26–24).

CONTOURS. Overcontoured crowns and restorations tend to accumulate plaque and possibly prevent the self-cleaning mechanisms of the adjacent cheek, lips, and tongue[3, 47, 56, 89] (Fig. 26–25). Previous claims that undercontouring of crowns may also have a deleterious effect due to lack of protection of the gingival margin during mastication have not been proved.[89]

Inadequate or improperly located proximal contacts and failure to reproduce the normal protective anatomy of the occlusal marginal ridges and developmental grooves lead to food impaction. Failure to re-establish adequate interproximal embrasures fosters the accumulation of irritants.

OCCLUSION. Restorations that do not conform to the occlusal patterns of the mouth cause occlusal disharmonies that may be injurious to the supporting periodontal tissues.

MATERIALS. Restorative materials are not by themselves injurious to the periodontal tissues.[3, 42] One exception to this may be self-curing acrylics.[87]

Restorative materials differ in their capacity to retain plaque,[87] but all can be adequately cleaned if they are polished[58, 73] and accessible to brushing. The composition of plaque formed on all types of restorative materials is similar, with the exception of that formed on silicate.[58] Plaque formed at the margins of restorations is similar to that formed on adjacent tooth surfaces.

DESIGN OF REMOVABLE PARTIAL DENTURES. Several investigations have shown that after the insertion of partial dentures there is an increase in mobility of the abutment teeth, gingival inflammation, and periodontal pocket

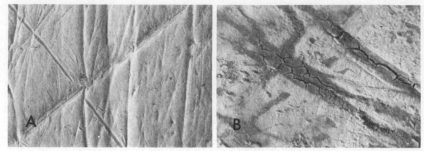

Figure 26–21 *A*, A polished gold alloy crown demonstrates surface scratches. *B*, A gold alloy crown that had been in the mouth for several years has scratches filled with deposits. (From Silness, J.: Dent. Clin. North Am., *24*:317, 1980.)

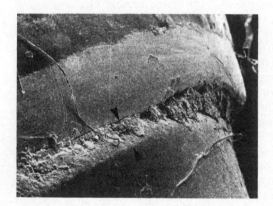

Figure 26–22 After cementation, luting material prevents approximation of the crown margin and the finishing line, leaving part of the prepared tooth uncovered (between arrows). (From Silness, J.: Dent. Clin. North Am., *24*:317, 1980.)

Figure 26–23 Craters have formed after dissolution and disintegration of the luting material. Spherical bodies are not identified. C, crown; R, root, (From Silness, J.: Dent. Clin. North Am., *24*:317, 1980.)

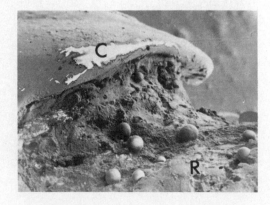

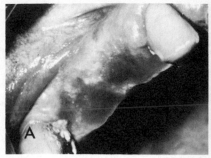
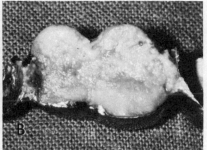

Figure 26–24 *A,* Red, inflamed soft tissues (dark area on the ridge) were found beneath the pontics after removal of a bridge that had been in the mouth for 12 years. *B,* The undersurfaces of the pontics were covered with a thick layer of plaque. (From Silness, J.: Dent. Clin. North Am., *24*:317, 1980.)

formation.[10, 16, 77] This is due to the fact that partial dentures favor the accumulation of plaque, particularly if they cover the gingival tissue. Partial dentures that are worn night and day induce more plaque formation than those used only during the day.[10]

These observations emphasize the need for careful and personalized oral hygiene instruction in order to avoid harmful effects of partial dentures on the remaining teeth.[9]

The presence of removable partial dentures induces not only quantitative changes in dental plaque[25] but also qualitative changes, promoting the development of spirilla and spirochetes.[26]

DENTAL PROCEDURES. The use of rubber dam clamps, copper bands, matrix bands, and disks in such a manner as to lacerate the gingiva results in varying degrees of inflammation. Although for the most part such transient injuries undergo repair, they are needless sources of discomfort to the patient. Injudicious tooth separation and excessively vigorous condensing of gold foil restorations are sources of injury to the supporting tissues of the periodontium which may be attended by acute symptoms such as pain and sensitivity to percussion.

PERIODONTAL PROBLEMS ASSOCIATED WITH ORTHODONTIC THERAPY

RETENTION OF PLAQUE. Orthodontic appliances tend to retain bacterial plaque and food debris, resulting in gingivitis (Fig. 26–26). Patients should be taught proper oral hygiene methods when appliances are inserted, and their importance should be stressed. The condition of the periodontium should be checked regularly during orthodontic treatment, and periodontal care should be instituted at the earliest sign of disease. Water irrigation under pressure is a helpful oral hygiene aid for these patients.

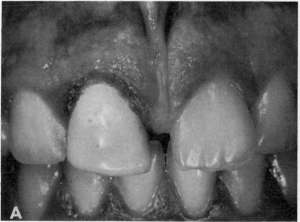
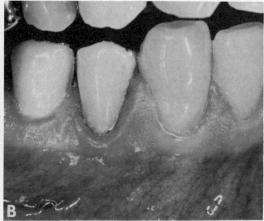

Figure 26–25 *A,* **Gingival Inflammation and Recession** associated with accumulated irritants on rough margin of crown. *B,* **Inadequate Mesioproximal Contour on First Premolar Restoration** leads to accumulation of irritants and gingival inflammation.

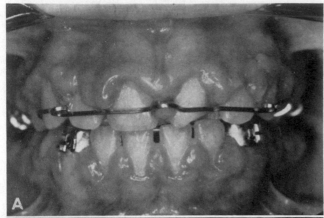
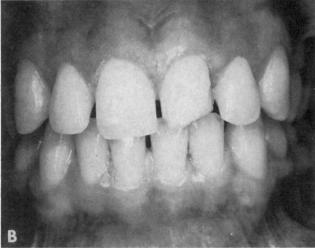

Figure 26–26 Gingival Inflammation and Enlargement Associated with Orthodontic Appliance and Poor Oral Hygiene. *A,* Gingival disease with orthodontic appliance in place. *B,* After removal of the appliance and periodontal treatment.

IRRITATION FROM ORTHODONTIC BANDS. Orthodontic treatment is often started at a stage of tooth eruption when the junctional epithelium is still on the enamel. The bands should not extend into the gingival tissues beyond the level of attachment. Forceful detachment of the gingiva from the tooth followed by apical proliferation of the junctional epithelium results in the increased gingival recession sometimes seen in orthodontically treated patients.[63] If gingival inflammation is present, the gingival margin is prevented from following the migrating epithelium, and pocket formation results.

TISSUE RESPONSE TO ORTHODONTIC FORCES. Orthodontic tooth movement is possible because the periodontal tissues are responsive to externally applied forces.[68, 76] The bone is remodeled by an increase in osteoclasts and bone resorption in areas of pressure and by increased osteoblastic activity and bone formation in areas of tension. Orthodontic forces also produce vascular changes in the periodontal ligament that may influence the bone resorptive and bone formative patterns.[18, 27]

TISSUE INJURY FROM ORTHODONTIC FORCES. From the periodontal viewpoint, it is important to avoid excessive force and too rapid tooth movement in orthodontic treatment. Excessive force may produce necrosis of the periodontal ligament and adjacent alveolar bone, which ordinarily undergo repair. However, destruction of the periodontal ligament at the crest of the alveolar bone may lead to irreparable damage. If the periodontal fibers beneath the junctional epithelium are destroyed by excessive force and the epithelium is stimulated to proliferate along the root by local irritants, *the epithelium will cover the root and prevent re-embedding of the periodontal fibers in the course of repair. Absence of functional stimulation from the periodontal fibers may result in atrophy of the crest of the alveolar bone.* Excessive orthodontic forces also increase the risk of apical root resorption.

It has been reported that the marginal and attached gingivae are "pulled" when teeth are orthodontically rotated[20] and that relapse of the occlusion after orthodontic treatment can be reduced by surgical resection or removal of free gingival fibers, combined with a brief retention period.[12, 55] Temporary separation of the reduced enamel epithelium on the tension side of orthodontically moved teeth and displacement and folding of the interdental papillae on the pressure side have also been noted.[6] Zachrisson and Alnaes[90, 91] found a statistically significant greater loss of attachment and of alveolar bone after orthodontic treatment.

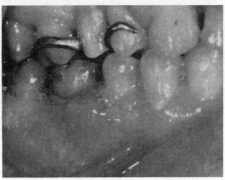

Figure 26–27 Gingival Inflammation and Abscess Formation associated with food impaction between the mandibular second premolar and molar.

FOOD IMPACTION

Food impaction is the forceful wedging of food into the periodontium by occlusal forces. It may occur interproximally or in relation to the facial or lingual tooth surfaces. Food impaction is a very common cause of gingival inflammation. Far too frequently, failure to recognize and eliminate food impaction is responsible for the unsuccessful outcome of an otherwise thoroughly treated case of periodontal disease.

The Mechanism of Food Impaction

The forceful wedging of food normally is prevented by the integrity and location of the proximal contacts, the contour of the marginal ridges and developmental grooves, and the contour of the facial and lingual surfaces. An intact, firm proximal contact relationship prevents the forceful wedging of food interproximally. The location of the contact is also important in protecting the tissues against food impaction. The optimal cervico-occlusal location of the contact is at the longest mesiodistal diameter of the tooth, close to the crest of the marginal ridge. The proximity of the contact point to the occlusal plane reduces the tendency toward food impaction in the smaller occlusal embrasure. The absence of contact or the presence of an unsatisfactory proximal relationship is conducive to food impaction (Fig. 26–27).

The contour of the occlusal surface established by the marginal ridges and related developmental grooves normally serves to deflect food away from the interproximal spaces (Fig. 26–28). As the teeth wear down and flattened surfaces replace the normal convexities, the wedging effect of the opposing cusp into the interproximal space is exaggerated (Fig. 26–28), and food impaction results. Cusps that tend to forcibly wedge food interproximally are known as *plunger cusps*. The plunger cusp effect may occur with wear, as indicated above, or may be the result of a shift in tooth position following the failure to replace missing teeth.

Excessive anterior overbite is a common cause of food impaction. The forceful wedging of food into the gingiva on the facial surfaces of the mandibular anterior teeth and the lingual surfaces of the maxillary teeth produces varying degrees of periodontal involvement. Gingival changes in the mandibular anterior region, associated with excessive anterior overbite, are easily detectable (Fig. 26–29). Unless they are severe, however, the effects of food impaction on the lingual surface of the maxilla are often overlooked. It should be stressed that inflammation caused by lingual food impaction may spread to the contiguous facial gingival margin. The possibility that lingual food impaction may be a contributory factor should always be explored when the etiology of gingival disease in the anterior maxilla is being considered.

A classic analysis of the factors leading to food impaction has been made by Hirschfeld.[34] He recognized the following factors: uneven occlusal wear, opening of the contact point due to loss of proximal support or to extrusion, congenital morphologic abnormalities, and improperly constructed restorations (Figs. 26–30 to 26–35). However, the presence of the above-mentioned abnormalities does not necessarily lead to food impaction and periodontal disease. A study of interproximal contacts and marginal ridge relationships in three groups of periodontally healthy males revealed that from 61.7 to 76 per cent of the proximal contacts were defective and 33.5 per cent of adjacent marginal ridges were uneven.[60]

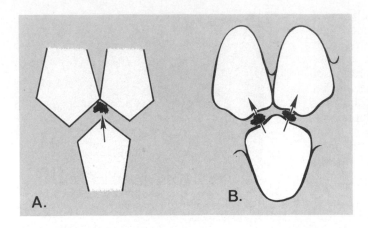

Figure 26–28 Food Impaction. *A,* Wedging effect upon food bolus (arrow) which results from wearing away of normal occlusal convexities and protective marginal ridges (after Hirschfeld[34]). *B,* Food impaction corrected by restoring occlusal convex surfaces and marginal ridges and directing food onto the occlusal surface (arrows).

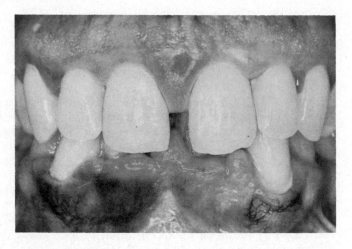

Figure 26–29 Inflammatory Gingival Enlargement in the mandibular anterior region associated with overbite and food impaction.

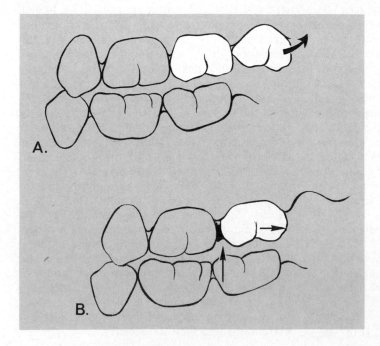

Figure 26–30 Food Impaction. *A,* Removal of maxillary third molar (arrow) permits second molar to be forced distally when teeth contact in occlusion. *B,* Bolus of food forced interproximally (arrow) as maxillary second molar is wedged distally (arrow).

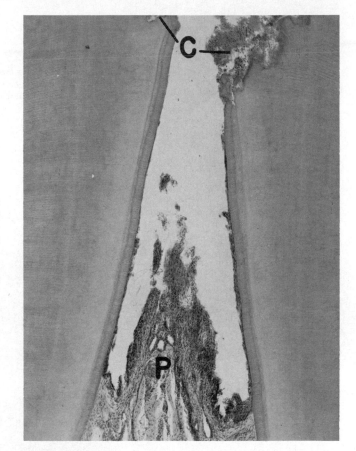

Figure 26–31 Mesiodistal section through mandibular premolars showing loss of proximal contact because of caries (C), which results in food impaction and inflammation of the interdental gingiva (P).

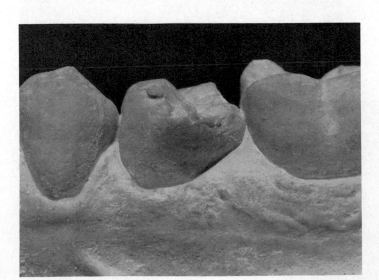

Figure 26–32 Improper Proximal Contact Relationship Associated with Malposed Premolar. Note inclined "plateau" which directs food from occlusal surface of the premolar into the distal interdental space.

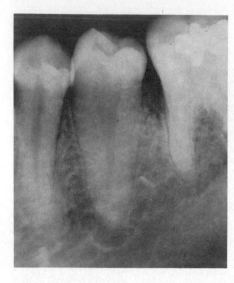

Figure 26–33 Bone Loss in area of food impaction associated with improper contact between mandibular second premolar and molar.

Figure 26–34 Malposed Teeth with food impaction and gingival inflammation.

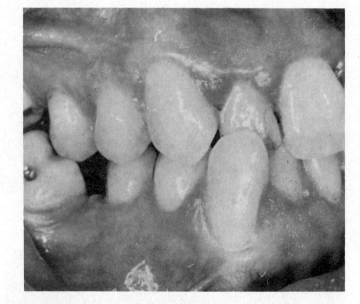

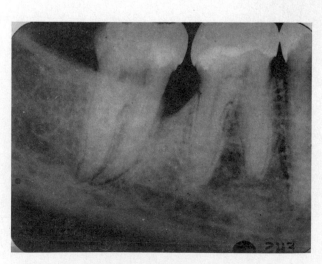

Figure 26–35 Food Impaction and bone loss associated with restorations that fail to restore and maintain proximal contact.

LATERAL FOOD IMPACTION. In addition to food impaction due to occlusal forces, lateral pressure from the lips, cheeks, and tongue may force food interproximally. This is more likely to occur when the gingival embrasure is enlarged by tissue destruction in periodontal disease or by recession. Impaction results when food forced into such an embrasure during mastication is retained instead of passing through.

Sequelae of Food Impaction

Food impaction serves to initiate gingival and periodontal disease and aggravates the severity of pre-existent pathologic changes. The following signs and symptoms occur in association with food impaction:

1. Feeling of pressure and the urge to dig the material from between the teeth.
2. Vague pain, which radiates deep in the jaws.
3. Gingival inflammation with bleeding and a foul taste in the involved area.
4. Gingival recession.
5. Periodontal abscess formation.
6. Varying degrees of inflammatory involvement of the periodontal ligament with an associated elevation of the tooth in its socket, prematurity in functional contact, and sensitivity to percussion.
7. Destruction of alveolar bone.
8. Caries of the root.

UNREPLACED MISSING TEETH

Failure to replace extracted teeth initiates a series of changes producing varying degrees of periodontal disease.[19, 35] In isolated cases, spaces created by tooth extraction may not cause undesirable sequelae. However, the frequency with which periodontal disease results from the failure to replace one or more missing teeth points to the advisability and prophylactic value of early prosthesis.

The ramifications of the failure to replace the first molar are sufficiently consistent to be recognized as a clinical entity. When the mandibular first molar is missing, the initial change is a mesial drifting and tilting of the mandibular second and third molars and extrusion of the maxillary first molar. The distal cusps of the mandibular second molar are elevated and act as plungers, impacting food into the interproximal space between the extruded maxillary first molar and the maxillary second molar (Fig. 26–36). If there is no maxillary third molar, the distal cusps of the mandibular second molar act as a wedge which breaks the contact between the maxillary first and second molars and deflects the maxillary second molar distally. This results in food impaction, gingival inflammation, and bone loss in the interproximal area between the maxillary first and second molars. Tilting of the mandibular molars and extrusion of the maxillary molars alter the respective contact relationships of these teeth, thereby favoring food impaction. Bone loss and pocket formation are commonly seen in relation to the extruded and tilted teeth (Figs. 26–37 to 26–39).

Tilting of the posterior teeth also results in reduction in the vertical dimension and accentuation of the anterior overbite. The mandibular anterior teeth slide gingivally along the palatal surfaces of the maxillary anterior teeth, resulting in a distal shift in the position of the mandible. In addition, there is food impaction and pocket formation in relation to the anterior teeth and a tendency toward labial migration and diastema formation in the maxilla. Distal drifting of the second premolar with food impaction and pocket formation in relation to the opened interproximal space between the premolars may be further complications. The aforementioned changes are accompanied by alterations in the functional relationships of the inclined cusps, with resultant occlusal disharmonies injurious to the periodontium.

The combination of changes associated with the unreplaced mandibular first molar does not occur in all cases, nor are all the changes identified with failure to replace other teeth in the arch. In general, however, drifting and tilting of the teeth, with alterations in proximal contact, result from failure to replace teeth that have been extracted. These changes are common factors in the etiology of periodontal disease.

MALOCCLUSION

Depending upon its nature, malocclusion exerts a varied effect in the etiology of gingivitis and periodontal disease.[54, 71] Irregular alignment of teeth will make plaque control difficult or even impossible. Several authors have found a positive correlation between crowding and periodontal disease[13, 62, 86] others, however, have found no correlation.[24] Uneven marginal ridges of contiguous posterior teeth have been found to have a low

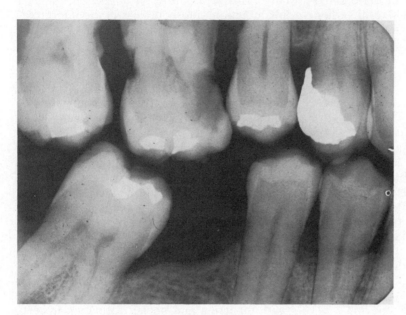

Figure 26–36 Tilted Mandibular Molar and Extruded Maxillary Molar associated with unreplaced tooth. Note caries in maxillary molar.

Figure 26–37 Extrusion of Maxillary First Molar into space created by unreplaced mandibular molar.

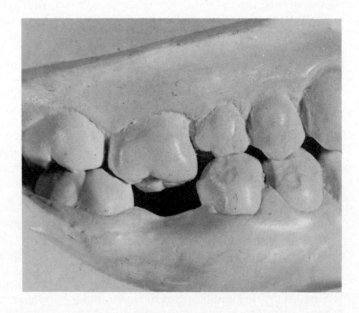

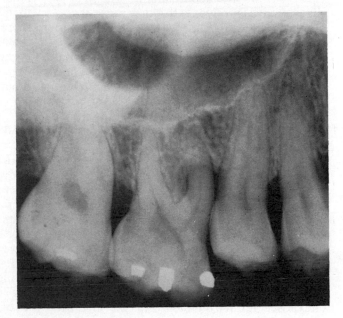

Figure 26–38 Extruded Maxillary First Molar with Trifurcation Involvement.

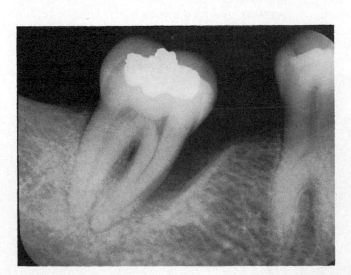

Figure 26–39 Angular Bone Loss on the Mesial Surface of Tilted Molar.

correlation with pocket depth, loss of attachment, plaque, calculus, and gingival inflammation.[44]

Gingival recession is associated with facially displaced teeth (Fig. 26–40). Occlusal disharmony associated with malocclusion results in injury to the periodontium.[57, 61] The incisal edges of the anterior teeth often cause irritation to the gingiva in the opposing jaw in patients with a severe overbite. Open bite relationships lead to unfavorable periodontal changes caused by accumulation of plaque and an absence of or diminution in function (Fig. 26–41).[14, 45] The prevalence and severity of periodontal disease are increased in children with bimaxillary protrusions.[36]

MOUTH BREATHING

Gingivitis is often associated with mouth breathing.[50] The gingival changes include erythema, edema, enlargement, and a diffuse surface shininess in the exposed areas. The maxillary anterior region is the common site of such involvement. In many cases the altered gingiva is clearly demarcated from the adjacent unexposed normal mucosa (Fig. 26–42). The exact manner in which mouth breathing affects gingival changes has not been demonstrated. Its harmful effect is generally attributed to irritation from surface dehydration. However, comparable changes could not be produced by air drying the gingivae of experimental animals.[46]

Several studies have shown conflicting evidence with respect to the association of mouth breathing and gingivitis. The following findings have been reported; mouth breathing has no effect on the prevalence or extent of gingivitis except in patients with considerable calculus[1]; mouth breathers have more severe gingivitis than non–mouth breathers with similar plaque scores[38]; there is no relationship between mouth breathing and prevalence of gingivitis except a slight increase in severity[86]; crowding of teeth is associated with gingivitis only in mouth breathers.[39]

HABIT

Habit is an important factor in the initiation and progression of periodontal disease. Frequently, the presence of an unsuspected habit is revealed in patients who have failed to respond to periodontal therapy. Habits of significance in the etiology of periodontal disease have been classified as follows by Sorrin[83]:

1. *Neuroses,* such as lip biting and cheek biting, which lead to extrafunctional positioning of the mandible; toothpick biting and wedging between the teeth; "tongue thrusting;" fingernail biting; pencil and fountain pen biting; and occlusal neuroses.

2. *Occupational habits,* such as the holding of nails in the mouth as practiced by cobblers, upholsterers, or carpenters; thread biting; and pressure of a reed during the playing of certain musical instruments.

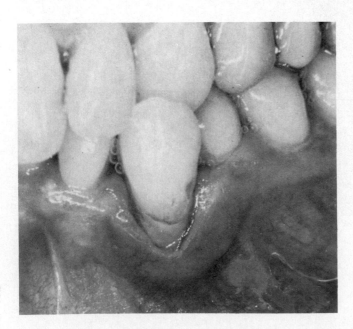

Figure 26–40 Gingival Recession and Inflammation on Malposed Canine.

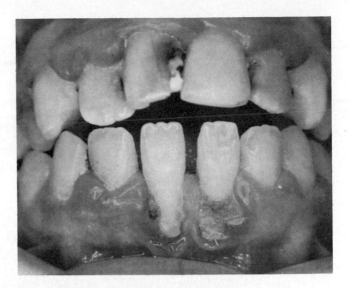

Figure 26–41 Chronic Gingivitis associated with open bite and accumulation of plaque and food debris.

3. *Miscellaneous,* such as pipe (Fig. 26–43) or cigarette smoking, tobacco chewing, incorrect methods of toothbrushing, mouth breathing, and thumb sucking.

Tongue-Thrusting

Special mention should be made of tongue-thrusting because it is so frequently undetected. It entails persistent, forceful wedging of the tongue against the teeth, particularly in the anterior region. Instead of the dorsum of the tongue being placed against the palate with the tip behind the maxillary teeth during swallowing, the tongue is thrust forward against the mandibular anterior teeth, which tilt and also spread laterally (Fig. 26–44).

Ray and Santos[67] divided patients with tongue-thrusting into two groups: (1) those in whom tongue-thrusting is part of a syndrome including a *hyposensitive palate* and *macroglossia,* and (2) those in whom the tongue-thrusting is a habit acquired in childhood or adult life. Tongue-thrusting is generally associated with abnormal swallowing habits (reverse swallow). These habits usually develop in infancy, and some suspect that they arise from bottle feeding with improperly designed nipples.[2, 85] Nasopharyngeal disease and allergy have also been implicated as possible causes of tongue-thrusting.

Tongue-thrusting causes excessive lateral pressure, which may be traumatic to the periodontium.[17, 80] It also causes spreading and tilting of the anterior teeth, with an open bite anteriorly, posteriorly, or in the premolar area (Fig. 26–44).

Numerous secondary sequelae may develop from tongue-thrusting. The altered inclination of the maxillary anterior teeth results in a change in the direction of the functional forces

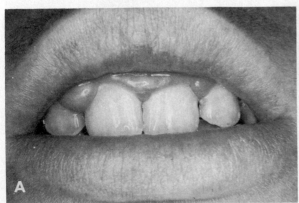
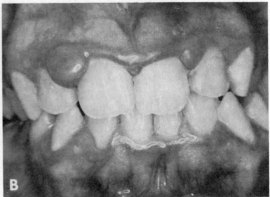

Figure 26–42 Gingivitis in Mouth Breather. *A,* High lip line in mouth breather. *B,* Gingivitis and inflammatory gingival enlargement in exposed area of gingiva.

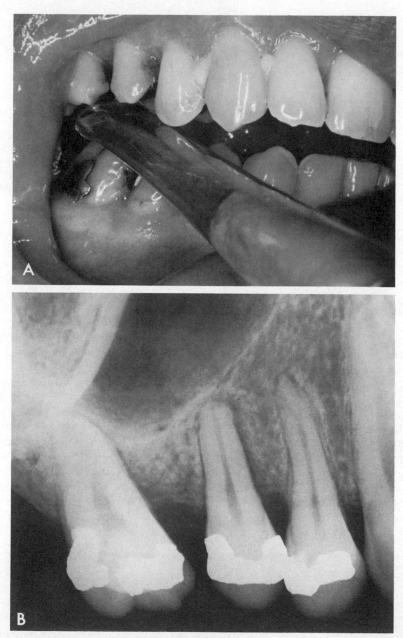

Figure 26–43 Trauma Associated with Holding Pipe in Fixed Position. *A*, Pipe held by maxillary first and second premolars and molar. Note the intruded second premolar and tilted molar. *B*, Radiograph showing intruded second premolar with apical resorption and widened periodontal ligament and angular bone destruction on the mesial surface. Note the widened periodontal ligament on the first premolar and the tilted molar.

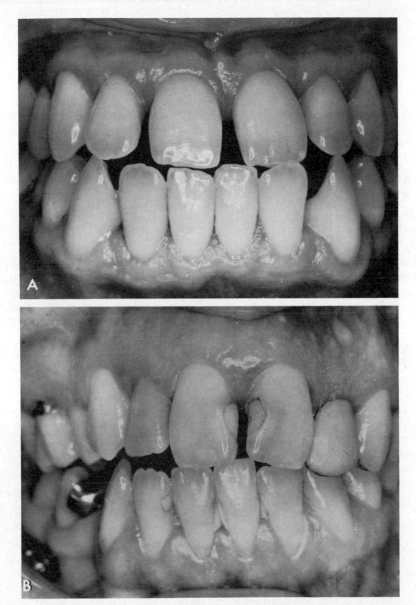

Figure 26–44 Tongue-thrusting. *A*, Tilting and spreading of anterior teeth associated with tongue-thrusting. *B*, Hypo-occlusion of lateral incisor, canine, and premolar associated with tongue-thrusting.

so that lateral pressure against the crowns is increased. This aggravates the labial drift and undesirable labiolingual rotational forces. The antagonism between forces that direct the tooth labially and inward pressure from the lip may lead to tooth mobility. The altered inclination of the teeth also interferes with food excursion and favors the accumulation of food debris at the gingival margin. The loss of proximal contact leads to food impaction. Tongue-thrusting is an important contributing factor in pathologic tooth migration.[17, 19]

Bruxism, Clenching, and Tapping

See Chapter 27.

Tobacco

Ordinarily, smoking does not lead to striking gingival changes. However, heat and the accumulated products of combustion are local irritants that are particularly undesirable in periods of posttreatment healing. The following oral changes may occur in smokers:

1. Brownish, tar-like deposits and discoloration of tooth structure.
2. Diffuse grayish discoloration and leukoplakia of the gingiva.
3. "Smoker's palate," characterized by prominent mucous glands with inflammation of the orifices and a diffuse erythema or by a wrinkled "cobblestone" surface.

The correlation between tobacco smoking and acute necrotizing ulcerative gingivitis has been clearly shown,[5] although a cause-and-effect relationship has not been proved. Both smoking and acute necrotizing ulcerative gingivitis may be the result of underlying anxiety and tension.

The influence of tobacco smoking on chronic gingivitis and plaque accumulation is still controversial. When smokers and nonsmokers are matched with regard to age and oral hygiene levels, no difference is found in the degree of gingival inflammation and periodontal breakdown.[49, 66, 79] Several authors, however, have found more severe gingivitis and periodontitis in smokers,[4, 23, 85] probably because of increased plaque accumulation, although some have found that tobacco smoking has little or no effect on the rate of plaque formation.[8]

It has been noted that women from the ages of 20 to 39 and men from 30 to 59 who smoke cigarettes have about twice the chance of having periodontal disease or becoming edentulous as do nonsmokers.[82] More calculus has been reported in pipe smokers than in cigarette smokers.[23, 64, 65]

A specific type of gingivitis termed "gingivitis toxica,"[65] characterized by destruction of the gingiva and underlying bone, has been attributed to the chewing of tobacco.

Keratinized cells in the gingiva are increased in smokers,[15] but no changes other than altered oxygen consumption can be detected in the buccal mucosa. The mucosal response to irritation from tobacco may be modified by experimentally induced systemic disturbance.[48] Daily application of cigarette smoke to the cheek pouch of hamsters for up to 20 months failed to produce any significant change other than occasional slight epithelial hyperplasia.[72] Oral polymorphonuclear leukocytes from smokers show a reduced ability to phagocytize particles.[43]

TOOTHBRUSH TRAUMA

Alterations in the gingiva as well as abrasions of the teeth may result from aggressive brushing in a horizontal or rotary fashion. The deleterious effect of abusive brushing is accentuated when excessively abrasive dentifrices are used.

The gingival changes attributable to toothbrush trauma may be acute or chronic. The acute changes are varied in appearance and

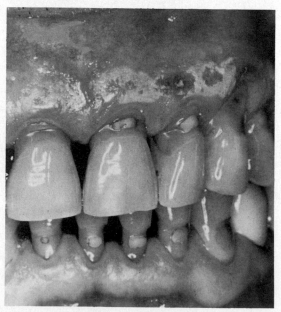

Figure 26–45 Toothbrush Trauma. Surface erosion and hyperkeratosis caused by abusive toothbrushing.

duration and include scuffing of the epithelial surface with denudation of the underlying connective tissue to form a painful gingival bruise (Fig. 26–45). Punctate lesions are produced by penetration of the gingiva by perpendicularly aligned bristles. Painful vesicle formation in traumatized areas is also seen. Diffuse erythema and denudation of the attached gingiva throughout the mouth may be a striking sequel of overzealous brushing. The acute gingival changes noted above commonly occur when the patient uses a new brush. A toothbrush bristle forcibly embedded and retained in the gingiva is a common cause of the acute gingival abscess (see Chapter 10).

Chronic toothbrush trauma results in gingival recession with denudation of the root surface. Often the gingival margin is enlarged and appears "piled up," as if it were molded in conformity with the strokes of the toothbrush. Linear grooves that extend from the marginal to the attached gingivae may be present. The gingiva in such areas is usually pink and firm.

Improper use of dental floss, toothpicks, or wooden interdental stimulators may result in gingival inflammation. The creation of interproximal spaces by destruction of the gingiva from overzealous use of toothpicks leads to the accumulation of debris and inflammatory changes.

CHEMICAL IRRITATION

Acute gingival inflammation may be caused by chemical irritation, as the result of either sensitivity or nonspecific tissue injury. In allergic inflammatory states, the gingival changes range from simple erythema to painful vesicle formation and ulceration. Severe reactions to ordinarily innocuous mouthwashes, dentifrices, or denture materials are often explainable on this basis.

Acute inflammation with ulceration may be produced by the nonspecific injurious effect of chemicals upon the gingival tissues. The indiscriminate use of strong mouthwashes (Figs. 26–46 and 26–47), application of aspirin tablets (Fig. 26–48) to alleviate toothache, injudicious use of escharotic drugs, and accidental contact with drugs such as phenol or silver nitrate are examples of the manner in which chemical irritation of the gingiva is commonly produced.

Gingival irritation is also seen in workers in various industries in which chemicals are employed.[74] Gases such as ammonia, chlorine, and bromine, acid fumes, and metallic dust are common offenders. The chemical irritation in such occupations is usually of long duration and is not necessarily productive of spectacular gingival changes. However, in patients with persistent gingival disease that is refractory to treatment, the occupational background should always be explored.

RADIATION

Gingival ulceration, bleeding, and suppuration, periodontitis, denudation of roots and bone, and loosening and loss of teeth have been noted following treatment with external and internal radiation in patients with malignancies of the oral cavity and adjacent regions.[7, 21, 84] Periodontal disease is a possible portal of entry for infection and the development of osteoradionecrosis following radiation therapy. Changes that vary in severity from edema and bleeding of the gingiva and

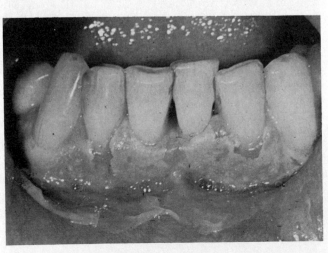

Figure 26–46 Chemical Burn. Necrosis and sloughing produced by undiluted mouthwash.

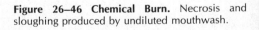

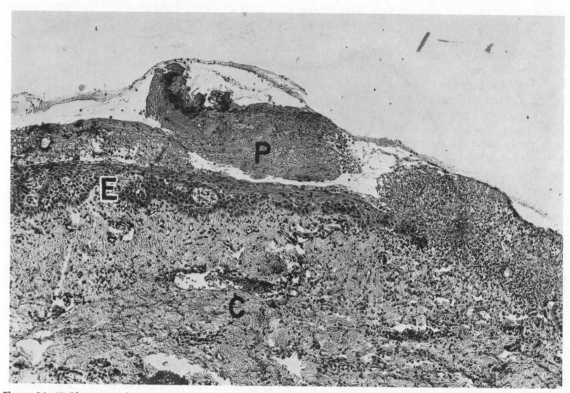

Figure 26–47 Biopsy Specimen of Necrotic Area Produced by Chemical Burn. Note inflamed connective tissue (C) and surface pseudomembrane (P). Of particular clinical importance is the newly formed sheet of epithelial cells (E), which undermines the necrotic pseudomembrane and separates it from the underlying connective tissue. This is an important feature of the healing process.

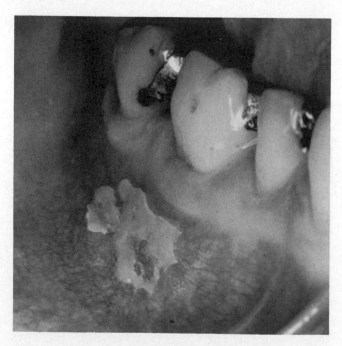

Figure 26–48 Aspirin Burn. Necrosis of mucosa produced by repeated use of aspirin tablets to relieve toothache.

widening of the periodontal ligament with disrupted deposition of cementum to necrosis of the gingiva and periodontal ligament and resorption of alveolar bone, loosening and shedding of the teeth, and the necrosis and sloughing of the oral mucosa have been reported in experimental animals exposed to single and multiple head or total-body roentgen radiation in individual doses of 10 R to 3000 R, to a total dosage of 11,000 rads.[22, 30, 31, 51, 52, 75]

REFERENCES

1. Alexander, A. G.: Habitual mouth breathing and its effect on gingival health. Parodontologie, 24:49, 1970.
2. Anderson, W. S.: The relationship of the tongue-thrust syndrome to maturation and other factors. Am. J. Orthod., 49:264, 1963.
3. App, G. R.: Effect of silicate, amalgam and cast gold on the gingiva. J. Prosthet. Dent., 11:522, 1961.
4. Arno, A., Schei, O., Lovdal, A., and Waerhaug, J.: Alveolar bone loss as a function of tobacco consumption. Acta Odontol. Scand., 17:3, 1959.
5. Arno, A., Waerhaug, J., Lovdal, A., and Schei, O.: Incidence of gingivitis as related to sex, occupation, tobacco consumption, toothbrushing, and age. Oral Surg., 11:587, 1958.
6. Atherton, J. D., and Kerr, N. W.: Effect of orthodontic tooth movement upon the gingivae. Br. Dent. J., 124:555, 1968.
7. Aub, J. C., Evans, R. D., Hempelmann, L. H., and Martland, H. S.: The late effects of internally-deposited radioactive material in man. Medicine (Baltimore), 31:221, 1952.
8. Bastian, R. J., and Waite, I. M.: Effects of tobacco smoking on plaque development and gingivitis. J. Periodontol., 49:480, 1978.
9. Bergman, B., Hugoson, A., and Olsson, C.: Periodontal and prosthetic conditions in patients treated with removable partial dentures and artificial crowns. Acta Odontol. Scand., 29:621, 1971.
10. Bissada, M. F., Ibrahim, S. I., and Barsoum, W. M.: Gingival response to various types of removable partial dentures. J. Periodontol., 45:651, 1974.
11. Bjorn, A. L., Bjorn, H., and Grcovic, B.: Marginal fit of restorations and its relation to periodontal bone level. Odont. Revy, 20:311, 1969.
12. Brain, W. E.: The effect of surgical transsection of free gingival fibers on the regression of orthodontically rotated teeth in the dog. Am. J. Orthod., 55:50, 1969.
13. Buckley, L.: The relationship between malocclusion and periodontal disease. J. Periodontol., 43:415, 1972.
14. Burwasser, P., and Hill, T. J.: The effect of hard and soft diets on the gingival tissues of dogs. J. Dent. Res., 18:389, 1939.
15. Calonius, P. E. B.: A cytological study on the variation of keratinization in the normal oral mucosa of young males. J. Western Soc. Periodontol., 10:69, 1962.
16. Carlsson, G. E., Hedegard, B., and Koivumaa, K.: Studies in partial dental prosthesis. IV. Final results of a four-year longitudinal investigation of dentogingivally supported partial dentures. Acta Odontol. Scand., 23:443, 1965.
17. Carranza, F. A., Sr., and Carraro, J. J.: El empuje lingual como factor traumatizante en periodoncia. Rev. Asoc. Odontol. Argent., 47:105, 1959.
18. Castelli, W. A., and Dempster, W. T.: The periodontal vasculature and its responses to experimental pressures. J. Am. Dent. Assoc., 70:891, 1965.
19. Chaikin, B. S.: Anterior periodontal destruction due to the loss of one or more unreplaced molars. Dent. Items Int., 61:17, 1939.
20. Edwards, J. G.: A study of the periodontium during orthodontic rotation of teeth. Am. J. Orthod., 54:441, 1968.
21. Ellinger, F.: Effects of ionizing radiation on the oral cavity. In Ellinger, F. (ed.): Medical Radiation Biology. Springfield, Ill., Charles C Thomas, 1957.
22. Frandsen, A. M.: Periodontal tissue changes induced in young rats by roentgen irradiation of the molar regions of the head. Acta Odontol. Scand., 20:393, 1962.
23. Frandsen, A. M., and Pindborg, J. J.: Tobacco and gingivitis. III. Difference in the action of cigarette and pipe smoking. J. Dent. Res., 28:404, 1949.
24. Geiger, A., Wasserman, B., and Turgeon, L.: Relationship of occlusion and periodontal disease. VIII. Relationship of crowding and spacing to periodontal destruction and gingival inflammation. J. Periodontol., 45:43, 1974.
25. Ghamrawy, E.: Quantitative changes in dental plaque formation related to removable partial dentures. J. Oral Rehabil., 3:115, 1976.
26. Ghamrawy, E.: Qualitative changes in dental plaque formation related to removable partial dentures. J. Oral Rehabil., 6:183, 1979.
27. Gianelly, A. A.: Force-induced changes in the vascularity of the periodontal ligament. Am. J. Orthod., 55:5, 1969.
28. Gilmore, N., and Sheiham, A.: Overhanging dental restorations and periodontal disease. J. Periodontol., 42:8, 1971.
29. Gorzo, I., Newman, H. N., and Strahan, J. D.: Amalgam restoration, plaque removal and periodontal health. J. Clin. Periodontol., 6:98, 1979.
30. Gowgiel, J. M.: Experimental radio-osteonecrosis of the jaws. J. Dent. Res., 39:176, 1960.
31. Greulich, R. C., and Ersho, B. M.: Delayed effects of multiple sublethal doses of total body x-irradiation on the periodontium and teeth of mice. J. Dent. Res., 10:1211, 1961.
32. Hakkarainen, K., and Ainamo, J.: Influence of overhanging posterior tooth restorations of alveolar bone height in adults. J. Clin. Periodontol., 7:114, 1980.
33. Highfield, J. E., and Powell, R. N.: Effects of removal of posterior overhanging metallic margins of restorations upon the periodontal tissues. J. Clin. Periodontol., 5:169, 1978.
34. Hirschfeld, I.: Food impaction. J. Am. Dent. Assoc., 17:1504, 1930.
35. Hirschfeld, I.: Individual missing tooth. J. Am. Dent. Assoc., 24:67, 1937.
36. Holden, S., Harris, J. E., and Ash, M. M., Jr.: Periodontal disease in Nubian children. I.A.D. R. Abstr., 48th General Meeting, 1970, p. 65.
37. Huttner, G.: Follow-up study of crowns and abutments with regard to the crown edge and the marginal periodontium. Dtsch. Zahnärztl. Z., 26:724, 1971.
38. Jacobson, L.: Mouth breathing and gingivitis. J. Periodont. Res., 8:269, 1973.
39. Jacobson, L., and Linder-Aronson, S.: Crowding and gingivitis: a comparison between mouth breathers and non-mouth breathers. Scand. J. Dent. Res., 80:500, 1972.
40. Jeffcoat, M. K., and Howell, T. H.: Alveolar bone destruction due to overhanging amalgam in periodontal disease. J. Periodontol., 51:599, 1980.
41. Karlsen, K.: Gingival reactions to dental restorations. Acta Odontol. Scand., 28:895, 1970.
42. Kawakara, H., Yamagani, A., and Nakamura, M., Jr.: Biological testing of dental materials by means of tissue culture. Int. Dent. J., 18:443, 1968.
43. Kenney, E. B., Kraal, J. H., Saxe, S. R., and Jones, J.: The effect of cigarette smoke on human oral polymorphonuclear leukocytes. J. Periodont. Res., 12:227, 1977.
44. Kepic, T. J., and O'Leary, T. J.: Role of marginal ridge relationships as an etiologic factor in periodontal disease. J. Periodontol., 49:570, 1978.
45. King, J. D., and Gimson, A. P.: Experimental investigations of paradontal disease in the ferret and related lesions in man. Br. Dent. J., 83:126, 1947.
46. Klingsberg, J., Cancellaro, B. A., and Butcher, E. O.: Effects of air drying on rodent oral mucous membrane: a histologic study of simulated mouth breathing. J. Periodontol., 32:38, 1961.
47. Koivamaa, K. K., and Wennstrom, A.: A histological investigation of the changes in gingival margins adjacent to gold crowns. Odont. T., 68:373, 1960.
48. Kreshover, S. J.: The effect of tobacco on the epithelial tissues of mice. J. Am. Dent. Assoc., 45:528, 1952.
49. Leon, A. R.: Amalgam restorations and periodontal disease. Br. Dent. J., 140:377, 1976.
50. Lite, T., et al.: Gingival pathosis in mouth breathers. A clinical and histopathologic study and a method of treatment. Oral Surg., 8:382, 1955.

51. Mayo, J., Carranza, F. A., Jr., Epper, C. E., and Cabrini, R. L.: The effect of total-body irradiation on the oral tissues of the Syrian hamster. Oral Surg., *15*:739, 1962.

52. Medak, H., and Burnett, G. W.: The effect of x-ray irradiation on the oral tissues of the macacus Rhesus monkey. Oral Surg., *7*:778, 1954.

53. Meyer, J., Shklar, G., and Turner, J.: A comparison of the effects of 200 KV radiation and dental structure of the white rat. Oral Surg., *15*:1098, 1962.

54. Miller, J., and Hobson, P.: The relationship between malocclusion, oral cleanliness, gingival conditions and dental caries in school children. Br. Dent. J., *111*:43, 1961.

55. Moffett, B. C.: Remodeling changes of the facial sutures, periodontal and temporomandibular joints produced by orthodontic forces in Rhesus monkeys. Bull. Pacific Coast Soc. Ortho., *44*:46, 1969.

56. Morris, M. L.: Artificial crown contours and gingival health. J. Prosthet. Dent., *12*:1146, 1962.

57. Mühlemann, H. R., et al.: Okklusion und Artikulation im Atiologiekomplex Parodontaler Erkrankungen. Parodontologie, *11*:20, 1957.

58. Norman, R. D., Mehia, R. V., Swartz, M. L., and Phillips, R. W.: Effect of restorative materials on plaque composition. J. Dent. Res., *51*:1596, 1972.

59. Normann, W., Regolati, B., and Renggli, H. H.: Gingival reaction to well-fitted subgingival proximal gold inlays. J. Clin. Periodontol., *1*:120, 1974.

60. O'Leary, T. J., and Sosa, C. E.: Signs of periodontal breakdown in patients with malocclusion. J. Dent. Educ., *10*:172, 1955.

61. O'Leary, T. J., Badell, M., and Bloomer, R.: Interproximal contact and marginal ridge relationships in periodontally healthy young males classified as to orthodontic status. J. Periodontol., *46*:6, 1975.

62. Paunio, K.: The role of malocclusion and crowding in the development of periodontal disease. Int. Dent. J., *23*:420, 1973.

63. Pearson, L. E.: Gingival height of lower central incisors, orthodontically treated and untreated. Angle Ortho., *38*:337, 1968.

64. Pindborg, J. J.: Tobacco and gingivitis. I. Statistical examination of the significance of tobacco in the development of ulceromembranous gingivitis and in the formation of calculus. J. Dent. Res., *26*:261, 1947.

65. Pindborg, J. J.: Tobacco and gingivitis. II. Correlation between consumption of tobacco, ulceromembranous gingivitis and calculus. J. Dent. Res., *28*:461, 1949.

66. Preber, H., Kant, T., and Bergstrom, J.: Cigarette smoking, oral hygiene and periodontal disease in Swedish army conscripts. J. Clin. Periodontol., *7*:106, 1980.

67. Ray, H. G., and Santos, H. A.: Consideration of tongue-thrusting as a factor in periodontal disease. J. Periodontol., *25*:250, 1954.

68. Reitan, K.: Tissue changes following experimental tooth movement as related to the time factor. Dent. Record, *73*:559, 1953.

69. Renggli, H. H.: The influence of subgingival proximal filling borders on the degree of inflammation of the adjacent gingiva. A clinical study. Schweiz. Monatsschr Zahnheilkd., *84*:181, 1974.

70. Renggli, H. H., and Regolati, B.: Gingival inflammation and plaque accumulation by well-adapted supragingival and subgingival proximal restorations. Helv. Odontol. Acta, *16*:99, 1972.

71. Rosenzweig, K. A., and Langer, A.: Oral disease in yeshiva students. J. Dent. Res., *40*:993, 1961.

72. Salley, J. J., and Kreshover, S. J.: Further studies of the effect of tobacco on oral tissues. J. Dent. Res., *37*:979, 1958.

73. Sanchez-Sotres, L., Van Huysen, G., and Gilmore, H. W.: A histologic study of gingival tissue response to amalgam, silicate and resin restorations. J. Periodontol., *42*:8, 1969.

74. Schour, I., and Sarnat, B. G.: Oral manifestations of occupational origin. J.A.M.A., *120*:1197, 1942.

75. Schule, H., and Betzold, J.: Experimental investigations on the effect of x-ray irradiation on marginal periodontal tissues. Dtsch. Zahnärztl. Z., *24*:140, 1969.

76. Schwartz, A. M.: Tissue changes incidental to orthodontic tooth movement. Ortho., Oral Surg., Rad., Int. J., *18*:331, 1932.

77. Seeman, S.: Study of the relationship between periodontal disease and the wearing of partial dentures. Aust. Dent. J., *8*:206, 1963.

78. Severson, H. M.: The effect of cigarette smoking on plaque formation. J. Periodontol., *50*:146, 1979.

79. Sheiham, A.: Periodontal disease and oral cleanliness in tobacco smokers. J. Periodontol., *42*:259, 1971.

80. Sheppard, I. M.: Tongue dynamics. Dent. Digest, *59*:117, 1953.

81. Silness, J.: Fixed prosthodontics and periodontal health. Dent. Clin. North Am., *24*:317, 1980.

82. Solomon, H., Priore, R., and Bross, I.: Cigarette smoking and periodontal disease. J. Am. Dent. Assoc., *77*:1081, 1968.

83. Sorrin, S.: Habit: An etiologic factor of periodontal disease. Dent. Digest, *41*:290, 1935.

84. Stafne, E. C., and Bowing, H. H.: The teeth and their supporting structures in patients treated by irradiation. Am. J. Orthod., *33*:567, 1947.

85. Summers, C. J., and Oberman, A.: Association of oral disease with twelve selected variables. I. Periodontal disease. J. Dent. Res., *47*:457, 1968.

86. Sutcliffe, P.: Chronic anterior gingivitis: an epidemiological study in school children. Br. Dent. J., *125*:47, 1968.

87. Waerhaug, J., and Zander, H. A.: Reaction of gingival tissue to self-curing acrylic restorations. J. Am. Dent. Assoc., *54*:760, 1957.

88. Wise, M. D., and Dykema, R. W.: The plaque retaining capacity of four dental materials. J. Prosthet. Dent., *33*:178, 1975.

89. Yuodelis, R. A., Weaver, J. D., and Sapkos, S.: Facial and lingual contours of artificial complete crowns and their effect on the periodontium. J. Prosthet. Dent., *29*:61, 1973.

90. Zachrisson, B. W., and Alnaes, L.: Periodontal condition in orthodontically treated and untreated individuals. I. Loss of attachment, gingival pocket depth and clinical crown height. Angle Orthod., *43*:402, 1973.

91. Zachrisson, B. W., and Alnaes, L.: Periodontal condition in orthodontically treated and untreated individuals. II. Alveolar bone loss: radiographic findings. Angle Orthod., *44*:48, 1974.

chapter twenty-seven

The Role of Morphofunctional Occlusal Factors in Periodontal Disease and Temporomandibular Disorders

OCCLUSAL INTERFERENCES AND OCCLUSAL DISORDERS

Occlusal interferences and occlusal disorders tend to destabilize the occlusion. As discussed in Chapter 5, occlusal interferences and disorders promote reduced muscle contraction at the involved occlusal position, muscle hyperactivity at the postural position, and incoordination in the timing and length of muscle contraction during function.[29, 36] Occlusal interferences may incite muscle activity in an effort to wear away the obstructing tooth surfaces; this activity becomes repetitive and develops into bruxing, clamping, or clenching habits.[14, 22, 37] These habits may increase the magnitude and/or modify the direction and frequency of the forces exerted upon the teeth, resulting in traumatic periodontal lesions with destruction of the periodontium and loosening of the teeth (see Chapter 19). They also deflect the pathway of the mandible[58] (Fig. 27–1).

When the periodontium has previously been reduced by marginal periodontitis, the effect of the forces generated by occlusal interferences is magnified by the reduced resistance of the periodontium to those forces. This is the so-called secondary trauma from occlusion described in Chapter 19. In addition, significant functional and structural disorders of the temporomandibular joints and of the mandibular body may result.

The fact that most people have occlusal prematurities without necessarily suffering their harmful effect is indicative of the adaptability of the oral tissues.[55] Bruxism and temporomandibular disorders and their treatment are covered here particularly as concerns the concepts of form and function. A review of reflex and other responses involving occlusal interferences is found in Chapter 5; for discussion of the definition, recognition, and treatment of occlusal interferences, the reader should refer to Chapter 47.

MALOCCLUSION. Abnormalities in the position of the teeth are not the same as occlusal interferences. In fact, malocclusions often result in an adaptive functional state free of obvious occlusal interferences. Localized occlusal interferences (tooth-to-tooth interferences) acquired from *dental malocclusion* can be identified and recorded as (1) prematurities disrupting uniform posterior contact in the intercuspal position (ICP), (2) prematurities preventing a coordinated, symmetrical glide from the retruded contact position (RCP) to the ICP; and (3) working and nonworking supracontacts on the molar teeth. Skeletal malocclusions generate maxillomandibular effects such as deep bite, crossbite, and open bite. While these conditions are not always associated with localized tooth-to-tooth interferences, they are often expressed as *occlusal disorders* since they are associated with adverse reflex loading response in the masticatory system.[29] In a sense, the whole malocclusion can be characterized as an occlusal interference.

The evaluation of malocclusions for occlusal interferences should be threefold: (1) visualization and measurement of tooth-to-tooth occlusal interferences (using dental casts registered in an articulator, if necessary); (2) analysis of the relationship of occlusal interferences to observed disturbances in functional movement capacity, and (3) consideration of the need for orthodontic diagnosis.

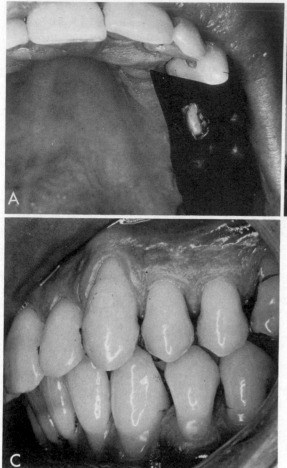

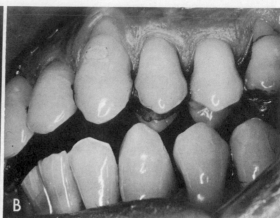

Figure 27–1 Retrusive Prematurity. *A*, Premature contact on the mesiolingual cusp of the maxillary first premolar, encountered when the mandible moves on the terminal hinge path of closure. *B*, Retrusive prematurity prevents closure into a multipointed retruded contact position. *C*, Upon full closure, the mandible is deflected anteriorly into the intercuspal position.

LOSS OF TEETH. The loss of posterior teeth, especially the first or second molar, and subsequent tooth migration lead to an occlusal disorder termed "collapsed bite." In cases of uncontrolled tooth migration, the teeth often develop inclinations conducive to tooth-to-tooth interferences. Disturbance in the ICP contact is usually transitory, but during uncontrolled migration subtle changes in mandibular loading take place, setting the stage for muscular and temporomandibular joint maladaptations. Tooth loss has been clinically linked to temporomandibular disorders and osteoarthrosis.[18, 23] Given these considerations, the practice of maintaining unreplaced molar spaces on the grounds of "conservation" should be seriously re-examined.

FAULTY RESTORATIONS. Restorative dentistry is fraught with possibilities for technical errors which result in immediate or progressive development of occlusal interferences. Progressive occlusal interferences develop secon-dary to restorations lacking occlusal contact in the ICP or when the contact results in tooth migration along unstable inclines. For example, nonworking interferences on second molars often occur subsequent to placement of a relatively large amalgam restoration, since these restorations are often left out of occlusion in the "carve-in" stage. When the tooth erupts into occlusion, there is a relative increase in the height of the cusp inclines, and these inclines then become nonworking interferences. Whereas some occlusal discrepancies occur at random owing to lapses in the clinician's attention to detail, others are systematic: e.g., the policy of placing the new restoration "slightly out of centric" to reduce chair time at insertion. Clinicians may fail to appreciate that the temporomandibular joint can undergo upward movement when the most posterior stop is released during preparation of the tooth, especially in second molar crown restorations. Failure to recognize this phenomenon results in supracontacts in the restoration, which may then cause periodontal complications. The choice of restorative material sometimes leads to uneven wear and interferences on teeth in areas remote to the restorations. By design, the single tooth restoration should include coupled vertical stops, when possible, and should allow for adequate overbite and overjet relationships to ensure smooth articulation in all excursions. The clinician seeking to alter faulty posterior restorations should be cognizant of the contact tolerances of the posterior teeth, as many cases of disturbed bite arise when excessive anterior tooth contact has inadvertently developed after selected occlusal adjustment of the posterior teeth.

FAULTY ORTHODONTICS. A controversy exists regarding the culpability of orthodontics in causing periodontal disease. On the other hand, it is generally accepted that an important reason for performing orthodontic therapy is to promote the health of the periodontium. Sadowsky and BeGole tested these two beliefs in a controlled study and failed to demonstrate major positive relationships.[45] These results notwithstanding, the clinician becomes aware of orthodontic pitfalls that jeopardize the periodontal health of individual patients. The most frequent problems include (1) lack of well-distributed occlusal stops at the ICP, (2) overlap discrepancies of the anterior and posterior teeth that lead to interferences on closure and in excursion, and (3) nonworking-side interferences resulting from uncontrolled second molar relationships. This usually occurs because the second molars were not banded during the orthodontic treatment. Often the discrepancies in the occlusion are accompanied by asymmetrical and complicated relationships between the RCP and the ICP. Patients who have had premolars extracted often have post-treatment occlusal problems, a complication that points not only to the inherent difficulty of extraction techniques, but also to the reality that extraction cases have the most serious maxillomandibular discrepancies and therefore pose more problems in obtaining an acceptable occlusal result. It can be suggested that occlusal adjustment should be considered for all orthodontic patients at some time in the retention stages.

FAULTY OCCLUSAL ADJUSTMENT. The literature abounds with conflicting viewpoints on the advantages and pitfalls of occlusal adjustment (equilibration). Most problems with oc-clusal adjustment are fundamental: they involve the lack of a biologic approach to adjustment procedures and failure to understand the principles of technique. The rationale for and technique of occlusal adjustment are discussed in Chapter 47. Faulty occlusal adjustment can result in a subjective complaint, usually because of a lack of informed consent and also due to premature intraoral adjustment in difficult cases, undertaken without the benefit of a trial grinding on articulated dental casts. So-called spot grinding, without consideration of total maxillomandibular function, is the most common cause of problems involving faulty occlusal adjustment. Since localized tooth adjustments are integral in many periodontal cases, the clinician should take care to review the potential consequences of such adjustment. Ironically, a significant complication of incomplete occlusal adjustment is that the occlusal discrepancies can increase, thus subjecting the anterior teeth to trauma from occlusion.

The most alarming complication of occlusal therapy is the problem of positive occlusal sense or "phantom bite." Recognition of these cases is important, because further occlusal adjustment should be terminated in favor of psychotherapeutic consultation. Correct dental management of these cases avoids reinforcement of the patient's exaggerated concept that something is mechanically wrong with his or her jaw. Phantom bite can be suspected in those patients in whom the subjective complaints are high but the physical discrepancies are low. Phantom bite should also be suspected in cases of nonresponse to appropriately carried out occlusal adjustment procedures. Endless and repetitive occlusal adjustment of a dentition in the face of a volatile subjective response is contraindicated.

Occlusal adjustment on patients having clicking and intermittent locking can cause an increase in temporomandibular joint symptoms; for this reason, the indications for occlusal therapy should be carefully evaluated in these patients.

OCCLUSAL HABITS. Biting the soft tissues and foreign objects creates localized occlusal disorders that lead to unstable intercuspal contact. Examples of occlusal habits are nail biting, cheek biting, and biting foreign objects such as pencils, pipes, and hairpins. Occlusal habits are often associated with faulty prosthetic appliances. In these cases muscular stabilization with the tongue and other perioral musculature is substituted for the faulty occlusal stabilization.

INFLAMMATORY OR NEOPLASTIC DISPLACEMENT OF THE TEETH. Displacement of the teeth secondary to inflammatory or neoplastic disease calls for a comprehensive diagnosis of occlusal discrepancies, whatever their cause. In many cases the cause is obvious, but in the slower-developing tumors the change in occlusions can be subtle. Information about ICP contact distribution can be very helpful in affected patients; therefore, such data should be collected during the initial periodontal examination.

DENTAL WEAR AND TEAR

Attrition is the term used in English-speaking countries for wear and tear caused by *teeth against teeth*.[51] Such physical wearing patterns may occur on incisal, occlusal, and approximal tooth surfaces. A certain amount of tooth wear is physiologic, but intensified or even pathologic wear may prevail with abnormal anatomic or unusual functional factors. **Abrasion** implies *teeth against foreign substances*—it is the involvement of an extraneous foreign substance independent of masticatory function per se, as in wear from a hard bristle toothbrush, coarse toothpowder, the excessive use of toothpicks, or ritual customs.[51]

Excessive wear may result in obliteration of the cusps and the formation of either a flat or a cupped-out occlusal surface and reversal of the occlusal plane of the premolars and first and second molars (Fig. 27–2). Occlusal wear increases with age and is characterized by a reduction in cusp height and inclination and by the formation of facets. Tooth surfaces worn by attrition are hard, smooth, and shiny (facets), and if dentin is exposed, a yellowish-

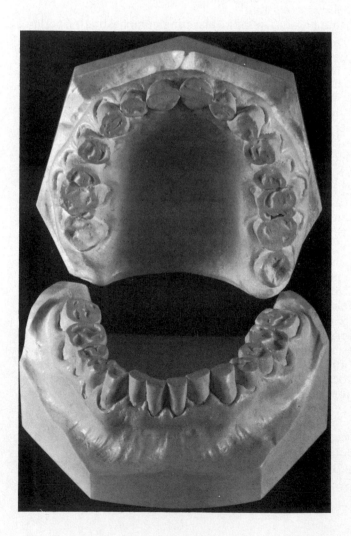

Figure 27–2 Reversed Faciolingual Occlusal Plane (Curve of Pleasure). The normal occlusal plane is sometimes reversed by excessive wear, so that in the mandible the occlusal surfaces slope facially instead of lingually, and in the maxilla they are inclined lingually. The third molars are not usually affected.

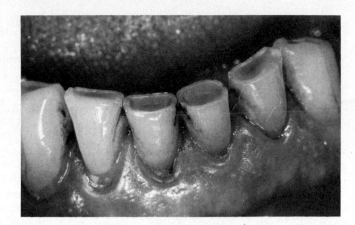

Figure 27–3 Occlusal Wear. Flat, shiny, discolored surfaces produced by occlusal wear.

brown discoloration frequently is present (Fig. 27–3). Facets generally represent occlusal wear from parafunctional tooth contacts such as bruxism and from premature tooth contacts, but may also be produced through mastication.

Facets vary in size and location, depending upon whether they are produced by physiologic or abnormal wear[3, 4, 62] (Fig. 27–4). They have been reported in 98 per cent of adults and in 83 per cent of all teeth examined.[63] Facets are usually not sensitive to thermal and tactile stimulation. Unworn teeth in a mouth with generalized cuspal wear are often sites of premature occlusal contact.

The angle of the facet upon the tooth surface is of potential significance to the periodontium. Horizontal facets tend to direct forces in the vertical axis of the teeth, to which the periodontium can adapt most effectively. *Angular facets direct occlusal forces laterally and increase the risk of periodontal injury.*

Erosion, excluding the idiopathic variety, is unique in being anatomically smooth and clean and in having more or less clear-cut causative factors, such as those related to the digestive system, medicinal therapy, field of occupation (e.g., acid battery workers), and dietary habits (e.g., baking products, citrus fruits, and carbonated drinks). **Idiopathic dental erosion** has long been the subject of much confusion. Some of these cases may be related to **frictional ablation,** a process caused by physical juxtaposition of natural or artificial dental surfaces and hyperfunctional oral soft tissues.[50, 51] Frictional ablation is actually a traumatic activity of the soft tissue against the dentition. It is generated through the vestibular pressures of suction, swallowing, tongue motions, and the intervening forced flow of saliva.[51]

All of the above forms of dental wear exert influences which should be considered in the control and prevention of periodontal disease.

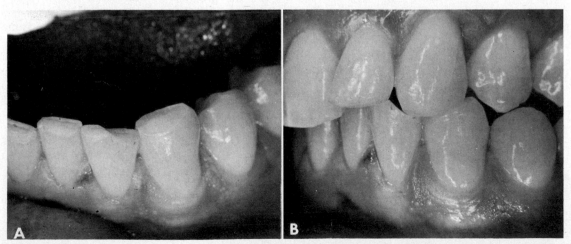

Figure 27–4 Wear Facets. *A,* Flat facets worn on incisal edges of anterior teeth. Note notch on lateral incisor also produced by wear. *B,* Maxillary canine fits into notch on lateral incisor produced by parafunctional mandibular movements.

BRUXISM

Bruxism is the clenching or grinding of the teeth when the individual is not chewing or swallowing.[39] **Clenching** is the continuous or intermittent closure of the jaws under vertical pressure. *Tapping* and *toothsetting* involve repetitive mandibular movement or placement at isolated contact locations. Bruxism often occurs without any neurologic disorders or defects and can be viewed as a phenomenon present in healthy individuals, provided some other factors eliciting this behavior are present.

Most people are not aware of a bruxism habit until it is brought to their attention. Bruxing can be very loud, or it can be silent. Individuals who brux generally begin with the teeth in an ICP.[23] They may also lift the teeth apart and press on a more distant contact. If bruxism involves forceful "tooth grinding" with the production of sounds, accelerated wear develops. Wear from bruxism can be observed as facet patterns. The typical pattern is suggestive of side-to-side movements, but small, asymmetrical retrusive movements or longer movements protrusively along the lingual surfaces of the maxillary anterior teeth are also common.

Little is known about the prevalence of bruxism in normal populations. It has been reported to be as high as 5 to 20 per cent in some populations, with about equal occurrence in men and women.[48, 55] In a clinical population, however, bruxists were more often women.[33] Since nighttime bruxism is likely to be underreported, the prevalence of all bruxism is probably greater.

Etiology

There seems to be a hereditary predisposition to bruxism in certain types of individuals. It has been reported that children of bruxist parents are more apt to be bruxists than children of nonbruxist parents.[1] Olkinuora classified bruxists into two categories: (1) those whose bruxism was associated with stressful events, and (2) those whose bruxism had no such association.[33] He concluded that hereditary bruxism was much more common in the non–stress-related bruxism group. Evaluations from psychometric and health inventories suggest that "stress" bruxists have more muscular symptoms and seem more emotionally disturbed.

Sleep studies[31, 41, 47] have shown that bruxism occurs in any stage of sleep, but mostly in Stage II. Moreover, bruxism is *not* correlated with rapid eye movement (REM) sleep. Satoh and Harada observed that bruxism tended to occur during the transition from a deeper stage of sleep to a lighter stage of sleep.[47] Thus, bruxism was associated with an arousal phenomenon. These investigators were able to elicit bruxism in sleeping subjects with an auditory stimulus.

There are only a few controlled studies of relationships between bruxism and psychologic variables. Bruxism has been considered a multifactorial psychosomatic phenomenon, with individuals displaying "aggressive, controlling, precise, energetic personality types on the one hand (non-stress bruxists) and anxious, tense types on the other (stress bruxists)."[32] It is likely that these psychologic characteristics fall within the normal limits of personality structure.[40] *There is no evidence to suggest that bruxists have personality derangements or are mentally ill.*

The relationship between emotional states and muscle tension appears better understood. Reports have demonstrated that increased masseter muscle tension is directly related to stress situations during the day.[70] One study demonstrated that increased stress levels (as measured by urinary epinephrine content) were strongly correlated with increased levels of masseter muscle activity at night.[9] These studies have consistently shown a strong interrelationship between nonfunctional masseter muscle activity (bruxism) and stress.

Another interesting aspect of bruxism concerns the perception of stress by bruxism patients. One study suggests that those patients with the greatest amount of bruxism have a diminished ability to recognize when they are under stress.[10] This may occur because chronic bruxism subjects are constantly overreacting to stress and therefore cannot determine when it increases. Alternatively, it may be that the bruxism subject simply has never learned to recognize or attend to the physiologic changes which occur in the body during stressful situations.

Attempts to demonstrate the relationship between stress and bruxism in the natural environment have involved the use of portable electromyographic recording devices. The recordings indicate that bruxist behavior may vary greatly from night to night and is correlated with the previous day's stress level (Fig. 27–5).[44] Overall, it may be concluded that mental strain and predisposing oral factors may act together to produce bruxism.[31]

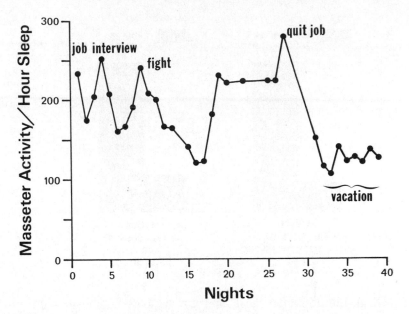

Figure 27–5 Electromyographic Data Collected on Bruxism Patient. Nocturnal electromyographic recordings indicate that bruxist behavior may vary greatly from night to night and is correlated with the previous day's stress level. (From Rugh, J. D., and Solberg, W. K.: Oral Sci. Rev., *1*:3, 1976.)

Not enough is known to say conclusively whether occlusal factors are a direct cause of bruxism. It has been suggested that occlusal malrelationships or interferences may precipitate bruxism when combined with nervous tension.[48] In one study, bite splint therapy significantly reduced bruxism levels while the splints were worn, but bruxism returned to previous levels after splint removal.[54] Continuing investigations indicate that the response of bruxism subjects to occlusal therapy is likely to be variable.

Effects of Bruxism Habits

Although bruxism is widespread, it need not be pathologic. Indeed, bruxism can be compatible with states of normal function. In bruxism, the muscles move the mandible over tooth contacts where there is a potential for large forces. Most subjects brux by just playing on the teeth, without much forceful contraction. However, under general neuromuscular tension, increased tooth contact pressure will result. Over an extended period, this pressure may exceed the threshold of the periodontal pressor-receptors, and the patient will no longer be aware of increased muscle activity.[23] The muscles involved will be unable to relax, resulting in fatigue, tenderness, and limited opening of the mouth (Fig. 27–6).

When muscles contract *isometrically* they are stressed to a greater degree than during *isotonic* contraction. This stress is even worse when the muscle is lengthened while it is

contracting tension, as in lateral disclosing movements. As a habit, bruxism takes on further significance because as the response strengthens the likelihood of functional disorders increases. The mechanism for the pain and tenderness is likely to be ischemic.[29] Bruxism can be especially harmful if the threshold of resistance is lowered by persistent neuromuscular tension or structural weakness from previous pathology.

Treatment of Bruxism

Bruxism* is common, but not all patients with the habit are necessarily injured by it. Those who are suffer from microtrauma in the periodontium, musculature,[6–8, 30] and temporomandibular joints. Occlusal prematurities, excessive muscle tension, and emotional factors, singly or together, are the accepted causes of bruxism, but opinions differ as to which is the primary or most critical factor.

There are three general modalities by which the patient with bruxism can be treated. The **behavioral modality** is initiated by the dentist through *explanation* and *arousal* of the patient to the habit. Specific behavioral therapies such as biofeedback, hypnosis, and negative practice may be prescribed.[43] The **emotional modality** may be initiated in the form of psychologic guidance.[30, 45, 49, 57] The **interceptive modality** consists of prescribing a bite guard appliance (maxillary stabilization splint) to

---

*Includes clamping and clenching habits.

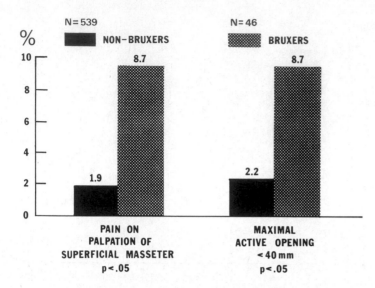

Figure 27–6 Prevalence of Masseter Muscle Tenderness and Limited Opening in Bruxers and Nonbruxers (young adult non patient population). There was a significant association between bruxism and these symptoms. (From Solberg, W. K., Woo, M., and Houston, J. B.: J. Am. Dent. Assoc., *98*:25, 1979.)

protect the tooth surfaces and to dissipate forces built up in the musculoskeletal system through bruxism.[35] There is evidence that these appliances effect a significant decrease in the bruxism habit of some individuals.[54] In application, the bite guard is more practical for treating *nocturnal* bruxism than daytime clenching habits.

Occlusal adjustment plays a role in treating bruxism when prematurities are obvious, especially when they occur in connection with recently placed dental restorations. More invasive occlusal alterations, in the form of reconstruction or orthodontic treatment, are sometimes necessary.

Occlusal therapies, even when combined with psychologic guidance and behavioral therapies, may not be effective in all patients. In unresponsive patients bite guards become more significant in the management of the destructive effects of bruxism.

TEMPOROMANDIBULAR PAIN AND DYSFUNCTION

Temporomandibular (TM) disorders are characterized by **impaired function** *and* **pain.** At present, there is agreement that the definitional symptoms include one or more of the following: (1) **pain and tenderness** in the region of the muscles of mastication and temporomandibular joints, (2) **sounds** during condyle movement, and (3) **limitation** of mandibular movement.[11, 15, 44, 54, 71] Recurrent headache appears to merit consideration as a symptom because of its demonstrated association with TM disorders.[26] The symptom complex defined

above is the musculoskeletal component of a larger group of microtraumatic signs and symptoms, all of which are manifestations of generalized injury-producing activity called dysfunction (occlusal traumatism).[44]

The term *myofascial pain-dysfunction (MPD) syndrome* has been advocated to identify a subgroup of temporomandibular joint pain and dysfunction.[24] The criteria for inclusion in this subgroup are the triad of symptoms listed above along with the following negative characteristics: (1) absence of clinical or radiographic evidence of organic changes in the temporomandibular joints, and (2) lack of tenderness in the temporomandibular joint when this area is palpated in the external auditory meatus.

The term "syndrome" may be a misnomer, because the symptoms are more apt to be sequential than concurrent, as in the classic syndromes. The usual sequence of temporomandibular pain and dysfunction is clicking and incoordination followed by acute pain and/or locking at two finger breadths of opening. Limitation and chronic pain are the final complications. Syndromes classically have a specific etiology; most evidence suggests that temporomandibular pain and dysfunction are multicausal.

Temporomandibular disorders may not be a specific entity, even though patients may display similar symptoms.[16, 27, 44] Therefore, the tendency to lump all "TMJ patients" into one group should be avoided. *Careful examination and analysis of patients with temporomandibular pain and dysfunction will reveal that the origin of most complaints can be found in one or more of the following areas:* (1) within the temporomandibular joints, (2) within the masticatory muscles, and (3) from the neck (referred pain). Individual emotional factors can add an additional diagnostic dimension concerning the development and/or persistence of temporomandibular pain and dysfunction.[44]

Clinical Features

The most common causes of *jaw restriction* are intracapsular derangement,[20] capsular contracture and adhesions,[59] muscle spasms, and bony impingement. Therefore, the examiner must attempt to develop a differential diagnosis. Intracapsular restriction usually affects only the sliding function of the condyle. Therefore, most patients with temporomandibular joint problems will be able to hinge their jaws at least two finger breadths (26 mm). If the active mouth opening is greater than 35 mm, there is increasing likelihood that the problem is mainly muscular in origin, rather than due to intracapsular restriction. Movement in which full rotation of the condyles (26 mm) is prevented suggests restriction from the temporalis and masseter muscles.

Joint sounds occur as *clicking* (popping, snapping) or *crepitus* (grating). Clicking may be produced by disc displacements influenced by muscular disharmony and a compromised integrity of the disc. The disc may be in a persistent prolapsed relationship at the closed position, which is characteristically identified by clicks on opening and closing. The clicking sound is produced as the condyle bumps over the thickened posterior border of the articular disc on opening and, in closing, as the disc and condyle destabilize to the prolapsed disc relationship.[1] Failure of this disc-condyle relationship to self-reduce results in an abrupt limitation of jaw motion (at about 26 to 30 mm), termed *locking*. The thickening and flattening process of these changes probably causes a binding effect during condyle translation (through the mechanism of overstretching the lateral ligament).

Pain from temporomandibular disorders may be limited to the preauricular area, or it may radiate to the jaw, teeth, temples, and ear. The symptoms are usually unilateral, but the unaffected joint is progressively affected. The pain may be constant or recurrent. It is usually precipitated by movement of the mandible; this is the hallmark of the TM disorder. It may be elicited by digital pressure on the muscle or the capsular structures. Tenderness experienced during joint palpation via the external auditory meatus can be considered capsular pain as opposed to muscular tenderness palpated elsewhere. Painless limitation of joint movement does occur, but infrequently. *Pain referred to the ear and face from the cervical muscles often complicates the clinical picture of temporomandibular pain.*

Prevalence

The vast majority (70 to 90 per cent) of patients with temporomandibular pain and dysfunction are women between the ages of 20 and 40.[13] Symptoms of dysfunction are very common in otherwise normal populations. Several studies of normal populations have demonstrated that levels of signs and symptoms approach 25 to 50 per cent.[18] Five per cent of the total patient population of a dental school were treated for temporomandibular joint disorders,[19] suggesting a significant prevalence of this problem among dental patients.

Etiology

Conclusive evidence that there is one major cause for temporomandibular joint disorders is absent, even though there are abundant claims to the contrary. The symptoms reported by any one patient develop from a unique set of psychologic, structural, and functional factors. Weakness or instability in gnathic structure which makes an individual unusually susceptible to temporomandibular joint dysfunction may be inherited, developmental, the result of prior injury, or the result of poor restoration of the occlusion. The possibility that an occlusal interference may activate bruxism cannot be overlooked. It is possible that occlusal interferences as well as traumatic or extensive dental work may focus the subject's attention on the mouth and jaws, making these a vulnerable potential outlet for emotional tension. *The following factors are thought to be the most significant in the multicausal etiology of temporomandibular pain and dysfunction:*

MACROTRAUMA. *Macrotrauma is a sudden exterior force with subsequent reflex contraction of muscle.* External blows to the jaws or whiplash injuries are frequently elicited in the history. Macrotrauma frequently leads to a compromised posterior attachment of the disc and is followed by suboptimal healing of the tissues. Unguarded or excessive forces on the temporomandibular joints during dental procedures are frequently associated with the onset of clinical symptoms. Overstretching or prolonged opening can be macrotraumatic, especially for the individual with incipient dysfunction.

MICROTRAUMA. *Microtrauma is a continuing or repetitive mechanical stress.* In this process, muscle tonus can be abnormally increased by an interplay of emotional tension, pain, and occlusal interferences.[38] Even the normal forces of function can cause microtrauma in cases of disturbed occlusal support and guidance.

DEGENERATIVE JOINT DISEASE. Deviations in joint contours and lesions of the articular surfaces disturb articular and synovial function and can be associated with production of joint symptoms. The temporomandibular joint is not an uncommon site of focus if the individual is afflicted by rheumatoid arthritis.[5]

EMOTIONAL TENSION. Evidence indicates that emotional factors may play a significant role in the etiology of temporomandibular disorders.[44] Emotional states such as anxiety, frustration, fear, and anger cause increased activity in the masticatory muscles, thereby causing prolonged muscle tension and symptoms characteristic of temporomandibular pain and dysfunction.

Treatment of Temporomandibular Joint Disorders

Except for conditions caused by other recognizable joint[46] and myofascial diseases, **temporomandibular pain and dysfunction can usually be treated by allowing normalization of what is essentially an acute or poorly healed traumatic injury.** The notion that most temporomandibular joint disorders are caused solely by occlusal factors should be viewed with caution. The probability that a given patient will present with dysfunctional symptoms is clearly dependent upon a staggering number of factors, many of which are not well understood. The one cause–one disease–one treatment concept must therefore be discarded in favor of the more applicable polytherapeutic concept (i.e., several therapeutic factors act upon an organ system at the same time).[44] *It should be realized that some affected patients will not get well despite the use of treatments that have been successful for others.* This is especially true in patients with long-standing pain. Chronic pain associated with temporomandibular joint disorders eventually complicates management and can potentiate emo-

tional disturbances and untoward behavioral changes in some individuals. In effect, these patients will continue to have intermittent or chronic musculoskeletal rheumatism. For these patients, data gathering and patient monitoring techniques take on added importance, as does the need to attain a practical end point in therapy.[56]

Clinical History and Examination

The *history* should focus on the categorical complaints seen in temporomandibular pain and dysfunction: (1) **decreased mobility of the mandible,** (2) **joint incoordination,** and (3) **muscle and joint pain.** The relationship of these symptoms to macrotrauma, dental treatment, or bruxism should be noted. Symptoms aggravated by emotional stress are significant.[25] Preauricular pain is characteristic of periarticular problems, whereas masseter pain is more apt to be associated with bruxism.

Muscle and joint function is examined first; then these findings are correlated with features of the occlusion.[23, 52] *Mouth opening* is meas-

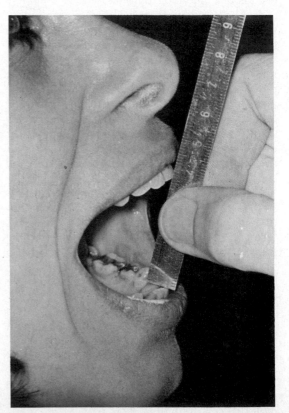

Figure 27–7 Maximum Mouth Opening Measured Interincisally. Less than 40 mm is considered abnormal. (From Clark, J. [ed.]: Clinical Dentistry. Vol. 2, Chapter 35. New York: Harper & Row, 1976.)

ured (less than 40 mm, abnormal range[2]), and the path of opening is observed (Fig. 27–7). Protrusive and lateral test excursions are made (less than 8 mm, abnormal range[2]). If the mandible deviates to the side of the painful joint, malfunction of the muscles or condyle on that side may be responsible. Preauricular pain when the mandible is moved to the contralateral side could be caused by inflammation of the temporomandibular joint or the lateral pterygoid muscle. If the mandible deviates to the side opposite the painful joint, malfunction of the medial pterygoid may be the cause. Simultaneous shortening of the masseter and medial pterygoid on the same side restricts mandibular movement without deflection. In evaluating *joint incoordination*, the forefingers are placed *lightly* over the joint area, and an attempt is made to detect clicking or crepitation (grating) on opening and closing of the

mouth. These two sounds do not have the same clinical significance and should be differentiated. Clicking is symptomatic of a destabilized disc-condyle complex having more to do with soft tissue conditions than with bony changes. Crepitation is correlated with osteoarthritis.[52] Early clicks on opening are more clinically significant than clicks at full mouth opening, which are more easily treated by avoidance. Early, reciprocal clicks (those occurring repeatedly on opening and closing) are associated with anterior disc displacement. Closed locking is a form of unresolved disc displacement and may also result from adhesions within the joints.

In testing for *tenderness,* the temporomandibular joints are palpated bimanually with point pressure on the lateral and dorsal (posterior) aspects of the joint capsule (Fig. 27–8). Posterior tenderness (Fig. 27–8A) suggests

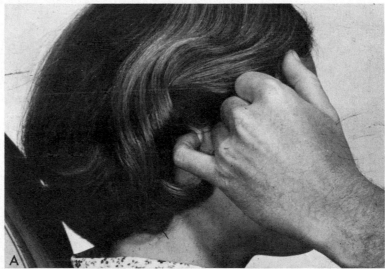

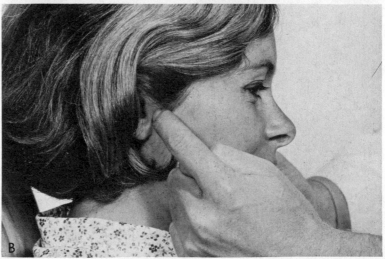

Figure 27–8. *A,* Posterior capsular tenderness suggests that **periarticular inflammation** is present. *B,* Lateral tenderness may be temporomandibular joint inflammation or may result from the lateral pterygoid muscle spasm. (*From* Clark, J. [ed.]: Clinical Dentistry. Vol. 2, Chapter 35. New York: Harper & Row, 1976.)

periarticular inflammation. The masticatory muscles generally are palpated near their musculotendinous junctions. The posterior cervical, trapezius, and sternocleidomastoid muscles are included in the muscle palpation, as these muscles refer pain to the ear, temporomandibular joint, and head.[61] It is helpful if a diagram is used (Fig. 27–9) to chart tenderness.

The main feature of the occlusal examination should involve testing the zones of *ICP contact, occlusal instability,* or *bite collapse* and *asymmetrical relationships between RCP and ICP.* Interferences disturbing free and smooth gliding contact movement should also be identified, in addition to gross features involving occlusal plane, overjet, and overbite. An effort should be made to detect active facet patterns caused by bruxism.

Radiographic Examination

Radiographs of the joints are useful but show only the position and structure of the subchondral bony parts. Since many of the problems of clinical temporomandibular pain and dysfunction involve noncalcified tissues of the joint, radiographs are not conclusive. Indeed, most radiographs of patients with temporomandibular pain and dysfunction appear remarkably normal. There are many special techniques for joint radiographs.[12, 42, 64] Panoramic projections (e.g., Panorex) are useful for identifying gross pathologic conditions of

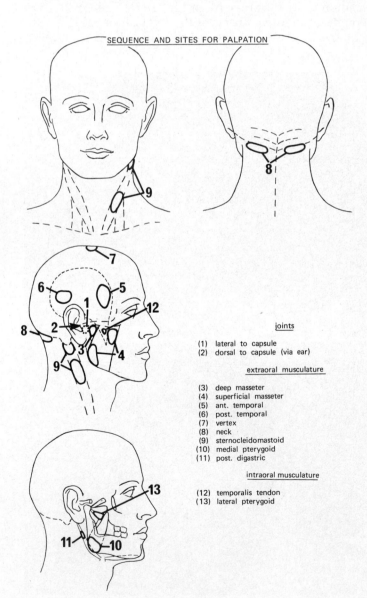

SEQUENCE AND SITES FOR PALPATION

joints

(1) lateral to capsule
(2) dorsal to capsule (via ear)

extraoral musculature

(3) deep masseter
(4) superficial masseter
(5) ant. temporal
(6) post. temporal
(7) vertex
(8) neck
(9) sternocleidomastoid
(10) medial pterygoid
(11) post. digastric

intraoral musculature

(12) temporalis tendon
(13) lateral pterygoid

Figure 27–9 Suggested Areas for Muscle and Joint Palpation.

the condyle. The lateral oblique transcranial projections[34] are the most common projections taken on the temporomandibular joints. Tomography,[12, 21, 34] however, is most reliable for detecting changes in structure and condyle position. Lateral views of the temporomandibular joints are best obtained with the teeth fully together and at maximum jaw opening. Frontal tomograms taken with the jaw protruded contribute greatly to the descriptive process.

Osteoarthritis (degenerative joint disease) of the temporomandibular joints most often involves the articulating surface of the temporal bone and the articular disc. Remodeling (deviation in form) is most common in the condyle.[17] For this reason, radiographic changes (flattening and lipping) seen in the condyle do not necessarily imply the condition of osteoarthritis.[17] Asymmetrical condyle-fossa

TABLE 27–1 CONDITIONS COMMONLY ENCOUNTERED IN PATIENTS WITH FACIAL PAIN AND MANDIBULAR DYSFUNCTION*

I. Traumatic and Degenerative Disorders
A. *Temporomandibular Joints*
1. Traumatic derangement (clicking, subluxation, and closed locking)
2. Traumatic capsulitis (pain, contracture, no history of clicking or locking)
3. Degenerative joint disease (crepitation)
4. Open dislocation (luxation)
5. Fibrosis
B. *Myofascial Structures*
1. Myofascitis (interstitial myofibrosis)
(a) Latent myofascial tenderness
(b) Active myofascial trigger points and referred pain
(1) masticatory muscles
(2) neck muscles
2. Contracture (fibrosis, mechanical shortening)
3. Dyskinesia (weakness, incoordination)
4. Muscle spasm (acute muscle splinting)
C. *Oro-dental Structures*
1. Accelerated tooth wear, uncontrolled migration of teeth
2. Trauma from occlusion
3. Trauma to the lips, cheeks, and tongue.
II. Atypical (Idiopathic) Symptoms Affecting the Head and Neck
A. *Chronic facial pain (emotional and behavior problems prominent)*
B. *Positive occlusal sense (uncomfortable bite)*
C. *Atypical facial neuralgias*
III. Arthritis
A. *Polyarthritis (rheumatoid arthritis)*
B. *Infectious*
C. *Other*

*Does not include pathologic entities such as cranial nerve neuralgias, organ-related disease (sinuses, ears), regional tumors, headache (vascular, migraine), fracture, or bony impingement.

relationships are frequently associated with clinical temporomandibular joint dysfunction.[28, 66] Some clinicians treat these condyle malrelationships by altering the mandibular occlusal position.[65] Frequently, this is accomplished by means of a repositioning splint.

Arthrography of the temporomandibular joint has been employed as a means of identifying disorders of the articular disc.[67] In this technique, a radiopaque contrast medium is injected into the upper and lower joint compartments, allowing visualization of the articular parts. Perforation, hyperplasia, and anterior displacements are the most common findings reported from arthrographic investigations.[67] Clinically, these conditions have been associated with clicking, subluxation, and closed locking. Investigations of several aspects of temporomandibular joint conditions suggest that intracapsular pathology is more common in patients with "TMJ syndrome" than previously thought.

Diagnosis

Diagnosis of temporomandibular pain and dysfunction includes the delineation of potential problems within the *temporomandibular joints* and the *masticatory muscles* and *referred pain from the neck muscles*. Conditions commonly encountered in patients with facial pain and mandibular dysfunction are categorized in Table 27–1.

Subluxation of the Temporomandibular Joint

It is within the normal range for the condyle to move anterior to the articular eminence. However, if the condyle becomes momentarily locked open in this position, the condition is referred to as subluxation or, when persistent, open dislocation (luxation). Subluxation of the mandible is self-reducing, incomplete dislocation of the temporomandibular articulation. Acute trauma, previous dislocation of the mandible, or excessive manipulation of the jaw during a dental procedure may cause abnormal looseness of the capsule and recurrent subluxation or luxation. Reduction of acute dislocation of the mandible often may be accomplished by applying downward pressure on the mandibular buccal shelf while applying upward pressure under the chin. Unresolved cases may be relieved by local anesthetics, immobilization, or surgical arthroplasty.

Treatment

Conservative treatment of temporomandibular and myofascial pain is formulated using the three-part conceptual treatment program outlined in Table 27–2. Overall, **this program aims at eliminating abnormal function and does no more than provide conditions favorable for the normal processes of repair and resolution.** Using this system, the best prognosis can be given when treatment is started before irreversible pathologic changes have occurred in the musculoskeletal or dental structures. The three-part treatment is an approach of *escalation,* which begins with generalized therapy, mobilization techniques, and removable splints. Temporomandibular joint surgery, intracapsular injections, or irreversible "spot grinding," intended as a quick solution to temporomandibular pain and dysfunction, can result in unnecessary problems and generally should be considered only after conservative, reversible therapy has been attempted.

PART 1. NEUTRALIZING SELF-DESTRUCTIVE BEHAVIOR. *Undoubtedly, the most important and universal treatment for controlling temporomandibular pain and dysfunction is some form of arousal and behavior modification.*[44] The patient is made aware of excessive and inappropriate oral habits. This orientation sets the stage for the patient to relearn specific behavior that will allow the tissues to normalize. The axis-opening exercise is the basis for retraining or relearning mandibular movements.[68] This exercise involves making symmetrical opening and closing movements with the jaw in a centered hinge position. When appropriate, ample time should be taken to discuss the role of emotional stress in creating muscle tension in the gnathic system. In so doing, the dentist demonstrates that healing and health maintenance depend upon the patient's input and willingness to participate actively in the therapy process. Diazepam (Valium) may be prescribed to induce muscle relaxation and decrease anxiety. The dosage should be individualized (2 to 10 mg two to four times per day) and prescribed for short durations.

PART 2. MOBILIZATION. Many physical modalities have a beneficial effect on abnormal muscular and capsular tissues, e.g., heat, cold, medications, electrostimulation, acupuncture, and vapocoolant sprays. Even though these modalities soothe the muscles and joints, they do not give physiologic restoration of function and therefore are not sufficient in themselves.[53, 61] *Therapeutic mobilization is the key to restoring and perpetuating normal musculoskeletal function.* The *spray-stretch technique*[60] is a common method for mobilization of muscles and joints. Fluori-Methane* is sprayed on the skin over the tender area, resulting in momentary desensitization of muscles and joints (Fig. 27–10). During this period the jaws are actively or passively stretched to gain increased opening. The rationale of this technique is that muscles brought to their physiologic resting length will cease to be painful. Continuous joint and muscle pains are relieved at home by applying moist heat, by means of a towel soaked in hot water, for 15 minutes two or three times a day. Prescribed retraining exercises or gentle range-of-motion stretching

*Gebauer Chemical Company, Cleveland, Ohio 44104.

TABLE 27–2   TEMPOROMANDIBULAR AND MYOFASCIAL DISORDERS: THREE-PART TREATMENT PROGRAM

	Problem	Treatment Goal
1. Neutralization	a. Abrupt condyle translation	Prescribed condyle rotation
	b. Neuromuscular tension	Graded relaxation; coordinated motion
	c. Chronic overuse	Neutralization of habits
2. Mobilization	a. Myofascial referred pain (active trigger points) Muscles shortened	Desensitize trigger points; stretch muscles to physiologic resting length
	b. Inelastic muscles and capsular tissues	Range-of-motion exercises
	c. Uncoordinated movement	Symmetrical coordinated motion
	d. Weakened muscles	Prescribe strengthening exercises
*3. Stabilization**	a. Muscular stabilization	Occlusal stabilization
	b. Asymmetrical joint relationships	Symmetrical condylar relationships
	c. Disturbed closure	One functional end-point of closure

*Axial tomographic radiographs may reveal obvious condyle malpositioning. Decision to reposition condyle(s) by altering normal intercuspal closure position on splint may be made immediately or following evaluation of standard splint therapy. This type of splint is termed a *repositioning splint.*

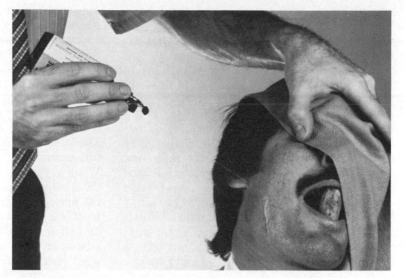

Figure 27–10 Fluori-Methane spray is used to desensitize the skin and underlying muscle trigger points temporarily. Following application, the muscles are stretched.

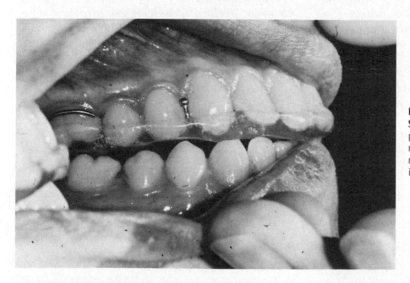

Figure 27–11 Removable Full-Arch Stabilization Splint used for bruxism patients and patients with temporomandibular joint disorders. The splint may be constructed for either the maxillary or the mandibular arch.

Figure 27–12 The Occlusal Contact Scheme Established for the Maxillary Full-Arch Stabilization Splint. Large black dots denote posterior vertical stops of positive contact in the intercuspal position. Dotted lines denote light incisal contact. Clear areas are the pathways of protrusive and lateral guidance. Note that there is freedom from lateral or protrusive posterior contact. If heavy lateral and protrusive facets are observed at the follow-up visit, these areas should be reduced. Wrought-wire ball clasps (between canines and premolars) and retentive arms (molars) are used to aid retention.

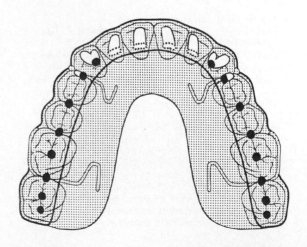

should follow the application of moist heat. With recovery, the muscles should be exercised under light to moderate loads (resistance exercises). The chief cause of failure of the correct spray-stretch procedure is inability to secure full muscle length because of subordination of the reflex mechanisms of trigger point pain to fibrosis or some other pathologic condition of the temporomandibular joint.

PART 3. STABILIZATION. The majority of patients with temporomandibular pain and dysfunction are helped by removable full-arch maxillary stabilization splints (Fig. 27–11). The purpose of the splint is threefold: (1) to allow the muscles of mastication to function without spasm at their proper physiologic length from origin to insertion; (2) to allow normalization of temporomandibular joint derangements, particularly those related to disc-condyle malrelationships and synovitis; and (3) to achieve a precise functional end point of closure compatible with joint and occlusal harmony. The occlusal criteria for splinting are summarized in Table 27–3. The prescribed contact scheme is shown in Figure 27–12.

Occlusal adjustment without prior splint therapy is performed only when an obvious connection can be made between the symptoms and recent occlusal changes (e.g., dental treatment, tooth migration). If initial occlusal adjustment is done, the patient should be warned of the possibility that a removable splint may be necessary at a later date.

The splint is placed and carefully adjusted according to the criteria listed in Table 27–3. The patient is instructed to wear the splint constantly, day and night, even when eating. The patient is seen at 2- or 3-week intervals for evaluation and adjustment of the splint. When symptoms disappear, an evaluation of the occlusion will reveal discrepancies from the musculoskeletal readjustment. The dentist must use judgment in determining: (1) whether immediate permanent occlusal adjustment is advisable, (2) whether the splint should be worn indefinitely at night, or (3) whether the splint therapy should be stopped with no occlusal change. To repeat, *occlusal therapy following splint therapy is not mandatory unless clear-cut occlusal problems are evident.*[69] The evident multifactorial causes for temporomandibular pain and dysfunction argue against such dogmatic treatment procedures.[44]

TABLE 27–3 CRITERIA FOR MAXILLARY STABILIZATION SPLINT*

Occlusal Criteria
1. *Appliance:* stable.
2. *RCP, ICP:* stable, multi-pointed, widely distributed contacts.
3. *ICP:* posterior vertical stops in firm contact; incisor teeth in slight infracontact.
4. *RCP–ICP relationship:* RCP and ICP in same sagittal plane; ICP and RCP are nearly identical.
5. Smooth gliding contact in all excursions (incisal and/or canine disclusion optional).
6. *MCP:* stable, repeatable.

Technique for Verification of Criteria

Criterion 1 (Split Stability)	No hint of movement to tipping forces.
Criterion 2 (RCP)	Red inked ribbon on dry surface.
Criterion 3 (Vertical Stops)	Mylar strips held firmly by telling subject, "Close your back teeth, both sides at the same time."
Criterion 4 (RCP–ICP)	No slide from RCP to ICP.
Criterion 5 (Guidance)	Use full arch red-blue paper. Mark excursion in RED, then vertical stops in BLUE.
Criterion 6 (MCP)	"Solid" MCP tapping by patient in upright position; patient verifies "even" contact.

*RCP = retruded contact position; ICP = intercuspal position; MCP = muscular contact position.

REFERENCES

1. Abe, K., and Shimakawa, M.: Genetic and developmental aspects of sleeptalking and teeth-grinding. Acta Paedopsychiatr., *33*:336, 1966.
2. Agerberg, G.: On Mandibular Dysfunction and Mobility. Umea University Odontological Dissertation. Abstract No. 3, 1974.
3. Arstad, T.: The Capsular Ligaments of the Temporomandibular Joint and Retrusion Facets of the Dentition in Relationship to Mandibular Movements. Oslo, Academisk Forlag, 1954.
4. Beyron, H. L.: Occlusal changes in the adult dentition. J. Am. Dent. Assoc., *48*:674, 1954.
5. Chalmers, I. M., and Blair, G. S.: Rheumatoid arthritis of the temporomandibular joint. Q. J. Med., *42*:369, 1973.
6. Christensen, L. V.: Facial pain from the masticatory system induced by experimental bruxism. Tandlaegebladet, *71*:1171, 1967.
7. Christensen, L. V.: Facial pain from experimental tooth clenching. Tandlaegebladet, *74*:175, 1970.
8. Christensen, L. V.: Facial pain in negative and positive work of human jaw muscles. Scand. J. Dent. Res., *84*:327, 1976.
9. Clark, G. T.: The relationship between stress, nocturnal masseter muscle activity and symptoms of masticatory dysfunction. Master's thesis, University of Rochester, 1977.
10. Clark, G. T., et al.: Stress perception and nocturnal masseter muscle activity. Int. Assoc. Dent. Res. Prog., Abstract No. 436, 1977.
11. DeBoever, J. A.: Functional disturbances of the temporomandibular joints. Oral Sci. Rev., *2*:100, 1973.
12. Eckerdal, O.: Tomography of the temporomandibular joint. Acta Radiol., 1(Suppl.):329, 1973.
13. Franks, A. S.: The social character of temporomandibular joint dysfunction. Dent. Practit. Dent. Rec., *15*:94, 1964.
14. Funakoshi, M., Fujita, N., and Takehana, S.: Relations between occlusal interference and jaw muscle activities in responses to changes in head position. J. Dent. Res., *55*:684, 1976.

15. Greene, C. S., and Laskin, D. M.: Splint therapy for the myofascial pain-dysfunction (MPD) syndrome: a comparative study. J. Am. Dent. Assoc., *84*:624, 1972.

16. Greene, C. S., Lerman, M. D., Sutcher, H. D., and Laskin, D. M.: The TMJ pain-dysfunction syndrome: heterogeneity of the patient population. J. Am. Dent. Assoc., *79*:1168, 1969.

17. Hansson, T.: Temporomandibular Joint Changes: Occurrence and Development. Dissertation. University of Lund, 1977.

18. Helkimo, M.: Epidemiological surveys of dysfunction of the masticatory system. Oral Sci. Rev., *1*:54, 1976.

19. Helöe, B., and Helöe, L. A.: Characteristics of a group of patients with temporomandibular joint disorders. Community Dent. Oral Epidemiol., *3*:72, 1975.

20. Ireland, V. E.: The problem of the clicking jaw. R. Soc. Med., *44*:363, 1951.

21. Klein, I. E., Blatterfein, L., and Miglino, J. C.: Comparison of the fidelity of radiographs of mandibular condyles made by different techniques. J. Prosthet. Dent., *24*:419, 1970.

22. Kloprogge, M. J., and van Griethuysen, A. M.: Disturbances in contraction and coordination pattern of the masticatory muscles due to dental restoration. J. Oral Rehabil., *3*:207, 1976.

23. Krogh-Poulsen, W. G., and Olsson, A.: Management of the occlusion of the teeth. *In* Schwartz, L., and Chayes, C. (eds.): Facial Pain and Mandibular Dysfunction. Philadelphia, W. B. Saunders Company, 1968.

24. Laskin, D. M.: Etiology of the pain-dysfunction syndrome. J. Am. Dent. Assoc., *79*:148, 1969.

25. Lupton, D.: Psychological aspects of temporomandibular joint dysfunction. J. Am. Dent. Assoc., *79*:131, 1969.

26. Magnusson, T., and Carlsson, G. E.: Comparison between two groups of patients in respect of headache and mandibular dysfunction. Swed. Dent. J. *2*:85, 1978.

27. Marbach, J. J.: Arthritis of the temporomandibular joints and facial pain. Bull. Rheum. Dis., *27*:918, 1977.

28. Marcovic, M. A., and Rosenberg, H. M.: Tomographic evaluation of 100 patients with temporomandibular joint symptoms. Oral Surg., *42*:838, 1976.

29. Møller, E.: The myogenic factor in headache and facial pain. *In* Kawzmura, Y., and Dubner, R. (eds.): Oral-Facial Sensory and Motor Functions. Tokyo, Quintessence, 1982, p. 225.

30. Nadler, S.: The importance of bruxism. J. Oral Med., *23*:142, 1968.

31. Olkinuora, M.: Bruxism as a psychosomatic phenomenon. Academic dissertation. Forssan Kirjapaino Oy-Forssa. Helsinki, 1972.

32. Olkinuora, M.: Psychosocial aspects in a series of bruxists compared with a group of non-bruxists. Proc. Finn. Dent. Soc., *68*:200, 1972.

33. Olkinuora, M.: A psychosomatic study of bruxism with emphasis on mental strain and familial predisposition factors. Proc. Finn. Dent. Soc., *68*:110, 1972.

34. Omnell, K.-A., and Petersson, A.: Radiography of the temporomandibular joint utilizing oblique lateral transcranial projection. Odont. Rev., *27*:77, 1976.

35. Posselt, V., and Wolff, I. B.: Treatment of bruxism by bite guards and bite plates. J. Can. Dent. Assoc., *29*:773, 1963.

36. Pruzansky, S.: Applicability of electromyographic procedures as a clinical aid in the detection of occlusal disharmony. Dent. Clin. North Am., *4*:117, 1960.

37. Ramfjord, S. P.: Bruxism, a clinical and electromyographic study. J. Am. Dent. Assoc., *62*:21, 1961.

38. Ramfjord, S. P., and Ash, M. M., Jr.: Occlusion. 2nd ed. Philadelphia, W. B. Saunders Company, 1971.

39. Ramfjord, S. P., Kerr, D. A., and Ash, M. M.: World Workshop in Periodontics. Ann Arbor, University of Michigan Press, 1966.

40. Reding, G., Zrpelin, H., and Monroe, L.: Personality study of nocturnal tooth grinders. Percept. Mot. Skills, *26*:523, 1960.

41. Reding, G., et al.: Sleep pattern of bruxism: revision. Psychophysiology, *4*:396, 1967–1968.

42. Ricketts, R. M.: Laminagraphy in the diagnosis of temporomandibular joint disorders. J. Am. Dent. Assoc., *46*:620, 1953.

43. Rugh, J. D., and Solberg, W. K.: Electromyographic evalua-

44. Rugh, J. D., and Solberg, W. K.: Psychological implications in temporomandibular pain and dysfunction. Oral Sci. Rev., *1*:3, 1976.

45. Sadowsky C., and BeGole, E. A.: Long-term effects of orthodontic treatment on periodontal health. Am. J. Orthod., *80*(2):156, 1981.

46. Sarnat, B. G., and Laskin, D. M.: Diagnosis and surgical management of diseases of the temporomandibular joint. Springfield, Ill.: Charles C Thomas, 1962.

47. Satoh, T., and Harada, Y.: Tooth grinding during sleep as an arousal reaction. Experientia, *27*:785, 1971.

48. Schärer, P.: Bruxism. Front. Oral Physiol., *1*:293, 1974.

49. Shapiro, S., and Shannon, J.: Bruxism—as an emotional reactive disturbance. Psychosomatics, *6*:427, 1965.

50. Sognnaes, R.: Frictional ablation—a neglected factor in the mechanisms of hard tissue destruction? *In* Kuhlencordt, F., and Kruse, H. P. (eds.): Calcium Metabolism, Bone and Metabolic Bone Diseases. Berlin, Springer-Verlag, 1975.

51. Sognnaes, R.: Periodontal significance of intraoral frictional ablation. J. Western Soc. Periodontol., *25*:112, 1977.

52. Solberg, W. K.: Occlusion related pathosis and its clinical evaluation. *In* Clark, J. (ed.): Clinical Dentistry. Hagerstown, Md.: Harper & Row, 1976, vol. 2, chap. 35.

53. Solberg, W. K.: Myofascial pain and dysfunction. *In* Clark, J. (ed.): Clinical Dentistry. Hagerstown, Md.: Harper & Row, 1976, vol. 2, chap. 37.

54. Solberg, W. K., Clark, G. T., and Rugh, J. D.: Nocturnal electromyographic evaluation of bruxism patients undergoing short term splint therapy. J. Oral Rehabil., *2*:215, 1975.

55. Solberg, W. K., Woo, M., and Houston, J. B.: Prevalence of mandibular dysfunction in young adults. J. Am. Dent. Assoc., *98*:25, 1979.

56. Taylor, R. C., Ware, W. H., and Horowitz, M. J.: The importance of determining the end point in treatment of patients with temporomandibular joint syndrome. J. Oral Med., *22*:3, 1967.

57. Thaller, J. L., Rosen, G., and Saltzman, S.: Study of the relationship of frustration and anxiety to bruxism. J. Periodontol., *38*:193, 1967.

58. Thielemann, K.: Biomechanik der Paradentose ins besondere Artikulationsausgleich durch Einschleifen. 2nd ed. Munchen, Barth, 1956.

59. Toller, P. A.: The synovial apparatus and temporomandibular joint function. Br. Dent. J., *111*:335, 1961.

60. Travell, J.: Temporomandibular joint pain referred from muscles of the head and neck. J. Prosthet. Dent., *10*:745, 1960.

61. Travell, J.: Myofascial trigger points: clinical view. *In* Bonica, J., and DeAlbe-Fessards, D. (eds.): Advanced Pain Research and Therapy. New York, Raven Press, 1976.

62. Weinberg, L. A.: Diagnosis of facets in occlusal equilibration. J. Am. Dent. Assoc., *52*:26, 1956.

63. Weinberg, L. A.: The prevalence of tooth contact in eccentric movements of the jaw: its clinical implications. J. Am. Dent. Assoc., *62*:402, 1961.

64. Weinberg, L. A.: Technique for temporomandibular joint radiographs. J. Prosthet. Dent. *27*:284, 1972.

65. Weinberg, L. A.: Temporomandibular joint function and its effect on centric relations. J. Prosthet. Dent., *30*:176, 1973.

66. Weinberg, L. A.: Posterior bilateral condylar displacement: its diagnosis and treatment. J. Prosthet. Dent., *36*:426, 1976.

67. Wilkes, C. H.: Alterations in structure and function of the temporomandibular joint in patients with the TMJ syndrome. Minn. Med., *61*:645, 1978.

68. Yavelow, I., Forster, I., and Winniger, M.: Mandibular relearning. Oral Surg., *36*:632, 1973.

69. Yemm, R.: Some experimental evidence of the aetiology and pathology of masticatory dysfunction. J. Dent. Assoc. S. Afr., *30*:213, 1975.

70. Yemm, R.: Neurophysiological studies of temporomandibular joint dysfunction. Oral Sci. Rev., *1*:31, 1976.

71. Zarb, G. A., and Thompson, G. W.: The treatment of patients with temporomandibular joint pain dysfunction syndrome. J. Can. Dent. Assoc., *7*:410, 1975.

chapter twenty-eight

Nutritional Influences in the Etiology of Periodontal Disease

The majority of opinions and research findings on the effects of nutrition on oral and periodontal tissues point to the following:

1. There are nutritional deficiencies that produce changes in the oral cavity; these changes include alterations of the lips, oral mucosa, and bone, as well as of the periodontal tissues. These changes are considered periodontal or oral manifestations of nutritional disease.

2. There are no nutritional deficiencies which by themselves can cause gingivitis or periodontal pockets. There are, however, nutritional deficiencies that can affect the condition of the periodontium and thereby aggravate the injurious effects of local irritants and excessive occlusal forces.

Theoretically, it can be assumed that there may be a "border zone" in which local irritants of insufficient severity could cause gingival and periodontal disorders if their effect upon the periodontium were aggravated by nutritional deficiencies. On the basis of this, some clinicians enthusiastically adhere to the theory that would assign a key role in periodontal disease to nutritional deficiencies and imbalances. Although research conducted up to the present does not in general support this view, it has been pointed out that numerous problems in experimental design and data interpretation may render those research findings inadequate.[2]

This chapter will analyze the existing knowledge in the field of nutrition as it relates to periodontal disease, and reference will also be made to other oral changes of nutritional origin.

PHYSICAL CHARACTER OF THE DIET

Numerous experiments in animals have shown that the physical character of the diet may play some role in the accumulation of plaque and the development of gingivitis.[30] Soft diets, although nutritionally adequate, may lead to plaque and calculus formation.[6, 13, 14, 16, 26] Hard and fibrous foods provide surface cleansing action and stimulation, which result in less plaque and gingivitis,[8, 31] even if the diet is nutritionally inadequate.[13] On the other hand, studies in humans have been unable to demonstrate reduced plaque formation when hard foods are consumed.[16, 34] The difference may be related to differences in tooth anatomy and to the fact that hard-consistency foods are fed to experimental animals as the only diet, whereas humans also consume soft foods. Human diets also have a high sucrose content, which favors the production of a thick plaque.

THE EFFECT OF NUTRITION UPON ORAL MICROORGANISMS

With increased interest in the role of bacterial plaque in periodontal disease, attention has been directed to a relatively unexplored aspect of nutrition—namely, its effect upon the oral microorganisms. Although dietary intake is generally thought of in terms of sustaining the individual, it inadvertently is also the source of bacterial nutrients.

By its effects upon the oral bacteria, the composition of the diet may influence the relative distribution of types of organisms, their metabolic activity, and their pathogenic potential, which in turn affects the occurrence and severity of oral disease. Consideration of the role of nutrition upon the oral flora and of its possible implications in oral disease is in its early stages. Morhart and Fitzgerald[25] present an excellent analysis of this subject.

It may be that the oral changes considered to be the result of nutritional deficiencies upon the oral tissues could be manifested first as an effect upon the oral microorganisms, so that their products become increasingly injurious to the oral tissues.

Sources of nutrients for the microorganisms can be endogenous and exogenous. Among the exogenous factors, the influence of the sugar content of the diet has been extensively studied; it has been demonstrated that the amount and type of carbohydrates in the diet and the frequency of intake can influence bacterial growth.[7] The mechanisms of attachment and subsequent colonization of the tooth surface by certain microorganisms may also be made possible by components of the diet.

VITAMIN A DEFICIENCY

Deficiency of vitamin A results in keratinizing metaplasia of the epithelium; increased susceptibility to infection[11]; disturbances in bone growth, shape, and texture[18]; abnormalities in the central nervous system[36]; and ocular manifestations—which include night blindness (nyctalopia), xerosis of the conjunctiva, and xerosis of the cornea with subsequent corneal turbidity, ulceration, and keratomalacia.[15]

Oral Findings in Experimental Animals

The following changes have been reported in vitamin A–deficient rats: widening of the periodontal ligament of the molars and incisors, degeneration of the principal fibers, thickening of the cementum of the molars,[29] apical hypercementosis with imperfect root formation, retarded eruption, and malposition of the teeth.[29] Hyperkeratosis of the oral epithelium produced by vitamin A deficiency in experimental animals is comparable to that resulting from prolonged administration of estrogen.[38] Alveolar bone changes in vitamin A–deficient animals include increased density with fewer marrow spaces,[19] hypercalcification with retardation in the rate of bone deposition,[29] resorption with fibrosis, atrophy with resorption (most pronounced in the furcation areas),[24] osteophytic formation,[5] and osteoporosis and resorption of the crest of the alveolar bone, which may be the result of the deficiency or may occur secondary to gingival changes.[12]

Vitamin A Deficiency and Periodontal Disease

Some studies in experimental animals suggest that vitamin A deficiency may predispose to periodontal disease.[4, 20, 22] Loss of neurotrophic stimulation as a result of peripheral nerve degeneration[12, 23] and atrophy of the salivary glands[4] have been suggested as causative factors.

The gingiva shows epithelial hyperplasia and hyperkeratinization with proliferation of the junctional epithelium.[5, 12, 19] The life cycle of the epithelial cells is shortened, as evidenced by early karyolysis.[8] Gingival hyperplasia with inflammatory infiltration and degeneration,[20] pocket formation[4, 5] and the formation of subgingival calculus[12] also occur.

Local irritation is necessary before abnormal epithelial tendencies associated with vitamin A deficiency are manifested in the gingival sulcus.[10] Pocket formation does not occur in vitamin A–deficient animals in the absence of local irritation, but when local irritation is present, the pockets are deeper than in nondeficient animals and exhibit associated epithelial hyperkeratosis. Repair of gingival wounds is retarded in vitamin A–deficient animals,[9, 21] which are also subject to leukoplakia of the oral mucosa in areas other than the gingiva.[1]

In contrast with the abundance of evidence in experimental animals, there is little information regarding the effects of vitamin A deficiency upon the oral structures in humans. Low daily intake of vitamin A has been associated with periodontal disease.[27] Marshall-

Day[17] reported a possible correlation between the incidence of periodontal disease and dermatologic lesions characteristic of vitamin A deficiency, and Russell[28] reported that populations with a high incidence of periodontal disease tend to be deficient in vitamin A. However, several other studies carried out in the Far East, where vitamin A deficiency is common, and in Africa failed to demonstrate any relation between this vitamin and periodontal disease.[33]

Hypervitaminosis A

Large doses of vitamin A in young, growing rats produce generalized bone resorptive activity and osteoporosis, which result in multiple fractures. Developing dental tissues are not affected, but the alveolar bone shows marked resorption without repair.[37] Hypervitaminosis A may accelerate bone growth.[35] Furthermore, melanin-like pigmentation of the skin, scaling dermatosis, disturbed menstruation, itching, and exophthalmos have been identified with hypervitaminosis A in humans.[32]

REFERENCES

Physical Character of the Diet and Vitamin A

1. Abels, J. C., Rekers, P. E., Hayes, M., and Rhoads, C. P.: Relationship between dietary deficiency and occurrence of papillary atrophy of tongue and oral leukoplakia. Cancer Res., 2:381, 1942.
2. Alfano, M. C.: Controversies, perspectives and clinical implications of nutrition in periodontal disease. Dent. Clin. North Am., 20:519, 1976.
3. Behbehani, M. J., and Jordan, H. V.: Comparative colonization of human *Actinomyces* species in hamsters under different dietary conditions. J. Periodont. Res., 15:395, 1980.
4. Boyle, P. E.: Effect of vitamin A deficiency on the periodontal tissues. Am. J. Orthod., 33:744, 1947.
5. Boyle, P. E., and Bessey, O. A.: The effect of acute vitamin A deficiency on the molar teeth and paradontal tissues, with a comment on deformed incisor-teeth in this deficiency. J. Dent. Res., 20:236, 1941.
6. Burwasser, P., and Hill, T. J.: The effect of hard and soft diets on the gingival tissues of dogs. J. Dent. Res., 18:389, 1939.
7. Carlsson, J., and Egelberg, J.: Effect of diet on early plaque formation in man. Odont. Revy, 16:122, 1965.
8. Egelberg, J.: Local effect of diet on plaque formation and development of gingivitis in dogs. I. Effect of hard and soft diets. Odont. Revy, 16:31, 1965.
9. Frandsen, A. M.: Periodontal tissue changes in vitamin A deficient young rats. Acta Odontol. Scand., 21:19, 1963.
10. Glickman, I., and Stoller, M.: The periodontal tissues of the albino rat in vitamin A deficiency. J. Dent. Res., 27:758, 1948.
11. Green, H. N., and Mellanby, E.: Vitamin A as anti-infective agent. Br. Med. J., 2:691, 1928.
12. King, J. D.: Abnormalities in the gingival and subgingival tissues due to diets deficient in vitamin A and carotene. Br. Dent. J., 68:349, 1940.
13. King, J. D., and Glover, N. E.: The relative effects of dietary constituents and other factors upon calculus formation and gingival disease in the ferret. J. Pathol. Bacteriol., 57:353, 1945.
14. Krasse, B., and Brill, N.: Effect of consistency of diet on bacteria in gingival pockets in dogs. Odont. Revy, 11:152, 1960.
15. Kruse, H. D.: Medical evaluation of nutritional status. IV. The ocular manifestations of avitaminosis A, with especial consideration of the detection of early changes by biomicroscopy. Milbank Mem. Fund Q., 19:207, 1941.
16. Lindhe, J., and Wicen, P. O.: The effects on the gingivae of chewing fibrous foods. J. Periodont. Res., 4:193, 1969.
17. Marshall-Day, C. D.: Nutritional deficiencies and dental caries in northern India. Br. Dent. J., 76:143, 1944.
18. Mellanby, E.: A Story of Nutritional Research. Baltimore, Williams & Wilkins Company, 1950.
19. Mellanby, H.: Effect of maternal dietary deficiency of vitamin A on dental tissues in rats. J. Dent. Res., 20:489, 1941.
20. Mellanby, M.: Diet and the teeth: an experimental study. Part I. Dental structures in dogs. Med. Res. Council (Brit.) Spec. Rep. Series No. 140, London, 1929.
21. Mellanby, M.: Diet and the teeth: an experimental study. Part II. Diet and dental disease. B. Diet and dental structure in animals other than the dog. Med. Res. Council (Brit.) Spec. Res. Series No. 153, London, 1930.
22. Mellanby, M.: Dental research, with special reference to parodontal disease produced experimentally in animals. Dent. Record, 59:227, 1939.
23. Mellanby, M., and King, J. D.: Diet and the nerve supply to the dental tissues. Br. Dent. J., 56:538, 1934.
24. Miglani, D. C.: The effect of vitamin A deficiency on the periodontal structures of rat molars with emphasis on cementum resorption. Oral Surg., 12:1372, 1959.
25. Morhart, R. E., and Fitzgerald, R. J.: Nutritional determinants of the ecology of the oral flora. Dent. Clin. North Am., 20:473, 1976.
26. Pelzer, R.: A study of the local oral effect of diet on the periodontal tissues and the gingival capillary structure. J. Am. Dent. Assoc., 27:13, 1940.
27. Radusch, D. F.: Nutritional aspects of periodontal disease. Ann. Dent., 7:169, 1940.
28. Russell, A. L.: International nutrition surveys: a summary of preliminary dental findings. J. Dent. Res., 42:233, 1963.
29. Schour, I., Hoffman, M. M., and Smith, M. C.: Changes in incisor teeth of albino rats with vitamin A deficiency and effects of replacement therapy. Am. J. Pathol., 17:529, 1941.
30. Sreebny, L. M.: Effect of the physical consistency of food on the "crevicular complex" and the salivary glands. Int. Dent. J., 22:394, 1972.
31. Stralfors, A., Thilander, H., and Bergenholtz, A.: Caries and periodontal disease in hamsters fed cereal foods varying in sugar content and hardness. Arch. Oral Biol., 12:1681, 1967.
32. Sulzberger, M. B., and Lazar, M. P.: Hypervitaminosis A. J.A.M.A., 146:788, 1951.
33. Waerhaug, J.: Epidemiology of periodontal disease. Review of literature. In World Workshop in Periodontics, 1966, p. 181.
34. Wilcox, C. E., and Everett, F.: Friction on the teeth and the gingiva during mastication. J. Am. Dent. Assoc., 66:5, 1963.
35. Wolbach, S. B.: Vitamin A deficiency and excess in relation to skeletal growth. Proc. Inst. Med. Chicago, 16:118, 1946.
36. Wolbach, S. B., and Bessey, O. A.: Vitamin A deficiency and the nervous system. Arch. Pathol., 32:689, 1941.
37. Wolbach, S. B., and Bessey, O. A.: Tissue changes in vitamin deficiencies. Physiol. Rev., 22:233, 1942.
38. Ziskin, D. E., Rosenstein, S. N., and Drucker, L.: Interrelation of large parenteral doses of estrogen and vitamin A and their effect on the oral mucosa. Am. J. Orthod., 29:163, 1943.

VITAMIN B COMPLEX DEFICIENCY

The vitamin B complex includes the following substances: thiamine (vitamin B_1), riboflavin (vitamin B_2), nicotinic acid (niacin) or nicotinic acid amide (niacinamide), pantothenic acid, pyridoxine (vitamin B_6), biotin, para-aminobenzoic acid, inositol, choline, folic acid (folacin, pteroylglutamic acid), and vitamin B_{12} (cyanocobalamin).

Oral disease is rarely due to a deficiency in just one component of the B complex group. The deficiency is generally multiple. Oral changes common to deficiencies in the B complex group are gingivitis, glossitis, glossodynia, angular cheilitis, and inflammation of the entire oral mucosa. **The gingivitis in vitamin B deficiencies is nonspecific, as it is caused by local irritation rather than by the deficiency, but it is subject to the modifying effect of the latter.**[1]

Oral Findings Associated with Vitamin B Complex Deficiency

THIAMINE (VITAMIN B_1). The human manifestations of thiamine deficiency, called *beriberi,* are characterized by paralysis, cardiovascular symptoms (including edema), and loss of appetite. Frank beriberi is rare in the United States; however, less striking polyneuropathies do result from accompanying conditioning factors that interfere with the absorption or utilization of thiamine. Many animals, including man, have microorganisms in their intestinal tracts that have the capacity to synthesize thiamine, thus complicating experimental inducement of deficiency of this vitamin.

The following oral disturbances have been attributed to thiamine deficiency: hypersensitivity of the oral mucosa,[13] minute vesicles (simulating herpes) on the buccal mucosa, under the tongue, or on the palate; and erosion of the oral mucosa.[7] Glossitis could not be produced in humans by deprivation of thiamine.[21] Since thiamine is essential to bacterial and carbohydrate metabolism, it has been postulated that the activity of the oral flora is diminished in thiamine deficiency.[10]

RIBOFLAVIN (VITAMIN B_2). The symptoms of riboflavin deficiency (ariboflavinosis) include glossitis, angular cheilitis, seborrheic dermatitis, and a superficial vascularizing keratitis.[15, 16] The *glossitis* is characterized by a magenta discoloration and atrophy of the papillae. Disappearance of the papillae of the tongue varies, depending upon the severity of the deficiency. In mild to moderate cases, the dorsum presents a patchy atrophy of the lingual papillae[1] and engorged fungiform papillae, which project as pebble-like elevations.[8]

In severe deficiency, the entire dorsum is flat, having a dry and often fissured surface. The margin of the tongue presents a scalloped appearance, caused by contiguous indentations that conform to the pattern of the interdental spaces of the dentition.

Angular cheilitis is one of the changes most frequently identified with riboflavin deficiency. It begins as an inflammation of the commissure of the lips, followed by erosion, ulceration, and fissuring (Fig. 28–1). Riboflavin deficiency is not the only cause of angular cheilitis. Loss of vertical dimension, together with drooling of saliva into the angles of the lips, may produce a condition similar to angular cheilitis. Candidiasis may develop in the commissures of debilitated persons; this lesion has been termed "perlèche."[6]

Changes observed in riboflavin-deficient animals include severe lesions of the gingivae, periodontal tissues, and oral mucosa (including noma)[3, 18] *and retarded chondrogenic and osteogenic activity in the condylar growth center of the mandible.*[23]

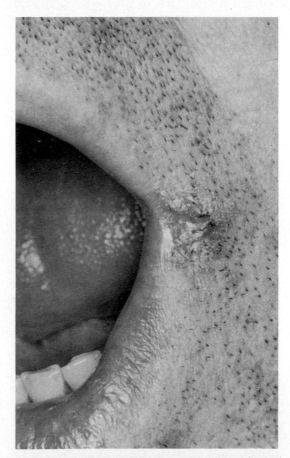

Figure 28–1 Angular Cheilitis in patient with conditioned vitamin B complex deficiency.

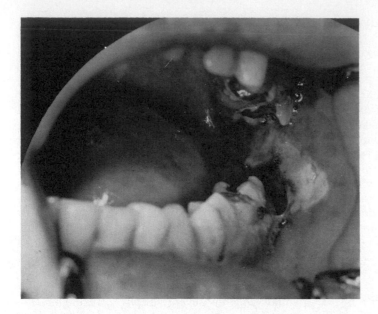

Figure 28–2 Ulceration of Buccal Mucosa in Patient with Nicotinic Acid Deficiency. Note sharp cusp of maxillary molar which initiated the irritation. (Courtesy of Dr. David Weisberger.)

NICOTINIC ACID (NIACIN). Nicotinic acid deficiency, or aniacinosis, results in *pellagra,* which is characterized by dermatitis, gastrointestinal disturbances, neurologic and mental disturbances (dermatitis, diarrhea, and dementia), glossitis, gingivitis, and generalized stomatitis.

Oral Changes. Glossitis and stomatitis may be the earliest clinical signs of nicotinic acid deficiency.[14] In the acute form, there is hyperemia of the tongue, enlargement of the papillae, and indentation of the margin, followed by atrophic changes and a resultant glazed surface. The tongue in acute nicotinic acid deficiency is "beefy red" and painful, with "burning" (glossopyrosis).[11] In chronic nicotinic acid deficiency the tongue is thinned and fissured, with surface crevices, marginal serrations, and atrophy of the fungiform and filiform papillae.

The gingiva may be involved in aniacinosis[9] with or without tongue changes. The most frequent finding is acute necrotizing ulcerative gingivitis, usually in areas of local irritation (Fig. 28–2).

Oral manifestations of vitamin B complex and nicotinic acid deficiencies in experimental animals include black tongue[1, 4] and gingival inflammation with destruction of the gingiva, periodontal ligament, and alveolar bone.[2] Necrosis of the gingiva and other oral tissues and leukopenia are terminal features of nicotinic acid deficiency in experimental animals.

PANTOTHENIC ACID. Oral changes caused by pantothenic acid deficiency have been identified in animals but not in humans. These include angular cheilitis, hyperkeratosis with ulceration and necrosis of the gingiva and oral mucosa, proliferation of the basal layer of the oral epithelium, and resorption of the crest of the alveolar bone.[20, 23] The absence of an inflammatory response is a striking finding. Radiographically, narrowing of the periodontal ligament space, alveolar bone loss, and rarefaction of bone may be observed.

The oral mucosa and lips are glistening red, sometimes with ulceration. In the early stages salivary flow is increased and accompanied by drooling, but the dehydration which occurs as the disease progresses leads to reduced salivary flow and dryness.

PYRIDOXINE (VITAMIN B$_6$). Anemia, cardiovascular disturbances, convulsions, retardation of growth,[22] and patchy atrophy of the dorsum of the tongue (similar to that observed in riboflavin deficiency) have been noted in experimental animals on diets deficient in pyridoxine.[1]

Humans with pyridoxine deficiency present angular cheilitis and glossitis with swelling, atrophy of the papillae, magenta discoloration, and discomfort. When experimentally created in humans, the deficiency results in glossitis resembling that of nicotinic acid deficiency, reddening with small ulcerations of the mucosa, and angular cheilitis.[19]

FOLIC ACID (FOLACIN, PTEROYLGLUTAMIC ACID). Folic acid deficiency results in macrocytic anemia with megaloblastic erythropoiesis, with oral changes and gastrointestinal lesions, diarrhea, and intestinal malabsorption.[5]

Oral Changes. Folic acid–deficient animals

present necrosis of the gingiva, periodontal ligament, and alveolar bone without inflammation.[16] The absence of inflammation is the result of deficiency-induced granulocytopenia.

In humans with sprue and other folic acid deficiency states there is generalized stomatitis, which may be accompanied by ulcerated glossitis and cheilitis. Ulcerative stomatitis is an early indication of a toxic effect of folic acid antagonists used in the treatment of leukemia.

In sprue, glossitis may be the presenting complaint; it usually occurs after the onset of steatorrhea. Swelling and redness at the tip and lateral margins of the tongue are the initial disorders, accompanied in some cases by painful minute ulcers on the dorsum. Disappearance of the filiform and fungiform papillae is followed by the development of a smooth, atrophic, red tongue. Painful burning symptoms and increased salivation accompany the oral changes.

VITAMIN B$_{12}$ (CYANOCOBALAMIN). Vitamin B$_{12}$, the antipernicious anemia factor, is the only vitamin which contains cobalt. It is a potent catalyst and is involved in the synthesis of nucleic acid and in folic acid metabolism. Pernicious anemia is the most severe form of vitamin B$_{12}$ deficiency. Other macrocytic anemias are thought to be mild forms of vitamin B$_{12}$ deficiency complicated by deficiency of folic acid. Oral changes in pernicious anemia are described in Chapter 30.

REFERENCES

Vitamin B Complex

 1. Afonsky, D.: Oral lesions in niacin, riboflavin, pyridoxine, folic acid and pantothenic acid deficiencies in adult dogs. Oral Surg., *8*:207, 315, 867, 1955.
 2. Becks, H., Wainwright, W. W., and Morgan, A. F.: Comparative study of oral changes in dogs due to deficiencies of pantothenic acid, nicotinic acid and unknowns of B vitamin complex. Am. J Orthod., *29*:183, 1943.
 3. Chapman, O. D., and Harris, A. E.: Oral lesions associated with dietary deficiencies in monkeys. J. Infect. Dis., *69*:7, 1941.
 4. Denton, J.: A study of tissue changes in experimental black tongue of dogs compared with similar changes in pellagra. Am. J. Pathol., *4*:341, 1928.
 5. Dreizen, S.: Oral manifestations of human nutritional anemias. Arch. Environ. Health, *5*:66, 1962.
 6. Goodman, M. H.: Perlèche: A consideration of its etiology and pathology. Bull. Johns Hopkins Hosp., *51*:263, 1932.
 7. Govier, W. M., and Grieg, M. E.: Prevention of oral lesions in B$_1$ avitaminotic dogs. Science, *98*:216, 1943.
 8. Jeghers, H.: Riboflavin deficiency. IV. Oral changes. Advances in Internal Medicine I. New York, Interscience Publishers, Inc., 1942, p. 257.
 9. King, J. D.: Vincent's disease treated with nicotinic acid. Lancet, *2*:32, 1940.
10. Kneisner, A. H., Mann, A. W., and Spies, T. D.: Relationship of dental caries to deficiencies of vitamin B group. J. Dent. Res., *21*:259, 1942.

11. Kruse, H. D.: Lingual manifestations of aniacinosis with especial consideration of detection of early changes by biomicroscopy. Milbank Mem. Fund Q., *20*:262, 1942
12. Levy, B. M.: The effect of riboflavin deficiency on the growth of the mandibular condyle of mice. Oral Surg., *2*:89, 1949.
13. Mann, A. W., Spies, T. D., and Springer, M.: Oral manifestations of vitamin B complex deficiencies. J. Dent. Res., *20*:269, 1941.
14. Manson-Bahr, P., and Ransford, O. N.: Stomatitis of vitamin B$_2$ deficiency treated with nicotinic acid. Lancet, *2*:426, 1938.
15. Sebrell, W. H., and Butler, R. E.: Riboflavin deficiency in man. Public Health Rep., *53*:2282, 1938; *54*:2121, 1939.
16. Shaw, J. H.: The relation of nutrition to periodontal disease. J. Dent. Res., *41*(Suppl. 1):264, 1962.
17. Sydenstricker, V. P.: Clinical manifestations of ariboflavinosis. Am. J. Public Health, *31*:344, 1941.
18. Topping, N. H., and Fraser, H. F.: Mouth lesions associated with dietary deficiencies in monkeys. Public Health Rep., *54*:416, 1939.
19. Vilter, R. W., et al.: The effect of vitamin B$_6$ deficiency induced by desoxypyridoxine in human beings. J. Lab. Clin. Med., *42*:335, 1953.
20. Wainwright, W. W., and Nelson, M.: Changes in oral mucosa accompanying acute pantothenic acid deficiency in young rats. Am. J. Orthod., *31*:406, 1945.
21. Williams, R. D., Masson, H. L., Wilder, R. M., and Smith, B. F.: Observations on induced thiamine deficiency in man. Arch. Intern. Med., *66*:785, 1940; *69*:721, 1942.
22. Wolbach, S. B., and Bessey, O. A.: Tissue changes in vitamin deficiencies. Physiol. Rev., *22*:233, 1942.
23. Ziskin, D. E., Stein, G., Gross, P., and Runne, E.: Oral, gingival and periodontal pathology induced in rats on a low pantothenic acid diet by toxic doses of zinc carbonate. Am. J. Orthod. (Oral Surg. Sec.), *33*:407, 1947.

VITAMIN C (ASCORBIC ACID) DEFICIENCY

Severe vitamin C deficiency in humans results in scurvy, a disease characterized by hemorrhagic diathesis and retardation of wound healing. The hemorrhages commonly occur in areas of trauma or marked function.[17] Clinical features of scurvy include fatigue, breathlessness, lethargy, loss of appetite, sallow complexion, fleeting pains in joints and limbs, skin petechiae (particularly around hair follicles), epistaxis, ecchymosis (mainly in lower extremities), hemorrhage into muscles and deeper tissues (scurvy siderosis), hematuria, edema of the ankles, and anemia.[22] Increased susceptibility to infection and impaired wound healing are also features of vitamin C deficiency.[4, 30]

Vitamin C deficiency (scurvy) results in defective formation and maintenance of collagen, mucopolysaccharide ground substance, and intercellular cement substance in mesenchymal tissues.[33] Its effect on bone is marked by retardation or cessation of osteoid formation, impaired osteoblastic function,[25] and osteoporosis.[8, 32] Vitamin C deficiency is also characterized by increased capillary permeability, susceptibility to traumatic hemorrhages, hyporeactivity of the contractile elements of the peripheral blood vessels, and sluggishness of blood flow.[17] Changes in liver cells and in

autonomic ganglia have been reported in chronic marginal vitamin C deficiency.[28]

Possible Etiologic Relationships of Ascorbic Acid and Periodontal Disease

It has been suggested that ascorbic acid may play a role in periodontal disease by one or more of the following mechanisms[34]:

1. Low levels of ascorbic acid influence the metabolism of collagen within the periodontium, thereby affecting the ability of the tissue to regenerate and repair itself. There is no experimental evidence to support this view of the role of ascorbic acid; furthermore, it has been shown that collagen fibers in the periodontal ligament of scorbutic monkeys are the last affected prior to the death of the animals.[31]

2. Ascorbic acid deficiency interferes with bone formation, leading to loss of periodontal bone. However, changes which do occur in alveolar bone and other bones due to failure of the osteoblasts to form osteoid take place very late in the deficiency state.[9] Osteoporosis of alveolar bone in scorbutic monkeys occurs as a result of increased osteoclastic resorption and is not associated with periodontal pocket formation.[31]

3. Ascorbic acid deficiency increases the permeability of the oral mucosa to tritiated endotoxin and tritiated inulin[1, 2] and the permeability of normal human crevicular epithelium to tritiated dextran.[18] Optimum levels of this vitamin, therefore, would maintain the epithelium's barrier function to bacterial products.

4. Increasing levels of ascorbic acid enhance both the chemotactic and the migratory action of leukocytes without influencing their phagocytic activity.[12] Megadoses of vitamin C seem to impair the bactericidal activity of leukocytes.[27] The significance of these findings for the pathogenesis and treatment of periodontal diseases is not understood.

5. An optimum level of ascorbic acid is apparently required to maintain the integrity of the periodontal microvasculature, as well as the vascular response to bacterial irritation and wound healing.[4]

6. Depletion of vitamin C may interfere with the ecologic equilibrium of bacteria in plaque and thus increase the pathogenicity of plaque. However, there is no evidence to demonstrate this effect.

EPIDEMIOLOGIC STUDIES. Several studies in large populations have analyzed the relation between gingival or periodontal status and ascorbic acid levels. The studies employed different methods for the biochemical analysis of ascorbic acid and various indices for the assessment of periodontal changes. These studies were made in different parts of the world, with populations of different socioeconomic status, different races, and various ages. All the epidemiologic surveys failed to establish a causal relationship between levels of vitamin C and the prevalence or severity of periodontal disease.[3, 7, 24]

GINGIVITIS. The legendary association of severe gingival disease with scurvy led to the presumption that vitamin C deficiency is an etiologic factor in gingivitis, which is so common at all ages.

Gingivitis, with enlarged, hemorrhagic, bluish-red gingiva, is described as one of the classic signs of vitamin C deficiency (see Chapter 10), **but gingivitis is not caused by vitamin C deficiency per se.** Nor do all vitamin C–deficient patients necessarily have gingivitis; it does not occur in the absence of local irritants. **If gingivitis is present in a vitamin C–deficient patient, it is caused by bacterial plaque.** Vitamin C deficiency may aggravate the gingival response to plaque and worsen the edema, enlargement, and bleeding,[13] and the severity may be reduced by correcting the deficiency, but gingivitis will remain as long as bacterial irritation is present.

PERIODONTITIS. Changes in the supporting periodontal tissues and gingiva in vitamin C deficiency have been documented extensively in experimental animals.[9, 14, 15, 31, 32] **Acute vitamin C deficiency results in edema and hemorrhage in the periodontal ligament, osteoporosis of the alveolar bone, and tooth mobility; hemorrhage, edema, and degeneration of collagen fibers occur in the gingiva, but acute vitamin C deficiency does not cause or increase the incidence of gingivitis.**[10]

The periodontal fibers that are least affected by vitamin C deficiency are those just below the junctional epithelium and above the alveolar crest, which explains the infrequent apical downgrowth of the epithelium.[31] **Local irritation must be present for gingivitis to occur in experimental animals with acute vitamin C deficiency.**[9, 10] **The deficiency alters the response to irritation so that the gingiva is enlarged, edematous, and hemorrhagic. Vitamin C deficiency also retards gingival healing.**[5, 30]

Vitamin C deficiency does not cause periodontal pockets; local irritating factors are required for pocket formation to occur. However, when pocket formation does occur in a patient with vitamin C deficiency, it is of greater depth than that normally produced under comparable local conditions. The occurrence of pocket formation and destruction of underlying tissues in vitamin C deficiency is not attributable to the deficiency alone, but indicates the presence of a complicating local factor.

Acute vitamin C deficiency alters the response of the supporting periodontal tissues to the extent that the destructive effect of gingival inflammation upon the underlying periodontal ligament and alveolar bone is accentuated.[10] The exaggerated destruction results partly from inability to marshal a defensive delimiting reaction to the inflammation and partly from destructive tendencies caused by the deficiency itself. Factors contributing to the destruction of the periodontal tissues in vitamin C deficiency include inability to form a peripheral delimiting connective tissue barrier, reduction in inflammatory cells, diminished vascular response, inhibition of fibroblast formation and differentiation to osteoblasts, impaired formation of collagen and mucopolysaccharide ground substance.

Experimental studies have been conducted in humans. In 1940, Crandon et al.[6] had one human subject follow a vitamin C–free diet for 6 months. The leukocyte-platelet ascorbic acid level was 0 from day 83 onward. Although "the gums were slightly more boggy on pressure" and some discontinuity in the periodontal lamina dura was seen in the radiographs, there was no gingival bleeding, and no other clinical gingival changes were seen. The human studies of Restarski and Pijoan[23] and of Hodges et al.[13] also failed to show the dramatic clinical changes that have traditionally been described in scurvy. None of these human experimental studies, however, contained a thorough, well-controlled analysis of the periodontal condition.

In summary, analysis of the literature[34] indicates that the microscopic signs of vitamin C deficiency are quite different from those which occur in plaque-induced periodontal disease in humans. Patients with acute or chronic vitamin C–deficient states and no plaque accumulation show minimal, if any, changes in their gingival health status.

REFERENCES

Vitamin C

1. Alfano, M. C., Miller, S. A., and Drummond, J. F.: Effect of ascorbic acid deficiency on the permeability and collagen biosynthesis of oral mucosal epithelium. Ann. N.Y. Acad. Sci., *258*:253, 1975.

2. Alvares, O., and Siegel, I.: Permeability of gingival sulcular epithelium in the development of scorbutic gingivitis. J. Oral Pathol., *10*:40, 1981.

3. Buzina, R., et al.: Epidemiology of angular stomatitis and bleeding gums. Int. J. Vitam. Nutr. Res., *43*:401, 1973.

4. Cabrini, R. L., and Carranza, F. A., Jr.: Adenosine triphosphatase in normal and scorbutic wounds. Nature, *200*:1113, 1963.

5. Cabrini, R. L., and Carranza, F. A., Jr.: Alkaline and acid phosphatase in gingival and tongue wounds in normal and vitamin C deficient animals. J. Periodontol., *34*:74, 1963.

6. Crandon, J. H., Lund, C. C., and Dill, D. B.: Experimental human scurvy. N. Engl. J. Med., *223*:353, 1940.

7. Enwonwu, C. O., and Edozien, J. C.: Epidemiology of periodontal disease in western Nigerians in relation to socioeconomic status. Arch. Oral Biol., *15*:1231, 1970.

8. Follis, R. H.: The Pathology of Nutritional Disease. Springfield, Ill., Charles C Thomas, Publisher, 1948, p. 134.

9. Glickman, I.: Acute vitamin C deficiency and periodontal disease. I. The periodontal tissues of the guinea pig in acute vitamin C deficiency. J. Dent. Res., *27*:9, 1948.

10. Glickman, I.: Acute vitamin C deficiency and the periodontal tissues. II. The effect of acute vitamin C deficiency upon the response of the periodontal tissues of the guinea pig to artificially induced inflammation J. Dent. Res., *27*:201, 1948.

11. Glickman, I., and Dines, M. M.: Effect of increased ascorbic acid blood levels on the ascorbic acid level in treated and nontreated gingiva. J. Dent. Res., *42*:1152, 1963.

12. Goetzl, E. J.: Enhancement of random migration and chemotactic response of human leukocytes by ascorbic acid. J. Clin. Invest., *53*:813, 1974.

13. Hodges, R. E., et al.: Experimental scurvy in man. Am. J. Clin. Nutr., *22*:535, 1969.

14. Höjer, J. A.: Studies in scurvy. Acta Paediatr., *3*:(Suppl.):119, 1924.

15. Hoher, J. A., and Westin, G.: Jaws and teeth in scorbutic guinea pig. Dent. Cosmos, *67*:1, 1925.

16. Keller, S. E., Ringsdorf, W. M., and Cheraskin, E.: Interplay of local and systemic influences in the periodontal diseases. J. Periodontol., *34*:259, 1963.

17. Lee, R. E., and Lee, N. Z.: The peripheral vascular system and its reactions in scurvy: an experimental study. Am. J. Physiol., *149*:465, 1947.

18. Mallek, H., and Miller, S. A.: Role of ascorbic acid in barrier function of human crevicular gingiva. I.A.D.R. Abstr., J. Dent. Res., *58A*:351, 1979.

19. O'Leary, T. J., Rudd, K. D., Crump, P. P., and Kruase, R. E.: The effect of ascorbic acid supplementation on tooth mobility. J. Periodontol., *40*:284, 1969.

20. Parfitt, G. J., and Hand, C. D.: Reduced plasma ascorbic acid levels and gingival health. J. Periodontol., *34*:347, 1963.

21. Perlitsh, M., Nielsen, A. G., and Stanmeyer, W. R.: Ascorbic acid plasma levels and gingival health in personnel wintering over in Anatarctica. J. Dent. Res., *40*:789, 1961.

22. Ralli, E. P., and Sherry, S.: Adult scurvy and the metabolism of vitamin C. Medicine, *20*:251, 1941.

23. Restarski, J. S., and Pijoan, M.: Gingivitis and vitamin C. J. Am. Dent. Assoc. *31*:1323, 1944.

24. Russell, A. L.: International nutrition surveys: a summary of preliminary dental findings. J. Dent. Res., *42*:233, 1963.

25. Salter, W. T., and Aub, J. C.: Studies of calcium and phosphorus metabolism. IX. Deposition of calcium in bone in healing scorbutus. Arch. Pathol., *11*:380, 1931.

26. Shannon, I., and Gibson, W. A.: Intravenous ascorbic acid loading in subjects classified as to periodontal status. J. Dent. Res., *44*:355, 1965.

27. Shilotri, P. G., and Bhat, K. S.: Effect of megadoses of vitamin C on bactericidal activity of leukocytes. Am. J. Clin. Nutr., *30*:1077, 1977.

28. Sulkin, N. M., and Sulkin, D. F.: Tissue changes induced by marginal vitamin C deficiency. Ann. N.Y. Acad. Sci., *258*:317, 1975.

29. Thomas, A. E., Busby, M. C., Ringsdorf, W. M., and Cheraskin, E.: Ascorbic acid and alveolar bone loss. Oral Surg., *15*:555, 1962.

30. Turesky, S., and Glickman, I.: Histochemical evaluation of gingival healing in experimental animals on adequate and vitamin C deficient diets. J. Dent. Res., *33*:273, 1954.

31. Waerhaug, J.: Effect of C-avitaminosis on the supporting structures of the teeth. J. Periodontol., *29*:87, 1958.

32. Wolbach, S. B., and Bessey, O. A.: Tissue changes in vitamin deficiencies. Physiol. Rev., *22*:233, 1942.
33. Wolbach, S. B., and Howe, P. R.: Intercellular substances in experimental scorbutus. Arch. Pathol., *1*:1, 1926.
34. Woolfe, S. N., Hume, W. R., and Kenney, E. B.: Ascorbic acid and periodontal disease: a review of the literature. J. Western Soc. Periodontol., *28*:44, 1980.

VITAMIN D (CALCIUM AND PHOSPHORUS) DEFICIENCY

Vitamin D, a fat-soluble vitamin, is essential for the absorption of calcium from the gastrointestinal tract, for the maintenance of the calcium-phosphorus balance, and for the formation of teeth and bones. The metabolism of calcium and phosphorus and metabolism of vitamin D are interrelated. The effects of variations in the calcium, phosphorus, and vitamin D intake upon the skeletal and dental structures are influenced by numerous other factors, such as parathyroid function, the presence of carbohydrate, fat, and such inorganic elements as strontium and beryllium, and age. Deficiency in vitamin D and/or imbalance in the calcium-phosphorus intake results in *rickets* in the very young and *osteomalacia* in adults. Their effect upon the periodontal tissues of experimental animals has been described as follows:

Vitamin D deficiency with normal dietary calcium and phosphorus in young dogs is characterized by osteoporosis of alveolar bone[5]; osteoid formed at a normal rate, but remaining uncalcified; failure of osteoid to resorb, leading to its excessive accumulation; reduction in the width of the periodontal space; a normal rate of cementum formation, but defective calcification and some cementum resorption[16]; and distortion of the growth pattern of alveolar bone. In young rats the periodontium is unaltered in vitamin D deficiency, provided that the diet is adequate in minerals.[13]

In osteomalacic animals there is rapid, generalized, severe osteoclastic resorption of alveolar bone, proliferation of fibroblasts which replace bone and marrow and new bone formation around remnants of unresorbed bony trabeculae.[7] Radiographically, there is generalized partial to complete disappearance of the lamina dura and reduced density of the supporting bone, loss of trabeculae, increased radiolucence of the trabecular interstices, and increased prominence of the remaining trabeculae. Microscopic and radiographic changes in the periodontium are almost identical with those seen in experimentally induced hyperparathyroidism.

In *vitamin D and calcium deficiency with normal dietary phosphorus,* there is generalized bone resorption in the jaws, fibro-osteoid hemorrhage in the marrow spaces, and destruction of the periodontal ligament.[4] The pattern is suggestive of changes in hyperparathyroidism.

Vitamin D and phosphorus deficiency with normal dietary calcium presents rachitic changes characterized by marked osteoid deposition.[11]

In *calcium and phosphorus deficiency with normal dietary vitamin D,* there is excessive bone resorption[1, 4]; resorption of alveolar bone and cementum occurs in adult animals on a calcium-deficient diet.[10]

In *phosphorus deficiency with normal dietary vitamin D and calcium,* jaw growth is disturbed and tooth eruption and condylar growth are retarded,[6, 15] accompanied by malocclusion.

Calcium deficiency in young rats produces osteoporosis and reduction in the number and diameter of periodontal fibers and increased cemental resorption.[13]

Hypervitaminosis D

Hypervitaminosis D in humans is characterized by nausea, vomiting, diarrhea, epigastric fullness, polyuria, polydipsia, albuminuria, impaired renal function, hypercalcemia, and hyperphosphatemia. It may prove fatal. In experimental animals, Follis[9] observed that excessive doses of vitamin D (125,000 units of vitamin D given daily for 9 days) resulted in marked osteoblastic activity and production of large quantities of osteoid about the trabeculae in the shafts of long bones. Baker[2] noted that guinea pigs maintained on hypervitaminotic D diets develop generalized osteoporosis and metastatic calcifications. Weinmann and Sicher[17] suggested that the bone-destructive effect of hypervitaminosis D is a phenomenon secondary to renal damage, which would create a condition of hyperparathyroidism.

The periodontal findings in experimental hypervitaminosis D include osteosclerosis characterized by marked endosteal and periosteal bone formation (or deposition of an amorphous, highly calcified material), osteoporosis and resorption of alveolar bone,[8] dystrophic calcification in the periodontal ligament and gingiva, severe calculus formation, deposition of a cementum-like substance on the root surfaces (resulting in hypercementosis and the ankylosis of many teeth), and extensive periodontal disease.[3, 5]

Nomura found deposits of dystrophic calcification in the collagen fiber bundles,[12] whereas Shoshan et al. reported calcification only when hypervitaminosis D and osteolathyrism occurred together, not when the vitamin deficiency occurred alone.[14]

REFERENCES

Vitamin D (Calcium and Phosphorus) Deficiency

1. Arnim, S. S., Clarke, M. F., Anderson, B. G., and Smith, A. H.: Dental changes in rats consuming diet poor in organic salts. Yale J. Biol. Med., *9*:117, 1936.
2. Baker, S. L.: The general pathology of bone. *In* Shanks, S. C., and Kerley, P. (eds.): A Textbook of X-ray Diagnosis. 2nd ed. Philadelphia, W. B. Saunders Company, 1950.
3. Becks, H.: Dangerous effects of vitamin D overdosage on dental and paradental structure. J. Am. Dent. Assoc., *29*:1947, 1942.
4. Becks, H., and Weber, M.: Influence of diet in bone system with special reference to alveolar process and labyrinthine capsule. J. Am. Dent. Assoc., *18*:197, 1931.
5. Becks, H., Collins, D. A., and Freytog, R. M.: Changes in oral structures of the dog persisting after chronic overdoses of vitamin D. Am. J. Orthod., *32*:463, 1946.
6. Burrill, D. Y.: The effect of low phosphorus intake on the growth of the jaws in dogs. J. Am. Dent. Assoc., *30*:513, 1943.
7. Dreizen, S., Levy, B. M., Bernick, S., Hampton, J. K., Jr., and Kraintz, L.: Studies on the biology of the periodontium of marmosets. III. Periodontal bone changes in marmosets with osteomalacia and hyperparathyroidism. Israel J. Med. Sci., *3*:731, 1967.
8. Fahmy, H., Rodgers, W. E., Mitchell, D. F., and Brewer, H. E.: Effects of hypervitaminosis D on the periodontium of the hamster. J. Dent. Res., *40*:870, 1961.
9. Follis, R. H., Jr.: The influence of essential nutrients and hormones on cartilage and bone. Trans. Josiah Macy Jr. Foundation Conference on Metabolic Interrelations, *2*:221, 1950.
10. Henrikson, P.: Periodontal disease and calcium deficiency: an experimental study in the dog. Acta Odontol. Scand., *26*(Suppl. 50):1, 1968.
11. MacCollum, E. V., Simmonds, N., Shipley, P. G., and Park, B. A.: The production of rickets by diets low in phosphorus and fat soluble. A. J. Biol. Chem., *47*:507, 1921.
12. Nomura, H.: Histopathological study of experimental hypervitaminosis D₂ on the periodontium of the rat. Shikwa Gaku, *69*:1, 1969.
13. Oliver, W. M.: The effect of deficiencies of calcium, vitamin D, or calcium and vitamin D and of variations in the source of dietary protein on the supporting tissues of the rat molar. J. Periodont. Res., *4*:56, 1969.
14. Shoshan, S., Pisanti, S., and Sciaky, I.: The effect of hypervitaminosis D on the periodontal membrane collagen in lathyritic rats. J. Periodont. Res., *2*:121, 1967.
15. Weinmann, J. P.: Rachitic changes of the mandibular condyle of the rat. J. Dent. Res., *25*:509, 1946.
16. Weinmann, J. P., and Schour, I.: Experimental studies in calcification. Am. J. Pathol., *21*:821, 1047, 1945.
17. Weinmann, J. P., and Sicher, H.: Bone and Bones. St. Louis, C. V. Mosby Company, 1948, p. 147.

VITAMIN E, VITAMIN K, AND VITAMIN P DEFICIENCIES

VITAMIN E. No relationship has been demonstrated between deficiencies in vitamin E and oral disease.[5] Extirpation of the submaxillary and sublingual glands in vitamin E–deficient animals results in gingival bleeding, loosening and exfoliation of the molars, and purulent discharge from the sockets.[2] In humans, a favorable response to vitamin E therapy has been reported in patients who have severe periodontal disease, with a minimum of local irritating factors.[4]

VITAMIN K. Vitamin K is necessary for the production of prothrombin in the liver; vitamin K deficiency results in a hemorrhagic tendency. It may cause excessive gingival bleeding after toothbrushing or spontaneously. In humans vitamin K is synthesized by bacteria in the intestinal tract. Antibiotics and sulfa drugs which inhibit the bacterial action may interfere with this synthesis. Bile salts are important in the absorption of vitamin K; obstruction of the biliary tract may lead to hypoprothrombinemia. Vitamin K is used for the prevention and control of oral hemorrhage.

VITAMIN P (CITRIN). Vitamin P is involved in the maintenance of capillary integrity and the prevention of capillary fragility.[1, 6] It has been used therapeutically to control hemorrhage and in the treatment of blood dyscrasias.[7] Kreshover and Burket[3] suggested that the capillary fragility frequently encountered in patients with periodontal disease may be due in part to vitamin P deficiency. This is based on the finding of normal blood ascorbic acid levels in patients who manifested a high petechial count in capillary fragility testing. The use of citrin in the treatment of gingival disease is still in the experimental stage.

REFERENCES

Vitamin E, Vitamin K, and Vitamin P Deficiencies

1. Bourne, G.: Vitamin P deficiency in guinea pigs. Nature, *152*:659, 1943.
2. Goldbach, H.: Success of vitamin E therapy in periodontal disease. Z. Stomatol., *43*:379, 1946.
3. Kreshover, S., and Burket, L.: Cited in Burket, L.: Oral Medicine. Philadelphia, J. B. Lippincott Company, 1946, p. 411.
4. Lieb, H., and Mathis, H.: The treatment of periodontal disease with vitamin E. Z. Stomatol., *47*:358, 1950.
5. Nelson, M. A., and Chaudhry, A. P.: Effects of tocopherol (vitamin E) deficient diet on some oral, para-oral and hematopoietic tissues of the rat. J. Dent. Res., *45*:1072, 1966.
6. Rusznyák, S., and Szent-Györgyi, A.: Vitamin P: flavonals as vitamins. Nature, *138*:27, 1936.
7. Scarborough, H.: Vitamin P. Biochem. J., *33*:1400, 1939.

PROTEIN DEFICIENCY

Protein depletion results in hypoproteinemia with many pathologic changes, including muscular atrophy, weakness, weight loss, anemia, leukopenia, edema, impaired lactation, decreased resistance to infection, slow wound healing, lymphoid depletion, and reduced ability to form certain hormones and enzyme systems.[2] *Kwashiorkor,* a protein deficiency disease of children that has a high mortality rate, is fairly widespread in malnourished populations.[12]

Protein deprivation causes the following changes in the periodontium of experimental animals[4, 6, 9]**: degeneration of the connective tissue of the gingiva and periodontal ligament, osteoporosis of alveolar bone,**[3] **retardation in the deposition of cementum, delayed wound healing**[14] **(Fig. 28–3), and atrophy of the tongue epithelium.**[16] **Similar changes occur in the periosteum and bone in other areas. Osteoporosis results from reduced deposition of osteoid, reduction in the number of osteoblasts, and retardation in the morphodifferentiation of connective tissue cells to form osteoblasts, rather than from increased osteoclasis.**

These observations are of interest in that they reveal a loss of alveolar bone that is the result of the inhibition of normal bone-forming activity rather than of the introduction of destructive factors.

Protein deficiency accentuates the destructive effects of local irritants[15] and occlusal trauma[11] upon the periodontal tissues, but the initiation of gingival inflammation and its severity depend upon the local irritants. Tryptophan deficiency in rats results in osteoporosis of alveolar bone.[1]

Combined Protein-Vitamin Deficiencies

Protein deficiency commonly produces anemia. However, protein deficiencies are always accompanied by deficiencies of hematopoietic

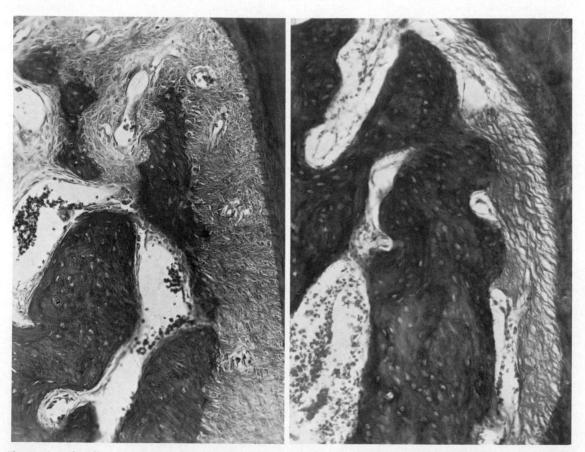

Figure 28–3 The Effect of Protein Deprivation upon the Periodontium of the Albino Rat. *Left,* **Control Animal.** Periodontal ligament and alveolar bone between the molar roots, showing dense collagen fibers. Note continuity of the collagen fibrils of the periodontal ligament with the matrix of the bone and polyhedral cells along the bone margin between the periodontal fibers. *Right,* **Protein Deprivation.** Periodontal ligament and alveolar bone between the molar roots. Note degeneration of the periodontal ligament marked by reduction in number and wavy outline of collagen fibrils. A clear-cut demarcation is seen between the bone matrix and the periodontal ligament (compare with control).

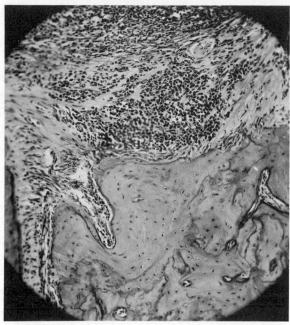

Figure 28–4 Margin of Alveolar Bone beneath area of artificially induced inflammation in albino rat on adequate diet. The bone surface in relation to the leukocytic infiltration presents lacunar resorption and an adjacent layer of osteoid lined with osteoblasts.

vitamins and iron, and vitamin deficiencies include some degree of disturbed protein metabolism, so that anemia is often the result of combined protein-vitamin deficiency.[5] Such deficiency can produce macrocytic anemia with hematologic and oral changes identical with those of pernicious anemia (see Chapter 30). Several types of anemia occur in kwashiorkor, and the oral changes resemble those of pellagra, which is a mixed protein-vitamin deficiency state with severe oral manifestations.

STARVATION

The term "hunger osteopathy" connotes skeletal disturbances that occur in individuals in famine areas. Such disturbances are characterized by a reduction in the amount of normally calcified bone and have been attributed to deficiencies in calcium, phosphorus, vitamin D, and protein and to associated hormonal dysfunction. In a study of controlled semistarvation in young adults,[10] there were no changes in the oral cavity or skeletal system despite a 24 per cent loss of body weight. Another study, however, showed reduction in plaque index scores and a considerable increase in gingival index scores as the fasting period lengthened.[13]

In experimental animals acute starvation results in osteoporosis of alveolar bone and other bones, reduction in the height of alveolar bone,

and accentuated bone loss associated with gingival inflammation[6] **(Figs. 28–4 and 28–5). Furthermore, bone formation associated with extrusion of teeth following the extraction of functional antagonists is impaired by acute starvation.**[7]

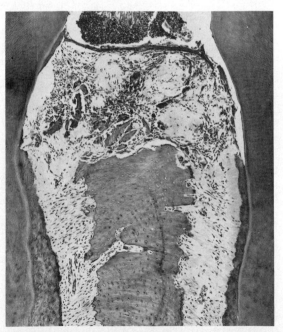

Figure 28–5 Interdental Bony Septum subjacent to artificially induced gingival inflammation in albino rat on starvation diet. The bone presents lacunar resorption without any evidence of new bone formation. (Compare with Fig. 28–4.)

REFERENCES

Protein Deficiency

1. Bavetta, L. A., and Bernick, S.: Effect of tryptophane deficiency on bones and teeth of rats. III. Effect of age. Oral Surg., *9*:308, 1956.
2. Cannon, P. R.: Some Pathologic Consequences of Protein and Amino Acid Deficiencies. Springfield, Ill., Charles C Thomas, Publisher, 1948.
3. Carranza, F. A., Jr., Cabrini, R. L., Lopez Otero, R., and Stahl, S. S.: Histometric analysis of interradicular bone in protein deficient animals. J. Periodont. Res., *4*:292, 1969.
4. Chawla, T. N., and Glickman, I.: Protein deprivation and the periodontal structures of the albino rat. Oral Surg., *4*:578, 1951.
5. Dreizen, S.: Oral manifestations of human nutritional anemias. Arch. Environ. Health, *5*:66, 1962.
6. Frandsen, A. M., et al.: The effects of various levels of dietary protein on the periodontal tissues of young rats. J. Periodontol., *24*:135, 1953.
7. Glickman, I.: The effect of acute starvation upon the apposition of alveolar bone associated with the extraction of functional antagonists. J. Dent. Res., *24*:155, 1945.
8. Glickman, I., Morse, A., and Robinson, L.: The systemic influence upon bone in periodontoclasia. J. Am. Dent. Assoc., *31*:1435, 1944.
9. Goldman, H. M.: Protein deprivation in rats. J. Dent. Res., *39*:690, 1960.
10. Keys, A., et al.: The Biology of Human Starvation. Vol. 1. Minneapolis, University of Minnesota Press, 1950, Chapter 12.
11. Miller, S. C., Stahl, S. S., and Goldsmith, E. D.: The effects of vertical occlusal trauma on the periodontium of protein deprived young adult rats. J. Periodontol., *28*:87, 1957.
12. Scrimshaw, N. S., and Béhar, M.: Protein malnutrition in young children. Science, *133*:2039, 1961.
13. Squire, C. F., and Costley, J. M.: Gingival status during prolonged fasting for weight loss. J. Periodontol., *47*:98, 1976.
14. Stahl, S. S.: The effect of a protein-free diet on the healing of gingival wounds in rats. Arch. Oral Biol., *7*:551, 1962.
15. Stahl, S. S., Sandler, H. C., and Cahn, L.: The effects of protein deprivation upon the oral tissues of the rat and particularly upon the periodontal structures under irritation. Oral Surg., *8*:760, 1955.
16. Stein, G., and Ziskin, D.: The effect of protein free diet on the teeth and the periodontium of the albino rat. J. Dent. Res., *28*:529, 1949.

MINERAL DEFICIENCIES AND TOXICITIES

IRON. Pallor of the oral cavity and tongue is the most common and sometimes the only oral manifestations of iron deficiency anemia. The tongue may also be swollen, with a blotchy or total atrophy of the papillary epithelium.[9, 28] Petechial hemorrhages in the mucosa and angular cheilitis occur in some cases.

Deutsch et al.[10] produced chronic iron deficiency anemias in rats by feeding them liquid and powdered milk diets; blood studies confirmed the anemic state. Changes observed in the periodontium, however, were related to the physical consistency of the diet and not to the anemia.

FLUORIDE. Observations in populations using fluoridated water supplies do not agree regarding the effects, if any, of ingested fluoride upon the condition of the periodontium (see Chapter 23). Findings in experimental animals vary, with some investigators reporting that fluoride increases periodontal disease[26, 30] and others that it decreases[8] or protects against periodontal disease.[27] It has also been shown that fluoride reduces the severity of cortisone-induced alveolar bone resorption,[34] prevents adverse effects of hypervitaminosis D,[14] and inhibits bone resorption in tissue culture.[17] Fluoride in drinking water in levels used to prevent tooth decay presents no health hazards, although at much higher concentrations fluoride may affect the skeletal system adversely and produce spondylosis deformans, which is characterized by progressive osteosclerosis, ossification of tendon and ligament insertions, and spinal rigidity.[22] In experimental animals fluoride intoxication results in extensive periosteal bone deposition at sites of muscular insertion and generalized osteoporosis of the jaws.[4] Periodontal disease with loss of alveolar bone appeared to be associated with increased fluorine intake in South African natives.[1] Based upon the increased bone density associated with high levels of ingested fluoride, as much as 100 mg per day of sodium fluoride has been tried in the treatment of osteoporosis.[21] (See Chapter 45 for a discussion of the use of fluorides in periodontal therapy.)

OTHER INTOXICATIONS. Reduction in the rate of alveolar bone formation,[11] widening of the periodontal ligament,[11, 23] retarded tooth eruption, and gingival enlargement with connective tissue hyperplasia have been observed in **magnesium-deficient animals.**[6] Other changes include altered alveolar bone architecture (with the formation of a mosaic pattern[7]), increased resorption, fibrosis of the marrow, calculus formation, and loosening of the teeth. **Molybdenum toxicity** in experimental animals causes mandibular exostoses, cemental spurs, hypercementosis, and disorganization of the odontoblastic layer.[29]

Beryllium and strontium intoxications result in a hyperproduction of bone and cementum and dentin matrix that do not calcify, leading to a rickets-like lesion.[19]

OSTEOLATHYRISM

Lathyrism is a disease of the nervous system in man and domestic animals caused by the ingestion of certain types of peas, such as *Lathyrus sativus*. It does not produce changes in the jaws or oral tissues. Animals fed diets rich in *Lathyrus odoratus* peas, or administered certain aminonitriles such as aminoacetonitrile, aminopropionitrile, or methyleneaminonitrile, develop osteolathyrism, a disease which bears no resemblance to lathyrism in humans.[31] Osteolathyrism is characterized by oral as well as systemic changes.

Exostoses occur on the jaws in areas of muscle attachment, and the condylar cartilage is enlarged. The fibroblasts of the periodontal ligament exhibit increased cytoplasmic basophilia and palisading, and the collagen fibers are fine, disoriented, and embedded in amorphous eosinophilic material.[12, 25] Hydroxyproline activity and conversion of soluble collagen to the insoluble type are decreased, according to some authors,[33] but in tissue culture studies with a lathyrogenic agent the synthesis and degradation of collagen are unaffected.[18] The alveolar bone is osteoporotic, and there is pronounced hypercementosis and loosening of teeth.[13] Mechanical force is an important contributing factor in the development of osteolathyritic changes in the jaws,[24] and systemic conditioning agents modify their severity.[15]

The electron microscope shows mottling of the bone matrix and disturbed development of osteoblasts.[3]

CALCIPHYLAXIS

Calciphylaxis is a condition of induced systemic hypersensitivity described by Selye,[32] in which tissues respond to appropriate challenging agents with precipitous, sometimes evanescent local calcification. Substances which predispose to calciphylaxis are known as sensitizers; agents which precipitate the calciphylaxis phenomenon are known as challengers. *Sensitizers* include dihydrotachysterol (DHT), vitamin D, parathormone, and sodium acetylsulfathiazole, among many calcium salts and phosphates.

Challengers may be *direct* or *indirect*. Direct challengers include mechanical trauma and various chemical agents (salts of iron, chromium, aluminum, zinc, manganese, and cesium) which cause calcification at the site of application and may elicit some form of systemic calciphylaxis when administered intravenously or intraperitoneally. Indirect challengers have little or no effect at the site of application and produce diverse systemic syndromes of calcification and sclerosis.

Prolonged administration of DHT in rats produces a *chronic intoxication syndrome* with the following severe changes in the periodontium: **osteosclerosis, pronounced osteoid formation, bulbous distortion in the shape of the bone, and degeneration of the marrow and the periodontal ligament.** Intraperitoneal administration of ferric dextran (Fe-Dex) induced calciphylaxis, which reduced the toxic effects of DHT upon the periodontium.[16]

DISTURBANCES OF THE ACID-BASE BALANCE

The acid-base balance refers to the state of equilibrium that normally exists between the acid and base components of the tissues and fluids of the body. Acidosis is an abnormal state in which there is accumulation of acids or loss of alkali in the blood; it may be accompanied by changes in bone.[2] Acidosis from renal tubular insufficiency without glomerular insufficiency may result in osteomalacia in adults. Osteoporosis of the jaws has been described associated with acidosis in experimental animals.[5] Alkalosis is an abnormal state in which there is an accumulation of alkali or loss of acid. Retrograde changes in alveolar bone have been described in animals maintained on alkaline diets.[20]

REFERENCES

Mineral Deficiencies and Toxicities

1. Abrahams, L. C.: Masticatory apparatus of the people of Calvinia and Namaqualand in the North-Western Cape of the Union of South Africa. J. Dent. Assoc. South Africa, *1*:5, 1946.
2. Albright, F., and Reifenstein, E. C.: The Parathyroid Glands and Metabolic Bone Disease. Baltimore, Williams & Wilkins Company, 1948, p. 241.
3. Amemiya, A.: Electron microscopic study of periosteal hyperostosis in rats with lathyrism induced by aminoacetonitrile. Bull. Tokyo Med. Dent. Univ., *13*:319, 1966.
4. Bauer, W. H.: Experimental chronic fluorine intoxication: effects on bones and teeth. Am. J. Orthod., *31*:700, 1945.
5. Bauer, W. H., and Haslhofer, L.: Veränderung der Kiefer und Zähne durch Zuckerverabreichung. Z. Stomatol., *31*:1359, 1933.
6. Becks, H., and Furuta, W. J.: Effect of magnesium deficient diets on oral and dental tissues. II. Changes in the enamel structure. J. Am. Dent. Assoc., *28*:1083, 1941.
7. Becks, H., and Furuta, W. J.: The effects of magnesium deficient diets on oral and dental tissues. III. Changes in dentine and pulp tissue. Am. J. Orthod., *28*:1, 1942.
8. Costich, E. R., Hein, J. W., Hodge, H. C., and Shourie, K. L.: Reduction of hamster periodontal disease by sodium fluoride and sodium monofluorophosphate in drinking water. J. Am. Dent. Assoc., *55*:617, 1957.
9. Darby, W. J.: The oral manifestations of iron deficiency. J.A.M.A., *130*:830, 1946.
10. Deutsch, C. M., Dreizen, S., and Stahl, S. S.: The effects of chronic deficiency anemia on the periodontium of the adult rat. J. Periodontol., *40*:736, 1969.

11. Gagnon, J. A., Schour, I., and Patras, M. C.: Effect of magnesium deficiency on dentin apposition and eruption in incisor of rat. Proc. Soc. Exp. Biol. Med., *49*:662, 1942.

12. Gardner, A. F.: Morphologic study of oral connective tissue in lathyrism. J. Dent. Res., *39*:24, 1960.

13. Gardner, A. F.: Alterations in mesenchymal and ectodermal tissues during experimental lathyrism. Apposition and calcification of cementum. Parodontologie, *20*:111, 1966.

14. Gedalia, I., and Binderman, I.: Effect of fluoride on hypervitaminosis D in rats. J. Dent. Res., *45*:825, 1966.

15. Glickman, I., Selye, H., and Smulow, J. B.: Systemic factors which influence the manifestations of osteolathyrism in the periodontium. J. Dent. Res., *42*:835, 1963.

16. Glickman, I., Selye, H., and Smulow, J. B.: Reduction by calciphylaxis of the effects of chronic dihydrotachysterol overdose upon the periodontium. J. Dent. Res., *44*:374, 1965.

17. Goldhaber, P.: The inhibition of bone resorption in tissue culture by nontoxic concentrations of sodium fluoride. Israel J. Med. Sci., *3*:617, 1967.

18. Golub, L., Stern, B., Glimcher, M., and Goldhaber, P.: The effect of a lathyrogenic agent on the synthesis and degradation of mouse bone callagen in tissue culture. Arch. Oral Biol., *13*:1395, 1968.

19. Gravina, O., Cabrini, R. L., and Carranza, F. A., Jr.: Effect of a strontium-containing diet on periodontal tissues of rat molars. J. Periodontol., *41*:174, 1970.

20. Jones, M. R., and Simonton, F. V.: Mineral metabolism in relation to alveolar atrophy in dogs. J. Am. Dent. Assoc., *15*:881, 1928.

21. Jowsey, J., Schenk, R. K., and Reutter, F. W.: Some results of the effect of fluoride on bone tissue in osteoporosis. J. Clin. Endocrinol. Metab., *28*:869, 1968.

22. Kemp, F. H., Murray, M. M., and Wilson, D. C.: Spondylosis deformans in relation to fluorine and general nutrition. Lancet, *243*:93, 1942.

23. Klein, H., Orent, E. R., and McCollum, E. V.: Effects of magnesium deficiency on teeth and their supporting structures in rats. Am. J. Physiol., *112*:256, 1935.

24. Krikos, G. A., Beltran, R., and Cohen, A.: Significance of mechanical stress on the development of periodontal lesions in lathyritic rats. J. Dent. Res., *44*:600, 1965.

25. Krikos, G. A., Morris, A. L., Hammond, W. S., and McClure, H. H.: Oral changes in experimental lathyrism (odoratism). Oral Surg., *11*:309, 1958.

26. Kristoffersen, T., Bang, G., and Meyer, K.: Lack of effect of high doses of fluoride in prevention of alveolar bone loss in rats. J. Periodont. Res., *5*:127, 1970.

27. Likins, R. C., Pakis, G., and McClure, F. J.: Effect of fluoride and tetracycline on alveolar bone resorption in the rat. J. Dent. Res., *42*:1532, 1963.

28. Monto, R. W., Rizek, R. A., and Fine, G.: Observations on the exfoliative cytology and histology of the oral mucous membranes in iron deficiency. Oral Surg., *14*:965, 1961.

29. Ostram, C. A., Van Reen, R., and Miller, C. W.: Changes in the connective tissue of rats fed toxic diets containing molybdenum salts. J. Dent. Res., *40*:520, 1961.

30. Ramseyer, W. F., Smith, C. A. H., and McCay, C. M.: Effect of sodium fluoride administration on body changes in old rats. J. Gerontol., *12*:14, 1957.

31. Selye, H.: Lathyrism. Rev. Can. Biol., *16*:3, 1957.

32. Selye, H.: Calciphylaxis. Chicago, University of Chicago Press, 1962.

33. Smith, D. J.: Biochemical aspects of repair in lathyrism. J. Dent. Res., *45*:500, 1966.

34. Zipkin, I., Bernick, S., and Menczel, J.: A morphological study of the effect of fluoride on the periodontium of the hydrocortisone-treated rat. Periodontics, *3*:111, 1965.

chapter twenty-nine

Endocrinologic Influences in the Etiology of Periodontal Disease

HORMONAL INFLUENCES ON THE PERIODONTIUM

Hormones are organic substances produced by the endocrine glands. They are secreted directly into the blood stream and exert an important physiologic influence upon the functions of certain cells and systems. The significance of hormonal disturbances in the causation of periodontal disease is presented here.

Hypothyroidism

The effects of hypothyroidism vary with the age at which it occurs. The basal metabolic rate is depressed, and growth is retarded. Cretinism, juvenile myxedema, and adult myxedema are the three clinical syndromes that result from hypothyroidism.

Cretinism is the manifestation of hypothyroidism that is either congenital or occurs shortly after birth. Delayed physical and mental development is characteristic of the disease.

Juvenile myxedema occurs between the ages of 6 and 12 years and may be related to iodine deficiency or other injurious influences on the thyroid gland.

Hypothyroidism in the adult results in *myxedema*. The patient is easily fatigued and usually gains weight in spite of lack of appetite. The characteristic nonpitting edema of subcutaneous tissues is seen. The basal metabolic rate and blood pressure are low, the pulse is slow, and the blood cholesterol is elevated.

HYPOTHYROIDISM AND THE PERIODONTIUM. Aside from impaired development, no notable changes in the periodontal tissues have been attributed to cretinism. Chronic periodontal disease with severe bone loss has been described in patients with myxedema,[3, 8, 9] with the suggestion that the latter condition contributes to periodontal destruction. Degenerative changes in the gingiva have been reported in thyroidectomized animals.[1, 20]

In animals with thiouracil-induced hypothyroidism, apposition of alveolar bone is retarded[6] and the size of the haversian systems is reduced,[4] but there is no evidence of periodontal disease.[5] Animals with experimentally induced myxedema present hyperparakeratosis with some keratosis of the gingival epithelium, edema, and disorganization of the collagen bundles in the connective tissue; hydropic degeneration and fragmentation of the fibers of the periodontal ligament; and osteoporosis of the alveolar bone.[11]

Hyperthyroidism

Hyperfunction of the thyroid gland is common in young and middle-aged adults. Among the symptoms are cardiovascular effects (increased pulse rate, hypertension, and cardiac enlargement), nervousness and emotional instability, loss of weight, and exophthalmos. Infants with this disorder show increased growth and development (in contrast to those with a hypothyroid condition), with early eruption of the teeth. The teeth and jaws are well formed and present no unusual irregularities. Alveolar bone appears somewhat rarefied and partially decalcified. In the adult, salivary flow is increased owing to sympathetic hyperstimulation, but there are no notable oral changes.[13]

HYPERTHYROIDISM AND THE PERIODONTIUM. Osteoporosis of the alveolar bone, lacunar resorption, and an increase in the size of the marrow spaces (with fibrosis of the marrow and an increase in the width and vascularity of the periodontal ligament) have been described in experimental animals fed thyroid extract over a period of 1 to 16 weeks.[1]

Thyroid feeding accentuates the osteoporosis of alveolar bone induced in animals by tryptophan deficiency.[2]

Hypopituitarism

Hypopituitarism, a deficiency in the secretion of the anterior pituitary lobe, is marked by a retardation in the growth of all tissues. The earlier in life the condition occurs, the more severe the clinical changes. Hypopituitarism in children results in dwarfism.

In dwarfism, the cranium and face develop very slowly, resembling those of a much younger child. The face is relatively small compared with the cranium, and the sinuses are underdeveloped, especially the frontal sinuses. Retardation in the development of the teeth and jaws has been noted by many observers. There is delayed resorption in the formation and eruption of the permanent teeth. The growth of the maxilla and mandible is arrested, with the mandible showing the greater degree of change. Retarded growth of the ramus, causing failure in increase of the vertical height of the mandible, reduced intermaxillary space, crowding of the teeth, and a tendency toward a distal relationship of the mandible have been attributed to hypopituitarism.

HYPOPITUITARISM AND THE PERIODONTIUM. The following is a summary of the microscopic changes observed in the periodontal tissue of experimental animals with artificially induced hypopituitarism:

Resorption of cementum in the molar furcation areas, reduced apposition of cementum, and resorption of alveolar bone in animals with a short postoperative life, with sclerosis and the suggestion of a mosaic pattern. The vascularity of the periodontal ligament is reduced, and there is degeneration of the ligament with cystic degeneration and calcification of many of the epithelial rests. The junctional epithelium is often atrophic or ab-

sent. It has been suggested that the changes observed in these animals may not be specific for hypophysectomy, but may be attributable to an associated reduction in the blood supply, caused either by the hypophysectomy or by resulting changes in other endocrine glands.[12, 14]

Hyperpituitarism

Hyperpituitarism, an increase in the secretion of the anterior lobe of the pituitary, results in gigantism or acromegaly, depending upon the age at which it occurs. Hyperpituitarism before the age of 6 years results in *gigantism*, characterized by unusual height and disproportion. When hyperpituitarism occurs after the age of 6, *juvenile acromegaly* is the result, with abnormal height, huge hands and feet, long face, and prognathious jaw.

In *adults*, hyperpituitarism results in *acromegaly*, which is characterized by a disproportionate overgrowth of the facial bones, with overdeveloped sinuses. The face is large with coarse features. The lips are greatly enlarged, and localized areas of hyperpigmentation are often seen along the nasolabial folds. **A marked overgrowth of the alveolar process causes an increase in the size of the dental arch and consequently affects the spacing of the teeth. This may affect the periodontium by introducing the irritation of food impaction. Hypercementosis is another feature of the increased rate of growth.**

Hypoparathyroidism

Hypoparathyroidism results from accidental removal of the glands in thyroidectomy or from deficiencies occurring early in life. There is a hypocalcemia and a resultant increased excitability of the nervous system. The condition is known as *parathyroid tetany*.

If the condition occurs in infancy, it causes enamel hypoplasia and disturbances in the calcification of dentin.

Hyperparathyroidism

Parathyroid hypersecretion produces generalized demineralization of the skeleton, the formation of bone cysts and giant cell tumors, increased osteoclasis, occasional osteoid for-

mation, and proliferation of the connective tissue in the marrow spaces and the haversian canals. Serum calcium is increased, serum phosphorus is decreased, and serum phosphatase may be normal or elevated.[19]

HYPERPARATHYROIDISM AND THE PERIODONTIUM. Different investigators report the number of patients with hyperparathyroidism who present oral changes as 25 per cent,[15] 45 per cent,[10] and 50 per cent.[16]

The oral changes include malocclusion and tooth mobility, radiographic evidence of alveolar osteoporosis with closely meshed trabeculae, widening of the periodontal space, absence of the lamina dura, and radiolucent cyst-like spaces.

Loss of the lamina dura and giant cell tumors in the jaws are late signs of hyperparathyroid bone disease, which in itself is uncommon. Complete loss of the lamina dura does not occur often, and there is a danger of attaching too much diagnostic significance to it. Other diseases in which it may occur are Paget's disease, fibrous dysplasia, and osteomalacia.

In hyperparathyroidism associated with renal insufficiency, Weinmann[18] reported extensive resorption of lamellated bone and its replacement by immature coarse fibrillar spongy bone and fibrosis of the bone marrow. In experimental animals,[19] small doses of parathormone induce a short period of osteoclasis, followed by osteoblastic activity and osteosclerosis of the alveolar bone; massive doses lead to resorption of the bone and its replacement by connective tissue.

A relationship has been suggested between periodontal disease in dogs and hyperparathyroidism secondary to calcium deficiency in the diet.[7] This has not been confirmed by other studies.[17]

REFERENCES

1. Baume, L. J., and Becks, H.: The effect of thyroid hormone in dental and paradental structures. Paradentologie, 6:89, 1952.
2. Bavetta, L. A., Bernick, S., and Ershoff, B.: The influences of dietary thyroid on the bones and periodontium of rats on total and partial tryptophan deficiencies. J. Dent. Res., 36:13, 1957.
3. Becks, H.: Systemic background of paradentosis. J. Am. Dent. Assoc., 28:1447, 1941.
4. English, J. A.: Experimental effects of thiouracil and selenium on the teeth and jaws of dogs. J. Dent. Res., 28:172, 1949.
5. Fisher, R. L., and Mitchell, D. F.: Induced hypothyroidism on the periodontium of the hamster. I.A.D.R. Abstracts, 1962, p. 67.
6. Glickman, I., and Pruzansky, S.: Propyl-thiouracil hypothyroidism in the albino rat. J. Dent. Res., 26:471, 1947.
7. Henrikson, P. A.: Periodontal disease and calcium deficiency in the dog. Acta Odontol. Scand., 26(Suppl. 50), 1968.
8. Hutton, J. H.: Relation of endocrine disorders to dental disease. J. Am. Dent. Assoc., 23:226, 1936.
9. Lewis, A. B.: Oral manifestations of endocrine disturbances—myxedema. Dent. Cosmos, 77:47, 1935.
10. Rosenberg, E. H., and Guralnick, W. C.: Hyperparathyroidism. Oral Surg., 15(Suppl. 2):84, 1962.
11. Rosenberg, E. H., Goldman, H. M., and Garber, E.: The effects of experimental thyrotoxicosis and myxedema on the periodontium of rabbits. J. Dent. Res., 40:708, 1961.
12. Schour, I.: The effects of hypophysectomy on the periodontal tissues. J. Periodontol., 5:15, 1934.
13. Schour, I., and Massler, M.: Endocrines and dentistry. J. Am. Dent. Assoc., 30:595, 763, 943, 1943.
14. Shapiro, S., and Shklar, G.: The effect of hypophysectomy on the periodontium of the albino rat. J. Periodontol., 33:364, 1962.
15. Silverman, S., Gordan, G., Grant, T., Steinbach, H., Eisenberg, E., and Manson, R.: The dental structures in primary hyperparathyroidism. Oral Surg., 15:426, 1962.
16. Strock, M. S.: The mouth in hyperparathyroidism. N. Engl. J. Med. 224:1019, 1945.
17. Svanberg, G., Lindhe, J., Hugoson, A., and Grondahl, H. G.: Effect of nutritional hyperparathyroidism on experimental periodontitis in the dog. Scand. J. Dent. Res., 81:155, 1973.
18. Weinmann, J. P.: Bone changes in the jaw caused by renal hyperparathyroidism. J. Periodontol., 16:94, 1945.
19. Weinmann, J. P., and Schour, I.: The effect of parathyroid hormone on the alveolar bone and teeth of the normal and rachitic rat. Am. J. Pathol., 21:857, 1945.
20. Ziskin, R. D., and Stein, G.: The gingiva and oral mucous membrane of monkeys in experimental hypothyroidism. J. Dent. Res., 21:296, 1942

Diabetes

As long ago as 1862, Seiffert described an association between diabetes mellitus and pathologic changes in the oral cavity.

Diabetes is a metabolic disease characterized by hypofunction or lack of function of the beta cells of the islets of Langerhans in the pancreas, leading to high blood glucose levels and excretion of sugar in the urine. It is a complicated biochemical disease; the metabolic regulation of carbohydrates involves not only the beta cells, which secrete the insulin that reduces glycemia, but also the alpha cells of the pancreas (which secrete glucagon), the corticoadrenal hormones, and the anterior pituitary hormones, all of which increase glycemia.

Two basic types of diabetes have been described: (1) insulin dependent and (2) non–insulin dependent.

Insulin-dependent diabetes is also known as juvenile diabetes or juvenile-onset diabetes, although it may sometimes appear at older ages. This type of diabetes is very unstable, is difficult to control, has a marked tendency toward ketosis and coma, is not preceded by obesity, and requires insulin to be controlled. The disease presents the symptoms traditionally associated with diabetes, such as polyphagia, polydipsia, polyuria, predisposition to infections, and anorexia.

The **non-insulin-dependent** type of diabetes is the adult type (onset usually occurs after age 45). It generally occurs in obese individuals and can often be controlled by diet or by oral hypoglycemic agents. The development of ketosis and coma is not common. Adult-onset diabetes has the same symptoms as juvenile diabetes but in a less severe form.

In these two types of diabetes, a genetic predisposition appears to be so important that the following conditions have been described in normal people with a family history of diabetes: (1) **prediabetes** (normal fasting blood sugar, normal glucose tolerance test, and normal stress glucose tolerance test), (2) **subclinical** or **suspected diabetes** (normal fasting blood sugar, normal glucose tolerance test, and abnormal stress glucose tolerance test), and (3) **latent** or **chemical diabetes** (normal fasting blood sugar and abnormal glucose tolerance test).

Other types of diabetes, classified as **secondary diabetes**, are those associated with other diseases that involve the pancreas and destroy the insulin-producing cells. Endocrine diseases such as acromegaly and Cushing's syndrome, tumors, pancreatectomy, and drugs and chemicals that cause hyperinsulinism are included in this group. Experimentally induced types of diabetes generally belong in this category rather than with the classic types of disease.

Control of diabetes may be attained by diet or by the administration of insulin and/or other drugs.

Oral Manifestations of Diabetes

Oral manifestations in uncontrolled and controlled diabetics will be described.

UNCONTROLLED DIABETICS. The following findings have been described in the oral mucosa: cheilosis and a tendency toward drying and cracking[29]; burning sensations[7]; decrease in salivary flow[39]; and alterations in the flora of the oral cavity, with greater predominance of *Candida albicans*, hemolytic streptococci, and staphylococci.[1] These changes, however, are not specific, and terms such as "diabetic stomatitis" should not be used.[40] Other findings reported include altered eruption patterns of the teeth,[1] increased tooth sensitivity to percussion, increased incidence of enamel hypoplasia, and increased incidence of caries.

Perhaps the most striking changes in uncontrolled diabetes are the reduction in defense mechanisms and the increased susceptibility to infections leading to destructive periodontal disease. This topic will be dealt with in a subsequent section.

CONTROLLED DIABETICS. In the well-controlled diabetic, none of the above-mentioned changes is found. There is a normal tissue response, no increase in the incidence of caries, a normally developed dentition and a normal defense against infections. However, the possibility that the control of the disease may be inadequate makes it advisable to exercise special care in the periodontal treatment of controlled diabetics (see Chapter 36).

Diabetes and the Periodontium

Opinions still differ regarding the exact relationship of diabetes and periodontal disease. A variety of periodontal changes have been described in diabetic patients, such as a tendency toward abscess formation, "diabetic periodontoclasia," enlarged gingiva, "sessile or pedunculated gingival polyps,"[30] polypoid gingival proliferations, and loosened teeth.[51]

Periodontal changes in diabetics will be described with reference to human and animal studies.

STUDIES IN HUMANS. *Clinical Aspects.* Despite the generalized increased susceptibility to infection[49] and severe inflammation[43] in diabetes, some investigators[9, 37, 46, 48] recognize no relationship between diabetes and oral disease and maintain that, when the two conditions exist together, it is a coincidence rather than a specific cause-and-effect relationship. Others report increased severity of gingivitis[16] and periodontal disease in diabetes, with increased tooth mobility not related to increased local irritants[5] and an associated increase in tooth loss (Fig. 29-1).

Most of the above-mentioned studies have been highly subjective. However, the utilization of indices to measure local irritants and clinical manifestations of disease has permitted a more rigorous analysis of the relation between periodontal disease and diabetes. The majority of these studies show a higher prevalence and severity of periodontal disease in diabetics than in nondiabetics with similar local irritation.[7, 13, 20] However, other studies have not found a correlation between the diabetic state and the periodontal condition. Probably the different degrees of diabetic involvement and control of the disease in patients examined and the diversity of indices and patient sampling are responsible for this lack of consistency.

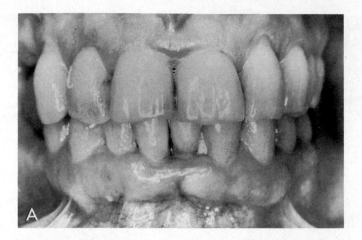

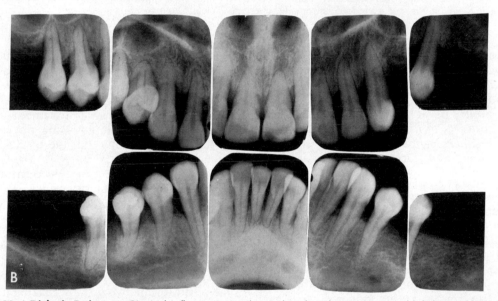

Figure 29–1 Diabetic Patient. *A,* Gingival inflammation and periodontal pockets in 34-year-old diabetic of long duration. *B,* Extensive generalized bone loss in patient shown in *A.* Failure to replace posterior teeth adds to the occlusal burden of the remaining dentition.

In general, the rate of periodontal destruction appears to be similar for diabetics and nondiabetics up to the age of 30,[25, 58] and after 30 there is a greater degree of destruction in diabetics. Patients showing overt diabetes over a period of more than 10 years have greater loss of periodontal structures than those with diabetic history of less than 10 years.[25]

The extensive literature on this subject and the overall impressions of clinicians point to the fact that *periodontal disease in diabetics follows no consistent pattern.* Very severe gingival inflammation, deep periodontal pockets, and frequent periodontal abscesses often occur in patients with poor oral hygiene. In juvenile diabetics, there is often extensive periodontal destruction, which is noteworthy because of their age. However, in many other diabetic patients, juvenile and adult, the gingival changes and bone loss are not unusual.

According to Cianciola et al.,[14] periodontitis in insulin-dependent diabetics appears to start after age 12. The prevalence of periodontitis is 9.8 per cent in 13- to 18-year-olds, increasing to 39 per cent in those 19 years and older. The same authors found that insulin-dependent diabetic children tend to have more destruction around the first molars and incisors than elsewhere, but the destruction becomes more generalized at older ages.[14]

The distribution and severity of local irritants affect the severity of periodontal disease

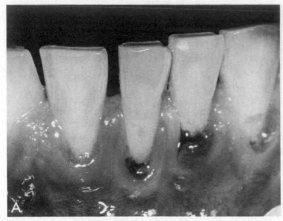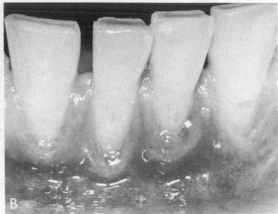

Figure 29–2 *A,* **Adult Diabetic Patient,** blood glucose level 400 mg per 100 ml. Note gingival inflammation, spontaneous bleeding, and edema. *B,* After 4 days of insulin therapy (glucose level less than 100 mg per 100 ml) the clinical periodontal picture has improved in the absence of local therapy. (Courtesy of Dr. Joan Otomo.)

in diabetes. *Diabetes does not cause gingivitis or periodontal pockets, but there are indications that it alters the response of the periodontal tissues to local irritants* (Fig. 29–2) *and that it hastens bone loss in periodontal disease and retards postsurgical healing of the periodontal tissues. Frequent periodontal abscesses appear to be an important feature of periodontal disease in diabetics.*

Microscopic Aspects. **Microscopic changes in the gingiva include the following: hyperplasia with hyperkeratosis,**[62] **or a change from a stippled to a smooth surface with diminished keratinization; intranuclear vacuolization in the epithelium; increased intensity of inflammation; fatty infiltration in the inflamed tissue**[23] **an increase in calcified foreign bodies**[47]**; widening of the basement membrane of capillaries and precapillary arterioles,**[11, 31, 33] **but no osteosclerotic changes**[32]**; periodic acid–Schiff and fuchsinophilic thickening of small blood vessels**[33]**; and reduced staining of acid mucopolysaccharides. Oxygen consumption in the gingiva and the oxidation of glucose are reduced.**[12]

Arteriolar changes consisting of increased fuchsinophilia, thickened walls, narrowed lumen, medial degeneration, and vacuolization have been reported in the gingiva of patients with diabetes and/or hypertensive cardiovascular disease.[57]

Among the microscopic changes described, *thickening of the basement membrane of capillaries* warrants special attention, because (1) this change in the vessel walls may hamper the transport of nutrients necessary for the maintenance of gingival tissues, and (2) it has been

suggested that gingival biopsies may be an important aid in the detection of prediabetic and diabetic states. These procedures have also been used in other tissues.[22] The thickness of capillary and arteriolar wall basement membranes has been measured using optical[31, 32] and electron microscopy, but the results have been inconsistent.

Listgarten et al.[36] used the electron microscope to study gingival biopsy specimens from 10 diabetic and 10 nondiabetic subjects; each group was composed of five normal and five inflamed gingivae. A statistically significant increase in the thickness of the basement membrane of capillaries was found in diabetics. However, there was considerable overlapping of the result for the two groups, making it very difficult to use this as a diagnostic aid. Frantzis et al.[21] reported greater differences in the thickness of the basement membrane between diabetics and control subjects and also suggested that this may have diagnostic importance. The thickness of the basement membrane was found to be unrelated to inflammation, age, and duration of diabetes.[36]

Biochemical Studies. Comparison of the salivary and blood sugar levels with the periodontal condition of diabetics revealed that salivary glucose levels (1 hour after breakfast) were higher in diabetics, but not to a degree which could be diagnostic.[42]

In another study,[19] the glucose content of gingival fluid and blood was found to be higher in diabetics than in nondiabetics with a similar plaque and gingival index scores; the protein content was found to be similar in the two groups.[19] The increased glucose in the gingival fluid and blood of diabetics could change the environment of the microflora, inducing qualitative changes in bacteria that could affect periodontal changes.

Gingival fluid from diabetics contains a reduced level of cyclic adenosine monophosphate (cyclic AMP) compared with that of nondiabetics. Since cAMP reduces inflammation, this is another possible mechanism that could lead to increased severity of gingival inflammation in diabetics.

Microbiologic Studies. Massler in 1949 reported 40 per cent more *Staphylococcus aureus* in the gingival and pharyngeal mucosa of diabetics than in those of nondiabetics. Sanchez Cordero et al. found a highly significant difference in the incidence of staphylococci in diabetics as compared with nondiabetics and predominance of *S. saprophyticus* in nondiabetics and *S. epidermidis* in diabetics.[54] The role of these bacteria in periodontitis is unknown.

Immunologic Studies. The increased susceptibility of diabetics to infection has been hypothesized as being due to polymorphonuclear leukocyte deficiencies resulting in impaired chemotaxis,[44] defective phagocytosis,[61] or impaired adherence.[24] Robertson and Polk[50] found no alteration of immunoglobulins A, G, or M in diabetics.

STUDIES IN ANIMALS. There have been many studies of the periodontium in animals with diabetes induced by injection of the drug alloxan[26] or partial pancreatectomy[10] and in hamsters[17, 55] and mice[18] that developed the disease spontaneously. Animals in which diabetes is induced develop a secondary type of the disease, some features of which may differ from those of the spontaneous type.

The following has been reported:

Osteoporosis and reduction in the height of alveolar bone occur in diabetic animals, with comparable osteoporosis in other bones.[26] The periodontal ligament and cementum are not affected, but glycogen is depleted in the gingiva. Others report that gingival inflammation and bone destruction associated with local irritants are more severe in diabetic than in nondiabetic animals.[8]

Generalized osteoporosis, resorption of the alveolar crest, and gingival inflammation and periodontal pocket formation associated with calculus have been described in Chinese hamsters with hereditary diabetes under insulin replacement therapy,[55] whereas no periodontal changes were observed in other animals with autosomal recessive diabetes.

Periodontal injury produced by excessive occlusal forces[28] and periodontal atrophy resulting from insufficient forces[35] are worsened in experimental diabetes, and postsurgical gingival healing is retarded.[29]

REFERENCES

1. Adler, P., Wegner, H., and Bohatka, A.: Infuence of age and duration of diabetes on dental development in diabetic children. J. Dent. Res., 52:535, 1973.
2. Anapolle, S. F., Albright, J. T., and Craft, F. O.: Ultrastructure of the gingiva in the diabetic mouse. Microvasc. Res., 4:132, 1972.
3. Anapolle, S. F., Albright, J. T., and Craft, F. O.: Continued study of the ultrastructure of the gingiva in the diabetic mouse. Microvasc. Res., 6:44, 1973.
4. Anapolle, S. F., Albright, J. T., and Craft, F. O.: Microvascular lesions of gingival and cheek pouch tissue in the diabetic Chinese hamster. J. Periodontol., 48:341, 1977.
5. Belting, C. M. Hinicker, J. J., and Dummett, C. O.: Influence of diabetes mellitus on the severity of periodontal disease. J. Periodontol., 35:476, 1964.
6. Benveniste, R., Bixler, D., and Cornally, P. M.: Periodontal disease and diabetes. J. Periodontol., 38:271, 1967.
7. Bernick, S. M., Cohen, D. W., Baker, L., and Laster, L.: Dental disease in children with diabetes mellitus. J. Periodontol., 46:241, 1975.
8. Bissada, N. F., Schaffer, E. M., and Laarow, A.: Effect of alloxan diabetes and local irritating factors on the periodontal structures of the rat. Periodontics, 4:233, 1966.
9. Boenheim, F.: The endocrine system in periodontal disease. *In* Miller, S. C. (ed.): Textbook of Periodontia. 2nd ed. Philadelphia, Blakiston Company, 1943, p. 545.
10. Borghelli, R. F., Devoto, F. C. H., Foglia, V., and Erausquin, J.: Periodontal changes and dental caries in experimental prediabetes. Diabetes, 16:804, 1967.
11. Campbell, M. J. A.: An electron microscope study of the basement membrane of the small vessels from the gingival tissue of the diabetic and non-diabetic patient. J. Dent. Res., 46:1302, 1967.
12. Campbell, M. J. A.: The oxygen utilization and glucose oxidation rate of gingival tissue from non-diabetic and diabetic patients. Arch. Oral Biol., 15:305, 1970.
13. Campbell, M. J. A.: Epidemiology of periodontal disease in the diabetic and the non-diabetic. Aust. Dent. J., 17:274, 1972.
14. Cianciola, L. J., et al.: Prevalence of periodontal disease in insulin-dependent diabetes mellitus (juvenile diabetes). J. Am. Dent. Assoc., 104:653, 1982.
15. Cohen, B., and Fosdick, L. S.: Chemical studies in periodontal disease. VI. The glycogen content of gingival tissues in alloxan diabetes. J. Dent. Res., 29:48, 1950.
16. Cohen, D. W., Friedman, L. A., Shapiro, J., and Kyle, G. C.: Studies on periodontal patterns in diabetes mellitus. J. Periodont. Res., 4(Suppl.):35, 1969.
17. Cohen, M. M., Shklar, G., and Yerganian, G.: Periodontal pathology in a strain of Chinese hamster with hereditary diabetes mellitus. Am. J. Med., 31:864, 1961.
18. El Geneldy, A. K., Stallard, R. E., Fillios, L. C., and Goldman H. M.: Periodontal and vascular alterations: their relationship to the changes in tissue glucose and glycogen in diabetic mouse. J. Periodontol., 45:394, 1974.
19. Ficara, A. I., Levin, M. P., Grover, M. F., and Kramer, G. D.: A comparison of the glucose and protein content of gingival fluid from diabetics and non-diabetics. J. Periodont. Res., 10:171, 1975.
20. Finestone, A. J., and Boorujy, S. R.: Diabetes mellitus and periodontal disease. Diabetes, 16:336, 1967.
21. Frantzis, T. G., Reeve, C. M., and Brown, J. R.: The ultrastructure of capillary basement membranes in the attached gingiva of diabetic and non-diabetic patients with periodontal disease. J. Periodontol., 42:406, 1971.
22. Friederici, H. H. R., Tucker, W. R., and Schwartz, T. B.: Observations on small blood vessels in normal and diabetic patients. Diabetes, 15:233, 1966.

23. Gescheff, G.: Einige Lipoiduntersuchungen des Paradentium bei Diabetes. Berlin, Frankfurt am Main Verlangen, 1931, p. 8.

24. Gillman, A., et al.: Decreased phagocytosis associated with surface hydrophobicity of neutrophils of children with chronic infections. Fed. Proc., 35:227, 1976.

25. Glavind, L., Lund, B., and Löe, H.: The relationship between periodontal state and diabetes duration, insulin dosage and retinal changes. J. Periodontol., 39:341, 1968.

26. Glickman, I.: The periodontal structure in experimental diabetes. N. Y. J. Dent., 16:226, 1946.

27. Glickman, I., Smulow, J., and Moreau, J.: Effect of alloxan diabetes upon the periodontal response to excessive occlusal forces. J. Periodontol., 37:146, 1966.

28. Glickman, I., Smulow, J., and Moreau, J.: Post-surgical periodontal healing in alloxan diabetes. J. Periodontol., 38:93, 1967.

29. Gottsegn, R.: Dental and oral considerations in diabetes mellitus N. Y. J. Med., 62:389, 1962.

30. Hirschfeld, I.: Periodontal symptoms associated with diabetes. J. Periodontol., 5:37, 1934.

31. Hove, K. A., and Stallard, R. E.: Diabetes and the periodontal patient. J. Periodontol., 41:713, 1970.

32. Keene, J. J., Jr.: Observations of small blood vessels in human nondiabetic and diabetic gingiva. J. Dent. Res., 48:967, 1969.

33. Keene, J. J., Jr.: An alteration in human diabetic arterioles. J. Dent. Res., 41:569, 1972.

34. Khandari, K. C., et al.: Investigations into the causation of increased susceptibility of diabetics to cutaneous infections. Indian J. Med. Res., 57:1295, 1969.

35. Koronori, A.: Histological studies of the influence of occlusal function on the periodontal tissues of alloxan diabetic rate. Bull. Tokyo Med. Univ., 11:207, 1964.

36. Listgarten, M. A., et al.: Vascular basement lamina thickness in the normal and inflamed gingiva of diabetics and non-diabetics. J. Periodontol., 45:676, 1974.

37. MacKenzie, R. S., and Millard, H. O.: Interrelated effects of diabetes, arteriosclerosis and calculus on alveolar bone loss. J. Am. Dent. Assoc., 66:191, 1963.

38. Maider, M. Z., Abelson, D. C., and Mandel I. D.: Salivary alterations in diabetes mellitus. J. Periodontol., 46:567, 1975.

39. Mascola, B.: The oral manifestations of diabetes mellitus: a review. N. Y. Dent. J., 36:139, 1970.

40. McCarthy, P., and Shklar, G.: Diseases of the Oral Mucosa. 2nd ed. Philadelphia, Lea & Febiger, 1980.

41. McMullen, J., Gottsegen, R., and Camerini-Davalos, R.: PAS fuchsinophilic thickening of small blood vessels in diabetic gingiva due to accumulation in the periendothelial area. J. Periodontol., 5:61, 1967.

42. Mehrotia, K. K., Chawla, T. N., and Kumar, A.: Correlation of salivary sugar and blood sugar with periodontal health and oral hygiene status among diabetics and non-diabetics. J. Indian Dent. Assoc., 40:287, 1968.

43. Menkin, V.: Biochemical factors in inflammation and diabetes mellitus. Arch. Pathol., 34:182, 1942.

44. Mowat, B., et al.: Chemotaxis of PMN leukocytes from patients with diabetes mellitus. New Engl. J. Med., 28:621, 1971.

45. Nichols, C., Laster, A. A., and Bodak-Gyovai, L. Z.: Diabetes mellitus and periodontal disease. J. Periodontol., 49:85, 1978.

46. O'Leary, T. M., Shannon, I., and Prigmore, J. R.: Clinical and systemic findings in periodontal disease. J. Periodontol., 32:243, 1962.

47. Ray, H. G., and Orban, B.: The gingival structures in diabetes mellitus. J. Periodontol., 21:85, 1950.

48. Reeve, C. M., and Winklemann, R. K.: Glycogen storage in gingival epithelium of diabetic and non-diabetic patients. I. A. D. R. Abstracts, 1962, p. 31.

49. Richardson, R.: Influence of diabetes on the development of antibacterial properties in the blood. J. Clin. Invest., 12:1143, 1933.

50. Robertson, H. D., and Polk, H. C., Jr.: The mechanism of infection in patients with diabetes mellitus. A review of leukocyte malfunction. Surgery, 75:123, 1974.

51. Rudy, A., and Cohen, M. M.: The oral aspects of diabetes mellitus. N. Engl. J. Med., 219:503, 1938.

52. Rutledge, C. E.: Oral and roentgenographic aspects of the teeth and jaws in juvenile diabetics. J. Am. Dent. Assoc., 27:1740, 1940.

53. Saadoun, A. P.: Diabetes and periodontal disease: a review and update. J. Western Soc. Periodontol., 28:116, 1980.

54. Sanchez Cordero, S., Hoffman, H., and Stahl, S. S.: Occurrence of *Staphylococcus* in periodontal pockets of diabetic and nondiabetic adults. J. Periodontol., 50:1979.

55. Shklar, G., Cohen, M. M., and Yerganian, G.: Periodontal disease in the Chinese hamster with hereditary diabetes. J. Periodontol., 33:14, 1962.

56. Siperstein, M. A., Unger, R. H., and Madison, L. L.: Studies of muscle, capillary basement membrane in normal subjects, diabetics and prediabetic patients. J. Clin. Invest., 47:1973, 1968.

57. Stahl, S. S., Witkin, G. J., and Scopp, I. W.: Degenerative vascular changes observed in selected gingival specimens. Oral Surg., 15:1495, 1962.

58. Sznajder, N., Carraro, J. J., Rugna, S., and Sereday, M.: Periodontal findings in diabetic and non-diabetic patients. J. Periodontol., 49:445, 1978.

59. Williams, J. B.: Diabetic periodontoclasia. J. Am. Dent. Assoc., 15:523, 1928.

60. Williams, R., and Mahan, C. J.: Periodontal disease in diabetic young adults. J.A.M.A., 72:776, 1960.

61. Yoon, J. W., et al.: Isolation of virus from the pancreas of a child with diabetic ketoacidosis. N. Engl. J. Med., 300:1173, 1979.

62. Ziskin, D. E., Loughlin, W. C., and Seigel, E. H.: Diabetes in relation to certain oral and systemic problems. Part II. Am. J. Orthod., 30:758, 1944.

The Gonads

Identification of several types of gingival disease with altered secretion of sex hormones has led to increased interest in hormonal effects upon the periodontal tissues and upon periodontal wound healing. There are several types of gingival disease in which modification of the sex hormones is considered to be either the initiating or a complicating factor; these types of gingival alterations are characterized by their association with physiologic hormonal changes, by a marked hemorrhagic tendency, and by nonspecific inflammatory changes with a predominant vascular component.

Experimental Studies

Progesterone alone produces dilatation of the gingival microvasculature, which increases susceptibility to injury and exudation, but it does not affect the morphology of the gingival epithelium.[22] *Estrogen* injections counteract tendencies toward hyperkeratosis of the gingival epithelium and fibrosis of the vessel walls in castrated female animals.[55] Locally applied progesterone, estrogen, and gonadotropin appear to reduce the acute inflammatory response to chemical irritation.[34]

Repeated injections of estrogen cause increased endosteal bone formation in the jaws,[43, 58] and decreased polymerization of mucopolysaccharide protein complexes in the bone ground substance.[1] Estrogen also stimulates bone formation and fibroplasia, which compensate for destructive changes in the periodontium induced by the systemic administration of cortisone.[18]

Elevated levels of *estrogen and progesterone* increase gingival exudation in female animals with and without gingivitis, most likely because of hormone-induced increased permeability of the gingival vessels.[35]

Ovariectomy results in osteoporosis of alveolar bone, reduced cementum formation, and reduced fiber density and cellularity of the periodontal ligament[17] in young adult mice, but not in older animals,[48] and fibrosis of periodontal blood vessels.[54] There is also thinning and reduced cellular activity in the epithelium of the buccal mucosa, but not that of the gingiva.[36] The gingival epithelium is atrophic in estrogen-deficient animals.[64]

Systemic administration of *testosterone* retards the downgrowth of sulcular epithelium over the cementum,[53] stimulates osteoblastic activity in alveolar bone, increases the cellularity of the periodontal ligament,[59] and restores osteoblastic activity which is depressed by hypophysectomy.[60] The healing of oral wounds is accelerated by castration in males and is unaffected by ovariectomy.[4]

The Gingiva in Puberty

Puberty is frequently accompanied by an exaggerated response of the gingiva to local irritation.[29, 61] Pronounced inflammation, bluishred discoloration, edema, and enlargement result from local irritants that would ordinarily elicit a comparatively mild gingival response (Fig. 29–3). Excessive anterior overbite aggravates these cases because of the complicating effects of food impaction and injury to the gingiva on the labial aspect of the mandibular teeth and the palatal aspect of the maxillary teeth.[7]

As adulthood is approached, the severity of the gingival reaction diminishes, even when local irritants are still present. However, complete return to normal requires their removal. Although the prevalence and severity of gingival disease are increased in puberty, it should be understood that gingivitis is not a universal occurrence during this period; with proper care of the mouth it can be prevented.

Gingival Changes Associated with the Menstrual Cycle

As a general rule, the menstrual cycle is not accompanied by notable gingival changes, but occasional problems do occur. During the menstrual period the prevalence of gingivitis increases.[29] The patient may complain of bleeding gums or a bloated, tense feeling in the gums in the days preceding menstrual flow. Horizontal tooth mobility does not change significantly during the menstrual cycle.[15] The salivary bacterial count is increased during menstruation and at ovulation 11 to 14 days earlier.[49] The exudate from inflamed gingiva is increased during menstruation, suggesting that existent gingivitis is aggravated by menstruation, but the crevicular fluid of normal gingiva is unaffected.[21]

A variety of oral changes have been reported associated with the menstrual cycle; usually they appear several days before the menstrual

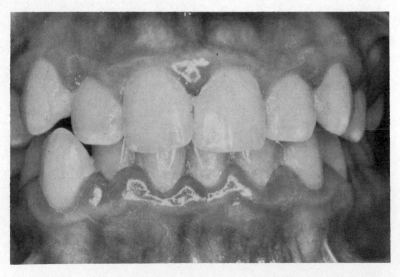

Figure 29–3 Gingivitis in Puberty, with edema, discoloration, and enlargement.

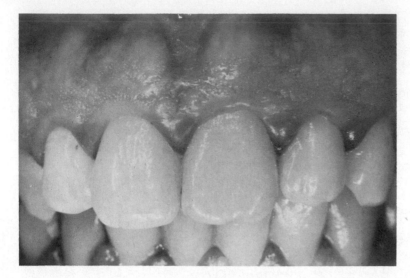

Figure 29–4 Early Changes in the Interdental Papillae in Pregnancy.

period. These include ulcerations of the oral mucosa that seem to have a familial trend,[8, 46] aphthae, vesicular lesions, and vicarious bleeding in the oral cavity[57]; "menstruation gingivitis" characterized by periodic recurrent hemorrhage with bright red and rose-colored proliferations of the interdental papillae; and persistent ulceration of the tongue and buccal mucosa that worsens just before the menstrual period. Microscopic examination of the gingiva in a patient with a cyclic recurrent gingivitis revealed desquamation of epithelial cells from the stratum granulosum and the surface.[42]

Periodically recurring ulcers of the mouth and occasionally of the vulva may accompany or precede the menstrual period. The oral lesions heal in 3 to 4 days and the vaginal tenderness disappears after menstruation and for the remainder of the cycle.

The lesions do not appear if the patient becomes pregnant, but they recur post partum. Improvement has been reported with systemic estrogen[24] or anterior pituitary hormone.[64]

Cyclic gingival changes associated with menstruation have been attributed to hormonal imbalances and in some instances are accompanied by a history of ovarian dysfunction.[5] Rhythmic changes in capillary fragility associated with the menstrual cycle and an increased tendency to capillary hemorrhage immediately before and during menstruation[3] may affect bleeding of the gingiva. Periodic agranulocytic

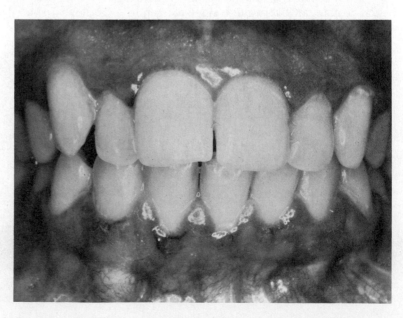

Figure 29–5 Gingiva in Pregnancy, showing edema, discoloration, and bleeding.

leukopenia, which may be a factor in the production of oral changes, has also been associated with the menstrual cycle.[23]

Gingival Disease in Pregnancy

Pregnancy itself does not cause gingivitis. Gingivitis in pregnancy is caused by local irritants, just as it is in nonpregnant individuals. Pregnancy accentuates the gingival response to local irritants and produces a clinical picture different from that which occurs in nonpregnant individuals (Figs. 29–4 to 29–6). No notable changes occur in the gingiva during pregnancy in the absence of local irritants. *Local irritants cause the gingivitis; pregnancy is a secondary, modifying factor.*

The severity of gingivitis is increased during pregnancy beginning from the second or third month. Patients with slight chronic gingivitis which attracted no particular attention before the pregnancy become aware of the gingiva because previously inflamed areas become excessively enlarged and edematous and more noticeably discolored. Patients with a slight amount of gingival bleeding before pregnancy become concerned about an increased tendency to bleed.

Gingivitis becomes more severe by the eighth month and decreases during the ninth, and plaque accumulation follows a similar pattern.[37] Some report the greatest severity between the second and third trimesters.[26] The correlation between gingivitis and the quantity of plaque is closer after parturition than during pregnancy.[27] This suggests that pregnancy introduces other factors which aggravate the gingival response to local irritants.

The reported incidence of gingivitis in pregnancy—38 per cent,[2] 45.4 per cent,[39] 52 per cent,[37] 53.8 per cent,[14] 85.9 per cent,[20] 100 per cent[29, 37]—varies according to the group studied and the method used. The incidence appears to be increased in pregnancy,[56] but this is a difficult determination to make. Pregnancy affects the severity of previously inflamed areas; it does not alter healthy gingiva. Impressions of increased incidence may be created by the aggravation of previously inflamed but unnoticed areas.[52, 57] Also increased in pregnancy are tooth mobility,[50] pocket depth, and gingival fluid.[22, 31]

CLINICAL FEATURES. Pronounced vascularity is the most striking clinical feature. The gingiva is inflamed and varies in color from a bright red to a bluish red sometimes described as "old rose."[65, 68] The marginal and interdental gingivae are edematous, pit on pressure, appear smooth and shiny, are soft and pliable, and sometimes present a raspberry-like appearance. The extreme redness results from marked vascularity, and there is an increased tendency to bleed. The gingival changes are usually painless unless complicated by acute infection, marginal ulceration, and pseudomembrane formation. In some cases the inflamed gingiva forms discrete "tumor-like" masses, referred to as "pregnancy tumors" (described in Chapter 10).

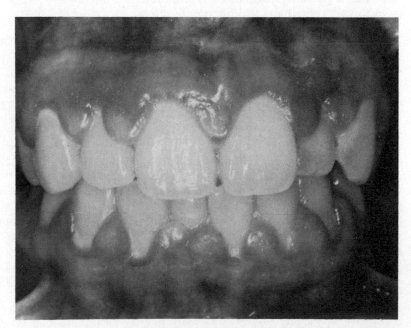

Figure 29–6 Gingiva in Pregnancy, showing edema, discoloration, and enlargement.

There is partial reduction in the severity of gingivitis by 2 months post partum, and after 1 year the condition of the gingiva is comparable to that of patients who have not been pregnant.[6] However, the gingiva does not return to normal so long as local irritants are present. Also reduced following pregnancy are horizontal tooth mobility, gingival fluid, and pocket depth. In a longitudinal investigation of the periodontal changes during pregnancy and 15 months post partum, no significant loss of attachment was observed.[6]

HISTOPATHOLOGY. The microscopic picture[39, 68] of gingival disease in pregnancy is one of nonspecific, vascularizing, proliferative inflammation. There is marked inflammatory cellular infiltration with edema and degeneration of the gingival epithelium and connective tissue. The epithelium is hyperplastic, with accentuated rete pegs and varying degrees of intracellular and extracellular edema and infiltration by leukocytes. Newly formed engorged capillaries are present in abundance. Surface ulcerations and pseudomembrane formation are occasional findings.

Histochemical studies reveal abnormal amounts of water- and alcohol-insoluble glycoprotein residues in the inflamed gingiva.[12] Comparable findings are observed in gingivitis in puberty and menstruation and in severe desquamative gingivitis. In an effort to differentiate changes caused by the pregnancy from those caused by local irritation, Turesky et al.[62] studied the attached gingiva that was uninvolved by inflammation, as distinguished from inflamed marginal and interdental areas. They reported that in pregnancy there is diminished surface keratinization, an increase in rete peg length, and an increase in glycogen in the epithelium. In the connective tissue, the basement layer is thinned and the carbohydrate-protein complexes and glycogen in the ground substance are reduced in density. Electrometric studies indicate a decrease in the density of glycoprotein in the gingiva in the early months of pregnancy, which returns to normal several months after parturition.[16]

The effect of pregnancy upon the gingival response to local irritants is explained on a hormonal basis. There is a marked increase in estrogen and progesterone during pregnancy and a reduction after parturition. The severity of gingivitis varies with the hormonal levels in pregnancy.[22] The aggravation of gingivitis has been attributed principally to the increased progesterone which produces dilatation and tortuosity of the gingival microvasculature, circulatory stasis, and increased susceptibility to mechanical irritation—all of which favor leakage of fluid into the perivascular tissues.[41, 44]

The gingiva is a target organ for female sex hormones. Formicola et al.[13] have shown that radioactive estradiol injected into female rats appears not only in the genital tract but also in the gingiva.

It has also been suggested that the accentuation of gingivitis in pregnancy occurs in two peaks: (1) during the first trimester, when there is overproduction of gonadotropins; and (2) during the third trimester, when estrogen and progesterone levels are highest.[37] Destruction of gingival mast cells by the increased sex hormones and the resultant release of histamine and proteolytic enzymes may also contribute to the exaggerated inflammatory response to local irritants.[33]

The possibility that bacterial-hormonal interactions may change the composition of plaque and lead to gingival inflammation has not been extensively explored. Kornman and Loesche[28] have reported that the subgingival flora changes to a more anaerobic flora as pregnancy progresses; the only microorganism whose proportions increase significantly during pregnancy is *Bacteroides melaninogenicus*, subspecies *intermedius*. This increase appears to be associated with elevations in systemic levels of estradiol and progesterone and to coincide with the peak in gingival bleeding.[28]

It has also been suggested that during pregnancy there is a depression of the maternal T-lymphocyte response that may be a factor in the altered tissue response to plaque.[45]

Hormonal Contraceptives and the Gingiva

Hormonal contraceptives aggravate the gingival response to local irritants in a manner similar to pregnancy,[10, 32] and, when taken for a period of over 1½ years, increase periodontal destruction.[26]

Although some brands of oral contraceptives produce more dramatic changes than others,[47] no correlation has been found to exist based on the differences in progesterone or estrogen content in the various brands.[25] Cumulative exposure to oral contraceptives apparently has no effect on gingival inflammation or oral debris index scores.[25]

Menopausal Gingivostomatitis (Senile Atrophic Gingivitis)

This condition occurs during the menopause or in the postmenopausal period. Mild signs and symptoms sometimes appear associated with the earliest menopausal changes. *Menopausal gingivostomatitis is not a common condition.* Its designation has led to the erroneous impression that it invariably occurs associated with the menopause, whereas the opposite is true. Oral disturbances are not a common feature of the menopause.[63]

CLINICAL FEATURES. The gingiva and remaining oral mucosa are dry and shiny, vary in color from abnormal paleness to redness, and bleed easily. There is fissuring in the mucobuccal fold in some cases,[51] and comparable changes may occur in the vaginal mucosa. The patient complains of a dry, burning sensation throughout the oral cavity, associated with extreme sensitivity to thermal changes; abnormal taste sensations described as "salty," "peppery," or "sour"[40]; and difficulty with removable partial prostheses.

HISTOPATHOLOGY. Microscopically, the gingiva presents atrophy of the germinal and prickle cell layers of the epithelium and, in some instances, areas of ulceration.

When menopausal gingivostomatitis occurs in edentulous patients, they cannot tolerate dentures very well. Normally, when full dentures are inserted there is an initial period of adaptation of the oral mucosa. Thickening of the epithelium is part of the physiologic adaptation that makes toleration of the denture possible. In patients with menopausal gingivostomatitis, the thin, atrophic epithelium offers very little protection. Consequently, the oral mucosa bruises easily in the presence of even slight surface abrasion. Thickening of the epithelium to accommodate the denture does not develop because of the atrophic tendency governing the epithelium. As a result, the patient is continually uncomfortable, even with well-fitting dentures in proper functional relation. The outline of the denture is clearly demarcated by the fiery-red and shiny appearance of the underlying sore mucosa.

The signs and symptoms of menopausal gingivostomatitis are in some degree comparable with those of chronic desquamative gingivitis. Signs and symptoms similar to those of menopausal gingivostomatitis occasionally occur following ovariectomy or sterilization by radiation in the treatment of malignant neoplasms.

REFERENCES

1. Bernick, S., and Ershoff, B. H.: Histochemical study of bone in estrogen-treated rats. J. Dent. Res., *42*:981, 1963.
2. Biro, S.: Studies regarding the influence of pregnancy upon caries. Vierteljahrschr. Zahnheilk, *14*:371, 1898.
3. Brewer, J. L.: Rhythmic changes in the skin capillaries and their relations to menstruation. Am. J. Obstet. Gynecol., *36*:597, 1938.
4. Butcher, E. O., and Klingsberg, J.: Age, gonadectomy and wound healing in the palatal mucosa. J. Dent. Res., *40*:694, 1961.
5. Calman, A. S.: Oral complications of pregnancy. Dent. Outlook, *17*:2, 1930.
6. Cohen, D. W., Shapiro, J., Friedman, L., Kyle, C. G., and Franlin, S.: A longitudinal investigation of the periodontal changes during pregnancy and fifteen months post-partum. J. Periodontol., *42*:653, 1971.
7. Cohen, M.: The gingiva at puberty. J. Dent. Res., *34*:679, 1955.
8. Dayton, A. C.: A case of metastasis of menstrual secretion from the uterus to mouth. Am. J. Dent. Sci., *10*:42, 1949.
9. Deasy, M. J., Grota, A. J., and Kennedy, J. E.: The effect of estrogen, progesterone and cortisol on gingival inflammation. J. Periodont. Res., *7*:111, 1972.
10. El-Ashiry, G. M., et al.: Comparative study of the influence of pregnancy and oral contraceptives on the gingivae. Oral Surg., *30*:472, 1970.
11. El Attar, T. M. A., and Hugoson, A.: Comparative metabolism of female sex steroids in normal and chronically inflamed gingiva of the dog. J. Periodont. Res., *9*:284, 1974.
12. Engel, M. B.: Hormonal gingivitis. J. Am. Dent. Assoc., *44*:691, 1952.
13. Formicola, A. J., Weatherford, T., and Grupe, H., Jr.: The uptake of H[3]-estradiol by the oral tissues in rats. J. Periodont. Res., *5*:269, 1970.
14. Fraser, G. A.: Pregnancy gingivitis. S. Afr. Dent. J., *10*:138, 1944.
15. Friedman, L. A.: Horizontal tooth mobility and the menstrual cycle. J. Periodont. Res., *7*:125, 1972.
16. Gans, B. J., Engel, M. B., and Joseph, N. R.: Electrometric studies of human gingiva in pregnancy. J. Dent. Res., *35*:566, 1956.
17. Glickman, I., and Quintarelli, G.: Further observations regarding the effect of ovariectomy upon the tissues of the periodontium. J. Periodontol., *31*:31, 1960.
18. Glickman, I., and Shklar, G.: The steroid hormones and the tissues of the periodontium. Oral Surg., *8*:1179, 1955.
19. Hartzer, R. C., Toto, P. D., and Gargiulo, A. W.: Immune reactions in the gingiva of the pregnant and non-pregnant female. J. Periodontol., *42*:239, 1971.
20. Heinemann, M., and Anderson, B. G.: Oral manifestations of certain systemic disorders. Yale J. Biol. Med., *17*:583, 1945.
21. Holm-Pederson, P., and Löe, H.: Flow of gingival exudate as related to menstruation and pregnancy. J. Periodont. Res., *2*:13, 1967.
22. Hugoson, A.: Gingival inflammation and female sex hormones. J. Periodont. Res., *5* (Suppl.), 1970.
23. Jackson, H., Jr., and Merril, D.: Agranulocytic angina associated with the menstrual cycle. N. Engl. J. Med., *210*:175, 1934.
24. Jones, O. V.: Cyclical ulcerative vulvitis and stomatitis. J. Obstet. Gynaecol. Br. Emp., *47*:557, 1940.
25. Kalkwarf, K. L.: Effect of oral contraceptive therapy on gingival inflammation in humans. J. Periodontol., *49*:560, 1978.
26. Knight, G. M., and Wade, A. B.: The effects of hormonal contraceptives on the human periodontium. J. Periodont. Res., *9*:18, 1974.
27. Kolodzinski, E., Muñoa, N., and Malatesta, E.: Clinical study of gingival tissue in pregnant women. J. Dent. Res., *53*:693, 1974 (abstract).
28. Kornman, K. S., and Loesche, W. J.: The subgingival microbial flora during pregnancy. J. Periodont. Res., *15*:111, 1980.
29. Kutzleb, H. J.: Changes in the oral mucosa in ovarian disturbances. Dtsch. Zahnärtzl. Wochenschr., *42*:906, 1939.
30. Larato, D., Stahl, S., Brown, R., Jr., and Witkin, G.: The effect of a prescribed method of toothbrushing on the fluctuation of marginal gingivitis. J. Periodontol., *40*:142, 1969.
31. Lindhe, J., and Attstrom, R.: Gingival exudation during the menstrual cycle. J. Periodont. Res., *2*:194, 1967.
32. Lindhe, J., and Bjorn, A. L.: Influence of hormonal contraceptives on the gingiva of women. J. Periodont. Res., *2*:1, 1967.

33. Lindhe, J., and Branemark, P. I.: Changes in microcirculation after local application of sex hormones. J. Periodont. Res., *2*:185, 1967.

34. Lindhe, J., and Sonesson, B.: The effect of sex hormones on inflammation II. Progestogen, oestrogen and chorionic gonadotropin. J. Periodont. Res., *2*:7, 1967.

35. Lindhe, J., Attstrom, R., and Bjorn, A.: Influence of sex hormones on gingival exudation in gingivitis—free female dogs. J. Periodont. Res., *3*:272, 1968.

36. Litwack, D., Kennedy, J. E., and Zander, H. A.: Response of oral epithelia to ovariectomy and estrogen replacement. I.A.D.R. Abstracts, No. 606, 1970, p. 100.

37. Loe, H.: Periodontal changes in pregnancy. J. Periodontol., *36*:209, 1965.

38. Looby, J. P.: Cited by Burket, K. W.: Oral Medicine. Philadelphia, J. B. Lippincott Company, 1946, p. 294.

39. Maier, A. W., and Orban, B.: Gingivitis in pregnancy. Oral Surg., *2*:234, 1949.

40. Massler, M., and Henry, J.: Oral manifestations during the female climacteric. Alpha Omegan, Sept., 1950, p. 105.

41. Mohamed, A. H., Waterhouse, J. P., and Friederici, H. H.: The microvasculature of the rat gingiva as affected by progesterone: an ultrastructural study. J. Periodontol., *45*:50, 1974.

42. Mühlemann, H. R.: Gingivitis intermenstrualis. Schweiz. Mschr. Zahnheilk., *58*:865, 1948.

43. Nutlay, A. G., et al.: The effect of estrogen on the gingiva and alveolar bone in rats and mice. J. Dent. Res., *33*:115, 1954.

44. Nyman, S.: Studies on the influence of estradiol and progesterone on granulation tissue. J. Periodont. Res., 7(Suppl.), 1971.

45. O'Neil, T. C. A.: Maternal T-lymphocyte response and gingivitis in pregnancy. J. Periodontol., *50*:178, 1979.

46. Pappworth, M. H.: Cyclical mucosal ulceration. Br. Med. J., *1*:271, 1941.

47. Perry, D. A.: Oral contraceptives and periodontal health. J. Western Soc. Periodontol., *29*:72, 1981.

48. Piroshaw, N., and Glickman, I.: The effect of ovariectomy upon the tissues of the periodontium and skeletal bones. Oral Surg., *10*:133, 1957.

49. Prout, R. E. S., and Hopps, R. M.: A relationship between human oral bacteria and the menstrual cycle. J. Periodontol., *41*:98, 1970.

50. Rateitschak, K. H.: Tooth mobility changes in pregnancy. J. Periodont. Res., *2*:199, 1967.

51. Richman, J. J., and Abarbanel, A. R.: Effects of estradiol, testosterone, diethylstilbestrol and several of their derivatives upon the human mucous membrane. J. Am. Dent. Assoc., *30*:913, 1943.

52. Ringsdorf, W. M., Powell, B. J., Knight, L. A., and Cheraskin, E.: Periodontal status and pregnancy. Am. J. Obstet. Gynecol., *83*:258, 1962.

53. Rushton, M. A.:Epithelial downgrowth: effect of methyl testosterone. Br. Dent. J., *93*:27, 1952.

54. Schneider, H.: Changes in the periodontium of the rat following ovariectomy. (Ger.) Parodontologie/Acad. Rev., *1*:106, 1967.

55. Schneider, H., and Pose, G.: The effect of estrogen on periodontal conditions in castrated rats. Dtschr. Stomatol., *19*:25, 1969.

56. Schour, I.: Endocrines and teeth. J. Am. Dent. Assoc., *21*:322, 1934.

57. Shelmire, B.: Certain diseases of oral mucous membrane and vermilion border of lips. Int. J. Orthod., *14*:817, 1928.

58. Shklar, G., and Glickman, I.: The effect of estrogenic hormone on the periodontium of white mice. J. Periodontol., *27*:16, 1956.

59. Shklar, G., Chauncey, H., and Peluso, D.: The effect of testosterone on the periodontium of the male albino rat. I.A.D.R. Abstracts, 1962, p. 68.

60. Shklar, G., Chauncey, H., and Shapiro, S.: The effect of testosterone on the periodontium of normal and hypophysectomy rats. J. Periodontol., *38*:203, 1967.

61. Sutcliffe, P.: A longitudinal study of gingivitis and puberty. J. Periodont. Res., *7*:52, 1972.

62. Turesky, S., Fisher, B., and Glickman, I.: A histochemical study of the attached gingiva in pregnancy. J. Dent. Res., *37*:1115, 1958.

63. Wingrove, F. A., Rubright, W. C., and Kerber, P. E.: Influence of ovarian hormone situation on atrophy, hypertrophy, and/or desquamation of human gingiva in premenopausal and postmenopausal women. J. Periodontol., *50*:445, 1979.

64. Ziserman, A. J.: Ulcerative vulvitis and stomatitis of endocrine origin. J.A.M.A., *104*:826, 1935.

65. Ziskin, D. E., and Blackberg, S. N.: A study of the gingivae during pregnancy. J. Dent. Res., *13*:253, 1933.

66. Ziskin, D. E., and Blackberg, S. N.: The effect of castration and hypophysectomy on the gingiva and oral mucous membranes of Rhesus monkeys. J. Dent. Res., *19*:381, 1940.

67. Ziskin, D. E., and Nesse, G. J.: Pregnancy gingivitis, history, classification, etiology. Am. J. Orthod., *32*:390, 1946.

68. Ziskin, D. E., Blackberg, S. N., and Stout, A.: The gingivae during pregnancy: an experimental study and a histopathological interpretation. Surg. Gynecol. Obstet., *57*:719, 1933.

Corticosteroid Hormones

In humans systemic administration of cortisone and adrenocorticotropic hormone (ACTH) appears to have no effect upon the incidence and severity of gingival and periodontal disease.[4] However, renal transplant patients who are receiving immunosuppressive therapy (prednisone or methyl prednisone and azathioprine or cyclophosphamide) have significantly less gingival inflammation than control subjects with similar amounts of plaque.[5, 13]

The systemic administration of cortisone in experimental animals results in osteoporosis of alveolar bone (Fig. 29–7), capillary dilatation and engorgement (with hemorrhage in the periodontal ligament and gingival connective tissue), degeneration and reduction in the number of collagen fibers of the periodontal ligament, and increased destruction of the periodontal tissues associated with inflammation caused by local irritation.[2] Loss of tooth-supporting bone has been noted in adrenalectomized animals.[2] Osteogenesis in alveolar bone, which is reduced in adrenalectomized animals, was restored by cortisone replacement.[9]

THE GENERAL ADAPTATION SYNDROME AND THE DISEASES OF ADAPTATION

Many forms of stress, such as trauma, cold, muscular fatigue, drug intoxication, and nervous stimuli, affect the body generally and produce interrelated, nonspecific tissue changes. The composite of the systemic reactions that result from continued exposure to stress is termed the *general adaptation syndrome* (GAS), which is described by Selye as the basis for the pathogenesis of many diseases previously considered to be of unrelated eti-

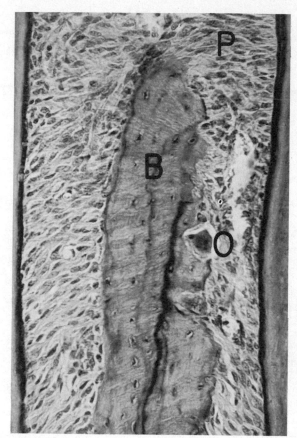 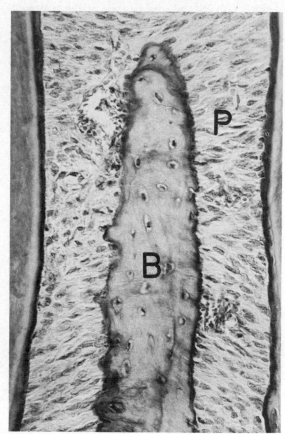

Figure 29–7 The Effects of Systemically Administered Cortisone upon the Periodontium. *Left,* **Control Animal, Interdental Septum.** There is a thin layer of newly formed osteoid bordered by a row of osteoblasts along one surface of the bone (B). The outer surface presents concavities of resorption with an occasional osteoclast (O). The periodontal ligament is shown at P. *Right,* **Cortisone-Injected Animal.** Note absence of normal osteoid and osteoblasts and irregularly indented deeply staining bone margin (B). The connective tissue cells of the periodontal membrane (P) are reduced in number. The collagen fibers appear fibrin-like and fragmented.

ology.[7, 8] According to Selye, the general adaptation syndrome is a generalized group of physiologic mechanisms which represent an attempt by the body to resist the damaging effect of stress.

Stress acts through the endocrine glands, particularly the anterior lobe of the pituitary gland and the adrenal cortex, to produce the morphologic and functional changes that comprise the general adaptation syndrome. Among these changes are enlargement of the adrenal cortex, with increased secretion of adrenocorticoid hormones; involution of the lymphatic organs; hyalinization and inflammatory changes in blood vessels with hypertension; gastrointestinal ulceration; and malignant nephrosclerosis. The "collagen" diseases of man are benefited by treatment with ACTH and cortisone, and they appear to be part of the general adaptation syndrome. Thus, the adaptive mechanism of the body in response to stress produces recognizable disease entities, referred to as the "diseases of adaptation."

The general adaptation syndrome develops in three stages: (1) the initial response—the "alarm reaction"; (2) the adaptation to stress—the "resistance stage"; and (3) a final stage marked by inability to maintain adaptation to the stress—the "exhaustion stage."

STRESS AND THE PERIODONTAL TISSUES. The following observations have been reported in stressed experimental animals:

In the alarm reaction,[11] no significant changes; in the late stage of the stress syndrome, osteoporosis of alveolar bone,[3] epithelial sloughing, degeneration of the periodontal ligament, and reduced osteoblastic activity[6]; in chronic stress, osteoporosis of alveolar bone, apical migration of the epithelial attachment, and formation of periodontal pockets.[10]

Stress results in delayed healing of the connective tissue and bone in artificially induced gingival wounds but does not affect the epithelium.[12]

REFERENCES

1. Applebaum, E., and Seelig, A.: Histologic changes in jaws and teeth of rats following nephritis, adrenalectomy and cortisone treatment. Oral Surg., *8*:881, 1955.
2. Glickman, I., Stone, I. C., and Chawla, T. N.: The effect of cortisone acetate upon the periodontium of white mice. J. Periodontol., *24*:161, 1953.
3. Gupta, O. P., Blechman, H., and Stahl, S. S.: The effects of stress on the periodontal tissues of young adult male rats and hamsters. J. Periodontol., *32*:413, 1960.
4. Krohn, S.: The effect of the administration of steroid hormones on the gingival tissues. J. Periodontol., *29*:300, 1958.
5. Oshrain, H. I., Mender, S., and Mandel, I. D.: Periodontal status of patients with reduced immunocapacity. J. Periodontol., *50*:185, 1979.
6. Ratcliff, P. A.: The relationship of the general adaptation syndrome to the periodontal tissues in the rat. J. Periodontol., *27*:40, 1956.
7. Selye, H.: The general adaptation syndrome and the diseases of adaptation. J. Clin. Endocrinol., *6*:117, 1946.
8. Selye, H.: The physiology and pathology of exposure to stress. Acta Endocrinol. (Montreal), 1950.
9. Shklar, G.: The effect of adrenalectomy and cortisone replacement on the periodontium of the rat. Periodontics, *3*:239, 1965.
10. Shklar, G.: Periodontal disease in experimental animals subjected to chronic cold stress. J. Periodontol., *37*:377, 1966.
11. Shklar, G., and Glickman, I.: The periodontium and the salivary glands in the alarm reaction. J. Dent. Res., *32*:773, 1953.
12. Stahl, S. S.: Healing gingival injury in normal and systemically stressed young adult male rats. J. Periodontol., *32*:63, 1961.
13. Tollefsen, T., Saltvedt, E., and Koppang, H. S.: The effect of immunosuppressive agents on periodontal disease in man. J. Periodont. Res., *13*:240, 1978.

chapter thirty

Hematologic and Other Systemic Disorders in the Etiology of Periodontal Disease

HEMATOLOGIC DISORDERS IN THE ETIOLOGY OF PERIODONTAL DISEASE

Oral changes are often the earliest indication of a hematologic disturbance, but they cannot be relied upon for the diagnosis of the patient's hematologic disorder. Oral findings suggest the existence of a blood disturbance; specific diagnosis requires a complete physical examination and a thorough hematologic study. Comparable oral changes occur in more than one form of blood dyscrasia, and secondary inflammatory changes produce a wide range of variation in the oral signs. For these reasons, gingival and periodontal disturbances associated with blood dyscrasias must be thought of in terms of fundamental interrelationships between the oral tissues and the blood and blood-forming organs, rather than in terms of a simple association of dramatic oral changes with hematologic disease.

Abnormal bleeding from the gingiva or other areas of the oral mucosa that is difficult to control is an important clinical sign suggesting a hematologic disorder. Hemorrhagic tendencies occur in hematologic disorders whenever the normal hemostatic mechanism is disturbed.[59]

Leukemia

The leukemias are "malignant neoplasias of white blood cell precursors, characterized by (1) diffuse replacement of the bone marrow with proliferating leukemic cells; (2) abnormal numbers and forms of immature white cells in the circulating blood; and (3) widespread infiltrates in the liver, spleen, lymph nodes and other sites throughout the body."[59] According to the type of white blood cell involved, leukemias can be lymphocytic, myelogenous, or monocytic. According to their evolution, these forms can be acute, which is rapidly fatal, subacute, or chronic. The replacement of the bone marrow elements by leukemic cells reduces normal white blood cell and platelet production, leading to anemia and bleeding disorders.

Periodontal Disease in Leukemia

Oral manifestations occur with greatest frequency in acute and subacute monocytic leukemia, less frequently in acute and subacute lymphatic and myelogenous leukemia, and seldom in chronic leukemia. Periodontal changes in leukemia can be (1) *primary changes,* those directly attributable to the hematologic disturbance; and (2) *secondary changes,* those superimposed upon the oral tissues by the almost omnipresent local factors, which induce a wide range of inflammatory changes.

ACUTE AND SUBACUTE LEUKEMIA. Clinical changes that may occur in acute and subacute leukemia include a diffuse, cyanotic, bluish-red discoloration of the entire gingival mucosa (the surface of which becomes shiny); a diffuse, edematous enlargement obliterating the details of the normal surface markings (see Chapter 10); a rounding and tenseness of the gingival margin; a blunting of the interdental papillae; and varying degrees of gingival inflammation with ulceration, necrosis, and pseudomembrane formation (Figs. 30–1 and 30–2).

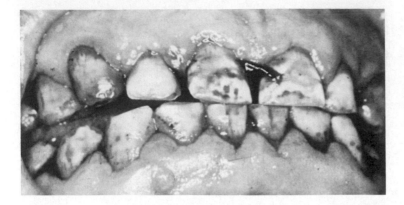

Figure 30–1 Acute Lymphocytic Leukemia. The gingiva is inflamed, edematous, and discolored and bleeds spontaneously.

Microscopically, the gingiva presents a dense, diffuse infiltration of predominantly immature leukocytes in the attached as well as the marginal gingiva. Occasional mitotic figures indicative of ectopic hematopoiesis may be seen. The normal connective tissue components of the gingiva are displaced by the leukemic cells (Fig. 30–3A). The nature of the cells depends on the type of leukemia. The cellular accumulation is denser in all the reticular connective tissue layer. In almost all cases, the papillary layer contains comparatively few leukocytes. The blood vessels are distended and contain predominantly leukemic cells. The red blood cells are reduced in number.

The epithelium presents a variety of changes. It may be thinned or hyperplastic. Degeneration associated with inter- and intracellular edema and leukocytic infiltration with diminished surface keratinization are common findings.

The microscopic picture of the marginal gingiva differs from that of the remainder of the gingiva in that it usually presents a notable inflammatory component in addition to the leukemic cells. Scattered foci of plasma cells and lymphocytes with edema and degeneration are common findings. The inner aspect of the marginal gingiva is usually ulcerated, and marginal necrosis with pseudomembrane formation may also be seen.

The periodontal ligament and alveolar bone

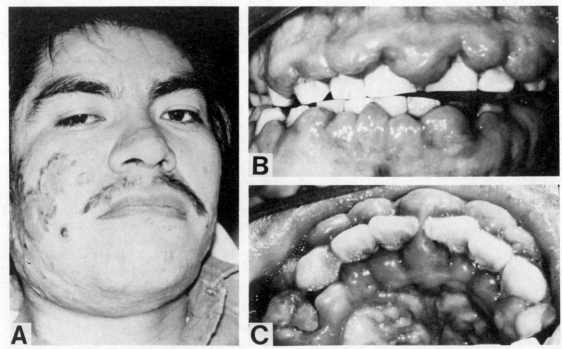

Figure 30–2 Acute Myelocytic Leukemia. *A,* Skin infection of the face. *B,* Frontal view of gingival enlargement. *C,* Occlusal view of upper anterior teeth. (Courtesy of Dr. Spencer Woolfe.)

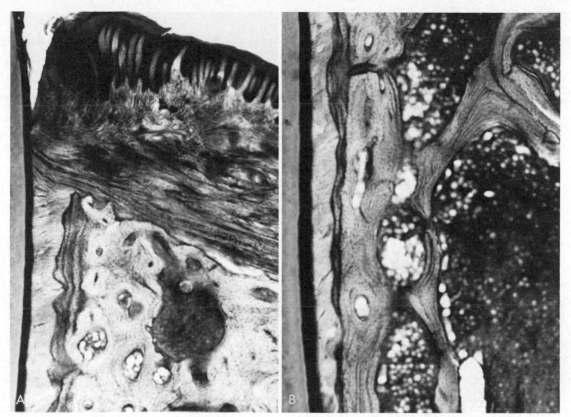

Figure 30–3 *A*, Leukemic infiltrate in gingiva and bone in a human autopsy specimen. *B*, Same case as *A*. Note the dense infiltrate in marrow spaces and lack of extension to the periodontal ligament.

may also be involved in acute and subacute leukemia (Fig. 30–3*B*). The periodontal ligament may be infiltrated with mature and immature leukocytes. The marrow of the alveolar bone presents a variety of changes, such as localized areas of necrosis, thrombosis of the blood vessels, infiltration with mature and immature leukocytes, occasional red blood cells, and replacement of the fatty marrow by fibrous tissue.[14, 30, 65]

In leukemic mice the presence of infiltrate in marrow spaces and the periodontal ligament results in osteoporosis of the alveolar bone with destruction of the supporting bone and disappearance of the periodontal fibers[13, 17] (Fig. 30–4).

Other Oral Mucous Membrane Changes. Areas of the oral mucous membrane other than the gingiva may be involved in acute or subacute leukemia. The site of involvement is generally an area subject to trauma, such as the buccal mucosa in relation to the line of occlusion or the palate. The lesion appears as a *severe ulceration* or *abscess* that is resistant to treatment and spreads rapidly. Because of

the difficulty of controlling the extension of infection and the severity of associated toxic complications, death occasionally results in such cases.

CHRONIC LEUKEMIA. In chronic leukemia there often are no clinical oral changes suggesting a hematologic disturbance. Tumor-like enlargement of the oral mucosa in response to local irritation,[18] generalized alveolar resorption, absence of the lamina dura, diffuse and irregular periodontal spaces, osteoporosis, subperiosteal elevation in the mental region, and analogous changes in other bones may occur in chronic leukemia.

The microscopic changes in chronic leukemia may consist of replacement of the normal fatty marrow of the jaws by islands of mature lymphocytes (Fig. 30–5) or lymphocytic infiltration of the marginal gingiva without dramatic clinical manifestations.

THE GINGIVAL BIOPSY AND LEUKEMIA. **The existence of leukemia is sometimes revealed by a gingival biopsy performed to clarify the nature of a troublesome gingival condition.** In such cases, the gingival findings must be

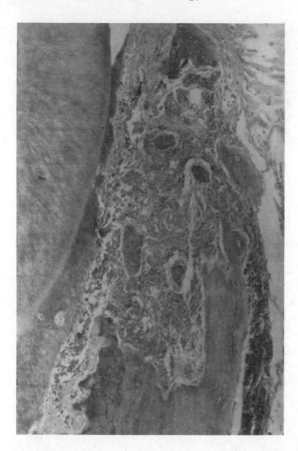

Figure 30–4 Leukemic infiltrate in alveolar bone in AKR mouse. Note the leukemic infiltrate producing destruction of bone and loss of periodontal ligament.

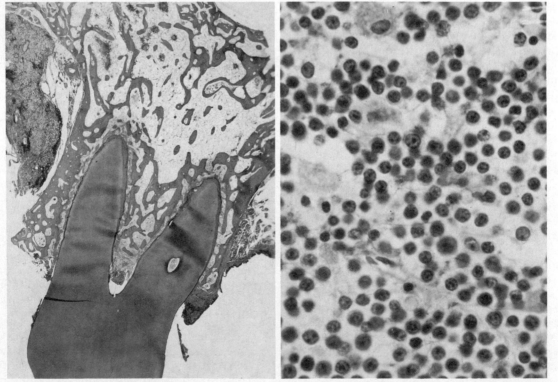

Figure 30–5 Chronic Lymphatic Leukemia. *Left,* Buccopalatal section through the maxilla (molar area) of a patient with chronic lymphatic leukemia, obtained at autopsy. *Right,* Detailed study of lymphocytes in the marrow of the maxilla.

corroborated by medical examination and hematologic study. The absence of leukemic involvement in a gingival biopsy does not rule out the possibility of leukemia. In chronic leukemia, the gingiva may simply present inflammatory changes, with no suggestion of a hematologic disturbance. In patients with recognized leukemia, the gingival biopsy indicates the extent to which leukemic infiltration is responsible for the altered clinical appearance of the gingiva. Although such findings are of interest, their benefit to the patient is insufficient to warrant routine gingival biopsy studies in known leukemic patients.

RELATION OF LOCAL IRRITATION TO GINGIVAL AND PERIODONTAL CHANGES IN LEUKEMIA. In leukemia, the response to irritation is altered, so the cellular component of the inflammatory exudate differs both quantitatively and qualitatively from that which occurs in nonleukemic individuals. There is pronounced infiltration of immature leukemic cells in addition to the usual inflammatory cells. With the cellular infiltration there is degeneration of the gingiva.

The inflamed gingiva differs clinically from that of the nonleukemic individual. It is a peculiar bluish red in color, markedly sponge-like and friable, and bleeds persistently upon the slightest provocation or even spontaneously. This markedly altered and degenerated tissue is extremely susceptible to bacterial infection. Because of the degenerated, anoxemic condition of the gingiva, the bacterial infection is so severe that acute gingival necrosis and pseudomembrane formation are comparatively common findings in acute and subacute leukemia. These oral changes produce associated disturbances that are a source of considerable difficulty to the patient, such as systemic toxic effects, loss of appetite, nausea, blood loss from persistent gingival bleeding, and constant gnawing pain.

There is considerable variation in the gingival and periodontal changes observed in acute and subacute leukemia. The severity of the leukemia affects the extent of cellular infiltration of the gingiva and supporting periodontal structures. The local irritants and the severity of infection account for more striking clinical changes, such as gingival ulceration and necrosis, pseudomembrane formation, and gingival bleeding. These are the secondary changes superimposed upon the oral tissues altered by the blood disturbance. Differences in the degree of local irritation account for the variation in the oral changes seen in different patients. They also modify the oral picture at different times in the same patient. **By eliminating local irritants it is possible to alleviate severe oral changes in leukemia.**

Anemia

Anemia refers to any deficiency in the quantity or quality of the blood as manifested by a reduction in the number of red blood cells and in the amount of hemoglobin. Anemia may be the result of blood loss, defective blood formation, or increased blood destruction. *Blood loss* may be acute, as in severe trauma; chronic, as in gastrointestinal ulcer; or excessive, as in abnormal menstrual bleeding.

Defective blood formation may be due to:

1. Deficiency of protein, iron, or the hematopoietically active vitamins folic acid, vitamin B_{12}, pyridoxine, vitamin C, or vitamin K.[23]

2. Depression of bone marrow activity by toxins, chemical substances such as the sulfonamides, physical agents such as roentgen rays, or mechanical interference such as neoplastic disease.

3. Unknown causes, as in "aplastic" anemia.

Increased blood destruction or hemolytic anemia may be due to infections, chemicals, or intrinsic causes.

The anemias are classified according to cellular morphology and hemoglobin content as (1) macrocytic hyperchromic anemia (pernicious anemia), (2) microcytic hypochromic anemia (iron deficiency anemia), (3) sickle cell anemia, and (4) normocytic normochromic anemia (hemolytic anemia or aplastic anemia).

MACROCYTIC HYPERCHROMIC ANEMIA (PERNICIOUS ANEMIA). Pernicious anemia is most frequently encountered in individuals past the age of 40. The sexes are affected equally. The disease, which has an insidious onset, is characterized by symptoms referable to the nervous, cardiovascular, and gastrointestinal systems. The usual triad of symptoms includes a numbness and tingling of the extremities, weakness, and a sore tongue. Macrocytic hyperchromic anemia is characterized by a severe decrease in the number of erythrocytes (1,000,000 per cu mm); an elevated color index (1.5); a decreased hemoglobin value; a decreased platelet count (40,000 per cu mm); a decrease in the number of white blood cells; anisocytosis, poikilocytosis, and polychromatophilia; and the presence of red blood cells containing nuclei or nuclear fragments.

Oral Changes. Changes occur in the gingiva, the remainder of the oral mucosa, the lips, and the tongue, the last of which is involved in 75 per cent of the cases. The earliest oral changes may be microscopic and consist of enlargement of the epithelial cells, with giant nuclei and nuclear pleomorphism.[12] **The gingiva and mucosa are pale and yellowish and susceptible to ulceration.** The tongue appears red, smooth, and shiny owing to the uniform atrophy of the fungiform and filiform papillae. The tongue is sensitive to hot or spicy foods, and swallowing is painful. The patient complains that the tongue feels raw, and there are sensations of burning and numbness. Atrophy of the tongue may be a manifestation of deficiency of vitamin B complex.[38] *Marked pallor of the gingiva* is a striking finding in pernicious anemia, and there is a wide variety of inflammatory changes, depending upon the nature of the local irritation (Figs. 30–6 and 30–7).

Pernicious anemia is cyclic, with intermittent symptom-free periods. Remissions may last for a short time or for years, but the glossitis of penicious anemia persists during all but the most complete remission. Exacerbation of the glossitis may be a signal of relapse.

MICROCYTIC HYPOCHROMIC ANEMIA (IRON DEFICIENCY ANEMIA). This form of anemia is caused by a deficiency in iron and other substances concerned with hemoglobin production, occurs in chronic blood loss, and is associated with inadequate iron ingestion or absorption. It is seen more often in females. Weakness, fatigue, and pallor are among the notable clinical features.

Microcytic hypochromic anemia is characterized by a moderate decrease in number of red blood cells (3,000,000 per cu mm), a lowered color index (0.5), an increased platelet count (500,000 per cu mm), and a decreased hemoglobin value.

Oral Changes. **Atrophy of alveolar bone, and inflammation of the gingiva occur in animals with experimentally induced anemia.** Not all patients with hypochromic anemia present oral changes.[53] When these do occur, the most conspicuous change is **pallor of the gingival mucosa and tongue,** followed by erythema of the lateral border of the tongue with papillary atrophy and loss of muscle tone.[22, 26] **Areas of gingival inflammation appear purplish red, in contrast to the adjacent gingival pallor.**

There is an initial erythema of the lateral border of the tongue, followed by pallor and papillary atrophy with loss of normal muscle tone.[22, 26] A correlation has been suggested between anemia and moderate to severe periodontal disease.[45] A syndrome consisting of glossitis, ulceration of the oral mucosa and oropharynx, and dysphagia, known as the *Plummer-Vinson syndrome,* may develop in patients with chronic anemia.

SICKLE CELL ANEMIA. This is a hereditary and familial form of chronic hemolytic anemia that occurs almost exclusively in blacks. It is

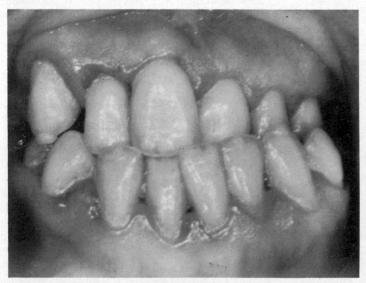

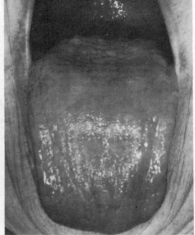

Figure 30–6   Figure 30–7

Figure 30–6 Diffuse Pallor of the Gingiva in Patient with Anemia. The discolored inflamed gingival margin stands out in sharp contrast to the adjacent pale attached gingiva.
Figure 30–7 Smooth Tongue in Patient with Pernicious Anemia.

characterized by pallor, jaundice, weakness, rheumatoid manifestations, leg ulcers, and acute attacks of pain. The blood picture is distinguished by peculiar sickle-shaped and oat-shaped red corpuscles, as well as signs of excessive blood destruction and active blood formation. Although not sex-linked, it occurs somewhat more frequently in females.

Oral changes include generalized osteoporosis of the jaws, reported in about 80 per cent of the cases, with a peculiar stepladder alignment of the trabeculae of the interdental septa,[60] **and pallor and yellowish discoloration of the oral mucosa.**[52]

NORMOCYTIC NORMOCHROMIC ANEMIA (HEMOLYTIC ANEMIA OR APLASTIC ANEMIA). In this group, the oral changes associated with beta-thalassemia in *Cooley's anemia* are noteworthy (see Chapter 21).

Thrombocytopenic Purpura

Thrombocytopenic purpura may be idiopathic (i.e., of unknown etiology, as in *Werlhof's disease*), or it may occur secondary to some known etiologic factor responsible for a reduction in the amount of functioning marrow and a resultant reduction in the number of circulating platelets. The latter conditions include aplasia of the marrow; crowding out of the megakaryocytes in the marrow, as, e.g., in leukemia; replacement of the marrow by tumor; destruction of the marrow by x-irradiation or radium or by drugs such as benzene, aminopyrine, and the arsenicals.

Thrombocytopenic purpura is characterized by a low platelet count, a prolonged clot retraction and bleeding time, and a normal or slightly prolonged clotting time.

In thrombocytopenic purpura there is spontaneous bleeding into the skin or from mucous membranes. **Petechiae and hemorrhagic vesicles occur in the oral cavity, particularly in the palate and the buccal mucosa. The gingiva is swollen, soft, and friable. Bleeding occurs spontaneously or upon the slightest provocation and is difficult to control. Special note should be made of the fact that the gingival changes represent an abnormal response to local irritation; the severity of the gingival condition is dramatically alleviated by removal of the local irritants (Fig. 30–8).**

Hemophilia

Hemophilia is an inherited sex-linked disease affecting only the male and transmitted by the female. The afflicted male does not transmit the disease to his male offspring. The defect is passed to the female offspring, who exhibits no symptoms of the disease but who transmits the defect to her son.

Hemophilia is characterized by prolonged hemorrhage from even slight wounds and by spontaneous bleeding into the skin. Spontaneous bleeding from mucous membranes is not a feature of the disease, but chronic marginal gingivitis in hemophiliac patients can constitute a serious complication because of the bleeding problem.

The clotting time is markedly prolonged, but the bleeding time remains normal. The prolonged clotting time is due to a deficiency of serum protein antihemophilic globulin (AHG; Factor VIII), which presumably results from platelet resistance to disintegration. The normal bleeding time may be explained on the following basis:

When a hemophiliac cuts himself, the capillary contracts as it would normally, with cessation of the bleeding. When the capillary later expands, however, there is no clot present

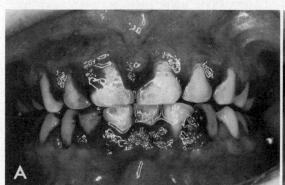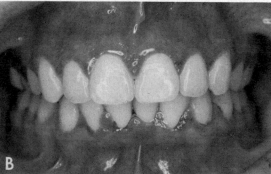

Figure 30–8 Thrombocytopenic Purpura. *A*, Hemorrhagic gingivitis in patient with thrombocytopenic purpura. *B*, Marked reduction in severity of gingival disease after removal of surface debris and careful scaling.

to plug the defect, and the bleeding starts again. (See Chapter 36 for special precautions in the management of hemophiliac patients.)

Christmas disease is characterized by abnormal bleeding tendencies that make it clinically indistinguishable from hemophilia. Another resemblance to hemophilia is that it is inherited by the male as a sex-linked recessive trait. It differs from hemophilia in that the hemostatic defect lies in the missing serum fraction, called plasma thromboplastin component (PTC, Factor IX), so named because it affects the production of thromboplastin, without which there is an abnormality in the clotting mechanism.

Mild Christmas disease may escape detection because the patient's bleeding time, coagulation time, and clot retraction time may be within normal limits. In patients with a history of abnormal bleeding, the prothrombin consumption test or the thromboplastin generation test may be necessary in order to rule out Christmas disease.[44]

Infectious Mononucleosis

This is a benign infectious disease of unknown etiology. It usually occurs in children or young adults. The suspicion that it is communicable has not been well substantiated. It is characterized by sudden onset, headache, fever, muscular ache, sore throat, malaise, nausea, vomiting, swelling and tenderness of the lymph nodes (particularly in the cervical area), occasional skin rash, and lymphocytosis.

Soreness of the mouth and throat is often the patient's initial complaint. The oral findings include **diffuse erythema of the entire mucosa with petechiae in some cases.**[21] **The marginal and interdental papillae are swollen and markedly reddened and bleed on the slightest provocation or even spontaneously.**

After 2 to 4 weeks the systemic symptoms usually begin to subside, but the oral changes may persist.

The diagnosis of infectious mononucleosis is based upon the hematologic findings. Leukopenia is seen in the early stages, followed by a marked lymphocytosis. Characteristic of the blood picture are typical "monocytoid" lymphocytes, or Downey cells. The heterophil antibody test (Paul-Bunnell test) is used as an aid in diagnosis. This test is based on the agglutination of sheep red blood cells by the patient's serum. Agglutination with serum dilution of 1:64 or above is diagnostic.

Agranulocytosis (Granulocytopenia)

Agranulocytosis is an acute disease characterized by extreme leukopenia and neutropenia and accompanied by ulceration of the oral mucosa, skin, and gastrointestinal tract.

Drug idiosyncrasy is the most common cause of agranulocytosis, but in some instances its etiology cannot be explained. It has been reported following the administration of drugs such as aminopyrine,[43, 58] barbiturates and their derivatives, benzene ring derivatives,[47] sulfonamides,[50] gold salts, or arsenicals. It generally occurs as an acute disease, but sometimes reappears in cyclic episodes (cyclic neutropenia) that may be correlated with the onset of the menstrual period.[71] It may be periodic with recurring neutropenic cycles.[70]

The onset of the disease is accompanied by fever, malaise, general weakness, and sore throat. Ulceration in the oral cavity, oropharynx, and throat is characteristic. The mucosa presents isolated necrotic patches that are black and gray and are sharply demarcated from the adjacent uninvolved areas.[41, 49] **The absence of a notable inflammatory reaction because of lack of granulocytes is a striking feature.** The gingival margin may or may not be involved. Gingival hemorrhage, necrosis, increased salivation, and fetid odor are accompanying clinical features.

Bauer[5] described the following microscopic changes in the periodontium: hemorrhage into the periodontal ligament with destruction of the principal fibers, osteoporosis of the cancellous bone with osteoclastic resorption; small fragments of necrotic bone in the hemorrhagic periodontal ligament, hemorrhage in the marrow adjacent to the teeth, areas in which the periodontal ligament is widened and consists of dense fibrous tissue with fibers parallel to the tooth surface, and the formation of new bony trabeculae. In cyclic neutropenia the gingival changes recur with recurrent exacerbation of the disease.[20]

Experimentally, neutropenia has been produced in dogs with heterologous antineutrophil serum. Neutrophilic granulocytes disappeared from the tissues, but ulcerative lesions and bacterial invasion were not observed, probably owing to the short duration of the experiment (4 days).[62]

Because infection is a common feature of agranulocytosis, differential diagnosis involves consideration of such conditions as acute necrotizing ulcerative gingivitis, diphtheria, noma, and acute necrotizing inflammation of the tonsils. Definitive diagnosis depends upon the hematologic findings of pronounced leukopenia and almost complete absence of neutrophils.

Arteriosclerosis

In aged individuals arteriosclerotic changes characterized by intimal thickening, narrowing of the lumen, thickening of the media, and hyalinization of the media and adventitia, with or without calcification, are common in vessels throughout the jaws as well as in areas of periodontal inflammation[56, 75] (Fig. 30–9). Periodontal disease and arteriosclerosis both increase with age, and it has been hypothesized

that the circulatory impairment induced by vascular changes may increase the patient's susceptibility to periodontal disease.[3]

In experimental animals partial ischemia of more than 10 hours' duration, created by arteriolar occlusion, produces changes in the oxidative enzymes and acid phosphatase activity and in the glycogen and lipid content of the gingival epithelium.[39] Focal necrosis, followed by ulceration, occurs in the epithelium, with the junctional epithelium least affected.[42] DNA duplication is depressed. Changes typical of periodontal disease do not occur. Ischemia is followed by hyperemia, accompanied by metabolic changes and increased DNA synthesis in the epithelium plus epithelial proliferation and thickening—all considered to be part of the gingival response to arteriolar occlusion.

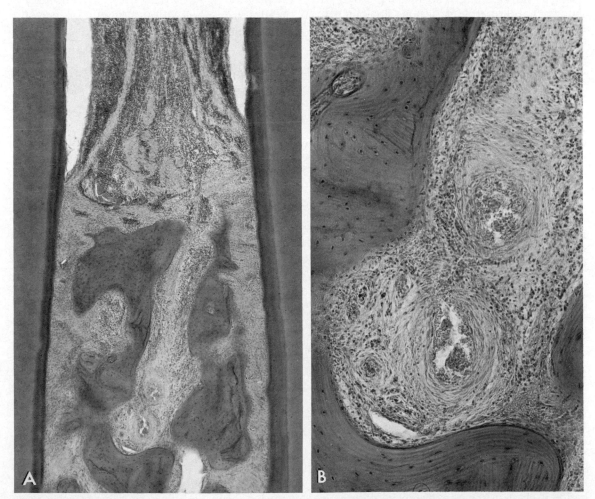

Figure 30–9 Vascular Changes in Aged Individual with Periodontal Disease. *A*, **Periodontitis,** showing inflammation extending from the gingiva into the interdental septum. *B*, Detailed view, showing arterioles with thickened walls in the marrow space of the interdental septum.

OTHER SYSTEMIC DISORDERS

Metal Intoxication

The ingestion of metals such as mercury, lead, and bismuth in medicinal compounds and through industrial contact may result in oral manifestations owing to either (1) intoxication or (2) absorption without evidence of toxicity.

BISMUTH INTOXICATION. Chronic bismuth intoxication is characterized by gastrointestinal disturbances, nausea, vomiting, and jaundice, as well as by an ulcerative gingivostomatitis, generally with pigmentation, accompanied by a metallic taste and a burning sensation of the oral mucosa. The tongue may be sore and inflamed. Urticaria, exanthematous eruptions of different types, bullous and purpuric lesions, and herpes zoster–like eruptions and pigmentation of the skin and mucous membranes are among the dermatologic lesions attributed to bismuth intoxication. Acute bismuth intoxication, which is less commonly seen, is accompanied by methemoglobin formation, cyanosis, and dyspnea.[36]

Bismuth Pigmentation in the Oral Cavity. **Bismuth pigmentation usually appears as a narrow bluish-black discoloration of the gingival margin in areas of pre-existent gingival inflammation** (see Chapter 9). Such pigmentation results from the precipitation of particles of bismuth sulfide associated with vascular changes in inflammation. It is not evidence of intoxication, but simply indicates the presence of bismuth in the blood stream. Bismuth pigmentation in the oral cavity also occurs in cases of intoxication. It assumes a linear form if the marginal gingiva is inflamed.

LEAD INTOXICATION.[40] The metal is slowly absorbed, and toxic symptoms are not particularly definitive when they do occur. There is pallor of the face and lips and gastrointestinal symptoms consisting of nausea, vomiting, loss of appetite, and abdominal colic. Peripheral neuritis, psychologic disorders, and encephalitis have been reported. Among the oral signs are salivation, coated tongue, a peculiar sweetish taste, gingival pigmentation, and ulceration. **The pigmentation of the gingiva is linear (burtonian line), steel gray, and associated with local irritation.** It may occur without toxic symptoms.

MERCURY INTOXICATION. Mercury intoxication is characterized by headache, insomnia, cardiovascular symptoms, pronounced salivation (ptyalsim), and a metallic taste. **Gingival pigmentation in linear form results from the deposition of mercuric sulfide. The chemical also acts as an irritant, which accentuates the pre-existent inflammation and commonly leads to notable ulceration of the gingiva and adjacent mucosa and destruction of the underlying bone.** Mercurial pigmentation of the gingiva also occurs in areas of local irritation in patients without symptoms of intoxication.

Other Chemicals

Other chemicals, such as *phosphorus,*[66] *arsenic,*[37] and *chromium,*[46] may cause necrosis of the alveolar bone with loosening and exfoliation of the teeth. Inflammation and ulceration of the gingiva are usually associated with destruction of the underlying tissues. *Benzene*[66] intoxication is accompanied by gingival bleeding and ulceration with destruction of the underlying bone.

DEBILITATING DISEASES AND THE PERIODONTIUM

Debilitating diseases such as *syphilis, chronic nephritis,* and *tuberculosis* may predispose the patient to periodontal disease by impairing tissue resistance to local irritants and creating a tendency toward alveolar bone resorption[63, 68] (see Chapter 12). A type of membranous stomatitis has been described associated with debilitation in uremia[8]; and a sore, dry mouth with edema, purulent inflammation, and bleeding of the gingiva has been noted in primary renal disease.[74] The absence of periodontal disease in chronically ill patients has been presented as evidence that in individual cases systemic disease may exert no deleterious effect upon the periodontium.[67]

A difference of opinion exists regarding the relationship of tuberculosis to periodontal disease. Although an increased incidence of gingivitis and chronic destructive periodontal disease, as well as of alveolar bone changes characterized by enlargement of the cancellous spaces, has been reported in tuberculous patients,[16, 57] these findings have not been corroborated in other studies.[32, 69] In patients with *leprosy* the chronic destructive periodontal disease has been described as nonspecific in nature, and no *Mycobacterium leprae* have been present in the gingiva.[72]

PSYCHOSOMATIC DISORDERS AND THE PERIODONTIUM

Harmful effects that result from psychic influences on the organic control of tissues are known as psychosomatic disorders.[33] There are two ways in which psychosomatic disorders may be induced in the oral cavity: (1) *through the development of habits which are injurious to the periodontium* and (2) *by the direct effect of the autonomic nervous system upon the physiologic tissue balance.* Giddon[29] has presented an excellent review of experimental evidence which relates psychologic factors to oral physiology.

Psychologically, the oral cavity is related directly or symbolically to the major human instincts and passions. In the infant, many oral drives find direct expression as oral-receptive and oral-aggressive trends and oral eroticism.[64] In the adult, most of the instinctual drives are normally suppressed by education and are satisfied in substitutive ways or are taken over by organs more appropriate than the mouth. **However, under conditions of mental and emotional duress, the mouth may subconsciously become an outlet for the gratification of basic drives in the adult.**

Gratification may be derived from neurotic habits, such as grinding or clenching the teeth,[15, 27] nibbling on foreign objects (such as pencils or pipes), nail biting, or excessive use of tobacco, which are potentially injurious to the periodontium. Correlations have been reported between psychiatric and anxiety states and the occurrence of periodontal disease,[2, 6, 48, 51] but these are questioned by some.[4] Psychologic factors in the etiology of acute necrotizing ulcerative gingivitis are discussed in Chapter 11.

It is necessary to correct local factors which may initiate harmful habits, but investigation of the psychic background is also indicated in difficult cases. Saul[64] describes a patient whose sore throat, bleeding gums, and ulceration of the buccal mucosa were traced to mouth breathing and bruxism associated with oral-aggressive dreams. Psychoanalysis resulted in elimination of the underlying difficulty and habit and relief of the oral disease.

Disorders of psychosomatic origin may be produced in the oral cavity by the influence of the autonomic nervous system upon the somatic control of the tissues.[11] Alterations in the vascular supply caused by autonomic stimulation may adversely affect the health of the periodontium by impairing tissue nutrition.[61]

Diminution in the secretion of saliva in emotional disorders may lead to xerostomia with painful symptoms. Weiss and English[73] outline the sequence of events whereby psychologic disturbances affect tissue alterations as follows:

Psychologic disturbance→ Functional impairment→ Cellular disease→ Structural alteration

Autonomic influences upon the muscles of mastication may result in impairment of mandibular movement, which resembles organically induced temporomandibular joint disorders. In such cases, psychiatric management may suffice for the restoration of the normal function of the mandible.

HEREDITY IN THE ETIOLOGY OF PERIODONTAL DISEASE

In experimental animals heredity appears to be a factor in calculus formation and periodontal disease.[54] Hypophosphatasia, an inherited disease characterized by rachitic-like skeletal changes, also presents premature loss of the deciduous incisors and the surrounding alveolar bone by 10 months of age, sometimes without the skeletal changes.[55]

Gancotti[28] concluded that an inherited tendency was a factor in 62 per cent of the cases of periodontal disease that he studied, whereas other investigators[19] found no indication that heredity affected gingival crevice depth or recession. Heinrich[35] noted that juvenile periodontitis was more common in the pyknic type of individual than in the asthenic type.

REFERENCES

1. Akers, L. H.: Ulcerative stomatitis following therapeutic use of mercury and bismuth. J. Am. Dent. Assoc., *23*:781, 1936.
2. Baker, E. G., Crook, G. H., and Schwabacher, E. D.: Personality correlates of periodontal disease. J. Dent. Res., *40*:396, 1961.
3. Barrett, R., Cheraskin, E., and Ringsdorf, W., Jr.: Alveolar bone loss and capillaropathy. J. Periodontol., *40*:131, 1969.
4. Barry, J. R., and Dutkovic, T. R.: Oral pathosis: exploration of psychological correlates. J. Am. Dent. Assoc., *67*:86, 1963.
5. Bauer, W. H.: Agranulocytosis and the supporting dental tissues. J. Dent. Res., *25*:501, 1946.
6. Belting, C. M., and Gupta, O. P.: The influence of psychiatric disturbances on the severity of periodontal disease. J. Periodontol., *32*:219, 1961.
7. Bender, I. B.: Bone changes in leukemia. A. J. Orthod., *30*:556, 1944.
8. Bereston, E. S., and Herb, H.: Membranous stomatitis with debilitation and uremia. Arch. Dermatol. Syph., *44*:562, 1941.
9. Bernick, S.: Age changes in the blood supply to human teeth. J. Dent. Res., *46*:544, 1967.
10. Bernick, S., Levy, B. M., and Patek, P. R.: Studies on the

biology of the periodontium of marmosets. VI. Arteriosclerotic changes in the blood vessels of the periodontium. J. Periodontol., *40*:355, 1969.

11. Biber, O.: Autonomic symptoms in psychoneurotics. Psychosom. Med., *3*:253, 1941.

12. Boen, S. T.: Changes in the nuclei of squamous epithelial cells in pernicious anemia. Acta Med. Scand., *159*:425, 1957.

13. Brown, L. R., et al.: Alveolar bone loss in leukemic and non-leukemic mice. J. Periodontol., *40*:725, 1969.

14. Burket, L. W.: A histopathologic explanation for the oral lesions in the acute leukemias. Am. J. Orthod., *30*:516, 1944.

15. Burstoen, M. S.: The psychosomatic aspects of dental problems. J. Am. Dent. Assoc., *33*:862, 1946.

16. Cahn, L. R.: Observations on the effect of tuberculosis on the teeth, gums and jaws. Dent. Cosmos, *67*:479, 1925.

17. Carranza, F. A., Jr., Gravina, O., and Cabrini, R. L.: Periodontal and pulpal pathosis in leukemic mice. Oral Surg., *20*:374, 1965.

18. Chaundry, A. P., et al.: Unusual oral manifestations of chronic lymphatic leukemia (report of a case). Oral Surg., *15*:446, 1962.

19. Ciancio, S., Hazen, S., and Cunat, J.: Periodontal observations in twins. J. Periodont. Res., *4*:42, 1969.

20. Cohen, D. W., and Morris, A. L.: Periodontal manifestations of cyclic neutropenia. J. Periodontol., *32*:159, 1961.

21. Cottrell, J. E.: Infectious mononucleosis. J. Periodontol., *9*:15, 1938.

22. Darby, W. J.: The oral manifestations of iron deficiency. J.A.M.A., *130*:830, 1946.

23. Dreizen, S.: Oral manifestations of human nutritional anemias. Arch. Environ. Health, *5*:66, 1962.

24. El Mostehy, M. R., and Stallard, R. E.: The Sturge-Weber syndrome: its periodontal significance. J. Periodontol., *40*:243, 1969.

25. Epstein, I. A.: Clinical indications for the use of blood examinations in the practice of periodontia. J. Periodontol., *6*:30, 1935.

26. Frantzell, A., et al.: Examination of the tongue. Acta Med. Scand., *122*:207, 1945.

27. Frohman, B. S.: Occlusal neuroses. Psychoanal. Rev., *19*:297, 1932.

28. Gancotti, M.: Hereditary factors in periodontal diseases. Ann. Stomatol. Roma, *5*:117, 1956.

29. Giddon, D. B.: Psychophysiology of the oral cavity. J. Dent. Res., *45*:1627, 1966.

30. Goldman, H. M.: Acute aleukemic leukemia. Am. J. Orthod., *26*:89, 1940.

31. Grant, D., and Bernick, S.: Arteriosclerosis in periodontal vessels of aging humans. J. Periodontol., *41*:170, 1970.

32. Gruber, I. E.: The condition of the teeth and the attachment apparatus in tuberculosis. J. Dent. Res., *28*:483, 1949.

33. Gupta, O. P.: Psychosomatic factors in periodontal disease. Dent. Clin. North Am., *10*:11, 1966.

34. Hall, J. F., and Robinson, H. B. G.: Alveolar atrophy in anemic dogs. J. Dent. Res., *16*:345, 1937.

35. Heinrich, E.: Report on sociologic and constitutional typologic examinations on paradentosis of 200 patients. Paradentium, *2*:32, 1933.

36. Higgins, W. H.: Systemic poisoning with bismuth. J.A.M.A., *66*:648, 1916.

37. Hudson, E. J.: Purpura hemorrhagica caused by gold and arsenical compounds with report of two cases. Lancet, *2*:74, 1935.

38. Hutter, A. M., Middleton, W. S., and Steenbock, H.: Vitamin B deficiency and the atrophic tongue. J.A.M.A., *101*:1305, 1933.

39. Itoiz, M. E., Litwack, D., Kennedy, J. E., and Zander, H. A.: Experimental ischemia in monkeys: III. Histochemical analysis of gingival epithelium. J. Dent. Res., *48*(2):895, 1969.

40. Jones, R. R.: Symptoms in early stages of industrial plumbism. J.A.M.A., *104*:195, 1935.

41. Kastlin, G.: Agranulocytic angina. Am. J. Med. Sci., *173*:799, 1927.

42. Kennedy, J. E., and Zander, H. A.: Experimental ischemia in monkeys. I. Effect of ischemia on gingival epithelium. J. Dent. Res., *48*(1):696, 1969.

43. Kracke, R. R.: Granulopenia as associated with amidopyrine administration. Report made at Annual Session of A.M.A., June, 1934.

44. Kramer, G., and Griffel, A.: Christmas disease (hemophilia B) in periodontal therapy. Oral Surg., *15*:1056, 1962.

45. Lainson, P., Brady, P., and Fraleigh, C.: Anemia, a systemic cause of periodontal disease. J. Periodontol., *39*:35, 1968.

46. Liberman, H.: Chrome ulcerations of the nose and throat. N. Engl. J. Med., *225*:132, 1941.

47. Madison, F. W., and Squier, T. L.: Primary granulocytopenia after administration of benzene chain derivatives. J.A.M.A., *102*:755, 1934.

48. Manhold, J. H.: Report of a study on the relationship of personality variables to periodontal conditions. J. Periodontol., *24*:248, 1953.

49. Mark, H. A.: Agranulocytic angina. Its oral manifestations. J. Am. Dent. Assoc., *21*:2119, 1934.

50. Meyer, A.: Agranulocytosis. Report of a case caused by sulfadiazine. California and West Med. J., *61*:54, 1944.

51. Miller, S. C., et al.: The use of the Minnesota Multiphasic Personality Inventory as a diagnostic aid in periodontal disease. A preliminary report. J. Periodontol., *27*:44, 1956.

52. Mittleman, G., Bakke, B. F., and Scopp, I. W.: Alveolar bone changes in sickle cell anemia. J. Periodontol., *32*:74, 1961.

53. Monto, R. W., Rizek, R., and Fine, G.: Observations on the exfoliative cytology and histology of the oral mucous membranes in iron deficiency. Oral Surg., *14*:965, 1961.

54. Moskow, B. S., Rennert, M. C., Wasserman, B. H., and Khurana, H.: Interrelationship of dietary factors and heredity in periodontal lesions in the gerbil. I.A.D.R. Abstracts, 1970, p. 134

55. Poland, C., III, Christian, J. C., and Bixler, D.: Hypophosphatasia: an inherited oral disease. I.A.D.R. Abstracts, 1970, p. 228.

56. Quintarelli, G.: Histopathology of the human mandibular artery and arterioles in periodontal disease. Oral Surg., *10*:1047, 1957.

57. Ramfjord, S.: Tuberculosis and periodontal disease, with special reference to the collagen fibers. J. Dent. Res., *31*:5, 1952.

58. Randall, C. L.: Granulocytopenia following barbiturates and amidopyrine. J.A.M.A., *102*:1137, 1934.

59. Robbins, S. L., and Cotran, R. S.: Pathologic Basis of Disease. 2nd ed. Philadelphia, W. B. Saunders Company, 1979.

60. Robinson, I. B., and Sarnat, B. G.: Roentgen studies of the maxillae and mandible in sickle cell anemia. Radiology, *58*:517, 1952.

61. Ryan, E. J.: Psychobiologic Foundation in Dentistry. Springfield, Ill., Charles C Thomas, Publisher, 1946, p. 27.

62. Rylander, H., Attstrom, R., and Lindhe, J.: Influence of experimental neutropenia in dogs with chronic gingivitis. J. Periodont. Res. *10*:315, 1975.

63. Sandler, H. C., and Stahl, S. S.: The influence of generalized diseases on clinical manifestations of periodontal disease. J. Am. Dent. Assoc., *49*:656, 1954.

64. Saul, L. J.: A note on the psychogenesis of organic symptoms. Psychoanal. Q., *4*:476, 1935.

65. Schonbauer, F.: Histological findings in the jaw in septicemia and leukemia. Z. Stomatol., *27*:804, 1929.

66. Schour, I., and Sarnat, B. G.: Oral manifestations of occupational origin. J.A.M.A., *120*:1197, 1942.

67. Scopp, I. W.: Healthy periodontium in chronically ill patients. J. Periodontol., *28*:147, 1957.

68. Stahl, S. S., et al.: The influence of systemic diseases on alveolar bone. J. Am. Dent. Assoc., *45*:277, 1952.

69. Tanchester, D., and Sorrin, S.: Dental lesions in relation to pulmonary tuberculosis. J. Dent. Res., *16*:69, 1937.

70. Telsey, B., Beube, F. E., Zegarelli, E. V., and Kutscher, A. H.: Oral manifestations of cyclical neutropenia associated with hypergammaglobulinemia. Oral Surg., *15*:540, 1962.

71. Thompson, W. P.: Observations on possible relation between agranulocytosis and menstruation with further studies on a case of cyclic neutropenia. N. Engl. J. Med., *210*:176, 1934.

72. Tochichara, Y.: Pyorrhea alveolaris in leprosy. Nippar No Shikai, *13*:165, 1933.

73. Weiss, E., and English, O. S.: Psychosomatic Medicine. 2nd ed. Philadelphia, W. B. Saunders Company, 1949.

74. Weller, C. V.: Constitutional factors in periodontitis. J. Am. Dent. Assoc., *15*:1081, 1928.

75. Wirthlin, M. R., Jr., and Ratcliff, P. A.: Arteries, atherosclerosis and periodontics. J. Periodontol., *40*:341, 1969.

chapter thirty-one

The Systemic Condition of Patients with Periodontal Disease

Systemic Findings in Periodontal Disease	**Hematologic Aspects**
Metabolism	**Focal Infection**
Endocrine	Periodontal Disease and Focal Infection
Blood Chemistry	**Bacteremia in Gingival and Periodontal Disease**
Gastric Chemistry	

Numerous clinical studies have been conducted to determine whether there are disorders that predispose to periodontal disease and also to determine the effect upon the patient of gingival and periodontal disease. The findings in such studies have been interpreted in the following ways:

1. There may be systemic disorders that predispose to periodontal disease.

2. Periodontal disease may predispose to certain systemic disorders.

3. There may be comparable factors that predispose patients to both periodontal disease and specific systemic disorders.

SYSTEMIC FINDINGS IN PERIODONTAL DISEASE

The following systemic aspects have been investigated in relation to periodontal disease. (Some studies differentiate between systemic findings in patients with periodontitis and those with juvenile periodontitis; others do not make this distinction.)

METABOLISM. Patients with periodontitis present no characteristic metabolic pattern.[6-8] In juvenile periodontitis the metabolism has been reported both as lowered[12] and as slightly elevated.[5, 52] Opinions differ as to whether a correlation exists between periodontal status and glucose tolerance levels.[38, 48]

ENDOCRINE. Dysfunction of the parathyroid and pituitary glands, ovaries and thyroid (particularly hyperthyroidism),[4, 5] and abnormal serum calcium levels have been reported in juvenile periodontitis.[13] Hypothyroidism was observed in 43 of 80 patients with periodontitis,[3] with and without other endocrine disorders (e.g., diabetes, hypogonadism, and pituitary dysfunction[50]), and reduced urinary estrogen levels have been correlated with increasing severity of periodontal disease.[23]

BLOOD CHEMISTRY. Elevated calcium,[51] lowered calcium with elevated phosphorus,[20] and elevated serum glycoprotein,[16] uric acid, glucose, cholesterol, citric acid, and bilirubin levels have been reported in the blood of patients with juvenile periodontitis.[25, 28, 47, 51] Serum glutamic oxaloacetic transaminase and serum glutamic pyruvic transaminase levels are not altered.[21]

In periodontitis, elevated blood calcium and lowered phosphorus,[2, 13, 19] elevated serum alkaline phosphatase[34] and citric acid,[43] and lowered blood catalase[15] levels have been described. Some investigators suggest the possibility of a relationship between dietary inadequacy and deviations in blood chemistry in patients with periodontal disease.[24] Others note no significant changes in periodontal disease. The levels of calcium, glucose, cholesterol, ascorbic acid,[22, 46] sodium and potassium,[34] chloride, inorganic phosphate, and urea nitrogen[31] in the blood are reported as unaltered. Serum total protein, albumin, globulin, and uric acid levels show no significant relationship to periodontal status.[39, 40] The level of serum free 17-hydroxycorticosterone is elevated in periodontal disease, but the significance of this finding has not been established. The glucose content of blood in the gingiva and the finger is the same in patients with periodontal disease,[25] but alkaline phosphatase is greater in gingival blood than in the general circulation.[32] C-reactive protein (CRP) (a nonspecific protein usually associated with disease causing inflammation and tissue breakdown and not found in healthy individuals) was noted in patients with severe periodontal disease.[41]

A laboratory study of 143 adult patients with advanced periodontal disease included evaluation of calcium, cholesterol, glucose, inorganic phosphorus, total protein, albumin, globulin, urea nitrogen, uric acid, protein-bound

487

iodine, and alkaline phosphatase; oral glucose tolerance tests (fasting, 30 minutes, and 1, 2, and 3 hours); and serum electrophoresis for albumin, alpha-1-globulin, alpha-2-globulin, beta-globulin, gamma-globulin, and total protein. There was no indication that the presence of advanced periodontal disease was in any way related to variations in the accepted normal values.[11]

GASTRIC CHEMISTRY. Gastric hyperacidity, hypoacidity, and anacidity[7, 35] occur in patients with periodontal disease. The contention of Broderick,[9] that periodontal disease results from alkalosis and that caries is caused by acidosis, has not been confirmed.

HEMATOLOGIC ASPECTS. Blood studies in patients with periodontal disease reveal the following: normal total and differential leukocyte counts and low red blood cell count,[42] elevated counts, frequent secondary anemia of the microcytic hypochromic type,[18] a decrease in hemoglobin values, and a low erythrocyte count, as well as a relative lymphocytosis and a decrease in polymorphonuclear leukocytes.[27] Blood type A was noted in 49 per cent of patients with periodontal disease, in contrast with 40 to 41.1 per cent of patients without periodontal disease,[33, 49] but no significant relationship between blood grouping and periodontal disease[1] or between arteriosclerosis and alveolar bone loss[26] has been established.

Comment

The preceding paragraphs are a review of investigations conducted for the most part in the thirties and forties, when the possibility of periodontal disease being of systemic origin was explored. At present, the infectious nature of periodontal disease has been shown; therefore, these studies are presented for their historic interest.

FOCAL INFECTION

According to the concept of focal infection, a primary site of infection in one part of the body may serve as the focus (Latin, *hearth*) from which the infection emanates to other parts of the body. Interest in focal infection has fluctuated considerably from the initial enthusiasm stimulated by the original investigation of Rosenow in 1917. With the introduction of chemotherapy, attention was again directed to the subject of focal infection.

In the early days of the focal infection concept, the oral cavity attracted attention because it harbored teeth with chronic apical disease. Physicians confronted with disease elsewhere in the body were drawn to the comparatively easily accessible "infected" teeth. The persistence of disease in other areas of the body even after all the "infected" teeth had been removed, coupled with the revelation that not all pathologic apical lesions are necessarily infected, exerted a somewhat sobering influence upon the medical and dental professions in regard to the problem of focal infection.

PERIODONTAL DISEASE AND FOCAL INFECTION. Interest in the oral cavity as a possible source of focal infection has shifted from the periapical areas to the periodontal pocket.[45] Within the limitations which govern the concept of focal infection, **the periodontal pocket represents a greater potential menace than periapical disease for the reasons shown in Table 31–1.**

The potential role of periodontal pathogens in *anaerobic* infections elsewhere in the body has been recently emphasized. Organisms associated with periodontal disease have been found in infected wounds, lung abscesses, subacute bacterial endocarditis, and other infections.

In patients with periodontal disease and a disturbance elsewhere in the body suspected of being of focal origin, **the responsibility for the decision regarding the fate of the teeth rests with the dentist.** It is reasonable to expect the dentist to understand more about the periodontal tissues than other medical specialists. The physician, on the other hand, is in a position to inform the dentist regarding the likelihood of the patient's medical problem being caused by infection elsewhere in the body. It should be borne in mind that, even in a patient with suppurative periodontal disease which the dentist might very well consider a potential focus of infection, there is no assurance that the patient's complaint is related to the oral condition.

BACTEREMIA IN GINGIVAL AND PERIODONTAL DISEASE

The literature consistently points to disease of the gingiva as a source of bacteremia following mechanical manipulation of the teeth.[10, 30, 36, 44] Murray and Moosnick[29] found positive blood cultures in 55 per cent of persons with

TABLE 31–1 THE PERIODONTAL POCKET VERSUS PERIAPICAL DISEASE

Periodontal Pocket	Periapical Disease
1. Infection is always present.	1. Infection is not necessarily present in long-standing periapical lesions.[10]
2. The bacterial as well as mycotic organisms are of great variety, considerably more numerous, and of greater pathogenic potential. They penetrate the soft tissue wall of the pocket.	2. The bacterial organisms are not as varied or numerous or of equal pathogenic significance.
3. Periodontal pockets are not circumscribed or walled off from the adjacent tissue.	3. Periapical areas are frequently well circumscribed within a fibrotic boundary.
4. Periodontal pockets are subject to constant mechanical stimulation in mastication, which could drive bacteria into the blood stream.	4. Periapical areas are located centrally in the bone, in a comparatively undisturbed environment.
5. Periodontal pockets are more prevalent in adults in age groups likely to be subject to ailments requiring medical attention.	5. Periapical disease is less prevalent than periodontal pockets.

varying degrees of dental caries and periodontal disease chewed paraffin cubes for 30 minutes. Fish and MacLean[17] reported positive blood cultures after tooth extractions in nine patients with periodontal disease. They assumed that luxation of the teeth in extraction caused alternate compression and stretching of the periodontal ligament and that streptococci were in this way pumped into the lymphatics and blood vessels. Okell and Elliott[30] reported 72 positive blood cultures following extraction in 100 patients with gingival disease. A significantly lower incidence of bacteremia was found in patients with no clinical periodontal disease. In addition, Elliott[14] found that, where marked gingival disease was present, rocking of the teeth alone sufficed to produce bacteremia in 86 per cent of the patients. Bacteremia occurred more frequently in association with deep periodontal pockets. The penetration of bacteria into the epithelium and connective tissue of the pocket wall may favor the bacteremia.[36] Burket and Burn[10] painted *Serratia marcescens* into the gingival sulcus prior to extraction and recovered it in postextraction blood cultures in 18 of 90 cases.

REFERENCES

1. Barros, L., and Witkop, C. S. J.: Oral and genetic study of Chileans 1960. III. Periodontal disease and nutritional factors. Arch. Oral Biol., 8:195, 1963.
2. Becks, H.: Newer aspects in paradentosis. Ann. Intern. Med., 6:65, 1932–1933.
3. Becks, H.: Systemic background of paradentosis. J. Ann. Dent. Assoc., 28:1447, 1941.
4. Boenheim, F.: Endokriner Status bei Paradentose. Zahnärztl. Rundsch., 37:1326, 1928.
5. Boenheim, F.: Ist das endokrine Druesensystem bei Paradentose gestoert? Paradentium, 3:91, 1930.
6. Boenheim, F.: Pyorrhea alveolaris as systemic disease. Br. Dent. J., 53:12, 1932.
7. Boenheim, F.: Pathogenic importance of the endocrine glands in paradontal disease. J. Dent. Res., 17:19, 1938.
8. Breuer, K.: Metabolic studies in disease of the paradentium. Z. Stomatol., 31:982, 1933.
9. Broderick, F. W.: Pyorrhea Alveolaris. London, John Bale Sons and Danielson, Ltd., 1931.
10. Burket, L. W., and Burn, G. G.: Bacteremia following dental extraction. Demonstration of source of bacteria by means of a non-pathogen. J. Dent. Res., 16:521, 1937.
11. Cattoni, M. and Shannon, I. L.: Laboratory study of patients with advanced periodontal disease. J. Western Soc. Periodontol., 24:172, 1976–1977.
12. Chiuminatto, L.: Investigation of metabolism in paradentoses. Stomatologie, 27:269, 1929.
13. Citron, J.: Die Paradentose als Symptom von Endokrinen. Z. Clin. Med., 108:331, 1928.
14. Elliott, S. D.: Bacteremia and oral sepsis. Proc. R. Soc. Med., 32:747, 1939.
15. Englander, H. R., et al.: The relationship of blood catalase activity and periodontal disease. J. Periodontol., 26:233, 1955.
16. Engle, M. B., Laskin, D. M., and Gans, B. J.: Elevation of a serum glycoprotein in periodontosis. J. Am. Dent. Assoc., 57:830, 1958.
17. Fish, E. W., and MacLean, L.: Distribution of oral streptococci in the tissues. Br. Dent. J., 61:336, 1936.
18. Goldstein, H.: Systemic and blood picture in several hundred periclasia-free and periclasia-involved individuals. J. Dent. Res., 16:320, 1937.
19. Grove, C. J., and Grove, C. T.: Blood phosphorus insufficiency in pyorrhea. J. Dent. Res., 13:191, 1933.
20. Hawkins, H. F., Nutritional influences on growth and development. Int. J. Orthod. 19:307, 1933.
21. Honjo, K., Nakamura, R., Tsunemitsu, A., and Matsummura, T.: Serum transaminases in periodontosis. J. Periodontol., 35:247, 1964.
22. Karshan, M., and Tenenbaum, B.: Blood studies in periodontoclasia. J. Dent. Res., 25:180, 1946.
23. Karshan, M., Tenenbaum, B., and Friedland, R.: Urinary estrogen in periodontosis. J. Dent. Res., 35:648, 1956.
24. Karshan, M., et al.: Studies in periodontal disease. J. Dent. Res., 31:11, 1952.
25. Landgraf, E., et al.: Investigations of uric acid blood level in periodontal disease. Z. Stomatol., 30:91, 1932.
26. Mackenzie, R. S., and Millard, H. D.: Interrelated effects of diabetes, arteriosclerosis, and calculus on alveolar bone loss. J. Am. Dent. Assoc., 66:191, 1963.
27. Martin, D.: The blood associated with pyorrhea alveolaris. Aust. Dent. J., 9:488, 1937.
28. Morelli, G.: The clinical and therapeutic evaluation of the results concerning constitutional factors in cases of paradentoses. Ann. Med., 41:648, 1935.
29. Murray, M., and Moosnick, F.: Incidence of bacteremia in patients with dental disease. J. Lab. Clin. Med., 26:801, 1941.
30. Okell, C. C., and Elliott, S. D.: Bacteremia and oral sepsis. Lancet, 2:869, 1935.
31. O'Leary, T. J., Shannon, I. L., and Prigmore, J. R.: Clinical and systemic findings in periodontal disease. J. Periodontol., 33:243, 1962.

32. Pelzer, R. H.: A method for plasma phosphatase determination for the differentiation of alveolar crest bone types in periodontal disease. J. Dent. Res., *19*:73, 1940.

33. Polevitsky, K.: Blood types in pyorrhea alveolaris. J. Dent. Res., *9*:285, 1929.

34. Rose, H. P., Kuna, A., and Kraft, E.: Systemic manifestations of periodontal disease. J. Periodontol., *34*:253, 1963.

35. Sagal, Z.: Pyorrhea alveolaris and gastric acidity. Dent. Cosmos, *68*:1145, 1926.

36. Saglie, R., Newman, M. S., Carranza, F. A., Jr., and Pattison, G. L.: Bacterial invasion of gingival tissue in advanced periodontitis in humans. J. Periodontol., *53*:217, 1982.

37. Sand, R.: Periodontal sepsis in relationship to systemic disease. J. Am. Dent. Assoc., *28*:710, 1941.

38. Shannon, I. L., and Gibson, W. A.: Oral glucose tolerance responses in healthy young adult males classified as to caries experience and periodontal status. Periodontics, *2*:292, 1964.

39. Shannon, I. L., and Gibson, W. A.: Serum total protein, albumin, and globulin in relation to periodontal status and caries experience. Oral Surg., *18*:399, 1964.

40. Shannon, I. L., Terry, J. M., and Chauncey, H. H.: Uric acid and total protein in serum and parotid fluid in relation to periodontal status. J. Dent. Res., *45*:1539, 1966.

41. Shklair, I., Loving, R., Leberman, O., and Rau, C.: C-reactive protein and periodontal disease. J. Periodontol., *39*:93, 1968.

42. Siegel, E.: Total erythrocyte, lymphocyte and differential white cell counts of blood in chronic periodontal disease. J. Dent. Res., *24*:270, 1945.

43. Simon, E., et al.: Citrate content of blood and saliva in relation to periodontal disease in man. Arch. Oral Biol., *13*:1243, 1968.

44. Stones, H. H.: Oral and Dental Diseases. Chronic Oral Sepsis and Relation to Systemic Diseases. Baltimore, Williams & Wilkins, 1948, Chap. 33.

45. Stortebecker, T. P.: Dental infectious foci and diseases of the nervous system. Acta Psychiatr. Neurol. Scand., *36*(Suppl. 157), 1961.

46. Tenenbaum, B., and Karshan, M.: Blood studies in periodontoclasia. J. Am. Dent. Assoc., *32*:1372, 1945.

47. Tsunemitsu, A., et al.: Citric acid metabolism in periodontosis. Arch. Oral Biol., *9*:83, 1964.

48. Tuckman, M. A., et al.: The relationship of glucose tolerance to periodontal status. J. Periodontol., *41*:513, 1970.

49. Weber, R., and Pastern, W.: Uber die Frage der Konstitutionellen Bereitschaft zur Sog. Alveolar Pyorrhoe (Alveolarpyorrhoe und Blutgruppen). Dtsch. Monatschr. Zahnheilk., *14*:704, 1927.

50. Weiner, R., Karshan, M., and Tenenbaum, B.: Ovarian function in periodontosis. J. Dent. Res., *35*:875, 1956.

51. Weinmann, J. P.: Study of metabolism in diffuse atrophy. Z. Stomatol., *25*:822, 1927.

52. Weinmann, J. P.: Investigation of metabolism in diffuse atrophy of the alveolar process. Z. Stomatol., *28*:1154, 1930.

THE TREATMENT OF PERIODONTAL DISEASE

Periodontal treatment requires the interrelationship of the care of the periodontium with other phases of dentistry. The concept of **total treatment** includes the following:

1. **The soft tissues**—elimination of gingival inflammation and the factors that lead to it (plaque accumulation favored by pocket formation, inadequate restorations, and areas of food impaction).

2. **The functional aspects**—establishment of optimal occlusal relationships for the entire dentition.

3. **The systemic aspects**—systemic adjuncts to local treatment and special precautions in patient management necessitated by systemic conditions.

All of these aspects are embodied in a **master plan,** which consists of a rational **sequence of dental procedures** that includes periodontal and other procedures necessary to create a well-functioning dentition in a healthy periodontal environment.

Part I

Diagnosis, Determination of the Prognosis, and the Treatment Plan

―――――――――― chapter thirty-two ――――――――――

Diagnosis

Proper diagnosis is essential for intelligent treatment. In addition to recognizing the clinical and radiographic features of different diseases, diagnosis requires an understanding of the underlying disease processes and their etiology. **Our interest is in the patient who has the disease and not simply in the disease itself.** Diagnosis must therefore include a general evaluation of the patient, as well as consideration of the oral cavity.

Diagnosis must be systematic and organized for specific purposes. It is not enough to assemble facts. The findings must be pieced together so that they provide a meaningful explanation of the patient's periodontal problem.

The diagnosis should provide answers to the following questions:

Which factors are responsible for plaque accumulation leading to gingival inflammation and periodontal pockets? Does the periodontium present evidence of trauma from occlusion? Are there occlusal relationships that account for the traumatic lesions? Are the gingival and periodontal changes explainable by the local factors or do they suggest the possibility of a contributing systemic etiology?

The following is a recommended sequence of procedures for the diagnosis of gingival and periodontal disease:

FIRST VISIT

Overall Appraisal of the Patient

From the first meeting, the operator should attempt an overall appraisal of the patient. This includes consideration of the patient's mental and emotional status, temperament, attitude, and physiologic age.

Systemic History

Most of the systemic history is obtained at the first visit and can be enlarged upon by pertinent questions at subsequent visits. The importance of the systemic history should be explained, because patients often omit information that they cannot relate to their dental problem. The systemic history will aid the operator in (1) **the diagnosis of oral manifestations of systemic disease,** (2) **the detection of systemic conditions that may be affecting the periodontal tissue response to local factors,** and (3) **the detection of systemic conditions that require special precautions and modifications in treatment procedures.** The systemic history should include reference to the following:

1. Is the patient under the care of a physician; if so, what is the nature and duration of the illness and the therapy? Special inquiry should be made regarding anticoagulants and corticosteroids—the dosage and duration of therapy.

2. History of rheumatic fever, rheumatic or congenital heart disease, hypertension, angina pectoris, myocardial infarction, nephritis, liver disease, diabetes, and/or fainting spells.

3. Abnormal bleeding tendencies such as nose bleeds, prolonged bleeding from minor cuts, spontaneous ecchymoses, tendency toward excessive bruising, and excessive menstrual bleeding.

4. Infectious disease, recent contact with infectious disease at home or at business, or recent chest x-ray.

5. Possibility of occupational disease.

6. History of allergy—hay fever, asthma, sensitivity to foods, and/or sensitivity to drugs such as aspirin, codeine, barbiturates, sulfonamides, antibiotics, procaine, and laxatives or to dental materials such as eugenol or acrylic resins.

7. Information regarding the onset of puberty and menopause and about menstrual disorders or hysterectomy, pregnancies, or miscarriages.

Dental History

Chief Complaint

The following are some of the symptoms in patients with gingival and periodontal disease: "bleeding gums," "loose teeth," "spreading of the teeth with the appearance of spaces where none existed before," "foul taste in the mouth," and "itchy feeling in the gums, relieved by digging with a toothpick." There may also be pain of varied types and duration, such as "constant dull gnawing pain," "dull pain after eating," "deep radiating pains in the jaws," "acute throbbing pain," "sensitivity to percussion," "sensitivity to heat and cold," "burning sensation in the gums," and "extreme sensitivity to inhaled air."

A preliminary oral examination is done to explore the source of the patient's chief complaint and to determine whether *immediate emergency care* is required.

The dental history should include reference to the following:

1. Visits to the dentist—frequency, date of last visit, and nature of the treatment. "Oral prophylaxis" or "cleaning" by a dentist or hygienist—frequency and date of last cleaning.

2. Toothbrushing—frequency, before or after meals, method, type of toothbrush and dentifrice, and interval at which brushes are replaced. Other methods for mouth care: mouthwashes, finger massage, interdental stimulation, water irrigation, and dental floss.

3. Orthodontic treatment—duration and approximate time of termination.

4. Pain "in the teeth" or "in the gums"—the manner in which it is provoked, its nature

and duration, and the manner in which it is relieved.

5. "Bleeding gums" when first noted, whether it occurs spontaneously, upon brushing or eating, at night, or with regular periodicity; whether it is associated with the menstrual period or other specific factors; and the duration of the bleeding and the manner in which it is stopped.

6. Bad taste in the mouth and areas of food impaction.

7. Tooth mobility—do the teeth feel "loose" or insecure? Is there difficulty in chewing?

8. History of previous "gum trouble"—the nature of the condition, previous treatment, duration, nature, and approximate period of termination.

9. Habits—"grinding the teeth," "clenching the teeth" during the day or night—do the teeth or muscles feel "sore" in the morning? Other habits, such as tobacco smoking or chewing, nail biting, and biting on foreign objects.

Intraoral Radiographic Survey

The radiographic survey should consist of a minimum of 14 intraoral films and posterior bite-wings (Fig. 32–1).

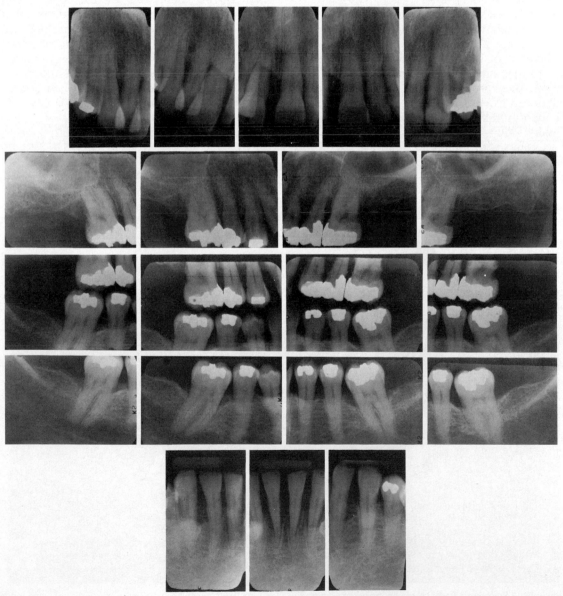

Figure 32–1 Full-mouth intraoral radiographic series (16 periapical films and 4 bite-wing films) used as an adjunct in periodontal diagnosis.

Panoramic radiographs are a simple and convenient method of obtaining a survey view of the dental arch and surrounding structures (Fig. 32–1). They are helpful for the detection of developmental anomalies, pathologic lesions of the teeth and jaws, and fractures (Fig. 32–2) and for dental screening examinations of large groups. They provide an informative overall radiographic picture of the distribution and severity of bone destruction in periodontal disease, but a *complete intraoral series is required for definitive diagnosis and treatment planning.*

Casts

Casts are extremely useful adjuncts in the oral examination. They indicate the position of the gingival margin and the position and inclination of the teeth, proximal contact relationships, and food impaction areas. In addition, they provide a view of lingual cuspal relationships. They are important records of the dentition before it is altered by treatment. Finally, they also serve as "visual aids" in discussions with the patient and are useful for pre- and posttreatment comparisons as well as for reference at checkup visits.

Clinical Photographs

Color photographs are not essential, but they are useful for recording the appearance of the tissue before and after treatment. Photographs cannot always be relied upon for comparing subtle color changes in the gingiva; they do depict changes in gingival morphology.

Review of Initial Examination

If no emergency care is required, the patient is dismissed and instructed when to report for the second visit. Before this visit, a correlated examination is made of the radiographs and casts to relate the radiographic changes to unfavorable conditions represented on the casts. The casts are checked for evidence of abnormal wear, plunger cusps, uneven marginal ridges, malposed or extruded teeth, crossbite relationships, or other conditions that could cause occlusal disharmony or food impaction. Such areas are marked on the casts, to be referred to in the detailed examination of the oral cavity to follow. The radiographs and casts are valuable diagnostic aids; however, it is the findings in the oral cavity that constitute the basis for diagnosis.

SECOND VISIT

Oral Examination

Oral Hygiene

The "cleanliness" of the oral cavity is appraised in terms of the extent of accumulated

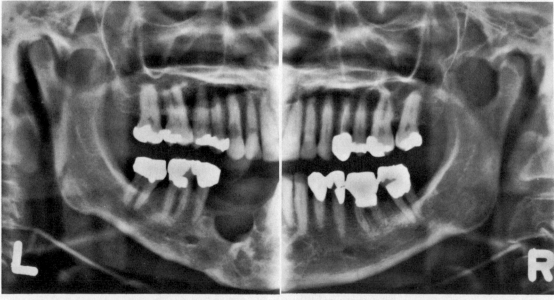

Figure 32–2 Panoramic Radiograph, showing temporomandibular joints and "cystic" spaces in the jaw. Areas of periodontal bone loss are not seen in detail. (Compare with Fig. 32–1.)

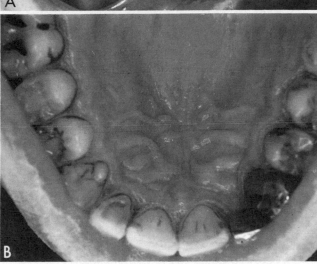

Figure 32–3 Poor Oral Hygiene. *A,* Gingival inflammation associated with plaque, materia alba, and calculus in a patient with hemophilia. *B,* Palatal view of the same patient showing only slight gingivitis because the mechanical action of the tongue and food excursion reduces the accumulation of local irritants.

food debris, plaque, materia alba, and tooth surface stains (Fig. 32–3). Disclosing solution should be used routinely to detect plaque that would otherwise be unnoticed.

Mouth Odors

Halitosis, also termed "fetor ex ore" or "fetor oris," is foul or offensive odor emanating from the oral cavity.[48] Mouth odors may be of diagnostic significance, and their origin may be either (1) local or (2) extraoral or remote.

LOCAL SOURCES. Local sources of mouth odors include the retention of odoriferous food particles on and between the teeth, coated tongue, acute necrotizing ulcerative gingivitis, dehydration states, caries, artificial dentures, smoker's breath, and healing surgical or extraction wounds. *The fetid odor characteristic of acute necrotizing ulcerative gingivitis is easily identified.* Chronic periodontal disease with

pocket formation may also cause unpleasant mouth odor from accumulated debris and the increased rate of putrefaction of the saliva.[8]

EXTRAORAL OR REMOTE SOURCES. These may include adjacent structures associated with rhinitis, sinusitis, or tonsillitis; disease of the lungs and bronchi, such as chronic fetid bronchitis, bronchiectasis, lung abscesses, gangrene of the lung, and pulmonary tuberculosis; and odors excreted through the lungs from aromatic substances in the blood stream, such as metabolites from ingested foods or excretory products of cell metabolism. Alcoholic breath, the acetone odor of diabetes, and the uremic breath accompanying kidney dysfunction are examples of the last group.

Examination of the Oral Cavity

The entire oral cavity should be carefully examined. The examination should include the lips, floor of the mouth, tongue, palate, and oropharyngeal region and the quality and quantity of saliva. Although these findings may not be related to the periodontal problem, the dentist should detect any pathology present in the mouth. Textbooks in oral medicine and oral diagnosis cover these topics in detail.

Lymph Nodes

Because periodontal, periapical, and other oral diseases may result in lymph node changes, the diagnostician should routinely examine and evaluate head and neck lymph nodes. Lymph nodes can become enlarged and/or indurated as a result of an infectious episode, malignant metastases, or residual fibrotic changes.

Inflammatory nodes become enlarged, palpable, tender, and fairly immobile. The overlying skin may be red and warm. Patients are frequently aware of the presence of "swollen glands." Acute herpetic gingivostomatitis, acute necrotizing ulcerative gingivitis, and acute periodontal abscesses may produce lymph node enlargement. After successful therapy, lymph nodes return to normal in a matter of days or a few weeks.

Examination of the Teeth

The teeth are examined for caries, developmental defects, anomalies of tooth form, wasting, hypersensitivity, and proximal contact relationships.

Wasting Disease of the Teeth

Wasting is defined as any gradual loss of tooth substance characterized by the formation of smooth, polished surfaces, without regard to the possible mechanism of this loss. The forms of wasting are erosion, abrasion, and attrition.

Erosion (cuneiform defect) is a sharply defined wedge-shaped depression in the cervical area of the facial tooth surface.[68] The long axis of the eroded area is perpendicular to the vertical axis of the tooth (Fig. 32–4). The surfaces are smooth, hard, and polished. Erosion generally affects a group of teeth. In the early stages, it may be confined to the enamel, but it generally extends to involve the underlying dentin, as well as the cementum and dentin of the root.

The etiology of erosion is not known. Decalcification by acid beverages[49] or citrus fruits and the combined effect of acid salivary secre-

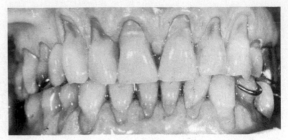

Figure 32–4 Erosion involving the enamel, cementum, and dentin.

tion and friction[50] are suggested causes. Sognnaes[84] refers to these lesions as "dentoalveolar ablations" and attributes them to forceful frictional actions between the oral soft tissues and the adjacent hard tissues. In patients with erosion the salivary pH, buffering capacity, and calcium and phosphorus content have been reported as normal, with the mucin level elevated.[46]

Abrasion refers to the loss of tooth substance induced by mechanical wear other than that of mastication. Abrasion results in saucer-shaped or wedge-shaped indentations with a smooth, shiny surface. Abrasion starts on exposed cementum surfaces rather than on the enamel and extends to involve the dentin of the root. Continued exposure to the abrasive agent, combined with decalcification of the enamel by locally formed acids, may result in a loss of the enamel, followed by loss of the dentin of the crown (Fig. 32–5).

Toothbrushing[35] with an abrasive dentifrice and the action of clasps are common causes of abrasion. The former is by far the more prevalent. According to Manly,[43, 45] the degree of tooth wear from toothbrushing depends upon the abrasive effect of the dentifrice and the angle of brushing. Horizontal brushing at right angles to the vertical axis of the teeth results in the severest loss of tooth substance. Occasionally abrasion of the incisal edges occurs as a result of habits such as holding a bobby pin or tacks between the teeth.

Attrition is the occlusal wear due to functional contacts with opposing teeth. It is described in Chapter 27.

Dental Stains

Pigmented deposits on the tooth surface are called *stains*. They are primarily esthetic problems. Stains result from the pigmentation of ordinarily colorless developmental and acquired dental coatings by chromogenic bacte-

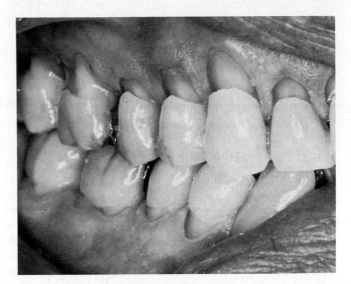

Figure 32–5 Abrasion Attributed to Aggressive Toothbrushing. Involvement of the roots is followed by undermining of the enamel.

ria, foods, and chemicals. They vary in color and composition and in the firmness with which they adhere to the tooth surface.

BROWN STAIN. This is a thin, translucent, acquired, usually bacteria-free, pigmented pellicle.[44, 93] It occurs in individuals who do not brush sufficiently or who use a dentifrice with inadequate cleansing action. It is found most commonly on the buccal surface of the maxillary molars and on the lingual surface of the mandibular incisors. The brown color is usually due to the presence of tannin.

TOBACCO STAIN. Tobacco produces tenacious dark brown or black surface deposits and brown discoloration of the tooth substance. Staining results from coal tar combustion products and from penetration of pits and fissures, enamel, and dentin by tobacco juices. Staining is not necessarily proportional to the amount of tobacco consumed, but depends to a considerable degree upon pre-existent acquired coatings which attach the tobacco products to the tooth surface.

BLACK STAIN. This usually occurs as a thin black line on the teeth facially and lingually near the gingival margin and as a diffuse patch on the proximal surfaces. It is firmly attached, tends to recur after removal, is more common in women, and may occur in mouths with excellent hygiene. The black stain that occurs on human primary teeth is typically associated with a low incidence of caries in affected children.[83, 88] Chromogenic bacteria have been implicated. The microflora of black stain is dominated by gram-positive rods, primarily *Actinomyces* species, and evidence implicates these bacteria as a probable cause. Isolated *Actinomyces* species can produce black pig-

mentation, and other in vitro investigations have demonstrated black pigment formation caused by *Actinomyces* in the dentin.[9, 58, 83] The chromogenic bacteria *Bacteroides melaninogenicus* account for less than 1 per cent of isolated bacteria and are not considered important for the cause of black stain.[83]

GREEN STAIN. This is a green or greenish-yellow stain, sometimes of considerable thickness, which is common in children (Plate IV). It is considered to be the stained remnants of the enamel cuticle, but this has not been substantiated.[3] The discoloration has been attributed to fluorescent bacteria and fungi such as *Penicillium* and *Aspergillus*.[4] Green stain usually occurs on the facial surface of the maxillary anterior teeth, in the gingival half, it occurs more often in boys (65 per cent) than in girls (43 per cent).[37] A high incidence has been reported in children with tuberculosis of the cervical lymph nodes and other tuberculous lesions.

ORANGE STAIN. Orange stain is less common than green or brown stains. It may occur on both the facial and lingual surfaces of anterior teeth. *Serratia marcescens* and *Flavobacterium lutescens* have been suggested as the responsible chromogenic organisms.[5]

METALLIC STAINS. Metals and metallic salts may be introduced into the oral cavity in metal-containing dust inhaled by industrial workers or through orally administered drugs. The metals combine with acquired dental coatings (usually pellicle), producing a surface stain, or penetrate the tooth substance and cause permanent discoloration. Copper dust produces a green stain and iron dust a brown stain. Iron-containing medicines cause a black iron sulfite deposit. Other occasionally seen metallic stains are manganese (black), mercury (greenish black), nickel (green), and silver (black).

CHLORHEXIDINE STAIN. Chlorhexidine was introduced as a general disinfectant with a broad antibacterial action against gram-positive and gram-negative bacteria and yeasts[20, 41] (Plate VI). It has been observed clinically that the continued use of chlorhexidine solution may promote discoloration in the mouth.[20, 21, 41, 55] In vivo experiments using radioactive carbon–labeled chlorhexidine have shown retention of chlorhexidine in the human oral cavity.[10, 20, 24] The retention is attributed to its affinity for sulfate and acidic groups such as those found in plaque constituents, carious lesions, pellicle, and bacterial cell walls.[10, 20, 31, 55] The retention of chlorhexidine is concentration- and time-dependent. It is not influenced by the temperature or pH of the rinsing solution.[10]

Chlorhexidine stain imparts a yellowish brown to brownish color to the tissues of the oral cavity.[14, 20, 21] The staining appears in the cervical and interproximal regions of the teeth, on restorations, in plaque, and on the surface of the tongue.[20, 21, 30, 41, 55] It appears that the presence of aldehydes and ketones, which are normally intermediates of both mammalian and microbial metabolism, are essential for formation of discoloration by chlorhexidine.[55] No permanent staining of the enamel or dentin is observed clinically, since toothbrushing with a dentifrice or professional prophylaxis can remove the stain accumulating on the teeth.[55] A similar stain occurs with the use of alexidine.

Hypersensitivity

Root surfaces exposed by gingival recession may be hypersensitive to thermal changes or tactile stimulation. Patients often direct the operator to the sensitive areas. These may be located by gentle exploration with a probe or cold air.

Proximal Contact Relations

Slightly open contacts permit food impaction. The tightness of contacts should be checked by means of clinical observation and with dental floss (Fig. 32–6). Abnormal contact relationships may also initiate occlusal changes such as a shift in the median line between the central incisors, labial version of the maxillary canine, buccal or lingual displacement of the posterior teeth, and an uneven relationship of the marginal ridges.

Tooth Mobility

All teeth have a slight degree of physiologic mobility, which varies in different teeth (highest in the central and lateral incisors) and at different times of the day.[56] It is highest upon arising in the morning and progressively decreases. The increased mobility in the morning is attributed to slight extrusion of the teeth because of limited occlusal contact during sleep. During the waking hours mobility is reduced by chewing and swallowing forces, which intrude the teeth in the sockets.

Tooth mobility beyond the physiologic range (pathologic or abnormal mobility) is increased in periodontal disease as the result of the loss of supporting tissues, in inflammation and trauma from occlusion, and in other conditions. Pathologic mobility is most common in the faciolingual direction; it is less frequent mesiodistally, and vertical mobility occurs only in extreme cases. (For a discussion of tooth mobility see Chapter 20.)

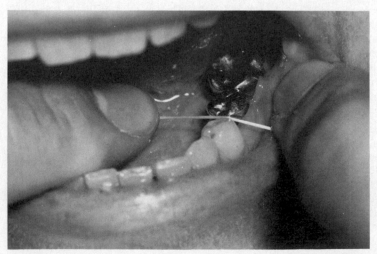

Figure 32–6 Tightness of contact points checked with dental floss.

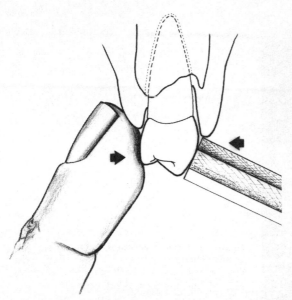

Figure 32–7 Tooth mobility checked with one metal instrument and one finger.

Mobilometers or *periodontometers* are mechanical or electronic devices for the precise measurement of mobility.[51, 57, 59] They are not widely used despite the fact that standardization of the grading of mobility would be helpful in the diagnosis of periodontal disease and in evaluating the outcome of treatment. As a general rule, mobility is graded clinically with a simple method such as the following.

The tooth is held firmly between the handles of two metal instruments or with one metal instrument and one finger (Fig. 32–7), and an effort is made to move it in all directions; abnormal mobility most often occurs faciolingually. Mobility is graded according to the ease and extent of tooth movement, assessed by the individual therapist as follows:

Physiologic mobility.

Pathologic mobility, grade 1—slightly more than physiologic.

Pathologic mobility, grade 2—moderately more than physiologic.

Pathologic mobility, grade 3—severe mobility faciolingually and/or mesiodistally combined with vertical displacement.

Sensitivity to Percussion

Sensitivity to percussion is a feature of acute inflammation of the periodontal ligament. Gently percussing a tooth at different angles to the long axis often aids in localizing the site of the inflammatory involvement. Percussion also serves as a method of "sounding" for detecting teeth with reduced periodontal support.

Pathologic Migration of the Teeth

Alterations in tooth position should be carefully noted, particularly with a view toward abnormal occlusal forces, tongue-thrusting, or other habits that may be contributing factors. Pathologic migration of anterior teeth in young persons is often a sign of juvenile periodontitis.

The Dentition with the Jaws Closed

Examination of the dentition with the jaws closed is not as revealing as examination with the jaws in function, but it does indicate conditions of periodontal significance.

Irregularly aligned teeth, extruded teeth, improper proximal contacts, and areas of food impaction are all important factors favoring the accumulation of bacterial plaque. Excessive overbite, seen most frequently in the anterior region, may cause impingement of the teeth upon the gingiva and food impaction, followed by gingival inflammation, enlargement, and pocket formation (Fig. 32–8). The real significance of excessive overbite on gingival health is, however, controversial.[1]

In open bite relationships, *abnormal vertical spaces exist between the maxillary and mandibular teeth.* The condition occurs most often in the anterior region, although posterior open bite is occasionally seen. Reduced mechanical cleaning by the passage of food may lead to accumulation of debris, calculus formation, and extrusion of teeth.

In crossbite, *the normal relationship of the mandibular teeth to the maxillary teeth is reversed, and the maxillary teeth are lingual to the mandibular teeth.* Crossbite may be bilateral or unilateral or may only affect a pair of antagonists. Trauma from occlusion, food impaction, spreading of the mandibular teeth, and associated gingival and periodontal disturbances may be caused by crossbite (Fig. 32–9).

Examination of Functional Occlusal Relationships

Examination of the functional occlusal relationships of the dentition is a critical part of the diagnostic procedure. Dentitions that appear normal when the jaws are closed may present marked functional abnormalities. Systematic procedures for the detection and correction of

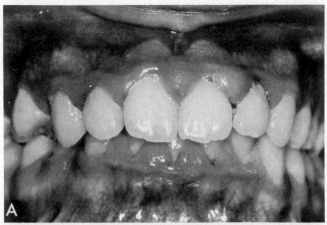

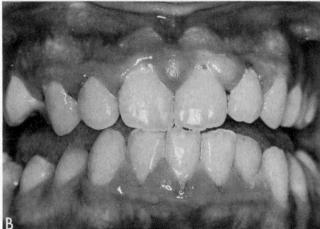

Figure 32–8 Excessive Anterior Overbite. *A*, Excessive anterior overbite with gingival inflammation and enlargement. *B*, Gingival enlargement in anterior region associated with overbite.

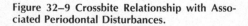

Figure 32–9 Crossbite Relationship with Associated Periodontal Disturbances.

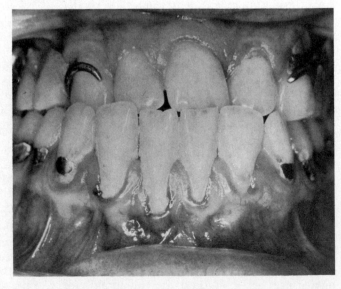

functional abnormalities are described in Chapter 47.

Examination of the Periodontium

It is important to look for the earliest signs of gingival and periodontal disease. The examination should be systematic, starting in the molar area in either the maxilla or the mandible and proceeding around the arch. This will avoid overemphasis of spectacular findings at the expense of other conditions which, though less striking, may be equally important.

Charts to record the periodontal and associated findings provide a guide for thorough examination and a record of the patient's condition (Fig. 32–10). They are also used for evaluating the response to treatment and for comparison at recall visits. However, excessively complicated mouth charting may lead to a frustrating maze of minutiae rather than to clarification of the patient's problem.

Plaque and Calculus

There are many methods of assessing plaque and calculus accumulation.[17] For the detection of **subgingival calculus** each tooth surface is carefully checked to the level of the gingival attachment with a sharp No. 17 or No. 3A explorer (Fig. 32–11). Warm air may be used to deflect the gingiva and aid in visualization of the calculus. The presence of supragingival calculus can be directly observed, and the amount can be measured with a calibrated periodontal probe.

The radiograph reveals heavy calculus deposits interproximally (Fig. 32–12) and sometimes on the facial and lingual surfaces of teeth, but *it cannot be relied upon for the thorough detection of calculus.*

Gingiva

The gingiva must be dried before accurate observations can be made (Fig. 32–13). Light reflection from moist gingiva obscures detail. In addition to visual examination and exploration with instruments, firm but gentle palpation should be used for detecting pathologic alterations in normal resilience, as well as for locating areas of pus formation.

Each of the following features of the gingiva should be considered: **color, size, contour, consistency, surface texture, position, ease of bleeding,** and **pain** (see Chapters 9 and 10).

No deviation from the normal should be overlooked. The distribution of gingival disease and its acuteness or chronicity should also be noted.

From a clinical point of view, gingival inflammation can produce two basic types of tissue response: (1) **edematous** and (2) **fibrotic.** *The edematous tissue response is characterized by a smooth, glossy, soft gingiva. In fibrotic gingiva some of the characteristics of normalcy persist; the gingiva is more firm, stippled, and opaque, although it is usually thicker and its margin appears rounded (Plate VI).*

The position of the gingiva warrants special mention. For accurate appraisal of recession, attention should be given to differentiating between the **apparent position and the actual position** of the gingival attachment on each tooth surface (see Chapter 9).

Use of Clinical Indices in Dental Practice

There has been a tendency in recent years to extend the use of indices originally designed for epidemiologic studies into dental practice. A detailed description of these indices can be found in Chapter 23. Of all the indices that have been proposed, the Gingival Index and the Sulcus Bleeding Index appear to be the two that can be most useful and most easily transferred to clinical practice.

The **Gingival Index of Löe and Silness** provides an assessment of the gingival inflammatory status that can be used in practice to compare gingival health before and after Phase I therapy or before and after surgical therapy; it can also be used to determine comparatively the gingival status at recall visits. It is important that good intra- and interexaminer calibration in the dental office is attained.[29]

The **Sulcus Bleeding Index of Mühlemann and Son** provides a very objective, easily reproducible assessment of the gingival status. It is extremely useful for detecting early inflammatory changes and the presence of inflammatory lesions located at the base of a periodontal pocket, an area inaccessible to visual examination.[27] Because it is easily understood by the patient, the Sulcus Bleeding Index can be used to enhance his or her motivation for plaque control (see Chapter 44).

Another method to assess gingival inflammation is **evaluation of the gingival exudate** (see Chapter 7). The amounts of gingival exudate are directly correlated with gingival clinical indices but may not be correlated with histologic indices obtained from biop-

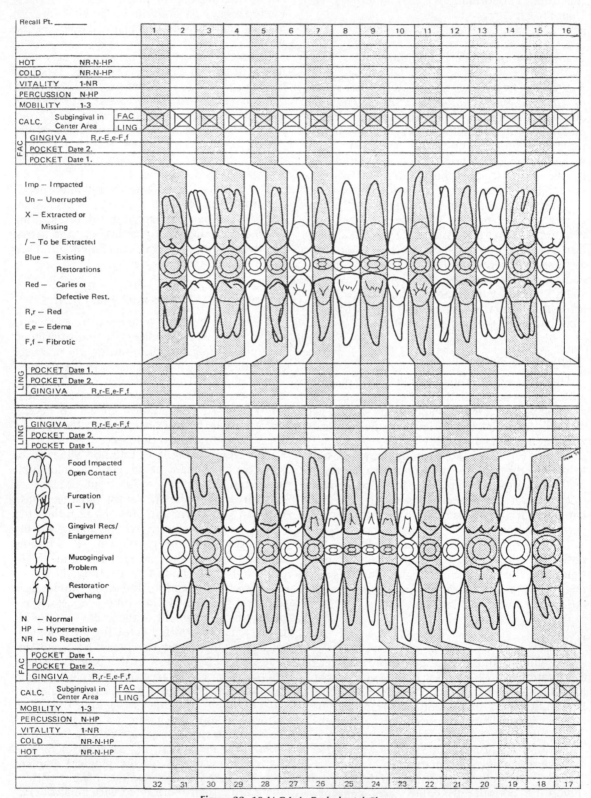

Figure 32–10 U.C.L.A. Periodontal Chart.

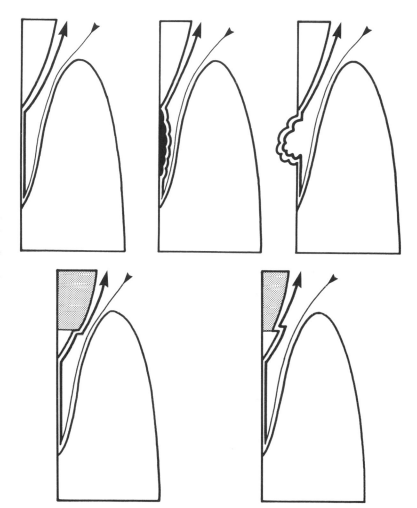

Figure 32–11 Detection of smoothness (*upper left*) or various irregularities on the root surface with outward motion of probe or explorer. *Upper center*, Calculus. *Upper right*, Carries. *Lower left and right*, Irregular margins of restorations.

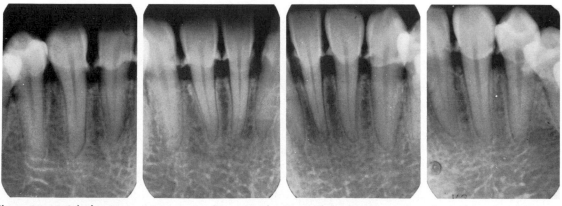

Figure 32–12 Calculus Appears Interproximally as Angular Spurs. The radiopaque image of calculus on the facial and lingual surface is superimposed on the teeth.

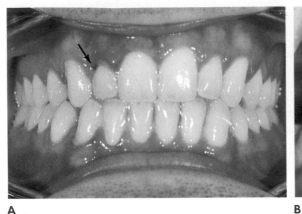

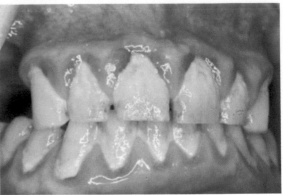

A

B

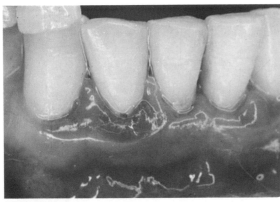

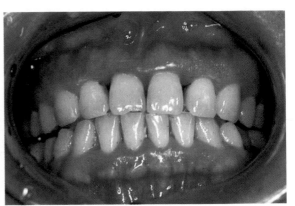

C

D

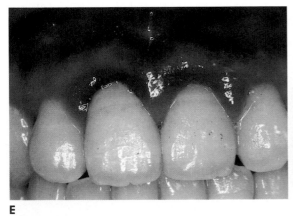

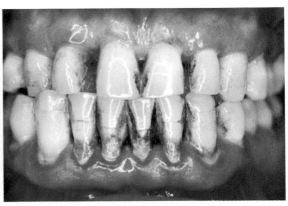

E

F

Plate VI

A, Incipient marginal gingivitis. Note slight puffiness and bleeding (*arrow*) around upper right lateral incisor.

B, Edematous type gingival inflammation. Note loss of stippling, increase in size, abundant plaque and materia alba, and change in color.

C, Close-up view of edematous type of gingival inflammation. Note the red, shiny, smooth gingiva.

D, Fibrotic type of gingival inflammation. Pockets of moderate depth are present, but the gingiva retains its stippling in some areas.

E, Severe generalized gingival inflammation and inflammatory gingival enlargement.

F, Fibrotic gingival inflammation. Note the abundant calculus and the gingival recession. The patient has pockets of moderate to severe depth in the mandibular anterior teeth and shallower pockets in the maxillary teeth.

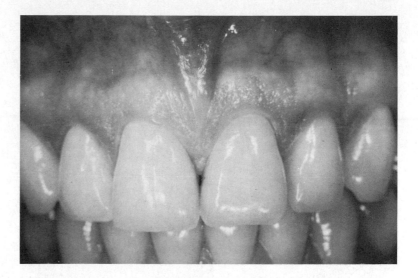

Figure 32–13 Normal Gingiva. Normal surface features are revealed by drying the gingiva.

sies.[12, 71, 77] This is because the histologic sections represent only a small part of the area from which the exudate derives. Different methods have been described for scoring gingival exudate. A brief description of them can be found in Chapter 7.

Periodontal Pockets

Examination for periodontal pockets should include consideration of the following: (1) presence and distribution on each tooth surface; (2) the type of pocket—whether it is suprabony or infrabony, and simple, compound, or complex; (3) pocket depth; and (4) level of the attachment on the root.

The only accurate method of detecting and evaluating periodontal pockets is careful exploration with a pocket probe. Pockets are not detected or measured by radiographic examination. The periodontal pocket is a soft tissue change. Radiographs indicate areas of bone loss where pockets may be suspected. They do not show whether pockets are present in these areas, nor do they reveal pocket depth or the location of the base of the pocket on the tooth surface.

Gutta percha points or calibrated silver points[33] can be used with the radiograph to assist in determining the level of the attachment of periodontal pockets and their relationship to the bone (Fig. 32–14). They may be used effectively for individual pockets, but their routine use throughout the mouth would be rather cumbersome. Clinical examination and probing are more direct and efficient.

POCKET PROBING. There are two different pocket depths: the biologic or histologic depth

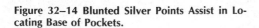

Figure 32–14 Blunted Silver Points Assist in Locating Base of Pockets.

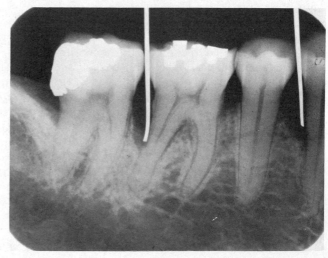

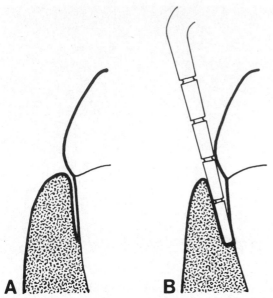

Figure 32–15 *A,* Biologic pocket depth. *B,* Probing or clinical pocket depth.

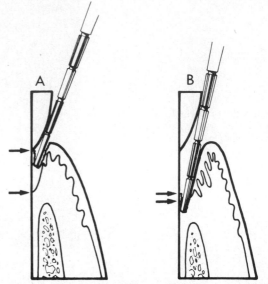

Figure 32–16 *A,* In a normal sulcus, with a long junctional epithelium (between arrows), probe penetrates about one third to one half the length of the junctional epithelium. *B,* In a periodontal pocket, with a short junctional epithelium (between arrows), the probe penetrates beyond the apical end of the junctional epithelium.

and the clinical or probing depth[38] (Fig. 32–15) (see Chapter 1).

The **biologic depth** is the distance between the gingival margin and the bottom of the pocket (the coronal end of the junctional epithelium). This can be measured only in carefully prepared histologic sections.

The **clinical** or **probing depth** is the distance to which an ad hoc instrument (probe) penetrates into the pocket. The depth of penetration of a probe in a pocket depends on factors such as the size of the probe, the force with which it is introduced, the direction of penetration, the resistance of the tissues, and the convexity of the crown.

Several studies have been made to determine the depth of penetration of a probe in a sulcus or pocket. Using "normal" probing forces, Sivertson and Burgett[81] and Listgarten et al.[40] showed that the probe tip penetrates to the coronal fibers of the connective tissue attachment. Armitage et al.[2] used beagle dogs to evaluate the penetration of a probe using a standardized force of 25 ponds.* They reported that in healthy specimens the probe penetrated the epithelium to about two thirds of its length, in gingivitis specimens it stopped 0.1 mm short of its apical end, and in periodontitis specimens the probe tip consistently went past the most apical cells of the junctional epithelium (Fig. 32–16).

---

*One pond is equal to 1 gram of absolute force.

The depth of penetration of the probe in the connective tissue apical to the junctional epithelium in a periodontal pocket is about 0.3 mm.[40, 72, 86] This is important in evaluating differences in probing depth before and after treatment, as the decreased penetrability of the tissues may play a significant role.[38, 42]

The probing forces have been explored by several investigators[19, 96]; forces of 0.75 N have been found to be well tolerated and accurate.[95] Interexaminer error (depth discrepancies between examiners) was reported to be as much as 2.1 mm, with an average of 1.5 mm in the same areas.[30]

Probing Technique. The probe should be inserted in line with the vertical axis of the tooth and "walked" circumferentially around each surface of each tooth to detect the areas of deepest probe penetration (Fig. 32–17). In addition, special attention should be directed to detecting the presence of interdental craters and furcation involvements. To detect an *interdental crater* the probe should be placed obliquely from both the facial and lingual surfaces so as to explore the deepest portion of the pocket located beneath the contact point (Fig. 32–18). In multirooted teeth the possibility of *furcation involvements* should be carefully explored. Sometimes in these cases probing with specially designed probes (Nabers probe) or with an explorer or curette may

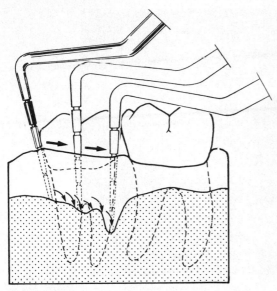

Figure 32–17 "Walking" the probe in order to explore the pocket in all its extent.

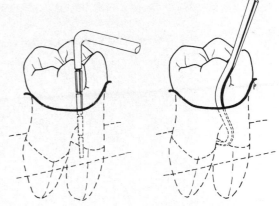

Figure 32–19 Exploring with a periodontal probe *(left)* may not detect furcation involvement; specially designed instruments (Nabers probe) *(right)* can enter the furcation area.

reveal lesions undetected with the probe (Fig. 32–19).

Level of Attachment Versus Pocket Depth. *The level of attachment of the base of the pocket on the tooth surface is of greater diagnostic significance than the depth of the pocket.* Pocket depth is simply the distance between the base of the pocket and the gingival margin. It may vary from time to time in untreated periodontal disease. For example, gingival bleeding caused by accidental mechanical irritation results in shrinkage of the pocket wall and some reduction in pocket depth. The level of attachment of the base of the pocket on the tooth surface affords a better indication of the severity of periodontal disease. **Shallow pockets attached at the level of the apical third of the roots connote more severe destruction than deep pockets attached in the coronal third of the roots** (see Chapter 14 and Figs. 14–26 and 14–27).

The level of attachment of the base of a periodontal pocket may vary on different surfaces of the same tooth and even in different areas of the same surface. Inserting the probe on all surfaces and in more than one area on individual surfaces reveals the depth and conformation of the pocket.

The level of attachment is determined in a gingival pocket by subtracting from the total depth the distance from the gingival margin to the cemento-enamel junction. When the gingival margin coincides with the cemento-enamel junction, the level of attachment and the pocket depth are equal; when the gingival margin is located apical to the cemento-enamel junction, the loss of attachment will be greater than the pocket depth. Drawing the gingival margin on the chart where pocket depths are entered will clarify this important point.

Suppuration

To determine whether pus is present in a periodontal pocket, the ball of the index finger is applied along the lateral aspect of the marginal gingiva and pressure is applied in a rolling motion toward the crown. Visual examination without digital pressure is not enough. Because the purulent exudate is formed on the inner pocket wall, the external appearance of the pocket may give no indication of its presence.

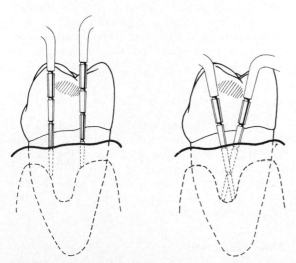

Figure 32–18 Vertical insertion of the probe *(left)* may not detect interdental craters; oblique positioning of the probe *(right)* reaches the depth of the crater.

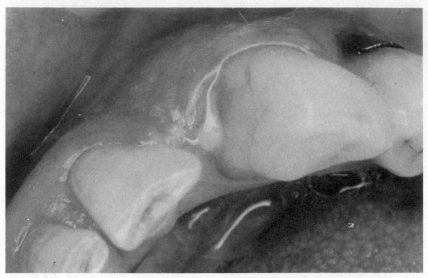

Figure 32–20 Pus Formation on the mesial surface of mandibular canine.

Pus formation does not occur in all periodontal pockets, but digital pressure often reveals it in pockets where it is not suspected (Fig. 32–20).

Amount of Attached Gingiva

It is important to establish the relation between the bottom of the pocket and the mucogingival line.

The width of the attached gingiva is the distance between the mucogingival junction and the projection on the external surface of the bottom of the gingival sulcus or the peri-

odontal pocket. It should not be confused with the width of the keratinized gingiva, since this includes the marginal gingiva (Fig. 32–21).

The width of the attached gingiva is determined by subtracting the sulcus or pocket depth from the total width of the gingiva (from the gingival margin to the mucogingival junction). This is done by stretching the lip or cheek in order to demarcate the mucogingival line while the pocket is probed (Fig. 32–22). It is generally considered that the amount of attached gingiva is insufficient when stretching the lip or cheek induces movement of the free gingival margin.

Other methods used to determine the amount of attached gingiva include pushing the adjacent mucosa coronally with a dull instrument and painting the mucosa with Schiller's potassium iodide solution, which stains keratin.

Palpation

Palpating the oral mucosa in the lateral and apical areas of the root is helpful in locating the origin of radiating pain which the patient cannot localize. Infection deep in the periodontal tissues and the early stages of periodontal abscess formation may also be detected by palpation.

Sinus Formation

In children a sinus orifice along the lateral aspect of a root is usually the result of periapical infection of a deciduous tooth. In the

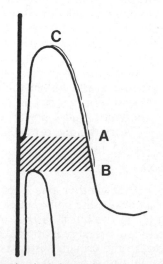

Figure 32–21 The shaded area shows the attached gingiva, which extends between the projection on the external surface of the bottom of the pocket (A) and the mucogingival junction (B). The keratinized gingiva may extend from the mucogingival junction (B) to the gingival margin (C).

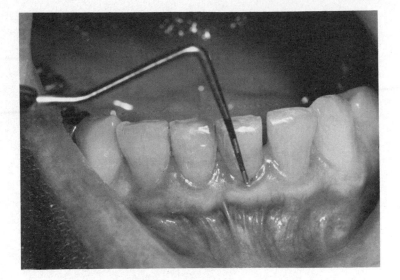

Figure 32–22 To determine the width of the attached gingiva, the pocket is probed at the same time that the lip (or cheek) is extended to demarcate the mucogingival line.

permanent dentition such an orifice may be caused by a periodontal abscess as well as by apical involvement. The orifice may be patent and draining or it may be closed and appear as a red, nodular mass (Fig. 32–23). Exploration of such masses with a probe usually reveals a pinpoint orifice that communicates with an underlying sinus.

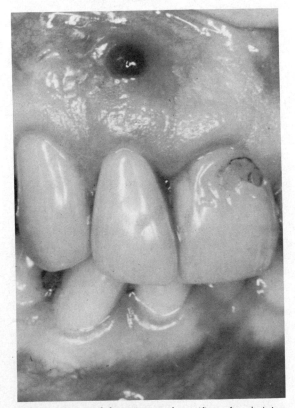

Figure 32–23 Nodular Mass at the orifice of a draining sinus.

Alveolar Bone Loss

Alveolar bone levels are evaluated by clinical and radiographic examination. Probing is helpful for determining the height and contour of the facial and lingual bone obscured on the radiograph by the dense roots and for determining the architecture of the interdental bone.

Transgingival probing, performed after the area is anesthetized, is a more accurate method of evaluation and provides additional information on bone architecture[26, 91] (see Chapter 54).

Trauma from Occlusion

Trauma from occlusion refers to *tissue injury* produced by occlusal forces—not to the occlusal forces themselves. The criterion that determines whether an occlusal force is injurious is whether it causes damage in the periodontal tissues; therefore, the diagnosis of trauma from occlusion is made from the condition of the periodontal tissues. The periodontal findings are then used as a guide for locating the responsible occlusal relationships.

Periodontal findings that suggest the presence of trauma from occlusion are the following: excessive tooth mobility, particularly in teeth showing radiographic evidence of a widened periodontal space (see Fig. 32–37); vertical or angular bone destruction (see Figs. 32–32 and 32–33); infrabony pockets; and pathologic migration, especially of the anterior teeth.

Additional findings which suggest the presence of abnormal occlusal relationships are neuromuscular disturbances such as impaired function of the masticatory musculature, which

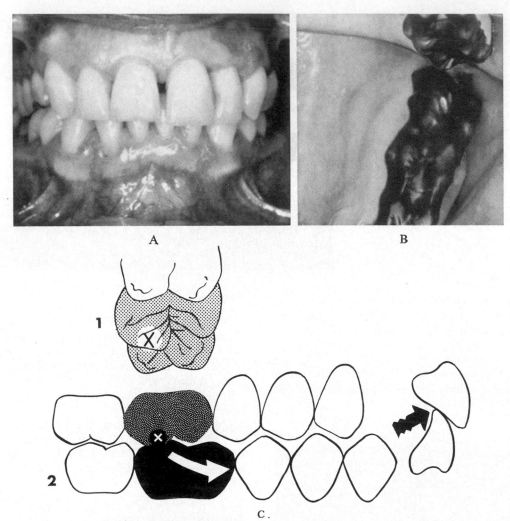

Figure 32–24 Pathologic Migration Associated with Trauma from Occlusion. *A,* Early pathologic migration of maxillary left central incisor. *B,* Mirror view of wax registration, showing prematurity on the mesiolingual incline of the maxillary molar, which deflects the mandible anteriorly and traumatizes the maxillary incisors. *C,* Diagrammatic representation showing (1) Prematurity (X) on the maxillary moiar and (2) anterior glide of the mandible (*arrow*) with impact against the maxillary incisors.

Illustration continued on the following page

in severe cases results in muscle spasm and temporomandibular joint disorders.

Special mention should be made of **pathologic migration of the anterior teeth** as a sign of trauma from occlusion. Premature tooth contacts in the posterior region that deflect the mandible anteriorly contribute to destruction of the periodontium of the maxillary anterior teeth and to pathologic migration (Figs. 32–24 and 32–25).

Determination of Activity or Inactivity of a Lesion

The determination of the depth of the pocket or the level of connective tissue attach-ment does not provide information on the presence of an active or inactive lesion. Al-though there is no sure method, at present, to determine activity or inactivity, the following indicators may be useful: bleeding, gingival fluid measurements, and microbial analysis of plaque.

An **inactive lesion** may show little or no bleeding upon probing and minimal amounts of fluid; the bacterial flora, as revealed by darkfield microscopy, consists mostly of coc-coid cells. **Active lesions** bleed more readily upon probing and have large amounts of fluid and exudate; their bacterial flora shows a greater number of spirochetes and motile bac-teria.[39]

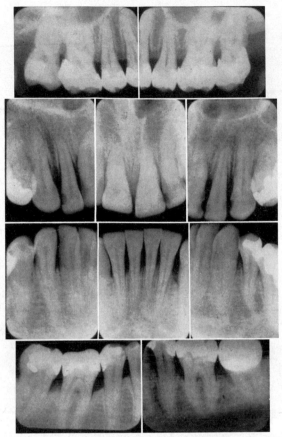

Figure 32–24 *Continued. D,* Radiographs of patient shown in *A.* Note the extensive bone destruction around the maxillary second molars and maxillary and mandibular incisors.

Other methods suggested for assessing the degree of gingival inflammation and activity of the lesions include the following: Hemastix strips which record the presence of hemoglobin derived from erythrocytes and myeloperoxidase derived from polymorphonuclear leukocytes,[89] colorimetric analysis of the protein content of gingival fluid,[12, 78] collagenolytic activity of crevicular fluid,[24] and temperature variations.[52, 53]

The precise determination of disease activity will have a direct influence on diagnosis, prognosis, and therapy. The goals of therapy may change, depending on the state of the periodontal lesion. None of the methods suggested heretofore, however, offers adequate, reliable information that can be used in the clinic.[29]

THE RADIOGRAPH IN THE DIAGNOSIS OF PERIODONTAL DISEASE

The radiograph is a valuable aid in the diagnosis of periodontal disease, the determination of the prognosis, and the evaluation of the outcome of treatment. *It is an adjunct to the clinical examination, not a substitute for it.* If a choice must be made, a more intelligent diagnosis can be made from the patient without the radiographs than from radiographs without the patient.

The radiographic image results from the superimposition of tooth, bone, and soft tissues in the pathway between the cone of the machine and the film. The radiograph reveals alterations in calcified tissue; it does not reveal current cellular activity, but shows the effects of past cellular experience upon the bone and roots. Showing changes in the soft tissues of the periodontium requires special techniques which are not yet in routine clinical usage.

Normal Interdental Septa

Because the facial and lingual bony plates are obscured by the relatively dense root structure, radiographic evaluation of bone changes in periodontal disease is based mainly upon the appearance of the interdental septa. The

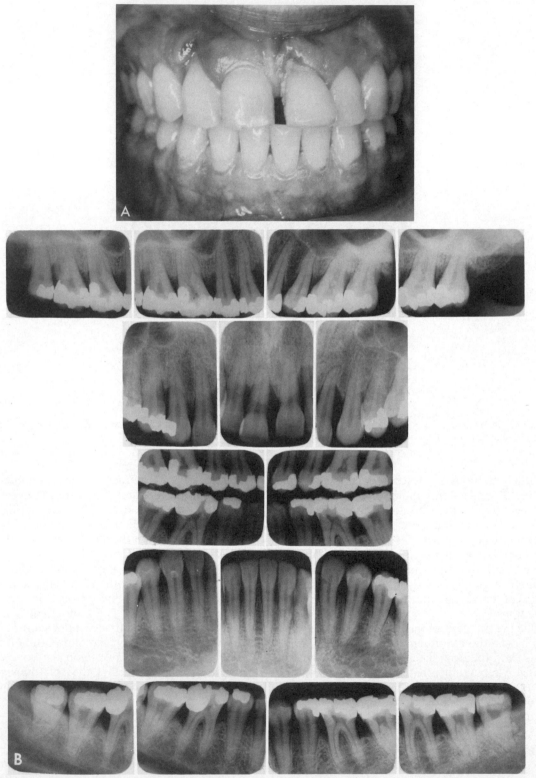

Figure 32–25 Periodontal Disease with Pathologic Migration of the Anterior Teeth. *A,* Periodontal inflammation and tissue loss and pathologic migration in the anterior maxilla. *B,* Radiograph showing generalized bone loss and the angular pattern of bone destruction in the anterior maxilla.

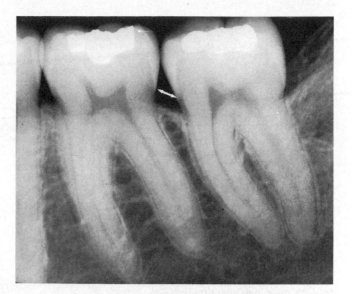

Figure 32–26 Crest of Interdental Septum Normally Parallel to a Line Drawn Between the Cemento-Enamel Junction of Adjacent Teeth *(arrow)*. Note also the radiopaque lamina dura around the roots and interdental septum.

interdental septum normally presents a thin radiopaque border, adjacent to the periodontal ligament and at the crest, referred to as the **lamina dura** (Fig. 32–26). This appears radiographically as a continuous white line, but it is perforated by numerous small foramina, containing blood vessels, lymphatics, and nerves, which pass between the periodontal ligament and the bone. **Since the lamina dura represents the bone surface lining the tooth socket, the shape and position of the root and changes in the angulation of the x-ray beam produce considerable variations in its appearance.**[47]

The width and shape of the interdental septum and the angle of the crest normally vary according to the convexity of the proximal tooth surfaces and the level of the cemento-enamel junction of the approximating teeth.[67] The interdental space and the interdental septum between teeth with prominently convex proximal surfaces are wider anteroposteriorly than are those between teeth with relatively flat proximal surfaces. The faciolingual diameter of the bone is related to the width of the proximal root surface. **The angulation of the crest of the interdental septum is generally parallel to a line between the cemento-enamel junctions of the approximating teeth** (Fig. 32–26). When there is a difference in the levels of the cemento-enamel junctions, the crest of the interdental bone is angulated rather than horizontal.

Distortion Produced by Variations in Radiographic Technique

Variations in x-ray technique produce artefacts which limit the diagnostic value of the radiograph. *The bone level, the pattern of bone destruction, the width of the periodontal ligament space,*[94] *and the radiodensity, trabecular pattern, and marginal contour of the interdental septum are modified by altering the exposure and development time, the type of film, and the x-ray angulation.*[60] Standardized, reproducible techniques are required to obtain reliable radiographs for pre- and posttreatment comparisons.[61, 64, 70] A grid calibrated in millimeters, superimposed upon the finished film, is helpful for comparing bone levels in radiographs taken under similar conditions[15] (Fig. 32–27).

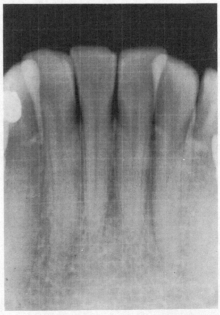

Figure 32–27 Radiograph with Superimposed Grid Calibrated in Millimeters.

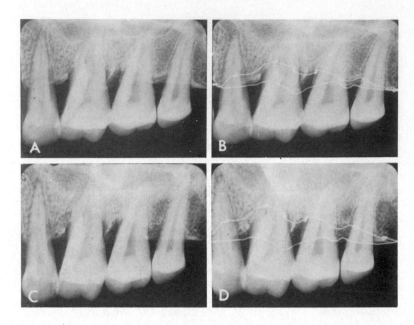

Figure 32–28 Long Cone Paralleling Technique and Bisection of the Angle Technique Compared. (Courtesy of Dr. Benjamin Patur.) *A,* Long cone technique. Radiograph of dried specimen. *B,* Long cone technique. Same specimen. The smooth wire is on the margin of the facial plate and the knotted wire is on the lingual plate to show their relative positions. *C,* Bisection of the angle technique. Same specimen. *D,* Bisection of the angle technique. Same specimen. Both bone margins are shifted toward the crown, the facial margin (smooth wire) more than the lingual margin (knotted wire), creating the illusion that the lingual bone margin has shifted apically.

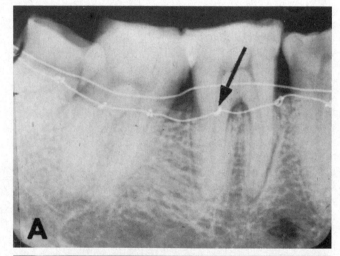

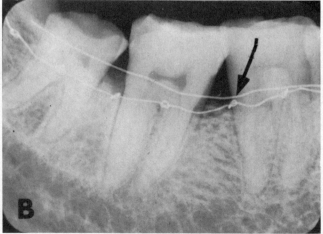

Figure 32–29 Distortion by Oblique Projection. *A,* **Long Cone Technique.** The smooth wire is on the facial bony plate, the knotted wire on the lingual. Note the knot *(arrow)* near the center of the distal root of the first molar, which shows bifurcation involvement. *B,* **Long Cone Technique. Cone is Placed Distally, Projecting the Rays Mesially and Obliquely.** The oblique projection shifts the image of all structures mesially. *The structures closest to the cone shift the most.* This creates the illusion that the knot *(arrow)* has moved distally. Note that the bifurcation involvement shown in *A* is obliterated in *B.*

The following are useful facts regarding the effects of angulation:

The long cone paralleling technique projects the most realistic image of the level of the alveolar bone[18] (Fig. 32–28). The bisection of the angle technique increases the projection and makes the bone margin appear closer to the crown; the level of the facial bone margin is distorted more than that of the lingual margin (Fig. 32–28). Shifting the cone mesially or distally without changing the horizontal plane projects the x-rays obliquely and changes the shape of the interdental bone, the width of the periodontal ligament space, and the appearance of the lamina dura and may distort the extent of furcation involvement (Fig. 32–29).

XERORADIOGRAPHY. This is a process by which x-ray images are recorded by means of a xerographic copying method. It does not involve wet chemical processing or the use of a darkroom. Instead of x-ray film, xeroradiography uses a uniformly charged selenium plate held in a light-tight cassette. Exposure to x-irradiation and adequate processing produce a real image on opaque paper which is viewed by reflected light rather than by transillumination.[97] Xeroradiography requires one third of the radiation of conventional radiography and, for periodontics, offers the advantage of an "edge-enhancement" effect that may permit better visualization of crestal height (Fig. 32–30). This technique is extensively used in the diagnosis of breast disease but is still in the initial stages of development for dental use.[25]

Bone Destruction in Periodontal Disease

Because the radiograph does not reveal minor destructive changes in bone,[6, 7, 65] periodontal disease that produces even slight radiographic changes has progressed beyond its earliest stages. The earliest signs of periodontal disease must therefore be detected clinically. The radiographic image tends to show less severe bone loss than that actually present.[90] The difference between the alveolar crest height and the radiographic appearance ranges from 0 to 1.6 mm,[66] mostly accounted for by x-ray angulation.

The Amount of Bone Loss

The radiograph is an indirect method for determining the amount of bone loss in periodontal disease. It indicates the amount of remaining bone rather than the amount lost. The amount of bone lost is estimated to be the

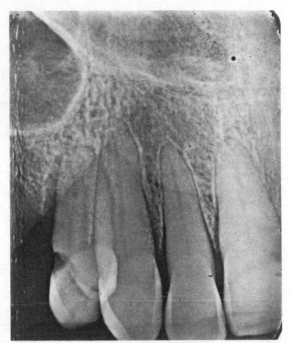

Figure 32–30 Xeroradiograph. (Courtesy of Dr. Barton Gratt.)

difference between the physiologic bone level of the patient and the height of the remaining bone.

The Distribution of Bone Loss

The distribution of bone loss is an important diagnostic sign. It points to the location of destructive local factors in different areas of the mouth and in relation to different surfaces of the same tooth.

The Pattern of Bone Destruction

In periodontal disease, the interdental septa undergo changes that affect the lamina dura, the crestal radiodensity, the size and shape of the medullary spaces, and the height and contour of the bone. The interdental septa may be reduced in height, with the crest horizontal and perpendicular to the long axis of the adjacent teeth (Fig. 32–31), *or they may present angular or arcuate defects* (Fig. 32–32). The former condition is called **horizontal bone loss,** the latter **angular or vertical bone loss** (see Chapter 16).

Radiographs do not indicate the internal morphology or depth of the crater-like interdental defects which appear as angular or vertical defects, nor do they reveal the extent of involvement on the facial and lingual surfaces. There

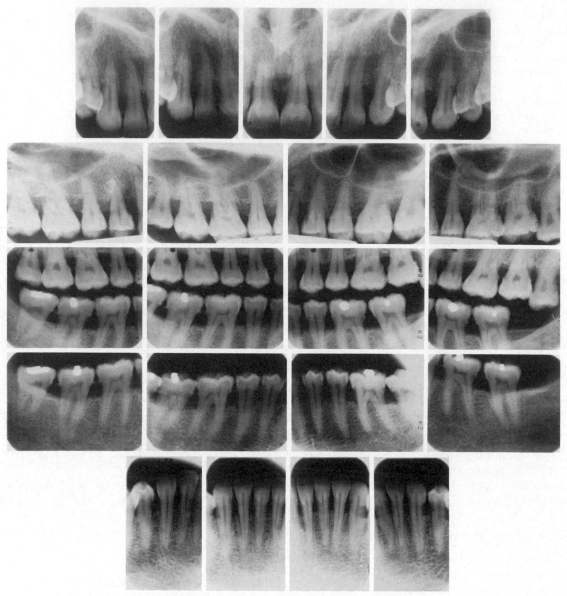

Figure 32–31 Generalized horizontal bone loss.

are several reasons for this. Facial and lingual surface bone destruction is obscured by the dense root structure, and bone destruction on the mesial and distal root surfaces may be partially hidden by a dense mylohyoid ridge (Fig. 32–33).

Dense cortical plates on the facial and lingual surfaces of the interdental septa obscure destruction which occurs in the intervening cancellous bone. This means that it is possible to have a deep crater in the bone between the facial and lingual plates without radiographic indications of its presence. In order for destruction of the interproximal cancellous bone to be recorded radiographically, the cortical bone must be involved. A reduction of only 0.5 or 1.0 mm in the thickness of the cortical plate is sufficient to permit radiographic visualization of destruction of the inner cancellous trabeculae.[62]

Passing a probe through the gingiva to the bone helps determine the architecture of osseous defects produced by periodontal disease. It also aids in the location of dehiscences and fenestrations. Gutta percha packed around the teeth increases the usefulness of the radiograph for detecting the morphology of osseous craters and involvement of the facial and lingual surfaces (Fig. 32–34). However, surgical exposure and visual examination provide the

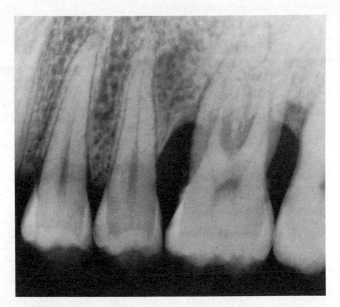

Figure 32–32 Angular Bone Loss on First Molar with Involvement of the Trifurcation.

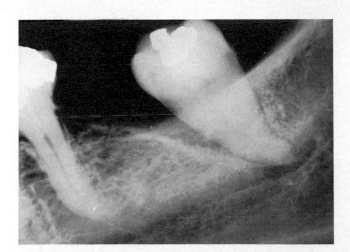

Figure 32–33 Angular Bone Loss on Mandibular Molar Partially Obscured by Dense Mylohyoid Ridge.

Figure 32–34 Gutta Percha Aids in Detecting Bone Defects. *A,* Gutta percha packed around teeth shows interproximal and facial and lingual bone loss. *B,* Same area without gutta percha gives little indication of the extent of bone involvement.

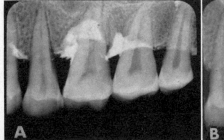
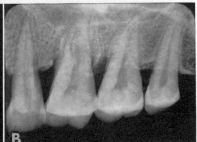

most definitive information regarding the bone architecture produced by periodontal destruction.[63]

Radiographic Changes in Periodontitis

The following is the sequence of radiographic changes in periodontitis and the tissue changes which produce them:

Fuzziness and a break in the continuity of the lamina dura at the mesial or distal aspect of the crest of the interdental septum have been described as the earliest radiographic changes in periodontitis (Fig. 32–35).

These result from the extension of inflammation from the gingiva into the bone and associated widening of the vessel channels and a reduction in calcified tissue at the septal margin.

No correlation has been found, however, between crestal lamina dura in radiographs and the presence or absence of clinical inflammation, bleeding upon probing, periodontal pockets, or loss of attachment.[28]

A wedge-shaped radiolucent area is formed at the mesial or distal aspect of the crest of the septal bone (Fig. 32–35B). The apex of the area is pointed in the direction of the root.

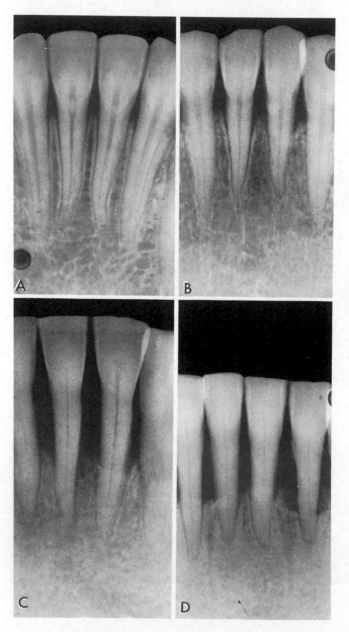

Figure 32–35 Radiographic Changes in Periodontitis. *A,* Normal appearance of interdental septa. *B,* Fuzziness and a break in the continuity of the lamina dura at the crest of the bone distal to the central incisor *(left).* There are wedge-shaped radiolucent areas at the crests of the other interdental septa. *C,* Radiolucent projections from the crest into the interdental septum indicate extension of destructive processes. *D,* Severe bone loss.

This is produced by resorption of the bone of the lateral aspect of the interdental septum, with an associated widening of the periodontal space.

The destructive process extends across the crest of the interdental septum and the height is reduced. Finger-like radiolucent projections extend from the crest into the septum (Fig. 32–35*C*)

The radiolucent projections into the interdental septum are the result of the deeper extension of the inflammation into the bone. Inflammatory cells and fluid, proliferation of connective tissue cells, and increased osteoclasis cause increased bone resorption along the endosteal margins of the medullary spaces. The radiopaque projections, separating the radiolucent spaces, are the composite images of the partially eroded bony trabeculae.

The height of the interdental septum (Fig. 32–35*D*) is progressively reduced by the extension of inflammation and the resorption of bone.

When inflammation is the sole destructive factor in periodontal disease, the crest of the interdental septum is usually horizontal; when the crest appears angular, the possible existence of trauma from occlusion should be explored.

Radiographic Changes in Juvenile Periodontitis

Juvenile periodontitis is characterized by a combination of the following radiographic features:

Loss of alveolar bone is localized in the early stages to a single tooth or group of teeth and tends to become generalized as the disease progresses. The bone loss occurs initially in the maxillary and mandibular incisor and first molar areas, usually bilaterally (Fig. 32–36). The interdental septa present vertical, arc-like, or angular destructive patterns. When the bone loss is generalized, it is least pronounced in the mandibular premolar areas.

A generalized alteration in the trabecular pattern of the alveolar bone consists of less clearly defined trabecular markings and an increase in the size of the cancellous spaces.

Radiographic Changes in Trauma from Occlusion

Trauma from occlusion can produce radiographically detectable changes in the lamina dura, in the morphology of the alveolar crest, in the width of the periodontal space, and in the density of the surrounding cancellous bone.

Traumatic lesions manifest themselves more

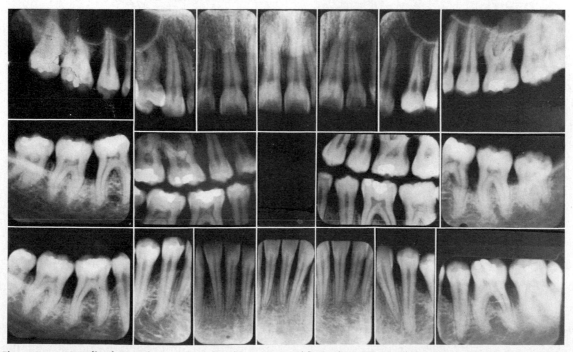

Figure 32–36 Localized Juvenile Periodontitis. The accentuated bone destruction in the anterior and first molar areas is considered characteristic of this disease, formerly called "periodontosis."

clearly in faciolingual aspects, since mesiodistally the tooth has the added stability provided by the contact areas with adjacent teeth. Therefore, slight variations in the proximal surfaces may indicate greater changes in the facial and lingual aspects. The radiographic changes listed below are not pathognomonic of trauma from occlusion and have to be interpreted in combination with clinical findings, particularly tooth mobility, presence of wear facets, pocket depth, and analysis of occlusal contacts and habits.

The *injury phase of trauma from occlusion* produces a loss of the lamina dura that may be noted in apices, furcations, and/or marginal areas. This loss of lamina dura will result in widening of the periodontal ligament space (Fig. 32–37). This change, particularly when incipient or very circumscribed, may easily be confused with technical variations due to angulation of the radiograph or malposition of

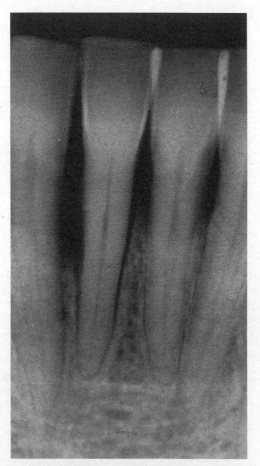

Figure 32–37 Widened Periodontal Space Caused by Trauma from Occlusion. Note the increased density of the surrounding bone caused by new bone formation in response to increased occlusal forces.

the tooth; it can be diagnosed with certainty only in radiographs of the highest quality.

The *repair phase of trauma from occlusion* will result in an attempt to strengthen the periodontal structures in order to better support the increased loads. Radiographically this is manifested by a widening of the periodontal ligament space, which may be generalized or localized.

Although microscopic measurements have determined that there are normal variations in the width of the periodontal space in the different regions of the root, these are not generally detected in radiographs. When variations in width between the marginal area and the midroot or between the midroot and the apex are detected, it means that the tooth is being subjected to increased forces.

Successful attempts to reinforce the periodontal structures by widening of the periodontal space will be accompanied by increased width of the lamina dura and sometimes by condensation of the perialveolar cancellous bone.

More advanced traumatic lesions may result in deep angular bone loss which, when combined with marginal inflammation, may lead to infrabony pocket formation. The very deep combined lesions will extend around the root apex, producing a wide radiolucent periapical image (cavernous lesions).

Root resorption may also occur as a result of excessive forces on the periodontium, particularly those caused by orthodontic appliances. Although trauma from occlusion produces many resorption areas, they are usually of a magnitude insufficient to be detected radiographically.

Additional Radiographic Criteria in the Diagnosis of Periodontal Disease

Radiopaque horizontal line across the roots. This line demarcates the portion of the root where the labial and/or lingual bony plate has been partially or completely destroyed from the remaining bone-supported portion (Fig. 32–38).

Vessel canals in the alveolar bone. Hirschfeld[32] described linear and circular radiolucent areas produced by interdental canals and their foramina, respectively (Fig. 32–39). These canals indicate the course of the vascular supply of the bone and are normal radiographic findings. The radiographic image of the canals is frequently so prominent, particularly in the anterior region of the mandible, that they

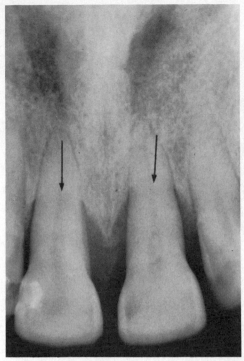

Figure 32–38 Horizontal Line across the roots of the central incisors *(arrows)*. The area of the roots below the horizontal lines is partially or completely denuded of the facial and/or lingual bony plates.

might be confused with radiolucence resulting from periodontal disease.

Differentiation between periodontal atrophy and chronic periodontal disease. In older persons it is sometimes necessary to determine whether the bone level is the result of periodontal atrophy or if destructive periodontal disease is a contributing factor. Clinical examination is the basic determinant. However, radiographically detectable alterations in the normal clear-cut peripheral outline of the septa are corroborating evidence of periodontal disease.

SKELETAL DISTURBANCES MANIFESTED IN THE JAWS

Skeletal disturbances may produce changes in the jaws that affect the interpretation of radiographs from the periodontal viewpoint. Included among the diseases in which destruction of tooth-supporting bone may occur are the following:

Osteitis fibrosa cystica (Recklinghausen's disease of bone) causes a diffuse granular mottling, scattered "cyst-like" radiolucent areas

throughout the jaws, and a generalized disappearance of the lamina dura.[69, 80]

In *Paget's disease*, the radiographic appearance of the jaws varies. The normal trabecular pattern may be replaced by a hazy, diffuse meshwork of closely knit, fine trabecular markings, with the lamina dura absent (Fig. 32–40), or there may be scattered radiolucent areas containing irregularly shaped radiopaque zones.[23]

Fibrous dysplasia may appear as a small radiolucent area at a root apex or as an extensive radiolucent area with irregularly arranged trabecular markings.[22] There may be enlargement of the cancellous spaces, with distortion of the normal trabecular pattern and obliteration of the lamina dura (Fig. 32–41).

In *Hand-Schüller-Christian disease*, the radiographic appearance is of single or multiple areas of radiolucency. Mobility of the teeth results from loss of bony support. *Letterer-Siwe disease and Gaucher's disease* may present comparable changes (Fig. 32–42).

Eosinophilic granuloma[73, 82] appears as single or multiple radiolucent areas, which may be unrelated to the teeth or entail destruction of the tooth-supporting bone.

Numerous radiolucent areas occur when the jaws are involved by *multiple myeloma*.

In *osteopetrosis* (marble-bone disease, Albers-Schönberg disease),[16] the outlines of the roots may be obscured by diffuse radiopacity

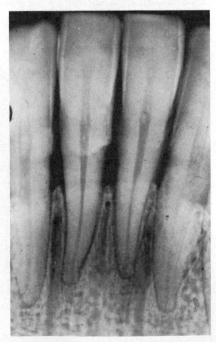

Figure 32–39 Prominent Vessel Canals in the Mandible.

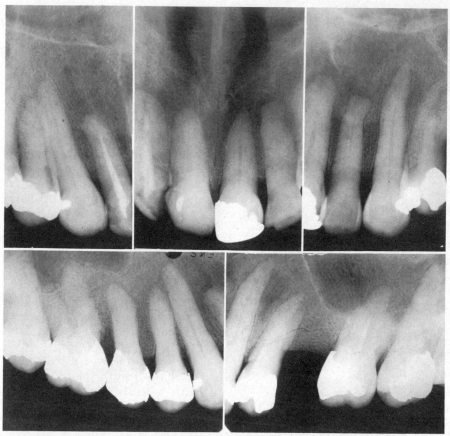

Figure 32–40 Altered Trabecular Pattern and Diminution in the Prominence of the Lamina Dura in Paget's Disease.

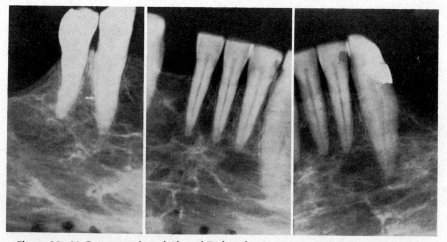

Figure 32–41 Osteoporosis and Altered Trabecular Arrangement in Fibrous Dysplasia.

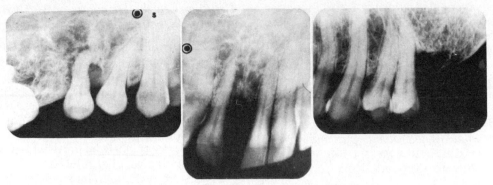

Figure 32–42 Osteoporosis in Gaucher's Disease.

of the jaws. In less severe cases, the increased density is confined to the bone in relation to the nutrient canals and the lamina dura.

In *scleroderma* (see Chapter 12), the periodontal ligament is uniformly widened at the expense of the surrounding alveolar bone (Fig. 32–43).

LABORATORY AIDS IN DIAGNOSIS

Biopsy

The Biopsy in the Diagnosis of Neoplasms

The diagnosis of neoplasms should be established by microscopic examination. If it is to serve the purpose for which it is intended, certain principles should govern the biopsy technique.

SITE OF THE BIOPSY. The guidelines for selecting the site of the biopsy are as follows:

1. Where the lesion is small, it should be totally excised. The excision should be wide enough and deep enough to include a border of healthy tissue along the entire cut surface.
2. Where the size of the lesion is such that complete excision is not possible or feasible, *obtain a specimen representative of the lesion*:
   a. *Select that portion of the lesion which demonstrates all of the pathologic*

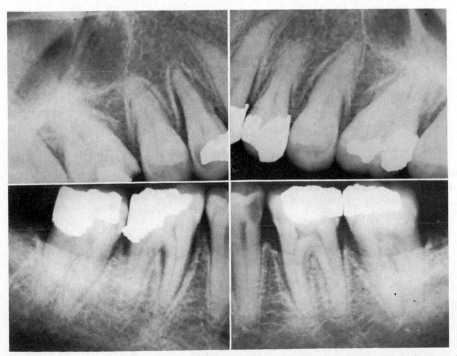

Figure 32–43 Scleroderma, showing typical uniform widening of the periodontal ligament and thickening of the lamina dura. (Courtesy of Drs. David F. Mitchell and Anand P. Chaudhry.)

*changes noted clinically.*If this is not possible with one biopsy specimen, select several areas.

b. *Take thin, deep sections rather than broad, shallow sections.* A small, superficial tab of tissue may show nothing more than degenerative, inflammatory, or necrotic changes.

c. *The section should include tissue at and beyond the lateral margins and base of the lesion.* In this way the transition from healthy to diseased tissue can be followed.

TECHNIQUES FOR OBTAINING THE TISSUE SPECIMEN. There are several biopsy techniques.

Incision. Incision can be performed with a scalpel or with a high-frequency cutting current. Removal of the tissue with a sharp blade appears to be the method of choice. Electrosurgery may be used to advantage in highly vascular tumors in which bleeding may be a difficult complication.

Punch Biopsy. This method is of limited value in the oral cavity. Its greatest applicability is in the removal of small tissue specimens from inaccessible areas, such as the maxillary sinus and the lateral or posterior pharyngeal walls.

Curettage. Tissue specimens are curetted from bony cavities and sinus tracts.

HANDLING OF THE TISSUE SPECIMEN.

1. The tissue should not be crushed or mutilated.

2. It should be placed in fixative immediately. Ten per cent formalin is an acceptable fixative. The volume of the fixative should be approximately 20 times the volume of the tissue specimen. If the pathologist to whom you submit biopsy specimens prefers another fixative, it would be wise to keep on hand several small bottles containing this fixative.

If the specimen is too thick, only the peripheral portions of the tissue will be completely infiltrated and fixed, and the central area will undergo degenerative changes.

3. The specimen bottle should be properly labeled. Indicate whether the tissue specimen is soft tissue only or contains bone and the time at which it was taken.

4. A brief history should accompany the specimen. This should include the name, age, and sex of the patient; a gross description of the lesion—its duration, location, and rate of growth or change in growth rate; and the method used to obtain the specimen.

The Biopsy in the Diagnosis of Gingival and Mucosal Disease

The gingival biopsy may be important in the diagnosis of some gingival disturbances. Microscopic study of gingival biopsy specimens is sometimes the only method of detecting local and systemic interrelationships that cannot be discerned by clinical examination. For example, amyloid is present in the gingiva of patients with amyloidosis, many of whom present no clinical gingival changes.

Tissues from the marginal and attached gingivae should be included in the biopsy specimen (Fig. 32–44). Inflammatory changes in the gingival margin tend to obscure any alterations that may be produced by a systemic disturbance. Inclusion of the attached gingiva, in which the effect of local irritants is less likely to be present, offers an opportunity to investigate tissue changes that may be produced by systemic disturbances.

In addition to differentiating between different types of gingival enlargement, gingival biopsy is indispensable when the presence of disease such as desquamative gingivitis, benign mucous membrane pemphigoid, pemphigus, or lichen planus is suspected.

Exfoliative Cytology

Exfoliative cytology is a diagnostic procedure consisting of the microscopic examination of cells obtained by scraping the surface of the suspected area or by rinsing the oral cavity. The former is preferred. Its reliability for the diagnosis of cancer is 86 per cent, as compared with the close to 100 per cent reliability of an

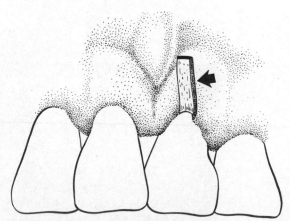

Figure 32–44 Rectangular Gingival Biopsy (*arrow*) **Includes Marginal and Attached Gingiva.**

oral biopsy.[79] Exfoliative cytology is not a substitute for biopsy, but it is valuable if a biopsy cannot be done for some reason and also in screening large groups of people for the presence of malignancy, provided it is used in conjunction with a careful oral examination. It is also helpful in the diagnosis of bullous and vesicular oral lesions.

To obtain a specimen, the entire surface of the abnormal mucosa is firmly scraped with the edge of a wooden tongue depressor. The material thus removed is spread directly on a glass slide, immediately fixed in 95 per cent alcohol, and submitted for microscopic diagnosis.[74]

OTHER AIDS USED IN THE DIAGNOSIS OF ORAL MANIFESTATIONS OF SYSTEMIC DISEASE

When unusual gingival or periodontal problems are present and cannot be explained by local causes, the possibility of contributing systemic factors must be explored. The dentist must understand the oral manifestations of systemic disease so that he or she can advise the physician regarding the type of systemic disturbance which may be involved in individual cases.

Numerous laboratory tests aid in the diagnosis of systemic diseases. Descriptions of the manner in which they are performed and the interpretation of findings are found in standard texts on the subject.[92] Those pertinent to the diagnosis of disturbances often manifested in the oral cavity are referred to briefly here.

Nutritional Status

If, when examining a patient, it is the dentist's impression that a nutritional deficiency exists, this suspicion must be corroborated by a medical evaluation of the patient's nutritional status. Nutritional therapy in the treatment of periodontal disturbances must be based on a demonstrated need, which is best determined by a nutritionist.

Nutrition refers to the complex relationship between the individual's total health status and the intake, digestion, and utilization of nutrients. *Nutritional deficiency connotes an inadequacy in the nutritional status of the tissue.* Malnutrition or poor nutrition may result from excessive food intake and improper nutrient

balance, as well as from an insufficiency of nutrients.

Nutritional deficiencies may be (1) *primary*, resulting from an overt insufficiency of nutrients; or (2) *secondary (conditioned)*, resulting from bodily conditions which interfere with the ingestion, transport, cellular uptake, or utilization of essential nutrients in the presence of adequate food intake. Nutritional deficiencies usually develop in stages as follows: (1) *depletion of the tissue nutrient reserve*, (2) *biochemical tissue lesions*, (3) *morphologic and functional abnormalities which are expressed as* (4) *clinical signs and symptoms,* and finally (5) *tissue death.*

Diagnosis of Nutritional Deficiency

A nutritional diagnosis is based upon four sequential routes of inquiry: (1) a medical and social history and a dietary history; (2) clinical examination; (3) laboratory tests; and (4) therapeutic trial.

MEDICAL AND SOCIAL HISTORY. Common complaints of patients with nutritional disorders include general weakness, chronic fatigue, failure of appetite, painful bleeding gums, sore lips, sore tongue and mouth, diarrhea, chronic nervousness, irritability, inability to concentrate, confusion, memory loss, dizziness, lethargy, photophobia, loss of manual dexterity, numbness, pain in the legs, and skin rashes.

Attention should be given to conditions which could lead to secondary nutritional deficiencies such as gastrointestinal disturbances which impair the digestion and absorption of nutrients, interferences with the utilization of foods, increased excretion of nutrients, factors which increase the nutritional requirements, and factors which interfere with the ingestion of food.

DIETARY HISTORY. The dietary history should provide information regarding the patient's usual dietary practices and should include questions regarding the following: (1) **length of time the present diet has been followed;** (2) **history of any special diet, its type and duration;** (3) **use of vitamins or other food supplements;** (4) **regularity of meals;** (5) **food likes, dislikes, and idiosyncrasies;** (6) **living conditions;** and (7) **economic status and education.**

After the desired information is obtained, the patient is given a "food diary," in which to record his or her daily food intake for at least 5 consecutive days which include a weekend.

EVALUATION OF THE DIET.[54] The adequacy of the diet is evaluated by transposing the information in the dietary history into the basic four food groups: (1) *milk,* (2) *meat,* (3) *vegetable and fruit,* and (4) *bread and cereal.* The *milk group* (milk, cheese) provides protein, calcium, riboflavin, vitamin A, and other nutrients; the *meat group* (meat, fish, poultry, eggs, dried beans, and peas) provides primarily protein, B complex vitamins, and iron; the *vegetable and fruit group* provide most of the vitamins A and C, as well as other minerals and vitamins; and the *bread and cereal group* furnishes B complex vitamins, iron, protein, and carbohydrate. Foods which provide only calories, such as sugar and sugar products, should be kept to a minimum. The same is true for fats, because they are usually contained in the milk and meat groups.

A person who consumes less food than the amounts recommended is not necessarily nutritionally deficient. The recommendations represent amounts considered desirable for maintaining good nutrition in healthy persons without bodily conditioning factors which interfere with food utilization. They represent goals to be strived for rather than requirements.

CLINICAL EXAMINATION. Certain signs and symptoms have been identified with different nutritional deficiencies.[75] However, many patients with nutritional disease do not exhibit classic signs of deficiency disorders, and different types of deficiency produce comparable clinical findings. Clinical findings are suggestive, but definitive diagnosis of nutritional deficiencies and their nature requires the combined information revealed by the history, clinical and laboratory findings, and therapeutic trial. *Clinical findings* identified with specific nutritional deficiencies and the *oral manifestations of nutritional disorders* are described in Chapter 28.

LABORATORY TESTS FOR NUTRITIONAL DEFICIENCY. Blood, serum, and urine tests reflect nutrient intake levels and absorption defects. The reader is referred to standard books on clinical nutrition for information on the different tests and their significance.

PATIENTS ON SPECIAL DIETS FOR MEDICAL REASONS. Patients on low-residue, nondetergent diets often develop gingivitis because the prescribed foods lack cleansing action and the tendency for plaque and food debris to accumulate on the teeth is increased. Because fibrous foods are contraindicated, special effort is made to compensate for the soft diet by emphasizing the patient's oral hygiene procedures. Patients on salt-free diets should not be given saline mouthwashes, nor should they be treated with saline preparations without consulting the patient's physician. Diabetes, gallbladder disease, and hypertension are examples of conditions in which particular care should be taken to avoid the prescription of contraindicated foodstuffs.

The Hemogram

Analyses of blood smears, red and white blood cell counts, white blood cell differential counts, and erythrocyte sedimentation rates are used to evaluate the presence of blood dyscrasias and of generalized infections. They may be useful aids in the differential diagnosis of certain types of periodontal diseases; the reader is referred to books on hematology,[98] which consider this point more fully.

Laboratory Tests for Determining the Etiology of Spontaneous or Excessive Bleeding

In infrequent instances one or more of the following tests may be required: coagulation time, bleeding time, clot retraction time, prothrombin time, capillary fragility test, and bone marrow studies. Discussions of their indications and the interpretation of their results can be found in books on clinical and laboratory diagnosis.

REFERENCES

1. Alexander, A. G., and Tipnis, A. K.: The effect of irregularity of teeth and the degree of overbite and overjet on the gingival health. Br. Dent. J., *128*:539, 1970.
2. Armitage, G. C., Svanberg, G. K., and Löe, H.: Microscopic evaluation of clinical measurements of connective tissue attachment levels. J. Clin. Periodontol., *4*:173, 1977.
3. Ayers, P.: Green stains. J. Am. Dent. Assoc., *26*:3, 1939.
4. Badanes, B. B.: The role of fungi in deposits upon the teeth. Dent. Cosmos, *75*:1154, 1933.
5. Bartels, H. A.: A note on chromogenic microorganisms from an organic colored deposit of the teeth. Int. J. Orthod., *25*:795, 1939.
6. Bender, I. B., and Seltzer, S.: Roentgenographic and direct observation of experimental lesions in bone. J. Am. Dent. Assoc., *62*:152, 1961.
7. Bender, I. B., and Seltzer, S.: Roentgenographic and direct observations of experimental lesions in bone. II. J. Am. Dent. Assoc., *62*:708, 1961.
8. Berg, M., Burrill, D. Y., and Fosdick, L. S.: Chemical studies in periodontal disease. IV. Putrefactive rate as index of periodontal disease. J. Dent. Res., *26*:67, 1947.
9. Björn, H., and Holmberg, K.: Radiographic determination of periodontal bone destruction in epidemiological research. Odont. Revy, *17*:232, 1966.

10. Bonesvell, D., Lokken, P., and Rolla, G.: Influence of concentration, time, temperature and pH on the retention of chlorhexidine in the human oral cavity after mouth rinses. Arch. Oral Biol., *19*:1025, 1974.
11. Daneshmand, H., and Wade, A. B.: Correlation between gingival fluid measurements and macroscopic and microscopic characteristics of gingival tissues. J. Periodontol., *11*:35, 1976.
12. Dombrowski, J. C., et al.: A rapid chairside test for the severity of periodontal disease using gingival fluid. J. Periodontol., *49*:391, 1978.
13. Easley, J.: Methods of determining alveolar osseous form. J. Periodontol., *38*:112, 1967.
14. Eriksen, H., and Gjermo, P.: Incidence of stained tooth surfaces in students using chlorhexidine-containing dentifrices. Scand. J. Dent. Res., *81*:533, 1973.
15. Everett, F. G., and Fixott, H. C.: Use of an incorporated grid in the diagnosis of oral roentgenograms. Oral Surg., *9*:1061, 1963.
16. Fairbank, H. A. T.: Osteopetrosis. J. Bone Joint Surg., *30*:339, 1948.
17. Fischman, S. L., and Picozzi, A.: Review of the literature: the methodology of clinical calculus evaluation. J. Periodontol., *40*:607, 1969.
18. Fitzgerald, G. M.: Dental radiography. IV. The voltage factor (k.p.). J. Am. Dent. Assoc., *41*:19, 1950.
19. Gabathuler, H., and Hassel, T. M.: A pressure sensitive periodontal probe. Helv. Odontol. Acta, *15*:114, 1971.
20. Gjermo, P.: Chlorhexidine in dental practice. J. Clin. Periodontol., *1*:143, 1974.
21. Gjermo, P., Basstad, K., and Rolla, G.: The plaque inhibiting capacity of eleven antibacterial compounds. J. Periodont. Res., *5*:102, 1970.
22. Glickman, J.: Fibrous dysplasia of alveolar bone. Oral Surg., *1*:895, 1948.
23. Glickman, I., and Glidden, S.: Paget's disease of the maxillae and mandible. Clinical analysis and case reports. J. Am. Dent. Assoc., *29*:2144, 1942.
24. Golub, L. M., Kaplan, R., Mulvihill, J. E., and Ramanurthy, N. S.: Collagenolytic activity of crevicular fluid and of adjacent gingival tissue. J. Dent. Res., *58*:2132, 1979.
25. Gratt, B. M., Sickles, E. A., and Armitage, G. C.: Use of dental xeroradiographs in periodontics: comparison with conventional radiographs. J. Periodontol., *51*:1, 1980.
26. Greenberg, J., Laster, L., and Listgarten, M. A.: Transgingival probing as a potential estimator of alveolar bone level. J. Periodontol., *47*:514, 1976.
27. Greenstein, G., Caton, J., and Polson, A. M.: Histologic characteristics associated with bleeding after probing and visual signs of inflammation. J. Periodontol., *52*:420, 1981.
28. Greenstein, G., et al.: Associations between crestal lamina dura and periodontal status. J. Periodontol., *52*:362, 1981.
29. Hancock, E. B.: Determination of periodontal disease activity. J. Periodontol., *52*:492, 1981.
30. Hassel, T. M., German, M. A., and Saxer, U. P.: Periodontal probing: inter-investigator discrepancies and correlations between probing force and recorded depth. Helv. Odontol. Acta, *17*:38, 1973.
31. Heyden, G.: Relation between locally high concentrations of chlorhexidine and staining as seen in the clinic. J. Periodont. Res., *8*(Suppl.):76, 1973.
32. Hirschfeld, I.: Interdental canals. J. Am. Dent. Assoc., *14*:617, 1927.
33. Hirschfeld, L.: A calibrated silver point for periodontal diagnosis and recording. J. Periodontol., *24*:94, 1953.
34. Karshan, M., Kutscher, A. H., Silver, H. G., Stein, G.., and Ziskin, D. E.: Studies in the etiology of idiopathic orolingual paresthesias. Am. J. Digest. Dis., *19*:341, 1952.
35. Kitchen, P. C.: The prevalence of tooth root exposure and the relation of the extent of such exposure to the degree of abrasion in differing age classes. J. Dent. Res., *20*:565, 1941.
36. Kutscher, A. H.: Experiences with a detailed color shade guide for use in the study of the oral mucous membranes in health and disease. Oral Surg., *15*:408, 1962.
37. Leung, S. W.: Naturally occurring stains on the teeth of children. J. Am. Dent. Assoc., *41*:191, 1950.
38. Listgarten, M. A.: Periodontal probing: what does it mean? J. Clin. Periodontol., *7*:165, 1980.
39. Listgarten, M. A., and Hellden, L.: Relative distribution of bacteria at clinically healthy and periodontally diseased sites in humans. J. Clin. Periodontol., *5*:115, 1978.
40. Listgarten, M. A., Mao, R., and Robinson, P. J.: Periodontal probing: the relationship of the probe tip to periodontal tissues. J. Periodontol., *47*:511, 1976.
41. Löe, H., and Schiott, C.: The effect of mouth rinses and topical application of chlorhexidine on the development of dental plaque and gingivitis in man. J. Periodont. Res., *5*:79, 1970.
42. Magnusson, I., and Listgarten, M. A.: Histological evaluation of probing depth following periodontal treatment. J. Clin. Periodontol., *7*:26, 1980.
43. Manly, R. S.: Abrasion of cementum and dentin by modern dentifrices. J. Dent. Res., *20*:583, 1941.
44. Manly, R. S.: A structureless recurrent deposit on teeth. J. Dent. Res., *22*:479, 1943.
45. Manly, R. S.: Factors influencing tests on the abrasion of dentin by brushing with dentifrices. J. Dent. Res., *23*:59, 1944.
46. Mannerberg, F.: Saliva factors in cases of erosion. Odont. Revy, *14*:156, 1963.
47. Manson, J. D.: The lamina dura. Oral Surg., *16*:432, 1963.
48. Massler, M., Emslie, R., and Bolden, T.: Fetor ex ore. Oral Surg., *4*:110, 1951.
49. McCay, C. M., and Wills, L.: Erosion of molar teeth by acid beverages. J. Nutr., *39*:313, 1949.
50. Miller, W. D.: Experiments and observations on the wasting of tooth tissue variously designated as erosion, abrasion, chemical abrasion, denudation, etc. Dent. Cosmos, *49*:1, 1907.
51. Mühlemann, H. R.: Tooth mobility: a review of clinical aspects and research findings. J. Periodontol., *38*:686, 1967.
52. Mukherjee, S.: The temperature of the gingival sulcus. J. Periodontol., *49*:580, 1978.
53. Ng, G. C., Compton, F. H., and Walker, T. W.: Measurement of human gingival sulcus temperature. J. Periodont. Res., *13*:295, 1978.
54. Nizel, A. E.: Nutrition in Preventive Dentistry: Science and Practice. 2nd ed. Philadelphia, W. B. Saunders Company, 1980.
55. Nordno, H.: Discoloration of human teeth by a combination of chlorhexidine and aldehydes or ketones in vitro. Scand. J. Dent. Res., *79*:356, 1971.
56. O'Leary, T. J.: Tooth mobility. Dent. Clin. North Am., *3*:567, 1969.
57. O'Leary, T. J., and Rudd, K. D.: An instrument for measuring horizontal tooth mobility. Periodontics, *1*:249, 1963.
58. Onisi, M., and Nuckolls, J.: Description of actinomycetes and other pleomorphic organisms recovered from pigmented carious lesions of the dentine of human teeth. Oral Surg., *11*:910, 1958.
59. Parfitt, G. J.: The dynamics of a tooth in function. J. Periodontol., *32*:102, 1961.
60. Parfitt, G. J.: An investigation of the normal variations in alveolar bone trabeculations. Oral Surg., *15*:1453, 1962.
61. Patur, B., and Glickman, I.: Roentgenographic evaluation of alveolar bone changes in periodontal disease. Dent. Clin. North Am., *4*:47, 1960.
62. Pauls, V., and Trott, J. R.: A radiological study of experimentally produced lesions in bone. Dent. Pract., *16*:254, 1966.
63. Prichard, J. F.: Role of the roentgenogram in the diagnosis and prognosis of periodontal disease. Oral Med., *14*:182, 1961.
64. Puckett, J.: A device for comparing roentgenograms of the same mouth. J. Periodontol., *39*:38, 1968.
65. Ramadan, A. B. E., and Mitchell, D. F.: A roentgenographic study of experimental bone destruction. Oral Surg., *15*:934, 1962.
66. Regan, J. E., and Mitchell, D. F.: Roentgenographic and dissection measurements of alveolar crest height. J. Am. Dent. Assoc., *66*:356, 1963.
67. Ritchey, B., and Orban, B.: The crests of the interdental septa. J. Periodontol., *24*:75, 1953.
68. Robinson, H. B. G.: Abrasion, attrition and erosion of teeth. Health Center J., Ohio State Univ., *3*:21, 1949.
69. Rosenberg, E. H., and Guralnick, W. C.: Hyperparathyroidism. Oral Surg., *15*:(Suppl. 2):84, 1962.
70. Rosling, B., Hollender, L., Nyman, S., and Olsson, G.: A radiographic method for assessing changes in alveolar bone height following periodontal therapy. J. Clin. Periodontol., *2*:211, 1975.

71. Rudin, H. J., Overdiek, H. F., and Rateitschak, K. H.: Correlation between sulcus fluid rate and clinical histological inflammation of the marginal gingiva. Helv. Odontol. Acta, 14:21, 1970.

72. Saglie, R., Johanson, J. R., and Flötra, L.: The zone of completely and partially destructed periodontal fibers in pathological pockets. J. Clin. Periodontol., 2:198, 1975.

73. Salman, I., and Darlington, C. G.: Eosinophilic granuloma, A.M. J. Orthopedics 31:89, 1945.

74. Sandler, H. C., Stahl, S. S. Cahn, L. R., and Freund, H. R.: Exfoliative cytology for the detection of early mouth cancer. Oral Surg., 13:994, 1960.

75. Sanstead, H. H., Carte, J. P., and Darby, W. J.: How to diagnose nutritional disorders in daily practice. Nutr. Today, 4:20, 1969.

76. Selikoff, I., and Robitzek, E.: Gingival biopsy for the diagnosis of generalized amyloidosis. Am. J. Pathol., 23:1099, 1947.

77. Shapiro, A., Goldman, H., and Bloom, A.: Sulcular exudate flow in gingival inflammation. J. Periodontol., 50:301, 1979.

78. Shapiro, L., et al.: Sulcular exudate protein levels as an indicator of the clinical inflammatory response. J. Periodontol., 51:86, 1980.

79. Shklar, G., Cataldo, E., and Meyer, I.: Reliability of cytologic smear in diagnosis of oral cancer. A controlled study. Arch. Otolaryngol., 91:158, 1970.

80. Silverman, S., Jr., Gordon, G., Grant, T., Steinback, H., Eisenberg, E., and Manson, R.: Dental structures in primary hyperparathyroidism. Oral Surg., 15:426, 1962.

81. Sivertson, J. F., and Burgett, F. G.: Probing of pockets related to the attachment level. J. Periodontol., 47:281, 1976.

82. Sleeper, E.: Eosinophilic granuloma of bone. Oral Surg., 4:896, 1951.

83. Slots, J.: The microflora of black stain on human primary teeth. Scand. J. Dent. Res., 82:484, 1974.

84. Sognnaes, R. F.: Periodontal significance of intraoral frictional ablation. J. Western Soc. Periodontol., 25:112, 1977.

85. Sponge, J. D.: Halitosis: a review of its causes and treatment. Dent. Pract., 14:307, 1964.

86. Spray, J. R., et al.: Microscopic demonstration of the position of periodontal probes. J. Periodontol., 49:148, 1978.

87. Stallard, H.: Residual food odors of the mouth. J. Am. Dent. Assoc., 14:1689, 1927.

88. Sutcliffe, P.: Extrinsic tooth stains in children. Dent. Pract., 17:175, 1967.

89. Tenuovo, J., and Anttonen, T.: Application of a dehydrated test strip. Hemastix for the assessment of gingivitis. J. Clin. Periodontol., 5:206, 1978.

90. Theilade, J.: An evaluation of the reliability of radiographs in the measurement of bone loss in periodontal disease. J. Periodontol., 31:143, 1960.

91. Tibbetts, L. S.: Use of diagnostic probes for detection of periodontal disease. J. Am. Dent. Assoc., 78:549, 1969.

92. Todd-Sanford Clinical Diagnosis by Laboratory Methods. Edited by Davidson, I., and Henry, J. B. 14th ed. Philadelphia, W. B. Saunders Company, 1969.

93. Vallotton, C. F.: An acquired pigmented pellicle of the enamel surface. J. Dent. Res., 24:161, 171, 183, 1945.

94. Van Der Linden, L. W. J., and Van Aken, J.: The periodontal ligament in the roentgenogram. J. Periodontol., 41:243, 1970.

95. Van Der Velden, U.: Probing force and the relationship of the probe tip to the periodontal tissues. J. Clin. Periodontol., 6:106, 1979.

96. Van Der Velden, U., and De Vries, J. H.: Introduction of a new periodontal probe. The pressure probe. J. Clin. Periodontol., 5:188, 1978.

97. White, S. C., Stafford, M. L., and Beeninga, L. R.: Intraoral xeroradiography. Oral Surg., 46:862, 1978.

98. Wintrobe, M. M.: Clinical Hematology. 5th ed. Philadelphia, Lea & Febiger, 1961, p. 105.

chapter thirty-three

Determination of the Prognosis

The prognosis is the prediction of the duration, course, and termination of a disease and the likelihood of its response to treatment. It must be determined before the treatment is planned. The prognosis of gingival and periodontal disease is critically dependent upon the patient—his attitude, his desire to retain his natural teeth, and his willingness and ability to maintain good oral hygiene. Without these, treatment will not succeed.

THE PROGNOSIS IN PATIENTS WITH GINGIVAL DISEASE

The prognosis of gingival disease depends upon the role of inflammation in the overall disease process. If inflammation is the only pathologic change, the prognosis is favorable, provided all local irritants are eliminated, gingival contours conducive to the preservation of health are attained, and the patient cooperates by maintaining good oral hygiene.

If inflammation is superimposed upon systemically caused tissue changes (such as in gingival enlargement associated with phenytoin therapy or in patients with nutritional, hematologic, or hormonal disorders), gingival health may be restored temporarily by local therapy alone, but the long-term prognosis depends upon the control or correction of the contributing systemic factors.

THE PROGNOSIS IN PATIENTS WITH PERIODONTAL DISEASE

There are two aspects to the determination of the prognosis in patients with periodontal disease: *the overall prognosis* and *the prognosis of individual teeth.*

The Overall Prognosis

The overall prognosis is concerned with the dentition as a whole. It answers the questions, "Should treatment be undertaken?" and "Is it likely to succeed?" The following factors are considered in determining the overall prognosis.

ASSESSMENT OF THE PAST BONE RESPONSE. The past response of the alveolar bone to local factors is a useful guide for predicting the bone response to treatment and the likelihood of arresting the bone-destructive process. Assessment of the past bone response entails consideration of the severity and distribution of the periodontal bone loss in terms of the following: the patient's age; the distribution, severity, and duration of local irritants such as plaque, calculus, and food impaction; occlusal abnormalities; and habits.

If the amount of bone loss can be accounted for by the local factors, local treatment can be expected to arrest the bone destruction; the overall prognosis for the dentition is good (Fig. 33–1).

If the bone loss is more severe than one would ordinarily expect at the patient's age in the presence of local factors of comparable severity and duration, factors other than those in the oral cavity are contributing to the bone destruction. In the last few years many of these rapidly destructive forms of periodontitis have been found to have an underlying defect in chemotaxis of the leukocytes (see Chapter 24).

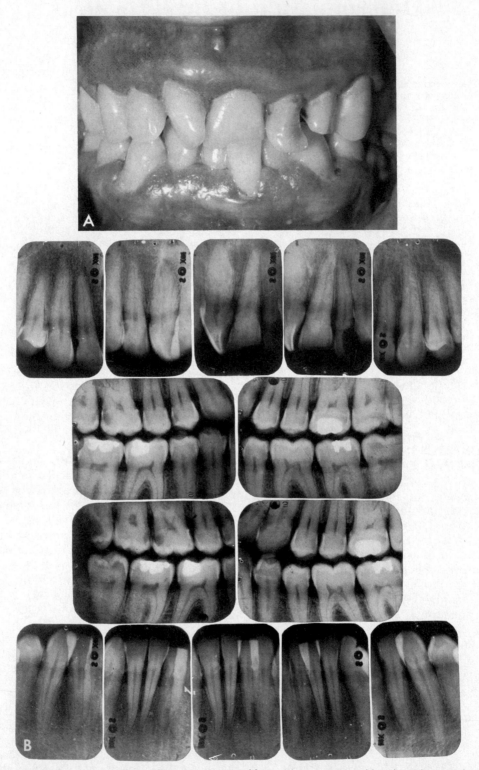

Figure 33–1 Good Bone Response, Overall Prognosis Favorable. A, Thirty-two-year-old male with generalized chronic marginal gingivitis, periodontal pocket formation, and excessive anterior overbite. B, Excellent bone picture despite unfavorable inflammatory and occlusal factors.

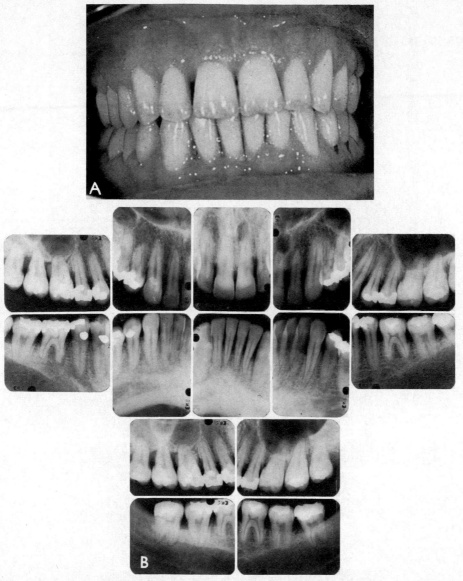

Figure 33–2 Poor Bone Response, Overall Prognosis Poor. *A,* Twenty-seven-year-old male with generalized chronic gingivitis and periodontal pocket formation. *B,* Bone destruction is in excess of that explainable by the local factors. The overall prognosis is poor.

The overall prognosis is generally poor, because of the difficulty encountered in determining the responsible systemic factor (Fig. 33–2). Local treatment can be relied upon to arrest bone destruction caused by the local factors, but unless the systemic etiologic factor is detected and corrected, bone loss may continue.

The prognosis is not necessarily hopeless even if the systemic defect has not been identified or cannot be treated, provided the disease is detected early and sufficient bone remains to support the teeth. In such cases, local treatment often can retain the dentition in useful function for many years by eliminating local destructive factors.

HEIGHT OF REMAINING BONE. The next question is, "Assuming bone destruction can be arrested, is there enough bone remaining to support the teeth?" The answer is readily apparent in extreme conditions, when there is so little bone loss that tooth support is not in jeopardy (Fig. 33–3) or when bone loss is severe and generalized and the remaining bone is obviously insufficient for proper tooth support (Fig. 33–4). Most patients, however, do not fit into the extreme categories. The height of the remaining bone lies somewhere in be-

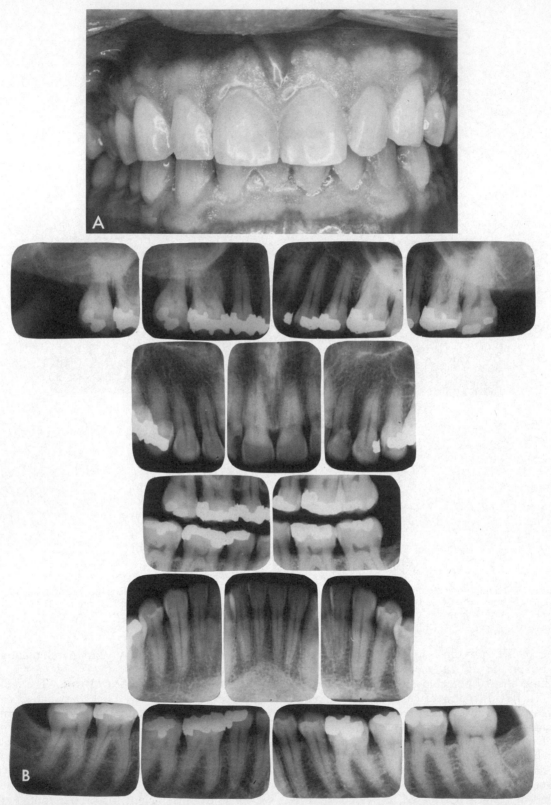

Figure 33–3 Good Bone Response in a 42-Year-Old Male. *A*, Gingival inflammation, poor oral hygiene, and pronounced anterior overbite. *B*, The bone loss is slight considering the age of the patient and the unfavorable local factors. This is a patient with a "positive bone factor."

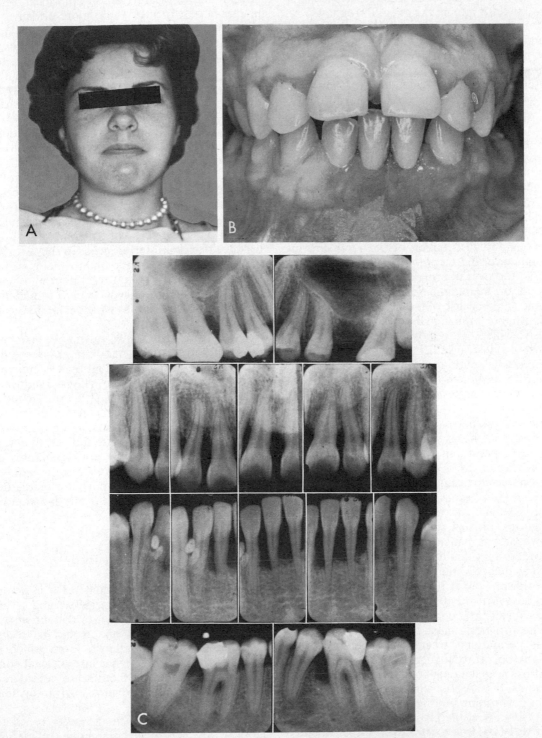

Figure 33–4 Poor Bone Response in a 17-Year-Old Female. *A,* Clinical appearance of patient. *B,* Gingival inflammation, periodontal pockets, and pathologic migration. *C,* Severe bone destruction exceeds that which ordinarily occurs in 17-year-old patient with comparable local factors. This patient has a "negative bone factor." The distribution of bone loss in the anterior and first molar areas is considered typical of juvenile periodontitis. Note the bifurcation and trifurcation involvement of three remaining first molars.

tween, making the bone level alone inconclusive for determining the overall prognosis.

PATIENT'S AGE. **All other factors being equal, the prognosis is better in the older of two patients with comparable levels of remaining alveolar bone.** The younger patient has suffered a more rapid bone destruction than the older patient because of the shorter period in which the bone loss has occurred. The younger person would ordinarily be expected to have a greater bone-reparative capacity and a better posttreatment prognosis. However, the fact that so much bone destruction has occurred in a relatively short period of time reflects unfavorably on the young patient's bone-reparative capacity.

NUMBER OF REMAINING TEETH. If the number and distribution of the teeth are inadequate for the support of a satisfactory prosthesis, the overall prognosis is poor. The likelihood of maintaining periodontal health is diminished because of the inability to establish a satisfactory functional environment. An extensive fixed or removable prosthesis constructed on an insufficient number of natural teeth creates periodontal injury which is more likely to hasten tooth loss than to provide a worthwhile health service.

PATIENT'S SYSTEMIC BACKGROUND. The patient's systemic background affects the overall prognosis in several ways. In patients with extensive periodontal destruction that cannot be accounted for by local factors alone, it is reasonable to assume a contributing systemic etiology, but because detection of the responsible systemic factors is usually difficult, the prognosis in such patients is usually poor. However, in patients with known systemic disorders that could affect the periodontium, such as diabetes, nutritional deficiency, hyperthyroidism, and hyperparathyroidism, the prognosis of the periodontal condition improves with their correction.

The prognosis must be guarded when surgical periodontal treatment is required but cannot be provided because of the patient's health. Incapacitating conditions (such as Parkinson's disease) which prevent the patient from performing oral hygiene procedures also adversely affect the prognosis.

GINGIVAL INFLAMMATION. Other factors being equal, the prognosis of periodontal disease is directly related to the severity of inflammation. In two patients with comparable bone destruction, the prognosis is better in the patient with the greater degree of inflammation. A larger component of the bone destruction is attributable to local irritation, and local treatment can be expected to be more effective in arresting the bone destruction.

PERIODONTAL POCKETS. The location of the base of periodontal pockets is more important than pocket depth in deciding the overall prognosis. Because pocket depth and the severity of bone loss are not necessarily related, a patient with deep pockets and little bone loss has a better prognosis than a patient with shallow pockets and severe bone destruction.

MALOCCLUSION. Irregularly aligned teeth, malformation of the jaws, and abnormal occlusal relationships may be important factors in the etiology of periodontal disease inasmuch as they may interfere with plaque control or produce occlusal interferences. In these cases, correction by orthodontic or prosthetic means is essential if periodontal treatment is to succeed. **The overall prognosis is poor in patients with occlusal deformities which cannot be corrected.**

THE PROGNOSIS OF JUVENILE PERIODONTITIS. In patients with periodontal disease diagnosed as juvenile periodontitis, systemic influences are considered to play a significant role in the periodontal destruction. Ideally, treatment should include correction of the responsible systemic conditions, along with local measures, but the former are difficult to determine. However, **except in advanced cases of juvenile periodontitis, in which the remaining bone is insufficient to support the teeth, the dentition can be retained in useful function by local treatment alone.**

The Prognosis of Individual Teeth

The prognosis of individual teeth is determined after the overall prognosis and is affected by it. For example, in a patient with a poor overall prognosis one would be disinclined to attempt to retain a tooth which is considered questionable because of local conditions. The following factors are considered in determining the prognosis of individual teeth:

MOBILITY. The principal causes of tooth mobility are loss of alveolar bone, inflammatory changes in the periodontal ligament, and trauma from occlusion. (Tooth mobility is discussed in detail in Chapter 20.) Tooth mobility caused by inflammation and trauma from occlusion is correctable.[9] Tooth mobility resulting from loss of alveolar bone alone is not likely to be corrected. **The likelihood of restoring tooth stability is inversely proportional to the extent to which it is caused by loss of alveolar bone.**

A longitudinal 8-year study of the response to treatment of teeth with different degrees of mobility revealed that pockets of clinically mobile teeth do not respond as well to periodontal therapy as those of firm teeth exhibiting the same initial disease severity.[5] Another study, however, in which an ideal control of plaque was attained, found similar healing in hypermobile and firm teeth.[11]

PERIODONTAL POCKETS. In suprabony pockets the location of the base of the pocket affected prognosis of individual teeth more than the pocket depth. **Proximity to frenum attachments and to the mucogingival line jeopardizes the prognosis unless corrective procedures are included in the treatment** (see Chapter 56).

Proximity of the Base of the Pocket to the Apex. The prognosis is adversely affected if the base of the pocket is close to the root apex, even if there is no evidence of apical disease. **The incidence of degenerative pulp changes is increased in teeth affected by periodontal disease, usually without clinical symptoms or pulp necrosis.** The pulp changes are attributed to irritation from bacterial products entering through the dentinal tubules of the exposed root surface wall of periodontal pockets and through lateral pulp canals. If the base of the pocket is closed to the root apex, injurious bacterial products may reach the pulp through the apical foramina. Root canal therapy is necessary in such cases to obtain optimal results from periodontal treatment.

When the periodontal pocket has extended to involve the apex, the prognosis is generally poor. However, striking apical and lateral bone repair is sometimes obtained by combining endodontic and periodontal therapy (see Chapter 55).

TOOTH MORPHOLOGY. The prognosis is poor in patients with short, tapered roots and relatively large crowns (Fig. 33–5). Because of the disproportionate crown-root ratio and the reduced root surface available for periodontal support,[7] the periodontium is more susceptible to injury by occlusal forces.

The **morphology of the tooth root** is a very important consideration in therapy.[6] Scaling and planing the root surface are fundamental if successful treatment is to be attained, and these can be hampered by bizarre root morphology. Oral hygiene by the patient is also

fundamental for maintenance of the healthy status reached in therapy; this too can be made very difficult by various root morphologies. The dentist should learn to recognize and evaluate such root forms, as their presence will sometimes play an essential role in treatment planning and the determination of the prognosis. These bizarre root findings offer no problems as long as they are apical to the epithelial attachment and therefore are not exposed to the lumen of the pocket. There is at this stage no need to scale the roots, nor later to clean them, since they are part of the attachment apparatus. But as soon as the disease progresses to uncover these areas, the problems appear.

Root concavities and the morphology of the furcation areas are essential features of interest. **Concavities** can vary from shallow flutings to deep depressions present in the proximal surfaces. They increase the attachment area and produce a root shape that is more resistant to torquing forces. Concavities appear more marked in the maxillary first premolars, the mesiobuccal root of the maxillary first molar, both roots of the mandibular first molars, and in the mandibular incisors[1, 2] (Fig. 33–6 and 33–7).

Access to the **furcation area** is sometimes very difficult to obtain (see Chapter 55). In 58 per cent of upper and lower first molars, the furcation entrance diameter is narrower than the width of commonly used periodontal curettes[1] (Fig. 33–8).

The presence of **developmental grooves,** which sometimes appear in the maxillary lateral incisors (palatogingival groove) (Fig. 33–9) or in the lower incisors, also creates an accessibility problem[3, 6] and worsens the prognosis.[13] Enamel projections extend into the furcation of 28.6 per cent of mandibular molars and 17 per cent of maxillary molars.[8] An intermediate bifurcation ridge has been described in 73 per cent of mandibular first molars, crossing from the mesial to the distal root at the midpoint of the bifurcation.[4]

TEETH ADJACENT TO EDENTULOUS AREAS. Teeth that serve as abutments are subjected to increased functional demands. More rigid standards are required in evaluating the prognosis of teeth adjacent to edentulous areas.

LOCATION OF REMAINING BONE IN RELATION TO THE INDIVIDUAL TOOTH SURFACES. When greater bone loss has occurred on one surface of a tooth, the bone height on the less involved surfaces should be taken into consid-

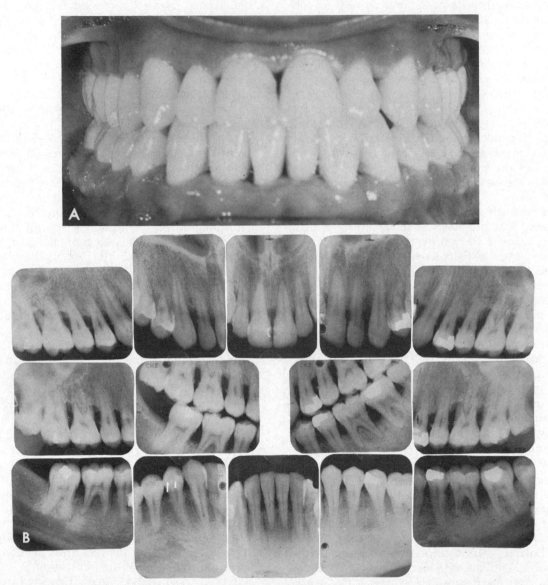

Figure 33–5 Poor Crown-Root Ratio, Overall Prognosis Unfavorable. A, Twenty-four-year-old patient with generalized gingivitis and periodontal pocket formation. B, Severity of bone destruction at this age indicates poor bone response. The contrast between the well-formed crowns and relatively short tapered roots worsens the unfavorable prognosis.

Figure 33–6. Root concavities in maxillary first molars sectioned 2 mm apical to the furca. (Data from Bower, R. C.: J. Periodontol., *50*:366, 1979). The furcal aspect of the root is concave in 94 per cent of the mesiobuccal (MB) roots, 31 per cent of the distobuccal (DB) roots, and 17 per cent of the palatal (P) roots. The deepest concavity is found in the furcal aspects of the mesiobuccal root (mean concavity, 0.3 mm). The furcal aspect of the buccal roots diverges toward the palate in 97 per cent of the teeth (mean divergence, 22°).

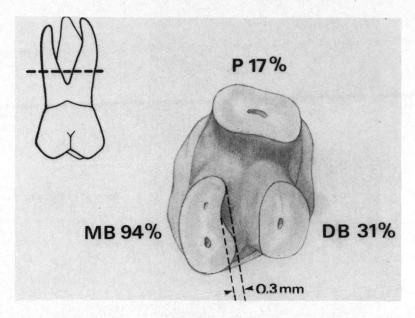

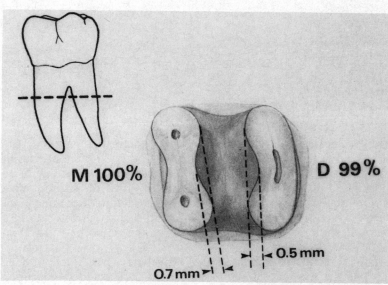

Figure 33–7 Root concavities in mandibular first molars sectioned 2 mm apical to the furca. (Data from Bower, R. C.: J. Periodontol., *50*:366, 1979). Concavity of the furcal aspect was found in 100 per cent of mesial (M) roots and 99 per cent of distal (D) roots. Deeper concavity was found in the mesial roots (mean concavity, 0.7 mm).

Figure 33–8 The furcation entrance is narrower than a standard curette in 58 per cent of first molars. (Data from Bower, R. C.: J. Periodontol., *50*:366, 1979.)

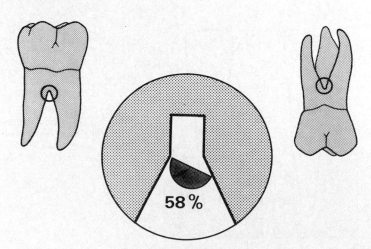

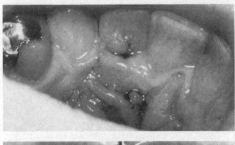

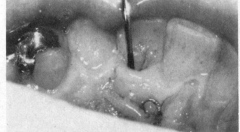

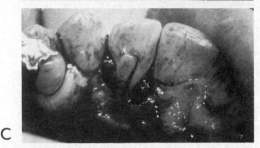

Figure 33–9 Palatogingival Groove. *A,* Gingival inflammation and exudate in area palatal to upper lateral incisor. *B,* Probing shows deep pocket. *C,* Area is flapped and the presence of a palatogingival groove is confirmed. (Courtesy of Dr. Robert Merin.)

eration in determining the prognosis. Because of the greater height of bone in relation to the latter surfaces, the center of rotation of the tooth will be nearer the crown (Fig. 33–10). The leverage upon the periodontium will therefore be more favorable than the bone loss on the most severely involved tooth surface suggests.

RELATION TO ADJACENT TEETH. In dealing with a tooth with a questionable prognosis, the chances of successful treatment should be weighed against the benefits that would accrue to the adjacent teeth if the tooth under consideration were extracted. **Heroic attempts to retain a hopelessly involved tooth jeopardize the adjacent teeth.** Extraction of the questionable tooth is followed by partial restoration of the bone support of the adjacent teeth (Fig. 33–11).

INFRABONY POCKETS. The likelihood of eliminating infrabony pockets depends upon several factors, critical among which are the

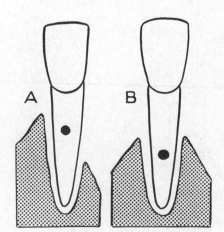

Figure 33–10 The Prognosis for Tooth A Is Better Than That for Tooth B, despite the fact that there is less bone on one of the surfaces. Because the center of rotation of tooth A is closer to the crown, the distribution of occlusal forces to the periodontium is more favorable than in B.

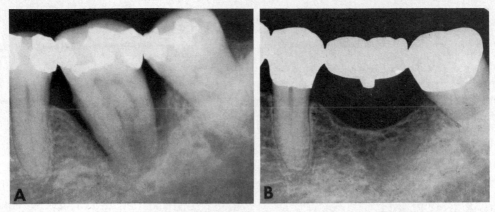

Figure 33–11 Extraction of Severely Involved Tooth to Preserve Bone on Adjacent Teeth. *A,* Extensive bone destruction around mandibular first molar. *B,* Eight and one-half years after extraction of first molar and replacement by prosthesis. Note the excellent bony support.

contour of the osseous defects and the number of the remaining bony walls (see Chapter 54).

FURCATION INVOLVEMENT. The presence of bifurcation or trifurcation involvement does not indicate a hopeless prognosis (see Chapter 55). However, when a lesion reaches the furcation it causes two additional important problems: the first is the difficulty of access to the area, both for scaling and root planing and for surgery; the second is the inaccessibility of the area to plaque removal by the patient. If both of these problems can be satisfactorily solved, the prognosis will be similar to or even better than that of single-rooted teeth with a similar degree of bone loss.

Upper first premolars offer the greatest difficulties, and therefore their prognosis is usually unfavorable when the lesion reaches the furcation. Upper molars also offer some degree of difficulty; sometimes their prognosis can be improved by resecting one of the buccal roots (either the mesiobuccal or the distobuccal), thereby improving access to the area. Lower first molars offer good access to the furcation area, and therefore their prognosis is usually better.

CARIES, NONVITAL TEETH, AND TOOTH RESORPTION. In teeth mutilated by extensive caries, the feasibility of adequate restoration and endodontic therapy should be considered before undertaking periodontal treatment. Extensive idiopathic root resorption jeopardizes the stability of teeth and adversely affects the response to periodontal treatment. **The periodontal prognosis of treated nonvital teeth is not different from that of vital teeth.** Reat-

tachment can occur to the cementum of nonvital or vital teeth. However, reattachment to exposed root dentin is not likely in nonvital teeth.[10]

REFERENCES

1. Bower, R. C.: Furcation morphology relative to periodontal treatment—furcation entrance architecture. J. Periodontol., *50*:23, 1979.
2. Bower, R. C.: Furcation morphology relative to periodontal treatment—furcation root surface anatomy. J. Periodontol., *50*:366, 1979.
3. Everett, F. G., and Kramer, G. N.: The disto-lingual groove in the maxillary lateral incisor, a periodontal hazard. J. Periodontol., *43*:352, 1972.
4. Everett, F. G., Jump, E. B., Holder, T. D., and Williams, G. C.: The intermediate bifurcational ridge: a study of the morphology of the bifurcation of the lower first molar. J. Dent. Res., *37*:162, 1958.
5. Fleszar, T. J., et al.: Tooth mobility and periodontal therapy. J. Clin. Periodontol., *7*:495, 1980.
6. Gher, M. E., and Vernino, A. R.: Root morphology—clinical significance in pathogenesis and treatment of periodontal disease. Am. Dent. Assoc., *101*:627, 1980.
7. Kay, S., Forscher, B. K., and Sackett, L. M.: Tooth root length-volume relationships. An aid to periodontal prognosis. I. Anterior teeth. Oral Surg., *7*:735, 1954.
8. Master, D. H., and Hoskins, S. W. P.: Projection of cervical enamel into molar furcations. J. Periodontol., *35*:49, 1964.
9. Morris, M. L.: The diagnosis, prognosis and treatment of the loose tooth. Oral Surg., *6*:1037, 1953.
10. Morris, M. L.: Healing of human periodontal tissues following surgical detachment and extirpation of vital pulps. J. Periodontol., *31*:23, 1960.
11. Rosling, B., Nyman, S., and Lindhe, J.: The effect of systematic plaque control on bone regeneration in infrabony pockets. J. Clin. Periodontol., *3*:38, 1976.
12. Slatten, R. W.: An evaluation of factors determining prognosis in inflammatory and retrogressive periodontal disease. J. Periodontol., *25*:30, 1954.
13. Withers, J. A., et al.: The relationship of palato-gingival grooves to localized periodontal disease. J. Periodontol., *52*:41, 1981.

The Treatment Plan

THE TREATMENT PLAN

After the diagnosis and prognosis have been established, the treatment is planned. *The treatment plan is the blueprint for case management.* It includes all procedures required for the establishment and maintenance of oral health, such as decisions as to teeth to be retained or extracted and decisions on techniques to be used for pocket therapy, the need for mucogingival or reconstructive surgical procedures and occlusal correction, the type of restorations to be employed, which teeth are to be used for abutments, and the indications for splinting.

Unforeseen developments during treatment may necessitate modification of the initial treatment plan. However, **it is axiomatic that, except for emergencies, no treatment should be started until the treatment plan has been established.**

Periodontal treatment requires long-range planning. **Its value to the patient is measured in years of healthful functioning of the entire dentition, not by the number of teeth retained at the time of treatment.** It is directed to establishing and maintaining the health of the periodontium throughout the mouth rather than to spectacular efforts to "tighten loose teeth."

The welfare of the dentition should not be jeopardized by a heroic attempt to retain questionable teeth. The periodontal condition of the teeth we decide to retain is more important than their number. Teeth that can be retained with a minimum of doubt and a maximum margin of safety provide the basis for the total treatment plan. Teeth on the borderline of hopelessness do not contribute to the overall usefulness of the dentition, even if they can be saved in a somewhat precarious state. Such teeth become sources of recurrent annoyance to the patient and detract from the value of the greater service rendered by the establishment of periodontal health in the remainder of the oral cavity.

THE MASTER PLAN FOR TOTAL TREATMENT

The aim of the treatment plan is *total treatment*—that is, the *coordination of all treatment procedures for the purpose of creating a well-functioning dentition in a healthy periodontal environment.* The "master plan" of periodontal treatment encompasses four different therapeutic objectives for each patient according to his or her needs.

1. THE SOFT TISSUE AREA. This entails the elimination of gingival inflammation, periodontal pockets, and the factors which cause them; the establishment of gingival contour and mucogingival relationships conducive to the preservation of periodontal health; restoration of carious areas; correction of the margins of existing restorations; and recontouring proximal, facial, and lingual surfaces and occlusal marginal ridges of existing restorations to provide proper proximal contacts and food excursion pathways.

2. THE FUNCTIONAL AREA. *An optimal occlusal relationship is one that provides the functional stimulation necessary to preserve periodontal health.* To obtain it may require occlusal adjustment; restorative, prosthetic, and orthodontic procedures; splinting; and the correction of bruxism, clamping, and clenching habits.

3. THE SYSTEMIC AREA. Systemic conditions may necessitate special precautions in the course of periodontal treatment, affect the tissue response to treatment procedures, or threaten the preservation of periodontal health after treatment is completed. Such situations should be taken care of in conjunction with the patient's physician. (For a discussion of systemic conditions which require special precautions, see Chapter 36.)

4. Case Maintenance. This entails all procedures for maintaining periodontal health after it has been attained. It consists of instruction in oral hygiene; recall of the patient at regular intervals according to his or her needs to check on the condition of the periodontium, the status of the restorative dentistry, and the need for further occlusal adjustment; and follow-up radiographs.

SEQUENCE OF THERAPEUTIC PROCEDURES

Periodontal therapy is an inseparable part of dental therapy. The sequence of procedures presented here includes periodontal procedures (marked with an asterisk) and other procedures not considered to be within the province of the periodontist.

Preliminary Phase

Treatment of emergencies
    Dental or periapical
    *Periodontal
    Other
Extraction of hopeless teeth and provisional replacement if needed (may be postponed to a more convenient time)

Phase I Therapy (Etiotropic Phase)

*Plaque control
  Diet control (in patients with rampant caries)
*Removal of calculus and root planing
*Correction of restorative and prosthetic irritational factors
  Excavation of caries and restoration (temporary or final, depending on whether a definitive prognosis for the tooth has been arrived at and on the location of caries)
*Occlusal therapy
*Minor orthodontic movement
*Provisional splinting

Evaluation of Response to Phase I

Rechecking
  *Pocket depth and gingival inflammation

Evaluation of Response to Phase I (continued)

  *Plaque and calculus caries

Phase II Therapy (Surgical Phase)

*Periodontal surgery
  Root canal therapy

Phase III Therapy (Restorative Phase)

Final restorations
Fixed and removable prosthodontics

Evaluation of Periodontal Response to Restorative Procedures

Phase IV Therapy (Maintenance Phase)

Periodic recalls, checking
  *Plaque and calculus
  *Gingival condition (pockets, inflammation)
  Caries
  *Occlusion, tooth mobility
  Other pathology

EXPLAINING THE TREATMENT PLAN TO THE PATIENT

The following are suggestions for explaining the treatment plan to the patient:

Be specific. Tell your patient: "You have gingivitis," or "You have periodontitis." Then, explain exactly what these conditions are, how they are treated, and the future for the patient's mouth after treatment. **Avoid vague statements** such as: "You have trouble with your gums," or "Something should be done about your gums." Patients do not understand the significance of such statements and disregard them.

Start your discussion on a positive note. Talk about the teeth which can be retained and the long-term service they can be expected to render. Do not start your discussion with the statement: "The following teeth have to be extracted." This creates a negative impression which adds to the erroneous attitude of hopelessness the patient already may have regarding his or her mouth.

Make it clear that every effort will be made to retain as many teeth as possible, **but do not dwell on the patient's loose teeth.** Emphasize the fact that the important purpose of the treatment is to prevent the other teeth from becoming as severely diseased as the loose teeth.

Present the entire treatment plan as a unit. Avoid creating the impression that treatment consists of separate procedures, some or all of which may be selected by the patient. **Make it clear that dental restorations and prostheses contribute as much to the health of the gums as does the elimination of inflammation and periodontal pockets.** Do not speak in terms of "having the gums treated" and "then taking care of the necessary restorations later" as if these were unrelated treatments.

Patients frequently seek guidance from the dentist with such questions as: "Are my teeth worth treating?" "Would you have them treated if you were I?" "Why don't I just go along the way I am until the teeth really bother me, and then have them all extracted?"

If the condition is treatable, make it clear that the best results are obtained by prompt treatment. If the condition is not treatable, the teeth should be extracted. Explain that "doing nothing" or holding onto hopelessly diseased teeth as long as possible is inadvisable for the following reasons:

In periodontal disease, proper mastication of food is impaired because of looseness of the teeth and discomfort incurred by chewing. This leads to the "bolting" of food, which complicates the digestive process and may lead to gastrointestinal disturbances.

Exudate from periodontal pockets spoils the taste of food. In addition, the incorporation of purulent material into the food may irritate the mucosa of the stomach and lead to gastritis. Infection in the periodontal area is also a potential source of bacteremia.

Inability to chew properly leads to habits of food selection with preference for soft foods, which are for the most part carbohydrates.

It is not feasible to place restorations or "bridges" on teeth with untreated periodontal disease, because the usefulness of the restoration is limited by the uncertain condition of the supporting structures.

Failure to eliminate a periodontal disease not only results in the loss of teeth already hopelessly involved, but also shortens the life span of other teeth which, with proper treatment, could serve as the foundation for a healthy, functioning dentition.

It is the dentist's responsibility to advise the patient of the importance of periodontal treatment. However, if treatment is to be successful, the patient must be sufficiently interested in retaining the natural teeth to maintain the necessary oral hygiene. Individuals who are not particularly perturbed by the thought of losing their teeth are generally not good patients for periodontal treatment.

Rationale for Periodontal Treatment

There are no forms of gingivitis or periodontal disease in which the removal of local irritants and prevention of their recurrence do not reduce the severity of the disease, lessen the rapidity of the destructive process, and prolong the usefulness of the natural dentition.

WHAT DOES PERIODONTAL THERAPY ACCOMPLISH?*

The effectiveness of periodontal therapy is made possible by the remarkable healing capacity of the periodontal tissues (Fig. 35–1). Periodontal therapy can restore chronically inflamed gingiva so that from a clinical and structural point of view it is almost identical with gingiva that has never been exposed to excessive plaque accumulation.[33]

Properly performed, periodontal treatment can be relied upon to accomplish the following: eliminate pain, eliminate gingival inflammation[51] and gingival bleeding, reduce periodontal pockets and eliminate infection, stop pus formation, arrest the destruction of soft tissue and bone,[52] reduce abnormal tooth mobility,[14] establish optimal occlusal function, restore tissue destroyed by disease in some instances, re-establish the physiologic gingival contour necessary for the preservation of periodontal health, prevent the recurrence of disease, and reduce tooth loss[45] (Fig. 35–2).

LOCAL THERAPY. The etiology of periodontitis and gingivitis is bacterial plaque accumulation on the tooth surface in close proximity to the gingival tissue. The accumulation of plaque can be favored by a variety of local factors, such as calculus, overhanging margins of restorations, food impaction, and so forth.

The removal of plaque and of all the factors that favor its accumulation is therefore the primary consideration in local therapy.

Abnormal forces on the tooth increase tooth mobility. The thorough elimination of plaque and the prevention of its new formation will, by themselves, maintain periodontal health, even if traumatic forces are allowed to persist.[31, 32] However, the elimination of trauma may increase the chances of bone regeneration and gain of attachment.[25] Although this point is not widely accepted,[47] it appears that creating occlusal relations that are more tolerable to the periodontal tissues increases the margin of safety of the periodontium to minor build-ups of plaque, in addition to reducing tooth mobility. It should be remembered that total plaque elimination as obtained in experimental studies may not be possible in all our human subjects.

SYSTEMIC THERAPY. Systemic therapy may be employed as an adjunct to local measures and for specific purposes, such as the control of systemic complications from acute infections, chemotherapy to prevent harmful effects of posttreatment bacteremia, supportive nutritional therapy, and the control of systemic diseases which aggravate the patient's periodontal condition or necessitate special precautions during treatment (see Chapter 36).

There are periodontal manifestations of systemic diseases (see Chapters 12, 28, 29, and 30) which are treated primarily by other than local measures. However, local therapy may still be indicated in order to reduce or prevent complications from gingival inflammation.

FACTORS WHICH AFFECT HEALING

In the periodontium, as elsewhere in the body, healing is affected by local and systemic factors.

---

*See Chapter 60 for a more detailed consideration of this topic.

LOCAL FACTORS. Systemic conditions which impair healing may reduce the effectiveness of local periodontal treatment and should be corrected prior to or along with local procedures. **However, it is the local factors, such as contamination by microorganisms, irritation from plaque, food debris, and necrotic tissue remnants, and trauma from occlusion, which are the most common deterrents to healing following periodontal treatment.** Healing is also delayed by excessive tissue manipulation during treatment, trauma to the tissues, and repetitive treatment procedures which disrupt the orderly cellular activity in the healing process. In addition, topically applied cortisone and ionizing radiation retard healing.[23]

Healing is improved by a local increase in temperature, débridement (the removal of degenerated and necrotic tissue), immobilization of the healing area, and pressure on the wound. The cellular activity in healing entails an increase in oxygen consumption, but healing of the gingiva is not accelerated by artificially increasing the oxygen supply beyond the normal requirements.[18]

SYSTEMIC FACTORS. The effects of systemic conditions upon healing have been extensively documented in animal experiments but are less clearly defined in humans. Healing capacity diminishes with age.[5, 21] Atherosclerotic vascular changes, which are common in aging, and the resultant reduction in blood circulation may be responsible. Healing is delayed in patients with generalized infections and in those with diabetes and other debilitating diseases.

The nutrient requirements of the healing tissues in minor wounds such as those created by periodontal surgical procedures are ordinarily satisfied by a well-balanced diet. Healing is retarded by insufficient food intake and by bodily conditions which interfere with the uti-

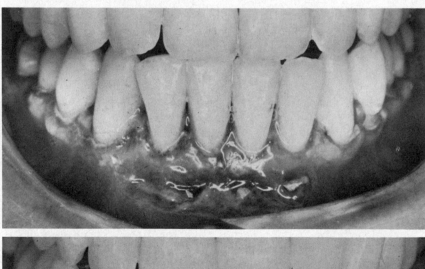
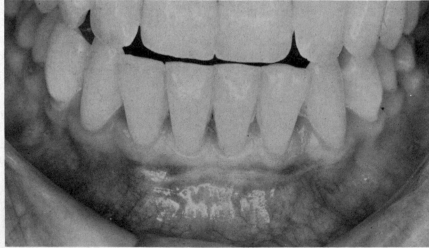

Figure 35–1 Excellent Healing Capacity of the Periodontium. *Above,* One week following periodontal surgery, after removal of periodontal dressing. *Below,* After 7 months, showing healed tissues and restoration of physiologic gingival contour.

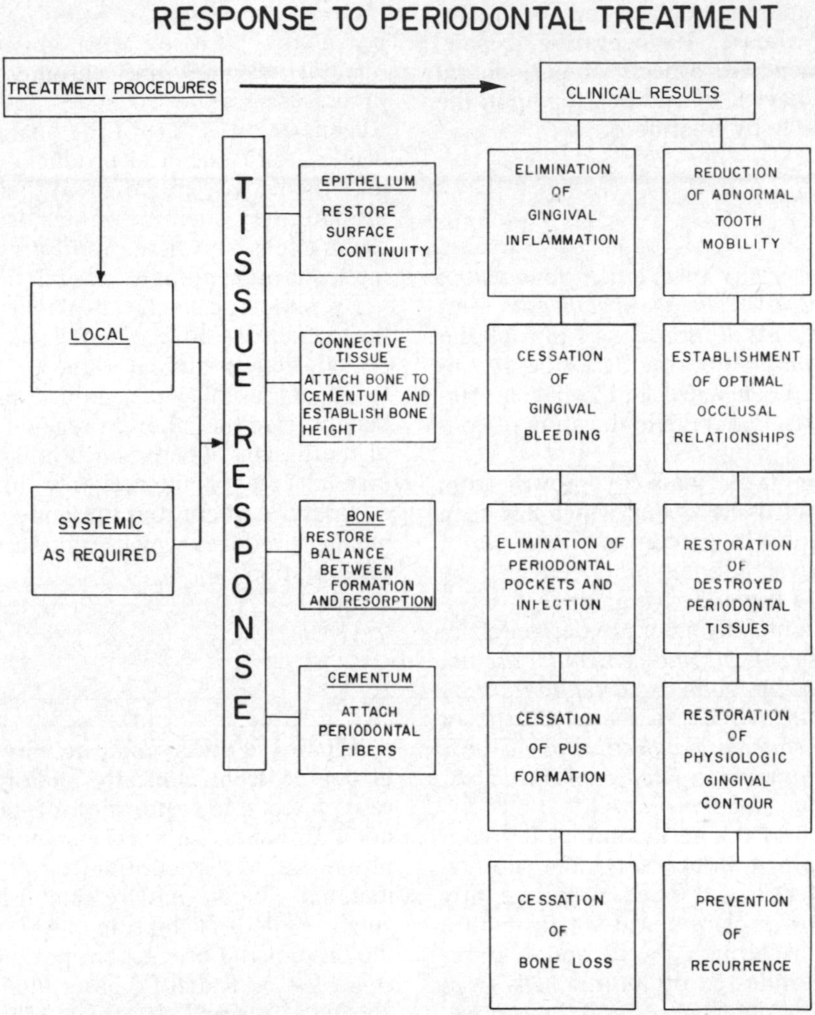

RESPONSE TO PERIODONTAL TREATMENT

TREATMENT PROCEDURES ──────────▶ CLINICAL RESULTS

TISSUE RESPONSE

LOCAL

SYSTEMIC
AS REQUIRED

EPITHELIUM
RESTORE
SURFACE
CONTINUITY

CONNECTIVE
TISSUE
ATTACH BONE TO
CEMENTUM AND
ESTABLISH BONE
HEIGHT

BONE
RESTORE
BALANCE
BETWEEN
FORMATION
AND RESORPTION

CEMENTUM
ATTACH
PERIODONTAL
FIBERS

ELIMINATION
OF
GINGIVAL
INFLAMMATION

CESSATION
OF
GINGIVAL
BLEEDING

ELIMINATION OF
PERIODONTAL
POCKETS AND
INFECTION

CESSATION
OF PUS
FORMATION

CESSATION
OF
BONE LOSS

REDUCTION
OF ABNORMAL
TOOTH
MOBILITY

ESTABLISHMENT
OF OPTIMAL
OCCLUSAL
RELATIONSHIPS

RESTORATION
OF
DESTROYED
PERIODONTAL
TISSUES

RESTORATION
OF
PHYSIOLOGIC
GINGIVAL
CONTOUR

PREVENTION
OF
RECURRENCE

Figure 35–2 Tissue Response and Clinical Results Following Periodontal Treatment.

lization of nutrients. Vitamin C deficiency[6, 71] delays healing by depressing collagen formation and altering the integrity of the capillary walls so that they are prone to rupture. Protein deficiency[64] retards healing by reducing the supply of sulfur-containing amino acids such as cystine and methionine. Healing is also retarded by vitamin A deficiency, by a fat-rich diet, and by overdose of vitamin D. The last causes necrosis and calcification in the arterioles of the granulation tissue.

Healing is affected by hormones. Systemically administered glucocorticoids such as cortisone hinder repair by depressing the inflammatory reaction or by inhibiting the growth of fibroblasts, the production of collagen, and the formation of endothelial cells. Systemic stress,[63] thyroidectomy, testosterone, adrenocorticotropic hormone (ACTH), and large doses of estrogen suppress the formation of granulation tissue and retard healing.[6] Proges-

terone increases and accelerates the vascularization of immature granulation tissue[30] and appears to increase the susceptibility of the gingiva to mechanical injury by causing dilatation of the marginal vessels.[22] Somatotropic hormone increases fibroplasia during gingival healing.[62]

Systemically administered antibiotics do not improve the epithelialization of gingival wounds in experimental animals,[65] nor do systemic antibiotics administered following gingivectomy in humans ("antibiotic umbrella") appear to prevent the occurrence of marked gingival inflammation.[68]

HEALING AFTER PERIODONTAL THERAPY

The basic healing processes are the same following all forms of periodontal therapy. They consist of the removal of degenerated tissue debris and the replacement of tissues destroyed by disease. **Regeneration, repair, and reattachment are aspects of periodontal healing which have a special bearing upon the results obtainable by treatment.**

Regeneration

Regeneration is the growth and differentiation of new cells and intercellular substances to form new tissues or parts. It consists of fibroplasia, endothelial proliferation, the deposition of interstitial ground substance and collagen, epithelial hyperplasia, and the maturation of connective tissue.

Regeneration takes place by growth from the same type of tissue as that which has been destroyed or from its precursor. In the periodontium, gingival epithelium is replaced by epithelium, and the underlying connective tissue and periodontal ligament are derived from connective tissue. *Bone and cementum are not replaced by existing bone or cementum but by connective tissue, which is the precursor of both. Undifferentiated connective tissue cells develop into osteoblasts and cementoblasts, which form bone and cementum.*

Regeneration of the periodontium is a continuous physiologic process. Under normal conditions new cells and tissues are constantly being formed to replace those which mature and die. This is termed "wear and tear repair."[27] It is manifested by mitotic activity in the epithelium of the gingiva[37] and the connective tissue of the periodontal ligament,[42] by the formation of new bone, and by the continuous deposition of cementum.

Regeneration is also going on during active periodontal disease. Most gingival and periodontal diseases are chronic inflammatory processes and, as such, are healing lesions. Regeneration is part of the healing. However, bacteria and bacterial products which perpetuate the disease process and the inflammatory exudate they elicit are injurious to the regenerating cells and tissues and prevent the healing from proceeding to completion.

By removing bacterial plaque and creating the conditions to prevent its new formation, periodontal treatment removes the obstacles to regeneration and enables the patient to benefit from the inherent regenerative capacity of the tissues. There is a brief spurt in regenerative activity immediately following periodontal treatment, but there are no local treatment procedures which promote or accelerate regeneration.

Repair

Repair is a microscopic activity which differs in degree from clinically and/or radiographically detectable restoration of destroyed periodontal tissues. In most instances, repair simply restores the continuity of the diseased marginal gingiva and re-establishes a normal gingival sulcus at the same level on the root as the base of the preexistent periodontal pocket (Fig. 35–3). Ratcliff[50] has called this process "healing by scar." It arrests bone destruction without necessarily increasing bone height. Restoration of the destroyed periodontium to a degree which is clinically and/or radiograph-

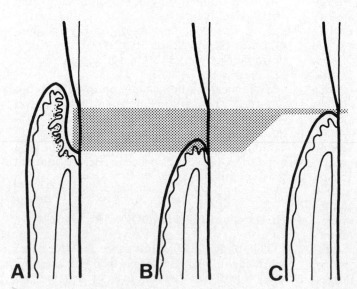

Figure 35–3 Two Possible Outcomes of Pocket Elimination. *A,* Periodontal pocket before treatment. *B,* Normal sulcus re-established at the level of the base of the pocket. *C,* Periodontium restored on the root surface previously denuded by disease. The latter is called reattachment. Shaded areas show denudation caused by periodontal disease.

ically detectable (see Fig. 35–6) occurs less frequently and is dependent upon reattachment.

Reattachment

Reattachment is the embedding of new periodontal ligament fibers into new cementum and the attachment of the gingival epithelium to a tooth surface previously denuded by disease (Fig. 35–3). The critical words in this definition are *"tooth surface previously denuded by disease"* (Fig. 35–4). Attachment of the gingiva or the periodontal ligament to areas of the tooth from which they may be removed in the course of treatment or during the preparation of teeth for restorations represents *simple healing* of the periodontium, not reattachment. The term *reattachment* has a unique usage in the periodontal field; it refers specifically to the restoration of the marginal periodontium, and not to repair of other areas of the root, such as that following traumatic tears in the cementum, tooth fractures, or the treatment of periapical lesions. Since it is not the

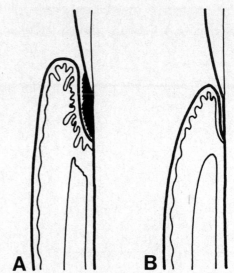

Figure 35–5 "Epithelial Adaptation" Following Periodontal Treatment. *A,* Periodontal pocket. *B,* After treatment. The pocket is closely adapted to, but not attached to, the root.

existing fibers that reattach but new fibers that are formed and attach to new cementum, there is a tendency to replace the term *reattachment* with *new attachment*. The two terms are used interchangeably in this text.

Epithelial adaptation is different from reattachment. The former is the close apposition of the gingival epithelium to the tooth surface without complete obliteration of the pocket.[4,28] The pocket space does not permit passage of a probe (Fig. 35–5). Although this may be a dangerous situation because bacteria could still penetrate the pocket, inducing further loss of attachment and even abscess formation, several clinical studies have shown that with an adequate maintenance phase of therapy these deep sulci lined by long, thin epithelium may be acceptable. The absence of bleeding or secretion upon probing, the absence of clinically visible inflammation, and the absence of stainable plaque on the root surface when the pocket wall is deflected from the tooth may indicate that the "deep sulcus" persists in an inactive state, causing no further loss of attachment.[7, 76] A posttherapy depth of 4 or even 5 mm may therefore be acceptable in these cases.

Opinions differ regarding the extent and conditions under which reattachment is attainable after periodontal treatment[29] (Fig. 35–6). It occurs more often following the treatment of infrabony pockets[8, 19, 20, 48, 73] than suprabony pockets,[29, 59, 72] except in patients with one-wall infrabony defects (for the treatment of infrabony pockets, see Chapter 54). It has been demonstrated histologically following the

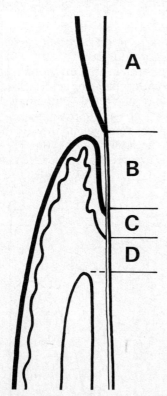

Figure 35–4 *A,* Enamel surface. *B,* Area of cementum denuded by pocket fomation. *C,* Area of cementum covered by junctional epithelium. *D,* Area of cementum apical to the junctional epithelium. The term "reattachment," or "new attachment," refers to a new junctional epithelium formed on zone B.

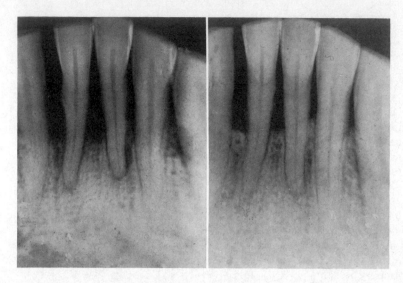

Figure 35–6 Bone Restored Following Periodontal Treatment. *Left,* Before treatment. *Right,* Five years later.

treatment of infrabony pockets,[1, 12, 58] but with suprabony pockets both positive[4, 16, 36, 56] and negative microscopic findings[26, 39] have been reported. Reattachment has been observed histologically in experimental animals following the healing of artificially created pockets[34, 35, 49] and marginal wounds[17, 57] and following the surgical removal of inflamed gingiva.

The following factors affect the likelihood of attaining reattachment:

REMOVAL OF THE JUNCTIONAL EPITHELIUM. Removal of the junctional epithelium in the treatment of deep suprabony and infrabony pockets increases the likelihood of obtaining reattachment. The posttreatment location of the junctional epithelium limits the height to which periodontal fibers become attached to the tooth. The level of attachment of the periodontal ligament in turn determines the maximum posttreatment height the bone can attain. *Leaving the junctional epithelium intact during periodontal treatment therefore automatically predetermines the posttreatment levels of the periodontal ligament and bone* (Fig. 35–7). *Removal of the junctional epithelium creates conditions in which connective tissue fibers could reattach to the tooth surface coronal to the pretreatment level* (Fig. 35–7) *and creates the potential for increased bone height and the repair of vertical defects.*

In the treatment of periodontal pockets, it cannot be determined by clinical examination whether the junctional epithelium has been completely removed. Some investigators report complete removal of the junctional epithelium,[39] the lateral epithelium.[2, 40] and some underlying inflamed connective tissue follow-

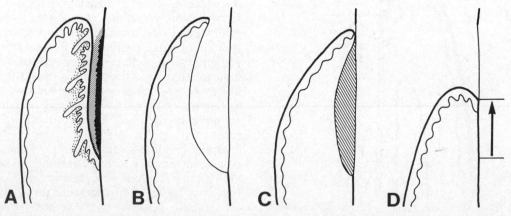

Figure 35–7 Removal of pocket epithelium and functional epithelium creates potential for post-treatment reattachment. *A,* Periodontal pocket. *B,* After scaling, root planing, and curettage. *C,* Blood clot formed between instrumented pocket wall and cementum surface. *D,* Reattachment has increased the height of gingival attachment.

ing gingival curettage, whereas others observe in situ remnants of the junctional epithelium and lateral epithelium.[56, 69, 72]

PREPARATION OF THE ROOT SURFACE. Changes in the tooth surface wall of periodontal pockets, such as the degeneration of remnants of Sharpey's fibers, accumulation of bacteria and their products, and disintegration of the cementum and dentin, interfere with reattachment. However, these obstacles to reattachment can be eliminated by thorough root planing.[24]

Several substances have been used in attempts to better condition the root surface for the attachment of new connective tissue fibers. They include the following:

Citric Acid. The acid demineralization of the root surface by means of citric acid has been extensively investigated in animals and humans. The following possible mechanisms for its action have been mentioned[15]: accelerating cementogenesis, widening dentinal tubules to allow for connective tissue ingress, exposing root dentinal collagen fibers, extracting endotoxin and other toxic plaque products, and inducing mesenchymal cell differentiation to osteoblasts or possibly cementoblasts. Studies in experimental animals have given encouraging results,[53, 54] especially for the treatment of furcation lesions,[11, 43, 44] but the results of studies in humans have been contradictory.[10, 52, 55, 67]

Fibronectin. This is the glycoprotein that fibroblasts require to attach to root surfaces. The addition of fibronectin to the root surface may promote reattachment.[13, 70] Clinical studies are not yet available.

Sodium Deoxycholate and Human Plasma Fraction Cohn IV. These agents can dissociate endotoxin into subunits and might thereby detoxify the diseased root surface. The human plasma fraction possibly contains fibronectin. Animal experiments using these agents have shown increased connective tissue attachment.[74, 75]

THE GRANULATION TISSUE. Granulation tissue adjacent to the pocket wall is removed to provide better visibility of and accessibility to the root surface. Its removal does not represent a sacrifice of tissue because it is replaced in the healing process.

THE CLOT. The clot forms the initial protective covering of the treated area. It is replaced by granulation tissue, which may extend up to the clot surface. The vascularity and bulk of the granulation tissue are reduced as it undergoes maturation to connective tissue. The height of the granulation tissue may affect the level at which the epithelium becomes attached to the root, because the proliferating epithelium is guided by the connective tissue surface along which it moves.

OTHER FACTORS. *Trauma from occlusion impairs posttreatment healing of the supporting periodontal tissues and reduces the likelihood of reattachment.* Widened periodontal spaces, angular bone defects, and tooth mobility often result when trauma persists during healing.

Reattachment is more likely to occur when the destructive process has been rapid, such as following the treatment of pockets complicated by the formation of acute periodontal abscesses and following the treatment of acute necrotizing ulcerative gingivitis.

The formation of new cementum and the embedding of periodontal ligament fibers can occur on the cementum and dentin of vital teeth; in nonvital teeth it can occur on cementum but is not likely to occur on exposed dentin.[40]

The likelihood of obtaining reattachment is increased by the elimination of infection and the correction of excessive tooth mobility.

Clinical techniques for reattachment are presented in Chapters 51 and 54.

REFERENCES

1. Beube, F. E.: A radiographic histologic study on reattachment. J. Periodontol., *23*:158, 1952.
2. Blass, J. L., and Lite, T.: Gingival healing following surgical curettage: a histopathologic study. N.Y. Dent. J., *25*:127, 1959.
3. Box, H. K.: Studies in periodontal pathology. Can. Dent. Res. Found. Bull. 7, May 1924, p. 75.
4. Box, H. K.: Treatment of the periodontal pocket. Toronto, University of Toronto Press, 1928, pp. 94, 105.
5. Butcher, E. O., and Klingsberg, J.: Age, gonadectomy, and wound healing in the palatal mucosa. J. Dent. Res., *40*:694, 1961.
6. Cabrini, R. L., and Carranza, F. A., Jr.: Adenosine triphosphatase in normal and scorbutic wounds. Nature, *200*:1113, 1963.
7. Caffesse, R. G., Ramfjord, S. P., and Nasjleti, C. E.: Reverse bevel periodontal flaps in monkeys. J. Periodontol., *39*:219, 1968.
8. Carranza, F. A., Sr.: A technique for treating infrabony pockets so as to obtain reattachment. Dent. Clin. North Am., *4*:75, 1960.
9. Cheraskin, E., et al.: Resistance and susceptibility to oral disease. II. A study in periodontometry and carbohydrate metabolism. Periodontics, *3*:296, 1965.
10. Cole, R., Nilveus, R., Ainamo, J., Bogle, G., Crigger, M., and Egelberg, J.: Pilot clinical studies on the effect of topical citric acid application on healing after replaced flap surgery. J. Periodont. Res., *16*:117, 1981.
11. Crigger, M., Bogle, G., Nilveus, R., Egelberg, J., and Selvig, K.: Effect of topical citric acid application in the healing of experimental furcation defects in dogs. J. Periodont. Res., *13*:538, 1978.
12. Cross, W. G.: Reattachment following curettage. A histological study. Dent. Pract., *7*:38, 1956.
13. Fernyhough, W., and Page, R. C.: Attachment, growth and synthesis of human gingival fibroblasts on demineralized or fibronectin-treated normal and diseased tooth roots. J. Periodontol., *54*:133, 1983.

14. Ferris, R. T.: Quantitative evaluation of tooth mobility following initial periodontal therapy. J. Periodontol., 37:190, 1966.
15. Fialkoff, B., and Fry, H. R.: Acid demineralization in periodontal therapy: a review of the literature. J. Western Soc. Periodontol., 30:52, 1982.
16. Fleming, W. E.: A clinical and microscopic study of periodontal tissues treated by instrumentation. Pac. Dent. Gazette, 24:568, 1926.
17. Glickman, I., and Lazansky, J. P.: Repair of the periodontium following gingivectomy in experimental animals. J. Dent. Res., 29:659, 1950 (abstract).
18. Glickman, I., Turesky, S. S., and Manhold, J.: The oxygen consumption of healing gingiva. J. Dent. Res., 29:429, 1950.
19. Goldman, H. M.: Subgingival curettage—a rationale. J. Periodontol., 19:54, 1948.
20. Gottlieb, B.: The new concept of periodontoclasia. J. Periodontol., 17:7, 1946.
21. Holm-Pedersen, P., and Löe, H.: Wound healing in the gingiva of young and old individuals. Scand. J. Dent. Res., 79:40, 1971.
22. Hugoson, A.: Gingival inflammation and female sex hormones. J. Periodont. Res., 5(Suppl.), 1970.
23. Itoiz, M. E., Cabrini, R. L., and Carranza, F. A., Jr.: Histochemical study of healing wounds: alkaline and acid phosphatase. J. Oral Surg., 27:641, 1969.
24. Jones, W. A., and O'Leary, T. J.: The effectiveness of "in vivo" root planing in removing bacterial endotoxin from the roots of periodontally involved teeth. J. Periodontol., 49:337, 1978.
25. Kantor, M., Polson, A. M., and Zander, H. A.: Alveolar bone regeneration after removal of inflammatory and traumatic factors. J. Periodontol., 47:687, 1976.
26. Kaplan, H., and Mann, J. B.: How is pyorrhea cured? J. Am. Dent. Assoc., 29:1471, 1942.
27. Leblond, C. P., and Walker, B. E.: Renewal of cell populations. Physiol. Rev., 36:255, 1956.
28. Leonard, H. J.: Conservative treatment of periodontoclasia. J. Am. Dent. Assoc., 26:1308, 1939.
29. Leonard, H. J.: In our opinion—reattachment. J. Periodontol., Suppl. to Jan., 1943, p. 5.
30. Lindhe, J., and Branemark, P. I.: The effect of sex hormones on vascularization of a granulation tissue. J. Periodont. Res., 3:6, 1968.
31. Lindhe, J., and Ericsson, I.: The influence of trauma from occlusion on reduced but healthy periodontal tissues in dogs. J. Clin. Periodontol., 3:110, 1976.
32. Lindhe, J., and Nyman, S.: The effect of plaque control and surgical pocket elimination on the establishment and maintenance of periodontal health. A longitudinal study of periodontal therapy in cases of advanced periodontal disease. J. Clin. Periodontol., 2:67, 1975.
33. Lindhe, J., Parodi, R., Liljenberg, B., and Fornell, J.: Clinical and structural alterations characterizing healing gingiva. J. Periodont. Res., 13:410, 1978.
34. Linghorne, W. J.: Studies in the reattachment and regeneration of the supporting structures of the teeth. IV. Regeneration in epithelialized pockets following the organization of a blood clot. J. Dent. Res., 36:4, 1957.
35. Linghorne, W. J., and O'Connell, D. C.: Studies in the reattachment and regeneration of the supporting structures of the teeth. II. Regeneration in epithelialized pockets. J. Dent. Res., 34:164, 1955.
36. McCall, J. O.: An improved method of inducing reattachment of the gingival tissues in periodontoclasia. Dent. Items Int., 48:342, 1926.
37. Meyer, J., Marwah, A. S., and Weinmann, J. P.: Mitotic rate of gingival epithelium in two age groups. J. Invest. Dermatol., 27:237, 1956.
38. Morris, M. L.: The removal of pocket and attachment epithelium in humans: a histological study. J. Periodontol., 25:57, 1954.
39. Morris, M. L.: Healing of naturally occurring periodontal pockets about vital human teeth. J. Periodontol., 26:285, 1955.
40. Morris, M. L.: Healing of human periodontal tissues following surgical detachment and extirpation of vital pulps. J. Periodontol., 31:23, 1960.
41. Moskow, B. S.: The response of the gingival sulcus to instrumentation. A histologic investigation. II. Gingival curettage. J. Periodontol., 35:112, 1964.

42. Mühlemann, H. R., Zander, H., and Halberg, F.: Mitotic activity in the periodontal tissues of the rat molar. J. Dent. Res., 33:459, 1954.
43. Nilveus, R., Johansson, O., and Egelberg, J.: The effect of autogenous cancellous bone grafts in healing in experimental furcation defects in dogs. J. Periodont. Res., 13:532, 1978.
44. Nilveus, R., Bogle, G., Crigger, M., Egelberg, J., and Selvig, K.: Effect of topical citric acid application in the healing of experimental furcation defects in dogs. 2. Healing after repeated surgery. J. Periodont. Res., 15:544, 1980.
45. Oliver, R. C.: Tooth loss with and without periodontal therapy. Periodont. Abstracts, 17:8, 1969.
46. Perez-Tamayo, R.: Mechanisms of Disease and Introduction to Pathology. Philadelphia, W. B. Saunders Company, 1961, p. 105.
47. Polson, A. M.: Interrelationship of inflammation and tooth mobility (trauma) in pathogenesis of periodontal disease. J. Clin. Periodontol., 7:351, 1980.
48. Prichard, J.: The infrabony technique as a predictable procedure. J. Periodontol., 28:202, 1957.
49. Ramfjord, S. P.: Experimental periodontal reattachment in Rhesus monkeys. J. Periodontol., 22:67, 1951.
50. Ratcliff, P. A.: An analysis of repair systems in periodontal therapy. Periodont. Abstracts, 14:57, 1966.
51. Rateitschak, K.: The therapeutic effect of local treatment on periodontal disease assessed upon evaluation of different diagnostic criteria. 2. Changes in gingival inflammation. J. Periodontol., 35:155, 1964.
52. Rateitschak, K., et al.: The therapeutic effect of local treatment on periodontal disease assessed upon evaluation of different diagnostic criteria. 3. Radiographic changes in appearance of bone. J. Periodontol., 35:263, 1964.
53. Register, A. A., and Burdick, F. A.: Accelerated reattachment with cementogenesis to dentin, demineralized in situ. 1. Optimum range. J. Periodontol., 46:646, 1975.
54. Register, A. S., and Burdick, F. A.: Accelerated reattachment with cementogenesis to dentin, demineralized in situ. 2. Defect repair. J. Periodontol., 47:497, 1976.
55. Renvert, S., and Egelberg, J.: Healing after treatment of periodontal intraosseous defects. II. Effect of citric acid conditioning of the root surface. J. Clin. Periodontol., 8:459, 1981.
56. Sato, M.: Histopathological study of the healing process after surgical treatment for alveolar pyorrhea. Bull. Tokyo Med. Dent. Univ., 1:71, 1960.
57. Schaffer, E. M., and Korn, N. A.: Comparison of curettage and gingivectomy in dogs. I.A.D.R. Abstracts, 40:69, 1962.
58. Schaffer, E. M., and Zander, H.: Histological evidence of reattachment of periodontal pockets. Paradentologie, 7:101, 1953.
59. Shapiro, M.: Reattachment in periodontal disease. J. Periodontol., 24:26, 1953.
60. Skillen, W. G., and Lundquist, G. R.: Experimental gingival injuries in dogs. J. Dent. Res., 15:165, 1935.
61. Skillen, W. G., and Lundquist, G. R.: An experimental study of peridental membrane reattachment in healthy and pathologic tissues. J. Am. Dent. Assoc., 24:175, 1937.
62. Stahl, S. S.: Effect of oral somatotrophic hormone injections upon gingival wounds in rats. J. Dent. Res., 38:725, 1959 (abstract).
63. Stahl, S. S.: Healing gingival injury in normal and systemically stressed young adult male rats. J. Periodontol., 32:63, 1961.
64. Stahl, S. S.: The effect of a protein-free diet on the healing of gingival wounds in rats. Arch. Oral Biol., 7:551, 1962.
65. Stahl, S. S.: The influence of antibiotics on the healing of gingival wounds in rats. I. Alveolar bone and soft tissue. J. Periodontol., 33:261, 1962.
66. Stahl, S. S.: Healing of gingival tissues following various therapeutic regimens—a review of histologic studies. J. Oral Therap. Pharmacol., 2:145, 1965.
67. Stahl, S., and Froum, S.: Human clinical and histologic repair responses following the use of citric acid in periodontal therapy. J. Periodontol., 48:261, 1977.
68. Stahl, S. S., Soberman, A., and DeCesare, A.: Gingival healing. V. The effects of antibiotics administered during early stages of repair. J. Periodontol., 40:521, 1969.
69. Stone, S., Ramfjord, S., and Waldron, J.: Scaling and gingival curettage. A radioautographic study. J. Periodontol., 37:415, 1966.

70. Terranova, V. P., and Martin, G. R.: Molecular factors determining gingival tissue interaction with tooth structure. J. Periodont. Res., *17*:530, 1982.

71. Turesky, S. S., and Glickman, I.: Histochemical evaluation of gingival healing in experimental animals on adequate and vitamin C deficient diets. J. Dent. Res., *33*:273, 1954.

72. Waerhaug, J.: Microscopic demonstration of tissue reaction incident to removal of subgingival calculus. J. Periodontol., *26*:26, 1955.

73. Williams, C. H. M.: Rationalization of periodontal pocket therapy. J. Periodontol., *14*:67, 1943.

74. Wirthlin, M. R., and Hancock, E. B.: Biologic preparation of diseased root surfaces. J. Periodontol., *51*:291, 1980.

75. Wirthlin, M. R., Hancock, E. B., and Gangler, R. W.: Regeneration and repair after biologic treatment of root surfaces in monkeys. I. Facial surfaces, maxillary incisors. J. Periodontol., *52*:729, 1981.

76. Yukna, R. A.: A clinical and histologic study of healing following the excisional new attachment procedure in Rhesus monkeys. J. Periodontol., *47*:701, 1976.

chapter thirty-six

Periodontal Treatment for Medically Compromised Patients

Cardiovascular Diseases	Parathyroid Disorders
Angina Pectoris	Adrenal Insufficiency
Arterial Bypass	Pregnancy
Cerebrovascular Accident	**Hemorrhagic Disorders**
Congestive Heart Failure	Coagulation Disorders
Hypertension	Thrombocytopenic Purpuras
Cardiac Pacemakers	Nonthrombocytopenic Purpuras
Infective (Bacterial) Endocarditis	**Blood Dyscrasias**
Renal Diseases	Leukemia
Pulmonary Diseases	Agranulocytosis
Immunosuppression and Chemotherapy	**Infectious Diseases**
Radiotherapy	Hepatitis
Endocrine Disorders	Sexually Transmitted Diseases
Diabetes	Tuberculosis
Thyroid Disorders	

Improvements in lifestyles, habits, and medical care have enhanced human longevity. They have also led to the creation of a population with chronic health problems that may require special precautions in dental therapy. The age range of the average periodontal patient increases the likelihood of underlying disease. Therefore, *our therapeutic responsibility includes identification of patients' medical problems in order to formulate proper treatment plans.*

Thorough medical histories are paramount. If significant findings are unveiled, consultation with or referral of the patient to an appropriate physician is required. Not only is the patient then correctly managed, but the clinician is covered medicolegally as well.

This chapter deals with some common medical problems and associated periodontal management. Understanding these problems will enable the clinician to treat the total patient, not merely the periodontal reflection of underlying disease. Because the coverage of the subject here is necessarily very general, the reader is urged to consult other texts regarding specific diseases.

CARDIOVASCULAR DISEASES

Health histories should be closely scrutinized for cardiovascular problems because an estimated 30 million Americans are affected by them. The following conditions may be de-

tected, and the periodontal treatment plan must be adjusted accordingly: history of angina pectoris, myocardial infarction, cerebrovascular accident or transient ischemic attacks, cardiac bypass surgery, and congestive heart failure. In most cases the patient's cardiologist should be consulted, and the following precautions should be taken to avoid stress: (1) schedule morning appointments, (2) maintain an open, concerned atmosphere during treatment, and (3) keep appointments short.

Angina Pectoris

Patients with a history of unstable angina pectoris (angina that occurs irregularly or on multiple occasions without predisposing factors) should be treated for emergencies only. Patients with stable angina (that which occurs infrequently, is associated with exertion or stress, and is easily controlled with medication and rest) can undergo elective dental procedures if the following precautions are taken:

1. Premedication as needed (diazepam [valium], nitrous oxide–oxygen, or a short-acting barbiturate such as pentobarbital [30 to 60 mg] or secobarbital [60 to 100 mg][13, 85]).
2. Adequate anesthesia (aspirate frequently and inject slowly).
3. Nitroglycerin premedication sublingually (1/200 grain) 5 minutes prior to a procedure that the patient feels is stressful.

The patient's medication (generally nitroglycerin) should be readily accessible on the dental tray. Also, note the date of the patient's nitroglycerin (which expires within a year), as well as the date of that in the office's emergency medical kit. If, during a periodontal procedure, the patient becomes fatigued or uncomfortable or has a sudden change in heart rhythm or rate, the procedure should be discontinued as soon as possible.

A patient who has an anginal episode in the dental chair should receive the following emergency medical treatment:

1. Discontinue the periodontal procedure.
2. Administer one tablet (0.3 to 0.6 mg) of nitroglycerin sublingually.
3. Reassure the patient.
4. Loosen restrictive garments.
5. Administer oxygen with the patient in a reclining position.
6. If the signs and symptoms cease within 3 minutes, complete the periodontal procedure if possible, making sure that the patient is comfortable. Terminate the procedure at the earliest convenient time.

If the anginal signs and symptoms do not resolve with this treatment within 2 to 3 minutes administer another dose of nitroglycerin, monitor the patient's vital signs, call his or her physician, and be ready to accompany the patient to the emergency room.

Arterial Bypass

Cardiac (aortocoronary) bypass, femoral artery bypass, and thromboendarterectomy have become common surgical procedures. The physician should be consulted prior to elective dental therapy if these procedures were performed recently. Although there has not been a statement regarding dental treatment of the bypass patient, it is advised that elective therapy *not* be performed until 6 months post bypass. Whether prophylactic antibiotics should be given to cardiac bypass and myocardial infarction patients has not yet been determined. Once again, the cardiologist should inform the dentist regarding the degree of heart damage or arterial occlusive disease, the stability of the patient's condition, and the potential for infective endocarditis or graft rejection. Patients who have had synthetic patches (e.g., Dacron) have an increased risk of bacterial colonization because of the surface discrepancies between normal arterial intima and the so-called prosthetic pseudointima.[52]

Cerebrovascular Accident

A cerebrovascular accident (CVA) occurs as a result of ischemic changes (e.g., cerebral thrombosis due to an embolus) or hemorrhagic phenomena. Hypertension and arteriosclerosis are predisposing factors to a CVA, and they should alert the clinician to evaluate the patient's medical history carefully for the possibility of early cerebrovascular insufficiency and to be aware of symptoms of the disease. A physician's referral should precede periodontal therapy if the signs and symptoms of early cerebrovascular insufficiency are evident.

Patients who are seen after a stroke should be treated following these guidelines:

1. No periodontal therapy (unless emergent) should be performed for 6 months because of the high risk of recurrence during this period.
2. After 6 months, periodontal therapy may be performed during short (maximum of 60 minutes), atraumatic appointments.
3. Mild sedation should be used only if the patient is extremely excitable or nervous.[57] General anesthetics and oversedation are contraindicated because of the impaired cerebral circulation. Malamed suggests using light levels of nitrous oxide–oxygen to reduce stress.[56]
4. Local anesthetics may be utilized with caution: aspirate, then inject slowly and carefully (not intravascularly). Epinephrine (1:100,000) may be used (maximum of 3 to 5 Carpules, depending upon the patient's age and weight).
5. Be aware that many poststroke patients have been placed on anticoagulant therapy. If this is the case
   a. Check prothrombin time prior to deep scaling or periodontal surgery
   b. Consult with the patient's physician to adjust the prothrombin time to not greater than 1.5 times normal
   c. Remember that anticoagulants have known interactions with other drugs, including those used in dental practice.
6. Monitor blood pressure carefully, for the post-CVA patient represents an "accident waiting to happen." Recurrence rates of CVAs are high, as are rates of associated functional deficits.
7. Know what to do in case of a recurrent CVA[56, 57]
   a. Know the signs and symptoms of a CVA
   b. Terminate the dental treatment

c. Make the patient comfortable in an upright position, if conscious
d. Loosen restrictive garments
e. Give oxygen only if respiratory difficulty develops
f. Monitor vital signs
g. Summon medical assistance
h. If the patient becomes unconscious, perform basic life support procedures, and place the patient in the supine position if cardiopulmonary resuscitation (CPR) is needed; the head should be elevated slightly if CPR is not required
i. Do not give medicines that elicit depression of the central nervous system.

Congestive Heart Failure

Congestive heart failure (CHF) begins with left ventricular failure caused by a "disproportion between the hemodynamic load and the capacity to handle the load."[54] It may be due to a chronic increase in workload (e.g., in hypertension or aortic, mitral, pulmonary, or tricuspid valvular disease), to direct damage to the myocardium (e.g., in myocardial infarction or rheumatic fever), or to an increase in the body's oxygen requirements (e.g., in anemia, thyrotoxicosis, or pregnancy). Left ventricular failure is related to pulmonary vascular congestion.

Patients with untreated congestive heart failure are not candidates for elective dental procedures. For patients with treated congestive heart failure, the clinician should consult with the physician regarding:

I. Medications
   A. Digitalis
      1. Watch for a tendency toward nausea and/or vomiting
      2. Watch for increased susceptibility to dysrhythmia
   B. Diuretics
      1. Watch for susceptibility to orthostatic hypotension
      2. Know the side effects of the prescribed diuretic
   C. Dicumarol: Prothrombin time should be 1.5 times normal (adjust with the physician)
   D. Analgesics: May increase prothrombin time
II. Degree of control of medical problem
III. Etiology of the disease process
IV. Presence of or potential for polycythemia, thrombocytopenia, or leukopenia in compensation for inadequate oxygen in the arterial system
   A. May require antibiotic coverage if the white blood cell count is low
   B. Potential for bleeding problems
   C. Do not dehydrate the patient
   D. Procedures should be shorter
   E. Do not place the patient in a flat reclining position
   F. Supplemental oxygen administration by nasal cannulas may be utilized
   G. Stress reduction should be emphasized; if the patient becomes fatigued or dyspneic, treatment should not begin or the procedure should be discontinued at the first opportune moment
   H. No saline rinses, owing to sodium absorption
   I. Understand the treatment steps for active developing CHF
      1. Administer oxygen 100 per cent by full face mask
      2. Position the patient sitting upright
      3. Record vital signs
      4. Apply rotating tourniquets high on the four extremities; this is a bloodless phlebotomy which will reduce the total circulating blood volume; release the tourniquets one at a time for 5 minutes every 30 minutes
      5. Reduce the patient's apprehension
      6. Call for medical assistance

Hypertension

At least one of every nine adults in the United States has hypertensive disease, which is defined as blood pressure elevated to 140/90 mm Hg or greater. Half of this population has not yet been diagnosed.[46, 70, 80] Of the 24 million people in the United States with hypertension, 21 million cases are undetected, untreated, or inadequately treated.[40, 96] The incidence among American black adults is estimated to be as high as 17 to 25 per cent.[70, 80] Therefore, the likelihood of encountering a patient with hypertensive disease in a dental practice occurs daily; it is even greater in a periodontal practice because of the observed increase in blood pressure levels with age.

Hypertension is divided into primary and secondary types. **Primary (essential) hypertension** occurs when no underlying pathologic abnormality can be found to explain the disease.[116] Approximately 70 to 90 per cent of all hypertension is essential. The remaining 10 to

30 per cent of hypertensives are **"secondary hypertensives,"** in whom an underlying etiology can be found and for whom surgical treatment may be possible. Examples of the conditions responsible for secondary hypertension are renal disease (e.g., polynephritis, polycystic disease of the kidney, and acute and chronic glomerulonephritis), endocrinologic changes (e.g., acromegaly, pheochromocytoma, adrenocortical hyperfunction, thyrotoxicosis, and pregnancy), and neurogenic disorders (e.g., tumors, CVAs, poliomyelitis, and psychogenic disorders).

The epidemiologic data demonstrate a graded relation between high blood pressure and a person's risk of subsequently developing a CVA, cardiac arrest, blindness, or renal failure. A Veterans Administration cooperative study indicates that, over a 5-year period, major complications from hypertension may be reduced from 55 to 18 per cent by treatment.[105] *The dental office may play a vital role in the detection and maintenance care of the patient with hypertensive disease.*[50, 60]

The periodontal recall system is an ideal method for hypertension detection. The first visit should include two blood pressure readings which are averaged and utilized as a baseline. Before referring a patient to a physician because of an elevated blood pressure, readings should be taken at a minimum of two appointments, unless the measurements are extremely high (i.e., diastolic pressure greater than 115 mm Hg). Also, in order to decide whether emergent changes in an individual's blood pressure are occurring, that particular patient's baseline levels must already have

been established. Periodontal procedures should not commence until accurate blood pressure measurements and a history have been taken to identify those patients with significant hypertensive disease. Note that patient position, cuff size, and sphygmomanometer calibration must be accurate. It should be noted that normal blood pressure increases from 70/45 mm Hg in infancy to 80/55 in early childhood and 100/75 in adolescence. In one third of the population, a transient increase in blood pressure may occur in early adulthood; an increase is the usual finding after age 60.[54]

The Joint National Committee on Detection, Evaluation, and Treatment of High Blood Pressure[61] has recommended the protocol shown in Figure 36–1 for evaluation and courses of action, depending upon the individual's initial blood pressure measurements. In addition, all adults with systolic blood pressures greater than 160 mm Hg should be advised to have their blood pressure rechecked.

If a patient is currently receiving hypertension therapy, consult his or her physician regarding current medical status, medications, the periodontal treatment plan, and patient management. Many physicians are not knowledgeable about the nature of specific periodontal procedures. It will be up to you to inform the physician regarding the stress, blood loss, length of the procedure, and complexity of the individualized treatment plan. Note that oral vascular changes have also been observed with hypertension.[17, 71, 73, 94, 95, 113] Saline rinses are contraindicated.

No periodontal treatment should be given to a patient who is hypertensive and not under

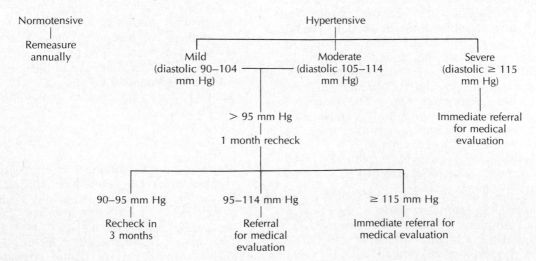

Figure 36–1 Protocol for evaluation and treatment of hypertension. (Note: Readings are determined by averaging two separate measurements.) (From Moser, M., et al.: J.A.M.A., 237:255, 1977.)

medical management. If the periodontal problem is an emergency, the treatment should be conservative (antibiotics and/or analgesics). Surgical procedures should be avoided because of the potential for excessive bleeding.

In treating hypertensive patients, one should not use a local anesthetic containing an epinephrine concentration greater than 1:100,000. Nor should a vasopressor to control local bleeding be utilized. Local anesthesia without epinephrine may be utilized for short procedures (less than 30 minutes). In a patient with hypertensive disease, however, it is important to reduce or eliminate pain by utilization of a local anesthetic to avoid an outpouring of endogenous epinephrine. Therefore, dosages should be titrated to be minimal, but should be adequate for pain control and stress minimization.

One should also be aware of the many side effects of the various antihypertensive medications. Depression is a common side effect of which many patients are unaware. Episodes of postural hypotension with or without syncope can be reduced by eliminating sudden positional changes in the dental chair. The chair should be slowly elevated to an upright position; then the patient should be allowed a few minutes to adjust to this position prior to standing up. One should also be aware of nausea secondary to antihypertensive medications.

Cardiac Pacemakers

Cardiac pacemakers are sustaining life for over 1 million patients in the United States today.[100] Since the first pacemaker was implanted in 1958, it has become apparent that particular attention must be paid to postimplantation patients in the dental environment.

Despite the lack of a definitive protocol for handling the pacemaker patient, there are precautions that should be utilized to enhance dental environmental safety. The clinician is medicolegally responsible for recognizing electrophysiologic problems attendant upon implantation of electronic circuits.[24]

These guidelines should be followed in treating patients with cardiac pacemakers:

1. *Health history:* A question should be included regarding pacemaker placement; if an affirmative response is given, further questioning should determine[20, 36, 66, 67, 69, 104]
   a. Location of the pacemaker
   b. Date of pacemaker placement
   c. Type of pacemaker
   d. Type of pacemaker electrode
   e. Reason for pacemaker placement (rule out the need for antibiotic prophylaxis)
   f. Level of pacemaker dependency
   g. Pulse rate setting.
2. *Consultation:* The patient's cardiologist should be consulted about the proposed periodontal treatment plan, the associated risks, the precautionary measures that should be taken, and the underlying cardiac reason for pacing.
3. *Positioning:* The patient should be positioned so as to minimize discomfort from strain on the lead wires or on the implant site. Shielding is best provided via a screen that acts as a Faraday cage to deflect electromagnetic forces. A lead shield may supplement this screen; however, pressure should be minimized over the area of the pacemaker apparatus. Positioning of the patients should be determined by their level of comfort. Some feel that a completely supine position could create breathing difficulties; these patients may be more comfortable in the semirecumbent position. Many patients do not find this to be a problem. (You may determine this by asking how many pillows the patient requires to sleep at night, then adjust the chair accordingly.)
4. *Leakage check:* All line-powered devices which come into contact with the patient should be measured for leakage. Any source of leakage greater than 10 microamperes can potentially interfere with pacemaker function.[75]
5. *Grounding:* All electrically powered dental equipment should be earth grounded.[66] Water pipe grounding is sufficient only if the pipe is not made of polyvinylchloride (PVC). Most cold water pipes are combinations of PVC and metal and thus are not sufficiently grounded because of PVC's capacity to interrupt current and eliminate the ground.
6. *Distance:* Try to keep all electrical equipment at least 1 foot (30 cm) from the patient.[75]
7. *Monitoring:* Continuous electrocardiographic monitoring should be utilized for all cardiac pacemaker patients. Variances in rhythm, rate, and wave form may signal impending complications.
8. *Limited use of electrical equipment:* Once again, many forms of dental equipment which apply an electrical current directly to

the patient may interfere with artificial pacemakers (e.g., ultrasonic and electrosurgical devices).[58, 68, 91, 108, 115] This external electromagnetic energy may mimic ventricular depolarization of the heart, thus inhibiting the pacemaker. Most pacemakers today, however, are adequately shielded to prevent the aforementioned changes in pacing.

Infective (Bacterial) Endocarditis

Bacterial endocarditis (BE) is a disease in which infective microorganisms colonize the damaged endocardium or heart valves. Although the incidence of BE is low (it occurs in approximately 1 per cent of all cardiac disorders[30, 53, 59, 72]), it is a serious disease with a poor prognosis despite modern therapy. BE has been divided into acute and subacute forms. The **acute form** involves virulent organisms, generally nonhemolytic streptococci and strains of staphylococci, which invade normal cardiac tissues, produce septic emboli, and run a rapid, generally fatal, course. The **subacute form,** on the other hand, occurs owing to colony formation on the damaged endocardium or heart valves by low-grade pathogenic organisms (the classic example is rheumatic carditis consequent to rheumatic fever). The organisms most commonly encountered in subacute BE are the alpha-hemolytic streptococci (e.g., *Streptococcus viridans*)[55] (Fig. 36–2).

Within the past few years it has been found that the original concept of bacterial endocarditis is changing.[28, 106, 112] Causative organisms and susceptible populations have been described that deviate from the original beliefs about the disease. Because of the isolation of fungi or viruses in infected tissues of patients with BE, many experts prefer to use the term "infective endocarditis" to describe the disease, rather than "bacterial endocarditis," which seems to imply a bacterial cause. The most susceptible population is people over 50,[99] owing to the increased occurrence of arteriosclerotic cardiovascular disease and open heart surgery in older people. Those defined as *highly susceptible* have a high risk of contracting BE subsequent to dental treatment, and the consequences of the disease are likely to be serious. This group includes people with a history of infective endocarditis and/or those with prosthetic heart valves.

Those defined as *susceptible* are people at risk for BE following dental treatment because they have congenital heart disease, rheumatic or other acquired valvular heart disease, idiopathic hypertrophic subaortic stenosis, a history of prosthetic or vascular repair surgery, a history of luetic heart disease, calcified aortic stenosis, calcified mitral anulus, mitral valve prolapse syndrome, or mitral insufficiency; this group also includes patients with permanent transvenous pacemakers and those addicted to drugs administered intravenously.[93]

The practice of periodontics is intimately concerned with the prevention of infective endocarditis. The American Heart Association Committee Report of June, 1977, states that "patients at risk to develop infective endocarditis should maintain the highest level of oral health to reduce potential sources of bacterial

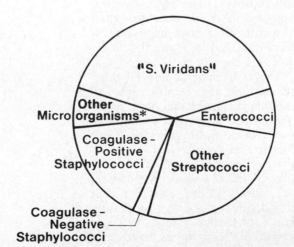

Figure 36–2 Infective endocarditis—implicated causative microorganisms.

*Mainly enteric gram-negative bacilli, fungi, pneumococci, diphtheroids, and H. influenzae.

seeding. Even in the absence of dental procedures poor dental hygiene or other dental diseases such as periodontal or periapical infections may induce bacteremia."[43] *The report recommended antibiotic prophylaxis for all dental procedures that are likely to cause gingival bleeding.* This includes almost all periodontal treatment procedures. In order to provide adequate preventive measures for BE, our major concern should be to reduce the microbial population in the oral cavity so as to minimize soft tissue inflammation and bacteremia.[78] Studies have confirmed that patients with periodontal disease have a greater and more frequent bacteremia than those without periodontal disease.[44, 55]

Preventive measures related to BE should consist of the following:

1. *Define the susceptible patient.* A careful medical history will disclose the aforementioned susceptible patients. Health questioning should cover rheumatic fever, rheumatic heart disease, cardiac murmurs, congenital heart defects, cardiac surgery, prosthetic heart valves, luetic heart disease, indwelling arteriovenous (A-V) shunts, ventriculoatrial shunts, and transvenous pacemakers. If in doubt, the patient's physician should be consulted.

2. *Oral hygiene instruction* should begin with gentle procedures, i.e., oral rinses and gentle toothbrushing with a soft brush. No antibiotic coverage for this procedure has been deemed necessary as yet. Of course, the bacteremia caused by oral hygiene procedures is dependent upon the degree of periodontal tissue inflammation. As the gingival health improves, more aggressive oral hygiene may be initiated. Because dental irrigation devices have been implicated in association with BE, their use should be discouraged in the susceptible population.[23, 42, 101] Oral hygiene should be practiced with methods that improve gingival health yet minimize bacteremia. Susceptible patients should be encouraged to maintain the highest level of oral hygiene once soft tissue inflammation is controlled.

3. *Currently recommended antibiotic prophylactic regimens should be practiced with all susceptible patients* (Table 36–1).[2, 21, 27] If there is any doubt regarding susceptibility, the patient's physician should be consulted.[44] Note that if patients have been receiving continuous oral penicillin for secondary prevention of rheumatic fever, penicillin-resistant alpha-hemolytic streptococci are occasionally found in the oral cavity. It

TABLE 36–1 PROPHYLAXIS OF INFECTIVE ENDOCARDITIS: ANTIBIOTIC REGIMENS FOR DENTAL PROCEDURES

Regimen A (Congenital Heart Disease, Rheumatic Heart Disease or Other Valvular Heart Disease, Idiopathic Hypertrophic Subaortic Stenosis, and Mitral Valve Prolapse)

1. Parenteral penicillin plus oral penicillin
   Adults: Aqueous crystalline penicillin G 1,000,000 units mixed with procaine penicillin G 600,000 units IM 30 minutes to 1 hour before the procedure; then penicillin V 500 mg orally every 6 hours for eight doses.
   Children: Aqueous crystalline penicillin G 30,000 units/kg mixed with procaine penicillin G 600,000 units IM; then penicillin V 500 mg (250 mg for children weighing less than 27 kg) orally every 6 hours for eight doses.

or

2. Oral penicillin
   Adults: Penicillin V 2.0 gm orally 30 minutes to 1 hour before the procedure; then 500 mg orally every 6 hours for eight doses.
   Children: For children weighing less than 27 kg, use 1.0 mg orally; then 250 mg orally every 6 hours for eight doses. (For children weighing over 27 kg, use adult doses.)

3. For patients allergic to penicillin, use either vancomycin (see Regimen B), *or*
   Adults: Erythromycin 1.0 gm orally 1–2 hours before the procedure; then 500 mg orally every 6 hours for eight doses.
   Children: Erythromycin 20 mg/kg orally; then 10 mg/kg every 6 hours for eight doses.

Regimen B (Prosthetic Heart Valves)

1. For patients not allergic to penicillin
   Adults: Aqueous crystalline penicillin G 1,000,000 units mixed with procaine penicillin G 600,000 units IM

   plus

   Streptomycin 1 gm IM 30 minutes to 1 hour before the procedure; then penicillin V 500 mg orally every 6 hours for eight doses.
   Children: Aqueous crystalline penicillin G 30,000 units/kg mixed with procaine penicillin G 600,000 units IM

   plus

   Streptomycin 20 mg/kg IM; then penicillin V 250 mg every 6 hours for eight doses.

   or

2. For patients allergic to penicillin
   Adults: Vancomycin 0.5–1.0 gm IV infused slowly over 1 hour before the procedure; then erythromycin 500 mg orally every 6 hours for eight doses.

is recommended, therefore, that regimen A (erythromycin) be followed instead (see Table 36–1). *Actinobacillus actinomycetemcomitans* has been found with increasing frequency in infective endocarditis[34] and is present in high numbers in periodontal pockets and tissues of patients with localized juvenile periodontitis (see Chapters 21 and 25). This organism is resistant to penicillin and to erythromycin but disappears from plaque samples for several weeks after tetracycline therapy (see Chapter 46). Therefore, Slots and co-workers[92] have suggested the following prophylactic regime for endocarditis-susceptible patients with localized juvenile periodontitis: first, systemic tetracycline, 250 mg four times daily for 14 days; second, conventional prophylactic protocol during the time of dental treatment.

4. *Periodontal treatment should be designed for susceptible patients to accommodate their particular degree of periodontal involvement.* The nature of periodontal therapy enhances the problems relating to the prophylaxis of subacute BE. We are faced with long-term therapy, healing periods that extend beyond a 3-day antibiotic regimen, multiple visits, and procedures that easily elicit gingival bleeding. The following guidelines should aid in the development of periodontal treatment planning for the patient susceptible to subacute BE:

   a. All periodontal treatment procedures (including probing) require antibiotic prophylaxis. Gentle oral hygiene methods are excluded from this prescription.

   b. In cases of delayed healing, it is prudent to provide additional doses of antibiotics. Also, periodontal suture removal may be performed more safely by extending antibiotic coverage to the fifth or sixth postoperative day or by placing resorbable sutures.

   c. Little and Falace recommend a concentrated 5- to 7-day oral hygiene/gross débridement program with antibiotic coverage.[54] If the patients do not seem able or willing to maintain oral hygiene, these authors feel that dentures should be considered. A similar recommendation was made regarding penicillin-allergic patients with diseased heart valves unless they are receiving in-hospital dental care. (Note, however, that edentulousness does not eliminate the risk of BE. Ulcerations from ill-fitting dentures have been associated with subacute BE.[64,83,99])

The severity of periodontal involvement should also influence decisions about edentulation.

   d. Dental extraction should be avoided in healthy mouths whenever possible. Endodontic therapy is the treatment of choice. Also, single extractions are preferred to multiple extractions.[55, 63]

   e. Severe periodontal disease and areas of periodontal suppuration or dental focus of infection require elimination.[48, 93]

   f. Avoid prolonged impingement on the gingival tissues, as with ligatures or tissue retractors. This would increase the opportunity for bacteremia.

   g. A 3-day antibiotic coverage should be used, with 10 to 14 days elapsing before starting a new coverage period if one is needed.[53, 103] An alternative, equally acceptable approach would be to rotate different antibiotics to minimize the emergence of resistant strains.

   h. Prior to surgical procedures, the gingival tissues should be cleansed. Several authors feel that antiseptics such as 1 to 5 per cent topical iodine should be applied preoperatively.[11, 55]

   i. All elective dental procedures should be postponed until the periodontal tissues approximate periodontal health. Rheumatic heart disease patients with recommended antibiotic coverage and no evidence of congestive heart failure may then receive any indicated dental treatment.

   j. Regular recall appointments, with an emphasis on oral hygiene reinforcement and the maintenance of periodontal health, are extremely important in this population.

Some authors recommend light scaling of a few teeth per appointment as preferable to heavy scaling. Also, electrosurgery or cryosurgery[55, 63] is thought by some authors to be preferable to gingivectomy with surgical blades. Further research is required to provide support for these recommendations.

Until more definitive information is available on prophylaxis of subacute bacterial endocarditis, it is better to err on the side of safety rather than the reverse.[102]

RENAL DISEASES

Eight million people in the United States are afflicted with some form of renal disease[38];

the most common causes of renal failure are glomerulonephritis, pyelonephritis, polycystic kidney disease, renovascular disease, drug nephropathy, obstructive uropathy, and hypertension.[29, 54] Because the dental management of the patient with renal failure is drastically altered, physician consultation is necessary in order to determine the stage of renal failure and the modality of the medical treatment prescribed and to plan periodontal treatment according to the stage of the disease and the type of associated medical treatment.[41, 79]

The patient in **chronic renal failure** has a progressive disease that may ultimately require renal transplantation or dialysis. *It is preferable to treat a patient dentally prior to rather than after transplant or dialysis.*[47] *The following treatment modifications should be utilized:*

1. Consult the patient's physician
2. Monitor blood pressure (patients in end-stage renal failure are usually hypertensive)[4]
3. Check laboratory values
   a. Partial thromboplastin time, prothrombin time, bleeding time, and platelet count
   b. Hematocrit
   c. Blood urea nitrogen (*do not* treat if > 60 mg per 100 ml)
   d. Serum creatinine (*do not* treat if > 1.5 mg per 100 ml)
4. Eliminate areas of oral infection because of enhanced susceptibility[15]:
   a. Oral hygiene should be good.
   b. Periodontal treatment should aim to provide easy maintenance. All questionable teeth should be extracted if medical parameters permit.
   c. Frequent recall appointments should be scheduled.
5. Drugs that are nephrotoxic or metabolized by the kidney should be eliminated: e.g., phenacetin, streptomycin, and tetracycline. Acetaminophen and acetylsalicylic acid may be used with caution.[7, 111]

The patient who is receiving **dialysis** requires treatment planning modifications.[4, 19, 22, 110] There are three modes of dialysis: hemodialysis, intermittent peritoneal dialysis (IPD), and chronic ambulatory peritoneal dialysis (CAPD). The pathophysiologic changes which may alter periodontal therapy among patients receiving hemodialysis are: (1) a high incidence of serum hepatitis, (2) a high incidence of anemia, (3) a significant incidence of secondary hyperparathyroidism, and (4) heparinization during hemodialysis.[12] For these reasons *the following should be added to the recommendations for treating patients with chronic renal disease:*

1. Screen for HB_sAg and anti-HB_s prior to any treatment.
2. Provide antibiotic prophylaxis to prevent endarteritis of the A-V fistula or shunt.
3. Prevent hypoxia.
4. Provide treatment on the day following dialysis because of heparinization. Dialysis treatments are generally done three times a week for 4 hours or twice a week for 5 hours. (Note that IPD and CAPD patients are not systemically heparinized; therefore, they do not usually have the bleeding problems potentially associated with hemodialysis.)
5. Establish a long-term maintenance system with frequent recalls.
6. Be careful to protect the dialysis shunt or fistula when the patient is in the dental chair. If the shunt or fistula is placed in the arm, do not cramp the limb; blood pressure readings should be taken from the other arm. Do not use the limb for the injection of medication. Patients with leg shunts should avoid sitting with the leg dependent for longer than 1 hour.[9] If appointments last longer, allow the patient to walk about for a few minutes, then resume therapy.
7. Refer the patient to the physician if uremic problems, such as uremic stomatitis, are noted to be developing.[18]

The **renal transplant patient's** greatest foe is infection. A periodontal abscess is potentially a life-threatening situation. For this reason, a dental team approach should be utilized before the transplantation to determine which teeth can be easily maintained. *Teeth with furcation involvements, periodontal abscesses, or extensive surgical requirements should be extracted, leaving an easily maintainable dentition.* In addition to the recommendations for chronic renal failure, the following should be considered for the renal transplant patient:

1. HB_sAg screening
2. Prophylactic antibiotics according to the American Heart Association recommendations. Some recommend an oral antibiotic mouthwash with nystatin (Mycostatin) 1 day before and continuing 2 days after the dental procedure.[9]

PULMONARY DISEASES

The periodontal treatment of a patient with pulmonary disease may require alteration, depending on the nature and the severity of the respiratory problem. Pulmonary diseases range from obstructive lung diseases such as asthma, emphysema, bronchitis, and acute obstruction to restrictive ventilatory disorders due to muscle weakness, scarring, obesity, or any condition that could interfere with effective lung ventilation. Combined restrictive-obstructive lung disease may also develop.[14]

The clinician should be aware of the signs and symptoms of pulmonary disease, such as (1) increased respiratory rate (the normal rate for adults is 12 to 16 breaths per minute), (2) central cyanosis, (3) clubbing of the fingers, (4) chronic cough, (5) chest pain, (6) hemoptysis, (7) dyspnea or orthopnea, and (8) wheezing.[54] Patients with these problems should be referred for medical evaluation and treatment.

Most patients with chronic lung disease may be seen for routine periodontal therapy if they are under adequate medical management. Caution should be taken in relation to the use of ultrasonics. Dried, retained secretions which result in partial airway obstruction may, because of their hydrophilic nature, cause complete obstruction when ultrasonic devices are used. Also, ultrasonic use may precipitate bronchospasms owing to the foreign body nature of aerosol droplets.[89] Similar reactions may occur with debris or aerosol from handpieces.

Caution should be practiced in relation to any treatment which may depress respiratory function. Patients with a history of chronic lung disease have a higher alveolar carbon dioxide partial pressure and a lower alveolar oxygen partial pressure. Acute respiratory distress may be caused, therefore, by slight airway obstruction or depression of respiratory function.[10] Because of their limited vital lung capacity, these patients also have a decreased cough effectiveness.[90] They must continually deal with the mental anxiety caused by air hunger and alter their position in attempts to improve their ventilatory efficiency.[33]

The following management should be utilized during periodontal therapy:

I. Identification and referral of patients with signs and symptoms of pulmonary disease
II. In patients with known pulmonary disease
   A. Consult with physician regarding
     1. Medications
       a. Antibiotics
       b. Steroids
       c. Chemotherapeutic agents
     2. Severity and degree of pulmonary disease
   B. Avoid elicitation of respiratory depression or distress
     1. Minimize the stress of a periodontal appointment
     2. Avoid medications that could cause respiratory depression (meperidine, morphine, sedatives, and general anesthetics)
     3. Do not give a bilateral mandibular block, which could cause increased airway obstruction
     4. Care should be performed when administering oxygen
       a. High oxygen concentrations at high flow levels may depress the ventilatory drive in a patient with chronic disease, resulting in acute hypercapnia
       b. Use extreme care with nitrous oxide–oxygen
     5. Care should be utilized with ultrasonic or rotary devices
     6. Position the patient to allow maximum ventilatory efficiency; many patients with chronic obstructive pulmonary disease should be semi- rather than fully reclined
     7. Be careful to prevent physical airway obstruction; keep the patient's throat clear; avoid excess periodontal packing, rubber dams, and so forth
   C. In patients with a history of asthma
     1. Make sure the patient's medication is available (e.g., isoproterenol [0.25 per cent] aerosol)
     2. Avoid complex dental procedures
   D. Patients with active fungal or bacterial diseases should not be treated unless the periodontal procedure is an emergency

IMMUNOSUPPRESSION AND CHEMOTHERAPY

Immunosuppressed patients possess impaired host defenses due to an underlying immunodeficiency or to drug administration (primarily related to organ transplantation or cancer chemotherapy).[3, 25, 77] Leukopenia, alterations in cellular immunity, disruption of intact integument, and alterations in the inflammatory response may facilitate secondary infection. Also, degrees of neutropenia which are dose dependent may occur. The oral cavity is an obvious reservoir for potential superinfection microorganisms. *Treatment in these pa-*

tients should, therefore, be directed toward the prevention of oral complications which could possibly be life threatening. The greatest potential for infection occurs during periods of high suppression; therefore, treatment should be conservative and palliative.

RADIOTHERAPY

The use of radiotherapy, alone or in conjunction with surgical resection, is common in the treatment of head and neck tumors. The side effects of ionizing radiation produce dramatic perioral changes of significant concern to dental health personnel.[8, 26] The extent and severity of mucositis, dermatitis, xerostomia, dysphagia, gustatory alteration, radiation caries, vascular changes, trismus, temporomandibular joint degeneration, and periodontal change are dependent upon a myriad of radiation factors[1, 26, 39, 82]: the type of radiation utilized, the fields of irradiation, the number of ports, the type of tissues in the fields, and the dosage.

Patients scheduled to receive radiation therapy require dental consultation at the earliest possible time in order to reduce the morbidity of the known perioral side effects. Preirradiation treatment depends upon the patient's prognosis, compliance, and residual dentition, in addition to the fields, ports, dose, and immediacy of radiotherapy. The initial visit should include panoramic and intraoral radiographs, a clinical dental examination, periodontal evaluation, and physician consultation. The physician should be asked about the number of rads to be administered, the extent and location of the lesion, the nature of any surgical procedures performed or to be performed, the number of radiation ports, the mode of radiation therapy, and the patient's prognosis (i.e., the likelihood of metastasis). Preirradiation treatment should commence immediately after the physician consultation. The first decision that should be made relates to possible extractions, as irradiation can cause side effects that interfere with healing. For head and neck squamous cell carcinomas, the dose is usually 5000 to 7000 rads of cobalt 60 delivered in a fractionated method (150 to 200 rads over a 6- to 7-week course). This is considered full-course radiation treatment, and the degree of perioral side effects will depend on the tissues irradiated. If this dose is administered to the salivary gland tissues, xerostomia will ensue.[87] The parotid is apparently the most

radiosensitive of the salivary glands; saliva may become extremely viscous or nonexistent, depending upon the dose delivered to the particular gland. Xerostomia will also cause a decrease in the normal salivary cleansing mechanisms, the buffering capacity of saliva, and the pH of oral fluids. Oral bacterial populations shift to predominantly cariogenic forms (*Streptococcus mutans, Actinomyces,* and *Lactobacillus*).[12] Another major concern regarding the decision about extractions involves the radiation dose to be received and the extent of involvement of the body of the mandible. The incidence of osteoradionecrosis of the mandible is directly related to its apparent lack of vascularity and to the higher incidence of carcinoma in mandibular areas (thus the associated increased frequency of irradiation). Therefore, the greater the glandular involvement and involvement of the body of the mandible, the greater the likelihood that there will be oral complications after radiation therapy.

If the patient is to receive full-course radiation therapy within the aforementioned fields, the required extractions should be performed a minimum of 10 days to 2 weeks prior to the initiation of radiation therapy, or not performed at all. If the periodontal support is less than half the root length, the teeth are nonrestorable or abscessed, or the patient's oral hygiene and motivation are poor, it is recommended that extractions be performed within the allocated time limit. Beumer feels that all teeth with furcation involvements should be extracted as well.[8] Extractions should be performed in a manner that allows primary closure. Mucoperiosteal flaps should be gently elevated; teeth should be extracted in segments; radical alveolectomy should be performed, allowing no rough osseous spicules; and primary closure should be provided without tension.[8] It is recommended that antibiotic coverage be provided for the initial 7- to 10-day healing period.[31]

The first visit should also include instruction in oral hygiene methods for maintenance of the remaining dentition. *During radiation therapy,* patients should receive weekly fluoride treatments, i.e., a 1-minute acidulated phosphofluoride rinse (1.23 per cent) followed by a 4-minute stannous fluoride (1.64 per cent) rinse unless it is irritating to a concurrent mucositis. Patients should be instructed to brush daily with stannous fluoride gels (0.4 per cent). All remaining teeth should receive thorough débridement (scaling and root planing).

The periodontal ligament has been reported to lose much of its cellularity and vascularity after radiation therapy; thus, its healing potential is severely compromised. Pulpal changes may become apparent as well.[1, 64] *During the course of radiation therapy, it is important to reinforce the patient's oral hygiene and to perform weekly professional plaque removal.* Simple restorations (alloys) should be placed where required.

Postirradiation morbidity may manifest as osteoradionecrosis (this occurs in 5 to 10 per cent of patients irradiated for head or neck carcinoma).[74] Osseous healing may progress slowly or not at all. A decreased vascular supply, along with damaged and diminished numbers of osteocytes and osteoblasts, contributes to this painful, often debilitating, pathologic response. Any trauma or infection may lead to osteoradionecrosis. An extraction or periodontal disease that exacerbates into an abscess may trigger osteoradionecrosis. For this reason, postirradiation periodontal care should be limited to routine scaling and root planing, oral hygiene reinforcement, and fluoride treatments. The teeth become somewhat brittle after full-course radiation therapy to the head or neck owing to the denaturation of their organic matrices.[32, 88] Periodontal care, therefore, should be limited to gentle hand instrumentation and fluoride treatment. Ultrasonic instrumentation is not recommended. Full-thickness flap techniques or periodontal procedures that could expose osseous structures should *not* be performed, especially on the mandible. *Periodontal care, therefore, should remain conservative for the duration of the patient's life.*

Postirradiation follow-up consists of palliative treatment, given as indicated. A 3-month recall interval is ideal. Viscous lidocaine may be prescribed for painful mucositis, or salivary substitutes may be given for xerostomia.[86] Patient monitoring in relation to systemic changes, as well as oral changes, is essential. It has been reported that 66 per cent of patients receiving radiation therapy for Hodgkin's disease (with head or neck lymphomas) had postirradiation thyroid dysfunction.[84] A final necessity of postirradiation management is that of supportive attitudes. Many patients undergo severe depression during radiotherapy and anxiety after therapy. They should be warned about perioral changes and return or loss of function, and their personal roles in decreasing postirradiation morbidity should be emphasized. Understanding and supportive encouragement are essential during this traumatic time in their lives.

ENDOCRINE DISORDERS

Diabetes

The diabetic patient requires special precautions prior to periodontal therapy. A full discussion of the role of diabetes in the etiology of periodontal disease is presented in Chapter 29. This section will outline periodontal therapy for the diabetic with respect to the diagnosis of glucose intolerance and the degree of disease control.

If signs of diabetes are noticed in a patient, further investigation via laboratory studies and history taking (e.g., hereditary predisposition) should be performed, because **periodontal treatment in the uncontrolled diabetic is contraindicated.**

If a patient is suspected to be diabetic, the following procedures should be performed:

1. Physician consultation
2. Analysis of laboratory tests (Table 36–2)
   a. Fasting blood glucose

TABLE 36–2 LABORATORY TESTS FOR DIABETES

Test	Value
Fasting blood glucose	50–100 mg/100 ml normal > 100 mg/100 ml suggestive > 130 mg/100 ml diagnostic
1- or 2-hour postprandial blood glucose	< 170 mg/100 ml 1 hour oral carbohydrate load < 120 mg/100 ml 2 hours oral carbohydrate load
Glucose tolerance test	Glucose load
	0 hour 100 mg/100 ml
	½ hour 170 mg/100 ml
	1 hour 170 mg/100 ml
	2 hours 120 mg/100 ml (diagnostic if >140 mg/100 ml)
	3 hours 110 mg/100 ml

b. Postprandial blood glucose
c. Glucose tolerance test
d. Urinary glucose
3. Rule out acute orofacial infection or severe dental infection; insulin and glucose requirements are altered in cases of infection; only antibiotic and analgesic care should be administered until a complete physical examination is performed and diabetic control is attained; if there is a periodontal condition that requires immediate care, antibiotic coverage is required prior to incision and drainage; the physician should monitor insulin requirements

If a patient is a "brittle" diabetic, one whose disease is difficult to control, optimal periodontal health is a necessity. Treatment of periodontal disease may reduce insulin requirements.[35] Glucose levels should be continuously monitored, and periodontal treatment should be performed when the patient is in a well-controlled state. Prophylactic antibiotics, started 2 days preoperatively and continued through the immediate postoperative therapy, should be administered. Penicillin is the drug of first choice. Periodontal recall maintenance appointments at frequent intervals are important to periodontitis and diabetes stabilization.[81] The clinician must also be able to recognize the signs of an oncoming diabetic coma or insulin reaction.

The well-controlled diabetic may, for the most part, be treated as an ordinary patient.[54] *There are, however, guidelines that should be followed to ensure diabetes control:*

1. Phase I therapy: Make certain that the prescribed insulin and later a meal have been taken. Morning appointments after breakfast are ideal because of optimal insulin levels.
2. Phase II therapy
   a. If general anesthesia, intravenous, or surgical procedures are performed that alter the patient's ability to maintain a normal caloric intake, postoperative insulin doses should be altered (Table 36–3). There is no agreement on medical management before and after periodontal therapy. Individual physician consultation is a prerequisite.
   b. Tissues should be handled as atraumatically and as minimally (< 2 hours) as possible.
   c. Endogenous epinephrine may increase insulin requirements; therefore, anxious patients may require preoperative sedation. The anesthetic should contain epinephrine in doses not greater than 1:100,000.
   d. Schedule morning appointments.
   e. Diet recommendations that enable the patient to maintain a proper glucose balance should be given. Dietary supplements may be prescribed if deemed necessary.
   f. There remains a controversy regarding antibiotic prophylaxis for the prevention of infection. If therapy is extensive, antibiotic coverage is recommended.
3. Maintenance therapy: Frequent recall appointments and fastidious home oral care should be stressed. Studies indicate that controlled diabetics and patients without diabetes have similar therapeutic responses.

Thyroid Disorders

Periodontal therapy in the patient with adequately managed thyroid disease requires minimal alterations. Patients with thyrotoxicosis and patients with inadequate medical management should not receive periodontal therapy until their condition is stabilized. Patients with a history of *hyperthyroidism* should be (1) carefully evaluated to determine the level of medical management, (2) carefully given medications (epinephrine, atropine, and other pressor amines should be given with caution owing to their overreactive effect in this population and should not be given in cases of thyrotoxicosis or poor control), and (3) treated so as to limit stress and infection.

Hypothyroid patients require careful administration of sedatives and narcotics because of their inability to tolerate drugs. One source states that only 25 per cent of the dose required for the euthyroid patient is needed for general anesthesia in the hypothyroid patients; also, levels of medical control should be watched.

Parathyroid Disorders

Once the patient with parathyroid disease has been identified and properly treated medically, routine periodontal therapy may be instituted. Those, however, who have not received medical care may have significant renal disease, uremia, and hypertension. Also, if hyper- or hypocalcemia is present, the patient

TABLE 36–3   INSULIN DOSE CHANGES PRIOR TO SURGICAL THERAPY

	Insulin		
	Short-acting	*Intermediate*	*Long-acting*
Degree of Dietary Restriction	*Regular (2–4 hours)* Semilente (2–4 hours)*	*NPH (6–12 hours) Lente (6–12 hours)*	*PZI (14–24 hours) Ultralente (18–24 hours)*
Minimal	None	None	None
Moderate	Stop A.M. dose	½ A.M. dose, meal given, then other ½ dose	½ A.M. dose
Severe (general anesthesia) No meals for 6 hours	Stop A.M. dose	Stop A.M. dose, followed by surgery in 2 hours	Stop A.M. dose

*Numbers in parentheses refer to peak activity.

may be more prone to cardiac arrhythmias. It is the role, therefore, of the dental practitioner to be attuned to the oral and dental changes occurring with hyperparathyroidism or hypoparathyroidism in order to provide astute detection and referral.

Adrenal Insufficiency

Acute adrenal insufficiency is associated with significant morbidity and mortality due to peripheral vascular collapse and cardiac arrest. One should, therefore, be aware of the clinical manifestations of (Table 36–4) and ways of preventing adrenal insufficiency in patients with a history of Addison's disease or in patients with normal adrenal cortices who have been given exogenous glucocorticosteroids.

Most commonly, adrenal insufficiency is witnessed in a person with a history of steroid therapy. Adrenal suppression occurs owing to adrenal cortical atrophy. Sustained hormonal therapy results in a variety of side effects, many of which resemble naturally occurring Cushing's syndrome. In addition, many of these patients cannot tolerate the stress caused by dental anxiety, surgical procedures, trauma, or infection.[117] The degree of suppression depends upon the drugs used, the dose, the duration of administration, the length of time

elapsed since steroid therapy was terminated, and the route of administration.

Treatment alterations in the aforementioned patients will differ according to whether they currently take steroids, have previously taken steroids, or are in an emergent situation. There is not a set protocol for steroid prophylaxis; therefore, endocrine consultation is advised. Medical histories should reveal diseases for which steroids are commonly prescribed, as well as a blanket question, "Have you ever received steroid therapy?"

For the patient who is currently receiving steroid therapy, the need for corticosteroid prophylaxis depends on the drug used because of the variance in equivalent therapeutic doses (Table 36–5). Most patients with Addison's disease receive a daily oral dose of 25.0 to 37.5 mg of cortisone (equivalent to 5.0 to 7.5 mg of prednisolone). This replaces the normal output of the adrenal cortex (which ranges from 20 to 30 mg per day). Treatment for rheumatoid arthritis, asthma, dermatologic diseases, and so forth may require greater doses and thus may readily suppress adrenal function if used for long periods of time. Note that the route of administration is important, for topical corticosteroids may have minimal

TABLE 36–4   MANIFESTATIONS OF ACUTE ADRENAL INSUFFICIENCY

Mental confusion, fatigue, and weakness
Nausea and/or vomiting
Hypertension
Syncope
Intense abdominal, lower back, and/or leg pain
Loss of consciousness
Coma

TABLE 36–5   EQUIVALENT DOSAGES OF CORTICOSTEROIDS

Corticosteroid	Equivalent Dose (mg)
Cortisone	25
Hydrocortisone	20
Prednisone	5
Prednisolone	5
Methylprednisone	5
Methylprednisolone	4
Triamcinolone	4
Dexamethasone	0.75
Bethamethasone	0.6

to no depressant effect.[4] Glucocorticosteroid coverage regimens vary; however, most provide a two- to fourfold increase in coverage, depending upon the stress produced by the procedure. Below are some examples:

A. Little and Falace[54]
  1. 30 to 60 mg hydrocortisone per day for at least 1 month
    a. Double normal dose on day of appointment
    b. Hospitalize patient for major procedures
  2. >60 mg hydrocortisone per day: No additional steroids required
  3. Topicals: Consult physician
B. Lenihan[51]: Two times normal steroid dose on the day prior to, the day of, and 2 days after the surgical appointment; then reinstitute normal dose
C. Malamed[56]: Two- or fourfold increase in dose on the day of stress
D. Glickman[16]: Patients on prolonged steroid therapy should be given 100 mg additional cortisone acetate or 20 mg prednisone orally 2 hours before periodontal surgery to prevent acute adrenal crisis; patients with Addison's disease ordinarily receive a daily dose of 25 to 37.5 mg of cortisone, which is equivalent to 5 to 7.5 mg of prednisone; for periodontal surgery, these patients should receive 100 to 200 mg of cortisone intramuscularly 18 to 24 hours before the operation (the regular oral dose is omitted); on the day of surgery, the patients receive 100 mg of cortisone intramuscularly; the next day they return to their regular daily oral dose

For the patient with a past history of steroid therapy, one should determine the degree of adrenal suppression. Malamed's "rule of two's" should alert the clinician to suspect adrenal suppression[56]: 20 mg of cortisone or its equivalent per day, via the oral or parenteral route, continuously over 2 weeks or longer, and within 2 years of dental therapy. Note that full regeneration of cortical function may occur within 9 to 12 months, but 2 years has also been reported. A minimum of 12 months should have passed since the last dose was taken before normal periodontal therapy is performed. Otherwise, steroid prophylaxis may be warranted.

The patient in an acute adrenal insufficiency crisis should receive the following therapy:

1. Terminate periodontal therapy.
2. Call for help.
3. Monitor vital signs.
4. Give oxygen.
5. Place the patient in a supine position.
6. Administer 100 mg of hydrocortisone sodium succinate (Solu-Cortef) intravenously over 30 seconds or intramuscularly.

Pregnancy

The aim of periodontal therapy for the pregnant patient is to minimize the potential exaggerated inflammatory response related to associated hormonal alterations. *Meticulous plaque control, scaling, root planing, and polishing should be the only nonemergent periodontal procedures performed.*

The second trimester is the safest time in which treatment may be performed. Long, stressful appointments, as well as periodontal surgical procedures, should be waived until post partum, however.

Owing to the "supine hypotensive syndrome of pregnancy" that occurs during the third trimester, performing elective periodontal treatment without taking precautions is not advised. Decreasing blood pressure, syncope, and then loss of consciousness may occur as a result of uterine pressure upon the inferior vena cava. Appointments should be short, and the patient should be allowed to change positions frequently. Fully reclining positioning should be avoided if possible.

Other precautions during pregnancy relate to the potential toxic or teratogenic effects of therapy on the fetus. Ideally no medications should be prescribed or radiographs taken unless the situation is emergent. Consultation with the patient's obstetrician should be secured if a drug could cross the placenta or cause respiratory depression.

HEMORRHAGIC DISORDERS

Patients with a history of bleeding problems caused by disease or drugs should be managed in a manner that minimizes risks. Identification of these patients via the health history, clinical examination, and clinical laboratory tests is paramount. Health questioning should cover: (1) history of bleeding after previous surgery or trauma, (2) past and present drug history, (3) history of bleeding problems among relatives, and (4) medical history to rule out possible illness associated with bleeding problems.

Clinical examinations should detect the existence of jaundice, ecchymosis, spider telangiectasias, hemarthrosis, petechiae, hemorrhagic vesicles, or gingival hyperplasia. Laboratory tests should include methods to measure the hemostatic, coagulation, or lytic phases of the clotting mechanism, depending upon clues regarding which phase is involved[5, 37, 76] (Table 36–6).

Patients who are "severe bleeders" should be referred for hematologic evaluation. If the history indicates "minor or equivocal bleeding tendencies," simple screening tests can be ordered, including the bleeding time, tourniquet test, complete blood count, prothrombin time, partial thromboplastin time, and coagulation time.

Bleeding disorders may be classified as: (1) coagulation disorders, (2) thrombocytopenic purpuras, and (3) nonthrombocytopenic purpuras. The most common of these disorders is due to acquired, iatrogenic bleeding affecting coagulation.

Coagulation Disorders

Periodontal care for patients on anticoagulation therapy should be altered depending on the medication utilized to reduce intravascular clotting. Drugs that perform this function include heparin, bishydroxycoumarin (dicumarol), sodium warfarin (Coumadin), phenindione derivatives, cyclocumarol, ethyl biscoumacetate, and aspirin.

Patients on Coumadin therapy have an inhibition of prothrombin or of vitamin K–dependent factors (Factors II, VII, IX, and X). Most are outpatients because the drug is administered orally. It is important to note that the duration of the action of Coumadin is a minimum of 6 days.

Periodontal treatment should be altered as follows:

1. Physician consultation to determine the nature of the underlying medical problem and the degree of required anticoagulation (the general therapeutic range is a prothrombin time between 1.5 and 3.0 times normal).
2. Periodontal scaling, surgery, and extractions require a prothrombin time < 1.5 times normal (25 to 30 per cent of normal).
   a. The physician should be consulted about discontinuing or reducing the dicumarol dosage until the desired prothrombin times are achieved.
   b. Changes in prothrombin time will not be apparent until 2 to 3 days after changing dosages.
   c. A prothrombin time measurement is required on the day of the procedure. If it is > 1.5 times normal, cancel the procedure and reschedule it for 1 to 3 days later. Remeasure the prothrombin time on the day of surgery.
3. After scaling and curettage, patients should not be dismissed until bleeding has stopped.
4. It is preferable to perform periodontal surgery in a hospital, but small segments of the mouth may be treated in the dental office if the following precautions are utilized:
   a. Minimize trauma.
   b. Prophylactic antibiotics are recommended to prevent postoperative infection that may lead to bleeding.[54]
   c. Use pressure hemostasis.
   d. Attempt to gain closure as close to primary as possible.
   e. There are no contraindications to local anesthesia with epinephrine; however, one should exercise caution with injections (especially blocks) owing to hematoma formation.
   f. Prior to periodontal pack placement, bleeding should be stopped by packing cotton pellets interproximally and pressure applied facially and lingually with a gauze sponge. The periodontal pack may then be placed over the cotton pellets.
5. Do not perform scaling or periodontal surgery if the patient has an acute infection.
6. Patients should return in 3 to 5 days to determine whether healing is normal; if so, the physician may resume the patient's anticoagulation therapy.

Patients on aspirin therapy should be screened by the bleeding time and partial thromboplastin time. Salicylates have been known to exert a Coumadin-like effect and interfere with normal platelet function. The effects are seen in patients on long-term and high-dose therapy. Note that aspirin should not be prescribed for patients known to be receiving anticoagulation therapy or who have illnesses known to be related to bleeding tendencies.

Heparin therapy is utilized only in hospital situations because of its parenteral route of administration. Its duration of action is 4 to 8 hours and may be variable up to 24 hours. Refer to the section on renal disease for dental treatment alterations.

Liver disease may affect all phases of blood clotting. Most of the coagulation factors are

TABLE 36–6 LABORATORY TESTS FOR COAGULATION AND BLEEDING DISORDERS

	Hemostatic			Lytic
	Vascular	*Platelet*	*Coagulation*	
Tests	1. Tourniquet test *N:* 10 petechiae *Abn:* > 10 petechiae 2. Bleeding time *N:* 1–6 minutes *Abn:* > 6 minutes	1. Platelet count *N:* 150,000–300,000/cu mm *Abn:* Clinical bleeding occurs at < 80,000/cu mm 2. Bleeding time 3. Clot retraction 4. Complete blood count	1. Prothrombin time (measures extrinsic and common pathways: Factors I, II, V, VII, and X) *N:* 11–14 seconds (depending upon laboratory) measured against a control *Abn:* > 1.5–2 times normal 2. Partial thromboplastin time (measures intrinsic and common pathways: Factors III, IX, XI, and low levels of Factors I, II, V, X, and XII) *N:* 25–40 seconds (depending upon laboratory) measured against a control *Abn:* > 1.5 times normal 3. Clotting (coagulation) time *N:* 30–40 minutes *Abn:* > 1 hour	1. Euglobin clot lysis time *N:* < 90 minutes *Abn:* > 90 minutes
Clinical disease association	Vascular (capillary) wall defect Rule out: Thrombocytopenia Purpuras Telangiectasia Aspirin therapy Leukemia Renal dialysis	Thrombocytopenia Rule out: Vascular wall defect Acute/chronic leukemia Aplastic anemia Liver disease Renal dialysis	All three tests: Liver disease Coumarin therapy Aspirin therapy Malabsorption syndrome or long-term antibiotic therapy (lack of vitamin K utilization) Prothrombin time: Factor VII deficiency Partial thromboplastin time: Hemophilia, renal dialysis	Increase in fibrinolytic activity

synthesized and removed by the liver. A long-term ethanol abuser or a jaundiced individual may have vascular wall alterations and platelet defects secondary to liver damage. *Dental treatment planning should include:*

1. Laboratory evaluations: prothrombin time, bleeding time, platelet count, and partial thromboplastin time (in later stages of liver disease)
2. Conservative, nonsurgical periodontal therapy
3. Evaluation of clinical symptoms
   a. Jaundice in mucous membranes and sclera is considered to be overt at a serum bilirubin level >2 mg per 100 ml, subclinical at 0.4 to 2.0 mg per 100 ml, and normal at 0.1 to 0.4 mg per 100 ml
   b. Clinical bleeding into tissues
   c. Fatigue
   d. Increased plasma volume
   e. Weight loss
4. General anesthesia is usually contraindicated because of cardiovascular compromise and the metabolism of barbiturates by the liver
5. Look for signs of disease associated with uncontrolled fibrinolysis (e.g., disseminated intravascular coagulation and thrombocytopenia)
6. If planning surgery (in hospital only)
   a. Prothrombin time should be at least 1.5 to 2.0 times normal and platelet count should exceed 80,000 cells per cu mm[13].
   b. If the prothrombin time is > 2.0 times normal, vitamin K may be effective in reducing it; if not, only smaller areas of the mouth should be treated in patients with advanced liver disease; daily intravenous doses of vitamin K (150 mg) may be tried, but the administration of fresh whole blood or plasma may also be required
   c. If platelets are low, concentrated platelets may be administered

Another disorder of coagulation is that of the inherited type, hereditary **hemophilia.** Periodontal procedures may be performed in hemophiliacs provided sufficient precautions are taken.[49, 62, 97] Conservative therapy and maintenance are preferable to surgery. If surgery is needed, treatment planning should be designed to maximize coordination of blood factor replacement, as determined by the variety of hemophilia and its severity (Table 36–7).

I. Consultation with hematologist as to the type of hemophilia, the level of factor deficiency, and the presence of factor inhibitors
II. Hospitalization for surgical procedures[6, 107]
   A. Replacement of coagulation factor (by hematologist)[109]
   B. Surgical technique
      1. Antibiotic coverage
      2. As atraumatic as possible
         a. Remove all sharp osseous spicules
         b. Treat soft tissues gingerly
         c. Remove all granulation tissue
      3. Maximum approximation of the wound edges
      4. Avoid suture strangulation and use of resorbable sutures
      5. Topical hemostatic agents may be applied
         a. Microfibrillar collagen, Gelfoam with thrombin, oxidized regenerated cellulose, or cotton pellets under pressure may be placed
         b. Periodontal pack should be placed only after bleeding has been controlled
      6. Postoperative follow-up
         a. Bleeding due to clot breakdown usually occurs 3 to 4 days after surgery
         b. Pressure hemostasis should be performed only if there is adequate replacement factor available to prevent subcutaneous bleeding from occurring
         c. Oral hygiene and 3-month maintenance are prerequisites
         d. No aspirin or aspirin products should be prescribed

Thrombocytopenic Purpuras

Bleeding due to a reduced number of platelets (thrombocytopenia) may be seen with idiopathic thrombocytopenic purpuras, radiation therapy, myelosuppressive drugs, leukemia, or infections. Normal platelet counts are 250,000 ± 100,000 cells per cu mm. Spontaneous bleeding occurs from 80,000 to 60,000 cells per cu mm. It may occur as a result of gingival irritation or inflammation caused by local factors. Periodontal therapy should be directed toward reducing local irritants to avoid the need for more aggressive therapy. *Patients who*

TABLE 36–7   Hemophilia: Tests and Treatment

Hemophilia Type	Prolonged	Normal	Treatment

A	Partial thromboplastin time	Prothrombin time
		Bleeding time
			Factor VIII cryoprecipitate,
			    fresh frozen plasma, or fresh
			    whole blood
			Epsilon aminocaproic acid

B	Partial thromboplastin time	Prothrombin time Bleeding time	Fresh frozen plasma Lyophilized Factor IX concentrates
von Willebrand's disease	Bleeding time Partial thromboplastin time Variable Factor VIII deficiency	Prothrombin time Platelet count	Cryoprecipitate or plasma

are candidates for periodontal therapy and are suspected of having a platelet abnormality should be treated as follows:

1. Physician referral for a definitive diagnosis and treatment of a platelet disorder.
2. Oral hygiene instruction—if the number of platelets is severely decreased, gentler oral hygiene products should be used (i.e., sponges).
3. Prophylactic treatment of potential abscesses. Frequent recall appointments are required.
4. No surgical procedures are indicated unless the platelet count is at least 80,000 cells per cu mm. A transfusion of platelets can be given prior to surgery.
   a. Surgical treatment should be as atraumatic as possible.
   b. Stents or thrombin-soaked cotton pellets placed interproximally with periodontal dressing should be utilized for clot formation and prevention of clot disruption.
   c. Gentle hydrogen peroxide mouthwashes may aid in controlling gingival hemorrhage.
   d. Close postsurgical follow-up should ensue.
5. Note that scaling and root planing may be carefully performed at low platelet levels (30,000 cells per cu mm).

Nonthrombocytopenic Purpuras

Nonthrombocytopenic purpuras occur as a result of either vascular wall fragility or platelet dysfunction (thrombasthenia). The former occurs owing to a multitude of causes: hypersensitivity reactions (immunologic connective tissue diseases), scurvy, infections, chemicals (phenacetin and aspirin), dysproteinemia, and several others. Thrombasthenia occurs in uremia, Glanzmann's disease, aspirin ingestion, and von Willebrand's disease.[98] Both kinds of nonthrombocytopenic purpuras may result in "immediate" bleeding following gingival injury. Treatment consists primarily of direct pressure for at least 15 minutes. This initial pressure should control the bleeding unless coagulation times are abnormal or reinjury should occur. Surgical therapy should be avoided unless the qualitative and quantitative platelet problems are resolved.

BLOOD DYSCRASIAS

Numerous disorders of red and white blood cells may affect the course of periodontal therapy. Alterations in wound healing, bleeding, tissue appearance, and susceptibility to infection may occur (see Chapter 29). Clinicians should be aware of the clinical signs and symptoms of blood dyscrasias, the availability of screening laboratory tests, and the need for physician referral.

Leukemia

The altered periodontal treatment for leukemic patients is based on their enhanced susceptibility to infection, their bleeding tendency, and the effects of chemotherapy:

I. Refer the patient for medical evaluation and treatment (close cooperation with the physician is required).
II. Prior to chemotherapy, a complete peri-

odontal treatment plan should be developed with a physician (see the section on treatment for patients receiving chemotherapy).

A. Monitor hematologic laboratory values daily: bleeding time, coagulation time, prothrombin time, and platelet count.

B. Cover with antibiotics prior to any periodontal treatment.

C. Extract all hopeless, nonmaintainable, or potentially infectious teeth a minimum of 10 days prior to the initiation of chemotherapy if systemic conditions allow.

D. Periodontal débridement (scaling and root planing) should be performed and thorough oral hygiene instructions given if the patient's condition allows. If there is an irregular bleeding time, careful débridement with cotton pellets soaked in 3 per cent hydrogen peroxide may be performed around the necks of the teeth.

III. *During the acute phases of leukemia,* patients should receive only emergency periodontal care.

A. *Persistent gingival bleeding* usually occurs deep in a periodontal pocket and should be treated as follows:

1. Cleanse the area with 3 per cent hydrogen peroxide.
2. Carefully explore the area and remove any etiologic local factors, making every effort to avoid gingival injury.
3. Recleanse the area with 3 per cent hydrogen peroxide.
4. Place a cotton pellet soaked in thrombin against the bleeding point.
5. Cover with gauze and apply pressure for 15 to 20 minutes.
6. If oozing persists after the removal of the gauze and pressure, replace the cotton pellet (saturated with 3 per cent hydrogen peroxide) firmly, then place a periodontal dressing over the area for 24 hours.

B. *Acute necrotizing ulcerative gingivitis* often complicates the oral picture in acute and subacute leukemia. Treatment should be designed to make the patient comfortable and to eliminate a source of systemic toxicity. Routine treatment procedures for acute necrotizing ulcerative gingivitis, described in Chapter 41, should be followed.

C. *Acute gingival or periodontal abscesses* are common sources of pain in these patients and are associated with regional adenopathy and systemic complications. Treatment is as follows:

1. Systemic antibiotics
2. Gentle incision and drainage
3. Cleanse the area with cotton pellets saturated with 3 per cent hydrogen peroxide.
4. Apply topical pressure with gauze for 15 to 20 minutes.

D. *Oral ulcerations* should be treated with antibiotics and bland mouth rinses.

1. Topical anesthetic rinses such as viscous lidocaine (Xylocaine) or promethazine hydrochloride syrup may be prescribed.
2. Topical protective ointments such as Orabase may be applied.
3. Sharp irritational areas (e.g., bony spicules) or appliances should be removed.

E. *Oral moniliasis* is common in the leukemic patient and can be treated with nystatin suspensions or vaginal suppositories (100,000 units per ml).

IV. In patients with *chronic leukemia* and those in remission, scaling and root planing can be performed without complication, but an effort should be made to avoid periodontal surgery.

A. Bleeding time should be measured on the day of the procedure. If it is low, postpone the appointment and refer the patient to a physician.

B. Plaque control and frequent recall visits should receive particular attention.

Agranulocytosis

Patients with agranulocytosis (cyclic neutropenia and granulocytopenia) are more susceptible to infection than unaffected subjects. There is a reduction in the total white blood cell count and a reduction or elimination of granular leukocytes. The periodontal response to inflammation is exaggerated; however, treatment should be performed only during remission of the disease. At that time, treatment should be conservative. Scaling, root

TABLE 36–8   Hepatitis A, B, and Non-A, Non-B

Features	Type A	Type B	Type Non-A, Non-B
Antigen	A virus (HAV)	B virus (HBV) B surface antigen (HB$_s$Ag) B core antigen (HB$_c$Ag) B e antigen (HB$_e$Ag)	Not specifically identified or characterized
Antibody	Antibody to A virus (anti-HAV)	Antibody to B surface antigen (anti-HB$_s$) Antibody to B core antigen (anti-HB$_c$) Antibody to B e antigen (anti-HB$_e$)	Not specifically identified or characterized
Incubation	15–40 days	50–180 days	15–180 days
Route of transmission	Fecal-oral (may occur parenterally)	Parenteral (has been found in all body fluids, however)	Parenteral
Virus in blood	Early acute and late incubation periods No carrier state	Acute phase and late incubation phase; may persist for months or years (5–10% carrier state)	Probably similar to type B
Age group	Children and young adults	All age groups	All age groups

planing, and oral hygiene instruction should be performed carefully under antibiotic prophylaxis. Because aminopyrines, barbiturates, and chloramphenicol have been implicated as potential causes of agranulocytosis, their use should be avoided.

INFECTIOUS DISEASES

Rarely does one contract or transfer an infectious disease if the necessary precautions have been taken. The undiagnosed, untreated patient who provides a poor medical history, however, is a potential hazard to the doctor, the staff, and other patients. This section will cover hepatitis, sexually transmitted diseases, and tuberculosis in relation to the precautions required in periodontal therapy.

Hepatitis

Hepatitis is divided into three clinically similar diseases (A, B, and non-A, non-B) that differ in their virology, epidemiology, and prophylaxis (Table 36–8). Because up to 75 per cent of individuals infected with hepatitis are undiagnosed, the clinician must be able to screen for and recognize the signs and symptoms of hepatitis (Table 36–9). The clinician

should be suspicious of patients in high-risk groups, such as renal dialysis patients, hospital (professional) personnel, blood bank personnel, morgue workers, homosexuals, obstetrics and gynecology personnel, immunosuppressed patients, drug users, and institutionalized patients. Because 10 to 15 per cent of hepatitis B patients may have chronic forms of the disease, one should carefully screen those who report a past history of hepatitis.

TABLE 36–9   SIGNS AND SYMPTOMS OF ACUTE VIRAL HEPATITIS

Phase	Signs and Symptoms
Preicteric phase: onset is acute in hepatitis A and insidious in hepatitis B	Fever Fatigue Anorexia Nausea, vomiting Abdominal pain Myalgia
Icteric phase: 4:1 an- icteric:icteric	Jaundice, biliuria Increased anorexia Increased nausea, vomiting Increased abdominal pain Mental depression Bradycardia Periarteritis
Posticteric phase:	Disappearance of signs and symptoms Hepatomegaly may persist

The following should be the framework for treating patients associated with hepatitis:

I. Diagnosis of history of hepatitis or active hepatitis
  A. If the disease is active, do not provide routine periodontal therapy unless the situation is an emergency; in that case, follow the protocol for HB$_s$Ag+ patients
  B. Past history of hepatitis
    1. Differentiate as to type according to the physician consultation, the course and length of the disease, the mode of transmission, and laboratory tests (Table 36–10)
    2. Type A
      a. Only emergency procedures should be performed if the disease is active
      b. If the patient has recovered, treat him or her as a routine periodontal patient
    3. Type B
      a. Emergency treatment only if the disease is active and acute
      b. If the patient has recovered, consult with the physician and order HB$_s$Ag and anti-HB$_s$ determinations (Fig. 36–3)
        (1) If HB$_s$Ag– and anti-HB$_s$– are negative but you are highly suspicious that HB virus is present, order another anti-HB$_s$ determination
        (2) If HB$_s$Ag+, the patient is probably infective; the degree of infectivity is measured via a HB$_e$Ag determination
        (3) If anti-HB$_s$+, the patient may be treated routinely

TABLE 36–10 LABORATORY TESTS FOR HEPATITIS

1. SGOT and SGPT*: determine hepatocellular necrosis (hepatitis A peaks at 40 days; hepatitis B peaks at 80–90 days)
2. Albumin: determines liver breakdown
3. Bilirubin: determines extent of liver dysfunction
4. Prothrombin time: determines clotting factors produced by the liver

*SGOT = serum glutamic-oxaloacetic transaminase; SGPT = serum glutamic-pyruvic transaminase.

II. Management precautions if a patient with HB$_s$Ag+ or active hepatitis requires emergency treatment
  A. Consult patient's physician regarding status
  B. If bleeding is likely, order a prothrombin time and bleeding time check and alter treatment accordingly
  C. All personnel in clinical contact with the patient should wear a mask, gloves, and glasses (or goggles); for surgical situations, disposable gowns should be utilized
  D. All instruments should be placed on a sheet of aluminum foil
  E. All disposable items (gauzes, floss, saliva ejectors, masks, gowns, gloves, and aluminum foil) should be placed in one lined wastebasket
  F. Minimize aerosol production by not using the cavitron, air syringe, or high-speed handpieces; remember that saliva is a distillate of the virus
  G. When the procedure is completed, all equipment should be scrubbed and sterilized
    1. Instruments should be moved on the aluminum foil to the sink and rinsed with dilute hypochlorite (1:3) for 10 minutes; next, they should be scrubbed, placed loosely in autoclave bags, and sterilized
    2. Handpieces should also be autoclaved
  H. The dental chair and unit should be wiped down with dilute hypochlorite
  I. Use as many disposable covers as possible; aluminum foil may be used for covering light handles, drawer handles, and bracket trays; headrest covers should also be used
  J. All disposable items should be gathered, bagged (in plastic), tied, labeled, and removed for proper disposal
  K. Aseptic technique should be practiced at all times
    1. Remove rings and arm jewelry
    2. Perform multiple vigorous hand lather and rinse cycles
    3. Some feel that patients should rinse with an oral antiseptic 30 seconds prior to periodontal procedures

III. If HB$_s$Ag–, the patient may be treated routinely

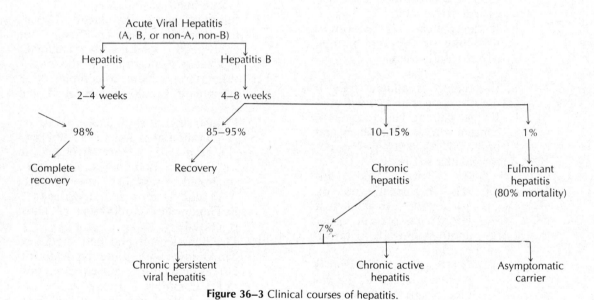

Figure 36–3 Clinical courses of hepatitis.

If you are exposed to a known HB_sAg+ patient, the currently available method of secondary prevention is immune globulin. Hepatitis B immune globulin (0.05 to 0.07 ml/kg of body weight) is administered within 7 days of exposure, and a second dose is given 25 to 30 days later. Immune serum globulin is effective in preventing hepatitis A if given within 2 weeks of exposure. A vaccine of hepatitis B surface antigen is available for immunization in three doses over a 6-month span. It is felt to be effective over a 5-year period and is indicated for the high-risk population.

Sexually Transmitted Diseases

The Public Health Service has categorized three groups of sexually transmitted diseases: syphilis, gonorrhea, and herpes. Those with active disease should receive emergency care only. Prophylactic measures as listed under hepatitis should be adhered to. Remember that oral lesions of primary and secondary syphilis, gonorrhea, and herpes are *infectious*.

Patients found to be free of disease may receive routine periodontal therapy. If one finds lesions or symptomatology suggestive of syphilis or gonorrhea, the patient should be referred for medical evaluation. The patient with herpetic lesions may receive treatment when the lesions resolve. One should, however, take precautionary measures if a history of recurrent lesions is given.

Tuberculosis

The patient with tuberculosis should be treated for emergency care only. One should follow the guidelines listed under hepatitis. If the patient has completed chemotherapy, his or her physician should be consulted regarding infectivity and the results of sputum cultures for *Mycobacterium tuberculosis*. When medical clearance has been given and the sputum cultures are negative, these patients may be treated normally. The patient who gives a history of poor medical follow-up (i.e., lack of yearly chest radiographs) or shows signs or symptoms indicative of tuberculosis should be referred for evaluation. Note that adequate treatment of tuberculosis requires a minimum of 18 months and that thorough posttreatment follow-up should include chest radiographs, sputum cultures, and a review of the patient's symptoms by the physician at least every 12 months.

REFERENCES

1. Adisman, I. K.: Characteristics of irradiated soft and hard tissues. J. Prosthet. Dent., *35*:549, 1976.
2. American Heart Association Committee: Report: prevention of bacterial endocarditis. Circulation, *56*:139A, 1977.
3. Armstrong, D.: Infection complications in cancer patients treated with chemical immunosuppressive agents. Transplantation Proc., *15*:1245, 1973.
4. Bailey, G. L. (ed.): Hemodialysis Principles and Practice. New York, Academic Press, 1972.
5. Beeson, P. B., and McDermott, W. (eds.): Textbook of Medicine. 14th ed. Philadelphia, W. B. Saunders Company, 1975.
6. Behrman, S. J., and Wright, I. S.: Dental surgery during continuous anticoagulation therapy. J. Am. Dent. Assoc., *62*:172, 1961.
7. Bennett, W. M., Singer, I., and Coggins, C. J.: A guide to drug therapy in renal disease. J.A.M.A., *230*:1544, 1974.
8. Beumer, J.: Maxillofacial Rehabilitation: Prosthodontic and Surgical Considerations. St. Louis, C. V. Mosby Company, 1979.
9. Bottomley, W. K., Cioffi, R. F., and Martin, A. J.: Dental management of the patient treated by renal transplantation: preoperative and postoperative considerations. J. Am. Dent. Assoc., *85*:1330, 1972.
10. Brashear, R. E., and Rhodes, H. L.: Chronic Obstructive Lung Disease: Clinical Treatment and Management. St. Louis, C. V. Mosby Company, 1978.
11. Brown, A. A.: Prevention of bacterial endocarditis. Ontario Dent., *54*:14, 1977.
12. Brown, L. R., et al.: Interrelations of oral microorganisms, immunoglobulins and dental caries following radiotherapy. J. Dent. Res., *57*:882, 1978.
13. Burkett, L. W.: Oral Medicine. 6th ed. Philadelphia, J. B. Lippincott Company, 1971.
14. Burton, G. G., Gee, G. N., and Hodgkin, J. E. (eds.): Respiratory Care: A Guide to Clinical Practice. Philadelphia, J. B. Lippincott Company, 1977.
15. Butler, D. L.: Team approach to oral health treatment of pre and post renal transplant patients. J. Hosp. Dent. Pract. *7*:144, 1973.
16. Carranza, F. A., Jr.: Glickman's Clinical Periodontology. 5th ed. Philadelphia, W. B. Saunders Company, 1979.
17. Castelli, W. A., Diaz-Perez, R., Nasjleti, C. E., and Caffesse, R. G.: Effect of renovascular hypertension on the morphology of oral blood vessels. Oral Surg., *46*:576, 1978.
18. Chambers, J. K.: Assessing the dialysis patient at home. Am. J. Nurs., *81*:750, 1981.
19. Charyton, C., Wasserman, B. S., and Russo, B.: The Dialysis Patient: An Informative Guide for the Dentist. Flushing, N.Y.: American Kidney Fund, Booth Memorial Medical Center.
20. Chung, E. K. (ed.): Artificial Cardiac Pacing: Practical Approach. Baltimore, Williams & Wilkins, 1978.
21. Corte, J. E.: Prophylaxis of endocarditis during surgical and dental procedures—medical staff conference, University of California, San Francisco. West. J. Med., *133*:141, 1980.
22. Donaldson, D.: Homologous serum hepatitis and the dental treatment of renal dialysis and kidney transplant patients. Br. Dent. J., *132*:391, 1972.
23. Drapkin, M. S.: Endocarditis after the use of an oral irrigation device. Ann. Intern. Med., *87*:455, 1977.
24. Dreifus, L. S., and Cohen, D.: Implanted pacemakers: medicolegal implications. Am. J. Cardiol., *36*:266, 1975.
25. Dreizen, S., et al.: Oral complications of cancer chemotherapy. Postgrad. Med., *58*:75, 1973.

26. Dreizen, S., et al.: Oral complications of cancer radiography. Postgrad. Med., *61*:85, 1977.

27. Durack, D. T.: Prophylaxis of infective endocarditis. *In* Mandell, G. L. (ed.): Principles and Practice of Infectious Diseases. 1st ed. New York, John Wiley & Sons, 1979.

28. Eggleston, D. J.: Teeth and infective carditis. Aust. Dent. J., *20*:375, 1975.

29. Epstein, F. H., and Merrill, J. P.: Chronic renal failure. *In* Thorn, G. W. (ed.): Harrison's Principles of Internal Medicine. 8th ed. New York, McGraw-Hill Book Company, 1977.

30. Falace, D. A., and Ferguson, T. W.: Bacterial endocarditis: survey of patients treated between 1963 and 1975. Oral Surg., *42*:189, 1976.

31. Fine, L.: Dental care of the irradiated patient. J. Hosp. Dent. Pract., *9*:127, 1975.

32. Frank, R. M., et al.: Acquired dental defects and salivary gland lesions after irradiation for carcinoma. Am. Dent. Assoc., *70*:868, 1965.

33. Frownfelter, D. L.: Chest Physical Therapy and Pulmonary Rehabilitation. Chicago, Year Book Medical Publishers, 1978.

34. Geraci, J. E., Wilson, W. R., and Washington, J. A.: Infective endocarditis caused by *Actinobacillus actinomycetemcomitans*. Report of four cases. Mayo Clin. Proc., *55*:415, 1980.

35. Goldman, H. M., and Cohen, D. W.: Periodontal Therapy. 6th ed. St. Louis, C. V. Mosby Company, 1980.

36. Griffiths, P. V.: The management of the pacemaker wearer during dental hygiene treatment. Dent. Hyg., *52*:573, 1978.

37. Harker, L. A.: Hemostasis Manual. 2nd ed. Philadelphia, F. A. Davis Company, 1974.

38. Heard, E., Jr., Staples, A. F., and Czerwinsku, A. W.: The dental patient with renal disease: precautions and guidelines. J. Am. Dent. Assoc., *96*:792, 1978.

39. Helman, J. C.: Dental care for the irradiated patient. Dent. Surv., *55*:40, 1979.

40. Hirschi, R. G.: Hypertension and the oral surgeon: a worldwide problem. Int. J. Oral Surg., *7*:416, 1978.

41. Hondrum, S. O., and Hays, G. L.: Renal disease relationship to dental and oral surgery. Dent. Surv., 48, Nov. 1979.

42. Kaplan, E. L., and Anderson, R. C.: Infective endocarditis after use of dental irrigation device. *Lancet*, *2*:810, 1977.

43. Kaplan, E. L., and Taranta, A. V. (eds.): Infective Endocarditis: An American Heart Association Symposium. Am. Heart Assoc. Monograph Series, 52, Dallas, 1977.

44. Kaye, D.: Prophylaxis of endocarditis. *In* Kaplan, E. L., and Taranta, A. V. (eds.): Infective Endocarditis. Baltimore, University Park Press, 1976.

45. Kieser, J. A.: Bacterial endocarditis—medicolegal or antibiotic cover? J. Dent. Assoc. S. Afr., *35*:28, 1980.

46. Kimura, T.: An epidemiological study of hypertension. Clin. Sci. Mol. Med., *43*:103, 1974.

47. Kirkpatrick, T. J., and Morton, J. B.: Factors influencing the dental management of renal transplant and dialysis patients. Br. J. Oral Surg., *9*:57, 1971.

48. Kraut, R. A., and Hicks, J. L.: Bacterial endocarditis of dental origin: report of a case. J. Oral Surg., *34*:1031, 1976.

49. Larson, C. E., Chang, J., Bleyaert, A. L., and Bedger, R.: Anesthetic considerations for oral surgery patients with hemophilia. J. Oral Surg., *38*:516, 1980.

50. Lavelle, C. L. B.: Hypertension and the dentist. J. Hosp. Dent. Prac., *11*:7, 1977.

51. Lenihan, J.: Considerations of systemic disease. *In* Steiner, R. B., and Thompson, P. D. (eds.): Oral Surgery and Anesthesia. Philadelphia, W. B. Saunders Company, 1977.

52. Lindeman, R. A., and Henson, J. L.: The dental management of patients with vascular groups placed in the treatment of arterial occlusive disease. J. Am. Dent. Assoc., *104*:625, 1982.

53. Little, J. W.: Management of the patient with a history of rheumatic fever in dental practice. J. Oral Med., *33*:47, 1978.

54. Little, J. W., and Falace, D. A.: Dental Management of the Medically Compromised Patient. St. Louis, C. V. Mosby Company, 1980.

55. Macedo-Sobrinho, B.: Infective endocarditis: is it being neglected within the dental profession? Clin. Prev. Dent., *1*:14, 1979.

56. Malamed, S. F.: Medical Emergencies in the Dental Office. St. Louis, C. V. Mosby Company, 1978.

57. McCarthy, T. M.: Emergencies in Dental Practice. 3rd ed. Philadelphia, W. B. Saunders Company, 1979.

58. McCormack, J.: Electrosurgical equipment and pacemaker: a possible hazard. Br. Dent. J., *139*:221, 1975 (letter).

59. Milford, M. L.: Bacterial endocarditis. J. Kans. State Dent. Assoc., *60*:26, 1976.

60. Modlinger, J. A.: Cardiology Update. Dent. Dimensions, *9*:5, 1975.

61. Moser, M., et al.: Report of the Joint National Committee on Detection, Evaluation, and Treatment of High Blood Pressure. J.A.M.A., *237*:255, 1977.

62. Mulkey, T. F.: Outpatient treatment of hemophiliacs for dental extractions. J. Oral Surg., *34*:428, 1976.

63. Munroe, C. O., and Lazarus, T. L.: Predisposing conditions of infective endocarditis. J. Can. Dent. Assoc., *42*:483, 1976.

64. Neutze, J. M., and Arter, W. J.: Bacterial endocarditis and the dentist. N. Z. Dent. J., *67*:79, 1971.

65. Nickens, G. E., et al.: Effect of cobalt-60 irradiation on the pulp of restored teeth. J. Am. Dent. Assoc., *94*:701, 1977.

66. Ore, D. E., and Shriner, W. A.: Doctor, don't shut off that pacemaker. CDS Rev., *67*:22, 1974.

67. Ore, D. E., and Shriner, W. A.: When your patient has a pacemaker. N.Y. J. Dent., *45*:227, 1975.

68. Oringer, M. J.: Electrosurgery in Dentistry. 2nd ed. Philadelphia, W. B. Saunders Company, 1975, p. 84.

69. Pacing Your Heart. Minneapolis, Medtronic, Inc., 1975.

70. Peart, W. S.: Arterial Hypertension. *In* Beeson, P. B., and McDermott, W. (eds.): Textbook of Medicine. 14th ed. Philadelphia, W. B. Saunders Company, 1975, pp. 981–992.

71. Perlstein, M. I., and Bissada, N. F.: Influence of Obesity and Hypertension on the Severity of Periodontitis in Rats. J. Dent. Res., *55*:B72, 1976 (abstract).

72. Pogre, M. A., and Welsky, P. D.: The dentist and prevention of infective endocarditis. Br. Dent. J., *139*:12, 1975.

73. Quart, D., Stahl, S. S., and Sorrin, S.: Gingival changes observed in arteriosclerotic men: a clinical and histologic study. Oral Surg. Oral Med., Oral Pathol., *13*:1181, 1960.

74. Rankow, R. W., and Weissman, B.: Osteoradionecrosis of the mandible. Ann. Otol. Rhinol. Laryngol., *80*:603, 1971.

75. Rezai, F. R.: Dental treatment of a patient with a cardiac pacemaker: review of the literature. Oral Surg., *44*:662, 1977.

76. Robbins, S. L., and Cotran, R. S.: Pathologic Basis of Disease. 2nd ed. Philadelphia, W. B. Saunders Company, 1979.

77. Rodriques, V.: Bacterial infection in immunosuppressed patients: diagnosis and management. Transplantation Proc., *5*:1249, 1973.

78. Rogosa, M., et al.: Blood sampling and cultural studies in the detection of post-operative bacteremias. J. Am. Dent. Assoc., *60*:171, 1960.

79. Rothwell, B. R.: The medically compromised patient. *In* Hooley, J. R., and Daun, L. G. (eds.): Hospital Dental Practice. St. Louis, C. V. Mosby Company, 1980.

80. Russel, R. P.: Systemic hypertension. *In* Harvey, A., (ed.): Osler's Principles and Practice of Medicine. 19th ed. New York, Appleton-Century-Crofts, 1976, pp. 370–392.

81. Saadoun, A. P.: Diabetes and periodontal disease: a review and update. J. Western Soc. Periodontol., *28*:116, 1980.

82. Santiago, A.: The role of the dentist in radiotherapy. J. Prosthet. Dent., *30*:196, 1973.

83. Santinga, J. T., et al.: Antibiotic prophylaxis for endocarditis in patients with a prosthetic heart valve. J. Am. Dent. Assoc., *93*:1001, 1976.

84. Schimpff, S. C., et al.: Radiation-related thyroid dysfunction: implications for the treatment of Hodgkin's disease. Ann. Intern. Med., *92*:91, 1980.

85. Scopp, I. W.: An overview of the heart patient in dental practice. N.Y. J. Dent., *49*:48, 1979.

86. Shannon, I. L.: A saliva substitute for use by xerostomic patients undergoing radiotherapy to the head and neck. Oral Surg., *44*:656, 1977.

87. Shannon, I. L., et al.: Effect of radiotherapy on whole saliva flow. J. Dent. Res., *56*:693, 1977.

88. Shannon, I. L., et al.: Laboratory study of cobalt-60 irradiated human dental enamel. J. Oral Med., *33*:23, 1978.

89. Shapiro, B. A.: Clinical Application of Respiratory Care. 2nd ed. Chicago, Year Book Medical Publishers, 1979.

90. Shapiro, B. A., et al.: Rehabilitation in chronic obstructive pulmonary disease: a two year prospective study. Respir. Care, *22*:1045, 1977.

91. Simon, A. B., Linde, B., Bonnette, G. H., and Schlentz, R. J.: The individual with a pacemaker in the dental environment. J. Am. Dent. Assoc., *91*:1224, 1975.

92. Slots, J., Rosling, B. G., and Genco, R. J.: Suppression of penicillin-resistant oral *Actinobacillus actinomycetemcomitans* with tetracycline. Considerations in endocarditis prophylaxis. J. Periodontol., *54*:193, 1983.

93. Spaulding, C. R., and Friedman, J. M.: Subacute bacterial endocarditis secondary to dental infection: case report. N.Y. State Dent. J., *41*:292, 1975.

94. Stahl, S. S., and Fox, L. M.: Histologic changes of the oral mucosa associated with certain chronic diseases. Oral Surg. Oral Med. Oral Pathol., *6*:339, 1953.

95. Stahl, S. S., Witkin, G. J., and Scopp, I. W.: Degenerative vascular changes observed in selected gingival specimens. Oral Surg. Oral Med. Oral Pathol., *15*:1495, 1962.

96. Stamler, J., and Stamler, R.: The challenge to conquer hypertension in the twentieth century. Urban Health, *5*:24, 1976.

97. Steiner, R. B., and Thompson, R. D. (eds.): Oral Surgery and Anesthesia. Philadelphia, W. B. Saunders Company, 1972.

98. Sydney, S. B., and Ross, R.: Periodontal surgery in a patient with von Willebrand's disease. J. Am. Dent. Assoc., *102*:660, 1981.

99. Sylvan, S. L., et al.: Bacterial endocarditis—changing concepts in dental management. J. Hosp. Dent., *12*:138, 1978.

100. Thalen, H. J., and Meere, C. C. (ed.): Fundamentals of Cardiac Pacing. Boston, Nyhoff Publishers, 1979.

101. Therapeutics Advisory Committee: Prevention of infective endocarditis associated with dental treatment and dental disease: report of the committee. Aust. Dent. J., *25*:51, 1980.

102. Trefez, B. R.: SBE prophylaxis reconsidered: rationale, questions, answers. Dent. Rev., *18*:7, 1978.

103. Tzuckert, A., et al.: Prevention of bacterial endocarditis resulting from dental treatment. Isr. J. Dent. Med., *27*:11, 1978.

104. Varriale, P., and Nacleio, E. A. (ed.): Cardiac Pacing: A Concise Guide to Clinical Practice. Philadelphia, Lea & Febiger, 1979.

105. Veterans Administration Cooperative Study: Effects of treatment on morbidity in hypertension. J.A.M.A., *213*:1143, 1970.

106. Waddy, J.: Bacterial endocarditis: a cardiologist's view of dental involvement. Oral Surg., *42*:240, 1976.

107. Waldrep, A. C., and McKelvy, L. E.: Oral surgery for patients on anticoagulation therapy. J. Oral Surg., *26*:374, 1968.

108. Walter, C.: Dental treatment of patients with cardiac pacemaker implants. Quint. Int., *8*:57, 1975.

109. Wells, T. J.: A new concept in the control of acute gingival hemorrhage. J. Am. Dent. Assoc., *102*:660, 1981.

110. Westbrook, S. D.: Dental management of patients receiving hemodialysis and kidney transplants. J. Am. Dent. Assoc., *96*:464, 1978.

111. Whitsett, T. L.: Modification of drug dosages in renal disease. J. Okla. State Med. Assoc., *65*:129, 1972.

112. Whittington, B. R.: Bacterial endocarditis: a clinical report. N.Z. Dent. J., *75*:39, 1979.

113. Williams, G.: Some considerations on the peripheral blood vessels in health and disease: a review. J. Periodontol., *43*:503, 1972.

114. Williams, L. F., Jr., and Wynne, G. F.: Fundamental Approach to Surgical Problems. Springfield, Ill., Charles C Thomas, Publishers, 1962, p. 127.

115. Woolley, L. H., Woodworth, J., and Dobbs, J. L.: A preliminary evaluation of the effects of electrical pulp testers on dogs with artificial pacemakers. J. Am. Dent. Assoc., *89*:1099, 1974.

116. Wright, A. D.: Ischaemic heart disease and hypertension. Br. Dent. J., *142*:226, 1977.

117. Zimmerman, B.: The endocrine glands. *In* Cole, W. H. (ed.): Textbook of Surgery. 8th ed. New York, Appleton-Century-Crofts, 1963, Chapter 39.

Part II

Instrumentation

chapter thirty-seven

The Periodontal Instrumentarium

Classification of Periodontal Instruments	**Surgical Instruments**
Periodontal Probes	Excisional and Incisional Instruments
Explorers	Periodontal Knives (Gingivectomy Knives)
Scaling and Curettage Instruments	Interdental Knives
Sickle Scalers (Superficial Scalers)	Surgical Blades
Curettes	Electrosurgery (Surgical Diathermy)
Hoe Scalers	Surgical Curettes and Sickles
Files	Periosteal Elevators
Chisel Scalers	Surgical Chisels and Hoes
Ultrasonic Instruments	Surgical Files
The EVA System	Scissors and Nippers
Cleansing and Polishing Instruments	

Periodontal instruments are designed for specific purposes, such as removal of calculus, planing of root surfaces, curettage of the gingiva, or removal of diseased tissue. Upon first examination, the number of instruments available for similar purposes appears confusing. With experience, however, one selects a relatively small set that fulfills all requirements.

CLASSIFICATION OF PERIODONTAL INSTRUMENTS

Periodontal instruments are classified according to the purposes they serve, as follows:

Periodontal probes are used to locate, measure, and mark pockets and determine their course on individual tooth surfaces.

Explorers are used to locate deposits and caries.

Scaling and curettage instruments serve the following purposes: removal of calcified deposits from the crown and root of a tooth; removal of necrotic, altered cementum from the subgingival root surface; and débridement of the soft tissue lining the pocket. Scaling and curettage instruments are classified as follows:

Sickle scalers are heavy instruments used to remove supragingival calculus.

Curettes are fine instruments used for subgingival scaling, root planing, and removal of the soft tissue lining the pocket.

Hoe, chisel, and file scalers are used to remove tenacious subgingival calculus and necrotic cementum. Their use is limited compared with curettes.

Ultrasonic instruments are used for scaling and cleansing tooth surfaces and curetting the soft tissue wall of the periodontal pocket.[10]

Cleansing and polishing instruments—rubber cups, brushes, portepolishers, and dental tape—are used to cleanse and polish tooth surfaces.

The wearing and cutting qualities of some types of steel used in periodontal instruments have been tested,[17, 18] but specifications vary among manufacturers. Each group of instruments has characteristic features; individual therapists often develop variations with which they operate most effectively. Small instruments are recommended to fit into pockets without injuring the soft tissues.[21, 26, 27]

The parts of each instrument, referred to as the *blade*, *shank*, and *handle*, are shown in Figure 37–1.

PERIODONTAL PROBES

Periodontal probes are used to measure the depth of pockets and to determine their configuration. The typical feature is a tapered rod-like portion calibrated in millimeters, with a

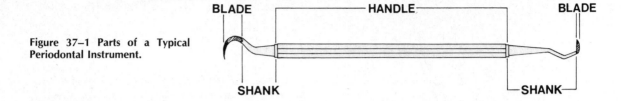

BLADE   **HANDLE**   **BLADE**

SHANK   **SHANK**

Figure 37–1 Parts of a Typical Periodontal Instrument.

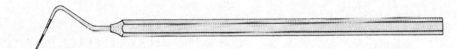

Figure 37–2 The periodontal probe is composed of the handle, the shank, and the calibrated working end.

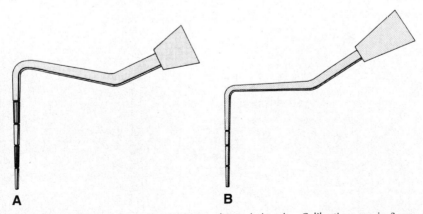

A   **B**

Figure 37–3 Types of Periodontal Probes. *A,* The Marquis color-coded probe. Calibrations are in 3-mm sections. *B,* The University of Michigan "O" probe.

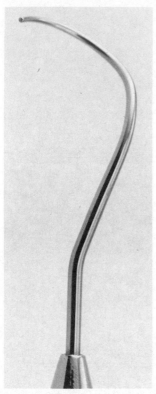

Figure 37–4 The Curved Nabers Probe for Detection of Furcation Areas.

blunt rounded tip (Fig. 37–2). There are several other designs with various millimeter calibrations (Fig. 37–3). Ideally, these probes are thin, and the shank is angled to allow easy insertion into the pocket. Furcation areas can best be evaluated by the curved Nabers probe (Fig. 37–4).

In measuring a pocket, the probe is inserted with a firm, gentle pressure to the bottom of the pocket. The shank should be aligned with the long axis of the tooth. Several measurements are made to determine the course of the pocket along the surface of the tooth.

EXPLORERS

Explorers are used to locate subgingival deposits and carious areas. They are also used to check the smoothness of the root surfaces after root planing. Explorers are designed with different shapes and angles for a variety of uses. Some of the most commonly used explorers are shown in Figure 37–5. Their uses and limitations are shown in Figure 37–6. The periodontal probe can also be very useful in the detection of subgingival deposits (Fig. 37–6).

SCALING AND CURETTAGE INSTRUMENTS

Scaling and curettage instruments are illustrated in Figure 37–7.

Sickle Scalers (Superficial Scalers)

The sickle scaler is used to remove supragingival deposits (Fig. 37–8). Because of the de-

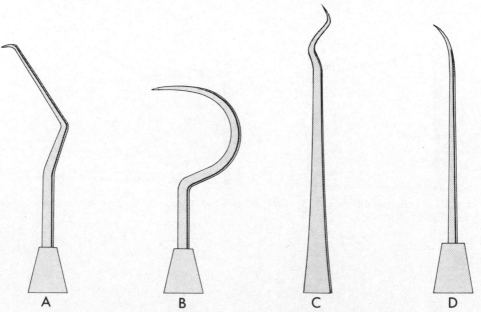

Figure 37–5 Four Typical Explorers. *A*, No. 17. *B*, No. 23. *C*, Pigtail. *D*, No. 3

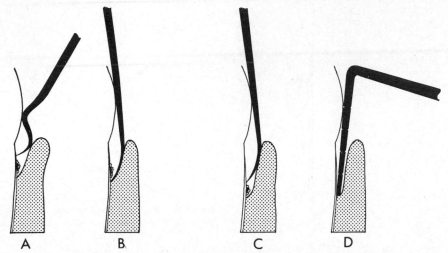

Figure 37–6 Insertion of Several Types of Explorers and a Probe in a Pocket for Calculus Detection. *A,* The limitations of the pigtail explorer in a deep pocket. *B,* Insertion of the No. 3 explorer. *C,* Limitations of the No. 3 explorer. *D,* Insertion of the probe.

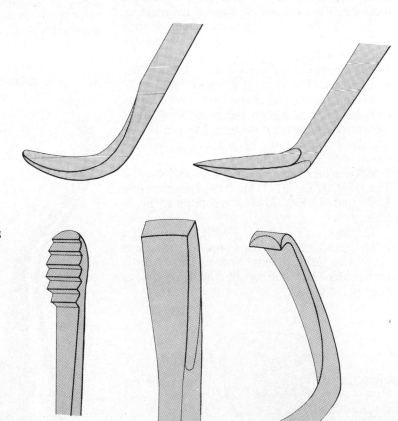

Figure 37–7 The Five Basic Scaling Instruments: curette, sickle, file, chisel, and hoe.

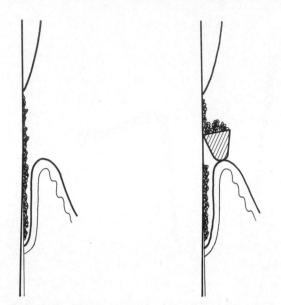

Figure 37–8 Use of Sickle Scaler for Removal of Supragingival Calculus.

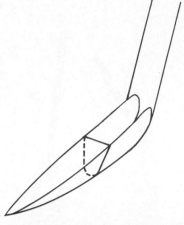

Figure 37–10 Basic Characteristics of Sickle Scaler: triangular shape, double cutting edge, and pointed tip.

It is important to note that sickle scalers with the same basic design can be obtained with different blade sizes and shank types to adapt to specific uses. The U15/30 and Ball sickles are very large. The Jaquette Nos. 1, 2, and 3 are medium-bladed. The Morse sickles, with their small blades (0, 00), are miniature instruments. The selection of these instruments should be based on the area to be scaled.

sign of this instrument, it would be difficult to insert the blade under the gingiva without damaging the surrounding gingival tissues (Fig. 37–9). The sickle scaler is triangular, with a pointed tip, and it has cutting edges on both sides of the blade (Fig. 37–10). It is used with a pull stroke. Both the sickle scaler and the curette consist of a handle, shank, and blade (see Fig. 37–1). The shank may have several sections, depending on the number of turns incorporated into the design. The portion of the shank closest to the blade is called the lower or working shank.

Sickle scalers have varying sizes and shapes. The U15/30 (Fig. 37–11) and the Jaquette Nos. 1, 2, and 3 (Fig. 37–12) are popular sickle scalers.

The Morse sickle (Fig. 37–13) is very useful in the mandibular anterior area when there is very little interproximal space. The blade is replaceable and can be obtained in various sizes (0, 00).

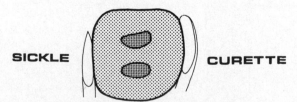

SICKLE   **CURETTE**

Figure 37–9 Subgingival adaptation around the root is better with the curette than with the sickle.

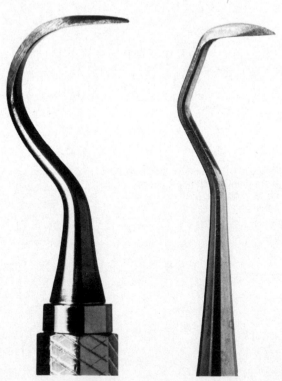

Figure 37–11 Both ends of a U15/30 scaler.

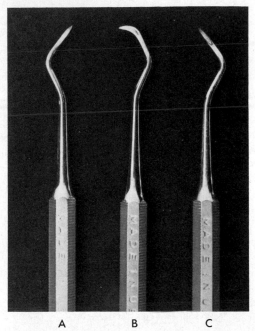

Figure 37–12 Jaquette Scalers. *A,* No. 2. *B,* No. 1. *C,* No. 3.

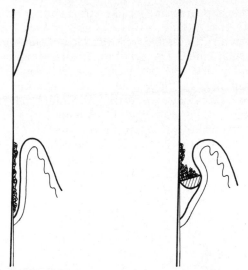

Figure 37–14 The curette is the instrument of choice for subgingival scaling and root planing.

Curettes

The curette is the instrument of choice for removing deep subgingival calculus, root planing the altered cementum, and removing the soft tissue lining the periodontal pocket (Fig. 37–14). It is finer than the sickle scalers and does not have any sharp points or corners other than the cutting edges of the blade (Fig. 37–15). Therefore, curettes provide better access to deep pockets with a minimum of soft tissue trauma (see Fig. 37–9). The design of the curette is such that in cross section, the

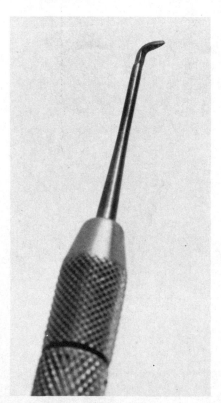

Figure 37–13 Morse Sickle Scaler. Blades are replaceable.

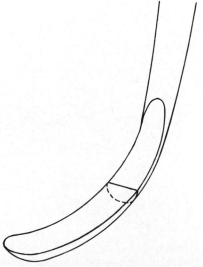

Figure 37–15 Basic Characteristics of a Curette: spoon-shaped blade and rounded tip.

blade appears semicircular with a convex base. The two lateral borders of the convex base form a cutting edge with the face of the semicircular blade. The tip of the blade is rounded, unlike that of the sickle scaler, which is pointed. The blade may have either one or two cutting edges, and the instrument may be single- or double-ended, depending on the preference of the operator.

As shown in Figure 37–9, the curved design of the curette allows the blade to hug the root surface, unlike the straight blade and pointed end of a sickle scaler.

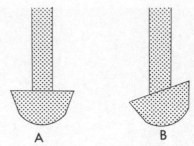

Figure 37–16 Principal Types of Curettes as Seen from the Toe of the Instrument. *A,* Universal curette. *B,* Gracey curette. Note the offset blade angulation of the Gracey curette.

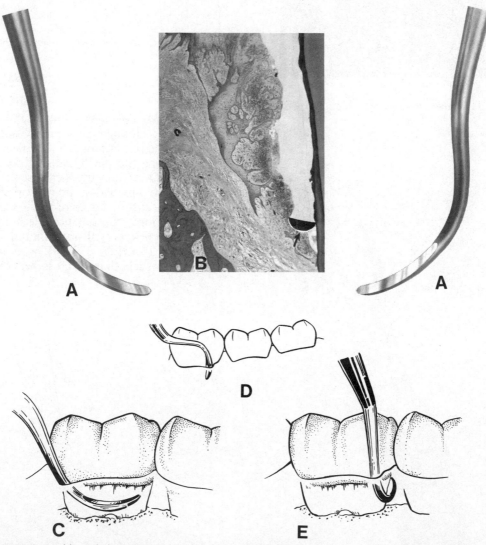

Figure 37–17 *A,* Double-ended curette for the removal of subgingival calculus. *B,* Cross section of the scaler blade *(arrow)* against cemental wall of a deep periodontal pocket. *C,* Curette in position at the base of a periodontal pocket on the facial surface of a mandibular molar. *D,* Curette inserted in pocket with tip directed apically. *E,* Curette in position at base of pocket on distal surface of mandibular molar.

The curettes are of two basic types, universal and specific. **Universal curettes** are designed so that they may be inserted in most areas of the dentition by altering and adapting the finger rest, the fulcrum, and hand position of the operator. The blade size and the angle and length of the shank may vary, but all universal curettes are at a 90° angle (perpendicular) to the lower shank when seen in cross section from the tip (Fig. 37–16*A*). The Barnhart Nos. 1–2 and 5–6 and the Columbia Nos. 13–14, 2R-2L, and 4R–4L (Figs. 37–17 and 37–18) are examples of universal curettes.

Gracey curettes are representative of the **specific curettes;** they are a set of several instruments designed and angled to adapt to specific anatomic areas of the dentition (Fig. 37–19). *These curettes are probably the best for subgingival scaling and root planing.* Double-ended Gracey curettes are paired in the following manner:

Gracey No. 1–2 ⎫
Gracey No. 3–4 ⎬ Anterior teeth

Gracey No. 5–6 ⎱ Anterior teeth and
⎰ bicuspids

Gracey No. 7–8 ⎱ Posterior teeth:
Gracey No. 9–10 ⎰ buccal and lingual

Gracey No. 11–12 ⎱ Posterior teeth: mesial
⎰ (Fig. 37–20)

Gracey No. 13–14 ⎱ Posterior teeth: distal
⎰ (Fig. 37–21)

Single-ended Gracey curettes can also be obtained, in which case a set would be composed of 14 instruments. Although these curettes are designed to be used in specific areas, as shown in the foregoing list, an experienced operator can adapt each instrument for use in several different areas by altering the position of his or her hand and the position of the patient.

The Gracey curette also differs from the universal curettes in that the blade is not at a 90° angle to the lower shank. The term *offset blade* is used for Gracey curettes, since they are angled approximately 60 to 70° from the lower shank (see Fig. 37–16*B*). This unique angulation allows the blade to be inserted in the precise position necessary for subgingival scaling and root planing, provided that the lower shank is parallel with the long axis of the tooth being scaled. Another difference in the blade is seen from the top. Specific curettes have a curved blade, whereas the blade of the universal curette is straight (Fig. 37–22). Thus, a pull stroke can be utilized. Some of the major differences between Gracey (specific)

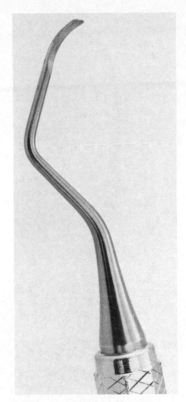

Figure 37–18 Columbia 4R–4L.

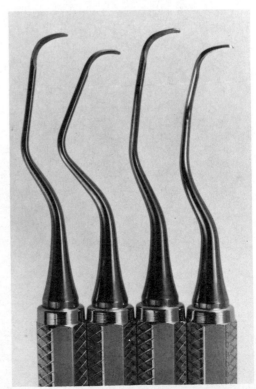

Figure 37–19 Reduced Set of Gracey Curettes. From left, No. 5–6, No. 7–8, No. 11–12 and No. 13–14.

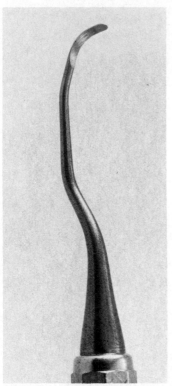

Figure 37–20 Gracey 11–12 Curette. Note the double turn of the shank.

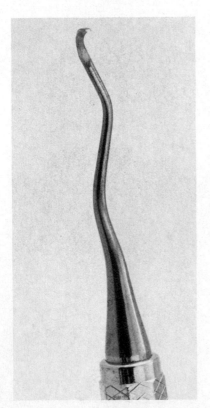

Figure 37–21 Gracey 13–14 Curette. Note the acute turn of the blade.

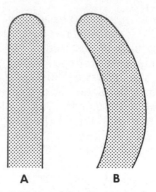

Figure 37–22 *A,* **Universal Curette as Seen from the Blade.** Note that blade is straight. *B,* **Gracey Curette as Seen from the Blade.** The blade is curved; only the convex cutting edge is used.

curettes and universal curettes are listed in Table 37–1).

Hoe Scalers

Hoe scalers are used for planing and smoothing root surfaces, which entails removal of calculus remnants and softened cementum (Fig. 37–23). The blade is bent at a 99° angle; the cutting edge is formed by the junction of the flattened terminal surface with the inner aspect of the blade. The cutting edge is beveled at 45°. The blade is slightly bowed so that it can maintain contact at two points on a convex surface. The back of the blade is rounded, and the blade has been reduced to minimum thickness to permit access to the roots of deep pockets without interference from the adjacent tissues.

Hoe scalers are used as follows:

1. The blade is inserted to the base of the periodontal pocket so that it makes two-point contact with the tooth (Fig. 37–23). This stabilizes the instrument and prevents nicking of the root.

2. The instrument is activated with a firm motion toward the crown, with every effort being made to preserve the two-point contact with the tooth.

McCall's hoe scalers Nos. 3, 4, 5, 6, 7, and 8 are a set of six hoe scalers designed to provide access to all tooth surfaces. Each instrument has a different angle between shank and handle.

Files

Files were popular at one time, but they are no longer used very much for scaling and root

TABLE 37–1   COMPARISON OF SPECIFIC (GRACEY) AND UNIVERSAL CURETTES*

	Gracey Curette	Universal Curette
Area of Use	*Area-specific.* Set of many designed for specific areas and surfaces.	*Universal.* One curette designed for all areas and surfaces.
Cutting Edge		
Use	*One cutting edge used.* Work with outer edge only.	*Both cutting edges used.* Work with either outer or inner edge.
Curvature	*Curved in two planes.* Blade curves up and to the side.	*Curved in one plane.* Blade curves up, not to side.
Blade Angle	*Offset blade.* Face of blade beveled at 60° to shank.	*Not offset.* Face of blade beveled at 90° to shank.

*Modified from Pattison, G., and Pattison, A.: Periodontal Instrumentation. Reston, Virginia: Reston Publishing Company, 1978.

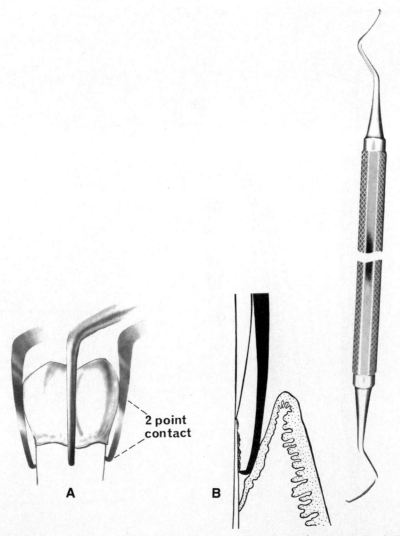

Figure 37–23 Hoe Scalers. *A,* Hoe scalers designed for different tooth surfaces, showing "two-point" contact. *B,* Hoe scaler in a periodontal pocket. The back of the blade is rounded for easier access. The instrument contacts the tooth at two points for stability.

planing because they gouge and roughen root surfaces.[15] They are sometimes used for removing overhanging margins of dental restorations.

Chisel Scalers

The chisel scaler, designed for the proximal surfaces of teeth too closely spaced to permit the use of other scalers, is usually used in the anterior part of the mouth. It is a double-ended instrument with a curved and a straight shank (Fig. 37–24); the blades are slightly curved with a straight cutting edge beveled at 45°.

The scaler is inserted from the facial surface. The slight curve of the blade makes it possible to stabilize it against the proximal surface, whereas the cutting edge engages the calculus without nicking the tooth. The instrument is activated with a push motion while the side of the blade is held firmly against the root.

Ultrasonic Instruments

Ultrasonic instruments may be used for scaling, curettage, and stain removal.[10] Their action is derived from physical vibrations of particles of matter, similar to sound waves, at frequencies ranging from 20,000 to many million cycles per second, above the range of human hearing ("cycles per second" are also referred to as Hertz or Hz). In periodontal instrumentation, tipped instruments producing up to 29,000 vibrations per second are used.

Ultrasonic tips of different shapes are available for scaling, curettage, root planing, and gingival surgery (Fig. 37–25). All tips are de-

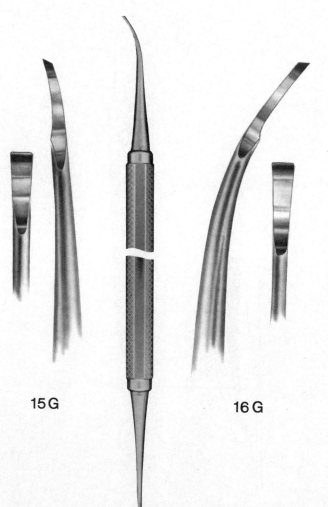

15 G   16 G

Figure 37–24 Chisel Scalers with Curved and Straight Shanks.

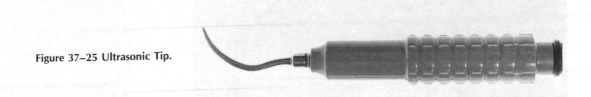

Figure 37–25 Ultrasonic Tip.

signed to operate in a wet field and have attached water outlets (Fig. 37–26). The spray is directed at the end of the tip to dissipate the heat generated by the ultrasonic vibrations.

The instrument is used with a light touch and a limited number of strokes per unit of area. Improper use may produce gouging and roughening of the root surfaces. The tips work best against hard tooth surfaces but can also be used against gingival tissue. The gingiva can be made more rigid by injecting anesthetic solution directly into it.[5] When placed against a tooth or soft tissue surface, the instrument mechanically débrides surface accumulations or necrotic tissue. The liquid sprayed on the vibrating tip reinforces the mechanical cleansing effect of the vibrations. The instrument should be kept away from bone to avoid the possibility of necrosis and sequestration. Ultrasonic instruments should not be used on young growing tissues; thus, their use in the treatment of children is not recommended.[10]

When applied to the gingiva of experimental animals, ultrasonic vibrations disrupt tissue continuity, lift off epithelium, dismember collagen bundles, and alter the morphology of fibroblast nuclei.[12] However, the simple application of ultrasonic vibrations to the gingiva produces no clinically discernible morphologic changes, and its use following gingivectomy does not appear to retard gingival healing.[11]

Ultrasound is effective for removing calculus[5, 14, 19, 21] and débriding the epithelial lining of periodontal pockets.[12] It produces a narrow band of necrotic tissue (microcauterization), which strips off from the inner aspect of the pocket. The Morse-type scaler and the rod-shaped instrument are used for this purpose. Some investigators find ultrasonic instruments as effective as manual instruments for curettage,[20] causing less inflammation but more pronounced disruption of the uppermost periodontal fibers.[29] When débriding the gingival wall of periodontal pockets, these instruments tend to remove less of the underlying connective tissue than manual instruments, but they do not smooth the root as well.[23] They tend to produce a stippled root with greater removal of tooth substance.[3] The volume and depth of tooth structure loss may be reduced by using a medium setting on the instrument and applying only slight tactile force.[6]

There are reports that ultrasonic instruments roughen dentin surfaces[4] and cause more goug-

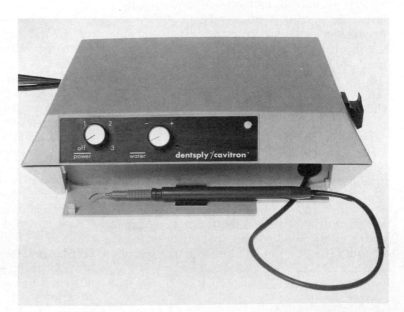

Figure 37–26 Ultrasonic Unit.

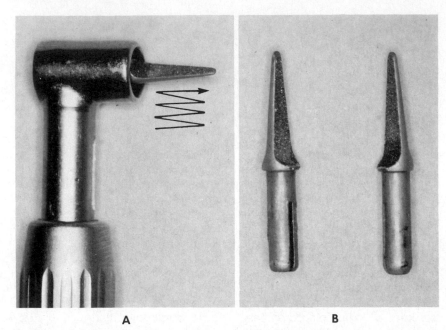

Figure 37–27 *A*, **EVA Handpiece.** Zig-zag arrow indicates direction of motion. *B*, **EVA Tips.**

ing and nicking of the roots than manual instruments[1, 14] and that they are not as effective as manual instruments for root planing.[24, 28] The roughness scores of teeth planed with ultrasound have been reported as twice those of teeth planed with hand curettes.[15] However, no significant differences were found in the clinical parameters of 4- to 6-mm pockets after ultrasonic root débridement and hand instrumentation.[25]

Opinions differ regarding the effectiveness of ultrasound for removing stains as compared with conventional methods of oral prophylaxis.[5, 14, 20] There is no significant difference between manual and ultrasonic instruments in the incidence of bacteremia following subgingival procedures.[2]

The EVA System

Probably the most efficient and least traumatic instruments for correcting overhanging or overcontoured proximal alloy and resin restorations are motor-driven diamond files (Fig. 37–27).* These files, which come in symmetric pairs, are made of aluminum in the shape of a wedge protruding from a shaft; one side of the wedge is diamond-coated, the other side is smooth. The files can be mounted on a special

---

*EVA prophylaxis instrument, designed by Dr. Per Axelsson, Karlstadt, Sweden.

dental handpiece attachment that generates reciprocating strokes of variable frequency. When the unit is activated interproximally, with the diamond-coated side of the file touching the restoration and the smooth side adjacent to the papilla, the oscillating file swiftly planes the contour of the restoration and reduces it to the desired shape.

CLEANSING AND POLISHING INSTRUMENTS

The rubber cup, portepolisher, bristle brush, and dental tape are employed in the dental office for cleansing and polishing the tooth surfaces.

Rubber cups consist of a rubber shell with or without web-shaped configurations in the hollow interior (Fig. 37–28). They are used in the handpiece with a special prophylaxis angle. There are many types of cleansing and polishing pastes, which should be kept moist to minimize frictional heat as the cup revolves. Aggressive use of the rubber cup may remove the layer of cementum, which is very thin in the cervical area.

The *portepolisher* is a hand instrument constructed to hold a wooden point with which polishing paste is applied to the tooth with a firm burnishing action. The Ivory straight portepolisher with the wood point set at an angle of 45° to the handle fulfills most needs

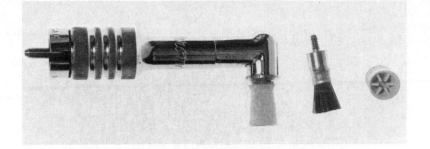

Figure 37–28 Prophylaxis Handpiece with Rubber Cup and Brush.

(Fig. 37–29). A contra-angle portepolisher, angulated at 60° for use in the posterior part of the mouth, is also available.

Bristle brushes are available in wheel and cup shapes (see Fig. 37–28). The brush is used in the handpiece with a polishing paste. Because the bristles are very stiff, use of the brush should be confined to the crown to avoid injuring the cementum.

Dental tape with polishing paste is used for polishing proximal surfaces inaccessible to the other polishing instruments. The tape is passed interproximally while being kept at a right angle to the long axis of the tooth and is activated with a firm labiolingual motion. Particular care is taken to avoid injury to the gingiva. The area should be cleansed with warm water to remove all remnants of paste.

SURGICAL INSTRUMENTS

Periodontal surgery is accomplished with numerous instruments. Figure 37–30 shows a typical surgical tray. Periodontal surgical instruments are classified as follows:
1. Excisional and incisional instruments
2. Surgical curettes and sickles
3. Periosteal elevators
4. Surgical chisels
5. Surgical files
6. Scissors
7. Hemostats and tissue forceps

Excisional and Incisional Instruments

PERIODONTAL KNIVES (GINGIVECTOMY KNIVES). The Kirkland knife is representative of those commonly used for gingivectomy. These knives can be obtained as either double- or single-ended instruments. The entire periphery of these kidney-shaped knives is a cutting edge (Fig. 37–31*A*).

INTERDENTAL KNIVES. The Orban No. 1–2 (Fig. 37–31*B*) and the Merrifield Nos. 1, 2, 3, and 4 are examples of knives that are used for the interdental areas. These spear-shaped knives have cutting edges on both sides of the blade and are designed with either double- or single-ended blades.

SURGICAL BLADES. Scalpel blades of different shapes and sizes are used in periodontal surgery. These blades are used in flap, mucogingival, and graft operations. The most commonly used blades are Nos. 11, 12, and 15 (Fig. 37–32). The blades are usually used once and are considered disposable.

ELECTROSURGERY (SURGICAL DIATHERMY)* The term *electrosurgery* is currently used to identify surgical techniques performed on soft tissue by using controlled high-frequency electrical (radio) currents in the range of 1.5 to 7.5 million cycles per second. Modern electronic research has produced a new gen-

---

*Section on electrosurgery contributed by Dr. John E. Flocken.

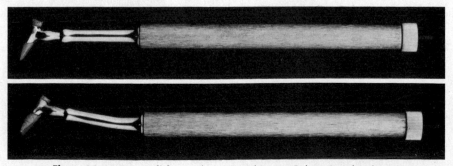

Figure 37–29 Portepolishers. *Above,* Straight type. *Below,* Angulated type.

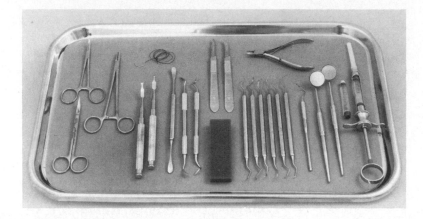

Figure 37–30 A Typical Surgical Instrument Tray.

eration of electrosurgical equipment capable of the precise, safe management of soft tissue (Fig. 37–33).

Since their initial use in 1900 for coagulation and in 1908 for tissue cutting, progress in the use of high-frequency currents has been very slow. Early electrosurgical units primarily developed for the medical and veterinary professions were overpowered and did not possess the refinement of current or currents required for the multitude of soft tissue procedures

performed within the oral cavity. Significant improvement in the equipment designed for dental use did not occur until the 1960s. In late 1973, filtered, fully rectified currents became available. The three types of current (partially rectified, fully rectified, and filtered, fully rectified) offer a wide range of control over tissue management and hemorrhage (Fig. 37–34).

There are three classes of active electrodes (Fig. 37–35): (1) single-wire electrodes for incising or excising, (2) loop electrodes for

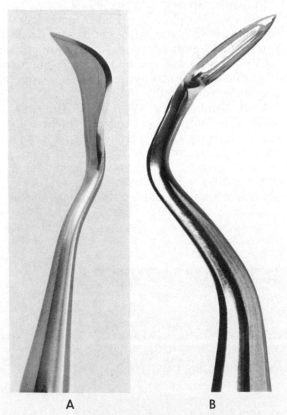

A   **B**

Figure 37–31 Gingivectomy Knives. *A,* Kirkland knife. *B,* Orban interdental knife.

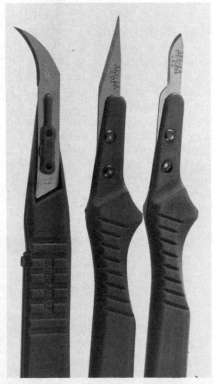

Figure 37–32 Surgical Blades. From left to right, Nos. 12, 11, and 15.

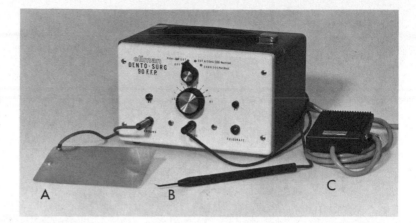

Figure 37–33 Electrosurgical Unit. *A,* Passive or conductive plate. *B,* Active electrode handle and tip electrode. *C,* Foot switch.

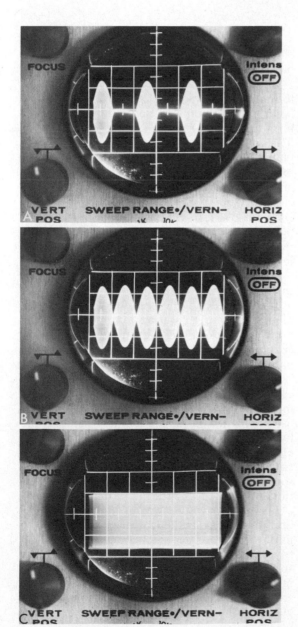

Figure 37–34 Oscilloscopic Views of Currents Used in Electrosurgery. *A,* Partially rectified current wave train. *B,* Fully rectified current. *C,* Filtered, fully rectified current wave train.

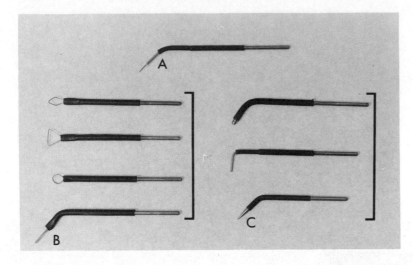

Figure 37–35 Active Electrodes. *A,* Single-wire cutting tip. *B,* Loop electrodes for planing. *C,* Coagulation electrodes.

planing tissue, and (3) heavy, bulkier electrodes for coagulation procedures.

Basically, there are four types of electrosurgical techniques:

Electrosection, also referred to as electrotomy or acusection, requires an undamped (fully rectified) or continuous (filtered, fully rectified) wave train. Three classes of procedures are included in electrosection: incisions, excisions, and planing. Incisions and excisions are performed with single-wire active electrodes that can be bent or adapted to perform any type of cutting procedure. Planing of tissue can be accomplished by selection of the appropriate loop electrode.

Electrocoagulation uses a damped or interrupted wave train such as the partially rectified current or the modified fully rectified current. A very wide range of coagulation or hemorrhage control can be obtained by utilizing the electrocoagulation current with different techniques. It must be clearly understood that electrocoagulation can *prevent* bleeding or hemorrhage at the initial entry into soft tissue. It cannot *stop* bleeding once blood is present. All forms of hemorrhage must be stopped first by some form of direct pressure: air, compress, or hemostat. Once bleeding has momentarily stopped, final sealing of the capillaries or large vessels can be accomplished by a short application of the electrocoagulation current. The active electrodes used for coagulation are much bulkier than the fine tungsten wire used for electrosection. There are three types of coagulation electrodes. Ball electrodes are used for general hemostasis, bar electrodes for controlling petechial or slight hemorrhage in restricted areas. The bar electrode can also be used to desensitize hypersensitive dentin. Cone electrodes can be used to control sulcular bleeding.

Electrosection and electrocoagulation are biterminal techniques that require the use of a large conductive plate electrode, which is referred to as the passive electrode (sometimes it is called the indifferent plate or dispersive plate or electrode). The closer the passive plate is to the operative site, the more effective any given current value will be. The passive plate is needed for predictable and refined cutting. Best results are obtained when the passive plate has direct contact with the skin, but it may be placed in a close but less obvious location for psychologic reasons.

Electrosection and electrocoagulation are the procedures most commonly used in all areas of dentistry. The two monoterminal techniques, electrofulguration and electrodesiccation, are seldom used. In monoterminal procedures, only the active electrode is used; the passive plate is not utilized.

Electrofulguration uses a high-voltage, low-current, damped wave train or, less often, an interrupted wave train. No passive plate is used. This technique somewhat resembles the hyprecator techniques of the 1950s. The active electrode is held just slightly out of tissue contact and moved over the tissue, spraying sparks to produce an eschar. Electrofulguration has limited application in dentistry.

Electrodesiccation, which employs a dehydrating current, is the least used as well as the most dangerous technique. The active electrode is inserted into the tissue, and the tissue surrounding the electrode is mass coagulated in situ. This procedure is useful in dermatology and cancer surgery and for cavernous hemangiomas.

It is well to remember that the electrosurgical unit is a radio transmitter. Just as a radio station must be fine-tuned for good reception, successful electrosurgical procedures also require fine-tuning. Each kind of body tissue has a different impedance or resistance value. Electrosurgical units, even from the same manufacturer, differ in wave form and output characteristics. Impedance and electrolyte content vary in different areas of the body and in different patients. Operatory environments differ in grounding potential. Also, current output varies with local demand for electrical energy. All these factors govern the outcome of electrosurgery.

The local heat generated in the tissues immediately lateral to the operative site is called *lateral heat*. It is directly under the control of the operator. Lateral heat is directly related to five controlling factors: the duration of current exposure to any one point, the dosage of current, the size and shape of the electrode, the type of current, and the tissue impedance. An excess of any one of these factors must be offset by a reduction of one or more of the other factors to prevent accumulation of destructive heat within the tissues.

The most important basic rule of electrosurgery is *always keep the tip moving.* Prolonged or repeated application of current to tissue induces heat accumulation and undesired tissue destruction, whereas interrupted application at intervals adequate for tissue cooling (5 to 10 seconds) reduces or eliminates heat build-up. Electrosurgery is *not* intended to destroy tissue; it is a controllable means of sculpturing or modifying oral soft tissue with the least discomfort and hemorrhage for the patient.

The advantages of electrosurgery are:
1. The active electrodes are flexible fine wires that:
   a. Can be bent or shaped to fit any requirement
   b. Never need sharpening
   c. Are self-sterilizing
   d. Require no pressure; in fact, pressure is contraindicated.
2. It permits any degree of hemorrhage control desired.
3. It prevents seeding of bacteria into the incision site.
4. It permits tissue planing—a procedure unique to electrosurgery.
5. It provides a better view of the operative site because bleeding is controlled and no pressure is needed for cutting.
6. It eliminates scar formation.

The disadvantages of electrosurgery are:
1. It is contraindicated for patients who have noncompatible or poorly shielded cardiac pacemakers.
2. It produces an odor and sometimes a taste that must be controlled.

The indications for electrosurgery in periodontal therapy and a description of wound healing after electrosurgery are presented in Chapter 52.

Surgical Curettes and Sickles

Larger and heavier curettes and sickles are often needed during surgery for the removal of granulation tissue, fibrous interdental tissues, and tenacious subgingival deposits. The Kramer Nos. 1, 2, and 3 (Fig. 37–36) and the Kirkland surgical instruments are heavy curettes, whereas the Ball scaler No. B2–B3 is a popular heavy sickle. The wider, heavier blades of these instruments make them suitable for surgical procedures.

Periosteal Elevators

These instruments are necessary to reflect and move the flap after the incision has been

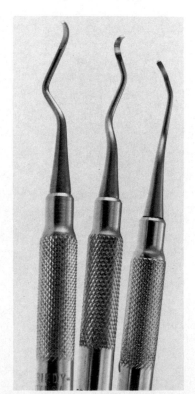

Figure 37–36 Kramer Heavy Surgical Curettes Nos. 1, 2, and 3.

made for flap surgery. The No. 24G (Fig. 37–37) and the Goldman-Fox No. 14 are two very well-designed periosteal elevators.

Surgical Chisels and Hoes

Chisels and hoes are used during periodontal surgery for removing and reshaping bone. The hoe has a curved shanked blade (Fig. 37–38), whereas the Wiedelstadt and Todd-Gilmore chisels are straight-shanked (Fig. 37–39A). The surgical hoe has a flattened, fishtail-shaped blade with a pronounced convexity in its terminal portion. The cutting edge is beveled with rounded edges and projects beyond the long axis of the handle to preserve the effectiveness of the instrument when the blade is reduced by sharpening. The surgical hoe is generally used for detaching pocket walls after the gingivectomy incision, but it is also useful for smoothing root and bone surfaces made accessible by any surgical procedure. The Ochsenbein No. 1–2 (Fig. 37–39B) is a very useful chisel with a semicircular indentation on both sides of the shank that allows the instrument to engage around the tooth into the interdental area. Surgical hoes are usually used with a pull

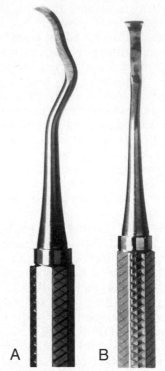

Figure 37–38 *A,* Lateral, and *B,* frontal view of a surgical hoe.

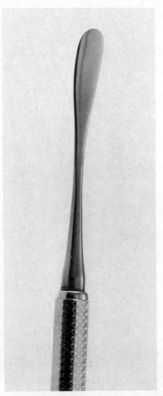

Figure 37–37 Glickman Periosteal Elevator No. 24G.

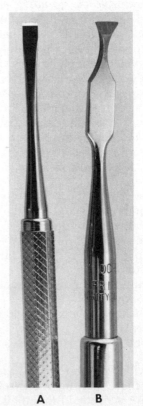

A   B

Figure 37–39 Surgical Chisels. *A,* Todd-Gilmore chisel. *B,* Ochsenbein chisel.

stroke, whereas chisels are engaged with a push stroke.

Surgical Files

Periodontal surgical files are used primarily to smooth rough bony ledges and to remove all areas of bone. The Schluger (Fig. 37–40) and Sugarman files are similar in design and can be used with a push-and-pull stroke, primarily in the interdental areas.

Scissors and Nippers

These are used in periodontal surgery for such purposes as removing tabs of tissue during gingivectomy, trimming the margins of flaps, enlarging incisions in periodontal abscesses, and removing muscle attachments in mucogingival surgery. There are many types; the choice is a matter of individual preference. Illustrated in Figure 37–41 is the Goldman-Fox No. 16 scissors with a curved beveled blade with serrations and the nippers.

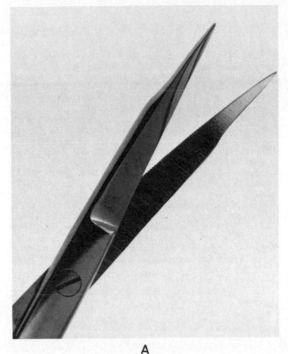

A

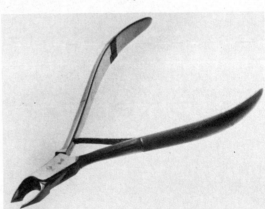

B

Figure 37–41 *A,* **Goldman-Fox No. 16 Scissors.** *B,* **Nippers.**

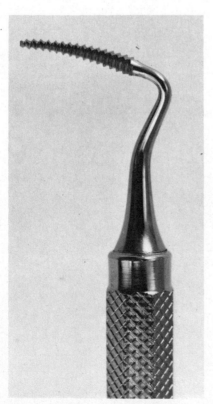

Figure 37–40 Schluger No. 9–10 Surgical File.

REFERENCES

1. Allen, E. F., and Rhoads, R. H.: Effects of high speed periodontal instruments on tooth surface. J. Periodontol., *34*:352, 1963.
2. Bandt, C. L., et al.: Bacteremias from ultrasonic and hand instrumentation. J. Periodontol., *35*:214, 1964.
3. Belting, C. M.: Effects of high speed periodontal instruments on the root surface during subgingival calculus removal. J. Am. Dent. Assoc., *69*:578, 1964.
4. Björn, H., and Lindhe, J.: The influence of periodontal instruments on the tooth surface. Odont. Revy, *13*:355, 1962.
5. Burman, L. R., Alderman, N. E., and Ewen, S. J.: Clinical application of ultrasonic vibrations for supragingival calculus and stain removal. J. Dent. Med., *13*:156, 1958.
6. Clark, S. M.: The effect of ultrasonic instrumentation on root surfaces. J. Periodontol., *39*:135, 1968.
7. Clark, S. M.: The ultrasonic dental unit: a guide for the

clinical application of ultrasonics in dentistry and in dental hygiene. J. Periodontol., *40*:621, 1969.

8. Everett, F. G., Foss, C. L., and Orban, B.: Study of instruments for scaling. Parodontologie, *16*:61, 1962.

9. Ewen, S. J.: The ultrasonic wound—some microscopic observations. J. Periodontol., *32*:315, 1961.

10. Ewen, S. J., and Glickstein, C.: Ultrasonic therapy in periodontics. Springfield, Ill., Charles C Thomas, 1968.

11. Frisch, J., et al.: Effect of ultrasonic instrumentation on human gingival connective tissue. Periodontics, *5*:123, 1967.

12. Goldman, H. M.: Histologic assay of healing following ultrasonic curettage versus hand instrument curettage. Oral Surg., *14*:925, 1961.

13. Green, E., and Ramfjord, S. J.: Tooth roughness after subgingival root planing. J. Periodontol., *37*:44, 1966.

14. Johnson, W. N., and Wilson, J. R.: The application of the ultrasonic dental units to scaling procedures. J. Periodontol., *28*:264, 1957.

15. Kerry, G. J.: Roughness of root surfaces after use of ultrasonic instruments and hand curettes. J. Periodontol., *38*:340, 1967.

16. Klug, R. G.: Gingival tissue regeneration following electrical retraction. J. Pros. Dent., *16*:955, 1966.

17. Lindhe, J.: Evaluation of periodontal scalers. II. Wear following standardized or diagonal cutting tests. Odont. Revy, *17*:121, 1966.

18. Lindhe, J., and Jacobson, L.: Evaluation of periodontal scalers. I. Wear following clinical use. Odont. Revy, *17*:1, 1966.

19. McCall, C. M., and Szmyd, L.: Clinical evaluation of ultrasonic scaling. J. Am. Dent. Assoc., *61*:559, 1960.

20. Nadler, H.: Removal of crevicular epithelium by ultrasonic curettes. J. Periodontol., *33*:220, 1962.

21. Orban, B., and Manella, V. B.: A macroscopic and microscopic study of instruments designed for root planing. J. Periodontol., *27*:120, 1956.

22. Romanelli, J. H.: Raspaje subgingival: su técnica. Rev. Odontol. (Buenos Aires), *36*:501, 1948; *37*:113, 277, 1949.

23. Sanderson, A. D.: Gingival curettage by hand and ultrasonic instruments—a histologic comparison. J. Periodontol., *37*:279, 1966.

24. Stende, G. W., and Schaffer, E. M.: A comparison of ultrasonic and hand scaling. J. Periodontol., *32*:312, 1961.

25. Torfason, T., Kiger, R., Selvig, K. A., and Egelberg, J.: Clinical improvement of gingival conditions following ultrasonic versus hand instrumentation of periodontal pockets. J. Clin. Periodontol., *6*:165, 1979.

26. Waerhaug, J., et al.: The dimension of instruments for removal of subgingival calculus. J. Periodontol., *25*:281, 1954.

27. Wentz, F. M.: Therapeutic root planing. J. Periodontol., *28*:59, 1957.

28. Wilkinson, R. F., and Maybury, J. E.: Scanning electron microscopy of the root surface following instrumentation. J. Periodontol., *44*:559, 1973.

29. Zach, L., and Cohen, G.: The histology of the response to ultrasonic curettage. J. Dent. Res., *40*:751, 1961.

chapter thirty-eight

Principles of Periodontal Instrumentation*

GENERAL PRINCIPLES OF INSTRUMENTATION

Effective instrumentation is governed by a number of general principles which are common to all periodontal instruments. Proper positioning of the patient and the operator, illumination and retraction for optimum visibility, and sharp instruments are fundamental prerequisites. A constant awareness of tooth and root morphology and of the condition of the periodontal tissues is also essential. Knowledge of instrument design enables the clinician efficiently to select the proper instrument for the procedure and the area in which it will be performed. In addition to all these principles, the basic concepts of grasp, finger rest, adaptation, angulation, and stroke must be understood before clinical instrumentation skills can be mastered.

Accessibility (Positioning of Patient and Operator)

Accessibility facilitates thoroughness of instrumentation. The position of the patient and operator should provide maximum accessibility to the area of operation. Inadequate accessibility impedes thorough instrumentation, prematurely tires the operator, and diminishes his effectiveness.

The clinician should be seated on a comfortable operating stool that has been posi-

tioned so that his feet are flat on the floor and his thighs parallel to the floor. The clinician should be able to observe the field of operation while keeping his back straight and his head erect.[18]

The patient should be in a supine position and placed so that the mouth is close to the resting elbow of the clinician. For instrumentation of the maxillary arch, the patient should be asked to raise his chin slightly to provide optimum visibility and accessibility. For instrumentation on the mandibular arch, it may be necessary to raise the back of the chair slightly and request that the patient lower his chin until the mandible is parallel to the floor. This will especially facilitate work on the lingual surfaces of the mandibular anterior teeth.

Visibility, Illumination, and Retraction

Whenever possible, direct vision with direct illumination from the dental light is most desirable (Fig. 38–1). If this is not attainable, indirect vision may be obtained by using the mouth mirror (Fig. 38–2), and indirect illumination may be obtained by using the mirror to reflect light to where it is needed (Fig. 38–3). Indirect vision and indirect illumination are often used simultaneously (Fig. 38–4).

Retraction provides visibility, accessibility, and illumination. The fingers, the mirror, or both are used for retraction, depending on the location of the area of operation. The mirror may be used for retraction of the cheeks or the tongue. The index finger is used for retraction of the lips or cheeks. The following illustrated methods are effective for retraction:

*Material in this chapter was drawn freely from Pattison, G., and Pattison, A.: Periodontal Instrumentation. Reston, Va., Reston Publishing Company, 1978.

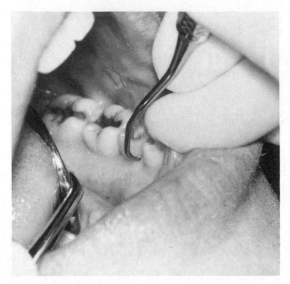

Figure 38–1 Direct Vision and Direct Illumination in the Mandibular Left Premolar Area.

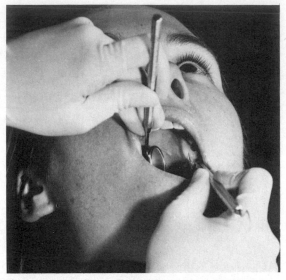

Figure 38–3 Indirect Illumination Using the Mirror to Reflect Light onto the Maxillary Left Posterior Lingual Region

1. Use of the mirror to deflect the cheek while the fingers of the nonoperating hand retract the lips and protect the angle of the mouth from irritation by the mirror handle (Fig. 38–5).
2. Use of the mirror alone to retract the lips and cheek (Fig. 38–6).
3. Use of the fingers of the nonoperating hand to retract the lips (Fig. 38–7).
4. Use of the mirror to retract the tongue (Fig. 38–8).
5. Combinations of the above.

When retracting, care should be taken to avoid irritation to the angles of the mouth. If the lips and skin are dry, softening the lips with petroleum jelly before beginning instru-

mentation is a helpful precaution against cracking and bleeding. Careful retraction is especially important for patients with a history of recurrent herpes labialis, because these patients may easily develop herpetic lesions following instrumentation.

Condition of Instruments (Sharpness)

Prior to any instrumentation, all instruments should be inspected to make sure that they are clean, sterile, and in good condition. The

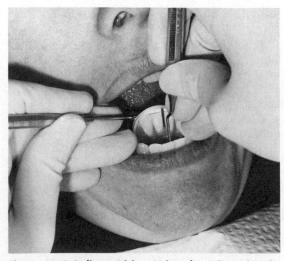

Figure 38–2 Indirect Vision Using the Mirror for the Lingual Surfaces of the Mandibular Anterior Teeth.

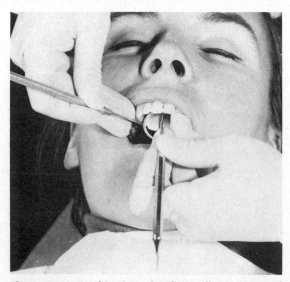

Figure 38–4 Combination of Indirect Illumination and Indirect Vision for the Lingual Surfaces of the Maxillary Anterior Teeth.

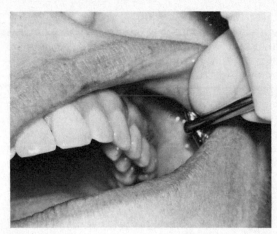

Figure 38–5 Retracting the Cheek with the Mirror and Fingers of the Nonoperating Hand.

working ends of pointed or bladed instruments must be sharp to be effective. *Sharp instruments enhance tactile sensitivity and allow the clinician to work more precisely and efficiently.* Dull instruments may lead to incomplete calculus removal and unnecessary trauma because of the excess force usually applied to compensate for their ineffectiveness (see Chapter 40).

Maintaining a Clean Field

Despite good visibility, illumination, and retraction, instrumentation can be hampered if the operative field is obscured by saliva, blood, and debris. The pooling of saliva interferes with visibility during instrumentation and impedes control because a firm finger rest cannot be established on wet, slippery tooth surfaces. Adequate suction with a saliva ejector or, if working with an assistant, an aspirator is essential.

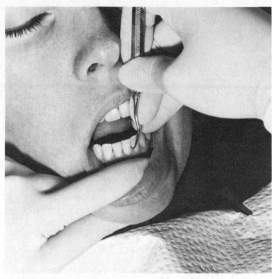

Figure 38–7 Retracting the Lip with the Index Finger of the Nonoperating Hand.

Gingival bleeding is an unavoidable consequence of subgingival instrumentation. In areas of inflammation this is not necessarily an indication of trauma from incorrect technique; rather, it is an indication of ulceration of the pocket epithelium. Blood and debris can be removed from the operative field with suction and by wiping or blotting with gauze squares. The operative field should also be flushed occasionally with water.

Compressed air and gauze squares can be used to facilitate visual inspection of tooth surfaces just below the gingival margin during instrumentation. A jet of air directed into the pocket will deflect a retractable gingival margin. Retractable tissue can also be deflected away from the tooth by gently packing the

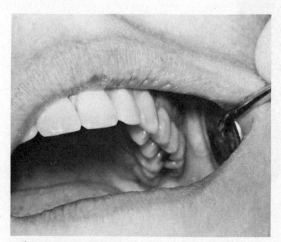

Figure 38–6 Retracting the Cheek with the Mirror.

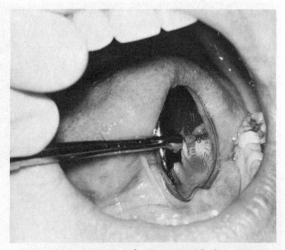

Figure 38–8 Retracting the Tongue with the Mirror.

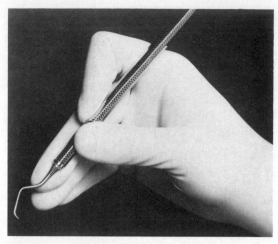

Figure 38–9 Modified Pen Grasp. Pad of the middle finger rests on the shank.

edge of a gauze square into the pocket with the back of a curette. Immediately after the gauze is removed, the subgingival area should be clean, dry, and clearly visible for a brief interval.

Instrument Stabilization

Stability of the instrument and the hand is the primary requisite for controlled instrumentation. Stability and control are essential for effective instrumentation and avoidance of injury to the patient or the clinician. The two factors of major importance in providing stability are the instrument grasp and the finger rest.

INSTRUMENT GRASP. A proper grasp is essential for the precise control of movements made during periodontal instrumentation. The most effective and stable grasp for all periodontal instruments is the **modified pen grasp** (Fig. 38–9). Although other grasps are possible, this modification of the *standard pen grasp* (Fig. 38–10) ensures the greatest control in performing intraoral procedures. *The thumb, index finger, and middle finger are used to hold the instrument as a pen is held, but the middle finger is positioned so that the pad rather than the side of the finger is resting on the instrument shank. The index finger is bent at the second joint from the fingertip and is positioned well above the middle finger on the same side of the handle. The pad of the thumb is placed midway between the middle and index fingers on the opposite side of the handle.* This creates a triangle of forces or *tripod effect* that enhances control because it counteracts the tendency of the instrument to turn uncontrollably between the fingers when scaling force is applied to the tooth. This stable modified pen grasp enhances control because it enables the clinician to roll the instrument in precise degrees against the index and middle fingers with the thumb in order to adapt the blade to the slightest changes in tooth contour. The modified pen grasp also enhances tactile sensitivity because slight irregularities on the tooth surface are best perceived when the tactile-sensitive pad of the middle finger is placed on the shank of the instrument.

The **palm and thumb grasp** (Fig. 38–11) is useful for stabilizing instruments during sharpening and for manipulating air and water syr-

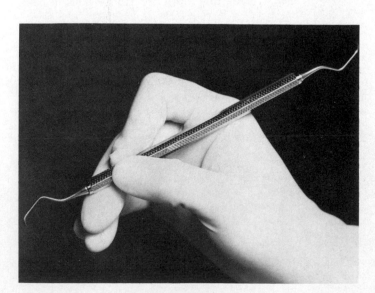

Figure 38–10 Standard Pen Grasp. Side of the middle finger rests on the shank.

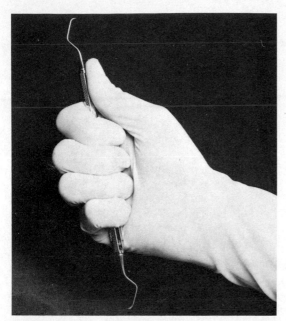

Figure 38–11 Palm and Thumb Grasp. Used for stabilizing instruments during sharpening.

inges, but it is not recommended for periodontal instrumentation. Maneuverability and tactile sensitivity are so inhibited by this grasp that it is unsuitable for the precise and controlled movements necessary during periodontal procedures.

FINGER REST. *The finger rest serves to stabilize the hand and the instrument by providing a firm fulcrum as movements are made to activate the instrument.* A good finger rest prevents injury and laceration of the gingiva and surrounding tissues by poorly controlled instruments. The fourth or ring finger is preferred by most clinicians for the finger rest. Although it is possible to use the third or middle finger for the finger rest, this is not recommended because it restricts the arc of movement during the activation of strokes and severely curtails the use of the middle finger for both control and tactile sensitivity. Maximum control is achieved when the middle finger is kept between the instrument shank and the fourth finger. This "built-up" fulcrum is an integral part of the wrist-forearm action that activates the powerful working stroke for calculus removal. Whenever possible, these two fingers should be kept together during scaling and root planing, to work as a one-unit fulcrum. The separation of the middle and fourth fingers during scaling strokes results in a loss of power and control because the separation of the fingers forces the clinician to rely solely on finger flexing for activation of the instrument.

Finger rests may be generally classified as *intraoral* finger rests or *extraoral* fulcrums. Intraoral finger rests on tooth surfaces are ideally established close to the working area. Variations of intraoral finger rests and extraoral fulcrums are utilized whenever good angulation and a sufficient arc of movement cannot be achieved by a finger rest close to the working area. The following examples illustrate the different variations of the intraoral finger rest:

1. *Conventional.* The finger rest is established on tooth surfaces immediately adjacent to the working area (Fig. 38–12).
2. *Cross-arch.* The finger rest is established on tooth surfaces on the other side of the same arch (Fig. 38–13).
3. *Opposite arch.* The finger rest is established on tooth surfaces on the opposite arch, e.g., a mandibular arch finger rest for instrumentation on the maxillary arch (Fig. 38–14).
4. *Finger-on-finger.* The finger rest is established on the index finger or thumb of the nonoperating hand (Fig. 38–15).

Extraoral fulcrums are essential for effective instrumentation of some aspects of the maxillary posterior teeth (see Chapter 39). When properly established, they allow optimal access and angulation while providing adequate stabilization. Extraoral fulcrums are not finger rests in the literal sense because the tips or pads of the fingers are not used for extraoral fulcrums as they are for intraoral finger rests. Instead, as much of the front or back surface of the fingers as possible is placed on the

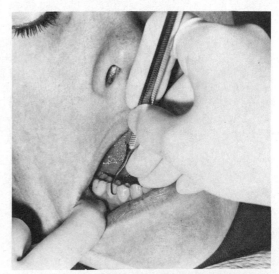

Figure 38–12 Intraoral Conventional Finger Rest. Fourth finger rests on the occlusal surfaces of adjacent teeth.

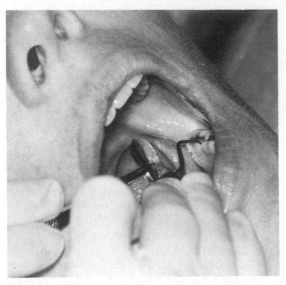

Figure 38–13 Intraoral Cross-arch Finger Rest. Fourth finger rests on the incisional surfaces of teeth on the opposite side of the same arch.

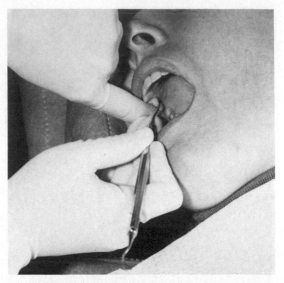

Figure 38–15 Intraoral Finger-on-finger Rest. Fourth finger rests on the index finger of nonoperating hand.

patient's face to provide the greatest degree of stability. The two most commonly used extraoral fulcrums are shown.

1. *Palm-up.* The fulcrum is established by resting the backs of the middle and fourth fingers on the skin overlying the lateral aspect of the mandible on the right side of the face (Fig. 38–16).
2. *Palm-down.* The fulcrum is established by resting the front surfaces of the middle and fourth fingers on the skin overlying

the lateral aspect of the mandible on the left side of the face (Fig. 38–17).

Both intraoral finger rests and extraoral fulcrums may be reinforced by applying the index finger or thumb of the nonoperating hand to the handle or shank of the instrument for added control and pressure against the tooth. The reinforcing finger is usually employed for opposite arch or extraoral fulcrums when precise control and pressure are compromised by the longer distance between the fulcrum and

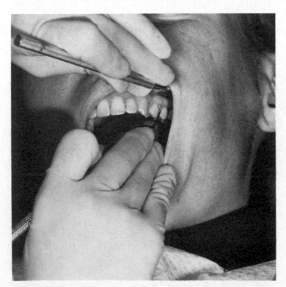

Figure 38–14 Intraoral Opposite Arch Finger Rest. Fourth finger rests on mandibular teeth while maxillary posterior teeth are instrumented.

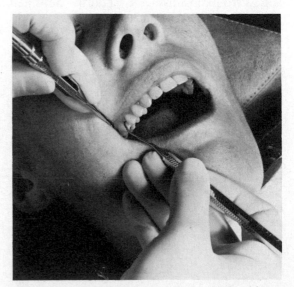

Figure 38–16 Extraoral Palm-up Fulcrum. Backs of fingers rest on right lateral aspect of mandible while maxillary right posterior teeth are instrumented.

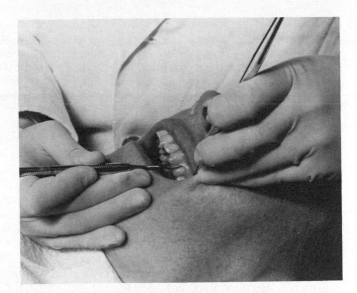

Figure 38–17 Extraoral Palm-down Fulcrum. Front surfaces of fingers rest on left lateral aspect of mandible while maxillary left posterior teeth are instrumented.

the working end of the instrument. Figure 38–18 shows the index finger reinforced, and Figure 38–19 shows the thumb reinforced.

Instrument Activation

ADAPTATION. *Adaptation* refers to the manner in which the working end of a periodontal instrument is placed against the surface of a tooth. The objective of adaptation is to make the working end of the instrument conform to the contour of the tooth surface. Precise adaptation must be maintained with all instruments to avoid trauma to the soft tissues and root surfaces and to ensure maximum effectiveness of instrumentation.

Correct adaptation of the probe is quite simple. The tip and side of the probe should be flush against the tooth surface as vertical strokes are activated within the crevice. Bladed instruments such as curettes and sharp-pointed instruments such as explorers are more difficult to adapt. The ends of these instruments are sharp and can lacerate tissue, so adaptation in subgingival areas becomes especially important. The lower third of the working end, which is the last few millimeters adjacent to

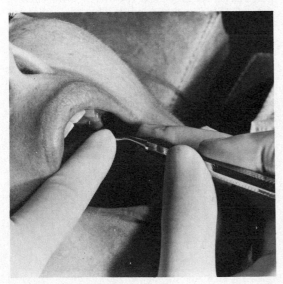

Figure 38–18 Index Finger Reinforced Rest. Index finger placed on shank for pressure and control in maxillary l∫ posterior lingual region.

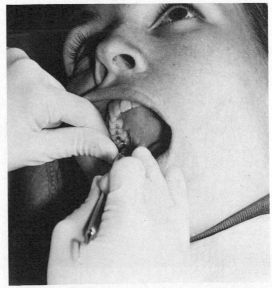

Figure 38–19 Thumb Reinforced Rest. Thumb placed on handle for control in maxillary right posterior lingual region.

the toe or tip, must constantly be kept in contact with the tooth while moving over varying tooth contours (Fig. 38–20). Precise adaptation is maintained by carefully rolling the handle of the instrument against the index and middle fingers with the thumb. This rotates the instrument in slight degrees so that the toe or tip leads into concavities and around convexities. On convex surfaces such as line angles, it is not possible to adapt more than 1 or 2 mm of the working end against the tooth. On broad, flat surfaces, however, more of the working end may be adapted.

If only the middle third of the working end is adapted on a convex surface, so that it contacts the tooth at a tangent, the toe or sharp tip will jut out into soft tissue, causing trauma and discomfort (Fig. 38–21). If the instrument is adapted so that *only* the toe or tip is in contact, the soft tissue can be distended or compressed by the back of the working end, also causing trauma and discomfort. A curette that is improperly adapted in this manner can be particularly damaging because the toe can gouge or groove the root surface.

ANGULATION. *Angulation* refers to the angle between the face of a bladed instrument and the tooth surface. It may also be called the "tooth-blade relationship."

Correct angulation is essential for effective calculus removal. For subgingival insertion of a bladed instrument such as a curette, angulation should be as close to 0° as possible (Fig.

38–22). The end of the instrument can be inserted to the base of the pocket more easily with the face of the blade flush against the tooth. *During scaling and root planing, optimal angulation is between 45 and 90°* (Fig. 38–22). The exact blade angulation depends on the amount and nature of the calculus, the procedure being performed, and the condition of the tissue. Blade angulation is diminished or closed by tilting the lower shank of the instrument toward the tooth. It is increased or opened by tilting the lower shank away from the tooth.

During scaling strokes on heavy, tenacious calculus, angulation should be just less than 90° so that the cutting edge "bites" into the calculus. With angulation of less than 45°, the cutting edge will not "bite" into or engage the calculus properly (Fig. 38–22). Instead, it will slide over the calculus, smoothing or "burnishing" it. If angulation is more than 90°, the lateral surface of the blade, rather than the cutting edge, is against the tooth and the calculus is not removed and may become burnished (Fig. 38–22). After the calculus has been removed, angulation of just less than 90° may be maintained or the angle may be slightly closed as the root surface is smoothed with light root planing strokes.

When gingival curettage is indicated, angulation greater than 90° is deliberately established so that the opposite cutting edge will engage and remove the pocket lining.

LATERAL PRESSURE. Lateral pressure refers to the pressure created when force is applied against the surface of a tooth with the cutting edge of a bladed instrument. The exact amount of pressure applied must be varied according

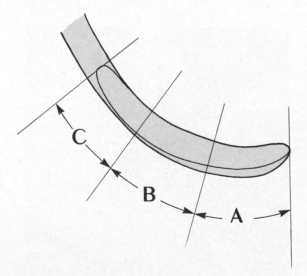

Figure 38–20 Gracey curette blade divided into three segments: the lower one third of the blade, consisting of the terminal few millimeters adjacent to the toe (A); the middle one third (B); and the upper one third, which is adjacent to the shank (C).

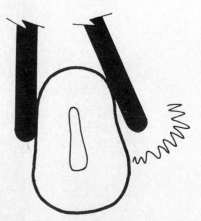

Figure 38–21 Blade Adaptation. The curette on the left is properly adapted to the root surface. The curette on the right is incorrectly adapted so that the toe juts out, lacerating the soft tissues.

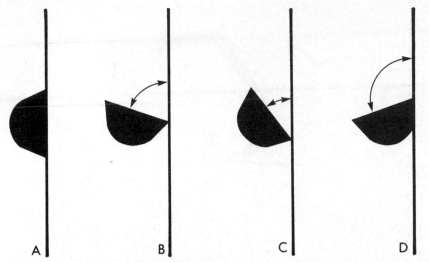

Figure 38–22 Blade Angulation. *A,* 0°—correct angulation for blade insertion. *B,* 45° to 90°—correct angulation for scaling and root planing. *C,* Less than 45°—incorrect angulation for scaling and root planing. *D,* More than 90°—incorrect angulation for scaling and root planing, correct angulation for gingival curettage.

to the nature of the calculus and according to whether the stroke is intended for initial scaling to remove calculus or for root planing to smooth the root surface.

Lateral pressure may be firm, moderate, or light. When removing calculus, firm or moderate lateral pressure is used initially and is progressively diminished until light lateral pressure is applied for the final root planing strokes. When insufficient lateral pressure is applied for the removal of heavy calculus, rough ledges or lumps may be shaved to thin, smooth sheets of burnished calculus that are very difficult to detect and remove. This burnishing effect often occurs in areas of developmental depressions and along the cemento-enamel junction.

Although firm lateral pressure is necessary for the thorough removal of calculus, the indiscriminate, unwarranted, or uncontrolled application of heavy forces during instrumentation should be avoided. Repeated application of excessively heavy strokes will neck or gouge the root surface.

The careful application of varied and controlled amounts of lateral pressure during instrumentation is an integral part of effective scaling and root planing technique and is absolutely critical to the success of both of these procedures.

STROKES. Three basic types of strokes are used during instrumentation: the exploratory stroke, the scaling stroke, and the root planing stroke. Any of these basic strokes may be activated by a pull or a push motion in a vertical, oblique, or horizontal direction (Fig. 38–23). Vertical and oblique strokes are used most frequently. Horizontal strokes are used selectively on line angles or deep pockets that cannot be negotiated with vertical or oblique strokes. The direction, length, pressure, and number of strokes necessary for either scaling or root planing are determined by four major factors: gingival position and tone, pocket depth and shape, tooth contour, and the amount and nature of the calculus or roughness.

The **exploratory stroke** is a light, "feeling" stroke that is used with probes and explorers to evaluate the dimensions of the pocket and to detect calculus and irregularities of the tooth surface. With bladed instruments such as the curette, the exploratory stroke is alternated with scaling and root planing strokes for these same purposes of evaluation and detection. The instrument is grasped lightly and adapted with light pressure against the tooth to achieve maximum tactile sensitivity.

The **scaling stroke** is a short, powerful *pull stroke* that is used with bladed instruments for the removal of both supragingival and subgingival calculus. The muscles of the fingers and hands are tensed to establish a secure grasp, and lateral pressure is firmly applied against the tooth surface. The cutting edge engages the apical border of the calculus and dislodges it with a firm movement in a coronal direction. The scaling motion should be initiated in the forearm and transmitted from the wrist to the hand with a slight flexing of the fingers. Rotation of the wrist is synchronized with movement of the forearm. The scaling stroke is not

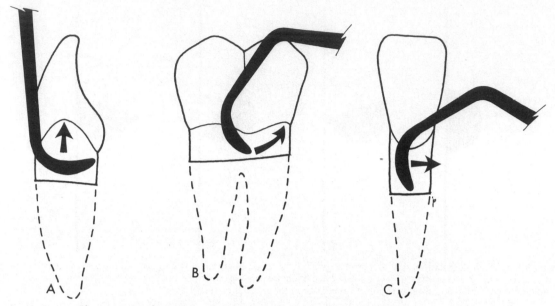

Figure 38–23 Three Basic Stroke Directions. *A,* Vertical. *B,* Oblique. C, Horizontal.

initiated in the wrist or fingers, nor is it carried out independently without the use of the forearm.

It is possible to initiate the scaling motion by rotating the wrist and forearm or by flexing the fingers. The use of wrist and forearm action versus the finger motion has long been debated among clinicians. Perhaps the strong feelings on both sides should be the most valid indication that there is a time and place for both. Neither method can be advocated exclusively because a careful analysis of effective scaling and root planing technique reveals that, indeed, both types of stroke activation are necessary for complete instrumentation. The wrist and forearm motion, pivoting in an arc on the finger rest, produces a more powerful stroke and is therefore preferred for scaling. Finger flexing is indicated for precise control over stroke length in areas such as line angles and when horizontal strokes are used on the lingual or facial aspects of narrow-rooted teeth.

The *push scaling motion* has been advocated by some clinicians. In the push stroke, the instrument engages the lateral or coronal border of the calculus and the fingers provide a thrust motion that dislodges the deposit. Because the push stroke may force calculus into the supporting tissues, its use, especially in an apical direction, is not recommended.

The **root planing stroke** is a moderate to light pull stroke that is used for final smoothing and planing of the root surface. Although hoes, files, and ultrasonic instruments have been used for root planing, curettes are widely acknowledged to be the most effective and versatile instruments for this procedure.[3, 5, 6, 8, 10, 12, 16, 19] The design of the curette, which allows it to be more easily adapted to subgingival tooth contours, makes curettes particularly suitable for root planing in periodontal patients who have deep pockets and furcation involvements. With a moderately firm grasp, the curette is kept adapted to the tooth with even lateral pressure. A continuous series of long, overlapping shaving strokes is activated. As the surface becomes smoother and resistance diminishes, lateral pressure is progressively reduced.

PRINCIPLES OF SCALING AND ROOT PLANING

Definitions and Rationale for Scaling and Root Planing

Scaling is the process by which plaque and calculus are removed from both supragingival and subgingival tooth surfaces. There is no deliberate attempt to remove tooth substance along with the calculus. **Root planing** is the process by which residual embedded calculus and portions of cementum are removed from the roots to produce a smooth, hard, clean surface.

The primary objective of scaling and root planing is to restore gingival health by completely removing from the tooth surface factors that provoke gingival inflammation: plaque, calculus, and altered cementum. Scaling and root planing are not separate procedures. All the principles of scaling apply equally to root planing. The difference between scaling and root planing is only a matter of degree. The nature of the tooth surface determines the degree to which the surface must be scaled or planed.

On enamel surfaces, plaque and calculus provoke gingival inflammation. Unless grooved or pitted, enamel surfaces are relatively smooth and uniform. When plaque and calculus form on enamel, the deposits are usually superficially attached to the surface and not locked into irregularities. Scaling alone is sufficient to completely remove plaque and calculus from enamel, leaving a smooth, clean surface.

Root surfaces exposed to plaque and calculus pose a different problem. Studies by Zander[20] and Moskow[9] have shown that *deposits of calculus on root surfaces are frequently embedded in cemental irregularities; scaling alone is therefore insufficient to remove them. A portion of the cementum itself must be removed to eliminate these deposits.* Furthermore, when cementum is exposed to plaque and the pocket environment, its surface is permeated by toxic substances, notably *endotoxins.*[1,2,7] Evidence suggests that this altered cementum is a source of gingival irritation and must be removed by root planing to produce a hard, clean, unaltered surface that is free of toxic substances.[1] The removal of the altered cementum may expose dentin. Although this is not the aim of treatment, it may be unavoidable.[12,16]

Scaling and root planing should not be thought of or practiced as separate procedures. It is apparent that scaling *without* root planing will often be inadequate to remove from root surfaces all the factors responsible for gingival inflammation.

As the rationale for scaling and root planing is thoroughly understood, it becomes apparent that mastery of these skills is essential to the ultimate success of any course of periodontal therapy. Of all clinical dental procedures, subgingival scaling and root planing in deep pockets are the most difficult and exacting skills to master. It has been argued that such proficiency in instrumentation cannot be attained; therefore, periodontal surgery is necessary to gain access to root surfaces. Others have argued that although proficiency is pos-sible, it need not be developed because access to the roots can be gained more easily with surgery. However, without mastering subgingival scaling and root planing skills, the clinician will be severely hampered and unable to treat adequately those patients for whom surgery is contraindicated.

Detection Skills

Good visual and tactile detection skills are required for the accurate initial assessment of the extent and nature of deposits and root irregularities before scaling and root planing. Valid self-evaluation upon completion of instrumentation depends on these detection skills.

Visual examination of supragingival calculus and of subgingival calculus just below the gingival margin is not difficult with good lighting and a clean field. Light deposits of supragingival calculus are often difficult to see when they are wet with saliva. Compressed air may be used to dry supragingival calculus until it is chalky white and readily visible. Air may also be directed into the pocket in a steady stream to deflect the marginal gingiva away from the tooth so that subgingival deposits near the surface can be seen.

Tactile exploration of the tooth surfaces in subgingival areas of pocket depth, furcations, and developmental depressions is much more difficult than visual examination of supragingival areas and requires the skilled use of a fine pointed explorer or probe. The explorer or probe is held with a light but stable modified pen grasp. This provides maximum tactile sensitivity for detection of subgingival calculus and other irregularities. The pads of the thumb and fingers, especially the middle finger, should perceive the slight vibrations conducted through the instrument shank and handle as irregularities in the tooth surface are encountered.

After a stable finger rest is established, the tip of the instrument is carefully inserted subgingivally to the base of the pocket. Light exploratory strokes are activated vertically up and down on the root surface. When calculus is encountered, the tip of the instrument should be advanced apically over the deposit until the termination of the calculus on the root is felt. The distance between the apical edge of the calculus and the bottom of the pocket usually ranges from 0.2 to 1.0 mm. The tip is adapted closely to the tooth to ensure the greatest degree of tactile sensitivity and to avoid tissue trauma. When exploring a proximal surface, strokes must be extended at least halfway across that surface past the contact area to ensure complete detection of interproximal deposits. When an explorer is used at line angles, convexities, and concavities, the handle of the instrument must be rolled slightly between the thumb and fingers to keep the tip constantly adapted to the changes in tooth contour.

Although exploring technique and good tactile sensitivity are very important, interpreting varying degrees of roughness and making clinical judgments based on these interpretations also require much expertise. The beginning student usually has difficulty detecting fine calculus and altered cementum. One must begin by recognizing ledges, lumps, or spurs of calculus, then smaller spicules, then slight roughness, and, finally, a slight graininess that feels like a sticky coating or film covering the tooth surface. Overhanging or deficient margins of dental restorations, caries, decalcification, and root roughness caused by previous instrumentation are all commonly found during exploration. These and other irregularities must be recognized and differentiated from subgingival calculus. Because this requires a great deal of experience and a high degree of tactile sensitivity, many clinicians agree that the development of detection skills is as important as the mastery of scaling and root planing technique.

Supragingival Scaling Technique

Supragingival calculus is generally less tenacious and less calcified than subgingival calculus. Since instrumentation is performed coronal to the gingival margin, scaling strokes are not confined by the surrounding tissues. This makes adaptation and angulation easier. It also allows direct visibility, as well as a freedom of movement that is not possible during subgingival scaling.

Sickles, curettes, and ultrasonic instruments are most commonly used for the removal of supragingival calculus. Hoes and chisels are less frequently used. To perform supragingival scaling, the sickle or curette is held with a modified pen grasp, and a firm finger rest is established on the teeth adjacent to the working area. The blade is adapted with an angulation of slightly less than 90° to the surface being scaled. The cutting edge should engage the apical margin of the supragingival calculus while short, powerful, overlapping scaling strokes are activated coronally in a vertical or oblique direction. The sharp pointed tip of the sickle can easily lacerate marginal tissue or gouge exposed root surfaces, so careful adaptation is especially important when this instrument is being used. The tooth surface is instrumented until it is visually and tactilely free of all supragingival deposits. If the tissue is retractable enough to allow easy insertion of the bulky blade, the sickle may be used slightly below the free gingival margin. If the sickle is used in this manner, final scaling and root planing with the curette should always follow.

Ultrasonic instrumentation for removal of supragingival calculus is described later in this chapter.

Subgingival Scaling and Root Planing Technique

Subgingival scaling and root planing are far more complex and difficult to perform than supragingival scaling. Subgingival calculus is usually harder than supragingival calculus, and it is often locked into root irregularities, making it more tenacious and therefore more difficult to remove.[9, 13, 20]

The overlying tissue creates significant problems in subgingival instrumentation. Vision is obscured by the bleeding that inevitably occurs during instrumentation, as well as by the tissue itself. The clinician must rely heavily on tactile sensitivity to detect calculus and irregularities, to guide the instrument blade during scaling and root planing, and to evaluate the results of instrumentation.

In addition, the direction and length of the strokes are limited by the adjacent pocket wall. The confines of the soft tissue make careful adaptation to tooth contours imperative in order to avoid trauma. Such precise adaptation cannot be accomplished without a thorough knowledge of tooth morphology. The clinician must form a mental image of the tooth surface to anticipate variations in contour, continually confirming or modifying the image in response to tactile sensations and visual cues like the position of the instrument handle and shank. The clinician must then instantaneously adjust the adaptation and angulation of the working end to the tooth. It is this complex and precise coordination of visual, mental, and manual skills that makes subgingival instrumentation one of the most difficult of all dental skills.

The curette is preferred by most clinicians for subgingival scaling and root planing because of the advantages afforded by its design. Its curved blade, rounded toe, and curved back allow the curette to be inserted to the base of the pocket and to be adapted to variations in tooth contour with a minimum of tissue displacement and trauma.

Hoes, files, and ultrasonic instruments are also used for subgingival scaling of heavy calculus but are not recommended for root planing. Although some delicate files may be inserted to the base of the pocket to crush or initially fracture tenacious deposits, heavier files, hoes, and ultrasonic instruments are bulky and cannot easily be inserted into deep pockets or where tissue is firm and fibrotic. Hoes and files are not able to produce as smooth a surface as curettes.[3, 12] Ultrasonic instruments are effective for the removal of readily accessible calculus, but curettes have been shown to be clearly superior for the removal of subgingival cementum.[16] Hoes, files, and ultrasonic instruments are all more hazardous than is the curette in terms of trauma to the root surface and surrounding tissues.[3, 10, 12]

Subgingival scaling and root planing are accomplished with either universal or area-specific (Gracey) curettes by the following basic procedure: The curette is held with a modified pen grasp, and a stable finger rest is established. The correct cutting edge is slightly adapted to the tooth, with the lower shank kept parallel with the tooth surface. The lower shank is moved toward the tooth so that the face of the blade is nearly flush with the tooth surface. The blade is then inserted under the gingiva and advanced to the base of the pocket by a light exploratory stroke. When the cutting edge reaches the base of the pocket, a working angulation between 45 and 90° is established, and pressure is applied laterally against the tooth surface. Calculus is removed by a series of controlled, overlapping, short, powerful strokes primarily utilizing wrist-arm motion (Fig. 38–24). As calculus is removed, resistance to the passage of the cutting edge diminishes until only a slight roughness remains. Longer, lighter root planing strokes are then activated with less lateral pressure until the root surface is completely smooth and hard. The instrument handle must be rolled carefully between the thumb and fingers to keep the blade adapted closely to the tooth surface as line angles, developmental depressions, and other changes in tooth contour are followed.

Scaling and root planing strokes should be confined to the portion of the tooth where calculus or altered cementum is found. This zone is known as the *"instrumentation zone."* Sweeping the instrument over the crown where it is not needed wastes operating time, dulls the instrument, and causes loss of control.

The amount of lateral pressure applied to the tooth surface depends on the nature of the calculus and on whether the strokes are for initial calculus removal or for final root planing. If heavy lateral pressure is continued after the bulk of calculus has been removed, and if the blade is repeatedly readapted with short, "choppy" strokes, the result will be a root surface roughened by numerous nicks and gouges, resembling the rippled surface of a washboard.[11] If heavy lateral pressure is continued with long, even strokes, the result will be excessive removal of root structure, producing a smooth but "ditched" or "riffled" root surface. To avoid these hazards of over-instrumentation, a deliberate transition from short, powerful scaling strokes to longer, lighter root planing strokes must be made as soon as calculus and the initial roughness have been eliminated.

Figure 38–24 Subgingival Scaling Procedure. *A,* Curette inserted with face of blade flush against tooth. *B,* Working angulation (45°–90°) is established at base of pocket. *C,* Lateral pressure is applied and scaling stroke is activated in coronal direction.

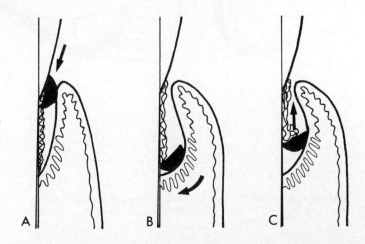

A   B   C

When scaling strokes are used to remove calculus, force can be maximized by concentrating the lateral pressure onto the lower third of the blade (see Fig. 38–20). This small section, the terminal few millimeters of the blade, is positioned slightly apical to the lateral edge of the deposit, and a short vertical or oblique stroke is used to split the calculus from the tooth surface. Without withdrawing the instrument from the pocket, the lower third of the blade is advanced laterally and repositioned to engage the next portion of the remaining deposit. Another vertical or oblique stroke is made, slightly overlapping the previous stroke. This process is repeated in a series of powerful scaling strokes until the entire deposit has been removed. The overlapping of these pathways or "channels" of instrumentation[11] ensures that the entire instrumentation zone is covered.

Engaging a large, tenacious ledge or piece of calculus with the entire length of the cutting edge is not recommended, because the force is distributed through a longer section of the cutting edge rather than being concentrated. Far more lateral pressure is required to dislodge the entire deposit in one stroke. Although some clinicians may possess the strength to remove calculus completely in this manner, the heavier forces that are required diminish tactile sensitivity and contribute to a

loss of control that results in tissue trauma. A single heavy stroke usually is not sufficient to remove calculus entirely. Instead, the blade skips over or skims the surface of the deposit. Subsequent strokes made with the entire cutting edge tend to shave the deposit down layer by layer, and when a series of these repeated whittling strokes is applied, the calculus may be reduced to a thin, smooth, burnished sheet that is very difficult to distinguish from the surrounding root surface.

A common error in instrumenting proximal surfaces is failing to reach the midproximal region apical to the contact because this area is relatively inaccessible and requires more instrumentation skill than do buccal or lingual surfaces. It is extremely important to extend strokes at least halfway across the proximal surface so that no calculus or roughness remains in the interproximal area. With properly designed curettes, this can be accomplished by keeping the lower shank of the curette parallel with the long axis of the tooth (Fig. 38–25). With the lower shank parallel with the long axis, the blade of the curette will reach the base of the pocket and the toe will extend beyond the midline as strokes are advanced across the proximal surface. This extension of strokes beyond the midline ensures the thorough exploration and instrumentation of these

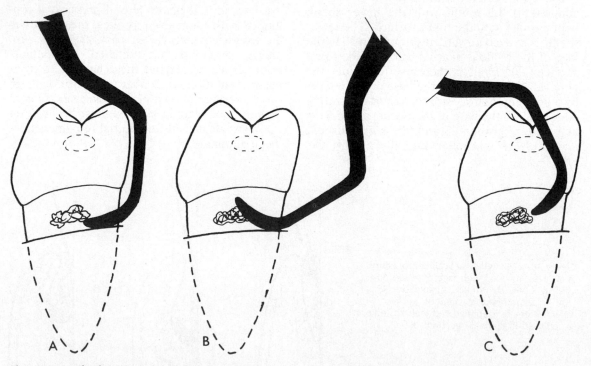

Figure 38–25 Shank Position for Scaling Proximal Surfaces. *A,* Correct shank position, parallel with the long axis of the tooth. *B,* Incorrect shank position, tilted away from tooth. *C,* Incorrect shank position tilted too far toward the tooth.

surfaces. If the lower shank is angled or tilted away from the tooth, the toe will move toward the contact area. Because this prevents the blade from reaching the base of the pocket, calculus apical to the contact will not be detected or removed. Strokes will be hampered because the toe tends to become lodged in the contact (Fig. 38–25). If the instrument is angled or tilted too far toward the tooth, the lower shank will hit the tooth or the contact area, preventing the extension of strokes to the midproximal region (Fig. 38–25).

The relationship between the location of the finger rest and the working area is important for two reasons. First, the finger rest or fulcrum must be positioned to allow the lower shank of the instrument to be parallel or nearly parallel with the tooth surface being treated. This parallelism is a fundamental requirement for optimal working angulation.

Second, the finger rest must be positioned to enable the operator to use wrist-arm motion to activate strokes. On some aspects of the maxillary posterior teeth, these requirements can be met only with the use of extraoral or opposite arch fulcrums. When intraoral finger rests are used in other regions of the mouth, the finger rest must be close enough to the working area to fulfill these two requirements. A finger rest that is established too far from the working area forces the clinician to separate the middle finger from the fourth finger in an effort to obtain parallelism and proper angulation. Effective wrist-arm motion is possible only when these two fingers are kept together in a "built-up" fulcrum. Separation of the fingers commits the clinician to the exclusive use of finger flexing for the activation of strokes.

As instrumentation proceeds from one tooth to the next, the location of the finger rest must be frequently adjusted or changed to allow parallelism and wrist-arm motion.

Instruments for Scaling and Root Planing

UNIVERSAL CURETTES. The working ends of the universal curette are designed in pairs so that all surfaces of the teeth can be treated with one double-ended instrument or a matched pair of single-ended instruments.

In any given quadrant, when approaching the tooth from the facial aspect, one end of the universal curette will adapt to the mesial surfaces and the other end will adapt to the distal surfaces. When approaching from the lingual aspect in the same quadrant, the double-ended universal curette must be turned end-for-end because the blades are mirror images. This means that the end that adapts to the mesial surfaces on the facial aspect also adapts to the distal surfaces on the lingual aspect and vice versa. Both ends of the universal curette are used to instrument the anterior teeth. On posterior teeth, however, owing to the limited access to distal surfaces, a single working end can be used to treat both mesial and distal surfaces by using both of its cutting edges. To do this, the instrument is first adapted to the mesial surface with the handle nearly parallel with the mesial surface. Because the face of the universal curette blade is honed at 90° to the lower shank, if the lower shank is positioned so that it is absolutely parallel with the surface being instrumented, the tooth-blade angulation is 90°. In order to close this angle and thus obtain proper working angulation, the lower shank must be tilted slightly toward the tooth. The distal surface of the same posterior tooth can be instrumented with the opposite cutting edge of the same blade. This cutting edge can be adapted at proper working angulation by positioning the handle so that it is *perpendicular* to the distal surface (Fig. 38–26).

When adapting the universal curette blade, as much of the cutting edge as possible should be in contact with the tooth surface, except on narrow convex surfaces such as line angles. Although the entire cutting edge should con-

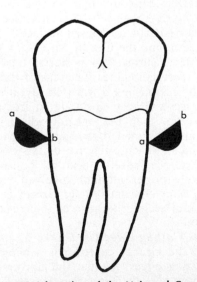

Figure 38–26 Adaptation of the Universal Curette on a Posterior Tooth. Cross-sectional representations of the same universal curette blade as its cutting edges are adapted to the mesial and distal surfaces of a posterior tooth.

tact the tooth, pressure should be concentrated on the lower third of the blade during scaling strokes. During root planing strokes, however, lateral pressure should be evenly distributed along the cutting edge.

The primary advantage of these curettes is that they are designed to be used universally on all tooth surfaces, in all regions of the mouth. However, universal curettes have a limited adaptability for the treatment of deep pockets in which apical migration of the attachment has exposed furcations, root convexities, and developmental depressions. For this reason, the Gracey curettes, which are area-specific and specially designed for subgingival scaling and root planing in periodontal patients, are preferred by many clinicians.

GRACEY CURETTES. Gracey curettes are a set of area-specific instruments that were designed by Dr. Clayton H. Gracey of Michigan in the mid-1930s.

Four design features make the Gracey curettes unique: (1) they are area-specific, (2) only one cutting edge on each blade is used, (3) the blade is curved in two planes, and (4) the blade is "offset." (These features have been summarized in Chapter 37 in Table 37–1.) Each of these features directly influences the manner in which the Graceys are used and should be discussed individually.

Area-Specificity. There are seven pairs of curettes in the set. The Gracey Nos. 1–2 and 3–4 are used on anterior teeth. The Gracey No. 5–6 may be used on both anterior and premolar teeth. The facial and lingual surfaces of posterior teeth are instrumented with the Gracey Nos. 7–8 and 9–10. The Gracey No. 11–12 is designed for mesial surfaces of posterior teeth, and the Gracey No. 13–14 adapts to the distal surfaces of posterior teeth. Although these guidelines for areas of use were originally established by Dr. Gracey, it is possible to use a Gracey curette in an area of the mouth other than the one for which it was specifically designed if the general principles regarding these curettes are understood and applied. Gracey curettes need not be reserved exclusively for periodontally involved patients. In fact, many clinicians prefer Gracey curettes for general scaling because of their excellent adaptability.

Single Cutting Edge Used. Like a universal curette, the Gracey curette has a blade with two cutting edges. Unlike the universal curette, however, the Gracey instrument is designed so that only one cutting edge is used. In order to determine which of the two is the

correct cutting edge to adapt to the tooth, the blade should be held face up and parallel with the floor. When viewed from this angle, the blade can be seen to curve to the side. One cutting edge forms a larger outer curve and the other forms a shorter, small inner curve. The larger outer curve, which has also been described as the inferior cutting edge or as the cutting edge farther away from the handle, is the correct cutting edge (Fig. 38–27).

Blade Curves in Two Planes. Like the toe of the universal curette, the toe of the Gracey curette curves upward. However, the toe of the Gracey curette also curves to the side, as previously mentioned. This unique curvature enhances the blade's adaptation to convexities and concavities as the working end is advanced around the tooth. Only the lower third or half of the Gracey blade is in contact with the tooth during instrumentation. The cutting edge of a universal curette blade, on the other hand, is straight and does not curve to the side. This makes it less adaptable to root concavities.

Offset Blade. Gracey curette blades are honed at an "offset" angle. This means that the face of the blade is not perpendicular to the lower shank as it is on a universal curette. Rather, Gracey curettes are designed so that *the tooth-blade working angulation is 60 to 70° when the lower shank is held parallel with the tooth surface.* Gracey curettes were originally designed to be used with push strokes and were beveled to provide tooth-blade angulation of 40° when the lower shank is parallel with the tooth surface. For many years, Graceys were available only in this form. Gracey curettes are now available not only in the original push design but also in a modified version to be used with pull strokes. It is important to understand this when purchasing

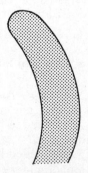

Figure 38–27 Determining the Correct Cutting Edge of a Gracey Curette. When viewed from directly above the face of the blade, the correct cutting edge is the one forming the larger, outer curve on the right.

Gracey curettes so as to avoid instruments that are not properly designed for pull strokes. When Graceys that are designed to be used with push strokes are used with pull strokes instead, they are very likely to burnish calculus rather than completely remove it. The design of the Gracey curette was modified to create an instrument that can be used with pull strokes in response to requests from clinicians who like the shank design and adaptability of the original Gracey instruments but were opposed to the use of push strokes for scaling and root planing. The push stroke is not recommended, especially for the novice clinician, because it is very likely to cause undue trauma to the junctional epithelium and to embed fragments of dislodged calculus in the soft tissues.

The general principles of use of the Gracey curettes are essentially the same as those for the universal curette. (Those italicized apply only to Gracey curettes.)

1. *Determine the correct cutting edge.* The correct cutting edge should be determined by visually inspecting the blade and confirmed by lightly adapting the chosen cutting edge to the tooth with the lower shank parallel with the surface of the tooth. With the toe pointed in the direction to be scaled (e.g., mesially with a No. 7–8 curette), only the back of the blade can be seen if the correct cutting edge has been selected (Fig. 38–28). If the wrong cutting edge has been adopted, the flat, shiny face of the blade will be seen instead (Fig. 38–29).

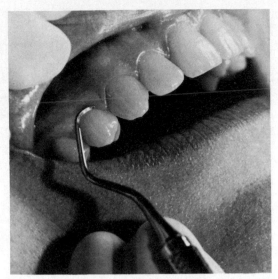

Figure 38–29 Incorrect Cutting Edge of a Gracey Curette Adapted to the Tooth.

2. *Make sure the lower shank is parallel with the surface to be instrumented.* The lower shank of a Gracey is that portion of the shank between the blade and the first bend in the shank. Parallelism of the handle or upper shank is not an acceptable guide with Graceys because the angulations of the shanks vary. On anterior teeth, the lower shank of the Gracey No. 1–2, 3–4, or 5–6 should be parallel with the mesial, distal, facial, or lingual surfaces of the teeth (Fig. 38–30). On posterior teeth, the lower shank of the No. 7–8 or 9–10 should be parallel with the facial or lingual surfaces of the teeth (Fig. 38–31), the lower shank of the No. 11–12 should be parallel with the mesial surfaces of the teeth (Fig. 38–32), and the lower shank of the No. 13–14 should be parallel with the distal surfaces of the teeth (Fig. 38–33).

3. When using intraoral finger rests, keep the fourth and middle fingers together in a "built-up" fulcrum for maximum control and wrist-arm action.

4. Use extraoral fulcrums or mandibular finger rests when working on the maxillary posterior teeth for optimal angulation.

5. *Concentrate on using the lower third of the cutting edge for calculus removal,* especially on line angles or when attempting to remove a calculus ledge by breaking it away in sections beginning at the lateral edge.

6. Allow the wrist and forearm to carry the burden of the stroke rather than flexing the fingers.

7. Roll the handle slightly between the thumb and fingers to keep the blade adapted

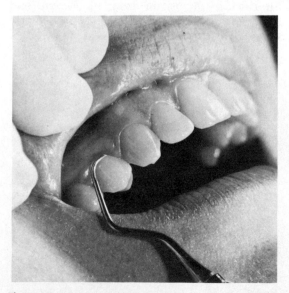

Figure 38–28 Correct Cutting Edge of a Gracey Curette Adapted to the Tooth.

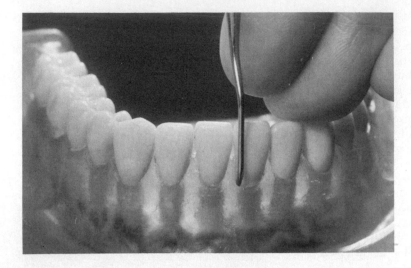

Figure 38–30 Gracey No. 5–6 Curette Adapted to an Anterior Tooth.

as the working end is advanced around line angles and into concavities.

8. Modulate lateral pressure from firm to moderate to light depending on the nature of the calculus, and reduce pressure as the transition is made from scaling to root planing strokes.

ULTRASONIC SCALING INSTRUMENTS. *When properly utilized, the ultrasonic scaling device is a useful adjunct to conventional hand instrumentation. Owing to several limitations, however, it should never be considered or utilized as a substitute for hand instruments in scaling and root planing.*

The vibrational energy produced by the ultrasonic instrument makes it useful for removing heavy, tenacious deposits of calculus and stain. Such deposits can be removed more quickly and with less effort than they can be manually. When ultrasonic instruments are properly manipulated, there is less tissue trauma and therefore less postoperative discomfort. This makes ultrasonic instrumentation useful for initial débridement in patients suffering from acute, painful conditions such as acute necrotizing ulcerative gingivitis.

Despite their effectiveness for gross supragingival scaling, ultrasonic instruments are significantly limited for subgingival scaling and root planing procedures. The working ends of the instruments are bulky and blunt. This makes subgingival insertion to the base of the pocket possible only when the tissue is extremely inflamed and retractable. It also greatly diminishes tactile sensitivity compared with hand instruments. The working end of the instrument must come into contact with the calculus deposit in order to fracture and remove it. Small pieces of calculus, particularly subgingival calculus, may easily be missed.

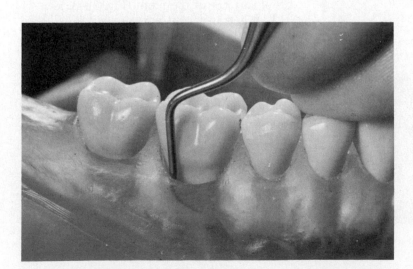

Figure 38–31 Gracey No. 7–8 Curette Adapted to the Facial Surface of a Posterior Tooth.

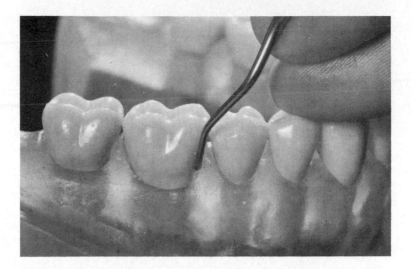

Figure 38–32 Gracey No. 11–12 Curette Adapted to the Mesial Surface of a Posterior Tooth.

It has been shown that ultrasonic instruments will remove root substance.[4] Although ultrasonic removal of cementum is possible in easily accessible areas, the curette has been established as a far more effective instrument for overall root planing.[5, 6, 8, 16]

Visibility is hampered by the constant water spray that is necessary for the operation of the instrument. During ultrasonic instrumentation the tooth surface should be frequently examined with an explorer to evaluate the completeness of calculus removal; and the use of ultrasonics should always be followed by hand instrumentation for the removal of residual deposits. These factors limit the use of ultrasonic instruments to the gross removal of heavy calculus, stain, and debris. Once this has been accomplished, curettes should be used to remove residual deposits and to plane the roots.

With these points in mind, the ultrasonic device is used in the following manner:

1. The instrument should be properly tuned to produce a light mist of water at the working tip. Adequate aspiration will be necessary to remove this water as it accumulates in the mouth. The power setting should be no higher than necessary to remove calculus. The clinician and the assistant should wear masks to minimize inhalation of the contaminated aerosol that is produced during instrumentation.

2. The instrument is grasped with a modified pen grasp, and a finger rest or fulcrum should be established as for conventional hand instrumentation.

The handle of the instrument is aligned with the long axis of the tooth and the working end is adapted to conform to the contour of the tooth surface.

3. The instrument is switched on by stepping on the foot pedal. Short, light, vertical strokes

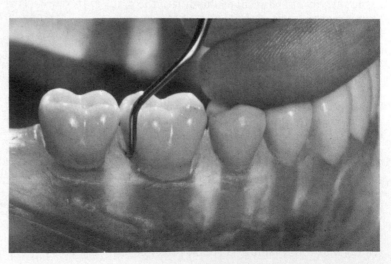

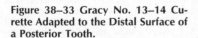
Figure 38–33 Gracy No. 13–14 Curette Adapted to the Distal Surface of a Posterior Tooth.

are activated and the working end is passed over the deposit. Heavy lateral pressure is unnecessary because it is the vibrational energy of the instrument that dislodges the calculus. However, the working end must touch the deposit for this to occur.

4. The working end should be kept in constant motion and the tip should never be held perpendicular to the surface of the tooth, as this would etch or groove the surface.

5. The foot pedal should be released periodically to allow for aspiration of water, and the tooth surface should be examined frequently with an explorer.

6. Scaling and root planing is completed with curettes or other hand instruments.

Evaluation of Scaling and Root Planing

The adequacy of scaling and root planing is evaluated when the procedure is performed and later, after a period of soft tissue healing.

Immediately following instrumentation, the tooth surfaces should be carefully inspected visually with optimum lighting and the aid of a mouth mirror and compressed air. They should also be examined with a fine explorer or probe. Subgingival surfaces should be hard and smooth. Although the complete removal of calculus is definitely necessary for the health of the adjacent soft tissue,[17] there is little documented evidence that root smoothness is necessary.[5] Nevertheless, relative smoothness is still the best immediate clinical indication that calculus and the altered cementum have been completely removed.[5]

Even though smoothness is the criterion by which scaling and root planing is immediately evaluated, the ultimate evaluation is based on tissue response.[17] Clinical evaluation of the soft tissue response to scaling and root planing, including probing, should not be conducted earlier than 2 weeks postoperatively. Re-epithelialization of the wounds created during instrumentation takes from 1 to 2 weeks.[14, 15] Until then, gingival bleeding on probing can be expected even when calculus has been completely removed, because the soft tissue wound is not epithelialized. Any gingival bleeding on probing that is noted after this interval is more likely to be due to persistent inflammation produced by residual deposits that were not removed during the initial procedure or to inadequate plaque control.

There may be times when the clinician finds that some slight root roughness remains after scaling and root planing. If sound principles of instrumentation have been followed, the roughness may not be calculus. Since calculus removal, *not* root smoothness per se, has been shown to be necessary for tissue health, it might be more prudent in such a case to stop short of perfect smoothness and re-evaluate the patient's tissue response after 2 weeks. This avoids overinstrumentation and removal of excessive root structure in the pursuit of smoothness for smoothness' sake. If the tissue is healthy after a 2-week interval, no further root planing is necessary. If the tissue is inflamed, the clinician must determine to what extent this is due to plaque accumulation or the presence of residual calculus and to what degree further root planing is necessary.

REFERENCES

1. Aleo, J., DeRenzis, F., and Farber, P.: In vitro attachment of human gingival fibroblasts to root surfaces. J. Periodontol., 46:639, 1975.
2. Aleo, J., DeRenzis, F., Farber, P., and Varboncoeur, A.: The presence and biological activity of cementum bound endotoxin. J. Periodontol., 45:672, 1974.
3. Barnes, J. E., and Schaffer, E. M.: Subgingival root planing: a comparison using files, hoes, and curets. J. Periodontol., 31:300, 1960.
4. Clark, S., Group, H., and Mabler, D.: The effect of ultrasonic instrumentation on root surfaces. J. Periodontol., 39:125, 1968.
5. Garrett, J. S.: Root planing: a perspective. J. Periodontol., 48:553, 1977.
6. Green, E., and Ramfjord, S. R.: Tooth roughness after subgingival root planing. J. Periodontol., 37:396, 1966.
7. Hatfield, C. G., and Baumhammers, A.: Cytotoxic effects of periodontally involved surfaces of human teeth. Arch. Oral Biol., 16:465, 1971.
8. Kerry, G. J.: Roughness of root surfaces after use of ultrasonic instruments and hand curets. J. Periodontol., 38:340, 1967.
9. Moskow, B. S.: Calculus attachment in cemental separations. J. Periodontol., 40:125, 1969.
10. Orban, B., and Manella, V.: Macroscopic and microscopic study of instruments designed for root planing. J. Periodontol., 27:120, 1956.
11. Parr, R., Green, E., Madsen, L., and Miller, S.: Subgingival Scaling and Root Planing. Berkeley, Calif., Praxis Publishing Company, 1976.
12. Schaffer, E. M.: Histologic results of root curettage on human teeth. J. Periodontol., 27:269, 1956.
13. Selvig, K.: Attachment of plaque and calculus to tooth surfaces. J. Periodont. Res., 5:8, 1970.
14. Stahl, S. S., Slavkin, H. C., Yamada, L., and Levine, S.: Speculations about gingival repair. J. Periodontol., 43:395, 1972.
15. Stahl, S. S., Weiner, J. M., Benjamin, S., and Yamada, L.: Soft tissue healing following curettage and root planing. J. Periodontol., 42:678, 1971.
16. Van Volkinburg, J., Green, E., and Armitage, G.: The nature of root surfaces after curette, cavitron, and alpha-sonic instrumentation. J. Periodont. Res., 11:374, 1976.
17. Waerhaug, J.: Healing of the dento-epithelial junction following subgingival plaque control. J. Periodontol., 49:1, 1978.
18. Wilkins, E. M.: Clinical Practice of the Dental Hygienist. 4th ed., Philadelphia, Lea & Febiger, 1976, pp. 49–50.
19. Wilkinson, R. F., and Maybury, J.: Scanning electron microscopy of the root surface following instrumentation. J. Periodontol., 44:559, 1973.
20. Zander, H. A.: The attachment of calculus to root surfaces. J. Periodontol., 24:16, 1953.

chapter thirty-nine

Instrumentation in Different Areas of the Mouth

Various approaches to instrumentation in different areas of the mouth are illustrated here in atlas form. The examples shown provide maximum efficiency for the clinician and comfort for the patient. For most areas, more than one approach is presented. Other approaches are possible and are acceptable if they provide equal efficiency and comfort.

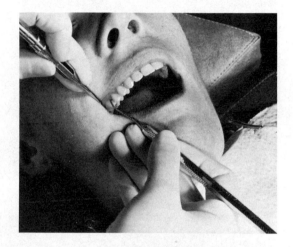

Figure 39–1 Maxillary Right Posterior Sextant; Facial Aspect.
Operator Position: Side position.
Illumination: Direct.
Visibility: Direct. Indirect for distal surfaces of molars.
Retraction: Mirror or index finger on nonoperating hand.
Finger Rest: Extraoral, palm-up. Backs of the middle and fourth fingers on the lateral aspect of the mandible on the right side of the face.

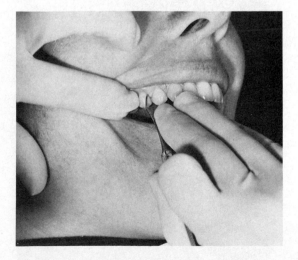

Figure 39–2 Maxillary Right Posterior Sextant; Facial Aspect.
Operator Position: Side or front position.
Illumination: Direct.
Visibility: Direct. Indirect for distal surfaces of molars.
Retraction: Mirror or index finger of nonoperating hand.
Finger Rest: Intraoral, palm-down. Fourth finger on incisal or facial surfaces of maxillary anterior teeth or on occlusal or facial surfaces of maxillary bicuspid teeth.

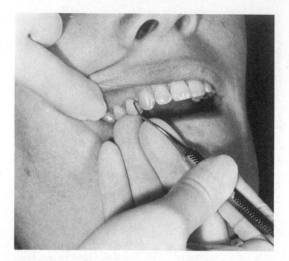

Figure 39–3 Maxillary Right Posterior Sextant, Premolar Region Only; Facial Aspect.

Operator Position: Side or back position.

Illumination: Direct.

Visibility: Direct.

Retraction: Mirror or index finger of nonoperating hand.

Finger Rest: Intraoral, palm-up. Fourth finger on the occlusal surfaces of the adjacent maxillary posterior teeth.

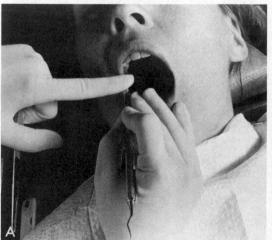

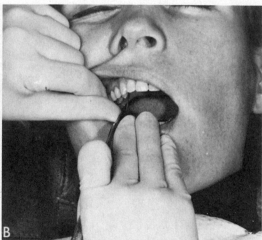

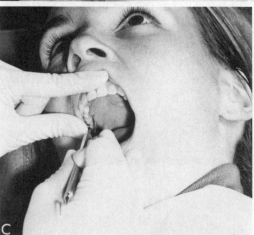

Figure 39–4 Maxillary Right Posterior Sextant; Lingual Aspect.

Operator Position: Front position.

Illumination: Direct.

Visibility: Direct.

Retraction: Index finger of nonoperating hand or no retraction.

Finger Rest: Intraoral, palm-down, opposite arch, reinforced. Fourth finger on incisal edges of mandibular anterior teeth, reinforced with the thumb or index finger of the nonoperating hand.

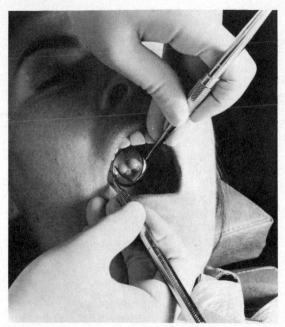

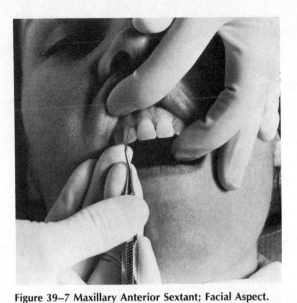

Figure 39–7 Maxillary Anterior Sextant; Facial Aspect.
Operator Position: Back position.
Illumination: Direct.
Visibility: Direct.
Retraction: Index finger of nonoperating hand.
Finger Rest: Intraoral, palm-up. Fourth finger on incisal
edges or occlusal surfaces of adjacent maxillary teeth.

Figure 39–5 Maxillary Right Posterior Sextant; Lingual Aspect.
Operator Position: Side or front position.
Illumination: Direct and indirect.
Visibility: Direct or indirect.
Retraction: None.
Finger Rest: Extraoral, palm-up. Backs of middle and
fourth fingers on the lateral aspect of the mandible on
the right side of the face.

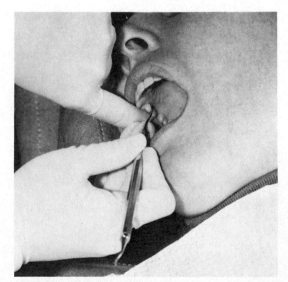

Figure 39–6 Maxillary Right Posterior Sextant; Lingual Aspect.
Operator Position: Front position.
Illumination: Direct.
Visibility: Direct.
Retraction: None.
Finger Rest: Intraoral, palm-up, finger-on-finger. Index
finger of nonoperating hand on occlusal surfaces of
maxillary right posterior teeth. Fourth finger of oper-
ating hand on index finger of nonoperating hand.

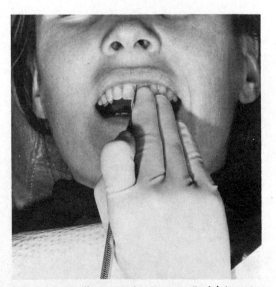

Figure 39–8 Maxillary Anterior Sextant; Facial Aspect.
Operator Position: Front position.
Illumination: Direct.
Visibility: Direct.
Retraction: Index finger of nonoperating hand.
Finger Rest: Intraoral, palm-down. Fourth finger on in-
cisal edges or occlusal or facial surfaces of adjacent
maxillary teeth.

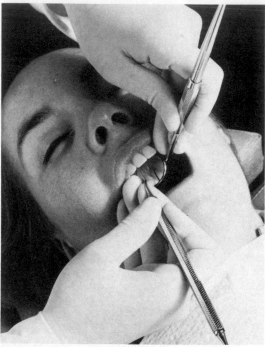

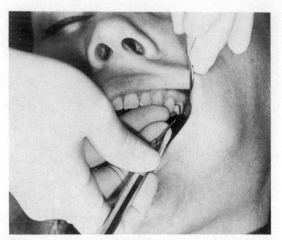

Figure 39–11 Maxillary Left Posterior Sextant; Facial Aspect.
Operator Position: Back or side position.
Illumination: Direct or Indirect.
Visibility: Direct or indirect.
Retraction: Mirror.
Finger Rest: Intraoral, palm-up. Fourth finger on incisal edges or occlusal surfaces of adjacent maxillary teeth.

Figure 39–9 Maxillary Anterior Sextant; Lingual Aspect.
Operator Position: Back position.
Illumination: Indirect.
Visibility: Indirect.
Retraction: None.
Finger Rest: Intraoral, palm-up. Fourth finger on incisal edges or occlusal surfaces of adjacent maxillary teeth.

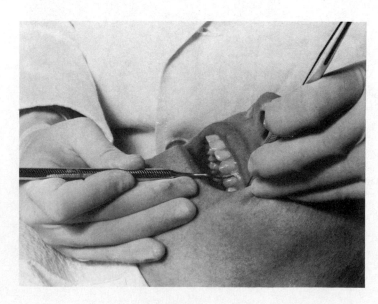

Figure 39–10 Maxillary Left Posterior Sextant; Facial Aspect.
Operator Position: Side or back position.
Illumination: Direct or indirect.
Visibility: Direct or indirect.
Retraction: Mirror.
Finger Rest: Extraoral, palm-down. Front surfaces of middle and fourth fingers on lateral aspect of mandible on left side of the face.

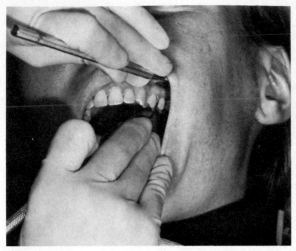

Figure 39–12 Maxillary Left Posterior Sextant; Facial Aspect.
Operator Position: Front positon.
Illumination: Direct or indirect.
Visibility: Direct or indirect.
Retraction: Mirror.
Finger Rest: Intraoral, palm-down, opposite arch. Fourth finger on incisal edges or occlusal or facial surfaces of mandibular left teeth.

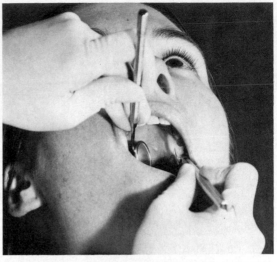

Figure 39–14 Maxillary Left Posterior Sextant; Lingual Aspect.
Operator Position: Front position.
Illumination: Direct and indirect.
Visibility: Direct and indirect.
Retraction: None.
Finger Rest: Intraoral, palm-down, opposite arch. Fourth finger on incisal edges of mandibular anterior teeth or facial surfaces of mandibular premolars. Nonoperating hand holds mirror in position for indirect illumination.

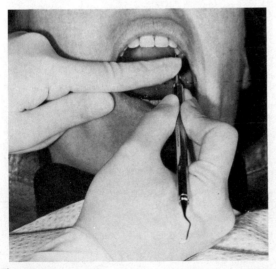

Figure 39–13 Maxillary Left Posterior Sextant; Lingual Aspect.
Operator Position: Front position.
Illumination: Direct.
Visibility: Direct.
Retraction: None.
Finger Rest: Intraoral, palm-down, opposite arch, reinforced. Fourth finger on incisal edges of mandibular anterior teeth or facial surfaces of mandibular premolars, reinforced with the index finger of the nonoperating hand.

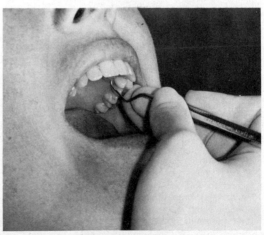

Figure 39–15 Maxillary Left Posterior Sextant; Lingual Aspect.
Operator Position: Side or front position.
Illumination: Direct.
Visibility: Direct.
Retraction: None.
Finger Rest: Intraoral, palm-up. Fourth finger on occlusal surfaces of adjacent maxillary teeth.

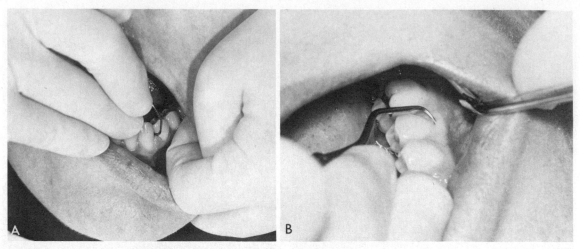

Figure 39–16 Mandibular Left Posterior Sextant; Facial Aspect.
Operator Position: Side or back position.
Illumination: Direct.
Visibility: Direct or indirect.
Retraction: Mirror or index finger of nonoperating hand.
Finger Rest: Intraoral, palm-down. Fourth finger on incisal edges or occlusal or facial surfaces of adjacent mandibular teeth.

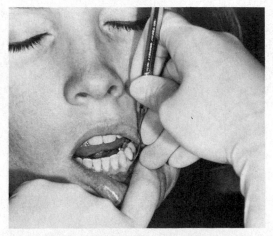

Figure 39–17 Mandibular Left Posterior Sextant, Premolar Region Only; Facial Aspect.
Operator Position: Front position.
Illumination: Direct.
Visibility: Direct.
Retraction: Index finger of nonoperating hand.
Finger Rest: Intraoral, palm-down, finger-on-finger. Index finger of nonoperating hand is placed in mandibular left vestibule. Fourth finger of operating hand rests on index finger of nonoperating hand.

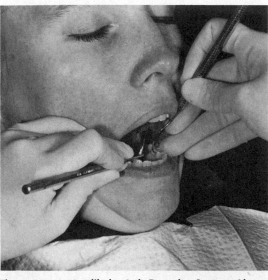

Figure 39–18 Mandibular Left Posterior Sextant; Lingual Aspect.
Operator Position: Front or side position.
Illumination: Direct and indirect.
Visibility: Direct.
Retraction: Mirror retracts tongue.
Finger Rest: Intraoral, palm-down. Fourth finger on incisal edges or occlusal surfaces of adjacent mandibular teeth.

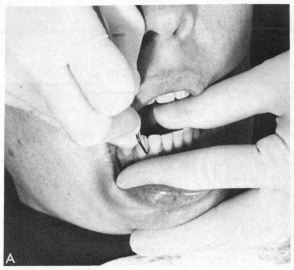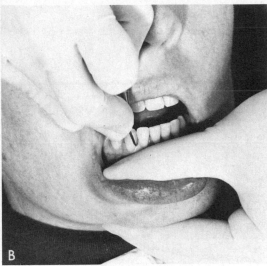

Figure 39–19 Mandibular Anterior Sextant; Facial Aspect.
Operator Position: Back position.
Illumination: Direct.
Visibility: Direct.
Retraction: Index finger or thumb of nonoperating hand.
Finger Rest: Intraoral, palm-down. Fourth finger on incisal edges or occlusal surfaces of adjacent mandibular teeth.

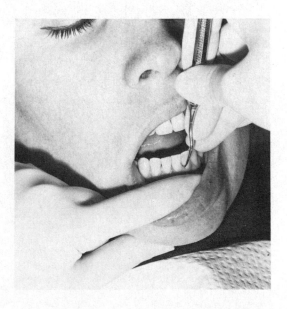

Figure 39–20 Mandibular Anterior Sextant; Facial Aspect.
Operator Position: Front position.
Illumination: Direct.
Visibility: Direct.
Retraction: Index finger of nonoperating hand.
Finger Rest: Intraoral, palm-down. Fourth finger on incisal edges or occlusal surfaces of adjacent mandibular teeth.

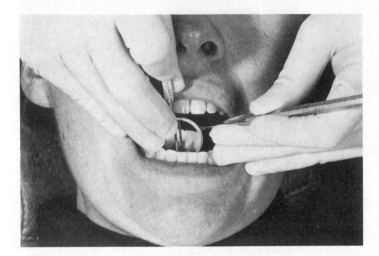

Figure 39–21 Mandibular Anterior Sextant; Lingual Aspect.
  Operator Position: Back position.
  Illumination: Direct and indirect.
  Visibility: Direct and indirect.
  Retraction: Mirror retracts tongue.
  Finger Rest: Intraoral, palm-down. Fourth finger on incisal edges or occlusal surfaces of adjacent mandibular teeth.

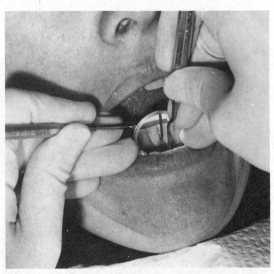

Figure 39–22 Mandibular Anterior Sextant; Lingual Aspect.
  Operator Position: Front position.
  Illumination: Direct and indirect.
  Visibility: Direct or indirect.
  Retraction: Mirror retracts tongue.
  Finger Rest: Intraoral, palm-down. Fourth finger on incisal edges or occlusal surfaces of adjacent mandibular teeth.

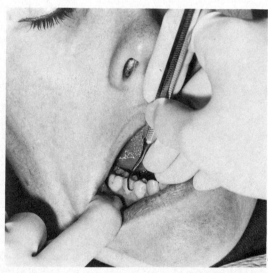

Figure 39–23 Mandibular Right Posterior Sextant; Facial Aspect.
  Operator Position: Side or front position.
  Illumination: Direct.
  Visibility: Direct.
  Retraction: Mirror or index finger of nonoperating hand.
  Finger Rest: Intraoral, palm-down. Fourth finger on incisal edges or occlusal surfaces of adjacent mandibular teeth.

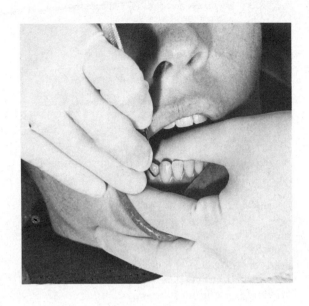

Figure 39–24 Mandibular Right Posterior Sextant, Premolar Region Only; Facial Aspect.

Operator Position: Back position.

Illumination: Direct.

Visibility: Direct.

Retraction: Index finger of nonoperating hand.

Finger Rest: Intraoral, palm-down, finger-on-finger. Index finger of nonoperating hand is placed in mandibular right vestibule. Fourth finger of operating hand rests on index finger of nonoperating hand.

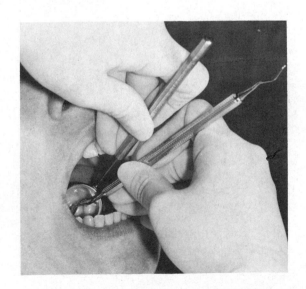

Figure 39–25 Mandibular Right Posterior Sextant; Lingual Aspect.

Operator Position: Front position.

Illumination: Direct and indirect.

Visibility: Direct and indirect.

Retraction: Mirror retracts tongue.

Finger Rest: Intraoral, palm-down. Fourth finger on incisal edges or occlusal surfaces of adjacent mandibular teeth.

Sharpening of Periodontal Instruments

It is impossible to carry out periodontal procedures efficiently with dull instruments. A sharp instrument cuts more precisely and quickly than a dull instrument. To do its job at all, a dull instrument must be held more firmly and pressed harder than a sharp instrument. This reduces tactile sensitivity and increases the possibility that the instrument will inadvertently slip. Therefore, *to avoid wasting time and operating haphazardly, one must be thoroughly familiar with the principles of sharpening and able to apply them to produce a keen cutting edge on the instruments one is using. Developing this skill requires patience and practice, but one cannot attain clinical excellence without it.*

SHARPNESS AND HOW TO EVALUATE IT

The cutting edge of an instrument is formed by the angular junction of two surfaces of its blade. The cutting edges of a curette, for example, are formed where the face of the blade meets the lateral surfaces (Fig. 40–1).

When the instrument is sharp, this junction is a fine line running the length of the cutting edge. As the instrument is used, metal is worn away at the cutting edge, and the junction of the face and lateral surface becomes rounded or dulled (Fig. 40–2).[1,3] Instead of an acute *angle,* the cutting edge is now a rounded *surface.* This is why a dull instrument cuts less efficiently and requires more pressure to do its job.[2]

Sharpness can be evaluated by sight and touch in one of the following ways:

1. When a dull instrument is held under a light, the rounded surface of its cutting edge reflects light back to the observer. It appears as a white line running the length of the cutting edge (Fig. 40–3). The acutely angled cutting edge of a sharp instrument, on the other hand, has no surface area to reflect light. When a sharp instrument is held under a light, no white line can be observed (see Fig. 40–1).

2. Tactile evaluation of sharpness is performed by drawing the instrument lightly across the thumbnail. A dull instrument will slide smoothly, without "biting" into the surface and raising a light shaving as a sharp instrument would.[5]

3. Tactile evaluation of sharpness can also be accomplished by gently drawing the pad of the thumb across the cutting edge.[2] A sharp instrument will produce a "grabbing" sensation on the skin. Naturally, care should be taken not to lacerate the thumb when using this method with extremely sharp periodontal knives.

SHARPENING STONES

Sharpening stones may be quarried from natural mineral deposits or produced artificially. In either case, the surface of the stone is made up of abrasive crystals that are harder than the metal of the instrument to be sharpened. Coarse stones have larger particles and cut more rapidly. They are used on instruments that are very dull. Finer stones with smaller crystals cut more slowly and are reserved for final sharpening to produce a finer edge and for sharpening instruments that are only slightly dull. India and Arkansas oilstones are examples of natural abrasive stones. Carborundum and ruby stones are man-made and are produced by impregnating nonmetallic substances with abrasive particles (Fig. 40–4).

Sharpening stones can also be categorized by their method of use.

MOUNTED ROTARY STONES. These stones are mounted on a metal mandrel and are used

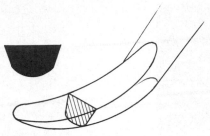

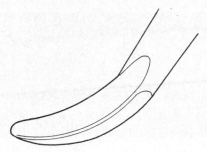

Figure 40–1 The cutting edge of a curette is formed by the angular junction of the face and lateral surfaces of the instrument. When the instrument is sharp, the cutting edge is a fine line.

Figure 40–3 Light reflected from the rounded cutting edge of a dull instrument appears as a white line.

in a motor-driven handpiece. They may be cylindrical, conical, or disc-shaped. These stones are generally not recommended for routine use because they are difficult to control precisely and can ruin the shape of the instrument, they tend to wear the instrument down quickly, and they can generate quite a bit of frictional heat which may affect the temper of the instrument.

UNMOUNTED STONES. These come in a variety of sizes and shapes. Some are rectangular with flat or grooved surfaces, whereas others are cylindrical or cone-shaped. Unmounted stones may be used in two ways: the instrument may be stabilized and held stationary while the stone is drawn across it, or the stone may be stabilized and held stationary while the instrument is drawn across it.

THE OBJECTIVE OF SHARPENING

The objective of sharpening is to restore the fine, thin linear cutting edge of the instrument. This is done by grinding the surfaces of the blade until their junction is once again sharply angular rather than rounded. For any given instrument, several sharpening techniques may produce this result. A technique is acceptable if it produces a sharp cutting edge without unduly wearing the instrument or altering its original design. To maintain the original design, the operator must understand the location and course of the cutting edges and the angles between the surfaces that form them. It is important to restore the cutting edge

without distorting the original angles of the instrument. When these angles have been altered, the instrument does not function as it was designed to function. This limits its effectiveness.

PRINCIPLES OF SHARPENING

1. Choose a stone suitable for the instrument to be sharpened, one that is of an appropriate shape and abrasiveness.

2. Use a sterilized sharpening stone if the instrument to be sharpened will not be resterilized before it is used on a patient.

3. Establish the proper angle between the sharpening stone and the surface of the instrument on the basis of an understanding of its design.

4. Maintain a stable, firm grasp of both the instrument and the sharpening stone. This ensures that the proper angulation is maintained throughout the controlled sharpening stroke. In this manner, the entire surface of the instrument can be reduced evenly, and the cutting edge will not be improperly beveled.

5. Avoid excessive pressure. Heavy pressure will cause the stone to grind the surface of the instrument more quickly and may shorten the instrument's life unnecessarily.

6. Avoid the formation of a "wire edge" with minute filamentous projections of metal extending as a roughened ledge from the sharpened cutting edge.[1, 2, 4, 5] When the instrument is used on root surfaces, these projections will produce a grooved rather than a smooth surface. A wire edge occurs when the direction of the sharpening stroke is away from, rather than into or toward, the cutting edge.[1, 4] When back-and-forth or up-and-down sharpening strokes are used, formation of a wire edge can be avoided by finishing with a down stroke toward the cutting edge.[3]

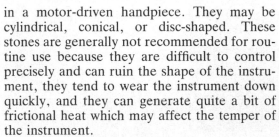

Figure 40–2 The cutting edge of a dull curette is rounded.

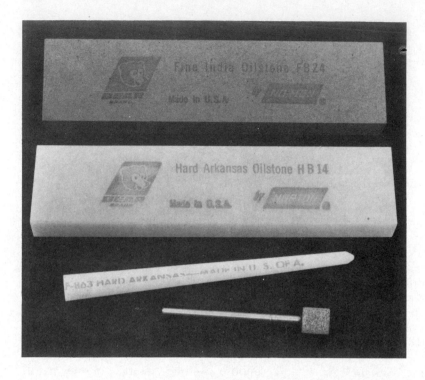

Figure 40–4 Sharpening Stones. At the top of the photograph is a flat India stone. Next is a flat Arkansas stone, and below that is a cone-shaped Arkansas stone. At the bottom is a mandrel-mounted ruby stone used in a handpiece.

7. Lubricate the stone during sharpening. This minimizes clogging of the abrasive surface of the sharpening stone with metal particles removed from the instrument.[2, 4, 5] It also reduces heat produced by friction. Use oil for natural stones and water for synthetic stones.

8. Sharpen instruments at the first sign of dullness. A grossly dull instrument is very inefficient and requires more pressure when used, which hinders control. Furthermore, sharpening such an instrument requires the removal of a great deal of metal to produce a sharp cutting edge. This shortens the effective life of the instrument.

SHARPENING INDIVIDUAL INSTRUMENTS

Universal Curettes

Several techniques will produce a properly sharpened curette. Whichever technique is employed, one must keep in mind that the angle between the face of the blade and the lateral surface of any curette is 70 to 80° (Fig. 40–5). This is the most effective design for calculus removal and root planing. Changing this angle distorts the design of the instrument and makes it less effective. A cutting edge of less than 70° is quite sharp but also very thin (Fig. 40–6). It wears down quickly and becomes dull. A cutting edge of 90° or more requires heavy lateral pressure to remove deposits. Calculus removal with such an instrument is often incomplete, and root planing cannot be done effectively (Fig. 40–6). *The following technique is recommended because it enables one to visualize the critical 70 to 80° angle easily, thereby consistently restoring an effective cutting edge.*

SHARPENING THE LATERAL SURFACE. When a flat hand-held stone is correctly applied to the lateral surface of a curette to maintain the 70 to 80° angle, the angle between the face of the blade and the surface of the stone will be 100 to 110° (see Fig. 40–5). This can best be visualized by holding the curette so that the face of the blade is parallel with the floor. Use a palm grasp and brace the upper arm against the body for support.

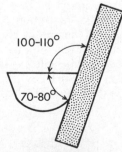

Figure 40–5 When the sharpening stone forms a 100 to 110° angle with the face of the blade, the 70 to 80° angle between the face and the lateral surface is automatically preserved.

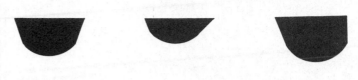

Figure 40–6 At the left is a properly sharpened curette that maintains a 70 to 80° angle between its face and lateral surface. The curette in the center has been sharpened so that one of its cutting edges is less than 70°. This fine edge is quite sharp but dulls easily. One of the cutting edges of the curette on the right has been sharpened to 90°. Heavy lateral pressure must be applied to the tooth to remove deposits with such an instrument.

1. Apply the sharpening stone to the lateral surface of the curette so that the angle between the face of the blade and the stone is 100 to 110° (Fig. 40–7; see also Fig. 40–5). If the curette is dull, there will be a gap between the face of the blade and the surface of the stone (Fig. 40–8).

2. Beginning at the shank end of the cutting edge and working toward the toe, activate the stone with short up-and-down strokes. Use consistent, light pressure and keep the stone continuously in contact with the blade. Make sure that the 100 to 110° angle is constantly maintained (Fig. 40–9). As metal is ground away from the lateral surface during sharpening, the gap between the cutting edge and the surface of the sharpening stone will gradually diminish until the stone reaches the cutting edge. If sharpening is then continued, a sludge of metal shavings and oil may develop on the face of the blade. These signs indicate that sharpening is nearly complete.

3. Check for sharpness as previously described, and continue sharpening as necessary. To prevent the toe of the curette from becom-ing pointed, sharpen the entire blade from shank end to toe. When approaching the toe, be sure to sharpen around it to preserve its rounded form (Fig. 40–10).

4. As the stone is moved along the cutting edge, finish each section with a down stroke into or toward the cutting edge. This will minimize the formation of a wire edge. Check the cutting edge under a light.

5. Sharpening the curette in this manner tends to flatten the lateral surface. This can be corrected by lightly grinding the lateral surface and the back of the instrument, away from the cutting edge, each time the instrument is sharpened.

6. When one edge has been properly sharpened, the opposite cutting edge can be sharpened in the same manner.

Some clinicians can produce the same result with curved up strokes or down strokes. Usually these are performed as a rapid series of separate strokes in which the stone is removed from the instrument at the end of each stroke and reapplied to begin a new stroke. Some clinicians will combine these up strokes and

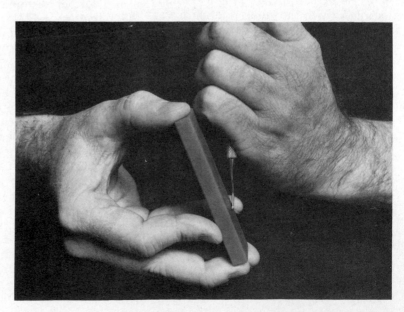

Figure 40–7 Using a palm grasp, the universal curette is held so that the face of the blade is parallel to the floor. The stone makes a 100 to 110 ° angle with the face of the blade.

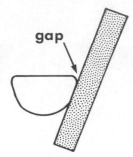

Figure 40–8 Note the gap between the face of the blade and the stone caused by the rounded cutting edge of a dull curette.

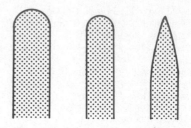

Figure 40–10 At the left is a new, unsharpened curette viewed from directly above the face of the blade. The curette in the center has been correctly sharpened to maintain the rounded toe. The curette at the right has been incorrectly sharpened, producing a pointed toe.

down strokes into a continuous series in which the stone never leaves the instrument (Fig. 40–11).

Performing these last sharpening operations properly requires a great deal of experience, because the angles cannot be directly seen during the sharpening movement. This, coupled with the fact that the angulation of the stone to the instrument is constantly changing during the sharpening stroke, leads to a tendency to produce a cutting edge that is 90° or more—a very inefficient curette design. Therefore, these sharpening methods are not recommended for novices or for anyone who cannot use them to produce a properly sharpened curette.

SHARPENING THE FACE OF THE BLADE. This may be done moving a hand-held cylindrical or cone-shaped stone back and forth across the face of the blade. A cylindrical or cone-shaped stone mounted in a handpiece may also be used by applying it to the face of the blade with the stone rotating toward the toe. These methods are not recommended for routine use for the following reasons: (1) The angulation between the instrument and the stone is difficult to maintain, and therefore the blade may be improperly beveled (Fig. 40–12).[1] (2) Sharpening the face of the blade narrows the working end from face to back. This weakens the blade and makes it likely to bend or break while in use (Fig. 40–12).[1, 3–5] (3) Sharpening the face of the blade with a hand-held stone using a back-and-forth motion

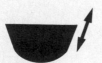

Figure 40–9 Maintaining the 100 to 110° angle, activate short up-and-down strokes.

will produce a wire edge that interferes with the sharpness of the blade.[1]

Gracey Curettes

Like a universal curette, a Gracey curette has an angle of 70 to 80° between the face and lateral surface of its blade. Therefore, the technique described for sharpening a universal curette can be used to sharpen a Gracey. However, there are several unique design features that distinguish a Gracey from a universal curette, and these must be understood to avoid distorting the design of the instrument while sharpening.

Gracey curettes have what is known as an offset blade, i.e., the face of the blade is not perpendicular to the shank of the instrument, as it is on a universal curette, but is offset at a 70° angle (Fig. 40–13). A Gracey curette is further distinguished by the curvature of its cutting edges. When viewed from directly above the face of the blade, the cutting edges of a universal curette extend in straight lines from shank to toe. Both cutting edges can be used for scaling and root planing. The cutting edges of a Gracey curette, on the other hand, curve gently from shank to toe. Only the larger, outer cutting edge is used for scaling and root planing (Fig. 40–14).

With these points in mind, a Gracey curette is sharpened in the following manner:

1. Hold the curette so that the face of the blade is parallel with the floor. Because the blade is offset, the shank of the instrument will not be perpendicular to the floor, as it is with universal curettes (Fig. 40–15).

2. Identify the edge to be sharpened. Remember that only one cutting edge is used, so only that edge needs to be sharpened. Apply the stone to the lateral surface so that the

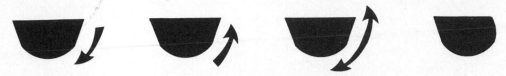

Figure 40–11 It is difficult to maintain proper angulation when a rapid series of curved up or down strokes is used to sharpen a blade. The result is often an instrument with a distorted cutting edge, as shown at the right.

angle between the face of the blade and the stone is 100 to 110°.

3. Activate short up-and-down strokes, working from the shank end of the blade to the curved toe. Finish with a down stroke.

4. Remember that the cutting edge is curved. Preserve the curve while sharpening from shank to toe by turning the stone. If the stone is kept in one place for too many strokes, the blade will be flattened (Fig. 40–16).

5. Evaluate sharpness as previously described. Continue sharpening as necessary.

Sickle Scalers

There are two types of sickle scalers, the straight sickle and the curved sickle. The face of the blade on a straight sickle is flat from shank to tip, whereas on the curved sickle the face of the blade forms a gentle curve (Fig. 40–17). The straight and curved sickle have similar cross-sectional designs, however. As in the curette, the angle between the face of the blade and the lateral surface of a sickle is 70 to 80° (Fig. 40–18). When a sharpening stone is correctly applied to the lateral surface to preserve this angle, the angle between the face of the blade and the surface of the stone is 100 to 110°. With this in mind, the sickler scaler can be sharpened in a manner very much like that described for the curette.

1. Grasp the sickle with a palm grasp so that the face of the blade is parallel with the floor.

2. Apply the sharpening stone to the lateral surface of the sickle so that the angle between the face of the blade and the surface of the stone is 100 to 110°.

3. Sharpen with short up-and-down strokes.

Use consistent, light pressure and keep the stone continuously in contact with the blade. On most sickles, the stone will contact the entire cutting edge from shank to toe. To sharpen a sickle whose blade is longer, begin sharpening at the shank end of the blade and work toward the toe. Sickles have a sharp, pointed toe. Do not make it rounded.

4. Look for a sludge of oil and metal shavings forming on the face of the blade. This indicates that sharpening is nearly complete. Finish with a down stroke to avoid producing a wire edge.

5. Check for sharpness as previously described. Continue sharpening as necessary.

6. When one edge has been properly sharpened, sharpen the opposite edge in the same manner.

7. A large flat stone may also be used to sharpen sickles (Fig. 40–19). The stone is stabilized on a table or cabinet with the left hand. The sickle is held in the right hand with a modified pen grasp and applied to the stone so that the angle between the face of the blade and the stone is 100 to 110°. The fourth finger is placed on the right-hand edge of the stone to stabilize and guide the sharpening movement. The right hand then pushes and pulls the sickle across the surface of the stone. To avoid a wire edge, finish with a pull stroke. Be sure that the proper angulation is always maintained.

A mounted stone can also be used to sharpen the lateral surface of a sickle. How-

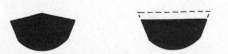

Figure 40–12 Angulation is difficult to control when sharpening the face of the blade and often results in unwanted beveling, as shown at the left. Sharpening the face also weakens the blade by narrowing it from face to back, as shown at the right.

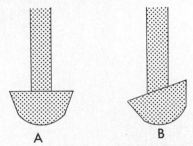

Figure 40–13 *A,* The face of a universal curette is at 90° to its shank. *B,* The face of a Gracey curette is offset, forming a 70° angle with its shank.

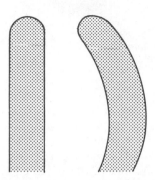

Figure 40–14 The cutting edges of a universal curette extend straight from shank to toe. The cutting edges of a Gracey curette gently curves from shank to toe. Only the larger, outer cutting edge at the right is used for scaling and needs to be sharpened.

Figure 40–15 Note that when held in proper sharpening position the shank of a Gracey curette is not perpendicular to the floor, owing to its offset blade angle. The stone meets the blade at an angle of 100 to 110°. Compare this position with the sharpening position of a universal curette in Figure 40–7.

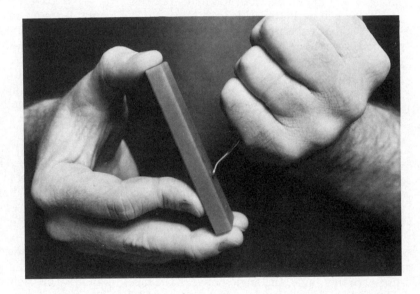

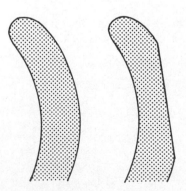

Figure 40–16 The Gracey curette on the left has been properly sharpened to maintain a symmetrical curve on its outer cutting edge. For the curette on the right the sharpening stone was activated too long in one place, thereby flattening the blade.

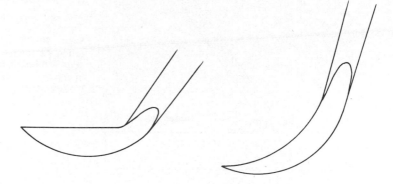

Figure 40–17 The face of the blade on a straight sickle is flat from shank to tip, whereas on the curved sickle the blade face forms a gentle arc.

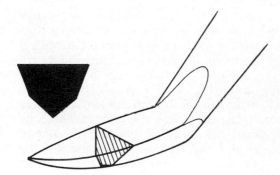

Figure 40–18 Like the curette, the sickle has an angle of 70 to 80° between the face of the blade and the lateral surface.

Figure 40–19 A large flat stone may also be used to sharpen the sickle. The stone is stabilized on a flat surface. The fourth finger of the right hand guides the sharpening stroke as the instrument is pulled across the face of the stone toward the operator.

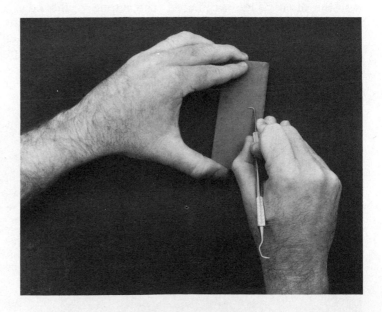

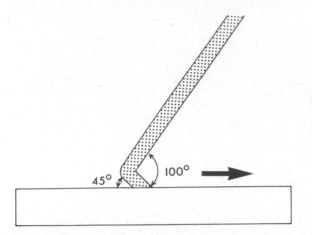

Figure 40–20 The angle between the face of the blade of a hoe and its shank is 100°. The 45° angle of the cutting edge will be maintained if the entire lateral surface is kept in contact with the stone as the instrument is pulled toward the operator.

ever, as with curettes, mounted stones are not recommended for routine use. Sickles can also be sharpened by grinding the face of the blade. Again, as with curettes, this is not recommended, because the proper angulation is difficult to maintain, leading to unwanted beveling of the face of the blade, and because sharpening the face narrows the instrument from face to back, thereby weakening the blade.

Hoe Scalers

Hoe scalers have a single straight cutting edge. The face of the hoe forms a 100° angle with the shank of the instrument. The cutting edge is formed by the juncture of the beveled lateral surface and the face of the blade, which meet at a 45° angle. The cutting edge is perpendicular to the shank of the instrument (Fig. 40–20).

To sharpen the hoe, stabilize a flat sharpening stone on a flat surface. Grasp the instrument with a modified pen grasp. Establish a finger rest with the pad of the third and fourth fingers against the straight edge of the sharpening stone (Fig. 40–21). Apply the flat beveled surface of the hoe to the surface of the stone. If the entire lateral surface is contacting the stone, the 45° angle between the lateral surface and the face of the blade will be maintained, and the instrument design will not be altered (see Fig. 40–20).

Using moderate, steady pressure with the hand and arm held rigid and the finger rest on the edge of the stone as a guide, pull the instrument toward you. Release pressure slightly and push the instrument back to its starting point. Repeat the sharpening stroke

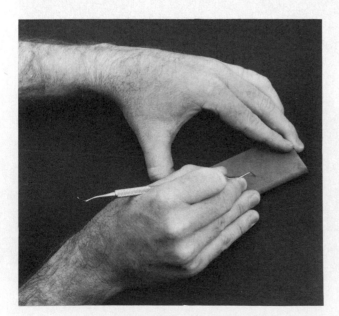

Figure 40–21 When sharpening a hoe, a large flat stone is stabilized on a flat surface. The instrument is applied to the stone at the proper angulation. The fourth finger on the side of the stone guides the sharpening motion as the instrument is pulled toward the operator.

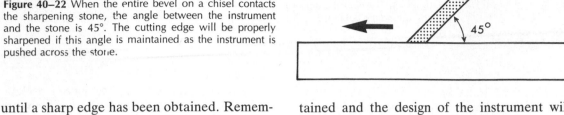

Figure 40–22 When the entire bevel on a chisel contacts the sharpening stone, the angle between the instrument and the stone is 45°. The cutting edge will be properly sharpened if this angle is maintained as the instrument is pushed across the stone.

until a sharp edge has been obtained. Remember to end with a pull stroke to prevent formation of a wire edge. Check for sharpness as previously described. Examine the instrument carefully to be sure its design has not been inadvertently altered.

Chisels

Chisels have a single straight cutting edge that is perpendicular to the shank. The face of the blade is continuous with the shank of the instrument, which may be directly in line with the handle or slightly curved. The end of the blade is beveled at 45° to form the cutting edge.

To sharpen a chisel, stabilize a flat sharpening stone on a flat surface. Grasp the instrument with a modified pen grasp. Establish a finger rest with the pad of the third and fourth fingers against the straight edge of the sharpening stone. Apply the flat beveled surface of the chisel to the surface of the stone. If the entire surface of the bevel is contacting the stone, the 45° angle between the beveled surface and the face of the blade will be maintained and the design of the instrument will not be altered (Figs. 40–22 and 40–23).

Using moderate, steady pressure, with the hand and arm acting as a unit and the finger resting on the edge of the stone as a guide, push the instrument across the surface of the sharpening stone. Release pressure slightly and draw the instrument back to its starting point. Repeat the sharpening stroke until a sharp edge has been obtained. Remember to finish with a push stroke to prevent formation of a wire edge. Check for sharpness as previously described. Examine the instrument carefully to be sure that its design has not been inadvertently altered.

Periodontal Knives

There are two general types of periodontal knives. The first are the disposable scalpel blades that come prepackaged. They are presharpened and sterilized by the manufacturer. These are not resharpened when they become dull but are discarded and replaced with a new blade.

A second group of periodontal knives are

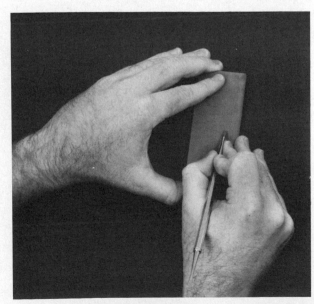

Figure 40–23 The chisel is also sharpened on a stationary flat sharpening stone.

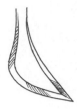

Figure 40–24 Flat-bladed gingivectomy knives like this Kirkland knife have a cutting edge that extends around the entire blade. The entire cutting edge must be sharpened.

reusable and must be sharpened when they become dull. The most commonly used knives in this group are the flat-bladed gingivectomy knives (of which the Kirkland Nos. 15K and 16K are examples) and the narrow, pointed interproximal knives.

FLAT-BLADED GINGIVECTOMY KNIVES. These knives have broad, flat blades that are nearly perpendicular to the lower shank of the instrument. The curved cutting edge extends around the entire outer edge of the blade and is formed by bevels on both the front and back surfaces of the blade (Fig. 40–24).

When sharpening these instruments, only the bevel on the back surface of the instrument need be ground. This can be done by drawing the blade across a stationary flat sharpening stone or by holding the instrument stationary and drawing the stone across its blade.

Stationary Stone Technique. Stabilize a flat sharpening stone on a flat surface. Grasp the handle of the instrument with a modified pen grasp. Apply the bevel on the back surface of the blade to the flat surface of the sharpening stone. With moderate pressure, pull the instrument toward you (Figs. 40–25 and 40–26). Release pressure slightly and return to the starting point. Begin at one end of the cutting

edge and continue around the blade by rolling the handle of the instrument slightly between the thumb and the first and second fingers. Finish each section of the blade with a pull stroke to prevent formation of a wire edge. Check for sharpness as described previously.

Stationary Instrument Technique. Grasp the instrument with the palm. Apply the flat surface of a hand-held sharpening stone to the bevel on the back surface of the blade. Begin at one end of the cutting edge and, with moderate pressure, draw the stone back and forth across the instrument. To prevent the formation of a wire edge, finish each section with a stroke into or toward the cutting edge. Proceed around the entire length of the cutting edge by gradually rotating the instrument and the stone in relation to one another.

Interproximal Knives

The blades of interproximal knives have two long, straight cutting edges that come together at the sharply pointed tip of the instrument. The cutting edges are formed by bevels on the front and back surfaces of the blade. The entire blade is roughly perpendicular to the lower

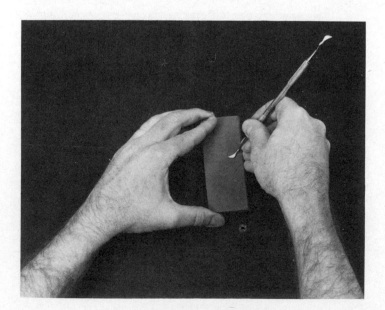

Figure 40–25 The gingivectomy knife may be sharpened on a stationary flat stone. The instrument is held with a modified pen grasp. The fourth finger guides the sharpening stroke as the instrument is rolled between the fingers so that all sections of the blade are sharpened.

Figure 40–26 This cross section of a gingivectomy knife shows the two short bevels that form the cutting edge. The bevel on the back of the blade is applied to surface of the stone, and the instrument is drawn toward the cutting edge.

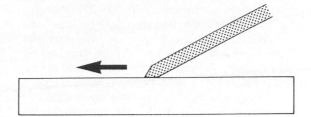

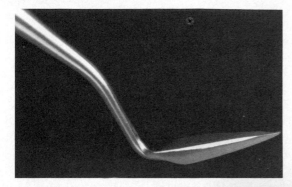

Figure 40–27 The two cutting edges of an interproximal knife are formed by bevels on the front and back surfaces of the blade.

Figure 40–28 The interproximal knife may be sharpened on a flat stationary stone. The blade is drawn toward the operator.

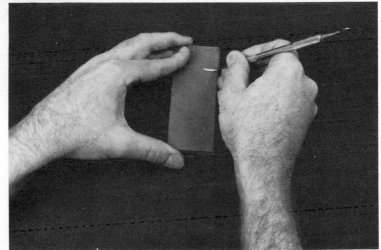

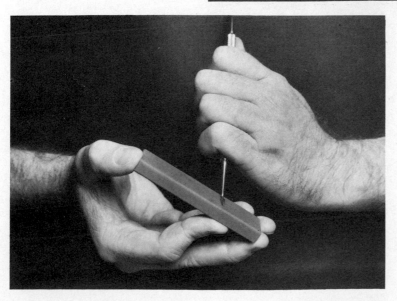

Figure 40–29 The interproximal knife may also be sharpened with a hand-held stone. The instrument is held with a palm grasp, and the stone is applied to the entire cutting edge.

shank of the instrument (Fig. 40–27). As with the flat-bladed gingivectomy knives, only the bevels on the back surface of the interproximal knives need be sharpened. Again, this can be accomplished by drawing the instrument across a stationary stone or by holding the instrument stationary and moving the stone across it.

Stationary Stone Technique. Grasp the instrument and stone as described for the flat-bladed gingivectomy knife. Apply the beveled cutting edge to the stone. Be sure the entire cutting edge is contacting the surface of the stone (Fig. 40–28). With moderate pressure, pull the instrument toward you. Release pressure slightly and return to the starting point. Continue until a sharp edge has been obtained. Be sure to finish with a pull stroke to prevent formation of a wire edge. Evaluate sharpness as previously described. When one cutting edge has been properly sharpened, sharpen the opposite edge.

Stationary Instrument Technique. Grasp the handle of the instrument with the palm. Apply a flat hand-held stone to the beveled cutting edge (Fig. 40–29). Sharpen the instrument using moderate pressure and up-and-down strokes. Be sure the entire cutting edge is contacting the surface of the stone. Finish with a down stroke to prevent a wire edge. Check for sharpness as before and proceed to the opposite cutting edge.

REFERENCES

1. Antonini, C. J., Brady, J. M., Levin, M. P., and Garcia, W. L.: Scanning electron microscope study of scalers. J. Periodontol., *48*:45, 1977.
2. Green, E., and Seyer, P. C.: Sharpening Curets and Sickle Scalers. 2nd ed. Berkeley, Calif., Praxis Publishing Company, 1972.
3. Lindhe, J., and Jacobson, L.: Evaluation of periodontal scalers. I. Wear following clinical use. Odontol. Rev., *17*:1, 1966.
4. Parquette, O. E., and Levin, M. P.: The sharpening of scaling instruments. I. An examination of principles. J. Periodontol., *48*:163, 1977.
5. Wilkins, E. M.: Clinical Practice of the Dental Hygienist. 4th ed. Philadelphia, Lea & Febiger, 1976.

Part III

Treatment of Emergencies

chapter forty-one

The Treatment of Acute Gingival Disease

The treatment of acute gingival disease entails the alleviation of the acute symptoms and the elimination of all other periodontal disease, chronic as well as acute, throughout the oral cavity. *Treatment is not complete so long as periodontal pathology or factors capable of causing it are still present.*

Acute necrotizing ulcerative gingivitis can occur in a mouth essentially free of any other gingival involvement or superimposed upon underlying chronic gingival disease. *The simplest part of clinical treatment is the alleviation of the acute symptoms; correction of the underlying chronic gingival disease requires more comprehensive procedures.*

The treatment of acute necrotizing ulcerative gingivitis consists of the following phases:

1. *Local:* Alleviation of the acute inflammation plus treatment of chronic disease either underlying the acute involvement or elsewhere in the oral cavity.
2. *Systemic:*
   a. Supportive Treatment: Alleviation of generalized toxic symptoms such as fever and malaise.
   b. Etiotropic Treatment: The correction of systemic conditions which contribute to the initiation or progress of the gingival changes.

Treatment should follow an orderly sequence, as described in the following paragraphs.

COMPREHENSIVE TREATMENT OF ACUTE NECROTIZING ULCERATIVE GINGIVITIS

At the **first visit** the dentist should obtain a general impression of the patient's background, including information regarding recent illness, living conditions, dietary background, type of employment, hours of rest, and mental stress. Observe the patient's general appearance, apparent nutritional status, and responsiveness or lassitude and *take the patient's temperature.* Palpate the submaxillary and submental areas to detect enlarged lymph glands.

Examine the oral cavity for the "characteristic lesion" of acute necrotizing ulcerative gingivitis (see Chapter 11), its distribution, and the possible involvement of the oropharyngeal region. Evaluate the oral hygiene; check for the presence of pericoronal flaps, periodontal pockets, and local irritants. A bacterial smear may be made from the material in the involved areas, but this is merely corroboratory and is not to be relied upon for diagnosis.

Examine the occlusion and check for bruxism, clamping, or clenching.

Question the patient regarding the history of the acute disease and its onset and duration. Is it recurrent? Are the recurrences associated with specific factors such as menstruation, particular foods, exhaustion, or mental stress? Has there been any previous treatment? When, and for how long? Inquire as to the type of treatment received and the patient's impression regarding its effect.

After the diagnosis is established, the patient is treated as either "nonambulatory" or "ambulatory," based upon the following criteria:

Nonambulatory Patients. These are patients with symptoms of generalized toxicity, such as high fever, malaise, and lassitude; bed rest is often necessary, and extensive office treatment should not be undertaken until the systemic symptoms subside.

Ambulatory Patients. In these patients, there may be localized adenopathy and a slightly elevated temperature but there are no serious systemic complications.

Preliminary Treatment for Nonambulatory Patients

DAY ONE. The following guidelines should be adhered to on the first day of preliminary treatment:

1. Local treatment is limited to gently removing the necrotic pseudomembrane with a pellet of cotton saturated with hydrogen peroxide.

2. The patient is advised to rest in bed and to rinse the mouth every 2 hours with a glassful of an equal mixture of warm water and 3 per cent hydrogen peroxide. For systemic antibiotic action, penicillin is administered either intramuscularly in a dose of 300,000 units or as 250-mg tablets every 4 hours. For penicillin-sensitive patients, other antibiotics, such as erythromycin (250 mg every 4 hours), are prescribed. Metronidazole (200 mg three times daily for 7 days), which is extensively used in Europe, is also very effective. Keep a carbon copy of the prescription in the patient's file for future reference. The patient is to report to the dentist after 24 hours.

Always stipulate the period for which the instructions are intended, and check the condition of the patient the next day. It is poor practice to place the patient on a home regimen for a protracted period of time. There may be a severe reaction to the antibiotic, and the hydrogen peroxide mouthwash may produce diffuse erythema, ulceration of the oral mucosa, and swelling of the tongue.

DAY TWO. If the patient's condition has improved, proceed to the treatment described under "Treatment for Ambulatory Patients." If there is no improvement at the end of 24 hours, a bedside visit should be made. *The instrumentarium required for this visit includes a mirror, an explorer, cotton pliers, a flashlight, a thermometer, a container of cotton pellets, and a glass-stoppered bottle of hydrogen peroxide.* At the bedside, the oral condition, the possibility of oropharyngeal involvement, and the patient's temperature are checked. The involved gingiva is again gently swabbed with hydrogen peroxide, and the instructions for the previous day are repeated. The patient is to communicate with the dentist after 24 hours.

DAY THREE. In most instances, the patient is improved by this time and is started on the treatment for ambulatory patients described below.

Treatment for Ambulatory Patients

The following is the procedure for ambulatory patients and for initially nonambulatory patients after their satisfactory response to the preliminary treatment:

DAY ONE. Instrumentarium: two dappen dishes, one containing topical anesthetic, the other containing 3 per cent hydrogen peroxide; cotton pellets and cotton rolls; a mirror; an explorer; cotton pliers; and superficial scalers.

Treatment is confined to the acutely involved areas, which are isolated with cotton rolls and dried. A topical anesthetic is applied, and after 2 or 3 minutes the areas are gently swabbed with a cotton pellet to remove the pseudomembrane and nonattached surface debris. Each cotton pellet is used in a small area and is then discarded; sweeping motions over large areas with a single pellet are not used. After the area is cleansed with warm water, the superficial calculus is removed. *Ultrasonic scalers are very useful for this purpose.*

Deep scaling and curettage are contraindicated at this time because of the possibility of extending the infection into deeper tissues and also of causing a bacteremia. Unless an emergency exists, procedures such as extractions or periodontal surgery are postponed until the patient has been symptom-free for a period of 4 weeks in order to minimize the likelihood of exacerbation of the acute symptoms.

The patient should be advised of the extent of the total treatment the condition requires and warned that treatment is not complete when the pain stops. He or she should be informed of the presence of chronic gingival and periodontal disease which must be eliminated in order to prevent recurrence of the acute symptoms. The patient is told to return in 24 hours.

Instructions to the Patient. The patient is dismissed with the following instructions:

Avoid tobacco, alcohol, and condiments. Heat and the products of tobacco irritate the inflamed tissue and retard healing. If the patient is a heavy smoker, it is preferable to recommend less smoking, rather than complete abstinence. A heavy smoker who might disregard a drastic order to discontinue smoking entirely may be more cooperative if permitted to indulge in tobacco occasionally. The occasional use of tobacco is obviously less harmful than would be total disregard of unacceptable instructions.

Rinse with a glassful of an equal mixture of 3 per cent hydrogen peroxide and warm water every 2 hours.

Pursue usual activities, but avoid excessive physical exertion or prolonged exposure to the sun as required in golf, tennis, swimming, or sunbathing.

Confine toothbrushing to the removal of surface debris with a bland dentifrice; overzealous brushing will be painful. Dental floss, interdental cleaners, and water irrigation under medium pressure are recommended.

DAY TWO. The patient's condition is usually improved; the pain is diminished or no longer present. The gingival margins of the involved areas are erythematous, but without a superficial pseudomembrane.

Scalers and curettes are added to the instrumentarium, and the procedures performed on day one are repeated. Shrinkage of the gingiva may expose previously covered calculus, which is removed during gentle curettage of the gingiva. The instructions to the patient are the same as on the previous day. If there have been undesirable effects of the hydrogen peroxide, warm water alone is used for rinsing.

DAY THREE. The patient is essentially symptom-free. There is still some erythema in the involved areas, and the gingiva may be slightly painful on tactile stimulation (Fig. 41–1). Scaling and curettage are repeated. The patient is instructed in plaque control procedures (described in Chapter 44), which are essential for the success of the treatment and the maintenance of periodontal health. The hydrogen peroxide rinses are discontinued.

DAY FOUR. Tooth surfaces in the involved areas are scaled and smoothed, and plaque control by the patient is checked and corrected if necessary.

DAY FIVE. *Unfortunately, treatment is often stopped at this time because the acute condition has subsided, but this is when comprehensive treatment of the patient's chronic periodontal problem should start. Appointments are scheduled for the treatment of chronic gingivitis,*

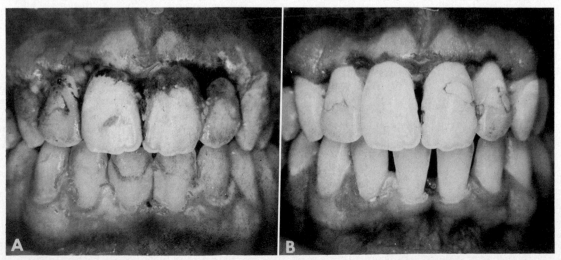

Figure 41–1 Initial Response to Treatment of Acute Necrotizing Ulcerative Gingivitis. *A,* Severe acute necrotizing ulcerative gingivitis. *B,* Third day. There is still some erythema, but the condition is markedly improved.

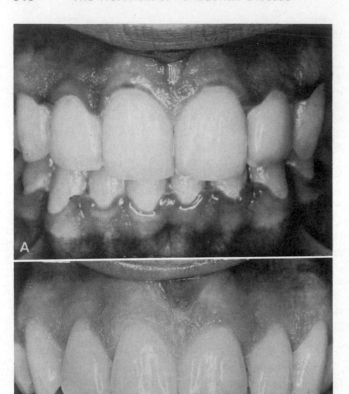

Figure 41–2 Treated Acute Necrotizing Ulcerative Gingivitis. *A,* Before treatment. Note the characteristic interdental lesions. *B,* After treatment, showing restoration of healthy gingival contour.

periodontal pockets, and pericoronal flaps and for the elimination of all forms of local irritation, plus occlusal adjustment if necessary.

Patients without gingival disease other than the treated acute involvement are dismissed for 1 week. If the condition is satisfactory at that time, the patient is dismissed for 1 month, at which time the schedule for subsequent recall visits is determined according to the patient's needs.

Gingival Changes with Healing

The characteristic lesion of acute necrotizing ulcerative gingivitis undergoes the following changes in the course of healing in response to treatment:

1. Removal of the surface pseudomembrane exposes the underlying red, hemorrhagic, crater-like depressions in the gingiva.

2. In the next stage the bulk and redness of the crater margins are reduced, but the surface remains shiny.

3. This is followed by the early signs of the restoration of normal gingival contour and color.

4. In the final stage the normal gingival color, consistency, surface texture, and contour are restored. Portions of the root exposed by the acute disease are covered by healthy gingiva (Figs. 41–2 and 41–3).

When the **menstrual period** occurs in the course of treatment, there is a tendency toward exacerbation of the acute signs and symptoms, giving the appearance of a relapse. Patients should be informed of this possibility and spared unnecessary anxiety regarding their oral condition.

CONTOURING THE GINGIVA AS AN ADJUNCTIVE TREATMENT PROCEDURE

Even in cases of severe gingival necrosis, healing ordinarily leads to restoration of the normal gingival contour (Fig. 41–4). However, if the teeth are irregularly aligned, healing sometimes results in the formation of a shelf-like gingival margin which favors the retention of food and the recurrence of gingival inflammation. This can be corrected by reshaping the gingiva with a periodontal knife or with electrosurgery (Fig. 41–5). Effective plaque control by the patient is particularly important to establish and maintain the normal gingival contour in areas of tooth irregularity.

SURGICAL PROCEDURES AND ACUTE NECROTIZING ULCERATIVE GINGIVITIS

Tooth extraction or extensive gingival surgery should be postponed until 4 weeks after the acute signs and symptoms of necrotizing ulcerative gingivitis have subsided. If emergency surgery is required in the presence of acute symptoms, prophylactic chemotherapy with penicillin or other antibiotics is indicated to prevent worsening or spreading of the acute disease. Penicillin is administered systemically either by the intramuscular injection of phe-noxymethyl penicillin (300,000 units once daily for 3 days beginning the evening before the surgical procedure) or by the oral administration of 250-mg tablets (one every 4 hours beginning the evening before the operation and continuing for 48 hours after it).

ROLE OF DRUGS IN THE TREATMENT OF ACUTE NECROTIZING ULCERATIVE GINGIVITIS

A large variety of drugs, some of which are listed in Table 41–1, have been used topically in the treatment of acute necrotizing ulcerative gingivitis.[3] **Topical drug therapy is only an adjunctive measure in the treatment of acute necrotizing ulcerative gingivitis; no drug, when used alone, can be considered complete therapy.**

Escharotic drugs such as phenol, silver nitrate, and chromic acid should not be used. They are necrotizing agents that alleviate the painful symptoms by destroying the nerve end-

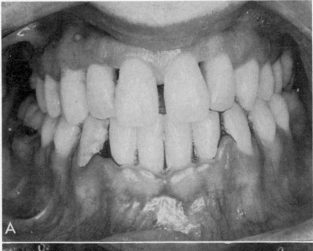
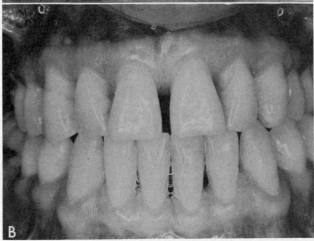

Figure 41–3 Physiologic Contour and Reattachment of Gingiva Following Treatment of Acute Necrotizing Ulcerative Gingivitis. *A*, Acute necrotizing ulcerative gingivitis showing the characteristic punched-out eroded gingival margin with surface pseudomembrane. *B*, After treatment. Note the restoration of physiologic gingival contour and reattachment of the gingiva to the surfaces of the mandibular teeth, which had been exposed by the disease.

A

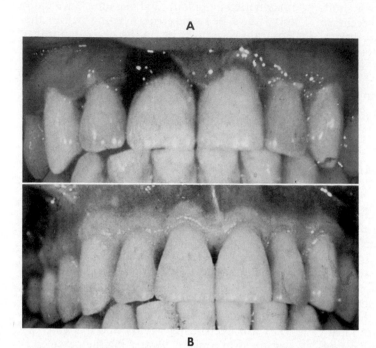

B

Figure 41–4 Gingival Healing Following Treatment. *A,* Before treatment. Severe acute necrotizing ulcerative gingivitis with crater formation. *B,* After treatment. Note the restored gingival contour.

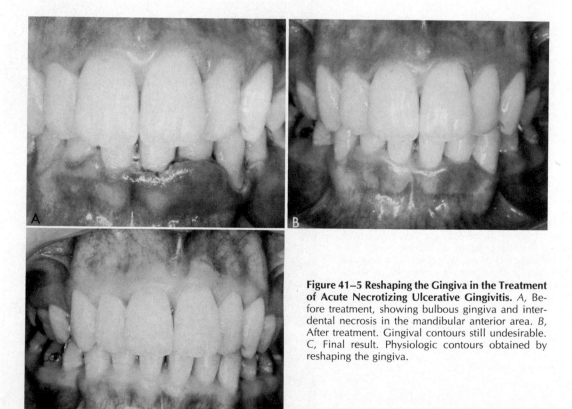

Figure 41–5 Reshaping the Gingiva in the Treatment of Acute Necrotizing Ulcerative Gingivitis. *A,* Before treatment, showing bulbous gingiva and interdental necrosis in the mandibular anterior area. *B,* After treatment. Gingival contours still undesirable. *C,* Final result. Physiologic contours obtained by reshaping the gingiva.

TABLE 41–1 TOPICALLY APPLIED DRUGS USED IN TREATMENT OF ACUTE
NECROTIZING ULCERATIVE GINGIVITIS

Oxygen-Liberating Agents	*Escharotics (Caustics)*
Zinc peroxide	Copper sulfate and zinc chloride
Hydrogen peroxide	Chromic acid 8%
Sodium perborate	Negatan
Potassium chlorate	Zinc chloride 8%
Potassium permanganate	Phenol 95%
Sodium peroxyborate[25]	Trichloroacetic acid 50%
	Iodine 16.5% and silver nitrate 35%
Mercurial Derivatives	*Aniline Dyes*
Tinct. Metaphen 1:200 (untinted)	Viogen (Berwick's solution)
Mercuric cyanide 1%	Acriviolet 1%
Merthiolate 1:1,000	Gentian violet 1%
Mercuric chloride 1:2,000	Acriflavine 1%
	Methylene blue 1%
Spirocheticides	*Other Agents*
Sodium carbonate 10% aqueous	Ascoxal[5]
Arsphenamine 10% aqueous	Copper sulfate, phenol, glycerin and water
Mapharsen	Metronidazole[7, 26]
Neoarsphenamine	Penicillin[8]
Fuadin	Sulfonamide in paraffin—especially sulfadiazine
	Surgical pack (zinc oxide–resin, eugenol)
	Vancomycin[6, 19]

ings in the gingiva. They also destroy the young cells necessary for repair and delay healing. Their repeated use results in the loss of gingival tissue, which is not restored when the disease subsides.[15]

SYSTEMIC ANTIBIOTICS IN THE TREATMENT OF ACUTE NECROTIZING ULCERATIVE GINGIVITIS

Antibiotics are administered systemically in patients with toxic systemic complications or local adenopathy but are not recommended for topical use because of the risk of sensitization. Phenoxymethyl (penicillin V) is the drug of choice. It may be administered as follows: (1) in tablet or capsule form, 250 mg every 4 hours (V-Cillin K, Pen-Vee, and other effective preparations), or (2) in intramuscular injections, 300,000 units, repeated at 24-hour intervals until the systemic symptoms subside. In penicillin-sensitive patients, other antibiotics, such as erythromycin (250 mg four times daily) or metronidazole (200 mg three times daily), may be used.

Antibiotics are continued until the systemic complications or local lymphadenopathy subsides. Systemic antibiotics also effect some reduction in the oral bacterial flora and a temporary alleviation of the oral symptoms,[26, 27] but it is only an adjunct to the complete local treatment the disease requires. Patients treated by systemic antibiotics alone should be cautioned that the acute painful symptoms may recur after the drug is discontinued.

SUPPORTIVE SYSTEMIC TREATMENT

In addition to systemic antibiotics, supportive treatment consists of copious fluid consumption and analgesics for relief of pain. Bed rest is necessary for patients with toxic systemic complications such as high fever, malaise, anorexia, and general debility.

NUTRITIONAL SUPPLEMENTS. The rationale for nutritional supplements in the treatment of acute necrotizing ulcerative gingivitis is based upon the following: (1) Lesions resembling those of acute necrotizing ulcerative gingivitis have been produced experimentally in animals with certain nutritional deficiencies (see Chapter 11). (2) It is possible that difficulty in chewing raw fruits and vegetables in a painful condition such as acute necrotizing ulcerative gingivitis could lead to the selection of a diet inadequate in vitamins B and C. Because these are water-soluble vitamins which are not stored in the body and which require continual replenishment, daily supplements may be needed to prevent a nutritional deficiency. (3) There are isolated clinical studies[17, 18] reporting fewer recurrences when local treatment of acute necrotizing ulcerative gingivitis is supplemented with vitamin B or vitamin C.

When the intake of water-soluble vitamins

B and C has been severely curtailed because of pain in acute necrotizing ulcerative gingivitis, nutritional supplements may be indicated along with local treatment in order to ward off deficiencies of the aforementioned vitamins. Under such circumstances the patient may be started on a standard multivitamin preparation combined with a therapeutic dose of vitamins B and C.

The patient should be placed on a natural diet with the required detergent action and nutritional content as soon as the oral condition permits. Nutritional supplements may be discontinued after 2 months.

Local procedures are the keystone of the treatment of acute necrotizing ulcerative gingivitis. Inflammation is a local conditioning factor which impairs the nutrition of the gingiva regardless of the systemic nutritional status. Local irritants should be eliminated in order to foster normal metabolic and reparative processes in the gingiva. Persistent or recurrent acute necrotizing ulcerative gingivitis is more likely to be caused by the failure to remove local irritants and by inadequate plaque control than by nutritional deficiency.

ETIOTROPIC SYSTEMIC TREATMENT

Etiotropic treatment consists of measures for the correction of systemic conditions which contribute to the initiation or progress of acute necrotizing ulcerative gingivitis. Since the role of systemic etiologic factors has not been established, the indications for and value of systemic therapy are not clearly defined.

SEQUELAE THAT MAY FOLLOW TREATMENT OF ACUTE NECROTIZING ULCERATIVE GINGIVITIS

PERSISTENT OR "NONRESPONSIVE" CASES. If the dentist finds it necessary to change from drug to drug in an effort to relieve a "stubborn" case of acute necrotizing ulcerative gingivitis, something is wrong with the overall treatment regimen which is not likely to be corrected by changing drugs. *When confronted with such a problem: (1) All local drug therapy should be discontinued so that the condition may be studied in an uncomplicated state. (2)* Careful differential diagnosis is undertaken to rule out diseases which resemble acute necrotizing ulcerative gingivitis (see Chapter 11). (3) A search is made for contributing local and systemic etiologic factors that may have been overlooked. (4) Special attention is given to instructing the patient in plaque control before undertaking comprehensive local treatment.

RECURRENT ACUTE NECROTIZING ULCERATIVE GINGIVITIS. The following factors should be explored in patients with recurrent acute necrotizing ulcerative gingivitis:

Inadequate Local Therapy. Too frequently, treatment is discontinued when the symptoms have subsided, without eliminating the chronic gingival disease and periodontal pockets which remain after the superficial acute condition is relieved. Persistent chronic inflammation causes degenerative changes which predispose the gingiva to recurrence of acute involvement.

Pericoronal Flap. Recurrent acute involvement in the mandibular anterior area is often associated with persistent pericoronal inflammation arising from difficult eruption of third molars.[12] The anterior involvement is less likely to recur after the third molar situation is corrected.

Anterior Overbite. Marked overbite is often a contributing factor in the recurrence of disease in the anterior region. When the incisal edges of the maxillary teeth impinge upon the labial gingival margin, or the mandibular teeth strike the palatal gingiva, the resultant tissue injury predisposes the gingiva to recurrent acute disease. Less severe overbite produces food impaction and gingival trauma. Correction of the overbite is necessary for the complete treatment of acute necrotizing ulcerative gingivitis.

Inadequate plaque control and heavy use of tobacco are also common causes of recurrent disease.

TREATMENT OF ACUTE PERICORONITIS

The treatment of pericoronitis depends upon the severity of the inflammation, the systemic complications, and the advisability of retaining the involved tooth. All pericoronal flaps should be viewed with suspicion. *Persistent symptom-free pericoronal flaps should be removed as a preventive measure against subsequent acute involvement.*

The following is the procedure for the treatment of acute pericoronitis:

VISIT ONE. Procedures for the first visit include the following:

1. The extent and severity of the involvement of adjacent structures and toxic systemic complications are determined (Fig. 41–6).

2. The area is gently flushed with warm water to remove superficial debris and surface exudate, and a topical anesthetic is applied.

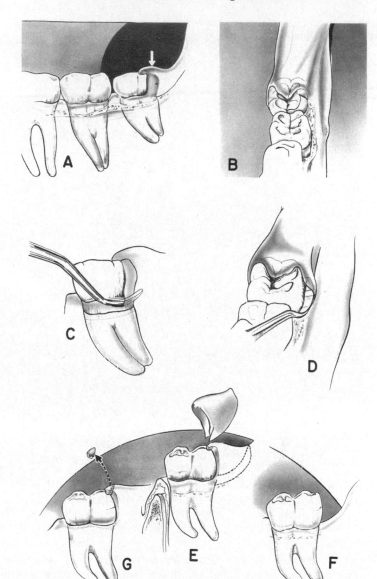

Figure 41–6 Treatment of Acute Pericoronitis. *A,* Inflamed pericoronal flap (*arrow*) in relation to the mandibular third molar. *B,* Anterior view of third molar and flap. *C,* Lateral view with scaler in position to gently remove debris under flap. *D,* Anterior view of scaler in position. *E,* Removal of section of the gingiva distal to the third molar, after the acute symptoms subside. The line of incision is indicated by the broken line. *F,* Appearance of the healed area. *G,* Incorrect removal of the tip of the flap, permitting deep pocket to remain distal to the molar.

3. The area is swabbed with antiseptic, and the flap is gently elevated from the tooth with a scaler. The underlying debris is removed, and the area is flushed with warm water (Fig. 41–6). Extensive curettage or surgical procedures are contraindicated at the initial visit. Instructions to the patient include hourly rinses with a solution of a teaspoonful of salt in a glass of warm water, rest, copious fluid intake, and systemic antibiotics if fever or other general symptoms are present. The patient is told to return in 24 hours.

4. If the gingival flap is swollen and fluctuant, an anteroposterior incision to establish drainage is made with a No. 15 Bard-Parker blade; followed by insertion of a ¼-inch gauze wick.

VISIT TWO. After 24 hours, the patient's condition is usually markedly improved. If a drain had been inserted, it is removed. The flap is gently separated from the tooth and the area flushed with warm water. The patient is told to continue with the instructions of the previous day and to return in 24 hours.

VISIT THREE. At this visit, a determination is made as to whether the tooth is to be retained or extracted. This decision is governed by the likelihood of further eruption into a good functional position. Bone loss on the distal surface of the second molars is a hazard following the extraction of partially or completely impacted third molars,[2] and the problem is significantly greater if the third molars are extracted after the roots are formed or in patients beyond their early twenties. *To reduce the risk of bone loss around second*

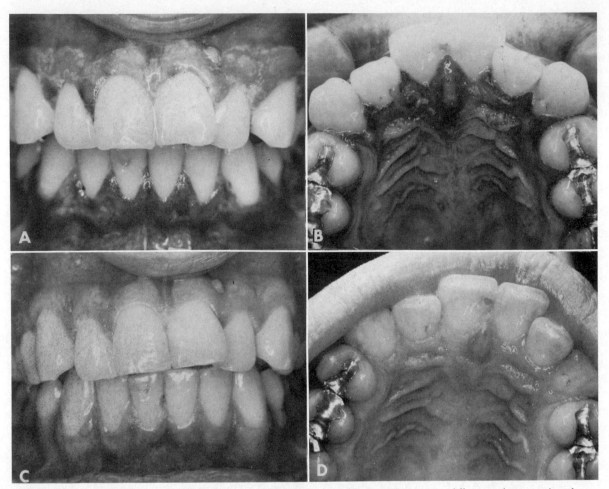

Figure 41–7 Treatment of Acute Herpetic Gingivostomatitis. *A,* Before treatment. Note diffuse erythema and surface vesicles. *B,* Before treatment, lingual view showing gingival edema and ruptured vesicle on palate. *C,* One month after treatment, showing restoration of normal gingival contour and stippling. *D,* One month after treatment, lingual view.

molars, partially or completely impacted third molars should be extracted as early as possible in their development.

If it is decided to retain the tooth, the necessary surgical procedures are performed at this visit, provided there are no acute symptoms. Periodontal knives or electrosurgery is used for this purpose. Under anesthesia, an incision is begun just anterior to the border of the ramus and brought downward and forward to the distal surface of the crown, as close as possible to the level of the cemento-enamel junction. This will detach a wedge-shaped section of tissue that includes the gingival flap (Fig. 41–6).

It is necessary to remove the tissue distal to the tooth as well as the flap on the occlusal surface. Incising only the occlusal portion of the flap leaves a deep distal pocket which invites recurrence of acute pericoronal involvement.

After the tissue is removed, a periodontal pack is applied. The pack may be retained by bringing it forward along the facial and lingual surfaces into the interproximal space between the second and third molars. The pack is removed after 1 week.

Pericoronitis and Acute Necrotizing Ulcerative Gingivitis

Pericoronal flaps which are chronically inflamed may become the sites of acute necrotizing ulcerative gingivitis. The disease is treated in the same manner as elsewhere in the mouth and, after the acute symptoms have subsided, the flap is removed. Pericoronal flaps are often referred to as "primary incubation zones" in acute necrotizing ulcerative gingivitis; their elimination is one of many measures required to minimize the likelihood of recurrent disease.

TREATMENT OF ACUTE HERPETIC GINGIVOSTOMATITIS

Various medications have been used in the treatment of this condition, including local applications of 8 per cent zinc chloride, camphorated phenol, spirits of camphor, Talbot's iodine, phenol, sulfonamide solutions, moccasin snake venom,[10] systemically administered yeast,[13] riboflavin, vitamin B complex,[4] thiamine, and radiation therapy. Aureomycin has been used successfully as a mouthwash,[1] applied topically in a 3 per cent ointment,[9] or administered systemically in the form of 250-mg capsules for a total dosage of 3 grams.[16] Vaccination with smallpox vaccine or a vaccine prepared from the contents of the herpetic vesicles has been described both as a therapeutic measure and as a measure for the prevention of recurrence,[11, 21] but the results are doubtful.

Treatment consists of palliative measures to make the patient comfortable until the disease runs its course (7 to 10 days).

Plaque, food debris, and superficial calculus are removed to reduce gingival inflammation, which complicates the acute herpetic involvement. Extensive periodontal therapy should be postponed until the acute symptoms subside so as to avoid the possibility of exacerbation (Fig. 41–7). The painful, swollen herpetic infection of a dentist's finger after preparing a crown in a patient with herpetic lesions on the lower lip has been reported.[23]

Relief of pain to enable the patient to eat comfortably is obtained with dyclonine hydrochloride (Dyclone), a topical anesthetic mouthwash[28] which is available in a 0.5 per cent solution which may be diluted 1:1 with water. It is held in the mouth for 1 or 2 minutes and swished around to produce an anesthetic effect that lasts for 40 minutes. It is helpful when used before meals, but may be used more often without toxic effects.

SUPPORTIVE TREATMENT. Supportive measures include copious fluid intake and systemic antibiotic therapy for the management of toxic systemic complications. For the relief of pain, systemically administered aspirin is usually sufficient. A dosage of 10 grains every 3 hours may be prescribed for adults, with smaller doses used for children.

REFERENCES

1. Arnold, H. L., Domzalski, C. A., and Austin, E. R.: Aureomycin mouthwash for herpetic stomatitis. Proc. Staff Meet. Honolulu, *15*:85, 1949.
2. Ash, M. M., Jr., Costich, E. R., and Hayward, J. R.: A study of periodontal hazards of third molars. J. Periodontol., *33*:209, 1962.
3. Burket, L. W.: Oral Medicine. 3rd ed. Philadelphia, J. B. Lippincott Company, 1946, p. 53.
4. Burket, L. W., and Hickman, G. C.: Oral herpes (simplex) manifestations: treatment with vitamin B complex. J. Am. Dent. Assoc., *29*:411, 1942.
5. Clausen, F. P.: Local treatment of acute necrotizing ulcerative gingivitis with ascoxal: clinical experiences from treatment of military personnel. Tandlaegebladet, *70*:1009, 1966.
6. Collins, J., and Hood, H. M.: Topical antibiotic treatment of acute necrotizing ulcerative gingivitis. J. Oral Med., *22*:59, 1967.
7. Duckworth, R., Waterhouse, J. P., Britton, D. E. R., Nuki, K., Sheiham, A., Winter, R., and Blake, G. C.: Acute ulcerative gingivitis: a double-blind controlled clinical trial of metronidazole. Br. Dent. J., *120*:599, 1966.
8. Emslie, R.: Treatment of acute ulcerative gingivitis. A clinical trial using chewing gum containing metronidazole or penicillin. Br. Dent. J., *122*:307, 1967.
9. Everett, F. G.: Aureomycin in the therapy of herpes simplex labialis and recurrent oral aphthae. J. Am. Dent. Assoc., *40*:555, 1950.
10. Fisher, A. A.: Treatment of herpes simplex with moccasin snake venom. Arch. Derm. Syph., *43*:444, 1941.
11. Frank, S. B.: Formalized herpes virus therapy and the neutralizing substance in herpes simplex. J. Invest. Dermatol., *1*:267, 1940.
12. Frankl, Z.: Dentitio difficilis and parodontosis. Paradentologie, *1*:107, 1947.
13. Gerstenberger, H J.: The etiology and treatment of herpetic (aphthous and aphthoulcerative) stomatitis and herpes labialis. Am. J. Dis. Child., *26*:309, 1923.
14. Glickman, I.: The use of penicillin lozenges in the treatment of Vincent's infection and other acute gingival inflammations. J. Am. Dent. Assoc., *34*:406, 1947.
15. Glickman, I., and Johannessen, L. B.: The effect of a six per cent solution of chromic acid on the gingiva of the albino rat– a correlated gross, biomicroscopic, and histologic study. J. Am. Dent. Assoc., *41*:674, 1950.
16. Jacobs, H. G., and Jacobs, M. H.: Aureomycin: its use in infections of the oral cavity. Oral Surg., *2*:1015, 1949.
17. King, J. D.: Nutritional and other factors in "trench mouth" with special reference to the nicotinic acid component of the vitamin B$_2$ complex. Br. Dent. J., *74*:113, 1943.
18. Linghorne, W. J., McIntosh, W. G., Tice, J. W., Tisdall, F. F., McCreary, J. F., Drake, T. G. H., Greaves, A. V., and Johnstone, W. M.: The relation of ascorbic acid intake to gingivitis. J. Can. Dent. Assoc., *12*:49, 1946.
19. Mitchell, D. F., and Baker, B. R.: Topical antibiotic control of necrotizing gingivitis. J. Periodontol., *39*:81, 1968.
20. Roth, H.: Vitamins as an adjunct in the treatment of periodontal disease. J. Am. Dent. Assoc., *32*:60, 1945.
21. Savitt, L. E., and Ayres, S., Jr.: Persistent multiple herpes-like eruption. Response to repeated intradermal injections of smallpox vaccine. Arch. Derm. Syph., *59*:653, 1949.
22. Shinn, D. L. S., Squires, S., and McFadzean, A.: The treatment of Vincent's disease with metronidazole. Dent. Practit., *15*:275, 1965.
23. Snyder, M. L., Church, D. H., and Rickles, N. H.: Primary herpes infection of right second finger. Oral Surg., *27*:598, 1969.
24. Stephen, K. W., McLatchie, M. F., Mason, D. K., Noble, H. W., and Stevenson, D. M.: Treatment of acute ulcerative gingivitis (Vincent's type). Br. Dent. J., *121*:313, 1966.
25. Wade, A. B., and Mirza, K. B.: The relative effectiveness of sodium peroxyborate and hydrogen peroxide in treating acute ulcerative gingivitis. Dent. Practit., *14*:185, 1964.
26. Wade, A. B., Blake, G., and Mirza, K.: Effectiveness of metronidazole in treating the acute phase of ulcerative gingivitis. Dent. Practit., *16*:440, 1966.
27. Wade, A. B., Blake, G. C., Manson, J. D., Berdon, J. K., Mathieson, F., and Bate, D. M.: Treatment of the acute phase of ulcerative gingivitis (Vincent's type). Br. Dent. J., *115*:372, 1963.
28. Weisberger, D.: Treatment of some diseases of the soft tissues of the mouth. Dent. Clin. North Am., *4*:215, 1960.

chapter forty-two

Treatment of the Periodontal Abscess

The Acute Periodontal Abscess
Drainage Through the Pocket
Drainage Through an External Incision

The Chronic Periodontal Abscess
Treatment by Gingivectomy
Treatment by Flap Operation

Periodontal abscesses may be acute or chronic. Acute abscesses are painful, edematous, red, shiny ovoid elevations of the gingival margin and/or attached gingiva. After their purulent content is partially exuded, they become chronic. Chronic abscesses may produce a dull pain and may at times become acute (see Chapter 18).

THE ACUTE PERIODONTAL ABSCESS

The purpose of treatment of an acute abscess is **to alleviate the pain, to control the spread of infection, and to establish drainage.**[1] After the case is diagnosed, the patient's general systemic response should be evaluated and his or her temperature taken. Drainage can be established through the pocket or by means of an incision from the outer surface. The former is preferable.

Drainage Through the Pocket

After application of a topical anesthetic, a flat instrument or a probe is carefully introduced into the pocket in an attempt to distend the pocket wall. A small curette or a Morse scaler can then be gently used to penetrate the tissue and establish drainage. When drainage cannot be easily established via the pocket or when the abscess can be seen pointing through the gingiva, an external incision will be indicated.

Drainage Through an External Incision

The abscess is isolated with gauze sponges and dried and swabbed with an antiseptic solution, followed by a topical anesthetic. Wait 2 or 3 minutes for the anesthetic to become effective; then the abscess is palpated gently to locate the most fluctuant area.

With the Bard-Parker No. 12 blade, a vertical incision is made through the most fluctuant part of the lesion, extending from the

mucogingival fold to the gingival margin (Fig. 42–1). If the swelling is on the lingual surface, the incision is started just apical to the swelling and extended through the gingival margin. The blade should penetrate to firm tissue to be sure of reaching deep purulent areas. After the initial extravasation of blood and pus, irrigate the area with warm water and gently spread the incision to facilitate draining.

If the tooth is extruded, it should be ground slightly so as to avoid contact with its antagonists. Stabilize the tooth with the index finger to reduce vibration and discomfort. It is often preferable to grind the teeth in the opposing jaw to avoid discomfort.

After the drainage stops, the area is dried and painted with an antiseptic. Patients without systemic complications are instructed to rinse hourly with a solution of a teaspoonful of salt in a glass of warm water and to return the next day. Penicillin or other antibiotics are prescribed for patients with elevated temperatures, in addition to the rinses (see Chapter 45). The patient is also instructed to avoid exertion and is put on a copious fluid diet. If necessary, bed rest is recommended. Analgesics are prescribed for pain.

The next day, the swelling is generally markedly reduced or absent, and the symptoms have subsided. If acute symptoms persist, the patient is instructed to continue the regimen prescribed the previous day and to return in 24 hours. The symptoms invariably disappear by then, and the lesion is ready for the usual treatment for a chronic periodontal abscess.

THE CHRONIC PERIODONTAL ABSCESS

Treatment by Gingivectomy*

After the acute symptoms have subsided, the treatment is the same as that employed if

---

*General principles of periodontal surgery are presented in Chapter 50, and the gingivectomy technique is described in detail in Chapter 52.

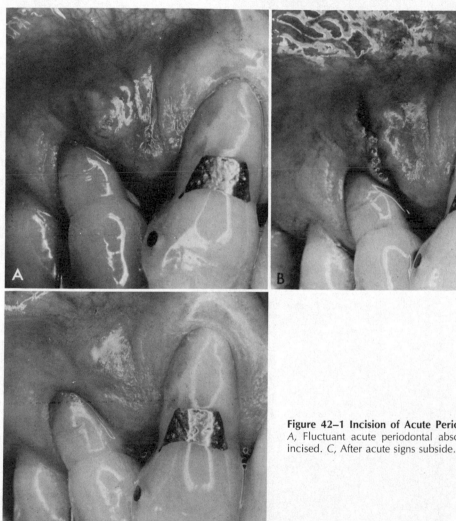

Figure 42–1 Incision of Acute Periodontal Abscess.
A, Fluctuant acute periodontal abscess. *B,* Abscess incised. *C,* After acute signs subside.

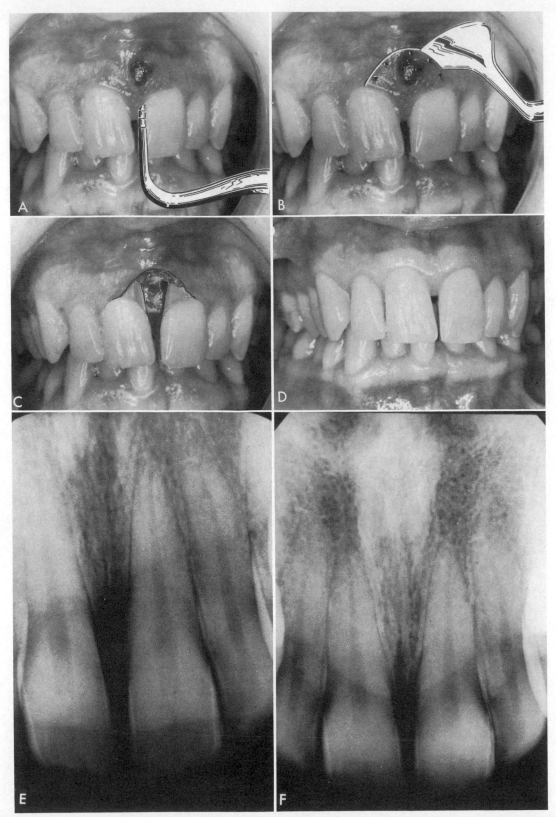

Figure 42–2 Chronic Periodontal Abscess Treated by Gingivectomy. *A,* Chronic periodontal abscess in the wall of a deep pocket is explored with periodontal probe (composite illustration). *B,* Semilunar incision approximately 2 mm apical to bleeding points made by pocket marker (composite illustration). *C,* Removal of pocket wall reveals abscess tract along incisor root (composite illustration). *D,* Appearance of healed gingiva after 1 year. *E,* Radiograph before treatment. *F,* Radiograph 1 year after treatment showing bone repair.

the patient presented initially with a chronic abscess.

The area is isolated, dried, and painted with an antiseptic solution and injected to ensure adequate anesthesia. The abscess is probed to determine the extent of involvement, and the pocket is marked with a pocket marker (Fig. 42–2*A*).

The supragingival calculus is removed, and a semilunar incision is made approximately 2 mm peripheral to the pinpoint markings with periodontal knives (Fig. 42–2*B*). The incised gingiva is removed with a surgical hoe, exposing the following: granulation tissue, calculus, and a tract of bone destruction along the root (Fig. 42–2*C*).

The granulation tissue and calculus are removed, and the roots are smoothed. The bone is not disturbed.

The area is cleansed with warm water and covered with a gauze pad until the bleeding stops, after which a periodontal pack is applied. Both the lingual and facial surfaces should be packed to provide better retention of the pack. The patient is dismissed with a list of instructions usually provided after surgery and instructed to return in 1 week, when the pack is removed. It is not necessary to replace the pack for another week unless the area is particularly sensitive. The patient is instructed in plaque control (see Chapter 44). Gingival health is restored within 6 to 8 weeks (Fig. 42–2*D*); bone repair may be observed radiographically after about 9 months (Fig. 42–2*E* and *F*).

Treatment by Flap Operation*

The area is isolated with gauze, dried, painted with antiseptic facially and lingually, and injected to ensure adequate anesthesia.

The first requirement is to determine the relative facial or lingual location of the purulent focus of the abscess. Lingual abscesses may produce swelling on the facial surface and vice versa. To locate the abscess area, probe around the gingival margin, following tortuous pockets to their termination. If a sinus is present, the abscess may be probed through it.

Because it offers better accessibility and visibility, the facial approach is preferred and is used unless the abscess is close to the lingual surface.

---

*The "flap technique" is presented in detail in Chapter 53.

After the approach is decided upon, the superficial calculus is removed and *two vertical incisions* are made from the gingival margin to the mucobuccal fold, outlining the field of operation. If the lingual approach is used, the incisions are made from the gingival margin to the level of the root apices. The operative field should be large enough to allow unhampered visibility and accessibility. A flap that is too narrow or too short jeopardizes the outcome of the treatment.

After the vertical incisions are made, a *mesiodistal incision is made across the interdental papilla* with a knife to facilitate detachment of the flap (Fig. 42–3*A*). A *full thickness flap* is raised with a periosteal elevator and held in position with a retractor. A flap on either the facial or lingual surface usually suffices. In the case of an abscess which was initially acute, the edges of the incision made the previous day are usually united so that the flap may be raised in one piece.

Elevation of the flap reveals some or all of the following conditions (Fig. 42–3*B*):

1. Granulation tissue at the gingival margin.
2. Calculus on the root surface.
3. Bony surfaces with multiple pinpoint bleeding areas.
4. A sinus opening on the external bone, which can be probed inwardly to the tooth.
5. Purulent spongy tissue in the orifice of the sinus.

After the field is carefully surveyed, the granulation tissue is removed with curettes to provide a clear view of the root. All deposits are scaled from the teeth, and the root surfaces are planed with hoe scalers and smoothed with curettes. If a sinus is present, it is explored and curetted (Fig. 42–3*D*).

The location of the sinus determines the manner in which the bone is managed. *The bone is not disturbed except in cases in which only a thin rim of bone separates the sinus from the crest of the alveolar bone* (Fig. 42–4). Thin marginal bridges of bone are removed, because they are usually pathologically involved and act as foreign bodies which impair healing.

The facial and lingual surfaces are covered with a piece of gauze shaped into a U, which is held in position until the bleeding stops. The gauze is then removed, and the flap is sutured and covered with a periodontal pack.

The patient is instructed not to rinse until the next day, when a pleasant-tasting mouthwash diluted 1:3 in warm water is used every 2 hours. The area should be cleansed gently with a soft toothbrush and water irrigation under medium pressure. The patient is to

A

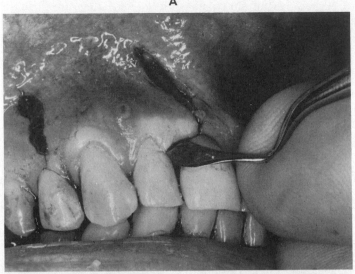

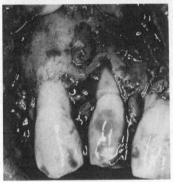

B

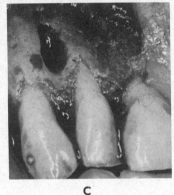

C

Figure 42–3 Simple Full Thickness Flap Operation for Periodontal Abscess. *A,* Operative field is outlined with two vertical incisions. Horizontal incision is being made across the interdental papilla with a periodontal knife preparatory to elevating a full thickness flap. Note how the knife is stabilized by the finger rest. *B,* Full thickness flap is elevated, showing granulation tissue at the gingival margin and sinus opening filled with spongy purulent tissue. *C,* Sinus curetted. Note the narrow marginal bridge of bone, which is usually infected and is removed to facilitate healing.

Figure 42–4 Various Levels at Which the Sinus from a Periodontal Abscess May Be Located. In the case of C, the narrow marginal bridge of bone is removed during treatment.

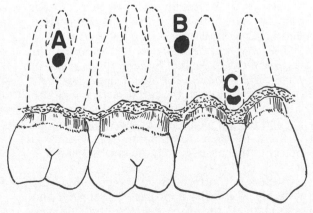

return in 1 week, at which time the pack and sutures are removed and the patient is instructed in plaque control. Repacking is usually not necessary.

The normal appearance of the gingiva is attained within 6 to 8 weeks; repair of the bone requires approximately 9 months. The prospects for bone repair and fill are better for osseous defects produced by rapidly destructive acute periodontal disease than for slowly progressing chronic lesions.[2]

REFERENCES

1. Manson, J. D.: Periodontics. 3rd ed. Philadelphia, Lea & Febiger, 1975.
2. Nabers, J. M., Meador, H. L., and Nabers, C. L.: Chronology, an important factor in the repair of osseous defects. Periodontics, 2:304, 1964.

Part IV

Phase I Therapy

The initial phase of periodontal therapy is directed at removing all local irritants that may cause gingival inflammation and instructing and motivating the patient in plaque control. A more proper name for this phase is the "etiotropic phase," since the treatment eliminates the etiologic factor in periodontal disease, but the terms "Phase I" or "initial phase" are in common use.

It is a common error to perform this phase of therapy, followed by the surgical phase when needed, and only then to place the patient in the maintenance phase. *The initial phase of therapy should be followed immediately by the maintenance phase; recall appointments should be scheduled and patient maintenance checked at regular intervals.* Periodontal surgical and restorative procedures are performed while the patient is on a maintenance schedule for nonoperated areas of the mouth (see Chapter 59).

_____ chapter forty-three _____

Preparation of the Tooth Surface

Rationale
Step 1: Limited Plaque Control Instruction
Step 2: Supragingival Removal of Calculus
Step 3: Recontouring of Defective Restorations
Step 4: Obturation of Carious Lesions

Step 5: Comprehensive Plaque Control Instruction
Step 6: Subgingival Root Treatment
Step 7: Tissue Re-evaluation

RATIONALE

Initial therapy or *Phase I therapy* is the first therapeutic step in the chronologic sequence of procedures that constitute periodontal treatment. The objective of the initial therapy is the reduction or elimination of gingival inflammation (Plate VII); this is achieved by the complete removal of calculus, correction of defective restorations, obturation of carious lesions, and institution of a comprehensive plaque control regimen.[4, 10, 24, 25, 42]

There has been considerable controversy regarding the necessity of an "initial preparation of the mouth" in cases requiring surgical therapy.[16] Preparatory therapy, especially prior to gingivectomy, does not seem to improve postoperative healing or gingival architecture[3, 15, 40] and subjects the patient twice, for each treated area, to the risk of

systemic complications caused by postoperative bacteremia.[19, 23] Current data from clinical research, however, indicate that, in the last analysis, the long-term success of periodontal treatment is dependent predominantly on maintaining the results achieved with Phase I therapy and much less on a specific surgical procedure.[26, 31, 36] In addition, Phase I therapy provides an opportunity for the periodontist to evaluate tissue response and a patient's attitude toward periodontal care, both of which are crucial to the prognosis of periodontal conditions.

The purpose of Phase I therapy is (1) to reduce or eliminate gingival inflammation, (2) to eliminate periodontal pockets produced by the edematous enlargement of inflamed gingiva, or (3) to achieve surgical manageability of the gingiva, i.e., firm consistency and minimal bleeding.

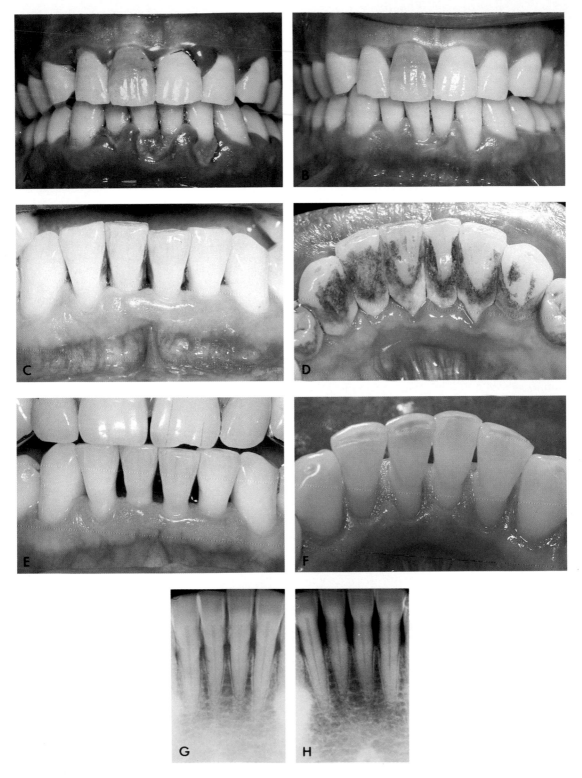

Plate VII Results of Phase I Therapy

   A, Heavy calculus deposits and severe gingival inflammation.

   B, Three weeks after elimination of irritants, gingival healing has resulted.

C–H, One case before and 1½ years after Phase I therapy. (Courtesy of Dr. Steven Levine.)

     C, and *D,* Clinical preoperative view. Note edematous gingival enlargement and abundant calculus.

      E and *F,* Clinical postoperative views after Phase I therapy and maintenance visits. Note excellent gingival contour and color.

     G and *H,* Radiographs taken before and 1½ years after treatment. Note presence of calculus in the preoperative radiograph and the clean root surface seen after treatment. Bone height remained unchanged.

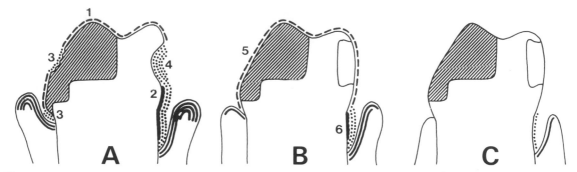

Figure 43–1 Steps in Phase I Therapy. *A,* Before starting therapy. Interrupted line (1) shows areas that can be cleaned by the patient. Dotted lines are areas that have to be prepared by the dentist before the patient can clean them; 2, calculus; 3, rough surfaces and overhanging margins of restorations; 4, caries. Parallel lines in the gingiva denote presence and degree of inflammation. *B,* After removal of supragingival calculus, correction of restoration, and removal and obturation of caries, the area that the patient can clean (interrupted line, 5) has been considerably extended. Inflammation (parallel lines in gingiva) is reduced. 6, subgingival calculus still not removed. *C,* After removal of subgingival calculus. Pocket persists and plaque accumulated in it cannot be removed by patient. Surgical pocket elimination may be indicated.

Based on the concept that microbial dental deposits (plaque) produce the primary pathogens of gingival inflammation, the specific aim of Phase I therapy is to facilitate the daily removal of such accretions from the teeth by eliminating rough and irregular contours from the tooth surfaces and then establishing a suitable plaque control regimen (see Chapter 44). As the institution of effective plaque control is the ultimate objective of every therapeutic periodontal procedure, Phase I therapy is primarily concerned with the fact that the presence of smooth and regular tooth surfaces is a major prerequisite for achieving this goal. Adequate plaque removal by the patient can be expected only if the tooth surfaces are free of rough deposits or irregular contours and readily accessible for oral hygiene aids.

After careful analysis of a case, the number of appointments needed to complete this phase of treatment is estimated. Patients with only slight amounts of calculus and relatively healthy tissues can be treated completely in one appointment. Most other patients will require several appointments. The dentist should estimate the number of appointments on the basis of number of teeth in the mouth, amount and location of calculus, depth of pockets, presence of furcation involvements, and so forth.

Step 1: LIMITED PLAQUE CONTROL INSTRUCTION (See Chapter 44.)

Introducing an oral hygiene program to the patient is of high priority in every periodontal treatment plan. Plaque control instructions should begin at the first therapeutic appoint-

ment. The patient is taught how to clean all smooth and regular surfaces of the teeth. When therapy is initiated, a number of tooth surfaces frequently are altered by calculus, defective restorations, carious lesions, or necrotic cementum (Fig. 43–1A), preventing sufficient access for oral hygiene aids. The patient should not be expected to remove plaque from such areas.

The toothbrush is often the only hygiene aid indicated at this stage of therapy. Dental floss should be used on *smooth* proximal tooth surfaces only, since flossing around sharp edges and coarse surfaces of calculus or overhanging restorations causes the floss to shred and break, leads to ineffective plaque removal as well as the persistence of inflammatory bleeding (see Fig. 43–4D), and is often a frustrating experience for the patient.

Step 2: SUPRAGINGIVAL REMOVAL OF CALCULUS

Dental calculus is a mineralized aggregate of nonvital microorganisms embedded in an intermicrobial matrix.[24] Although not injurious to the periodontium by itself,[2, 48] it provides a highly retentive surface for the oral microflora and thus promotes the accumulation of injurious dental plaque. Since adequate removal of plaque from calculus surfaces is not feasible with current oral hygiene techniques, calculus must be eliminated entirely in order to facilitate effective plaque control.

In the presence of inflamed, friable gingiva adjacent to deep periodontal pockets, calculus is first dislodged from all *supra*gingival tooth surfaces. This leads to a substantial improvement of the marginal gingiva. Removal of *sub*gingival calculus from these areas, prior to the resolution of pronounced marginal gingivitis, is not recommended, since it may produce undue laceration of the diseased gingiva and provoke an acute inflammatory tissue reaction.

Calculus is dislodged by scaling the tooth surfaces with instruments especially designed for that purpose (see Chapter 37). For supragingival calculus removal, ultrasonic scalers, hand scalers, and curettes are the instruments of choice.[38]

Scaling is performed with a pull motion, except on the proximal surfaces of closely spaced anterior teeth, where thin chisel scalers are used with a push motion. In the pull motion, the instrument engages the apical border of the calculus and dislodges it with a firm movement through the entire instrumentation zone in the direction of the crown (Fig. 43–2).

The scaling motion is initiated in the forearm and transmitted from the wrist to the hand with a slight flexing of the fingers. Rotation of the wrist is synchronized with movement of the forearm. The scaling motion is not initiated in the wrist or fingers, nor is it carried out independently without the use of the forearm.

In the push scaling motion, the fingers activate the instrument. This method is used with the chisel scaler on the proximal surfaces of crowded anterior teeth. The instrument engages the lateral border of the calculus and the fingers provide a thrust motion, which dislodges the calculus.

The removal of calculus is not a whittling operation. Calculus is dislodged in its entirety, starting below its border; it is not "pared down" until the tooth surface is reached. After calculus is removed from one section of the tooth, the instrument is moved laterally to engage the adjacent deposits.

Scaling is confined to a small area of the tooth on both sides of the cemento-enamel junction where the calculus and other deposits are located. Sweeping the instrument over the crown where scaling is not needed lengthens operating time, dulls the instrument, and is contrary to the careful attention to detail required for effective instrumentation.

Complete interproximal access for scaling instruments is often difficult, especially between incisor teeth with narrow embrasures. In those areas, sharp-pointed sickle scalers rather than round-ended curettes should be used to reach close to the contact zones. Crowding of anterior teeth frequently results in very long, tight contact zones and extremely narrow embrasures. This prevents adequate access even for sharp-pointed sickle scalers. Abrasive finishing strips inserted between the teeth can be used for effective removal of calculus and stain from such areas (Fig. 43–3).

Scaling invariably leaves the treated tooth, especially the cementum and dentin, with a rough and scratched surface that favors the quick re-establishment of plaque and calculus. Following calculus removal, the tooth surface must therefore be planed with suitable scalers or curettes[9, 12, 13, 17, 21, 29, 35, 45, 49] and polished with abrasive paste on a rotary rubber cup or brush. Smooth, polished tooth surfaces are highly conducive to effective plaque control and resist calculus formation considerably better than rough surfaces.[46]

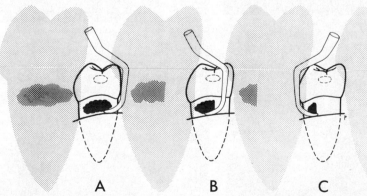

Figure 43–2 Instrumentation for Calculus Removal. *A,* Calculus is removed by engaging the apical border of movement with the cutting edge of the scaler; a vertical movement of the instrument will remove the fragment of calculus engaged by the instrument, as seen in the shaded drawing. *B,* The instrument is moved laterally and again engages the apical border of calculus, overlapping to some extent the previous stroke; the shaded drawing shows further removal. *C,* The final portion of the calculus is engaged and removed. Note how in an interdental space the operation is done entering facially and lingually.

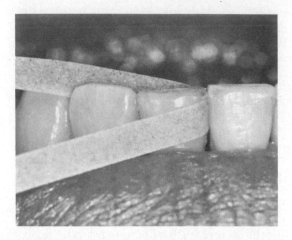

Figure 43–3 Finishing Strips are effective for removing stains and calculus from proximal tooth surfaces adjacent to tight contact areas and narrow embrasures.

Step 3: RECONTOURING OF DEFECTIVE RESTORATIONS

With few exceptions,[34] rough, overcontoured, overhanging, or smooth but subgingivally located restorations and orthodontic appliances are associated with pronounced accumulation of plaque[6, 8, 47, 48] and periodontal inflammation[1, 5, 18, 22, 30, 32, 33, 50] (Fig. 43–4), as well as loss of alveolar bone and periodontal attachment.[7, 14, 39, 44] Like calculus, such restorations or appliances interfere with efficient plaque control and must therefore be corrected or removed to allow the reduction or elimination of gingival inflammation. Correction of existing restorations is as important as the

A   B

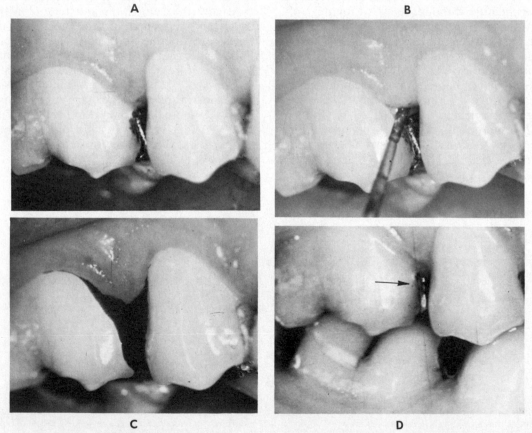

C   D

Figure 43–4 Effect on the Gingiva of an Overhanging Amalgam Restoration Mesial on the First Molar. *A,* Clinical aspect. *B,* Interproximal probing provokes profuse bleeding from the col area (C), a sign of gingival inflammation. *D,* Clinical aspect of recontoured restoration (*arrow*).

removal of calculus and should therefore be completed at the same time. *Adequate plaque control by the patient on teeth with restorations is feasible only if the restorations are well contoured and their surfaces are smooth* (see Fig. 43–6 *C* and *D*).

Defective restorations, especially overhanging margins, are detected clinically by running a fine explorer along their periphery, moving the explorer tip continuously back and forth across the margins of the restoration (Fig. 43–5). In the presence of an overhanging margin, a clicking sound is produced when the explorer is run from the restoration to the tooth, and a definitive catch is felt when moving the explorer from the tooth to the restoration. Bitewing radiography may be a helpful diagnostic adjunct in determining the approximate mesiodistal and occluso-apical dimension of a proximal overhang.

Special attention is given to restorations on root surfaces of molars and premolars. Frequently, the contours of such restorations do not reproduce the concave interradicular depressions usually found on these teeth. Instead, the restorations exhibit overhanging margins or overcontoured surfaces (Fig. 43–6A) that make it difficult for the patient to reach the subjacent tooth surface with an oral hygiene instrument (Fig. 43–6B).

Overhanging margins are eliminated either by replacing the entire restoration or by correcting the contour of the existing restoration. The latter, although often only a temporary measure, is preferred whenever feasible because it involves considerably less time and effort than does replacing an entire restoration. Thus, it does not unnecessarily prolong this phase of periodontal therapy.

Overhanging portions of *alloy* and *resin* restorations are removed with scalers or periodontal files (Fig. 43–7A), finishing burs (Fig. 43–7B), or diamond-coated files mounted on a special handpiece attachment that generates

reciprocating strokes of high frequency (see Fig. 37–27). These motor-driven files have recently been improved by the addition of a water spray to the handpiece and by offering a wider selection of diamond tips capable of recontouring composite, gold, and porcelain surfaces[27] (Fig. 43–7C).

Scalers and periodontal files are efficient for the gross removal of overhangs from accessible areas such as lingual and facial tooth surfaces or large interproximal embrasures. They leave a relatively rough surface on the restoration that needs to be smoothed with abrasive discs or finishing strips.

Finishing burs and handpiece-mounted files are more versatile owing to their small size, which makes narrow spaces accessible to them. Their high working speed allows them to remove large overhangs efficiently, leaving a relatively smooth restoration surface. When a bur is used, the instrument is pressed gently against the restoration and moved across the overhanging ledge to the tooth surface. The procedure is repeated until the overhang is eliminated. The bur should not be guided from the tooth toward the restoration, as this is likely to undermine the restoration and traumatize subjacent tooth structures. Final polishing of the recontoured restoration is accomplished with abrasive discs, finishing strips, or rubber cones (Fig. 43–7D). When a handpiece-mounted diamond file is used, it is centered with a continuous circular burnishing motion over the ledge of the restoration until all the excess material has been shaved down. For polishing, the procedure is repeated after replacing the file in the handpiece with a plastic tip of similar shape, coated with polishing paste. Since most polishing pastes tend to roughen restorative materials, especially conventional composites, they should be carefully selected.[37]

Overhanging *gold* restorations are corrected like alloy and resin restorations, but with thin,

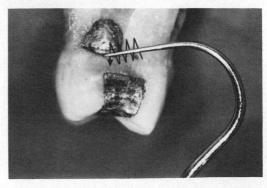

Figure 43–5 Identification of Defective Restorations. Rough surfaces and overhanging margins can be detected with the tip of a fine explorer.

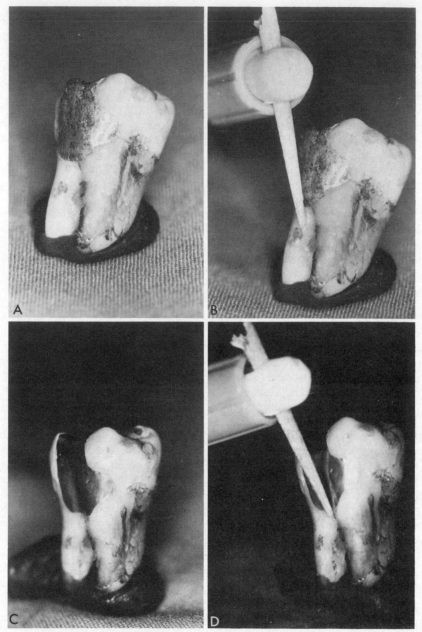

Figure 43–6 Effect of Restoration Contours on Plaque Control. *A,* Overcontoured amalgam restoration, causing *B,* poor accessibility for oral hygiene aid in furcation area. *C,* Recontoured restoration, providing *D,* adequate access for oral hygiene aid.

tapered *diamond* burs or diamond-coated files (Fig. 43–7*C*).

Step 4: OBTURATION OF CARIOUS LESIONS

Caries in the vicinity of the gingiva interferes with gingival health, even in the absence of adjacent calculus or defective restorations, because it acts as a large and usually inaccessible reservoir of microorganisms. The obturation of carious lesions is therefore an integral part of Phase I therapy. Complete removal of such lesions and permanent closure of the cavities are desirable whenever possible. Temporary restorations are also acceptable. However, their purpose in Phase I periodontal therapy is primarily to eliminate microbial reservoirs that are injurious to the gingiva, not to restore the form and function of the affected teeth. Therefore, temporary restorations should be placed only in cases in which (1) permanent restorative care is not immediately available to the patient, or (2) the prognosis of a decayed tooth depends upon the result of periodontal therapy.

In preparing a tooth to receive a temporary restoration, the main emphasis is on achieving a tight seal between tooth and restoration along the cavosurface line of the lesion. All carious material is eliminated from the tooth surface in immediate proximity to the cavity. A shallow carious lesion is removed entirely. In extensive lesions, the deepest portions of carious dentin are sometimes not removed completely in order to avoid potential complications, such as pulp exposure or fracture of undermined enamel, that would necessitate endodontic or restorative emergency care. The cavity is lined with a calcium hydroxide base and sealed with temporary restoration material. Fracture of a temporary restoration is best

prevented by undercontouring rather than overcontouring its surface, especially if reproducing the original tooth contour would leave large portions of the restoration unsupported by the tooth while under the forces of mastication. Final cavity preparation and replacement of the temporary filling with a permanent restoration should be performed as soon as periodontal therapy of the affected tooth is completed.

Step 5: COMPREHENSIVE PLAQUE CONTROL INSTRUCTION (See Chapter 44.)

Following removal of supragingival calculus, recontouring of defective restorations, and sealing of carious lesions, a dentition is restored to the point where a comprehensive plaque control regimen can be instituted. The patient is now expected to remove plaque from

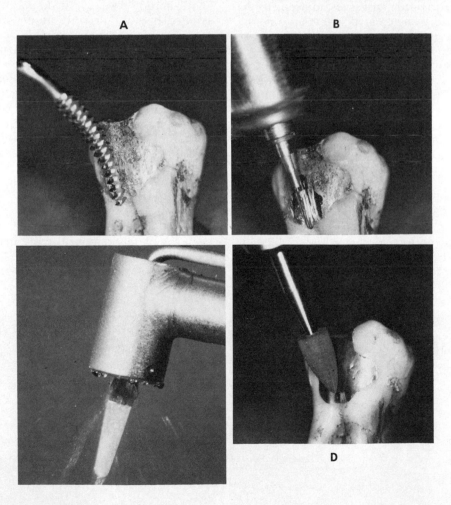

Figure 43–7 Instruments for Recontouring Existing Restorations. *A,* Periodontal file. *B,* Finishing bur. *C,* Diamond file mounted on a special handpiece. *D,* Rubber cone for final polishing.

the entire clinical crowns of all teeth except for root surfaces adjacent to deep periodontal pockets (see Fig. 43–1*B*).

Step 6: SUBGINGIVAL ROOT TREATMENT

When the patient is able to control supragingival plaque and marginal gingivitis, subgingival root treatment consisting of calculus removal, elimination of necrotic cementum, and root planing is initiated. This constitutes the final step in achieving smooth and regular contours on all oral tooth surfaces (see Fig. 43–1*C*).

Subgingival calculus is removed with curettes (see Chapters 37–39). Since these concrements are much harder and more tenacious than supragingival calculus, subgingival scaling requires considerable force and good control of the working instrument. Accidental injury to the soft periodontal tissues adjacent to the root surface being treated is not uncommon. Therefore, inflammation of the marginal gingiva should be under control before gingival root therapy is initiated; this reduces the friability of the tissue and the risk of severe tissue laceration during subgingival instrumentation.

The extent of the subgingival calculus should be appraised before an effort is made to remove it. This entails sliding a fine instrument (probe or explorer) gently along the calculus in the direction of the apex until the termination of the calculus on the root is felt. The distance between the apical edge of the calculus and the bottom of the pocket usually ranges from 0.2 to 1.0 mm. The operator should try to see the entire calculus mass by blowing warm air between the tooth and the gingival margin or by deflecting the gingiva with a probe or a small pellet of cotton. Although subgingival calculus is generally brown or dark gray and can be readily distinguished from the color of the tooth, it is often difficult to see calculus in deep pockets because of the bulk of the soft tissue wall.

The complete removal of subgingival calculus requires the development of a delicate sense of touch. With the toe of the curette sliding along the tooth surface, the instrument is gently inserted in the pocket and moved apically, beyond the deepest portion of the calculus (Fig. 43–8*A*). The curette should never be pushed hard in an apical direction, since this often forces calculus and other debris into the tissue and may elicit an acute inflammatory response. Calculus is dislodged from the tooth and the pocket by firmly pressing the tip of the curette sideways against the root surface and removing the instrument from the pocket with a long, swift stroke (Fig. 43–8*B*). Short, abrupt "sweeps" at the tooth should be avoided because they result in "nicking" of the root surface, which requires extensive planing, leads to undue loss of tooth structure, and causes postoperative sensitivity.

In the course of the scaling procedure, the smoothness of the root must be checked and rechecked with a fine probe or explorer (see Fig. 43–5). It should be borne in mind that there is often a slight vertical groove on proximal root surfaces of posterior teeth. Calculus lodged in these grooves often gives the root a regular contour, thus conveying the erroneous impression that the root surface is clean.

It is not enough to eliminate the calculus from the root surface. After subgingival calculus has been completely removed, there may be areas in which the root feels softened or rough (where the cementum has undergone necrotic

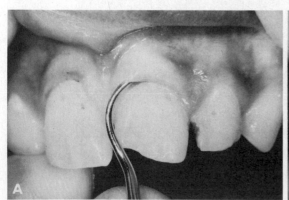 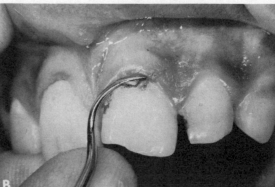

Figure 43–8 Removal of Subgingival Calculus. *A*, Currette inserted below gingival margin. *B*, Flint-like subgingival calculus removed.

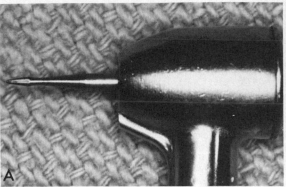
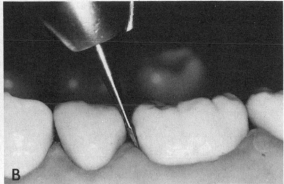

Figure 43–9 Rotary Scaler for Calculus Removal and Root Planing. *A*, Scaler tip inserted in high-speed handpiece. *B*, Scaler tip in position for calculus removal.

changes, or where heavy instrumentation has produced grooves and scratches in the surface). *The root must be planed until it is smooth. Smoothness of the root surface is essential for optimal plaque control and is one of the most reliable clinical signs for diagnosing the absence of calculus or necrotic cementum.*

Root planing requires the same instruments and procedures that are used for subgingival calculus removal. Initially, pull strokes with firm pressure against the tooth are indicated for the efficient removal of necrotic cementum or roughened dentin. As the surface becomes smoother, the pressure is gradually reduced while the length and frequency of the strokes are increased; in addition, vertical strokes are combined with oblique and horizontal strokes. This produces the required smoothness of the root. Manual scaling and root planing are strenuous procedures. The applicability of power-driven root surface instruments to these tasks has therefore gained increasing attention. Comparative studies indicate that ultrasonic and rotary scalers can be used safely and effectively in the débridement and planing of periodontally diseased root surfaces, although there is a high risk of tissue damage if they are used improperly[11, 28, 41, 43] (Fig. 43–9).

Within 3 to 4 weeks following removal of calculus, elimination of necrotic cementum, recontouring or planing of irregular tooth surfaces, and institution of plaque control, substantial reduction or elimination of gingival inflammation usually occurs. This healing process is frequently accompanied by transient root hypersensitivity, as well as by a marked recession of the gingival margin (Plate VII) that may have an unesthetic effect. The patient must be informed in advance of these therapeutic sequelae so as to prevent his or her potential distrust and loss of motivation regarding periodontal therapy.

Step 7: TISSUE RE-EVALUATION

The periodontal tissues are now re-examined to determine the need for further therapy. Pockets are reprobed to decide whether surgical treatment is indicated. However, further improvement of a periodontal condition following surgery can be expected only if Phase I therapy has been successfully completed. Therefore, surgical reduction or elimination of periodontal pockets should be attempted only if a patient is exercising effective plaque control and if the periodontal tissues are free of overt inflammation.

REFERENCES

1. Alexander, A. G.: Periodontal aspects of conservative dentistry. Br. J. Dent., *124*:111, 1968.
2. Allen, D. L., and Kerr, D. A.: Tissue response in the guinea pig to sterile and non-sterile calculus. J. Periodontol., *36*:121, 1965.
3. Ambrose, J. A., and Detamore, R. J.: Correlation of histologic and clinical findings in periodontal treatment. Effect of scaling on reduction of gingival inflammation prior to surgery. J. Periodontol., *31*:238, 1960.
4. Axelsson, P., and Lindhe, J.: The effect of a preventive programme on dental plaque, gingivitis and caries in school children. Results after one and two years. J. Clin. Periodontol., *1*:126, 1974.
5. Bergman, B., Hugoson, A., and Olsson, C-O.: Periodontal and prosthetic conditions in patients treated with removable partial dentures and artificial crowns. A longitudinal study. Acta Odontol. Scand., *29*:621, 1971.
6. Björby, A., and Löe, H.: The relative significance of different local factors in the initiation and development of periodontal inflammation. J. Periodont. Res., *2*:76, 1967.
7. Björn, A. L., Björn, H., and Grkovic, B.: Marginal fit of restorations and its relation to periodontal bone level. I. Metal fillings. Odontol. Rev., *20*:311, 1969.
8. Brebou, M., and Mühlemann, H. R.: The role of surface roughness of plastic foils in the collection of early calculus deposits. Helv. Odontol. Acta, *10*:137, 1966.
9. Burke, S. W., and Green, E.: Effectiveness of periodontal files. J. Periodontol., *41*:39, 1970.
10. Chawla, T. N., Nanda, R. S., and Kapoor, K. K.: Dental prophylaxis procedures in control of periodontal disease in Lucknow (rural) India. J. Periodontol., *46*:498, 1975.

11. Ellman, I. A.: Safe high-speed periodontal instrument. Dent. Survey, *36*:759, 1960.

12. Ewen, S. J.: A photomicrographic study of root scaling. Periodontics, *4*:273, 1966.

13. Ewen, S. J., and Gwinnett, A. J.: A scanning electron microscopic study of teeth following periodontal instrumentation. J. Periodontol., *48*:92, 1977.

14. Gilmore, N., and Sheiham, A.: Overhanging dental restorations and periodontal disease. J. Periodontol., *42*:8, 1971.

15. Glickman, I.: The effect of prescaling upon healing following periodontal surgery. A clinical and histologic study. J. Dent. Med., *16*:19, 1961.

16. Gottsegen, R.: Should the teeth be scaled prior to surgery? J. Periodontol., *32*:301, 1961.

17. Green, E., and Ramfjord, S. P.: Tooth roughness after subgingival root planing. J. Periodontol., *37*:396, 1966.

18. Gullo, C. A., and Powell, R. N.: The effect of placement of cervical margins of class II amalgam restorations on plaque accumulation and gingival health. J. Oral Rehab., *6*:317, 1979.

19. Gutverg, M., and Haberman, S.: Studies on bacteremia following oral surgery: some prophylactic approaches to bacteremia and the results of tissue examination of excised gingiva. J. Periodontol., *33*:105, 1962.

20. Karlsen, K.: Gingival reactions to dental restorations. Acta Odontol. Scand., *28*:895, 1970.

21. Kerry, G. J.: Roughness of root surfaces after use of ultrasonic instruments and hand curettes. J. Periodontol., *38*:340, 1967.

22. Koivumaa, K. K., and Wennstrom, A.: A histological investigation of the changes in gingival margins adjacent to gold crowns. Odontol. T., *68*:373, 1960.

23. Korn, N. A., and Schaffer, E. M.: A comparison of the postoperative bacteremias induced following different periodontal procedures. J. Periodontol., *33*:226, 1962.

24. Lightner, L. M., O'Leary, T. J., Drake, R. B., Crump, P., and Allen, M. F.: Preventive periodontics treatment procedures: results over 46 months. J. Periodontol., *42*:555, 1971.

25. Lindhe, J., and Koch, G.: The effect of supervised oral hygiene on the gingiva of children. Progression and inhibition of gingivitis. J. Periodont. Res., *1*:260, 1966.

26. Lindhe, J., and Nyman, S.: The effect of plaque control and surgical pocket elimination on the establishment and maintenance of periodontal health. A longitudinal study of periodontal therapy in cases of advanced disease. J. Clin. Periodontol., *2*:67, 1975.

27. Lutz, F., and Mörmann, W.: Interdentale Restorationsüberhänge—rationelle Entfernung mit neuentwickelten Maschineninstrumenten. Schweiz. Mschr. Zahnheilk., *91*:115, 1981.

28. Meyer, K., and Lie, T.: Root surface roughness in response to periodontal instrumentation studied by combined use of microroughness measurements and scanning electron microscopy. J. Clin. Periodontol., *4*:77, 1977.

29. Pameijer, C. H., Stallard, R. E., and Hiep, N.: Surface characteristics of teeth following periodontal instrumentation: a scanning electron microscope study. J. Periodontol., *43*:628, 1972.

30. Perel, M. L.: Axial crown contours. J. Prosthet. Dent., *25*:642, 1971.

31. Ramfjord, S. P., Knowles, J. W., Nissle, R. R., Burgett, F. G., and Shick, R. A.: Results following three modalities of periodontal therapy. J. Periodontol., *46*:522, 1975.

32. Renggli, H. H.: Reaktion der Gingiva auf überhängende Füllungsränder. Dtsch. Zahnärztl. Z., *27*:322, 1972.

33. Renggli, H. H.: Auswirkungen subgingivaler approximaler Füllungsränder auf den Etzündungsgrad der benachbarten Gingiva. Thesis, Dental Institute, Zürich, Switzerland, 1974.

34. Richter, W. A., and Ueno, H.: Relationship of crown margin placement to gingival inflammation. J. Prosthet. Dent., *30*:156, 1973.

35. Rosenberg, R. M., and Ash, M. M., Jr.: The effect of root roughness on plaque accumulation and gingival inflammation. J. Periodontol., *45*:146, 1974.

36. Rosling, B., Nyman, S., Lindhe, J., and Jern, B.: The healing potential of the periodontal tissues following different techniques of periodontal surgery in plaque-free dentitions. A 2-year clinical study. J. Clin. Periodontol., *3*:233, 1976.

37. Roulet, J. F., and Roulet-Mehrens, T. K.: The surface roughness of restorative materials and dental tissues after polishing with prophylaxis and polishing pastes. J. Periodontol., *53*:257, 1982.

38. Schaffer, E. M.: Periodontal instrumentation: scaling and root planing. Int. Dent. J., *17*:297, 1967.

39. Silness, J.: Periodontal conditions in patients treated with dental bridges. III. The relationship between the location of the crown margin and the periodontal condition. J. Periodont. Res., *5*:225, 1970.

40. Stahl, S. S., Witkin, G. J., Cantor, M., and Brown, R.: Gingival healing. II. Clinical and histologic repair sequences following gingivectomy. J. Periodontol., *39*:109, 1968.

41. Stewart, J. L., Briggs, R. L., Drisko, R. R., and Jamison, H. C.: Relative calculus and tooth structure loss with use of power-driven scaling instruments. J. Am. Dent. Assoc., *83*:840, 1971.

42. Suomi, J. D., Greene, J. C., Vermillion, J. R., Doyle, J., Chany, J. J., and Leatherwood, E. C.: The effect of controlled oral hygiene procedures on the progression of periodontal disease in adults: results after third and final year. J. Periodontol., *42*:152, 1971.

43. Torfason, T., Kiger, R., Selvig, K. A., and Egelberg, J.: Clinical improvement of gingival conditions following ultrasonic versus hand instrumentation of periodontal pockets. J Clin. Periodontol., *6*:165, 1979.

44. Valderhaug, J., and Birkeland, J. M.: Periodontal conditions in patients 5 years following insertion of fixed prostheses. I. Pocket depths and loss of attachment. J. Oral Rehabil., *3*:237, 1967.

45. Van Volkinburg, J. W., Green, E., and Armitage, G. C.: The nature of root surfaces after curette, cavitron and alpha sonic instrumentation. J. Periodont. Res., *11*:374, 1976.

46. Villa, P.: Degree of calculus inhibition by habitual tooth brushing. Helv. Odontol. Acta, *12*:31, 1968.

47. Waerhaug, J.: Tissue reactions around artificial crowns. J. Periodontol., *24*:172, 1953.

48. Waerhaug, J.: Effect of rough surfaces upon gingival tissue. J. Dent. Res., *35*:323, 1956.

49. Wilkinson, R. F., and Maybury, J. E.: Scanning electron microscopy of the root surface following instrumentation. J. Periodontol., *44*:559, 1973.

50. Wright, W. H.: Local factor in periodontal disease. Periodontics, *1*:163, 1963.

Plaque Control

Plaque control is the removal of microbial plaque[41, 48, 105, 152, 196] *and the prevention of its accumulation on the teeth and adjacent gingival surfaces.* Plaque control also retards the formation of calculus.[161, 201] Removal of microbial plaque leads to the resolution of gingival inflammation in its early stages.[34] Cessation of tooth cleaning leads to its recurrence.[104, 120] Thus, plaque control is an effective way of treating and preventing gingivitis and is therefore a critical part of all the procedures involved in the prevention of periodontal disease.[30, 33, 88, 112, 179]

To date, the most dependable mode of controlling microbial plaque is still by mechanical cleansing with a toothbrush and other hygiene aids. Considerable progress has also been made with chemical inhibitors of plaque incorporated in mouthwashes or dentifrices.

Plaque control is one of the keystones of the practice of dentistry. Without it oral health can be neither attained nor preserved, although there is probably a minimal plaque level that the gingiva can tolerate, beyond which plaque accumulation need not be reduced to prevent gingival and periodontal disease. *Every patient in every dental practice should be on a plaque control program.* For the patient with a healthy periodontium, plaque control means the preservation of health. For the patient with periodontal disease, it means optimal healing following treatment. For the patient with treated periodontal disease, plaque control means the prevention of recurrence of disease.

MANUAL TOOTHBRUSHES AND BRISTLES

The first bristle brush appeared about the year 1500 in China, was introduced to the Western world in 1640, and has since undergone very little change. Generally, toothbrushes vary in size and design, as well as in length, hardness, and arrangement of the bristles (Fig. 44–1).[23, 54] The American Dental Association has described the range of dimensions of acceptable brushes: these have a brushing surface from 1 to 1¼ inches (25.4 to 31.8 mm) long and 5/16 to 3/8 inch (7.9 to 9.5 mm) wide, two to four rows of bristles, and 5 to 12 tufts per row.[2] A toothbrush should be able to reach and clean efficiently most areas of the mouth. The choice is a matter of individual preference; there is no demonstrated superiority of any one type of brush. Ease of manipulation by the patient is an important factor in brush selection. The effectiveness of and potential injury from different types of brushes depend to a great degree on how the brushes are used.[32]

There are two kinds of bristle material used in toothbrushes, *natural* (hog bristle) and *artificial filaments* made predominantly of nylon. The cleaning effect of the two types seems to be equally satisfactory.[23] However, with regard to homogeneity of the material, uniformity of size, elasticity, resistance to fracture, and repulsion of water and debris, nylon filaments are clearly superior to natural bristles, which, because of their tubular form, are significantly more susceptible to fraying, breaking, contam-

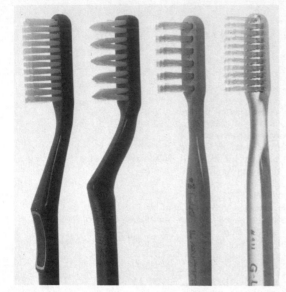

Figure 44–1 Types of manual brushes. The two brushes on the left have contra-angle shanks.

ination with diluted microbial debris, softening, and loss of elasticity. Patients accustomed to the softness of an old natural bristle brush often traumatize the gingiva when using new nylon bristles with comparable vigor. Careful instruction is therefore necessary when a patient changes from natural to nylon bristles.

The bristles are grouped in tufts that are usually arranged in three or four rows (Fig. 44–1). Four-row brushes (multitufted) contain more bristles and therefore tolerate more working pressure without flexing. Rounded bristle ends are assumed to be safer than flat-cut bristles with sharp ends. But this assumption has been questioned,[85] since cut bristle tips also round with regular use.[82] The question of the most desirable bristle hardness is not settled. Bristle hardness is proportional to the square of the diameter and inversely proportional to the square of bristle length.[79] Diameters of commonly used bristles range from 0.007 inch (0.2 mm) for soft brushes to 0.012 inch (0.3 mm) for medium brushes and 0.014 inch (0.4 mm) for hard brushes.[85] Soft bristle brushes of the type described by Bass[20] have gained wide acceptance. Bass recommended a straight handle, nylon bristles 0.007 inch (0.2 mm) in diameter and 13/32 inch (10.3 mm) long, with rounded ends arranged in three rows of tufts, six evenly spaced tufts per row, with 80 to 86 bristles per tuft (Fig. 44–1). For children, the brush is smaller, with thinner (0.005 inch or 0.1 mm) and shorter (11/32 inch or 8.7 mm) bristles.

Opinions regarding the merits of hard and soft bristles are based upon studies carried out under different conditions; these studies are often inconclusive and contradict each other.[86] Medium bristles seem to cleanse better than soft bristles.[43] Soft bristles are more flexible, cleanse beneath the gingival margin (sulcus cleansing),[21] and reach more of the proximal tooth surface, but they may not completely remove heavy plaque deposits.[64] Soft bristles, especially in a multitufted brush head, seem to cleanse better than hard bristles,[8] partly because of a "matting effect" produced by the combination of soft bristles and dentifrice,[26] partly because the close proximity of the bristles in a multitufted brush enables the user to generate significantly higher brushing forces against the teeth than would be possible with two- or three-row brushes.[35, 50] This increases tooth/dentifrice contact and adds to the cleansing action, but could also increase tooth abrasion.[79] However, the manner in which a brush is used and the abrasiveness of a dentifrice[1, 156] affect the cleansing action and abrasion to a greater degree than the bristle hardness itself.[134] It is commonly assumed that even rounded bristle tips are less injurious to oral tissues than irregularly cut filaments. Clinical research indicates that this assumption does not apply to wear on enamel surfaces.[162] With regard to the gingiva, the difference between round-ended and irregularly cut bristles is also of no clinical significance provided that only low brushing forces are applied.[10, 103] With vigorous brushing that generates a peak pressure against the gingiva of 500 grams and more, round-ended bristles cause 30 to 50 per cent less gingival trauma than coarse-tip filaments.[7]

Overzealous brushing can also lead to gingival recession; implantation of bristles into the gingiva, with ensuing abscess formation; overt bacteremia, especially in patients with pronounced gingivitis[63]; and wedge-shaped defects in the cervical area of root surfaces.[63, 162a]

Patients should be advised that, in order to benefit from the cleaning efficiency of a toothbrush, they must replace it as soon as the bristles begin to fray. Soft three-row brushes tend to wear out the fastest.[155] With conscientious, regular use of a brush, this should occur within 3 months. If a brush is "worn out" after 1 week, tooth cleaning is usually performed too vigorously; if the bristles are still straight after 6 months, the brushing is either done too gently, or the brush has not been used every day. Unfortunately, there is a tendency to use a brush "as long as it lasts," which is often long after the bristles have lost their cleaning effectiveness or have become injurious to the gingiva. National surveys have indicated that in the United States (population approximately

220 million people) only 50 million tooth-brushes are sold per year, and up to 80 per cent of the brushes in use are worn to the point of replacement.

Selecting the handle shape of a toothbrush is a matter of individual preference. A handle should be long enough to fit the palm of the hand. Straight handles are most common. Handles with contra-angle shanks (Fig. 44–1) may provide the grasping hand with a better feeling of touch, since the working surface of the brush, i.e., the bristle ends, is on the direct imaginary extension of the long axis of the handle. Also, the stretching of the lip when brushing facial molar surfaces is less with contra-angle handles than with straight handles. Recently, brushes with a 17° angle between the head and the handle have been introduced to improve access to the lingual surfaces of premolars and molars; reportedly, they clean these areas 10 per cent better than conventional brushes.[7]

For the routine patient, a short-headed brush with straight-cut, round-ended, soft-to-medium nylon bristles arranged in three or four rows of tufts is recommended.

POWERED TOOTHBRUSHES

In 1939, electrically powered toothbrushes were invented to make plaque control easier for the individual. There are many types of electric toothbrushes, some with a reciprocal arcuate or with a back-and-forth motion, others with a combination of both, some with a circular motion, and some with an elliptical motion (Fig. 44–2). The most recent develop-

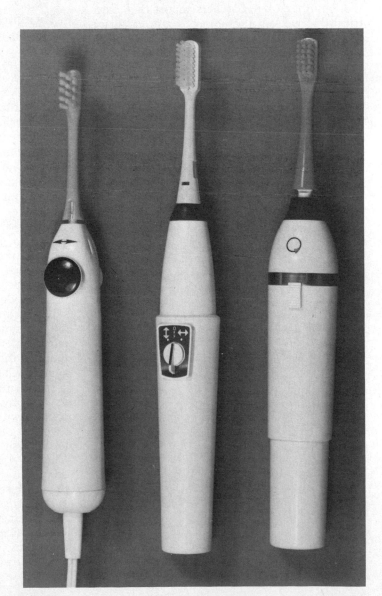

Figure 44–2 Types of powered brushes.

ment in powered tooth cleaners for home use is a dental prophylaxis handpiece with a rotary rubber cup, a tool which the dental profession has long since adopted as the most efficient mechanical means for cleaning teeth (Fig. 44–3). Regardless of the type, best results are obtained if the patient is instructed in its proper use.[14, 131] Patients who can develop the ability to use a toothbrush properly usually do equally well with a manual and an electric brush. Less diligent brushers do better with an electric toothbrush, which generates proper stroke motions automatically and requires minimal operator effort.[70] Electric brushes are recommended for (1) individuals lacking manual dexterity, (2) small children or handicapped or hospitalized patients who need to have their teeth cleaned by someone else, and (3) patients with orthodontic appliances.

A number of researchers report that electrically powered toothbrushes are superior to manual toothbrushes in terms of removing plaque, reducing calculus accumulation, and improving gingival health.[105, 112, 132, 152, 161] Others claim that manual and powered brushes are equally effective.[15, 70, 138, 198] Electric

brushes seem to produce less abrasion of tooth substance and restorative materials than manual brushes,[135, 137] unless the manual brush is used in a vertical rather than a horizontal direction.[79]

It is concluded that to date (1) no specific toothbrush can be singled out as superior for the routine removal of microbial deposits from the teeth; (2) toothbrush requirements differ greatly among individuals, depending on such factors as the morphology of each particular dentition, periodontal health, and manual dexterity; and (3) the one brush most commonly recommended by the dental profession appears to be a four-row, multitufted, soft nylon hand-held brush.[176]

DENTIFRICES

Dentifrices are aids for cleaning and polishing tooth surfaces. They are used mostly in the form of a paste. Tooth powders and liquids are also available. The cleansing effect of a dentifrice is related to its content of (1) abrasives such as calcium carbonate, calcium phosphate, calcium sulfate, sodium bicarbonate, sodium chloride, aluminum oxide, and silicate, and (2) detergents such as sodium lauryl sulfate and sodium lauryl sarcosinate. In addition, a paste contains humectants (glycerin, sorbitol), water, thickening agents (carboxymethylcellulose, alginate, amylose), flavoring, and coloring agents.

There is considerable interest in improving dentifrices by using them as vehicles for chemotherapeutic agents to inhibit plaque, calculus, caries, or root hypersensitivity. Except for the pronounced caries-prophylactic effect of fluorides incorporated in dentifrices,[136] substances such as chlorhexidine,[52] penicillin, dibasic ammonium phosphate, vaccines, vitamins, chlorophyll, formaldehyde, and strontium chloride have proved to be of little therapeutic value.

If a dentifrice is to be an effective adjunct to oral hygiene, it must come in intimate contact with the teeth. This is best achieved by placing the paste *between* the bristles of the toothbrush rather than on top of the bristles (Fig. 44–4), from which large portions of the dentifrice often are displaced before reaching the tooth surfaces.

Dentifrices should be sufficiently abrasive for satisfactory cleansing and polishing but should provide a margin of safety to protect the aggressive toothbrusher from wearing away tooth substance and soft restorative mate-

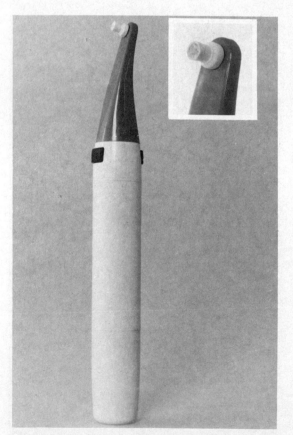

Figure 44–3 Powered tooth cleaner with rotary rubber cup.

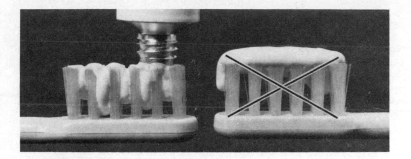

Figure 44–4 Correct and incorrect (×) application of dentifrice.

rials.[156, 165] Abrasives, commonly in the form of insoluble inorganic salts, make up 30 to 50 per cent of a dentifrice. The proper use of a dentifrice can enhance the abrasive action of a toothbrush as much as 40 times.[81, 134] Tooth powders contain about 95 per cent abrasives and are five times more abrasive than dentifrices. The abrasive quality of dentifrices affects enamel, but it is more of a concern in patients with exposed roots because dentin is abraded 25 times faster and cementum 35 times faster than enamel. This can lead to surface abrasion and root hypersensitivity.[187] Existing literature suggests that hard tissue damage from oral hygiene procedures is mainly due to abrasive dentifrices, whereas gingival lesions can be produced by a toothbrush alone.[162] However, the fact that abrasions are more prevalent on maxillary than on mandibular teeth and are found more frequently on the left than on the right half of the dental arch[53, 96] indicates that abrasion may be caused by a *number of factors*. Dentifrices that provide the cleansing effectiveness required for plaque control, with a minimum of abrasion, should be selected for periodontal patients. Inasmuch as the formulations of dentifrices are occasionally changed, the most current information should be obtained from the Council on Dental Therapeutics of the American Dental Association.[2]

TOOTHBRUSHING METHODS

There are many methods of toothbrushing.[22, 24, 40, 61, 84, 87, 178, 186] Numerous controlled studies have evaluated the effectiveness of the most common brushing techniques and have shown that no one method is clearly superior.[177] The scrub technique is probably the most popular method of brushing, whereas for patients with periodontal disease, the sulcular technique is the one most frequently recommended. The roll technique seems to be the least effective method,[177] conceivably because it generates only intermittent pressure against the teeth compared with the continuously sustained force applied with the sulcular and scrub techniques.[32] Depending on the individual morphology of a dentition, unconventional variations of accepted techniques, such as transversal scrubbing of mesial or distal tooth surfaces adjacent to edentulous areas, are frequently indicated.

Three methods of toothbrushing are presented here which, if properly performed, can accomplish the desired results. Each technique should be evaluated with regard to its feasibility in a given patient's dentition in order to arrive at a plaque control program that is tailored to the individual.

The Bass Method (Sulcus Cleansing)[22]

MAXILLARY TEETH: FACIAL AND FACIO-PROXIMAL SURFACES. Place the head of a soft-to-medium brush parallel with the occlusal plane with the "tip" of the brush distal to the last molar (Fig. 44–5). Place the bristles at the gingival margin, establish an apical angle of 45° to the long axis of the teeth, **exert gentle vibratory pressure in the long axis of the bristles,** and force the bristle ends into the facial gingival sulci (Fig. 44–6) as well as into the

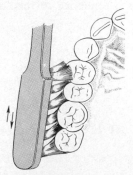

Figure 44–5 Bass Method. Position on facial and facio-proximal surfaces of maxillary molars.

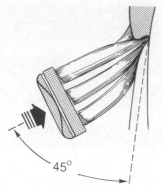

Figure 44–6 Bass Method. Intrasulcus position of brush at 45° angle to long axis of tooth.

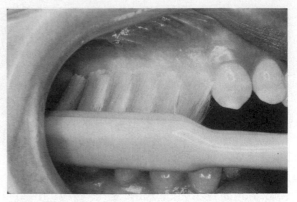

Figure 44–8 Bass Method. Correct application of brush should produce perceptible blanching of the gingiva.

interproximal embrasures (Fig. 44–7). This should produce perceptible blanching of the gingiva (Fig. 44–8). Activate the brush with a short back-and-forth motion *without dislodging the tips of the bristles*. Complete 20 such strokes in the same position. This cleans the teeth facially within the apical third of their clinical crowns, as well as within their adjacent gingival sulci and along their proximal surfaces as far as the bristles reach. Lift the brush, move it anteriorly, and repeat the process in the premolar and canine area (Fig. 44–9); place the brush so that its "heel" is still distal to the canine prominence. This cleans the premolars and the distal half of the canine. Then lift the brush and move it so that its "tip" is mesial to the canine prominence (Figs. 44–10 and 44–11). This cleans the mesial half of the canine and the incisors.

Continue on the opposite side of the arch, section by section, covering three teeth at a time, until the whole maxillary dentition is completed.

Common Errors. The following errors in the use of the brush often result in unsatisfactory cleansing or soft tissue injury:

1. When the arm holding the brush becomes tired, there is a tendency to relax and let the

brush slide down, creating an angle between the occlusal plane and the long axis of the brush (Fig. 44–12). This prevents the main bulk of the bristles from adequately penetrating interproximally and into the gingival sulci. The error is corrected by raising the elbow as far as necessary.

2. The bristles are placed on the attached gingiva rather than into the gingival sulci (Fig. 44–13). When the brush is activated, the gingival margin and the tooth surfaces are neglected, whereas the attached gingiva and the alveolar mucosa are traumatized (Fig. 44–14). The error is corrected by practicing correct positioning of the brush under visual guidance, using a dry brush without dentifrice.

3. The bristles are pressed sideways against the teeth rather than straight into the gingival sulci (Fig. 44–15). Activating the brush cleanses facial tooth surfaces but neglects the highly plaque-retaining areas interproximally and along the gingival margin. The error is corrected by practicing with a dry brush.

4. The brush is placed against the canine prominence (Fig. 44–16). This traumatizes the gingiva when the patient attempts to force the bristles into the interproximal embrasures of adjacent teeth and could lead to gingival recession at the canine prominence. The correct positions are shown in Figures 44–9 and 44–10.

MAXILLARY TEETH: PALATAL AND PALATOPROXIMAL SURFACES. Engage the brush at a 45° apical angle in the molar and premolar areas, covering three teeth at a time (Figs. 44–17 and 44–18). Clean each segment with 20 short back-and-forth strokes. To reach the palatal surface of the anterior teeth, insert the brush vertically (Figs. 44–19 and 44–20). Press the "heel" of the brush into the gingival sulci and interproximally at a 45° angle to the long

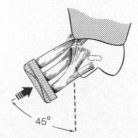

Figure 44–7 Bass Method. Interproximal position of brush at 45° angle to long axis of tooth.

Text continued on page 682

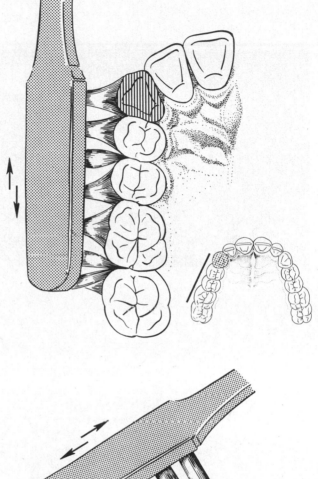

Figure 44–9 Bass Method. Position on facial and facioproximal surfaces of maxillary premolars and distal half of canine.

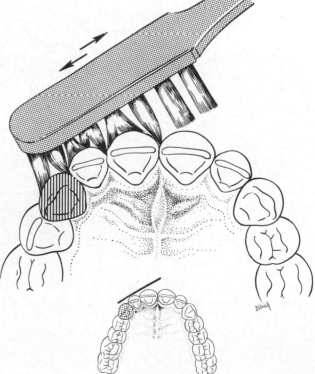

Figure 44–10 Bass Method. Position on facial and facioproximal surfaces of maxillary incisors and mesial half of canine.

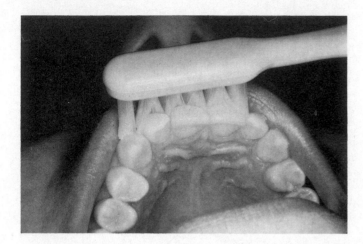

Figure 44–11 Bass Method. Clinical aspect of brush position on maxillary incisors.

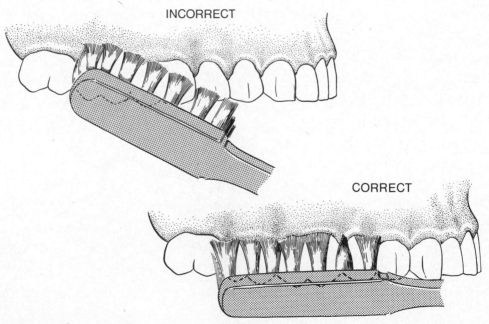

INCORRECT

CORRECT

Figure 44–12 Bass Method. Incorrect brush position *(top)* due to low position of elbow. Error corrected *(bottom)* by raising elbow.

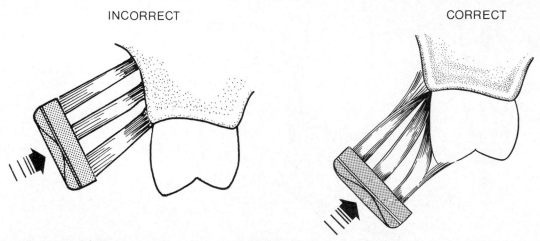

INCORRECT   CORRECT

Figure 44–13 Bass Method. Incorrect brush position *(left)* due to poor instruction. Position corrected *(right)* by practicing under visual guidance with a dry brush.

Figure 44–14 Bass Method. Scuffing of the gingiva produced by improper position of brush (see Figs. 44–13 and 44–15).

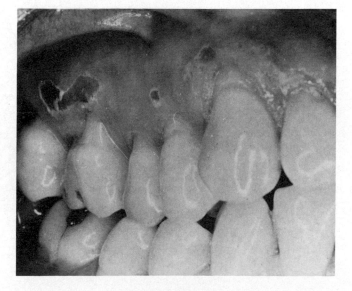

INCORRECT

CORRECT

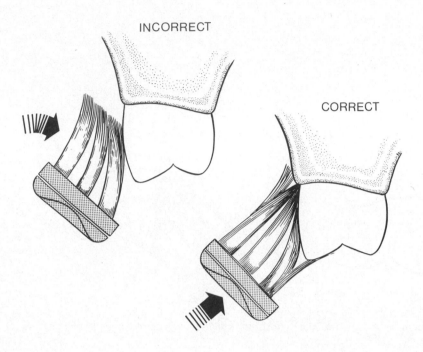

Figure 44–15 Bass Method. Incorrect brush position *(left)* due to poor instruction. Position corrected *(right)* by practicing under visual guidance with a dry brush.

INCORRECT

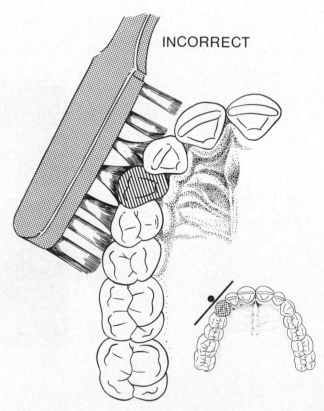

Figure 44–16 Bass Method. Incorrect brush position in facial canine area leads to mechanical trauma of the gingiva. Correct positions shown in Figures 44–9 and 44–10.

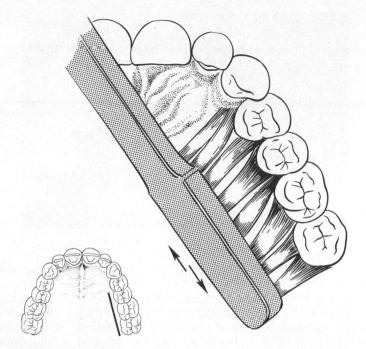

Figure 44–17 Bass Method. Palatal position on molars and premolars.

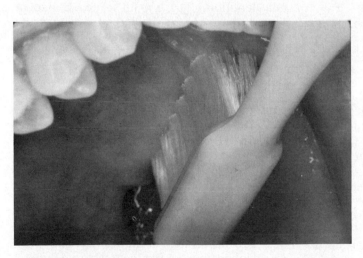

Figure 44–18 Bass Method. Clinical aspect of palatal position on molars and premolars.

Figure 44–19 Bass Method. Palatal position on incisors. Hard palate is used as guide plane for the brush.

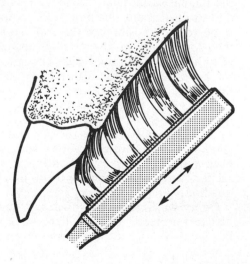

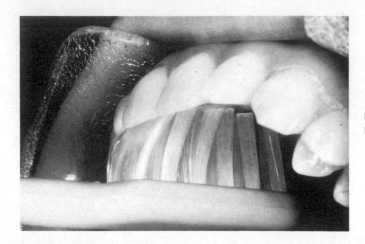

Figure 44–20 Bass Method. Clinical aspect of palatal position on incisors.

axis of the teeth, using the anterior portion of the hard palate as a guide plane. Activate the brush with 20 short up-and-down strokes. If the shape of the arch permits, the brush may be inserted horizontally between the canines with the bristles angulated into the gingival sulci of the anterior teeth (Fig. 44–21).

MANDIBULAR TEETH: FACIOPROXIMAL, LINGUAL, AND LINGUOPROXIMAL SURFACES. The mandibular teeth are cleaned in the same way as the maxillary teeth, section by section, 20 strokes in each position. In the anterior lingual region the brush is inserted vertically, using the lingual surface of the mandible as a guide plane, and with the bristles angulated into the gingival sulci (Fig. 44–22). If space permits, the brush may also be inserted horizontally between the canines (Fig. 44–23).

Common Error. The brush is placed on the incisal edge with the bristles on the lingual surface but not reaching into the sulci (Fig. 44–24). When the brush is moved back and forth, only the incisal edges and a portion of the lingual surfaces are cleaned. This error is due to insufficient opening of the mouth and a too relaxed position of the arm. To achieve the proper position, the mouth is opened wide and the elbow is raised high enough so that the hand holding the brush touches the tip of the nose.

OCCLUSAL SURFACES. Press the bristles firmly on the occlusal surfaces with the ends as deeply as possible into the pits and fissures (Fig. 44–25). Activate the brush with 20 short back-and-forth strokes, advancing section by section until all posterior teeth in all four quadrants are cleaned.

Common Error. The brush is "scrubbed" across the teeth in long horizontal strokes instead of short back-and-forth movements.

To reach the distal surface of the most distal molars, open the mouth wide and thrust the tip of the brush against that surface, 20 times for each molar (Fig. 44–26).

The Bass technique requires approximately 40 different toothbrush positions to cover a full dentition. The mouth of each patient should, therefore, be divided into sections and a systematic cleaning sequence individually prescribed, giving areas with high plaque retention priority over those with fewer deposits (Fig. 44–27).

The Bass method has the following distinct advantages over other techniques:

1. The short back-and-forth motion is **easy to learn** because it requires the same simple elbow movement familiar to most patients who are accustomed to the still popular long-stroke scrubbing technique. Except for the 45° sulcus position of the bristles and a considerably shorter stroke, there is no difference between the two methods.

2. It concentrates on the **cervical and interproximal portions of the teeth** where microbial plaque is most detrimental to the gingiva.

This technique can be **recommended for the routine patient** with or without periodontal involvement.

The Modified Stillman Method[87, 186]

A medium-to-hard two- or three-row brush is placed with the bristle ends resting partly on the cervical position of the teeth and partly on the adjacent gingiva, pointing in an apical direction at an oblique angle to the long axis of the teeth (Fig. 44–28). Pressure is applied laterally against the gingival margin so as to produce a perceptible blanching. The brush is

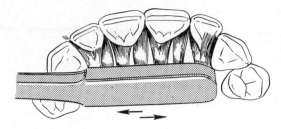

Figure 44–21 Bass Method. Variation of palatal brush position on incisors used if space permits.

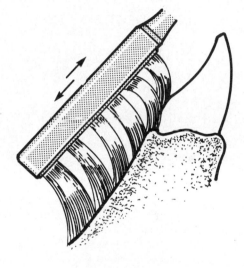

Figure 44–22 Bass Method. Lingual position on mandibular incisors. Lingual surface of mandible is used as guide plane for the brush.

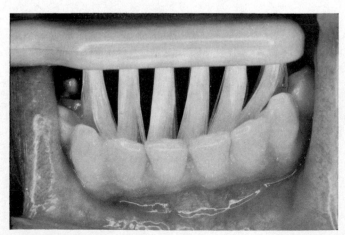

Figure 44–23 Bass Method. Variation of brush position to clean lingual surfaces of mandibular incisors.

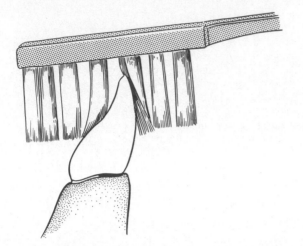

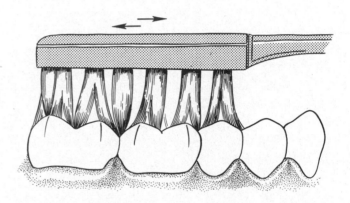

Figure 44–24 Bass Method. Incorrect application of brush due to insufficient opening of mouth and low elbow position. Error is corrected by opening wide and raising elbow.

INCORRECT

Figure 44–25 Brush position on occlusal surfaces used with the Bass, Stillman, or Charters method.

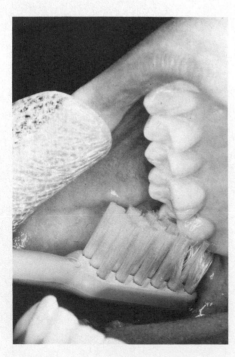

Figure 44–26 Bass Method. Position on distal surface of the most distal molars.

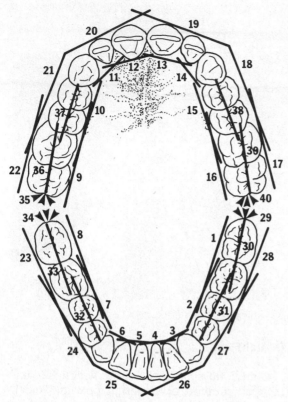

Figure 44–27 Bass Method. Recommended sequence of brush positions.

to the occlusal plane and penetrating deeply into the sulci and interproximal embrasures (see Fig. 44–25). With this technique, the sides rather than the ends of the bristles are used and penetration of the bristles into the gingival sulci is avoided. The Stillman method is therefore **recommended for cleaning in areas with progressing gingival recession** and root exposure in order to prevent abrasive tissue destruction.

The Charters Method[40]

A medium-to-hard two- or three-row brush is placed on the tooth with the bristles pointed toward the crown at a 45° angle to the long axis of the teeth (Fig. 44–29). To cleanse the occlusal surfaces, the bristle tips are placed in the pits and fissures and the brush activated with **short** back-and-forth strokes (see Fig. 44–25). The procedure is repeated until all chewing surfaces are cleansed, segment by segment.

The Charters method is **especially suitable for gingival massage.** When used in conjunction with a soft-to-medium brush, this technique is also recommended for temporary cleaning in areas of healing gingival wounds, e.g., following gingivectomy or flap surgery.

Methods of Cleaning with Powered Brushes

The various mechanical motions built into electric brushes do not require special tech-

activated with 20 short back-and-forth strokes and is simultaneously moved in a coronal direction along the attached gingiva, the gingival margin, and the tooth surface.

This process is repeated on all tooth surfaces, proceeding systematically around the mouth. To reach the lingual surfaces of the maxillary and mandibular incisors, the handle of the brush is held in a vertical position, engaging the "heel" of the brush.

The occlusal surfaces of molars and premolars are cleaned with the bristles perpendicular

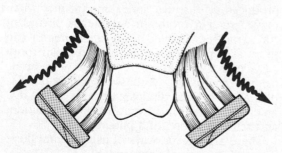

Figure 44–28 Modified Stillman Method. The sides of the bristles are pressed against teeth and gingiva while moving the brush with short back-and-forth strokes in a coronal direction.

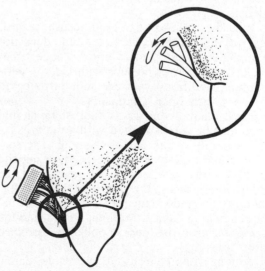

Figure 44–29 Charters Method. The bristles are pressed sideward against teeth and gingiva. The brush is activated with short circular on back-and-forth strokes.

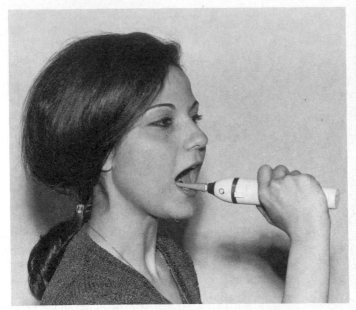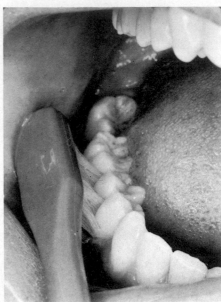

Figure 44–30 Powered toothbrushing using the Bass method.

niques of application provided the vibratory excursions of the bristle ends are small enough.

The three methods described for manual brushing are also suitable for powered tooth cleaning (Fig. 44–30).

INTERDENTAL CLEANSING AIDS

The majority of dental and periodontal disease appears to originate in interproximal areas (see Chapter 23), so interdental plaque removal conceivably is far more crucial to oral health than lingual, facial, and occlusal hygiene.

It has been shown that a toothbrush, regardless of the brushing method used, does not completely remove interdental plaque accumulation, either in persons with healthy periodontal conditions or in periodontally treated patients with open embrasures.[29, 67, 74, 170] For optimal plaque control, toothbrushing should therefore be supplemented with a more effective method of interdental cleaning. The specific aids required for this procedure depend upon various criteria such as the size of the interdental spaces, the presence of open furcations, the individual rate of plaque formation, smoking habits, tooth alignment, and the presence of orthodontic appliances or fixed prostheses.

Among the numerous aids available, dental floss and interdental cleansers such as wooden or plastic tips and interdental brushes are the most commonly used.

Dental Floss

Dental flossing is the most widely recommended method of cleansing proximal tooth surfaces.[66, 142] Floss is available as a multifilament nylon yarn that is either twisted or nontwisted, bonded or nonbonded, waxed or unwaxed, and thick or thin. Various individual factors, such as the tightness of tooth contacts, the roughness of tooth surfaces, and the patient's manual dexterity, determine the choice of dental floss, rather than the superiority of any one product. Clinical research so far has not been able to show any significant differences in the ability of the various types of floss to remove dental plaque.[58, 83, 91, 92, 162a] Individual conditions permitting, preference is given to unwaxed thin floss,[21] because it is often considerably finer than waxed floss and therefore passes more easily between teeth with tight contact areas. In addition, unwaxed floss produces a distinct squeaking sound when moved over a tooth surface that is devoid of soft deposits. This acoustic phenomenon can serve as a practical indicator of a clean tooth surface in areas where the effect of cleaning cannot be readily demonstrated with the use of a conventional disclosing agent. Thus, it is an effective aid for the motivation, instruction, and self-evaluation of a patient.

There are several ways of using dental floss. The following is recommended:

Cut a piece of floss about 1 foot long and tie the ends together to form a loop. Stretch the floss tightly between the thumb and fore-

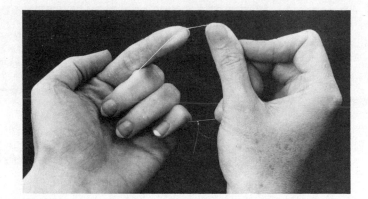

Figure 44–31 Dental flossing using the loop technique.

finger (Fig. 44–31) and pass it gently through each contact area with a firm sideward sawing motion. Do not forcibly snap the floss past the contact area, because this will injure the interdental gingiva. Wrap the floss around the proximal surface of one tooth, at the base of the gingival sulcus. Move the floss **firmly** along the tooth **up** to the contact area and **gently down** into the sulcus again, repeating this up-and-down stroke five or six times (Fig. 44–32). Displace the floss across the interdental gingiva and repeat the procedure on the proximal surface of the adjacent tooth. Continue through the whole dentition, including the distal surface of the last tooth in each quadrant. When the working portion of the floss becomes soiled or begins to shred, move the index finger and thumb along the loop to a fresh portion of floss.

The manipulation of dental floss can be simplified by using a floss holder (Fig. 44–33). Such a device, although considerably more time-consuming to use than the loop, is especially recommended for patients lacking manual dexterity and for nursing personnel assisting handicapped and hospitalized patients in cleaning their teeth. A floss holder should feature (1) one or two forks that are rigid enough to keep the floss taut even when it is moved past tight contact areas, and (2) an effective and simple mounting mechanism that holds the floss firmly in place yet allows quick rethreading of the floss whenever its working portion becomes soiled or begins to shred.

The purpose of flossing is to remove plaque, not to dislodge fibrous threads of food wedged in between two teeth or impacted in the gingiva. Chronic food impaction should be treated by correcting proximal tooth contacts and "plunger" cusps. Removing impacted food with dental floss simply provides temporary relief but permits the condition to become worse.

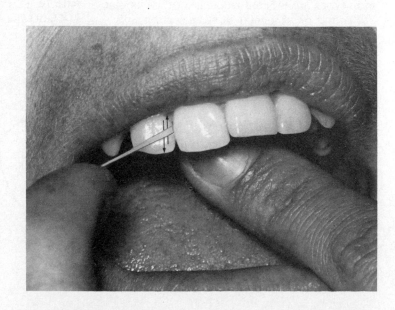

Figure 44–32 Dental Flossing. The floss is wrapped around each proximal surface and activated with repeated up-and-down strokes.

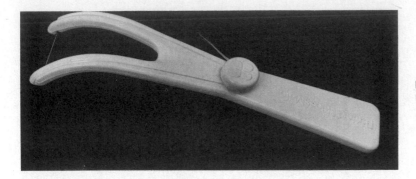

Figure 44–33 Floss Holder. It simplifies the manipulation of dental floss.

Interdental Cleansers

For cleaning in narrow gingival embrasures that are occupied by intact papillae and bordered by tight contact zones, dental floss is probably the most effective dental hygiene aid. Proper manipulation of the floss requires good dexterity, intensive instruction, and repeated monitoring. However, concave root surfaces and furcations cannot be reached with dental floss (Fig. 44–34A). Therefore, special cleaning devices that are easy to handle and that adapt themselves to irregular tooth surfaces better than does dental floss (Fig. 44–34B) are recommended for proximal cleaning of teeth with large or open interdental spaces such as those found in periodontally treated dentitions.

A wide variety of interdental cleansers are available for removing soft debris from tooth surfaces that are not accessible to a full-size toothbrush (Fig. 44–35). Clinical research has documented the effectiveness of interdental cleansers on proximal as well as on lingual and facial tooth surfaces.[27, 171, 203] The most common types are tapered wooden toothpicks that are round or triangular in cross section, mini-ature bottle brushes, and unitufted brushes. Many interdental cleansers can be attached to a handle for convenient manipulation around the teeth.

INTERDENTAL BRUSHES. These are cone-shaped brushes made of bristles or plastic disks mounted on a handle (Fig. 44–35C and D), unitufted brushes (Fig. 44–35E), or miniature bottle brushes (Fig. 44–35F). Interdental brushes are particularly suitable for cleaning large, irregular, or concave tooth surfaces adjacent to wide interdental spaces. They are inserted interproximally and activated with short back-and-forth strokes in a linguofacial direction. For best cleansing efficiency, the diameter of the brush should be slightly larger than the gingival embrasures so that the bristles or plastic disks can exert pressure on the tooth surfaces. The unitufted brushes are highly effective on the lingual surface of mandibular molars and premolars, where a regular toothbrush often interferes with the tongue and does not reach the gingival third of the crowns.

WOODEN TIPS. Wooden tips are used either with (e.g., Perio-Aid) or without (e.g., Stim-U-Dent) the aid of a special holder.

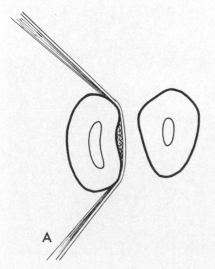
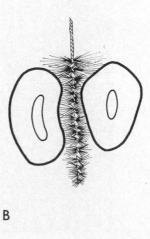

A   B

Figure 44–34 Cleaning of concave or irregular proximal tooth surfaces. Dental floss (A) is less effective than an interdental brush (B).

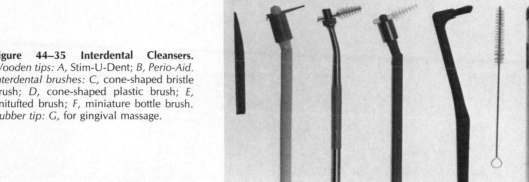

Figure 44–35 Interdental Cleansers. *Wooden tips: A, Stim-U-Dent; B, Perio-Aid. Interdental brushes: C, cone-shaped bristle brush; D, cone-shaped plastic brush; E, unitufted brush; F, miniature bottle brush. Rubber tip: G, for gingival massage.*

A *Stim-U-Dent* (Fig. 44–35*A*) consists of a soft wooden tip that is triangular in cross section. Held between middle finger, index finger and thumb, it is introduced in the interdental spaces in such a way that the base surface of the triangle rests tangentially on the interproximal gingiva and the sides are in contact with the proximal tooth surfaces (Fig. 44–36). The Stim-U-Dent is then repeatedly forced in and out of the embrasure, removing soft deposits from the teeth and mechanically stimulating the papillary gingiva.

The *Perio-Aid* (see Fig. 44–35*B*) consists of a round, tapered end of a toothpick that is inserted in a handle for convenient application. Deposits are removed by using either the side (Fig. 44–37*A*) or the end of the tip (Fig. 44–37*B*). This device is particularly efficient for cleaning along the gingival margin[170] and within gingival sulci or periodontal pockets. The small dimensions of the tip allow for exceptionally good visibility of the tooth surface being cleaned, which contributes substantially to the effectiveness of the Perio-Aid.

Selection of Interdental Cleansing Aids

For the purpose of selecting the most adequate interdental cleansing device, three types of interproximal embrasures can be distinguished.

Type I embrasures are totally occupied by the interdental papillae. **Type II** embrasures are characterized by a slight to moderate recession of the interdental papillae. **Type III** embrasures are created by extensive recession or complete loss of the interdental papillae.

In Type I embrasures, dental floss should be used (Fig. 44–38*A*). It is the only device that can be passed through such narrow spaces without forcing the papillae apically, which could induce undesired gingival recession.

In Type II embrasures, small interdental brushes (e.g., PROXABRUSH) should be used (Fig. 44–38*B*). Dental floss is less effective in these cases because interproximal gingival recession usually leads to the exposure of concave root depressions (see Fig. 44–34). Wooden tips can also be used.

In Type III embrasures, larger brushes such as a unitufted brush are recommended (Fig. 44–38*C*).

In general, the largest applicable device should always be selected.

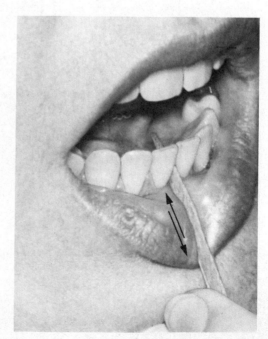

Figure 44–36 Wooden Tip (Stim-U-Dent). Interproximal cleaning and massage with the tip inserted tangentially to the facial surface of the gingival papilla.

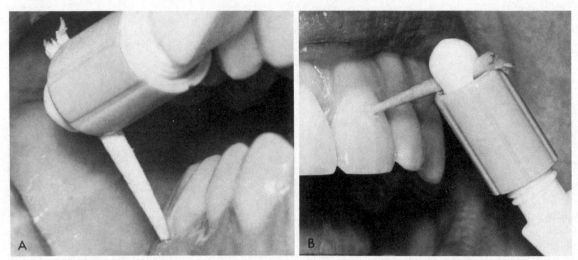

Figure 44–37 Wooden Tip (Perio-Aid). *A,* Side of tip is used to clean along gingival margins and subgingivally. *B,* Frayed end of tip cleans large surface areas.

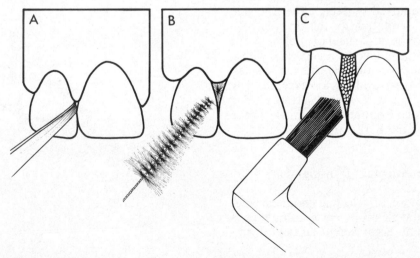

Figure 44–38 Interproximal Embrasure Types and Corresponding Interdental Cleansers. *A,* Type I—no gingival recession: dental floss. *B,* Type II—moderate papillary recession: interdental brush. *C,* Type III—complete loss of papillae: unitufted brush.

GINGIVAL MASSAGE

Massaging the gingiva with a toothbrush or interdental cleansers produces epithelial thickening, increased keratinization, and increased mitotic activity in the epithelium and connective tissue.[31, 36, 38, 39, 73, 158, 183, 184] It is claimed that massage improves blood circulation, the supply of nutrients and oxygen to the gingiva, tissue metabolism, and the removal of waste products.[150, 186] *Whether epithelial thickening, increased keratinization, and improved blood circulation provide substantial protection against microorganisms and other local irritants and are therefore beneficial or necessary for gingival health is questionable.*[72, 129] Since keratinization occurs in the oral gingiva and not in the sulcular gingiva, which is more vulnerable to microbial attack, it appears that the improved gingival health provided by toothbrushing and other oral hygiene procedures results predominantly from the removal of microbial pathogens and not from gingival massage. In addition, studies with chemotherapeutic mouth rinses have demonstrated that gingival health can be maintained in the absence of mechanical oral hygiene procedures.[119]

Gingival massage is recommended as an aid to stimulate and accelerate the re-establishment of firm and keratinized gingiva following surgical interventions such as gingivectomies or flap procedures. It is administered with a toothbrush by placing the side of the bristles against the gingival surface (see Figs. 44–28 and 44–29), with stimulators such as Stim-U-Dents (see Fig. 44–35*A*), or with rubber tips which are inserted in the handle of a toothbrush (see Fig. 44–35*G*) or are mounted on a separate holder. A stimulator is inserted interdentally with the end of the tip slanted toward the occlusal surface so that its side rests tangentially against the interdental gingiva (see Fig. 44–36). In this position, the tip is likely to create or preserve the normal slope of the interdental papillae. The brush or tip is activated with a rotary motion that is repeated 20 times, pressing the instrument into the interproximal space. Each interdental area is treated from both the facial and the lingual sides. This technique is also applicable to supragingival furcation areas. It is a common error to insert the Stim-U-Dent or rubber tip perpendicular to the long axis of the teeth. This creates flattened, cupped-out interdental gingival contours, which are less desirable esthetically and are more conducive to interproximal food trapping than is the sloped gingival surface produced by proper angulation of the instrument.

ORAL IRRIGATION DEVICES

Oral irrigators work by directing a high-pressure steady or pulsating stream of water through a nozzle to the tooth surfaces. The pressure is generated by a built-in pump or by attaching the device to a water faucet (Fig. 44–39). Oral irrigators clean nonadherent bacteria and debris from the oral cavity more effectively than toothbrushes and mouth rinses.[197] They are particularly helpful for removing nonstructured debris from inaccessible areas around orthodontic appliances and fixed prostheses. Also, gingival keratinization increases with the use of oral irrigators.[98] When used as adjuncts to toothbrushing, these devices can have a beneficial effect on periodontal health by retarding the accumulation of plaque and calculus[26, 49, 89, 113, 157] and reducing gingival inflammation and pocket depth.[37, 44, 100, 157] *However, water irrigation removes only negligible amounts of stainable plaque from tooth surfaces.*[57]

In the near future, oral irrigators may prove to be of considerable value as vehicles for administering chemotherapeutic agents that inhibit microbial growth, especially in inaccessible regions such as interdental areas or periodontal pockets.[3] Water irrigation may cause minimal damage to soft oral tissues[149] but does not induce bacteremia when the device is used according to the manufacturer's instructions in patients with health gingiva or gingivitis.[100, 194] Transient bacteremia following water irrigation in patients with periodontitis has been reported.[56] However, bacteremia as well as gingival trauma has also been found following toothbrushing.[148, 175]

CHEMICAL INHIBITORS OF PLAQUE AND CALCULUS

To date, mechanical tooth cleaning with manual or powered toothbrushes, interdental cleansing aids, and rotary brushes or rubber cups is still the most effective method available for controlling plaque, calculus, and ultimately periodontal disease. But since this is a tedious procedure that cannot be relaxed without risking the establishment of new accumulations and the onset of periodontal inflammation,

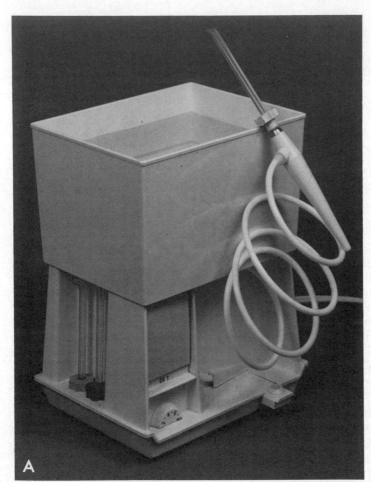

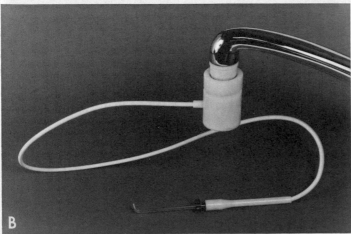

Figure 44–39 Oral Irrigation Devices. *A*, Type with built-in pump. *B*, Type which attaches to water faucet.

there is an increasing search for chemical aids which could prevent or significantly reduce plaque and inflammation, thus lessening our dependence upon mechanical cleansing.[5, 47, 133, 151, 173, 174, 188]

Many agents have been tested systemically or topically for their capability to inhibit the quantitative or qualitative development of microbial deposits, calculus, or periodontal inflammation.[123] Promising results have been reported with fluorides[125, 127]; chlorhexidine[65, 119]; alexidine[115, 180, 181]; antibiotics[122] such as erythromycin,[116] kanamycin,[124, 126] niddamycin (cc 10232),[202] penicillin,[207] spiramycin,[80] and vancomycin[141]; metronidazole and nitrimidazine[128]; urea[28, 144, 154]; bradosol,[94]; victamin C[94, 199, 200]; chlorides[94, 171] ascoxal[143]; sodium ricinoleate[174]; enzymes such as dextranase,[95, 114] mucinase,[6, 107, 185] and hyaluronidase[204]; and acetate compounds of zinc, manganese, and copper.[9] The most commonly used mode of applying these agents has been topical, in the form of mouthwashes, dentifrices, gels, lozenges, and chewing gum.

The agent that has attracted the most attention to date is **chlorhexidine,** a diguanidohexane with pronounced antiseptic properties. The initial finding that **two daily rinses with 10 ml of a 0.2 per cent aqueous solution of chlorhexidine gluconate** almost completely inhibit the development of dental plaque, calculus, and gingivitis[119] in the human model for experimental gingivitis[120] has been confirmed by a number of short term clinical investigations.[65, 117, 193] In most of the studies, a mouth rinse has been employed as the preferred mode of application.[65, 119, 174] Chlorhexidine incorporated into dentifrices, gels, and lozenges has proved so far to be considerably less, if at all, effective.[50, 59, 65, 78, 90, 164] This may be because of lower concentrations of chlorhexidine in, or partial inactivation of the agent by, these carriers.[68, 164]

Aside from some local, reversible side effects, such as brown staining of teeth, tongue, and silicate and resin restorations,[51, 59, 121] transient impairment of taste perception,[118, 173, 174] and discrete desquamation of the oral mucosa,[60] chlorhexidine appears to be one of the safest antiseptics known.[130, 145, 193] It has not so far shown any evidence of systemic toxic activity in humans[167], nor has it produced any appreciable resistance of oral microorganisms.[140, 166, 168]

Similarly promising results have been reported with alexidine, another bis-guanide that is closely related to chlorhexidine,[18, 115, 180, 181] with fluorides,[125, 127] and with other compounds.[205]

As evidence of a specific microbial etiology of inflammatory periodontal diseases is increasing (see Chapter 25), it seems likely that some antimicrobial agents that have so far proved to be effective against acute gingivitis may also be used to prevent or reduce the severity of chronic gingivitis and periodontitis.

DISCLOSING AGENTS

These are **solutions** and **wafers** capable of staining bacterial deposits on the surfaces of teeth, tongue, and gingivae. They are excellent oral hygiene aids because they provide the patient with a self-educational and self-motivational tool to improve his efficiency in plaque control (Fig. 44–40).[13]

Solutions

1. Basic fuchsin — 6 grams
   Ethyl alcohol, 95% — 100 ml
   Add two drops to water in a dappen dish

2. Potassium iodide — 1.6 grams
   Iodine crystals — 1.6 grams
   Water — 13.4 ml
   Glycerin — to make 30.0 ml

Solutions are applied to the teeth as concentrates on cotton swabs or as dilutes in mouthwashes. They usually produce heavy staining of bacterial plaque, gingivae, tongue, lips, fingers, and sink. Therefore, they are useful only in the dental office, where an impressive demonstration of bacterial deposits is desirable and excessive staining can be controlled or readily removed with prophylaxis instruments. Except for a sodium fluorescein dye, which produces a yellow glowing of dental plaque only when exposed to a light source of a certain wavelength,[42, 62, 102] solutions are not recommended for home use owing to this inconvenient intensive staining effect, which may act as a deterrent rather than as a motivator.

Wafers

FDC red #3 (erythrosine)	15 mg
Sodium chloride	0.747%
Sodium sucaryl	0.747%
Calcium stearate	0.995%
Soluble saccharin	0.186%
White oil	0.124%
Flavoring (FDA approved)	2.239%
Sorbitol	to make 7.0 grams

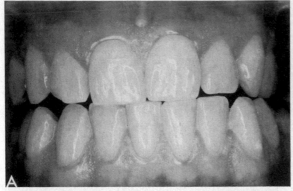

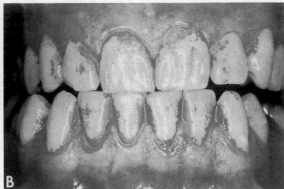

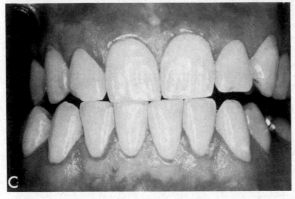

Figure 44–40 Effect of a Disclosing Agent. *A,* Unstained. *B,* Stained with a 6 per cent solution of basic fuchsin; plaque shows as dark particulate patches. *C,* Restained with basic fuchsin after thorough tooth cleaning.

Wafers are crushed between the teeth and swished around the mouth for about 30 seconds without swallowing. Because of the convenient mode of application, wafers are recommended specifically for home use.

It is obvious that the mere addition of disclosing agents to oral health instructions is not sufficient motivation for a patient to clean his teeth more effectively. Visual feedback can, however, be an important aspect of health education if used in conjunction with other methods.

FREQUENCY OF TOOTH CLEANING

In the controlled and supervised environment of clinical research, where well-trained individuals remove all visible plaque, gingival health can be maintained by one thorough cleaning exercise with brush, floss, and toothpicks every 24 to 48 hours.[93, 101, 119] In spite of such revealing data, clinical experience shows that routine oral hygiene falls far short of such perfection in the majority of patients. In an average cleaning exercise, lasting just 2 minutes every day, only 40 per cent of the deposits are removed, leaving 60 per cent to promote rapid regrowth of the microbiota.[45] Numerous studies have reported on improved periodontal

health associated with increasing frequency of brushing up to twice per day.[4, 76, 99, 139, 176, 189, 195] Higher cleaning frequencies, i.e., three or more times per day, did not produce significantly better periodontal conditions. For practical purposes, **two brushings per day,** one of them performed with detailed thoroughness, are recommended. Evidence that 80 to 90 per cent of educated people brush their teeth once or twice a day is encouraging only if it is ascertained that after brushing the teeth are clean.[50, 176]

In conclusion, emphasis must be placed on the efficiency rather than on the frequency of tooth cleaning.

STEP-BY-STEP PROCEDURE FOR PLAQUE CONTROL INSTRUCTION

In periodontal therapy, plaque control serves two important purposes: (1) to minimize gingival inflammation, and (2) to prevent the recurrence or progression of periodontal disease in the treated mouth. In view of many socioeconomic barriers still associated with the application of other successful modes of plaque control, such as professional tooth cleaning once every 2 to 4 weeks,[15, 16, 108, 110, 146, 159, 160] the daily mechanical removal of plaque by the patient appears to be the only practical means for improving oral hygiene on a long-term basis. The following step-by-step procedure to teach a patient this self-therapeutic approach to oral health is suggested.

Step I. Motivation

Motivation for effective plaque control is one of the most critical and most difficult elements of long-term success of periodontal therapy because, in most cases, it requires from a patient the following efforts: (1)**receptiveness,** i.e., understanding the concepts of the pathogenesis, the treatment, and the prevention of periodontal disease; (2) **change of habits**, i.e., adopting a self-administered *daily* plaque control regimen; and (3) **behavioral changes,** i.e., adjusting the hierarchy of one's beliefs, practices, and values so as to accommodate the required new oral hygiene habits.

A patient must understand what periodontal disease is, what its effects are, that he is susceptible to it, and what he can do to achieve and maintain oral health.[46] He must be willing and able to develop and use the manual skills that are necessary to establish a plaque-control regimen. He must then want to keep his mouth clean for his own benefit (and not only to please his dentist). If these efforts are not made by the patient, long-term failure of any individual plaque control program is inevitable and leads to frustration of the dentist and the patient. It should be recognized that effective long-range motivation from the dental office is often extremely difficult, if not impossible, to achieve. Therefore, the dentist should be prepared to alter his original treatment plan if a patient is not able to cooperate satisfactorily.

Step II. Education

Most patients think of toothbrushing only in terms of removing food debris and preventing tooth decay.[111] Its importance in the prevention and treatment of periodontal disease is rarely recognized and must therefore be explained. **Toothbrushing is the most important patient-administered preventive and therapeutic procedure.** In no other field of medicine can the patient so effectively assist in controlling a disease as can be done in relation to periodontitis by conscientious plaque control. If a person maintained good oral hygiene from 5 to 50 years of age, he very likely could avoid the destructive effects of periodontal disease during this major period of his life.[76, 109]

Patients must be informed that periodic scaling and cleansing of the teeth in the dental office are helpful protective measures against periodontal disease, but only if these are combined with daily oral hygiene procedures at home. Therefore, time spent in the dental office teaching the patient how to cleanse his teeth is as valuable a service as cleaning his teeth for him. It must be explained that dental visits 2 or 3 times a year are not nearly as effective as is daily oral home care. Only a combination of regular office visits with conscientious home care significantly reduces gingivitis and loss of supporting periodontal tissues.[109, 146, 192]

A periodontal patient should be shown that periodontal disease has manifested itself *in his own mouth*. Stained dental plaque, the bleeding of inflamed gingiva, and a periodontal probe inserted into a pocket are impressive and convincing documentation of the presence of pathogens and actual disease.[17] It is of even greater educational value to a patient to have his oral cleanliness and periodontal condition recorded periodically.[19]

He can utilize this as feedback information about his level of performance. The following indices are recommended:

PLAQUE CONTROL RECORD.[147] Disclosing solution is applied to all supragingival tooth surfaces. After the patient has rinsed, each tooth surface (except occlusal surfaces) is examined for the presence or absence of stained deposits at the dentogingival junction. If present, they are recorded by coloring the appropriate box in a diagram (Fig. 44–41). After all teeth have been scored, an index is calculated by dividing the number of surfaces with plaque by the total number of teeth scored.

PAPILLARY BLEEDING INDEX,[163] **MODIFIED.** A periodontal pocket probe is inserted facially into the mesial col area of each tooth. Keeping the tip in light touch with the bottom of the sulcus, the probe is gently drawn along the mesiofacial surface of the tooth and withdrawn at the mesiofacial line angle. In this way, the facial papilla mesial to each tooth is probed. When probing is completed in one arch, the margin of each probed papilla is scored as follows:

x = absence of corresponding tooth
0 = no bleeding
1 = minute blood spot
2 = large blood spot (or line)
3 = hemorrhagic oozing

Plaque Control Record

Previous Index _____   _____ Present Index

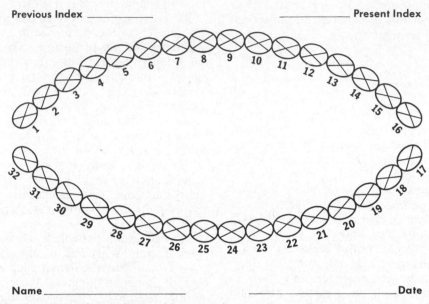

Name _____   _____ Date

Figure 44–41 The Plaque Control Record. An oral hygiene aid to patient motivation and instruction. (From O'Leary, T. J., Drake, R. B, and Naylor, J. E.: J. Periodontol., *43*:38, 1972.)

The scores are entered on an index chart (Fig. 44–42). The procedure is repeated in the opposite arch and the score tabulated for each quadrant. Five consecutive recordings spaced over the entire periodontal treatment period can be made on one chart. By teaching the patient how to probe with a thin toothpick, a weekly scoring of the anterior papillae can even be incorporated in his oral hygiene regimen as a self-educational tool.

The Papillary Bleeding Index is designed to demonstrate a clinical **effect,** i.e., bleeding gingiva, rather than the cause of periodontal inflammation. Since bleeding is commonly associated with trauma or disease, papillary bleeding can have a strong educational and motivational impact on a patient.

Step III. Instruction

With repeated instruction and supervision, patients can reduce the incidence of plaque and gingivitis far more effectively than with self-acquired oral hygiene habits.[75, 97, 169, 192, 205] However, instruction in how to clean teeth must be more than a cursory chairside demonstration of the use of a toothbrush and oral hygiene aids. It is a painstaking procedure that requires patient participation, careful supervision with immediate correction of developing mistakes, and reinforcement during return visits until the patient demonstrates that he has developed the necessary proficiency.[11, 17, 106]

At the **first instruction visit,** the patient is presented with a new toothbrush, an interdental cleanser, and a disclosing agent. First, the patient's plaque is located. Unstained, small amounts of bacterial deposits are difficult to see (see Fig. 44–40*A*); heavier accumulations of plaque and unstructured debris (materia alba) may be visible as gray, yellow, or white material on the teeth, along the gingival margin, and in faciolingual embrasures. Loose food debris and materia alba are washed off with a strong water spray. Then a disclosing agent (solution or wafer)[13] is applied to stain all otherwise invisible plaque. After a brief water rinse to remove stained saliva which would obscure the picture, the stained plaque and pellicle can now be clearly demonstrated to the patient (see Fig. 44–40*B*). Illuminated mouth mirrors especially designed for this purpose will give an impressive close-up view (Fig. 44–43). Polished dental restorations do not take up the stain, but the oral mucosa and the lips may retain it up to several hours. Covering the lips lightly with petrolatum (Vaseline) before using the stain is helpful.

Toothbrushing is now demonstrated on a cast, stressing the exact placement and activation of the bristles. This is followed by a

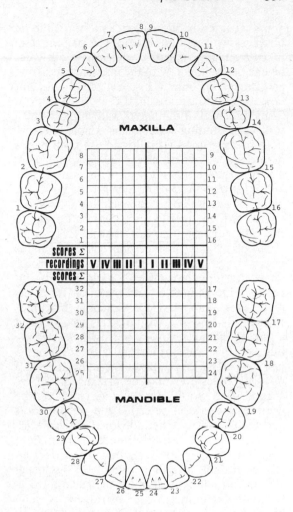

Figure 44–42 Papillary Bleeding Index. (Modified from Saxer, U. P., and Muhlemann, H. R.: Schweiz. Mschr. Zahnheilk., *85*:905, 1975.) Oral hygiene aid to patient motivation and instruction.

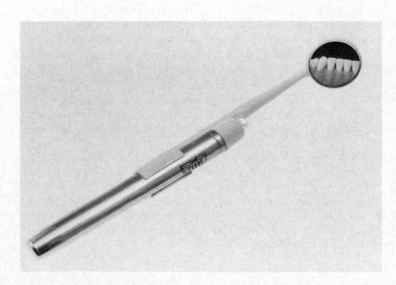

Figure 44–43 Illuminated Mouth Mirror. Oral hygiene aid for the patient to locate stained plaque.

demonstration in the patient's mouth while he observes with a hand mirror. The patient then takes over and repeats on his own teeth what he has been shown, with the instructor assisting and correcting him. This exercise should not be carried out in the dental chair but rather in front of a well-illuminated wall mirror and a sink with running water. This enables the patient to have good visibility, to use both hands if necessary, and to rinse the mouth freely. The procedure is repeated with dental floss and interdental cleansing aids according to the patient's needs. After one cleaning exercise is completed, the teeth are restained to evaluate the efficiency of plaque removal. Even after vigorous cleaning some stain usually remains on proximal surfaces. The instruction procedures are repeated until the patient is able to remove all stainable soft material from his teeth (see Fig. 44–40C). Teaching machines with film strips or transparencies can be used as an adjunct to person-to-person instruction—but not as a substitute for it. In addition, a person's ability to manipulate oral hygiene aids in a given fashion may be measured and recorded in the form of a skill index that can be used as a guide in selecting the proper tools and techniques for the individual patient[145]

When the first visit is terminated, the patient is given the hygiene aids that were demonstrated to him, including a supply of disclosing wafers for self-evaluation of his cleaning performance at home. He is instructed to clean his teeth at least once a day with thorough attention to all details. Such a cleansing exercise in a full dentition takes 5 to 10 minutes. The patient is advised to choose for his oral hygiene a convenient time and place in his daily schedule. Generally, bed time is considered not to be the best choice, since one's mental and physical state before retiring at night often is not conducive to a vigorous cleaning exercise.

Subsequent instruction visits are used to reinforce or modify previous instructions. The state of gingival health and oral cleanliness is recorded using first the Papillary Bleeding Index (see Fig. 44–42) and then the Plaque Control Record (see Fig. 44–41).

Following the recording of both indices, the patient is asked to remove the stained deposits, with special emphasis on areas that stained the heaviest. This exercise should be supervised. If corrections are indicated, they must be instituted immediately, making sure that the patient understands how and why they are made. During the first few weeks, a patient often has considerable technical or motivational difficulties with a new oral hygiene regimen. He should be encouraged to comment on his own experience so that potential deficiencies or aversions can be identified and corrected. Painful toothbrush lacerations of the gingiva (see Fig. 44–14) commonly occur with the use of a new toothbrush. They should not be overlooked. The patient is informed that the condition is transient and can be cured within a few days by temporarily cleaning with the sides rather than the ends of the bristles (see Fig. 44–29). If such a condition is overlooked, a patient could lose confidence in the new regimen and go back to his previous cleaning habits, often without telling the dentist about it.

A patient is not dismissed until he has demonstrated some improvement over his performance at the outset of the visit. However, instruction visits should not be longer than 10 minutes each. Long visits tend to tire the patient and may lead to embarrassment, frustration, and loss of motivation.

Subsequent instruction visits are scheduled, lengthening the intervals between them, until the patient attains the proficiency required to keep his mouth healthy. *Patience and repetition are the secrets of instruction in oral hygiene.*

PROFESSIONAL TOOTH CLEANING

Conscientious oral home care substantially inhibits the formation of plaque, stain, and calculus but cannot completely prevent their occurrence especially in patients with periodontal pockets and in heavy calculus formers. Therefore, periodic professional care consisting of complete mechanical removal of all stainable deposits and repeated hygiene instruction is an integral part of a comprehensive plaque control program. It must be emphasized, however, that professional tooth cleaning *alone* is insufficient for maintaining a healthy oral environment or preventing the progression of periodontal disease, even if administered once a month.[63, 190, 191] *Only a combination of professional tooth cleaning at regular intervals of up to 3 months, repeated enforcement of hygiene instructions, and conscientious daily plaque control by the patient* has proved to be successful for preserving periodontal health and arresting treated periodontal disease.[15, 16, 108–110, 145, 153, 159, 191]

During the past decades, little progress has been made in the area of mechanical plaque control. Nevertheless, reliable data from long-term clinical studies have now become available to prove that with regular assistance from the dental team, thorough daily removal of microbial deposits from the teeth by the individual patient can be effective in attaining or maintaining periodontal health.

REFERENCES

1. Abrasivity of Current Dentifrices: Report of the Council of Dental Therapeutics. J. Am. Dent. Assoc., 81:117, 1970.
2. Accepted Dental Therapeutics. 3rd ed. Chicago, American Dental Association, 1969–1970, p. 225.
3. Agerbaek, N., Melsen, B., and Rölla, G.: Application of chlorhexidine by oral irrigation systems. Scand. J. Dent. Res., 83:284, 1975.
4. Ainamo, J.: The effect of habitual tooth cleaning on the occurrence of periodontal disease and dental caries. Suom. Hammaslääk, 67:63, 1971.
5. Alderman, E. J., Jr., and Scallon, V. L.: An in vivo study of the effect of the prolonged use of a specific mouthwash on the oral flora. Chron. Omaha Dent. Soc., 28:284, 1965.
6. Aleece, A. A., and Forscher, B. K.: Calculus reduction with a mucinase dentifrice. J. Periodontol., 25:122, 1954.
7. Alexander, J. F., Saffir, A. J., and Gold, W.: The measurement of the effect of toothbrushes on soft tissue abrasion. J. Dent. Res., 56:722, 1977.
8. Allet, B., Regolati, B., and Mühlemann, H. R.: Die Rolle der Griffabwinkelung auf die Reinigungskraft einer Zahnbürste. Schweiz. Mschr. Zahnheilk., 82:452, 1972.
9. Amdur, B., Brudevold, F., and Messer, A. C.: Observations on the calcification of salivary sediment. I.A.D.R. Abstr., 1962, p. 18.
10. Anaise, J. Z.: Plaque removal by different types of toothbrush. Isr. J. Dent. Med., 25:19, 1976.
11. Anderson, J. L.: Integration of plaque control into the practice of dentistry. Dent. Clin. North Am., 16:621, 1972.
12. Annenroth. G., and Poppelman, A.: Histological evaluation of gingival damage by toothbrushing. An experimental study in dog. Acta Odontol. Scand., 33:119, 1975.
13. Arnim, S. S.: The use of disclosing agents for measuring tooth cleanliness. J. Periodontol., 34:227, 1963.
14. Ash, M. M.: A review of the problems and results of studies on manual and power toothbrushes. J. Periodontol., 35:202, 1964.
15. Axelsson, P., and Lindhe, J.: The effect of a preventive programme on dental plaque, gingivitis and caries in schoolchildren: results after one and two years. J. Clin. Periodontol., 1:126, 1974.
16. Axelsson, P., Lindhe, J., and Waseley, J.: The effect of various plaque control measures on gingivitis and caries in schoolchildren. Community Dent. Oral Epidemiol., 4:323, 1976.
17. Barkley, R. F.: Successful Preventive Practices. Macomb, Ill., Preventive Dentistry Press, 1972, pp. 75ff, 209ff.
18. Barnes, G. P., et al.: Dental plaque reduction with an antimicrobial mouth rinse. Part I. Oral Surg., 34:553, 1972.
19. Barrikman, R., and Penhall, O.: Graphing indexes reduce plaque. J. Am. Dent. Assoc., 87:1904, 1973.
20. Bass, C. C.: The optimum characteristics of toothbrushes for personal oral hygiene. Dent. Items Int., 70:696, 1948.
21. Bass, C. C.: Optimum characteristics of dental floss for personal oral hygiene. Dent. Items Int., 70:921, 1948.
22. Bass, C. C.: An effective method of personal oral hygiene. Part II. J. Louisiana State Med. Soc., 106:100, 1954.
23. Bay, I., Kardel, K., and Skougaard, M. R.: Quantitative evaluation of the plaque-removing ability of different types of toothbrushes. J. Periodontol., 38:526, 1967.
24. Bell, D. G.: Teaching home care to the patient. J. Periodontol., 19:140, 1948.
25. Belting, C. M., and Gordon, D. L.: In vitro effect of a urea containing dentifrice on dental calculus formation. II. J. Periodontol., 37:26, 1966.
26. Bergenholtz, A.: Mechanical cleaning. In Frandsen, A. (ed.): Oral Hygiene. Copenhagen, Munskgaard, 1971, pp. 27–60.
27. Bergenholtz, A., Bjorne, A., and Vikström, B.: The plaque-removing ability of some common interdental aids. J. Clin. Periodontol., 1:160, 1974.
28. Bergenholtz, A., Hugoson, A., and Sohlberg, F.: An evaluation of the plaque-removing ability of some aids to oral hygiene. Svensk. Tandlák. T., 60:447, 1967.
29. Bergenholtz, A., Hugoson, A., Lundgren, D., and Ostgren, A.: The plaque-removing ability of various toothbrushes used with the roll technique. Svensk. Tandlák. T., 62:15, 1969.
30. Berman, C. L., Hosiosky, E. N., Kutscher, A. H., and Kelly, A.: Observations of the effect of an electric toothbrush: preliminary report. J. Periodontol., 33:195, 1962.
31. Bertolini, A.: Experimental research on the effects of mechanical gingival massage. Parodontologie, 9:144, 1955.
32. Björn, H., and Lindhe, J.: On the mechanics of toothbrushing. Odont. Revy, 17:9, 1966.
33. Brandtzaeg, P.: The significance of oral hygiene in the prevention of dental diseases. Odont. T., 72:460, 1964.
34. Brandtzaeg, P., and Jamison, H. C.: The effect of controlled cleansing of the teeth on periodontal health and oral hygiene in Norwegian army recruits. J. Periodontol., 35:308, 1964.
35. Burgett, F. G., and Ash, M. M.: Comparative study of the pressure of brushing with three types of toothbrushes. J. Periodontol., 45:410, 1974.
36. Cantor, M. T., and Stahl, S. S.: The effects of various interdental stimulators upon the keratinization of the interdental col. Periodontics, 3:243, 1965.
37. Cantor, M. T., and Stahl, S. S.: Interdental col tissue responses to the use of a water pressure cleansing device. J. Periodontol., 40:292, 1969.
38. Carter, S. B.: The masticatory mucosa and its response to brushing: findings in the Merion rat, Meriones libycus, at different ages. Br. Dent. J., 101:76, 1956.
39. Castenfelt, T.: Toothbrushing and massage in periodontal disease. An experimental clinical histologic study. Stockholm, Nordisk Rotegravyr, 1952, p. 109.
40. Charters, W. J.: Eliminating mouth infections with the toothbrush and other stimulating instruments. Dent. Digest, 38:130, 1932.
41. Chilton, N. W., Didio, A., and Rothner, J. T.: Comparison of the clinical effectiveness of an electric and a standard toothbrush in normal individuals. J. Am. Dent. Assoc., 64:777, 1962.
42. Cohen, D. W., et al.: A comparison of bacterial plaque disclosants in periodontal disease. J. Periodontol., 43:333, 1972.
43. Conroy, C. W.: Comparison of automatic and hand toothbrushes: cleaning effectiveness. J. Am. Dent. Assoc., 70:921, 1965.
44. Crumley, P. J., and Sumner, C. F.: Effectiveness of a water pressure cleansing device. Periodontics, 3:193, 1965.
45. De la Rosa, M. R., Guerra, J. Z., Johnston, D. A., and Radike, A. W.: Plaque growth and removal with daily toothbrushing. J. Periodontol., 50:661, 1979.
46. Derbyshire, J. C.: Methods of achieving effective hygiene of the mouth. Dent. Clin. North Am., 8:231, 1964.
47. Dudding, N. J., et al.: Patient reactions to brushing teeth with water, dentifrice, or salt and soda. J. Periodontol., 31:386, 1960.
48. Elliot, J. R.: A comparison of the effectiveness of a standard and an electric toothbrush. J. Periodontol., 34:375, 1963.
49. Elliot, J. R., Bowers, G. M., Clemmer, B. A., and Rovelstad, G. H.: A comparison of selected oral hygiene devices in dental plaque removal. J. Periodontol., 43:217, 1972.
50. Engelmayer, H., and Lang, N. P.: Mundpflegegewohnheiten beieiner Gruppe von Schweizer Wehrmännern im Alter von 28 bis 32 Jahren. Schweiz. Mschr. Zahnheilk., 89:1103, 1979.
51. Eriksen, H. M., and Gjermo, P.: Incidence of stained tooth surfaces in students using chlorhexidine-containing dentifrices. Scand. J. Dent. Res., 81:533, 1973.

52. Eriksen, H. M., Gjermo, P., and Johansen, J. R.: Results from two years' use of chlorhexidine (CH)–containing dentifrices. Helv. Odontol. Acta, *17*:52, 1973.

53. Ervin, J. C., and Bucher, E. T.: Prevalence of tooth root exposure and abrasion among dental patients. Dent. Items Int., *66*:760, 1944.

54. Fanning, E. A., and Henning, F. R.: Toothbrush design and its relation to oral health. Aust. Dent. J., *12*:464, 1967.

55. Farleigh, C. M., McElhaney, J. H., and Heiser, R. A.: Toothbrushing force study. J. Dent. Res., *46*:209, 1967.

56. Felix, J. A., Rosen, S., and App, G. R.: Detection of bacteremia after the use of an oral irrigation device in subjects with periodontitis. J. Periodontol., *42*:785, 1971.

57. Fine, D. H., and Baumhammers, A.: Effect of water pressure irrigation on stainable material on the teeth. J. Periodontol., *41*:468, 1970.

58. Finkelstein, P., and Grossman, E.: The effectiveness of dental floss in reducing gingival inflammation. J. Dent. Res., *58*:1034, 1979.

59. Flötra, L.: Different modes of chlorhexidine application and related local side effects. J. Periodont. Res., *8*(Suppl. 12):41, 1973.

60. Flötra, L., et al.: A four-month study on the effect of chlorhexidine mouth washes on 50 soldiers. Scand. J. Dent. Res., *80*:10, 1972.

61. Fones, A. C.: Mouth Hygiene. 4th ed. Philadelphia, Lea & Febiger, 1934, p. 300.

62. Friedman, L., et al.: Bacterial plaque disclosure survey. J. Periodontol., *45*:435, 1974.

63. Gillette, W. B., and Van House, R. L.: Ill effects of improper oral hygiene procedures. J. Am. Dent. Assoc., *101*:476, 1980.

64. Gilson, C. M., Charbeneau, G. T., and Hill, H. C.: A comparison of physical properties of several soft toothbrushes. J. Michigan Dent. Assoc., *51*:347, 1969.

65. Gjermo, P.: Chlorhexidine in dental practice. J. Clin. Periodontol., *1*:143, 1974.

66. Gjermo, P., and Flötra, L.: The plaque-removing effect of dental floss and toothpicks: a group comparison study. J. Periodont. Res., *4*:170, 1969.

67. Gjermo, P., and Flötra, L.: The effect of different methods of interdental cleaning. J. Periodont. Res., *5*:230, 1970.

68. Gjermo, P., and Rölla, G.: The plaque-inhibiting effect of chlorhexidine-containing dentifrices. Scand. J. Dent. Res., *79*:126, 1971.

69. Gjermo, P., Baastad, K. L., and Rölla, G.: The plaque-inhibiting capacity of 11 antibacterial compounds. J. Periodont. Res., *5*:102, 1970.

70. Glass, R. L.: A clinical study of hand and electric toothbrushing. J. Periodontol., *36*:322, 1965.

71. Glavind, L.: Effect of monthly professional mechanical tooth cleaning on periodontal health in adults. J. Clin. Periodontol., *4*:100, 1977.

72. Glickman, I., Petralis, R., and Marks, R.: The effect of powered toothbrushing plus interdental stimulation upon the severity of gingivitis. J. Periodontol., *35*:519, 1964.

73. Glickman, I., Petralis, R., and Marks, R.: The effect of powered toothbrushing and interdental stimulation upon microscopic inflammation and surface keratinization of the interdental gingiva. J. Periodontol., *36*:108, 1965.

74. Goldman, H. M.: The effect of single and multiple toothbrushing in the cleansing of the normal and periodontally involved dentition. Oral Surg., *9*:203, 1956.

75. Gravelle, H. R., Shackelford, N. F., and Lovett, J. T.: The oral hygiene of high school students as affected by three different educational programs. J. Public Health Dent., *27*:91, 1967.

76. Gray, P. G., et al.: Adult dental health in England and Wales in 1968. London, H.M.S.O., 1970.

77. Greene, J. C.: Oral health care for the prevention and control of periodontal disease—review of literature. World Workshop in Periodontics, Ann Arbor, Michigan, June 6–9, 1966, p. 415.

78. Hansen, F., Gjermo, P., and Eriksen, H. M.: The effect of a chlorhexidine-containing gel on oral cleanliness and gingival health in young adults. J. Clin. Periodontol., *2*:153, 1975.

79. Harrington, J. H., and Terry, I. A.: Automatic and hand toothbrushing abrasion studies. J. Am. Dent. Assoc., *68*:343, 1964.

80. Harvey, R. F.: Clinical impressions of a new antibiotic in periodontics: spiramycine. J. Can. Dent. Assoc., *27*:576, 1961.

81. Hefferren, J. J.: A laboratory method of assessment of dentifrice abrasivity. J. Dent. Res., *55*:563, 1976.

82. Henschke, B., Lange, D. E., and Vahl, J.: Vergleichende raster-elektronenmikroskopische Untersuchungen von Zahnbürsten mit Kunststoff- und Naturborsten. Dtsch. Zahnärztl. Z., *33*:220, 1978.

83. Hill, H. C., Levi, P. A., and Glickman, I.: The effects of waxed and unwaxed dental floss on interdental plaque accumulation and interdental gingival health. J. Periodontol., *44*:411, 1973.

84. Hine, M. K.: The use of the toothbrush in the treatment of periodontitis. J. Am. Dent. Assoc., *41*:158, 1950.

85. Hine, M. K.: Toothbrush. Int. Dent. J., *6*:15, 1956.

86. Hiniker, J. J., and Forscher, B. K.: The effect of toothbrush type on gingival health. J. Periodontol., *25*:40, 1954.

87. Hirschfeld, I.: The toothbrush, its use and abuse. Dent. Items Int., *3*:833, 1931.

88. Hoover, D. R., and Lefkowitz, W.: Reduction of gingivitis by toothbrushing. J. Periodontol., *36*:193, 1965.

89. Hoover, D. R., Robinson, H. B. G., and Billingsley, A.: The comparative effectiveness of the Water-Pik in a noninstructed population. J. Periodontol., *39*:43, 1968.

90. Johansen, J. R., Gjermo, P., and Eriksen, H. M.: A longitudinal study on the effect of chlorhexidine containing dentifrices. J. Periodont. Res. *10*(Suppl.):36, 1972.

91. Keller, S. E., and Manson-Hing, L. R.: Clearance studies of proximal tooth surfaces. Part II. In vivo removal of interproximal plaque. Ala. J. Med. Sci. *6*:266, 1969.

92. Keller, S. E., and Manson-Hing, L. R.: Clearance studies of proximal tooth surfaces. Part III and IV. In vivo removal of interproximal plaque. Ala. J. Med. Sci., *6*:399, 1969.

93. Kelner, R. M., Wahl, B. R., Deasy, M. J., and Formicola, A. J.: Gingival inflammation as related to frequency of plaque removal. J. Periodontol., *45*:303, 1974.

94. Keyes, P. H., and McCabe, R. M.: The potential of various compounds to suppress microorganisms in plaques produced in vitro by streptococcus or an Actinomycete. J. Am. Dent. Assoc., *86*:396, 1973.

95. Keyes, P. H., et al.: Dispersion of dextranous bacterial plaques on human teeth with dextranase. J. Am. Dent. Assoc., *82*:136, 1971.

96. Kitchin, P.: The prevalence of tooth root exposure and the relation of the extent of such exposure to the degree of abrasion in different age classes. J. Dent. Res., *20*:565, 1941.

97. Koch, G., and Lindhe, J.: The effect of supervised oral hygiene on the gingiva of children. The effect of toothbrushing. Odont. Rev., *16*:327, 1965.

98. Krájewski, J., Giblin, J., and Gargiulo, A. W.: Evaluation of the water pressure cleansing device as an adjunct to periodontal treatment. Periodontics, *2*:76, 1964.

99. Kristofferson, T.: Periodontal conditions in Norwegian soldiers. An epidemiological and experimental study. Scand. J. Dent. Res., *78*:34, 1970.

100. Lainson, P. A., Berquist, J. J., and Fraleigh, C. M.: A longitudinal study of pulsating water pressure cleansing devices. J. Periodontol., *43*:444, 1972.

101. Lang, N. P., Cumming, B. R., and Löe, H.: Toothbrushing frequency as it relates to plaque development and gingival health. J. Periodontol., *44*:396, 1973.

102. Lang, N. P., Ostergaard, E. Q., and Löe, H.: A fluorescent plaque disclosing agent. J. Periodont. Res., *7*:59, 1972.

103. Lange, D. E.: Ueber den Einfluss verschiedener Zahnbürstentypen auf die Gingivaober fläche. Zahnärztl. Mitt., *12*:729, 1977.

104. Larato, D., Stahl, S., Brown, R., Jr., and Witkin, G.: The effect of a prescribed method of toothbrushing on the fluctuation of marginal gingivitis. J. Periodontol., *40*:142, 1960.

105. Lefkowitz, W., and Robinson, H. B. G.: Effectiveness of automatic and hand brushes in removing dental plaque and debris. J. Am. Dent. Assoc., *65*:351, 1962.

106. Less, W.: Mechanics of teaching plaque control. Dent. Clin. North Am., *16*:647, 1972.

107. Leung, S. W., and Draus, F. J.: Effect of certain enzymes on calculus deposition. J. Dent. Res., *38*:709, 1959 (abstract).

108. Lindhe, J., and Axelsson, P.: The effect of controlled oral

hygiene and topical fluoride application on caries and gingivitis in Swedish schoolchildren. Community Dent. Oral Epidemiol., *1*:96, 1973.

109. Lindhe, J., and Nyman, S.: The effect of plaque control and surgical pocket elimination on the establishment and maintenance of periodontal health. A longitudinal study of periodontal therapy in cases of advanced disease. J. Clin. Periodontol., *2*:67, 1975.

110. Lindhe, J., Axelsson, P., and Tollskog, G.: Effect of proper oral hygiene on gingivitis and dental caries in Swedish schoolchildren. Community Dent. Oral Epidemiol., *3*:150, 1975.

111. Linn, E. L.: Oral hygiene and periodontal disease: implications for dental health programs. J. Am. Dent. Assoc., *71*:39, 1965.

112. Lobene, R. R.: The effect of an automatic toothbrush on gingival health. J. Periodontol., *35*:137, 1964.

113. Lobene, R. R.: The effect of a pulsed water pressure cleaning device on oral health. J. Periodontol., *40*:667, 1969.

114. Lobene, R. R.: A clinical study of the effect of dextranase on human dental plaque. J. Am. Dent. Assoc., *82*:132, 1971.

115. Lobene, R. R., and Soparkar, P. M.: The effect of an alexidine mouthwash on human plaque and gingivitis. J. Am. Dent. Assoc., *87*:848, 1973.

116. Lobene, R. R., Brion, M., and Socransky, S. S.: Effect of erythromycin on dental plaque and plaque forming microorganisms of man. J. Periodontol., *40*:287, 1969.

117. Löe, H.: A review of the prevention and control of plaque. *In* McHugh, W. D. (ed.): Dental Plaque: A Symposium Held in the University of Dundee. Edinburgh, E. & S. Livingstone, 1969, p. 259.

118. Löe, H.: Does chlorhexidine have a place in the prophylaxis of dental disease? J. Periodont. Res., *8*(Suppl. 12):93, 1973.

119. Löe, H., and Schiött, C. R.: The effect of mouthrinses and topical application of chlorhexidine on the development of dental plaque and gingivitis in man. J. Periodont. Res., *5*:79, 1970.

120. Löe, H., Theilade, E., and Jensen, S. B.: Experimental gingivitis in man. J. Periodontol., *36*:177, 1965.

121. Löe, H., Schiött, C. R., Glavind, L., and Karring, T.: Two years oral use of chlorhexidine in man. I. General design and clinical effects. J. Periodont. Res., *11*:135, 1976.

122. Löe, H., et al.: Experimental gingivitis in man. III. The influences of antibiotics on gingival plaque development. J. Periodont. Res., *2*:282, 1967.

123. Loesche, W. J.: Chemotherapy of dental plaque infections. Oral Sci. Rev., *9*:65, 1976.

124. Loesche, W. J., and Nafe, D.: Reduction of supragingival plaque accumulations in institutionalized Down's syndrome patients by periodic treatment with topical kanamycin. Arch. Oral Biol., *18*:1131, 1973.

125. Loesche, W. J., Murray, R. J., and Mellberg, J. R.: The effect of topical fluoride on percentage of *Streptococcus mutans* and *Streptococcus sanguis* in interproximal plaque samples. Caries Res., *7*:283, 1973.

126. Loesche, W. J., et al.: Effect of topical kanamycin sulfate in plaque accumulation. J. Am. Dent. Assoc., *83*:1063, 1971.

127. Loesche, W. J., et al.: Effect of topical acidulated phosphate fluoride on percentage of *Streptococcus mutans* and *Streptococcus sanguis* in plaque. II. Pooled occlusal and pooled approximal samples. Caries Res., *9*:139, 1975.

128. Lozdan, J., et al.: The use of nitrimidazine in the treatment of acute ulcerative gingivitis. A double-blind controlled trial. Br. Dent. J., *130*:294, 1971.

129. Lyons, H.: Fiction and facts in periodontology: an appraisal. J. Am. Dent. Assoc., *39*:513, 1949.

130. MacKenzie, I. C., Nuki, K., Löe, H., and Schiött, C. R.: Two years oral use of chlorhexidine in man. V. Effects on stratum corneum of oral mucosa. J. Periodont. Res., *11*:165, 1976.

131. Manhold, B. S., Manhold, J. H., and Weisinger, E.: A study of total oral debris clearance. J. New Jersey State Dent. Soc., *38*:64, 1967.

132. Manhold, J. H.: Gingival tissue health with hand and power brushing: a retrospective with corroborative studies. J. Periodontol., *38*:23, 1967.

133. Manhold, J. H., Jr., Parker, L. A., and Manhold, B. S.: Efficacy of a commercial mouthwash: in vivo study. N.Y. J. Dent., *32*:165, 1962.

134. Manly, R. S., and Brudevold, F.: Relative abrasiveness of natural and synthetic toothbrush bristles on cementum and dentin. J. Am. Dent. Assoc., *55*:779, 1957.

135. Manly, R. S., Wiren, J., Manly, P. J., and Keene, R. C.: A method for measurement of abrasion of dentin by toothbrush and dentifrice. J. Dent. Res., *44*:533, 1965.

136. Marthaler, T. M.: Caries inhibition after seven years of unsupervised use of an amine fluoride dentifrice. Br. Dent. J., *124*:510, 1968.

137. McConnel, D., and Conroy, C. W.: Comparisons of abrasion produced by a stimulated manual versus a mechanical toothbrush. J. Dent. Res., *46*:1022, 1967.

138. McKendrick, A. J. W., Barbenel, L. M. H., and McHugh, W. D.: A two year comparison of hand and electric toothbrushes. J. Periodont. Res., *3*:224, 1968.

139. McKendrick, A. J. W., Barbenel, L. M. H., and McHugh, W. D.: The influence of time of examination, eating, smoking, and frequency of brushing on the oral debris index. J. Periodont. Res., *5*:205, 1970.

140. Mikkelsen, L., Jensen, S. B., Schiött, C. R., and Löe, H.: Studies on human plaque—Streptococci after two years of oral chlorhexidine hygiene. I.A.D.R., Scand. Div., Abstr. No. *23*:992, 1973.

141. Mitchell, D. F., and Holmes, L. A.: Topical antibiotic control of dentogingival plaque. J. Periodontol., *36*:202, 1965.

142. Mohammed, C.: Dental plaque removed by floss. J. New Jersey Dent. Soc., *36*:419, 1965.

143. Müller, E., et al.: The effect of two oral antiseptics on early calculus formation. Helv. Odontol. Acta, *6*:42, 1962.

144. Newman, M. G., Chaconas, S., and Newman, S. L.: Effect of oxygenating agents on the periodontium of orthodontic patients. J. Orthodont., *73*:108, 1978.

144a. Niederman, R., and Sullivan, T. M.: Oral hygiene skill achievement index. I. J. Periodontol., *52*:143, 1981.

145. Nuki, K., Schlenker, R., Löe, H., and Schiött, C. R.: Two years oral use of chlorhexidine in man. VI. Effect on oxidative enzymes in oral epithelia. J. Periodont. Res., *11*:172, 1976.

146. Nyman, S., Rosling, B., and Lindhe, J.: Effect of professional tooth cleaning on healing after periodontal surgery. J. Clin. Periodontol., *2*:80, 1975.

147. O'Leary, T. J., Drake, R. B., and Naylor, J. E.: The Plaque Control Record. J. Periodontol., *43*:38, 1972.

148. O'Leary, T. J., Shafer, W. G., Swenson, H. M., and Nesler, D. C.: Possible penetration of crevicular tissue from oral hygiene procedures. II. Use of the toothbrush. J. Periodontol., *41*:163, 1970.

149. O'Leary, T. J., Shafer, W. G., Swenson, H. M., Nesler, D. C., and Van Dorn, P. R.: Possible penetration of crevicular tissue from oral hygiene procedures. I. Use of oral irrigation devices. J. Periodontol., *41*:158, 1970.

150. O'Rourke, J. T.: The relation of the physical character of the diet to the health of the periodontal tissues. Am. J. Orthod., *33*:687, 1947.

151. Ostrolenk, M., and Weiss, W.: Effect of mouthwashes on the oral flora. Dent. Abstr., *5*:51, 1960.

152. Quigley, G. A., and Hein, J. W.: Comparative cleansing efficacy of manual and power brushing. J. Am. Dent. Assoc., *65*:26, 1962.

153. Ramfjord, S. P., Morrison, E. C., Burgett, I. G., Nissle, R. R., Shick, R. A., and Zann, G. J.: Oral hygiene and maintenance of periodontal support. J. Periodontol., *53*:26, 1982.

154. Reddy, J., and Salkin, L. M.: The effect of a urea peroxide rinse on dental plaque and gingivitis. J. Periodontol., *47*:607, 1976.

155. Robertson, N. A. E., and Wade, A. B.: Effect of filament diameter and density in toothbrushes. J. Periodont. Res., *7*:346, 1972.

156. Robinson, H. B. G.: Individualizing dentifrices: the dentist's responsibility. J. Am. Dent. Assoc., *79*:633, 1969.

157. Robinson, H. B. G., and Hoover, P. R.: The comparative effectiveness of a pulsating oral irrigator as an adjunct in maintaining oral health. J. Periodontol., *42*:37, 1971.

158. Robinson, H. B. G., and Kitchin, P. C.: The effect of massage with the toothbrush on keratinization of the gingiva. Oral Surg., *1*:1042, 1948.

159. Rosling, B., Nyman, S., and Lindhe, J.: The effect of

systematic plaque control on bone regeneration in infrabony pockets. J. Clin. Periodontol., *3*:38, 1976.
160. Rosling, B., Nyman, S., Lindhe, J., and Jern, B.: The healing potential of periodontal tissues following different techniques of periodontal surgery in plaque-free dentitions. A 2-year clinical study. J. Clin. Periodontol., *3*:233, 1976.
161. Sanders, W. E., and Robinson, H. B. G.: The effect of toothbrushing on deposition of calculus. J. Periodontol., *33*:386, 1962.
162. Sangnes, G.: Traumatization of teeth and gingiva related to habitual tooth cleaning procedures. J. Clin. Periodontol., *3*:94, 1976.
162a. Sangnes, G., and Gjermo, P.: Prevalence of oral soft and hard tissue lesions related to mechanical tooth cleaning procedures. Community Dent. Oral Epidemiol., *4*:77, 1976.
163. Saxer, U. P., and Mühlemann, H. R.: Motivation und Aufklärung. Schweiz. Mschr. Zahnheilk., *85*:905, 1975.
164. Saxer, U. P., and Schmid, M. O.: The plaque inhibiting effect of chlorhexidine lozenges. J. Western Soc. Periodontol., *24*:56, 1976.
165. Saxton, C. A.: The effects of dentifrices on the appearance of the tooth surface observed with the scanning electron microscope. J. Periodont. Res., *11*:74, 1976.
166. Schiött, C. R., Briner, W. W., and Löe, H.: Two years oral use of chlorhexidine in man. II. The effect on the salivary bacterial flora. J. Periodont. Res., *11*:145, 1976.
167. Schiött, C. R., Löe, H., and Briner, W. W.: Two years oral use of chlorhexidine in man. IV. Effect of various medical parameters. J. Periodont. Res., *11*:158, 1976.
168. Schiött, C. R., Briner, W. W., Kirkland, J. J., and Löe, H.: Two years oral use of chlorhexidine in man. III. Changes in sensitivity of the salivary flora. J. Periodont. Res., *11*:153, 1976.
169. Schmid, M. O., and Cuvilovic, Z.: Die Wirkung von Instruktion und Motivation auf die Mundhygiene. Schweiz. Mschr. Zahnheilk., *85*:457, 1975.
170. Schmid, M. O., Balmelli, O., and Saxer, U. P.: The plaque-removing effect of a toothbrush, dental floss and a toothpick. J. Clin. Periodontol., *3*:157, 1976.
171. Schmid, M. O., Schait, A., and Mühlemann, H. R.: Effect of a zinc chloride mouthrinse on calculus deposits formed on foils. Helv. Odontol. Acta, *17*:22, 1974.
172. Schmid, M. O., Zive, I., and Perry, D.: Cleaning effect of four different types of dental floss. J. Dent. Res., *60*(Suppl. A):341, 1981 (abstract).
173. Schroeder, H. E.: Formation and Inhibition of Dental Calculus. Berne, Hans Huber Publishers, 1969.
174. Schroeder, H. E., Marthaler, T. M., and Mühlemann, H. R.: Effect of some potential inhibitors on early calculus formation. Helv. Odontol. Acta, *6*:6, 1962.
175. Sconyers, J. R., Crawford, J. J., and Moriarty, J. D.: Study of bacteremia following toothbrushing using sensitive culture methods. I.A.D.R., Abstr. No. 757, 1971.
176. Sheiham, A.: Dental cleanliness and chronic periodontal disease: studies in British populations. Br. Dent. J., *129*:413, 1970.
177. Sheiham, A.: Prevention and control of periodontal disease. International Conference on Research in the Biology of Periodontal Disease. Chicago, June 12–15, 1977, p. 324.
178. Smith, T. S.: Anatomic and physiologic conditions governing the use of the toothbrush. J. Am. Dent. Assoc., *27*:874, 1940.
179. Smith, W. A., and Ash, M. M.: Effectiveness of an electric toothbrush. I.A.D.R., Abstr. No. 207, 1963.
180. Spolsky, V. W., and Forsyth, A. B.: Effects of alexidine mouthwash on plaque and gingivitis after six months. J. Dent. Res., *56*:805, 1977.
181. Spolsky, V. W., et al.: The effect of an antimicrobial mouthwash on dental plaque and gingivitis in young adults. J. Periodontol., *46*:685, 1975.
182. Stahl, S. S., and Goldman, H. M.: The incidence of gingivitis among a sample of Massachusetts school children. Oral Surg., *6*:707, 1953.
183. Stahl, S. S., Wachtel, N., DeCastro, C., and Pelletier, G.: The effect of toothbrushing on the keratinization of the gingiva. J. Periodontol., *24*:20, 1953.
184. Stanmeyer, W. R.: A measure of tissue response to frequency of toothbrushing. J. Periodontol., *28*:17, 1957.
185. Stewart, G. G.: Mucinase—a possible means of reducing calculus formation. J. Periodontol., *23*:85, 1952.
186. Stillman, P. R.: A philosophy of the treatment of periodontal disease. Dent. Digest, *38*:314, 1932.
187. Stookey, G. K., and Muhler, J. C.: Laboratory studies concerning the enamel and dentin abrasion properties of common dentifrice polishing agents. J. Dent. Res., *47*:524, 1968.
188. Strålfors, A., Thilander, H., and Bergenholtz, A.: Simultaneous inhibition of caries and periodontal disease in hamsters by disinfection, toothbrushing or phosphate addition. Arch. Oral Biol., *12*:1367, 1967.
189. Suomi, J. D.: Periodontal disease and oral hygiene in an institutionalized population: report of an epidemiology study. J. Periodontol., *40*:5, 1969.
190. Suomi, J. D., Smith, L. W., Chang, J. J., and Barbano, J. O.: Study of the effect of different prophylaxis frequencies on the periodontium of young adults. J. Periodontol., *44*:406, 1973.
191. Suomi, J. D., Greene, J. C., Vermillion, J. R., Doyle, J., Chang, J. J., and Leatherwood, E. E.: The effect of controlled oral hygiene procedures on the progression of periodontal disease in adults: results after third and final year. J. Periodontol., *42*:152, 1971.
192. Suomi, J. D., et al.: The effect of controlled oral hygiene procedures on the progression of periodontal disease in adults: results after two years. J. Periodontol., *40*:416, 1969.
193. Symposium on chlorhexidine in the prophylaxis of dental diseases. J. Periodont. Res., Suppl. No. 12, 1973.
194. Tamimi, H. A., Thomassen, P. R., and Moser, E. H., Jr.: Bacteremia study using a water irrigation device. J. Periodontol., *40*:424, 1969.
195. Todd, J. E., and Whitworth, A.: Adult Dental Health in Scotland, 1972. London, H.M.S.O., 1974.
196. Toto, P. D., and Farchione, A.: Clinical evaluation of an electrically powered toothbrush in home periodontal therapy. J. Periodontol., *32*:249, 1961.
197. Toto, P. D., Evans, C. L., and Sawinski, V. J.: Effects of water jet rinse and toothbrushing on oral hygiene. J. Periodontol., *40*:296, 1969.
198. Toto, P. D., Goljan, K. R., Evans, J. A., and Sawinski, V. J.: A study on the uninstructed use of an electric brush. J. Am. Dent. Assoc., *72*:904, 1966.
199. Turesky, S., Gilmore, N. D., and Glickman, I.: Calculus inhibition by topical application of the chloromethyl analogue of victamin C. J. Periodontol., *38*:142, 1967.
200. Turesky, S., Gilmore, N. D., and Glickman, I.: Reduced plaque formation by the chloromethyl analogue of victamin C. J. Periodontol., *41*:41, 1970.
201. Villa, P.: Degree of calculus inhibition by habitual toothbrushing. Helv. Odontol. Acta, *12*:31, 1968.
202. Volpe, A. R., et al.: Antimicrobial control of bacterial plaque and calculus and the effects of these agents on oral flora. J. Dent. Res., *48*:832, 1969.
203. Waerhaug, J.: The interdental brush and its place in operative and crown and bridge dentistry. J. Oral Rehabil., *3*:107, 1976.
204. Wasserman, B. H., Mandel, I. D., and Levy, B. M.: In vitro calcification of dental calculus. J. Periodontol., *29*:144, 1958.
205. Williford, J. W., Johns, C., Muhler, J. C., and Stookey, G. K.: Report of a study demonstrating improved oral health through education. J. Dent. Child., *34*:183, 1967.
206. Yankell, S. L., et al.: Effects of chlorhexidine and four antimicrobial compounds on plaque, gingivitis and staining in beagle dogs. J. Dent. Res., *61*:1089, 1982.
207. Zander, H. A.: The effect of penicillin dentifrice on caries incidence in schoolchildren. J. Am. Dent. Assoc., *40*:569, 1950.

chapter forty-five

Treatment of Uncomplicated Chronic Gingivitis

Treatment	Step Three
Step One	**Causes of Failure**
Step Two	

Uncomplicated chronic gingivitis is the most common disease of the gingiva. It affects the interdental and marginal gingivae. **It should be detected in its earliest stages and treated as soon as detected** (Figs. 45–1 and 45–2). Usually painless, it is the most common cause of gingival bleeding. Failure to treat it invites destruction of the underlying periodontal tissues and premature tooth loss.

Separation of the treatment of chronic gingivitis from the scaling and root planing technique described in Chapter 43 is somewhat artificial. However, chronic gingivitis is the initial stage of periodontitis and should be treated before pockets develop.

Chronic gingivitis is always caused by local irritation. Systemic conditions may aggravate the inflammation caused by local irritants and should be appropriately dealt with (see Chapter 28–30), but *no systemic conditions by themselves cause chronic gingivitis.*

TREATMENT

Treatment should be preceded by a careful examination to detect all sources of local irritation, such as dental plaque, calculus, food impaction, overhanging or improperly con- toured restorations, or irritating removable prostheses. The teeth should be stained with disclosing solution to reveal plaque and carefully probed with the No. 17 or No. 3A explorer to locate small particles of calculus.

STEP ONE. The treatment of uncomplicated gingivitis is started by explaining the importance of plaque control and teaching the patient how to achieve it. *This gives the patient a realistic perspective regarding the treatment of gingivitis: that it includes something he must do for himself, as well as something the dentist does for him.* It also provides an opportunity to demonstrate that plaque control really benefits the gums. After the patient is instructed in plaque control, an appointment for the next visit is made.

STEP TWO. The condition of the gums is reviewed with the patient, and improvement is pointed out. The teeth are stained with disclosing solution and plaque control is reviewed, with the patient demonstrating the various procedures used.

The teeth are scaled to remove all deposits, and all tooth surfaces are polished with a paste of fine pumice.

Polishing is an important preventive measure against the recurrence of gingivitis. Plaque, the

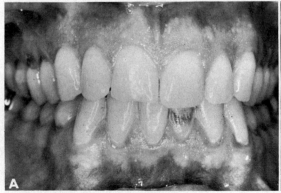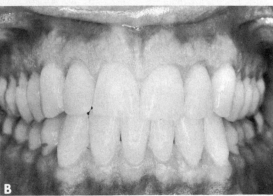

Figure 45–1 Uncomplicated Chronic Marginal Gingivitis. *A,* Before treatment. *B,* After treatment.

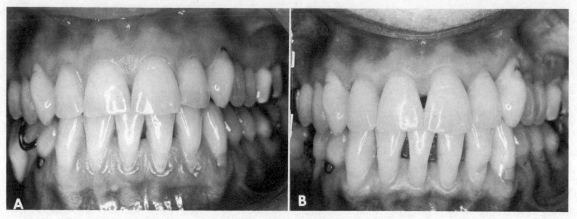

Figure 45–2 Chronic Marginal Gingivitis and Recession. *A,* Before treatment. *B,* After treatment.

most important cause of gingivitis and the initial stage in the formation of calculus, tends to form more readily on rough surfaces.

Other sources of local irritation listed earlier should also be eliminated.

STEP THREE. The gingivae are examined and plaque control is reviewed. Special attention is given to areas of persistent inflammation; this usually entails rescaling and emphasizing patient technique for cleansing the areas.

These procedure are repeated at subsequent visits until the gingivae are healthy. The patient is then placed on "recall," **with a careful explanation of the reasons for periodic visits and the importance of the care given the mouth in the intervening periods.**

CAUSES OF FAILURE

The treatment of chronic gingivitis should present no problems. However, if disease persists, the following are the most likely causes:

1. Failure to remove minute particles of calculus, often just beneath the cemento-enamel junction.

2. Failure to polish the tooth surfaces after deposits are removed.

3. Failure to eliminate sources of irritation other than deposits on the teeth. Food impaction is one of the frequently overlooked factors.

4. Inadequate plaque control because of one or more of the following: (a) insufficient patient instruction, (b) dismissal of the patient before he demonstrates competence in plaque control, or (c) lack of patient cooperation.

5. A tendency to seek a remote systemic etiology for persistent gingivitis caused by overlooked local irritants.

6. Dependence upon vitamins, mouthwashes, and topical application of drugs, particularly hormones, antibiotics, and oxidizing agents. *Except for topical anesthetics, drugs serve no significant purpose in the treatment of chronic gingivitis.*

chapter forty-six

Antimicrobial Agents in Periodontal Therapy

Systemic Administration of Antibiotics	Local Administration of Antibiotics and
Tetracyclines	Antimicrobials
Metronidazole	Antibiotics
Penicillin	Fluorides
Erythromycin	Other Agents
Spiramycin	**Treatment of Juvenile Periodontitis**

Antimicrobial agents have been used in periodontal therapy since early times.[31, 32, 59] In the last two decades, reports that systemically administered antibiotics are excreted via the saliva and/or the gingival fluid have triggered great interest in the subject.[1, 7] It has been shown in experimental animals that the systemic administration of antibiotics results in changes in the plaque flora, reduces gingivitis, and slows bone loss.[30, 36, 55] In humans, however, the use of antibiotics may present problems, such as the development of resistant strains of organisms and allergic manifestations.[16]

Antimicrobial agents can be used in patients with periodontitis for the following purposes:

1. In the treatment of systemic complications of the acute periodontal abscess or acute necrotizing ulcerative gingivitis. These topics are covered in Chapters 41 and 42.

2. For antibiotic coverage of patients with medical problems in order to prevent systemic complications. This is dealt with in Chapter 36.

3. As a mouthrinse used for plaque control and the prevention of gingivitis. This is discussed in Chapter 44.

4. As an adjunct in the treatment of the periodontal pocket. This use is covered in this chapter.

In conjunction with the pocket treatment, antimicrobial agents may be of importance in one or more of the following ways:

1. *Antimicrobials may be used as adjuncts to non-surgical therapy.* Antimicrobials may be valuable in reaching and killing bacteria that cannot be removed by scaling and curettage: e.g., bacteria that have penetrated into the tissues in advanced periodontitis[46] or localized juvenile periodontitis[9] or bacteria located on the root surface in inaccessible areas such as tortuous furcations or very deep pockets. The use of antimicrobials in conjunction with non-surgical therapy may reduce or eliminate the indications for periodontal surgery. Antimicrobials may also be useful in increasing the interval between two recall maintenance visits. Once bacteria have been removed from the pocket, it will be several weeks before a mature, aggressive plaque repopulates the pocket.[43] The use of antimicrobials during the initial scaling visit or subsequently by the patient may prolong this interval.

2. *Antimicrobials may enhance the success of new attachment and bone regenerating procedures.* The reinfection of the pocket area is probably one of the major factors working against reattachment.[8] The maintenance of a sterile area may favor the new attachment of the tissues and is also likely to improve the chances for success of osseous and nonosseous grafts.

The rationale for the use of antibiotics in the treatment of periodontal disease should be the same as for any infection. The causative microorganism(s) should be identified and the most effective agent selected. Although this appears simple, the difficulty lies primarily in the identification of the *specific etiologic microorganism(s)* rather than those simply *associated* with various periodontal disorders.[11]

According to Gibson, an *ideal* antibiotic for use in the prevention and treatment of periodontal disease should (1) act specifically on periodontal pathogens, (2) not be allergenic or toxic, (3) maintain activity in the oral environment or tissue for long periods, (4) not be in general use for treatment of other diseases, and (5) not be prohibitively expensive.[16]

Antibiotics have been evaluated both systemically and topically as plaque reducing agents. With some antibiotics the topical approach may be dangerous, since this is more likely to result in the development of hypersensitivity (see Chapter 24). The systemic route of administration provides bacteriostatic or bactericidal levels of some antibiotics in body fluids, including saliva and crevicular fluid.

The potential usefulness of antimicrobial agents in relation to pocket therapy requires considerably more investigation and development before such therapies can become a clinical reality.

SYSTEMIC ADMINISTRATION OF ANTIBIOTICS

The following antibiotics have been investigated:

TETRACYCLINES. Numerous studies have been made of the effect of tetracyclines on clinical and bacteriologic parameters of periodontal disease since Bader and Goldhaber demonstrated their excretion via the gingival sulcus.[1] Tetracyclines reach a concentration in the gingival sulcus 2 to 10 times that in the blood.[19]

Systemic tetracycline reduces plaque and gingival inflammation in dogs[36] and reduces bone loss in dogs[57] and rats.[55] Studies in humans have shown that the use of tetracycline as an adjunct to scaling and root planing enhances healing[36, 48] but does not result in an important gain of attachment.[36] One long-term study of patients taking low doses (250 mg per day for 2 to 7 years) showed the persistence of deep pockets that did not bleed on probing and contained high proportions of tetracycline-resistant gram-negative rods, mostly *Fusobacterium nucleatum;* after the antibiotic was discontinued, the flora returned to that characteristic of the disease.[29] A study in dogs reported that after 2 years of continuous systemic administration of tetracycline the beneficial effect of reducing the rate of bone loss may be lost.[26] Another study showed that tetracycline therapy increases the frequency of organisms resistant to tetracycline and to other antibiotics.[28]

The tetracycline derivative *minocycline* has been studied by Ciancio and co-workers, who reported reductions in total bacterial counts and the complete elimination of spirochetes for periods of up to 2 months and improvement in all clinical parameters after administration of 200 mg per day for 1 week.[12] The tetracyclines currently appear to be the antibiotic most likely to be of value in the United States for the treatment of certain forms of periodontitis.

Long-term use of low doses of tetracycline (250 mg per day) has been advocated in the past. However, this no longer appears advisable, owing to the various side effects that may occur, such as development of resistant strains.

METRONIDAZOLE. This drug is active against anaerobic organisms and has been used successfully in England in acute necrotizing ulcerative gingivitis.[14, 39, 47] Studies in experimental animals[22] and in humans[33, 35, 38] have shown the efficacy of metronidazole in the treatment of gingivitis and periodontitis. Administered systemically (800 to 1000 mg per day for 2 weeks), this drug suppresses the growth of anaerobic flora, including spirochetes, and results in disappearance of the clinical and histopathologic signs of periodontitis.[33, 35] Long-term studies to explore the effect of discontinuing the use of metronidazole are needed.

PENICILLIN. Penicillin is the drug of choice for the treatment of serious infections in humans; it also induces allergic reactions and bacterial resistance. Its use in periodontal therapy does not appear justified. See Chapter 50 for a discussion on the use of penicillin after periodontal surgery.

ERYTHROMYCIN. This antibiotic presents the drawbacks described for penicillin; therefore, it is not indicated for periodontal therapy.

SPIRAMYCIN. Spiramycin is a macrolide antibiotic active against gram-positive organisms; it is excreted in high concentrations in saliva. It is used as an adjunct to periodontal treatment in Canada and Europe, but its use has not been approved in the United States. Several studies have shown promising results when spiramycin is prescribed in advanced periodontal disease, as measured by the Gingival Index, the Plaque Index, pocket depth, and crevicular fluid flow.[42] In addition, it is a safe, nontoxic drug with few and infrequent side effects and is not in general use for medical problems.[16]

LOCAL ADMINISTRATION OF ANTIBIOTICS AND ANTIMICROBIALS

ANTIBIOTICS. The local delivery of antibiotics within the periodontal pocket is considered to have excellent potential as an adjunct to traditional periodontal therapy. The following local delivery systems have been tried for different agents: dentifrices, mouthrinses, and professional administration into the pocket by means of syringes, water irrigation devices, and hollow fibers.

Mouthrinses and dentifrices are inefficient delivery systems because of the transient period of contact of the drug with the tissue and the lack of penetration into the periodontal pocket. Direct irrigation using a syringe with a blunt needle has been tried by several investigators.[8, 49] Hardy et al. found penetration of the solution to the apical portion of the pocket if the needle tip is placed 3 mm within the pocket.[21] This method of administration appears to be an excellent way to enhance the results obtained with scaling and root planing at each recall visit (Fig. 46–1).

Goodson and co-workers have suggested that tetracycline-filled hollow fibers placed into the gingival sulcus would provide therapeutic effects with less than 1/1000 the amount of tetracycline used in systemic therapy.[18] The use of tetracycline in this manner has resulted in conflicting reports relative to the elimination of spirochetes and other motile microorganisms. However, the concept of a local delivery system for antibiotics deserves further investigation.[13]

FLUORIDES. Several studies have demonstrated the bactericidal effects of fluorides against plaque bacteria.[45] Stannous fluoride has a greater bactericidal effect than neutral sodium fluoride or acidulated phosphate fluoride.[60] Studies in animal model systems have shown beneficial effects of fluorides on plaque and gingivitis.[25, 28, 41] The antibacterial effect of fluoride mouthrinses in humans has also been shown.[51, 61] Mazza et al. described the effects of direct lavage of pockets in advanced periodontitis with 1.64 per cent stannous fluoride and found it to be effective in reducing Bleeding Index scores and in delaying the repopulation of the pocket by spirochetes and motile bacteria.[40]

OTHER AGENTS. The use of daily subgingival irrigation with chlorhexidine after one scaling and root planing session was evaluated by Wieder et al.[56] They found a reduction in periodontitis still apparent 2 months after the cessation of irrigation; the treatment permitted extension of the interval between recall visits.

Keyes et al. have described a method of periodontal therapy based on patient-applied hypertonic salts in an oxidative antiseptic for controlling plaque microorganisms.[27] Several studies have been made to evaluate this treatment modality,[20, 58] but the results are as yet inconclusive.

TREATMENT OF JUVENILE PERIODONTITIS

Discussion of the treatment of juvenile periodontitis is included in this chapter because of the important role played in it by antibiotics.

The prognosis in cases of juvenile periodontitis depends on whether the disease is gener-

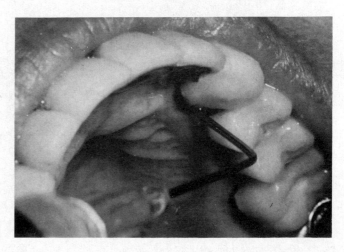

Figure 46–1 Placement of syringe into the pocket for irrigation after scaling and root planing.

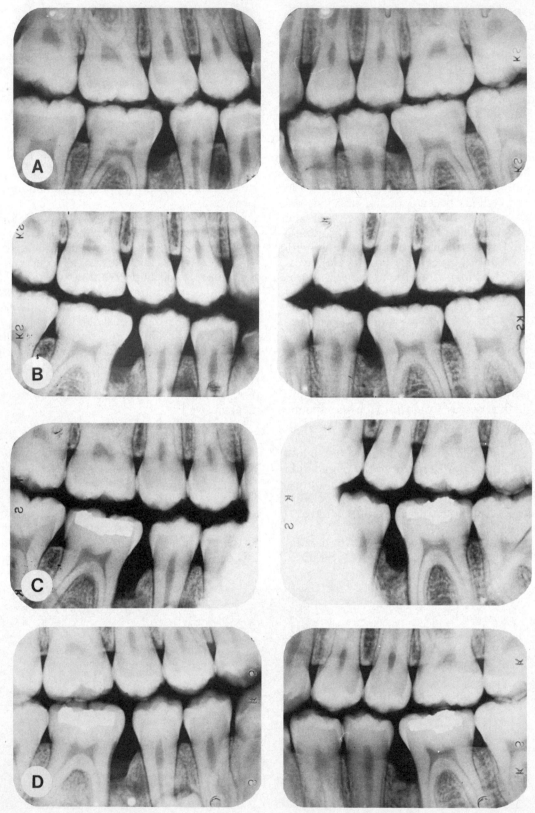

Figure 46–2 Radiographs depicting progression of the osseous lesion. *A*, January 29, 1979; *B*, August 16, 1979; *C*, February 22, 1980; *D*, May 15, 1981. Note the progressive deterioration of the osseous level. (From Barnett, M. L., and Baker, R. L.: J. Periodontol., *54*:148, 1983.)

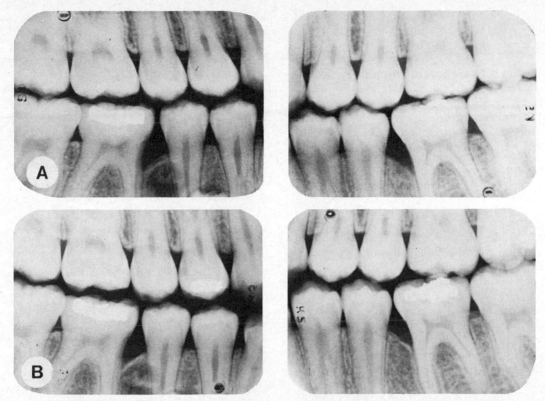

Figure 46–3 Postoperative radiographs of the patient in Figure 46–2. *A*, November 6, 1981; *B*, March 3, 1982. Treatment consisted of oral hygiene instruction; scaling and root planing concurrently with 1 gram of tetracycline per day for 2 weeks; and, finally, modified Widman flaps. (From Barnett, M. L., and Baker, R. L.: J. Periodontol., *54*:148, 1983.)

alized or localized and on the degree of destruction present at the time of examination. The generalized forms, usually associated with some systemic disease (see Chapter 22), have a worse prognosis than the localized forms. Juvenile periodontitis sometimes undergoes spontaneous remission. It is important, if possible, to obtain earlier radiographs in order to assess the stage of the disease. Numerous treatments for localized juvenile periodontitis have been attempted, with varying degrees of success:

1. Extraction. After the involved teeth, usually the first molars, have been extracted, uneventful healing ensues. The enlargement of the maxillary sinus has been mentioned as an unfavorable sequela that would make future treatment of neighboring teeth difficult.[2, 3]

2. Transplantation of developing third molars to the sockets of previously extracted first molars.[2] The developing donor tooth should have roots that are between one third and two thirds of their eventual length and should be seated in infraclusion. The transplanted tooth is splinted in place with crisscross sutures over the occlusal surface and periodontal packs.[4]

3. Standard periodontal therapy, including scaling and root planing, curettage, flap surgery with and without bone grafts, root amputations, hemisections, occlusal adjustment, and strict plaque control.[2, 5, 6, 34, 44, 50] However, the response is in general poor.

4. Frequent maintenance visits appear to be most important.[34, 44, 53, 54]

In recent years several authors have reported success using antibiotics as adjuncts to therapy. Genco et al. reported the treatment of localized juvenile periodontitis with scaling and root planing plus tetracycline (250 mg four times per day for 14 days) every 8 weeks.[15] Measurements of vertical defects were made at intervals up to 18 months after the initiation of therapy. Bone loss was stopped, and in one third of the defects there was an increase in bone level, whereas in the control group bone loss continued.

Liljenberg and Lindhe treated patients with localized juvenile periodontitis with tetracycline (250 mg four times per day for 2 weeks), modified Widman flaps, and periodic recall visits (one a month for 6 months, then every 3 months).[34] They reported that the lesions in patients with localized juvenile periodontitis healed more rapidly and more completely than similar lesions in other patients. Figures 46–2 and 46–3 show pretreatment destruction and bone repair in a patient treated by Barnett and Baker.[6]

The lack of response of juvenile periodontitis to scaling and root planing may be due to the fact that *Actinobacillus actinomycetemcomitans* is present in the tissues[9, 46] and remains after pocket therapy unless antibiotics or surgical elimination is employed.[10]

CONCLUSION

At the present time antimicrobial agents appear to be indicated for the treatment of the periodontal pocket in the following instances: (1) Stannous fluoride irrigation of the pocket in order to delay the bacterial repopulation of the pocket. This is particularly indicated in moderate and deep pockets and when access is difficult. (2) Tetracycline (250 mg four times per day for 1 to 2 weeks) or possibly minocycline or metronidazole administration as an adjunct to the treatment of juvenile periodontitis and rapidly destructive, nonresponsive forms of advanced periodontitis. The value of systemic antibiotics in enhancing the success of new attachment and bone regeneration procedures is still uncertain.

REFERENCES

1. Bader, H. I., and Goldhaber, P.: The passage of intravenously administered tetracycline into the gingival sulcus of dogs. J. Oral Therap. Pharmacol., *2*:324, 1968.
2. Baer, P. N., and Benjamin, S. D.: Periodontal disease in children and adolescents. Philadelphia, J. B. Lippincott Company, 1974.
3. Baer, P. N., and Everett, F. G.: The maxillary sinus as a problem in the therapy of periodontosis. J. Periodontol., *41*:476, 1970.
4. Baer, P. N., and Gamble, J. W.: Autogenous dental transplants as a method of treating the osseous defect in periodontosis. Oral Surg., *22*:405, 1966.
5. Baer, P. N., and Socransky, S. S.: Periodontosis: case report with long-term follow-up. Periodontal Case Reports, *1*:1, 1979.
6. Barnett, M. L., and Baker, R. L.: The formation and healing of osseous lesions in a patient with localized juvenile periodontitis. Case report. J. Periodontol., *54*:148, 1983.
7. Borzelleca, J., and Cherrick, H. M.: Excretion of drugs in saliva. J. Oral Therap. Pharmacol., *2*:180, 1965.
8. Carranza, F. A., Sr.: Experiencias clinicas sobre reinsercion. Ensayos con penicilina. Rev. Asoc. Odontol. Argent., *39*:55, 1951.
9. Carranza, F. A., Jr., Saglie, R., Newman, M. G., and Valentin, P.: Scanning and transmission electron microscopic study of tissue-invading microorganisms in localized juvenile periodontitis. J. Periodontol., in press.
10. Chrissterson, L. A., et al.: Demonstration of *Actinobacillus actinomycetemcomitans* in gingiva of localized juvenile periodontitis lesions. J. Dent. Res., *62*:198, 1983 (abstract).
11. Ciancio, S. G.: Use of antibiotics in periodontal therapy. *In* Newman, M. G., and Goodman, A. (eds.): Antibiotics in Dentistry. Chicago, Quintessence, 1983.
12. Ciancio, S. G., et al.: Clinical and microbiological evaluation of minocycline in treatment of periodontal disease. J. Dent. Res., *60*:527, 1981 (abstract).
13. Coventry, J., and Newman, H. N.: Experimental use of a slow release device employing chlorhexidine gluconate in areas of acute periodontal inflammation. J. Clin. Periodontol., *9*:129, 1982.
14. Duckworth, R., et al.: Acute ulcerative gingivitis. A double-blind controlled clinical trial of metronidazole. Br. Dent. J., *120*:599, 1966.
15. Genco, R. J., Ciancio, L. J., and Rosling, B.: Treatment of localized juvenile periodontitis. J. Dent. Res., *60*:527, 1981 (abstract).
16. Gibson, W.: Antibiotics and periodontal disease: a selective review of the literature. J. Am. Dent. Assoc., *104*:213, 1982.
17. Gold, S. I.: Combined therapy in the treatment of periodontosis: case report. Periodontal Case Reports, *1*:12, 1979.
18. Goodson, J. W., Haffajee, A., and Socransky, S. S.: Periodontal therapy by local delivery of tetracycline. J. Clin. Periodontol., *6*:83, 1979.
19. Gordon, J. M., et al.: Concentration of tetracycline in human gingival fluid after single doses. J. Clin. Periodontol., *8*:117, 1981.
20. Greenwell, H., et al.: Clinical and microbiological effectiveness of Keyes' method of oral hygiene on human periodontitis with and without surgery. J. Am. Dent. Assoc., *106*:457, 1983.
21. Hardy, J. H., Newman, H. N., and Strahan, J. D.: Direct irrigation and subgingival plaque. J. Clin. Periodontol., *9*:57, 1982.
22. Heijl, H., and Lindhe, J.: The effect of metronidazole on the development of plaque and gingivitis in the beagle dog. J. Clin. Periodontol., *6*:197, 1979.
23. Heiss, M. A., et al.: Antibiotic resistance of oral bacteria before and after administration of systemic tetracycline. J. Dent. Res., *60*:330, 1981 (abstract).
24. Hellden, L. B., Listgarten, M. A., and Lindhe, J.: The effect of tetracycline and/or scaling on human periodontal disease. J. Clin. Periodontol., *6*:222, 1979.
25. Hock, J., and Tinanoff, N.: Resolution of gingivitis in dogs following topical applications of 0.4% stannous fluoride and toothbrushing. J. Dent. Res., *58*:1652, 1979.
26. Jeffcoat, M. K., Williams, R. C., and Goldhaber, P.: Effect of tetracycline on gingival inflammation and alveolar bone resorption in beagles: an individual tooth by tooth analysis. J. Clin. Periodontol., *9*:489, 1982.
27. Keyes, P. H., Wright, W. E., and Howard, S. A.: The use of phase-contrast microscopy and chemotherapy in the diagnosis and treatment of periodontal lesions. An initial report. I and II. Quintessence Internat., *9*:51, 1978, *9*:69, 1978.
28. Keyes, P. H., Rowberry, S. A., Englander, H. A., and Fitzgerald, R. J.: Bio-assays of medicaments for the control of dento-bacterial plaque, dental caries and periodontal lesions in the Syrian hamster. J. Oral Therap. Pharmacol., *3*:157, 1966.
29. Kornman, K. S., and Karl, E. H.: The cultivable subgingival microflora of periodontitis patients on long term low dose tetracycline therapy. J. Dent. Res., *60*:604, 1981 (abstract).
30. Kornman, K. S., Caffesse, R. G., and Nasjleti, C. E.: The effects of intensive antibacterial therapy on the sulcular environment in monkeys. Changes in the bacteriology of the gingival sulcus. J. Periodontol., *51*:34, 1980.
31. Kritchevsky, B., and Seguin, P.: The pathogenesis and treatment of pyorrhea alveolaris. Dent. Cosmos, *60*:781, 1918. Translated from La Presse Medicale, Paris, May 13, 1918.
32. Krogh, H. W.: Reduction of the gingival flora preceding operation. J. Am. Dent. Assoc., *19*:659, 1932.
33. Lekovic, V., Kenney, E. B., Carranza, F. A., Jr., and Endres, B.: Effect of metronidazole on human periodontal disease. A clinical and microbiologic study. J. Periodontol., *54*:476, 1983.
34. Liljenberg, B., and Lindhe, J.: Juvenile periodontitis. Some microbiological, histopathological, and clinical characteristics. J. Clin. Periodontol., *7*:48, 1980.
35. Lindhe, J., Hiljenberg, B., Adielson, B., and Börjesson, I.: Use of metronidazole as a probe in the study of human periodontal disease. J. Clin. Periodontol., *10*:100, 1983.
36. Listgarten, M. A., Lindhe, J., and Parodi, R.: The effect of systemic antimicrobial therapy on plaque and gingivitis in dogs. J. Periodont. Res., *14*:65, 1979.

37. Loesche, W. J.: Chemotherapy of dental plaque infections. Oral Sci. Rev., *9*:65, 1976.

38. Loesche, W. J.: The treatment of periodontal patients according to the specific plaque hypothesis. *In* Carranza, F. A., Jr., and Kenney, E. B., (eds.): Prevention of Periodontal Disease. Chicago, Quintessence, 1981.

39. Lozdan, J., et al.: The use of metronidazole in the treatment of acute ulcerative gingivitis. A double-blind controlled trial. Br. Dent. J., *130*:194, 1971.

40. Mazza, J. E., Newman, M. G., and Sims, T. N.: Clinical and antimicrobial effect of stannous fluoride on periodontitis. J. Clin. Periodontol., *8*:203, 1981.

41. McDonald, J. L., Jr., Schemehorn, B. R., and Stookey, G. K.: Influence of fluoride upon plaque and gingivitis in the beagle dog. J. Dent. Res., *57*:899, 1978.

42. Mills, W. H., Thompson, G. W., and Beagrie, G. S.: Clinical evaluation of spiramycin and erythromycin in control of periodontal disease. J. Clin. Periodontol., *6*:308, 1979.

43. Mousques, T., Listgarten, M. A., and Phillips, R. W.: Effect of scaling and root planing on the composition of the human subgingival microbial flora. J. Clin. Periodontol., *15*:111, 1980.

44. Oshrain, H. I., and Kaslick, R. S.: Periodontosis—a sixteen year case report. Periodontal Case Reports, *3*:18, 1981.

45. Perry, D. A.: Fluorides and periodontal disease: a review of the literature. J. Western Soc. Periodontol., *30*:92, 1982.

46. Saglie, F. R., Carranza, F. A., Jr., Newman, M. G., Cheng, L., and Lewin, K. J.: Identification of tissue invading bacteria in human periodontal disease. J. Periodont. Res., *17*:452, 1982.

47. Shinn, D. H.: Metronidazole in acute ulcerative gingivitis. Lancet, *1*:1191, 1962.

48. Slots, J., Mashimo, P., Levine, M. J., and Genco, R. J.: Periodontal therapy in humans. I. Microbiological and clinical effects of a single course of periodontal scaling and root planing, and of adjunctive tetracycline therapy. J. Periodontol., *50*:495, 1979.

49. Soh, L. L., Newman, H. N., and Strahan, J. D.: Effects of subgingival chlorhexidine irrigation on periodontal inflammation. J. Clin. Periodontol., *9*:66, 1982.

50. Sugarman, M. M., and Sugarman, E. F.: Precocious periodontitis. a clinical entity and a treatment responsibility. J. Periodontol., *48*:397, 1977.

51. Tinanoff, N., Brady, J. M., and Gross, A.: The effect of NaF and SnF₂ mouthrinses on bacterial colonization of tooth enamel: TEM or SEM studies. Caries Res., *10*:415, 1976.

52. Tinanoff, N., Hock, J., Camosci, D., and Hellden, L.: Effect of stannous fluoride mouthrinse on dental plaque formation. J. Clin. Periodontol., *7*:232, 1980.

53. Waerhaug, J.: Plaque control in the treatment of juvenile periodontitis. J. Clin. Periodontol., *4*:29, 1977.

54. Waerhaug, J.: Subgingival plaque and loss of attachment in periodontosis as evaluated on extracted teeth. J. Periodontol., *48*:125, 1977.

55. Weiner, G. S., DeMarco, T. J., and Bissada, N. F.: Long term effects of systemic antimicrobial therapy on plaque and gingivitis in dogs. J. Periodontol., *50*:619, 1979.

56. Wieder, S. G., Newman, H. N., and Strahan, J. D.: Stannous fluoride and subgingival chlorhexidine irrigation in the control of plaque and chronic periodontitis. J. Clin. Periodontol., *10*:172, 1983.

57. Williams, R. C., et al.: Tetracycline treatment of periodontal disease in the beagle dog. I. Clinical and radiographic course over 12 months—maximal effect on rate of alveolar bone loss. J. Dent. Res., *16*:659, 1981.

58. Wolff, L. R., Bandt, C., Pihlstrom, B., and Brayer, H.: Phase contrast microscopic evaluation of subgingival plaque in combination with either conventional or antimicrobial home treatment of patients with periodontal inflammation. J. Periodont. Res., *17*:537, 1982.

59. Wright, B. L.: The treatment of pyorrhea alveolaris and its secondary systemic infections by deep muscular injections of mercury. Dent. Cosmos, *57*:1003, 1915.

60. Yoon, N. A., and Berry, C. W.: The antimicrobial effect on fluorides (acidulated phosphate, sodium and stannous) on *Actinomyces viscosus*. J. Dent. Res., *58*:1824, 1979.

61. Yoon, N. A., and Berry, C. W.: An in vivo study of the effects of fluoride (SnF₂ 0.4%, APF 1.23% and neutral NaF 0.5%) on levels of organisms resembling *Actinomyces,* gingival inflammation and plaque accumulation. J. Dent. Res., *58*:535, 1979.

62. Yoon, N. A., and Newman, M. G.: Antimicrobial effect of fluorides on *Bacteroides melaninogenicus* subspecies and *Bacteroides asaccharolyticus*. J. Clin. Periodontol., *7*:489, 1980.

Occlusal Adjustment

Occlusal therapy *is the establishment of functional relationships favorable to the periodontium by one or more of the following procedures: reshaping the teeth with grinding, dental restoration, tooth movement, tooth removal, or orthognathic surgery.* **Occlusal adjustment** (coronoplasty) is the selective reduction of occlusal areas with the primary purpose of influencing the mechanical conditions in contact situations and the neural pattern of sensory input.[24] It is a direct, permanent, and irreversible change of the occlusal scheme.[24] **There is a tendency to think of occlusal adjustment solely in a negative sense—namely, as a method of eliminating injurious occlusal forces, which indeed it should do. But its equally important purpose is to provide the functional stimulation necessary for the preservation of periodontal health, a positive dimension that occlusal adjustment adds to the practice of all phases of dentistry.**

ENVIRONMENTAL CONTROL AND THE PERIODONTIUM

THE LOCAL ENVIRONMENT OF THE PERIODONTIUM AND PERIODONTAL HEALTH. The local environment of the periodontium consists of two principal factors: (1) the saliva, with its microbial population; and (2) the occlusion. Two environmental pollutants adversely affect the periodontium: (1) dental plaque formed by oral bacteria, which leads to destructive periodontal inflammation; and (2) injurious occlusal forces, which damage the supporting periodontal tissues.

The establishment of a satisfactory local environment is essential in the treatment of periodontal disease and in the preservation of periodontal health. The urgency of controlling plaque is well recognized; occlusal adjustment to eliminate injurious forces and to create forces favorable to the periodontium is equally important.

THE RATIONALE OF OCCLUSAL ADJUSTMENT

Occlusal adjustment is based upon the premises that tissue damage and excessive tooth mobility[28, 45] caused by unfavorable occlusal forces undergo repair when the injurious forces are corrected[23] and that realigning occlusal forces by creating unobstructed functional contacts provides trophic stimulation beneficial to the periodontium, the muscles, and the temporomandibular joints.

FOR WHICH PATIENTS IS THE OCCLUSION ADJUSTED? The occlusion is adjusted for patients with evidence of microtrauma manifested in one or more of the following ways: (1) **periodontal injury** (excessive tooth mobility, angular thickening of the periodontal ligament, angular [vertical] bone destruction, infrabony pockets, some instances of furcation involvement, and migration of maxillary anterior teeth); (2) **muscular dysfunction;** and (3) **temporomandibular joint disorders.** Occlusal adjustment is also performed on individuals who complain of occlusal instability or bite discomfort following occlusal therapy.

Most people have retrusive prematurities in the permanent[3, 5, 15, 42] and deciduous[16] dentition, and prematurities in the intercuspal position (ICP) are also extremely common (Fig. 47–1, Group 1). Not all patients with occlusal prematurities have trauma from occlusion. It is assumed that trauma from occlusion is caused by repetitive parafunctional forces (bruxism, clamping, and clenching) more than

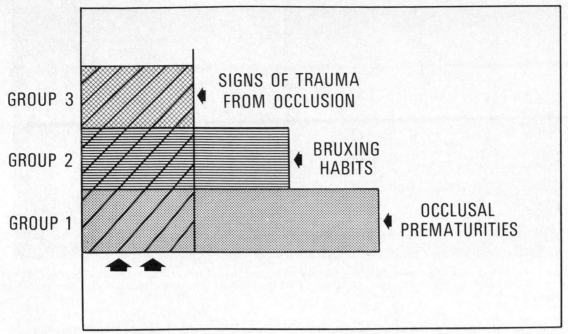

Figure 47–1 Occlusal Adjustment for Patients with Signs of Trauma from Occlusion. Group 1, Patients with occlusal prematurities. Group 2, Patients with prematurities who develop bruxing habits or abnormal function. Group 3, Patients with bruxing habits who develop trauma from occlusion. Occlusal adjustment is for patients in the cross-hatched vertical column *(double arrows)*.

by chewing and swallowing. This is because it has been estimated that teeth are in functional contact for approximately 17.5 minutes[12] in a 24-hour period, which would leave ample time for the periodontium to recover if it were injured by functional occlusal forces.

Occlusal prematurities are inciting causes of bruxism. Of the many people with occlusal prematurities, only some develop parafunctional habits (Fig. 47–1, Group 2). Bruxism* is common, but only some patients who brux develop trauma from occlusion (Fig. 47–1, Group 3).

The occlusion is adjusted for patients with occlusal prematurities who brux and present evidence of trauma from occlusion (the cross-hatched vertical column in Figure 47–1).

PREVENTIVE OCCLUSAL ADJUSTMENT. Preventive occlusal adjustment—the correction of what appear to be abnormal occlusal relationships in patients without signs of trauma from occlusion, for the ostensible purpose of preventing future damage—is not recommended. It is the tissue response in the periodontium, masticatory musculature, and temporomandibular joints that determines whether an occlusion is traumatic; the determination is not

made by the alignment of the teeth and the presence or absence of occlusal prematurities. The absence of tissue injury means that the occlusal forces are acceptable to the tissues despite the fact that the alignment and relationship of the teeth may appear abnormal. Changing the occlusion in anticipation of future injury, without any indication that it will necessarily occur, may upset the present satisfactory balance between the occlusion and the tissues. The occlusion must satisfy the needs of the periodontium, the musculature, and the temporomandibular joints, not the desires of the therapist.

WHEN TO ADJUST THE OCCLUSION IN THE SEQUENCE OF PERIODONTAL TREATMENT. We are often confronted with patients who have both inflammation and trauma from occlusion: it would be best to eliminate both at the same time. This is not always feasible, and when a choice must be made **the occlusion is usually adjusted after gingival inflammation and periodontal pockets have been eliminated, for the following reasons:**

1. Evidence related to the pathogenesis and healing aspects of trauma from occlusion[29, 30] suggests that the benefits of occlusal adjustment are not complete if inflammation is not eliminated first.

2. Teeth with periodontal disease often migrate. After the inflammation is eliminated,

---

*Used throughout the chapter to include clamping and clenching habits.

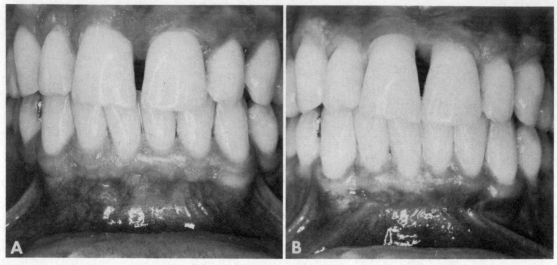

Figure 47–2 Change in Tooth Position Following Periodontal Treatment. *A*, Before treatment. Note the diastema between the maxillary central incisors. *B*, In the course of treatment the teeth return to their normal position following resolution of inflammation.

the teeth shift again, often in the direction of their original position (Fig. 47–2). If the occlusion is adjusted before the inflammation is alleviated, it will have to be readjusted after gingival health is restored.

The usual sequence of treatment is modified under the following conditions: **In infrabony pockets, excessive occlusal forces are important in determining the pattern of the osseous defects.** To provide optimal conditions for repair of the bony defect with or without the use of osseous and marrow implants, the occlusion is adjusted before or along with the pocket elimination procedures.[37] In mucogingival surgery, because occlusal forces affect the post-treatment contour of the facial bony plate,[11] and in cases of excessive tooth mobility, in which trauma from occlusion is a major causative factor, the occlusion is adjusted before or along with the treatment of the inflammation.

OCCLUSAL CONSIDERATIONS IN TREATMENT PLANNING

The main objective in occlusal therapy is to maintain or achieve mandibular stability. The first concern in occlusal treatment planning is whether to alter the mandibular position by instituting generalized occlusal changes. If the mandibular position is judged to be adequate, the goal is to maintain the existing occlusion and to remove isolated interferences in the course of therapy.

The decision to change the occlusal position should be based upon the positive results of an evaluation of the following two aspects of the patient's oral status:

1. GENERALIZED TRAUMA FROM OCCLUSION. *The presence or absence of signs of trauma from occlusion determines whether the patient's occlusal relationships merit perpetuation in periodontal therapy and ensuing re-*

TABLE 47–1 CHARACTERISTICS OF THERAPEUTIC OCCLUSION (NATURAL DENTITION)

1. **INTERCUSPAL POSITION** (ICP)—Bilateral, simultaneous, well-distributed contacts on the posterior teeth, providing arch stability.
2. **RETRUDED CONTACT POSITION** (RCP)—The RCP-ICP relationship is less than 1 mm along a forward (symmetrical) path measured at incisal levels.
3. **VERTICAL STOPS**—Stable, multiple contacts on the posterior teeth providing individual tooth stability. No buccal-lingual thrust or impact to any tooth in closure to ICP or RCP.
4. **LATERAL EXCURSIONS**—Smooth movement with disclusion controlled by the canine and first premolar on the laterotrusive (working) side. There is little or no contact on the mediotrusive (balancing) side.
5. **PROTRUSIVE EXCURSIONS**—Smooth movement with multiple contacts bilaterally distributed on the anterior teeth.
6. **INTERFERENCES**—Freedom from lateral or protrusive single tooth contacts on the molar teeth; freedom from mediotrusive (balancing) side contacts.
7. **ACCEPTABLE FREE WAY SPACE**—The normal range is 1 to 4 mm. If the free way space measures 8 mm., it then can be reduced. If there are symptoms that can be ascribed to overclosure, then it should be treated.

storative measures. If the trauma is limited to a single tooth or a few teeth, localized adjustment of interferences may suffice. No change in the mandibular position would be required. However, if there is generalized trauma from occlusion, faulty maxillomandibular relationships are often involved in the production of the trauma. *Normalization of these relationships involves major changes in the mandibular occlusal position in accordance with the standards of therapeutic occlusion* (Table 47–1). Under these conditions, the repetitive and excessive occlusal forces of dysfunction may be minimized.

2. OCCLUSAL RECONSTRUCTION. Coordinated periodontal and restorative therapy sometimes involves massive or total reconstruction of disorganized or unstable occlusion. *Attempts to preserve an acquired, eccentric occlusal position dictated by a few remaining teeth are unwarranted.* Since the re-establishment of a therapeutic occlusal position will involve a significant alteration in the existing intercuspal scheme anyway, a prescribed or "therapeutic" mandibular position is more practical. *That is, the occlusion and mandibular position may be coordinated according to standards of therapeutic occlusion* (Table 47–1). The initial phase of this mandibular reorientation often begins with occlusal adjustment during periodontal therapy.

To summarize, existing occlusal schemes and maxillomandibular relationships are altered when it is expected that the resulting changes will (1) normalize the lesions of generalized trauma from occlusion, and (2) facilitate occlusal stabilization (therapeutic occlusion) for future restorative or prosthetic procedures. The change in the mandibular position need not be permanent; it may be reversible, as in the case of removable bite guards and splints. **If a decision is made to maintain the existing ICP, then all occlusal treatments are conservative and are aimed at preserving relationships while removing only traumatic contacts in localized areas.** Three categories of patients can be identified with respect to the planning of occlusal positions and maxillomandibular relationships. These are noted in Table 47–2.

THERAPEUTIC OCCLUSION

Therapeutic occlusion is a treatment occlusion employed to counteract problems related to traumatic occlusion. It is also an occlusal scheme used in restoring or replacing teeth so that a minimum of adaptation is required of the individual and so that compensatory tissue changes are minimized.

By definition, "therapeutic" implies that there are no occlusal interferences and that the new occlusion will be coordinated with the most stable temporomandibular joint position. This ensures that jaw closure will be oriented to a functional end-point where both temporomandibular joints and teeth receive stresses with only a slight mesial component.[31] In constructing a therapeutic occlusion, the dentist will use prevailing principles formulated through his or her own clinical experience and evaluation of research reports. The basic characteristics of therapeutic occlusion are generally agreed upon and are summarized in Table 47–1.

Therapeutic occlusal alterations usually include stabilization of the retruded contact position (RCP) and smooth coordination of contacts between RCP and the intercuspal position (ICP). Also, smooth, interference-free lateral and protrusive excursions are facilitated from ICP. Disturbing posterior interferences along lateral border paths are usually lessened or removed. These alterations enable the dentist to help individuals with a low tolerance to

---

TABLE 47–2 OCCLUSAL TREATMENT PLANNING

1. Patient in **ORTHOFUNCTION** (normal function)	Treatments are aimed at preserving the existing occlusion and mandibular position. An effort is made, therefore, to *avoid introducing new occlusal interferences.*
2. Patient in **DYSFUNCTION**	Specific procedures are instituted to remove pathosis related to occlusal interferences. *Partial or total alteration of the occlusion is generally indicated with either reversible or permanent means.* Large scale alterations lead to a therapeutic mandibular position and occlusion.
3. Patient requiring **EXTENSIVE OCCLUSAL RECONSTRUCTION** for reasons other than traumatic occlusion	*Create new intercuspal position to therapeutic occlusal standards,* so that both joints and teeth receive stress with only a slight mesial component.

occlusal interferences or those who have occlusions weakened by bone loss.[33]

TECHNIQUES OF OCCLUSAL ADJUSTMENT*

There are many methods of occlusal adjustment, most of which fall into one of three categories:

1. **Functional method** (active jaw movement).[10, 13, 18-20] Functional movements made by the patient disclose the contacts to be reshaped or removed. This method develops intercuspal closure at the *muscular contact position* **(MCP),**† which in most cases is synonymous with the *intercuspal position* **(ICP)** and anterior to the *retruded contact position* **(RCP).** *The main feature of this technique is its dependence on the patient's neuromuscular control for determining the optimal occlusal position.*

2. **Border position method** (after Schuyler) (passive jaw manipulation).[38, 39] The dentist manipulates the mandible to disclose interferences at lateral and retrusive border positions and especially at the RCP. This method develops a new ICP coincident with RCP or at some point slightly anterior and sagittal to RCP. The postoperative ICP may be more *cranial* than the original one. *The main feature of this technique is its dependence upon the presumed stability and alignment of the temporomandibular joints to achieve an optimal occlusal position.*

3. **Myo-Monitor method**‡ (transcutaneous neural stimulation).[21] The masticatory muscles are "pulsed" by intermittent electrical stimulation, resulting in repetitive mandibular contact with the maxillary teeth (myocentric contact position). This method is reported to develop a new ICP anterior to both RCP and the previous ICP.[2, 22, 26, 34, 43] *This technique relies upon the effect of an artificially induced polymuscular contraction to achieve the prescribed occlusal (myocentric) position.*

WHICH TECHNIQUE OF OCCLUSAL ADJUSTMENT SHOULD BE SELECTED? Mandibular positions obtained with the *Myo-Monitor technique* have been compared with other reference positions in several studies.[2, 22, 26, 34, 43] These investigations reported that the "my-ocentric" mandibular position was anterior to both the RCP and the ICP. On the basis of these studies the Myo-Monitor technique appears questionable, since myocentric records position the condyles and the teeth anterior and inferior with respect to those intercuspal relationships[42] found in otherwise normal individuals.

Some clinicians favor *functional adjustment* to a neuromuscular closure (coordination of MCP and ICP) without attention to border positions, which they consider nonphysiologic parafunctional movements rather than regular features of chewing and swallowing.[14, 19] The advocates of functional adjustment claim that correction of prematurities at ICP and elimination of retrusive prematurities are sufficient to inhibit bruxing and dysfunctional habits (evidence is unsupported or inconclusive). Some advocates of the functional method do not adjust the retrusive range (RCP).

The *border position method* takes a more comprehensive approach and recommends adjustment of lateral and protrusive excursions which are often taken up by the bruxing patient. In this technique, minimal attention is given to the coordination of MCP and ICP. Whereas the functional method emphasizes intraborder adjustment (ICP), the border position method emphasizes the adjustment of border excursions and the development of a stable RCP. Dentists using either method routinely correct gross interferences such as extruded or tipped teeth, plunger cusps, uneven marginal ridges, and enlargement of flat areas due to occlusal wear.

Both the functional and the border position methods appear to have some advantages; i.e., **both intraborder and border adjustment are desirable.** *Intraborder* adjustment is logical, since there seems little doubt that the ICP is the most commonly used functional occlusion of the dentition.[10] *Border position* adjustment is practical because excursive interferences during gnashing and grinding of the teeth are traumatic (parafunctional).[32] The border method also provides the clinician with an objective method by which to align the mandible.

The occlusal adjustment technique suggested in this chapter consists of an integrated approach that can be progressively utilized to accomplish both limited and comprehensive occlusal adjustment. **The goal of this technique is to minimize occlusal interferences and to ensure that both the joints and the teeth are stabilized at a common functional end point at or centered slightly anterior to the RCP.**[31] The

---

*For detailed presentations of this subject, see Arnold, N. R., and Frumker, S. C.[1]; Dawson, P. E.[7]; Ramfjord, S. P.[32]; and Shore, N. A.[40]

†See Chapter 5 for definitions of nomenclature.

‡Myotronics Inc., Seattle, Washington.

occlusal alterations include stabilization of RCP and a coordination of the pathway between RCP and ICP. Also, smooth, interference-free lateral and protrusive excursions are facilitated from both RCP and ICP. Mediotrusive (balancing) interferences are reduced or eliminated. These features are expected to strengthen the adaptive capacity of individuals with a low tolerance to occlusal interferences or with occlusions weakened by bone loss.

OCCLUSAL ADJUSTMENT AND INTERNAL DERANGEMENTS OF THE TEMPOROMANDIBULAR JOINT (CLICKING, LOCKING JAW)

A number of concerns affecting the goals of occlusal adjustment have developed as a result of increased awareness of internal derangements of the temporomandibular joint (TMJ). Arthrography on patients with TMJ clicking has demonstrated anterior displacement of the articular disc occurring at the closed position; this corrects to its normal position with opening jaw movements.[4] Locking of the jaw (jaw restriction at midopening) occurs when the articular disc no longer can recover from its prolapsed position to a stable disc-condyle relationship.[4]

Clinically, TMJ derangements occur before the TMJ reaches the terminal stage of organic disease and are quite common in adults. Because internal derangements are often aggravated by vigorous jaw positioning, occlusal adjustment, particularly in the retruded position, should be performed with caution and only after appropriate informed consent is obtained. *Patients with clicking and locking usually should have occlusal splint therapy if significant changes in the occlusion are necessary in periodontal treatment.* Should patients develop bothersome clicking or locking as a result of occlusal adjustment, an evaluation for trial splint therapy should be made with the lower jaw in a slightly forward and open position, and any further occlusal adjustment should be carried out with a minimal decrease in the vertical dimension of occlusion.

RECOMMENDED TECHNIQUE FOR OCCLUSAL ADJUSTMENT

Objectives for Occlusal Adjustment

The practical objective of occlusal adjustment is to mechanically eliminate occlusal interferences involved in function and parafunction. Positive results of occlusal adjustment are:[24]

1. A change in the pattern and degree of afferent impulses.

2. A decreased tooth mobility, since stabilization of tooth position helps control the occlusal sensory input.

3. The creation of a multiple simultaneous contact spread over the occlusal scheme in order to create *occlusal stabilization* of the mandible (i.e., decrease *muscular stabilization*).

4. A change in the pattern of chewing or swallowing function.

5. The establishment of multidirectional mandibular movement patterns.

Casts and Occlusal Analysis

Casts should be made before the teeth are altered by occlusal adjustment. These records are useful during the procedure and for reference at follow-up visits. *When occlusal adjustment is to be performed in the mouth, a reasonable prediction of the biomechanical result by means of this approach is required.* Mounting the casts on a semi-adjustable articulator using a facebow transfer and a retruded position intermaxillary record assists in reaching this objective.[6] Many clinicians find that trial carving of the casts allows them to perform the occlusal adjustment with greater confidence and efficiency.

Armamentarium

It is best to combine the use of various products for identifying and marking tooth contact. Selected products are listed in Table 47–3 with recommendations for specific application in the occlusal adjustment process. Marking ribbon and marking paper work best on a dry tooth surface. Therefore, these products should be used in combination with adequate isolation. Blotting paper* and cotton rolls are useful for this purpose. The recommended armamentarium is shown in Figure 47–3*A* and *B*.

---

*Dri-Angles, Tru-Eze Manufacturing Company, Temecula, California 92390.

TABLE 47–3 RECOMMENDED MATERIALS FOR IDENTIFYING AND MARKING TOOTH CONTACT AND CONTACT MOVEMENT

Product	ICP Contact	RCP Contact	Protrusive and Lateral Contact	Intensity/Area of Contact
		Suggested Application of Product*		
Occlusal registration strips[a]	x		x	x
Occlusal indicator wax[b]	x	x		x
Marking ribbon[c] — red, green; blue Mylar ribbon[d]	x	x	x	
Articulating paper — blue[e]	x			

*ICP = intercuspal position; RCP = retruded contact position.
[a]Artus Corp., Englewood, New Jersey.
[b]Kerr Corp., Romulus, Michigan.
[c]Columbia Ribbon, Cucamonga, California.
[d]Parkel, Farmingdale, New Jersey.
[e]Holg Mark-Rite Interstate Dental Co., New Hyde Park, New York.

Classification of Supracontacts (Prematurities, Interferences)

Excursive interferences are classified according to the mandibular movement that caused the contact in question to take place (Fig. 47–4*A* and *B*). The reference point for this movement is the intercuspal position (ICP). For example, supracontacts occurring under retrusive excursion are called *retrusive* supracontacts. Supracontacts occurring under laterotrusion are termed *laterotrusive* supracontacts. *Note that excursive contacts are named exactly according to the way each functional segment of the mandible moves from ICP* (Fig. 47–4*A*).

Static prematurities at the ICP are not related to horizontal mandibular movements. They are identified as contact relationships in the frontal plane and are classified as follows:

CLASS I PREMATURITY. The buccal inclines of the buccal cusps of the mandibular molars and premolars against the lingual inclines of

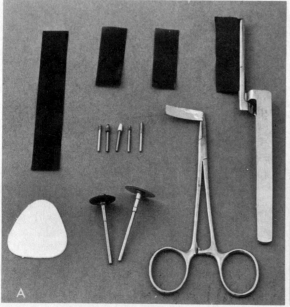
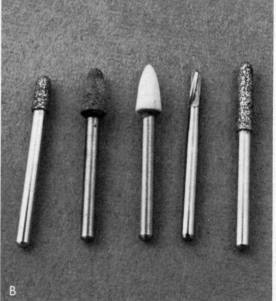

Figure 47–3 Instruments and Materials Used in Performing Occlusal Adjustment. *A, (Clockwise from lower right)* Mylar strip in hemostat, abrasive disk and wheel, blotting paper to reduce salivary flow, inked marking ribbon in ribbon holder, and *(center)* friction grip burs and stones. *B,* **Cutting and Abrasive Burs Used in Performing Occlusal Adjustment.** *(Left to right)* diamond, green stone, polystone, fluted carbide, and elongated diamond.

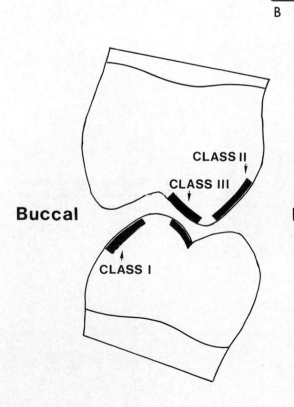

Figure 47–4 Excursive Interferences. These are named after the mandibular movement that caused the contact to occur. *A,* Note that the potential for interferences occurs over pathways determined by the rotating (working) condyle (C). M, mediotrusive interference. L, laterotrusive interference. *B,* **The Four Main Occlusal Interferences**. R, retrusive. P, protrusive. L, laterotrusive. M, mediotrusive. Open circle denotes the intercuspal position (ICP) contact area.

Maxillary Teeth

Maxillary

Mandibular

A

B

Buccal

Lingual

CLASS II

CLASS III

CLASS I

Figure 47–5 Prematurities at the intercuspal position (ICP) can be classified as Class I, Class II, and Class III.

the buccal cusps of the maxillary molars and premolars (Fig. 47–5); and the facial surfaces of the mandibular anterior teeth against the lingual surfaces of their maxillary antagonists.

CLASS II PREMATURITY. The lingual inclines of the lingual cusps of the maxillary molars and premolars against the buccal inclines of the lingual cusps of the mandibular molars and premolars (Fig. 47–5).

CLASS III PREMATURITY. The buccal inclines of the lingual cusps of the maxillary molars and premolars against the lingual inclines of the buccal cusps of the mandibular molars and premolars (Fig. 47–5).

How to Correct Supracontacts (Prematurities, Interferences)

The correction of occlusal prematurities after they have been located and marked on the teeth is a technique in itself. The objective is to reduce the prematurities so as to create unobstructed closure of cusps into fossae, while restoring and preserving original tooth anatomy. *It is not simply a matter of grinding down premature contacts*, which creates flattened planes that will further disrupt the occlusion. The correction of occlusal prematurities consists of: (1) **grooving,** (2) **spheroiding,** and (3) **pointing.**

Grooving consists of restoring the depth of developmental grooves made shallow by occlu-

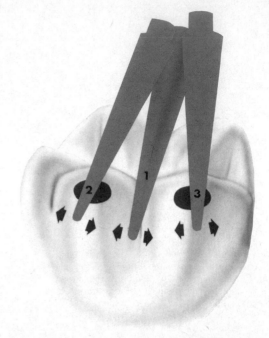

Figure 47–6 Grooving to Restore the Depth of Developmental Grooves on Worn Tooth Surfaces. A tapered diamond stone (1) is rotated slowly in the groove as indicated. After the desired depth is attained, the stone is moved (2 and 3) to spheroid the adjacent tooth surface.

sal wear. It is done with a tapered cutting tool until the desired depth is attained (Fig. 47–6).

Spheroiding consists of reducing the prematurity and restoring the original tooth con-

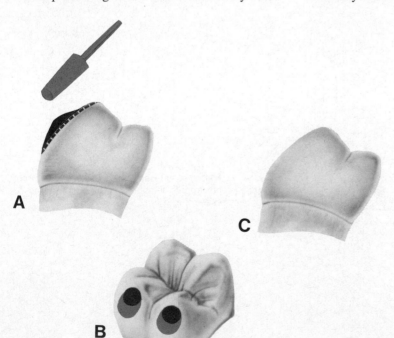

Figure 47–7 Spheroiding to Restore the Original Tooth Contour. *A,* Recontouring prematurity. *B,* Recontouring extends several millimeters below the black marking. *C,* Corrected contour.

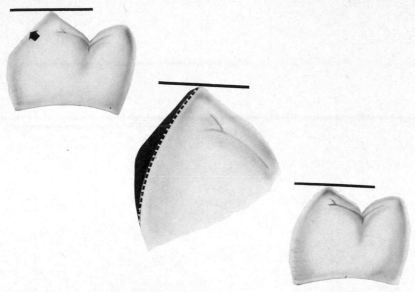

Figure 47–8 Correct Method of Spheroiding *(broken line)* and preserving the height of the buccal cusp *(horizontal line)*. The arrow points to the prematurity.

tour. Starting 2 or 3 mm mesial or distal to the prematurity, the tooth is recontoured from the occlusal margin to a distance 2 or 3 mm apical to the marking (Figs. 47–6 and 47–7). This is done with a light "paintbrush" stroke, gradually blending the area of the prematurity with the adjacent tooth surface. A special effort is made to preserve the occlusal height of the cusps (Figs. 47–8 and 47–9).

The purpose of spheroiding is not simply to narrow occlusal surfaces. When teeth are flattened by wear, the buccolingual diameter of the occlusal surface is increased. Spheroiding restores the buccolingual width of the occlusal

surface to what it was before wear occurred (Fig. 47–10).

Pointing consists of restoring cusp point contours (Fig. 47–11). It is done by reshaping the tooth with rotating cutting tools.

As a general rule, Class I prematurities are corrected on mandibular teeth. Class II and Class III prematurities are adjusted where feasible on both the maxillary and mandibular teeth. If doing all the correction on one jaw would entail mutilation of tooth anatomy, the opposing teeth are included in the correction process. The emphasis is always upon restoring and preserving tooth anatomy.

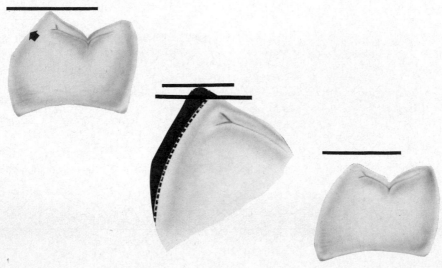

Figure 47–9 Incorrect Method of Spheroiding *(broken line)* results in excessive reduction in buccal cusp height *(horizontal line)*. The arrow points to the prematurity.

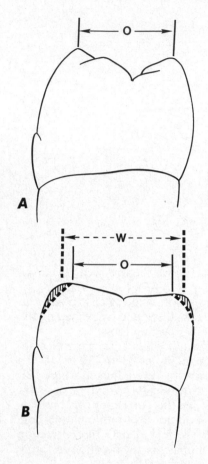

Figure 47–10 Flattened Occlusal Surface Restored to Unworn Width. *A*, Occlusal diameter (O) of unworn mandibular molar. *B*, Widened occlusal diameter (W) of worn molar restored to diameter of unworn surface (O) by recontouring *(shaded areas).*

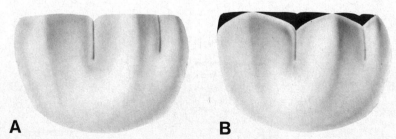

Figure 47–11 Pointing. *A*, Buccal margin of mandibular molar flattened by wear. *B*, Tooth recontoured to restore cusp points.

Schedule for Occlusal Adjustment

Occlusal adjustment can be accomplished using a variety of different sequences. A step-by-step approach is presented here for clarity, even though experienced clinicians tend to blend the steps together.

The occlusion is adjusted systematically according to the schedule in Table 47–4. The series of steps is normally accomplished over two or more appointments, with each visit limited to 30 minutes of adjustment. The number and duration of sessions may vary according to patient tolerance, but the sequence should not be changed.

Many situations in periodontal therapy require occlusal adjustment of only one or two teeth. Obviously, comprehensive occlusal adjustment is not warranted. In these cases, localized occlusal adjustment is often limited to intraborder reduction of Class I, II, and III supracontacts on the involved teeth (steps 1, 3, and 4).

The Ten Steps of Occlusal Adjustment

STEP 1. EXPLAIN OCCLUSAL ADJUSTMENT AND CREATE POSITIVE PATIENT ACCEPTANCE. Patients may be concerned that grinding their teeth will change their appearance, cause tooth decay, and increase tooth sensitivity. The operator should explain that the teeth are not going to be "ground down" but rather *reshaped* so that they will function better. The reshaping is done in areas where tooth decay rarely occurs. It should also be made clear that adjusting the occlusion is a necessary part of the total periodontal treatment, which benefits the periodontal tissues and prolongs the life of the teeth. The appearance of the teeth will not be spoiled; if anything, they may look better and feel more comfortable. Above all, the patient should understand that the teeth and the occlusion change with time and that the occlusion will be checked at periodic recall visits, at which time minor adjustments will be made, if necessary.

TABLE 47–4 SCHEDULE OF OCCLUSAL ADJUSTMENT*

Step 1. Explain; create positive patient acceptance.
Step 2. Remove retrusive prematurities and eliminate the deflective shift from RCP to ICP (the retrusive pathway prematurities are eliminated).
Step 3. Adjust ICP to achieve stable, simultaneous, multi-pointed, widely distributed contacts.
Step 4. Test for excessive contact (fremitus) on the incisor teeth.
Step 5. Remove posterior protrusive interferences and establish contacts bilaterally distributed on the anterior teeth.
Step 6. Remove or lessen mediotrusive (balancing) interferences.
Step 7. Reduce excessive cusp steepness on the laterotrusive (working) contacts.
Step 8. Eliminate gross occlusal disharmonies.
Step 9. Recheck tooth contact relationships.
Step 10. Polish all rough tooth surfaces.

*RCP = retruded contact position; ICP = intercuspal position.

STEP 2. REMOVE RETRUSIVE PREMATURITIES AND ELIMINATE THE DEFLECTIVE SHIFT FROM RCP TO ICP. The purpose of this step is to eliminate prematurities that interfere with hinge closure of the mandible to a stable RCP. When contact is located on terminal hinge closure, prematurities may cause the mandible to glide mesially into the ICP. This glide is termed the **shift from RCP to ICP** (Fig. 47–12). Retrusive adjustment will result in the elimination of the deflective RCP to ICP shift; in particular, it will neutralize or remove *asymmetrical shifts from RCP to ICP* (Fig. 47–13*A* and *B*). The normal areas of contact at RCP or ICP are referred to as *vertical (or centric) stops*.

How to Locate the RCP. Locating the RCP is the key to controlled occlusal adjustment. Begin by placing the patient in the supine position, which has been shown to reduce the activity of the protruder muscles most completely.[9, 25, 27] Test and rehearse hinge closure to RCP. Some patients allow their mandibles to be passively retruded quite easily; other patients defy experts! *Arriving at RCP is dependent upon specific verbal and motor actions*

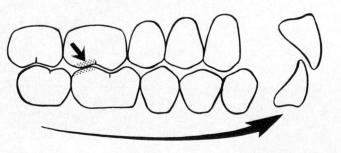

Figure 47–12 Shift from Retruded Contact Position (RCP) to Intercuspal Position (ICP). When contact is located on terminal hinge closure (RCP), prematurities may cause the mandible to glide mesially into the ICP.

Horizontal tracing

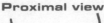
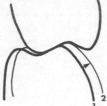

A

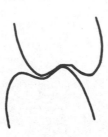

B

Proximal view

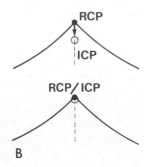

Figure 47–13 Shift from Retruded Contact Position (RCP) to Intercuspal Position (ICP). *A,* Before occlusal adjustment. Mandibular teeth shift from point 1 to point 2 (asymmetrical shift). The same movement is seen in the arrow point tracing in the horizontal plane. *B,* After occlusal adjustment. Asymmetrical shift from RCP to ICP is removed and resulting intercuspal position is nearer to or identical with RCP.

Figure 47–14 Methods of Locating Retruded Contact Position (RCP). *A,* Patient is supine. Forefinger and thumb are "butted" against the chin, with the other hand stabilizing the head. *B,* Dawson[7] method. All four fingers of each hand are placed on the lower border of the mandible. This places an upward pressure on the condyle during the manipulation. The thumbs are placed in the notch over the symphysis, exerting a downward pressure. The thumbs should touch each other.

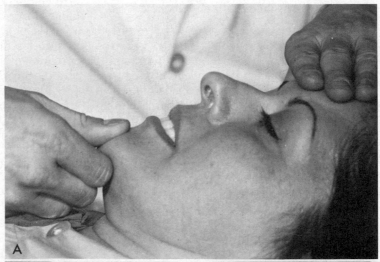

A

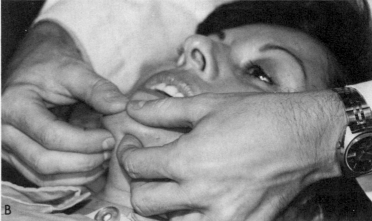

B

by the operator. Figure 47–14 shows two hand grasp methods that have proved effective for manipulation of the mandible.[7, 33] A common error is to grab the chin and nervously order the patient to "relax!" Ideally, the patient's mandible will fall passively to the RCP—the operator's main function is to create an arcing terminal hinge movement. Experience has shown that certain specific statements are better than others in obtaining the desired result:

1. With very light pressure, encourage small hinge movements and say, *"Let your mouth drop open."*

2. As the jaw falls downward and backward to the retruded position, exert more pressure and seek out the ligamentous resistance of the temporomandibular joints. You may encounter muscular resistance; when you sense this, remove your hands completely and begin the manipulation again. Talk in low tones, using repetitious phrases, e.g., *"Just let it go."* At this point you should have the jaw arcing. Then say, *"Let your jaw come together . . . just so you first touch."*

3. After the initial contact is perceived say, *"Squeeze."* The shift from RCP to ICP, if present, should be apparent. *Remember:* Locating RCP is dependent upon your ability to detect the "ligamentous signal" from the patient. A stiff wrist and forearm will improve your receptivity to the "ligamentous signal." Generally, if you cannot manipulate the mandible to RCP, an occlusal adjustment in the retruded position should not be attempted. Removable interocclusal splints are indicated for reducing the neuromuscular antagonism prior to occlusal adjustment.

4. Retrusive prematurities can be marked with either green wax or red marking ribbon. Red ribbon should be placed in a ribbon forceps* and inserted between the desired teeth after they are properly dried (Fig. 47–15). Occlusal registration wax is first placed on the maxillary or mandibular posterior quadrant, with the adhesive (shiny) surface pressed against the teeth (Fig. 47–16). The occlusal surface of the wax is moistened with a wet finger to prevent adherence of the opposing teeth. The mandible is manipulated to strike against the wax in short, interrupted closures. Mobile teeth are stabilized with the fingers so that prematurities will not be pushed aside. If there are no supracontacts on retruded closure

of the jaw, the wax will be uniformly transparent at the contact areas. Severe prematurities will cause perforation of the wax. The prematurities are marked on the teeth through the wax with a pencil, and the wax strips are removed (Fig. 47–17).

5. Question the patient as to which teeth seem to "hit first" as the jaws close. The patient's impression is often useful in locating the areas of premature contact. Common sites of prematurities are the mesial inclines of the lingual cusps and marginal ridges of the maxillary molars and premolars and their opposing tooth surfaces. The mesial inner incline of the lingual cusp of the maxillary first premolars is the most common initial prematurity.

Principles That Should Not Be Violated in the Retrusive Occlusal Adjustment. 1. Remove the inclines that cause interferences when the mandible moves from RCP to ICP. Do not remove the vertical stop or supporting cusp tip, only the incline between these two areas (Fig. 47–17C to E). These inclines, which are called retrusive prematurities, are usually found on *mesial facing inclines of the maxillary teeth and distal facing inclines of the mandibular teeth* (MUDL Rule).

2. Strive to achieve vertical stops at RCP on each tooth. Avoid losing them when grinding excursive interferences. If the vertical cusps are not aligned within the desired opposing fossa, corrections are made on the cusp slope or incline to place the cusp more nearly within the fossa. If the cusp and fossa are in alignment, either the fossa is deepened or the cusp is shortened—depending on which element is more out of harmony with the other like elements in the arch.[35]

3. Reshape, if possible, at the expense of the fossae, ridges, or cusp inclines. Preserve the marginal ridges; adjust the cusp tip as a last resort. Adjust worn facets to achieve point-to-surface rather than surface-to-surface contact.

4. Mobile teeth are stabilized with the fingers so that prematurities will be accurately registered; and not pushed aside. To avoid excessive grinding of one dental arch, do part of the correction on the other arch.

5. *Remove the lateral thrust in the RCP to ICP shift.* **In lateral shifts, the significant retrusive markings on the maxillary teeth face in the direction to which the mandible shifts from RCP to ICP.** Adjustment of these prematurities will eliminate the lateral component of the shift. This simple observation can be of great help in rapidly achieving the end point in retrusive range adjustment.

---

*Miltex Instrument Company, New York, New York 10010.

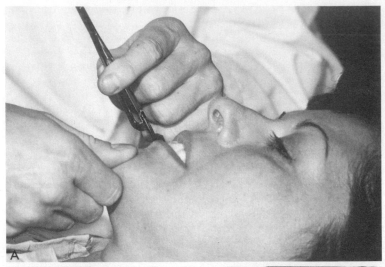

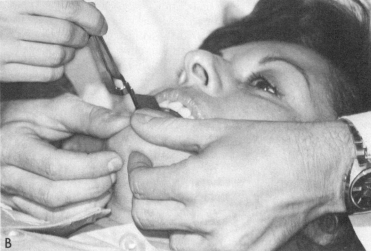

Figure 47–15 Techniques for Marking Retruded Contact Position (RCP) Contacts on the Teeth. *A,* Chin grasp technique. *B,* Technique after Dawson.[7]

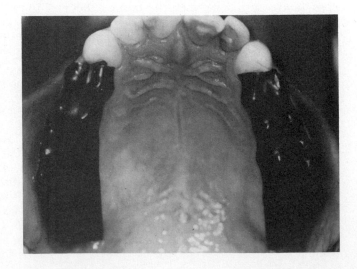

Figure 47–16 Wax Strips on the Maxillary Premolars and Molars. The anterior teeth are not covered.

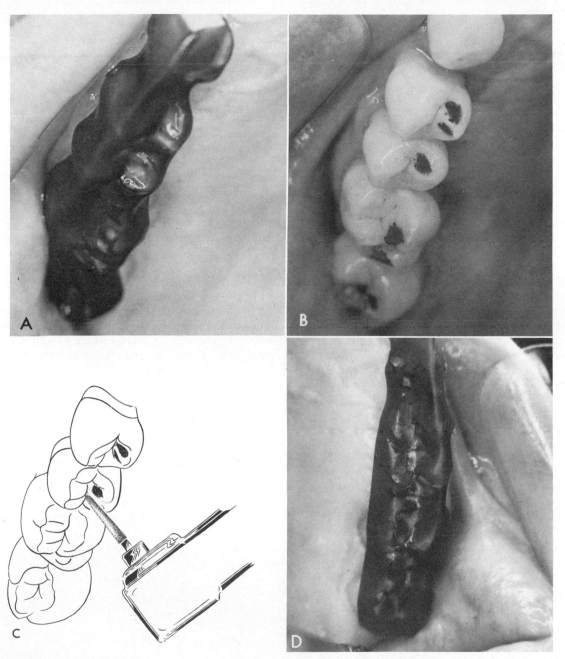

Figure 47–17 Correction of Retrusive Prematurities. *A,* Indentations in wax show retrusive prematurities on the mesial inner inclines of the maxillary lingual cusps. *B,* Retrusive prematurities marked on the teeth. *C,* Prematurities corrected with diamond point. *D,* After correction, wax shows evenly distributed contact on cusp tips and fossae.

Illustration continued on following page

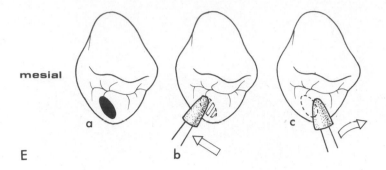

mesial

E

Figure 47–17 *Continued E*, Correction of retrusive interferences involves flat reduction (a and b) but should be followed by spheroiding (c).

6. Continue to adjust the RCP vertical stops so that they approach the same vertical level as the previous ICP. If the RCP stops appear stable but still require reduction to approach the same level as ICP, use the following guidelines: (a) reduce the cusp tip when supracontacts in excursions are associated with the movement of that cusp; and (b) otherwise, reduce the fossa, especially if it appears too shallow. Both the cusps and the fossae may eventually require adjustment to obtain RCP and ICP at the same level. Once this relationship is obtained, both the cranial and the lateral components of the RCP-ICP shift are removed. The therapeutic result is to allow sagittal movement between RCP and ICP at the same level; alternatively, RCP may be made slightly cranial to the preoperative ICP, in which case RCP and ICP may be nearly identical after occlusal adjustment.

7. The retrusive range adjustment is complete when the following conditions are achieved: (a) the contact pattern is bilateral with many-pointed contacts, (b) the deflective shift from RCP to ICP has been eliminated; (c) both RCP and ICP approach the same vertical dimension of occlusion; (d) the pathway from RCP to ICP, if present, is smooth and gliding; and (e) repeated closure of the teeth together in the hinge position produces a sharp, resonant sound.

STEP 3. ADJUSTMENT OF THE ICP. A task common to many dental procedures is the localized adjustment of ICP contacts on one or more teeth. The adjustment of ICP is also a major step involved with comprehensive occlusal adjustment. The purpose of this step is to achieve a stable ICP and to refine occlusal table relationships. **The main feature of this step is that the prematurities are identified without guidance by the operator's hand.** The reshaping is accomplished by progressive adjustment of Class I, II, and III prematurities during one or more visits. The posterior teeth are adjusted first, followed by the anterior teeth.

How to Locate Prematurities in ICP. Instruct the patient, *"Tap your back teeth together, both sides at the same time, slow and hard."* Have the patient repeat this process once or twice; the teeth normally will meet in the same position. This is the ICP or habitual

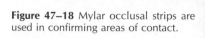

Figure 47–18 Mylar occlusal strips are used in confirming areas of contact.

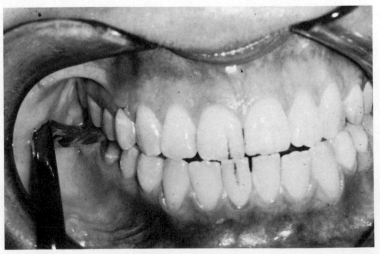

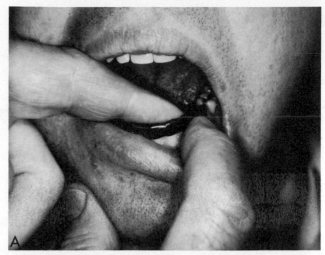

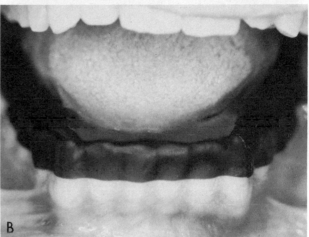

Figure 47–19 Correcting Prematurities in the Intercuspal Position (ICP). *A,* Placing the wax on the mandibular teeth. *B,* Wax in position.

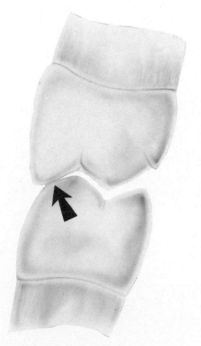

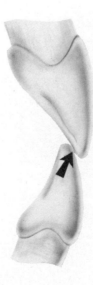

Figure 47–20 Class I Prematurities in the Intercuspal Position. Class I prematurities on the facial surface of the mandibular anterior and posterior teeth indicated by arrows.

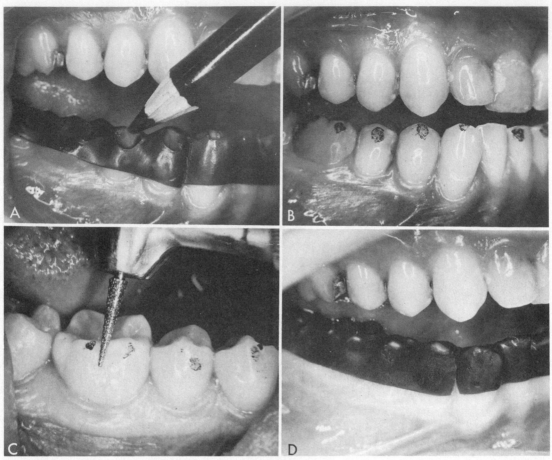

Figure 47–21 Correction of Class I Prematurities in Intercuspal Position (ICP). *A,* Prematurities are marked through the wax onto the teeth. *B,* Prematurities marked on the teeth. *C,* Grooving the buccal surface with a tapered diamond. *D,* After correction, contact is shown on the cusp tips.

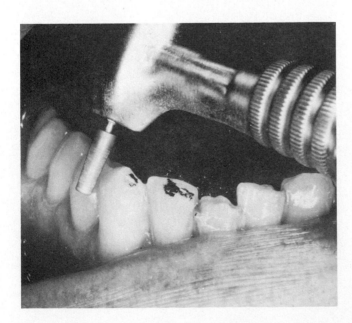

Figure 47–22 Spheroiding the Facial Surface of a Mandibular Premolar to Correct a Class I Prematurity in Intercuspal Position (ICP)

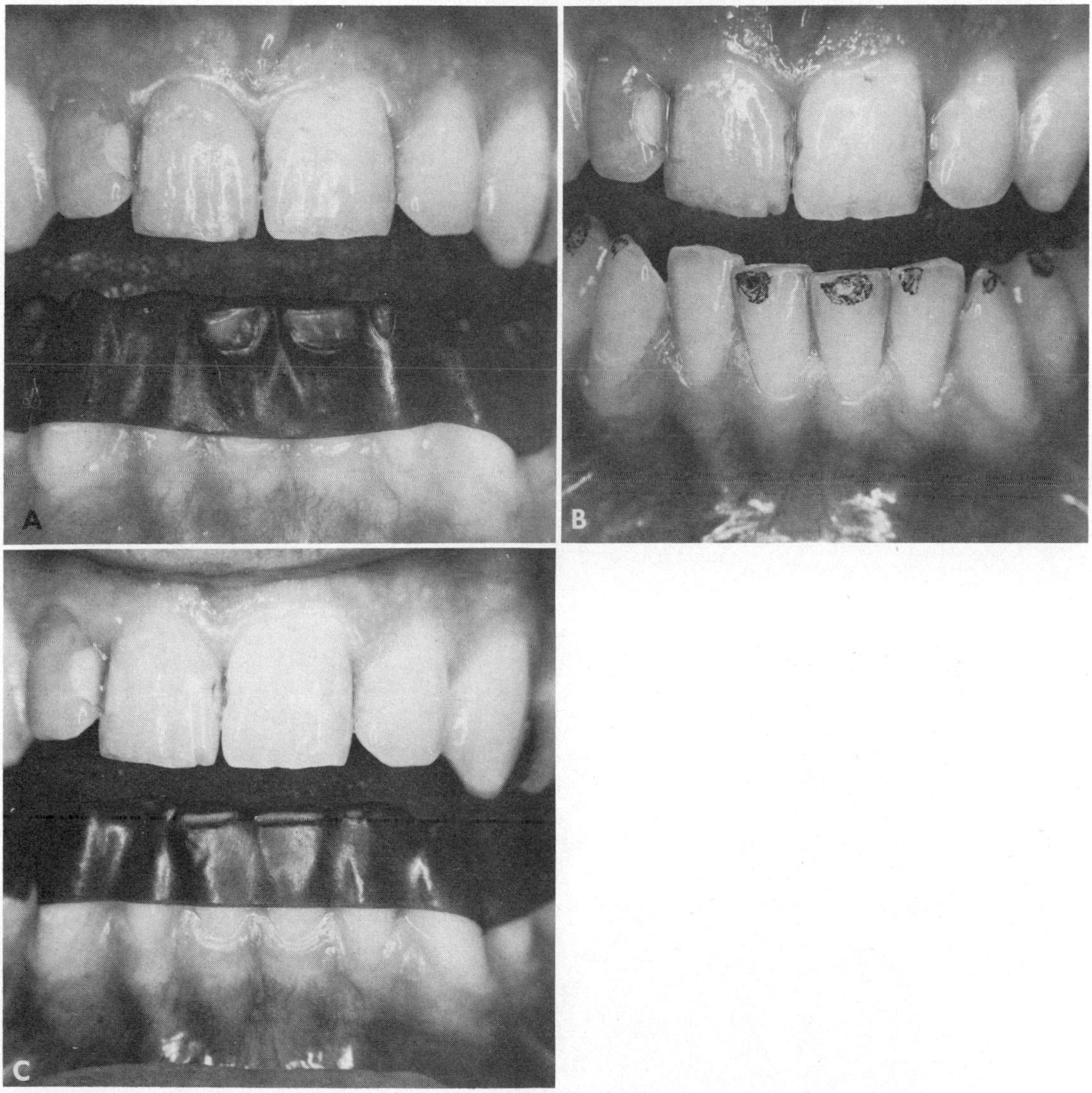

Figure 47–23 Correction of Class I Prematurities in Intercuspal Position (ICP) on the Mandibular Anterior Teeth. *A,* Class I prematurities on the facial surface registered in the wax. *B,* Prematurities marked on the teeth. *C,* After the prematurities are corrected, only the incisal edges contact the maxillary teeth.

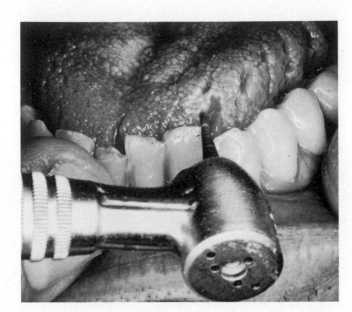

Figure 47–24 Reduction of Extruded Mandibular Incisors.

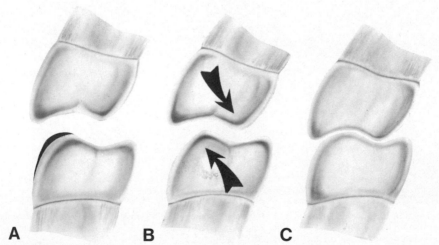

A   B   C

Figure 47–25 Eruption and Uprighting of Teeth After Correction of Class I Prematurities. *A*, Class I prematurity indicated in black. *B*, Direction of tooth movement after correction of prematurity. *C*, Teeth in adjusted position.

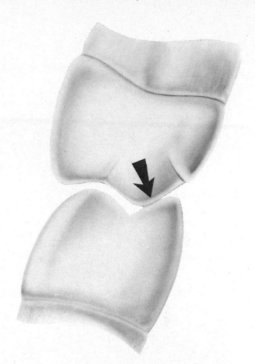

Figure 47–26 Class II Prematurity in the Intercuspal Position (ICP) on the Lingual Surface of Maxillary Molar indicated by arrow.

occlusion. Since relatively heavy muscular force is used, the choice of marking medium is less critical. The combined use of more than one medium for cross-comparison is advantageous. Occlusal indicator wax, blue marking paper, and marking ribbon work equally well. Actual ICP contact can be assessed by using Mylar occlusal indicator strips inserted between the closed teeth and tested with a "tugging" motion (Fig. 47–18). If wax is used, it is placed on the occlusal and incisal surfaces of the mandibular teeth (Fig. 47–19), and the patient is asked to open and close again as before. The translucent areas are marked on the mandibular teeth with a pencil, and the wax is removed.

Correction of Class I prematurities (Fig. 47–20) is started on the posterior teeth with contouring on the facial surface of the molars (Fig. 47–21), followed by spheroiding and pointing of the molars and premolars (Fig. 47–22). After the posterior segments are corrected, attention is directed to the anterior teeth (Fig. 47–23). The facial surfaces are spheroided mesiodistally to relieve the prematurities and at the same time to reduce the width of the worn incisal edges. Extruded teeth are reduced in the adjustment procedure (Fig. 47–24). Wax strips are placed on the teeth again, and correction is repeated until light transparencies appear only on the cusp tips and incisal edges

(Fig. 47–23C). This usually requires several applications of wax strips. If may be necessary to complete the correction on the opposing maxillary surfaces in order to avoid excessive reduction of the mandibular teeth. After the prematurities are eliminated, the teeth are smoothed and the patient is dismissed.

Teeth tend to right themselves and to erupt into the spaces created by the correction of Class I prematurities (Fig. 47–25). This reduces lateral stresses and redirects occlusal forces in the long axis of the teeth, but often creates new Class I prematurities, which are corrected at the next visit.

To locate *Class II prematurities* (Fig. 47–26) in ICP, the wax is applied to the maxillary posterior teeth (Fig. 47–27A). The patient again closes in habitual occlusion, and Class II prematurities are registered on the lingual surface of the lingual cusps (Fig. 47–27B and C). Prematurities are corrected by grooving and spheroiding (Fig. 47–27D), which are repeated until only the tips of the lingual cusps register in the wax (Fig. 47–27E).

To locate *Class III prematurities* (Fig. 47–28) in ICP, wax is placed on the maxillary posterior teeth. The patient closes in ICP, and the Class III prematurities are registered in the wax on the buccal surface of the lingual cusps. The Class III prematurities in ICP are corrected by grooving and pointing procedures

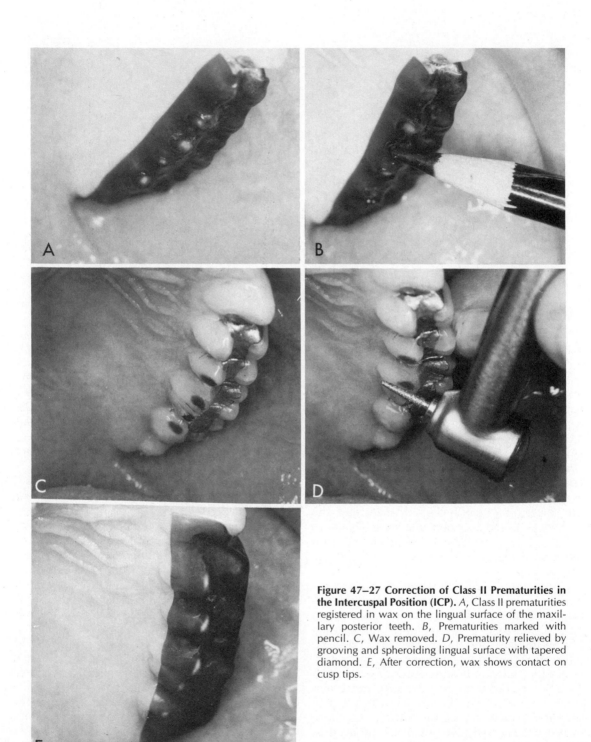

Figure 47–27 Correction of Class II Prematurities in the Intercuspal Position (ICP). *A*, Class II prematurities registered in wax on the lingual surface of the maxillary posterior teeth. *B*, Prematurities marked with pencil. *C*, Wax removed. *D*, Prematurity relieved by grooving and spheroiding lingual surface with tapered diamond. *E*, After correction, wax shows contact on cusp tips.

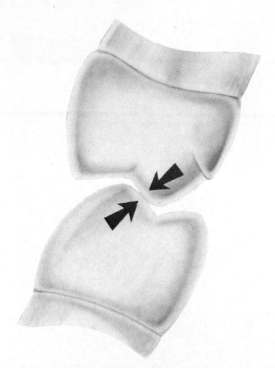

Figure 47–28 Class III Prematurity in the Intercuspal Position (ICP). The buccal surface of the lingual cusp of the maxillary molars and premolars, with the lingual aspect of the buccal cusps of the mandibular teeth.

described for correcting retrusive prematurities in the retruded position. It is desirable to achieve cross-tooth vertical stops in ICP wherever possible (Fig. 47–29).

STEP 4. TEST FOR EXCESSIVE CONTACT ON THE INCISOR TEETH IN ICP. The incisor teeth should be slightly out of contact or in light contact. The firmness of contact can be detected by using Mylar occlusal strips held by a hemostat. The Mylar strip should just slip through the incisor teeth when the patient clenches firmly in ICP. In addition, closing contacts should be tested for **fremitus**, *a vibration or displacement perceptible on palpation of the facial tooth surface with a moistened forefinger during repeated firm closure to ICP.* If a supracontact is present, it may be marked with wax or marking ribbon and reduced (see Fig. 47–23). No fremitus should be detectable on firm intercuspal closure of the teeth.

The ICP adjustment is complete when the following conditions are achieved:

1. The contact pattern is bilateral, stable, and many-pointed (Fig. 47–30*A* and *B*).

2. Each posterior vertical step holds a Mylar occlusal strip with equal resistance.

3. Sharp resonant sounds are heard when the patient taps his or her teeth together in ICP (stethoscope placed over the infraorbital skin area[46]) (Fig. 47–31).

4. Patient responds negatively to the following test: "Tap on your back teeth, slow and hard—do you feel any difference between the two sides?"

STEP 5. REMOVE POSTERIOR PROTRUSIVE INTERFERENCES—OBTAIN BILATERAL PROTRUSIVE GLIDE ON THE ANTERIOR TEETH. Protrusive excursion refers to the path of the mandible as it moves anteriorly or posteriorly between the ICP and the edge-to-edge relationship of the anterior teeth. The latter is called the **protrusive position.** Protrusive position and excursion are corrected separately.

Correction of Protrusive Position. The objective of this step is to attain bilateral, well-distributed contact on the incisal edges of the maxillary and mandibular incisor teeth. This is done as follows: From ICP contact, instruct the patient to protrude his or her mandible slowly. There should be bilateral contact in this segment with little or no deviant shift of the mandible. A deviant shift usually is caused by a molar interference or an asymmetrical incisal plane. Use finger pressure to help guide the patient's jaw along a *precise, symmetrical excursion* until the protrusive position is reached (Fig. 47–32*A*). The patient is instructed to open and close in this position with marking ribbon or wax strips between the teeth. Progressive adjustment of the marked areas permits the unmarked incisal edges to

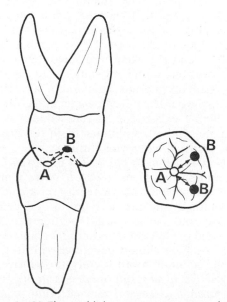

Figure 47–29 The establishment or preservation of cross-tooth contacts is a goal in occlusal adjustment. Cross-tooth contacts (A–B) are shown in proximal and occlusal views.

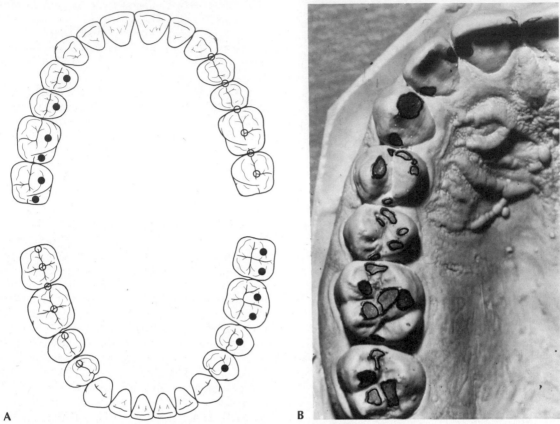

A **B**

Figure 47–30 Normal Zones of Contact in the Intercuspal Position (ICP). *A,* Open circles denote vertical (centric) stops; black circles denote centric cusps. *B,* Zones of contact in a natural dentition.

come into contact (Fig. 47–32*B* to *E*). Wherever possible, adjustment is confined to the maxillary teeth. The mandibular teeth are ground (a) when, because of pain, proximity to the pulp, or for esthetic reasons, the limit of grinding of the maxillary teeth has been reached; and (b) when individual mandibular teeth protrude either incisally of facially. It is important *not* to grind the mandibular teeth so that they would be out of contact in the various mandibular excursions. If such contact is not maintained, the mandibular teeth tend to extrude and re-create prematurities.

The production of flat, broad incisal surfaces by grinding should be avoided. After a maximum number of anterior teeth are in contact, the width of the incisal edges is reduced by grinding the facial margin of the maxillary teeth and the lingual margin of the mandibular teeth. Caution should be exercised in reshaping the anterior tooth merely to improve esthetics. *The ideal result of correction of protrusive position is several contact points equally distributed between the right and left anterior teeth.* This may not be fully attainable in cases of tooth irregularity.

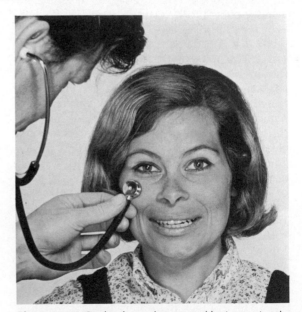

Figure 47–31 Occlusal sounds are tested by instructing the patient to tap *slowly* and *firmly* in intercuspal position (ICP). Ideally, the sounds should be sharp. Dull or mixed sounds are the result of discrepancy between the muscular contact position (MCP) and the ICP.[46] MCP-ICP discrepancies can be caused by occlusal prematurities or muscle imbalance or both.

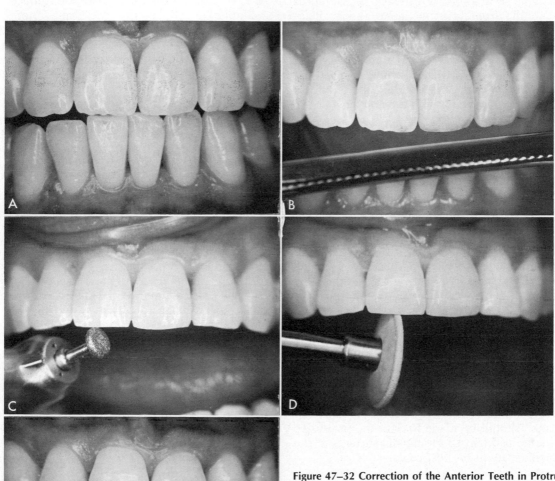

Figure 47–32 Correction of the Anterior Teeth in Protrusive Position. *A*, Before correction. *B*, Articulating paper in place to detect areas of contact. *C*, Marked areas on maxillary teeth reduced. *D*, Smoothing the ground surfaces with rubber wheel. *E*, Multipointed, bilateral contact of anterior teeth in protrusive position.

Correction of Protrusive Excursion. If any posterior teeth interfere or contact in the protrusive excursion, remove tooth structure from the offending cusps until all articulating contacts between the posterior teeth have been eliminated. Harmonious protrusive contact occurring during the first millimeter of jaw movement is permissible. Protrusive interferences are on the *distal facing* inclines of the maxillary teeth and the *mesial facing* inclines of the mandibular teeth. A practical method for marking excursive contact is the **two-color method.** The protrusive contacts are first marked by drying and isolating the teeth, inserting **red** marking ribbon, and having the patient produce several protrusive glides. The vertical stops are then marked with **blue** marking paper by having the patient tap his or her teeth together in ICP. As a result, the unwanted protrusive (red) interferences are clearly distinguished from the vertical stops (blue), which are to be preserved. *It is important not to disturb the cusp tips and vertical stops required for maintenance of the ICP.* Mobile teeth should be stabilized by the operator's fingers to prevent them from moving away from the forces of contact. Confirm the absence of posterior protrusive interferences by the use of occlusal Mylar strips.

The lingual surfaces of the maxillary teeth also are marked using the two-color method (protrusive gliding contacts in red; ICP stops, if present, in blue). The protrusive contacts are reduced to provide a bilateral, smooth contact glide along the path approaching the previously established protrusive position. Attempts should be made to limit the protrusive glide adjustment to the lingual surfaces of the maxillary teeth in most cases.

There are several types of problems that require the use of clinical judgment in the protrusive excursion adjustment. Occasionally, an open-bite situation will not permit edge-to-edge contact of the anterior teeth. The posterior teeth then must be recruited to play a role in the protrusive guidance, i.e., the preservation of smooth protrusive posterior contact.

Similarly, the anterior teeth may not be suitable for use as sole discluders of the teeth on protrusive excursion because of loss of bony support. In such instances, the anterior and posterior teeth should be brought into contact during the protrusive glide (especially the first 2 mm of contact movement). Attempts should also be made to evaluate habitual incisal "lock and key" bruxism facets. Any significant facets on teeth in the anterior segment should be rounded over without shortening the clinical crowns.

STEP 6. REMOVE OR LESSEN MEDIOTRUSIVE (BALANCING) INTERFERENCES. Mediotrusive (balancing) interferences complicate the correction of the laterotrusive (working) guidance. They even may prevent laterotrusive side guidance. Mediotrusive interferences are routinely observed as oblique facets on the first and second molar teeth (the inner inclines of the mandibular buccal cusps and the inner inclines of the maxillary lingual cusps) (Fig. 47–33). *Mediotrusive interferences should be lessened or removed to facilitate a dominant disclusion on the laterotrusive side.* It is recommended that both habitual excursion and passive (border) manipulation of the mandible be employed in order to detect mediotrusive interferences originating both from ICP and RCP. To record for reduction, mark the mediotrusive contact with red marking ribbon,

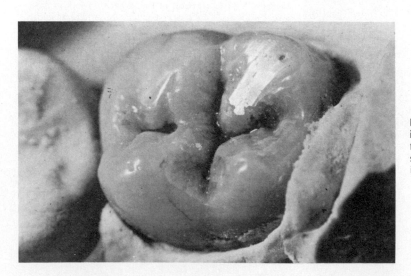

Figure 47–33 Mediotrusive (Balancing) Interferences appear as oblique facets on the molar teeth. Example shows extracted mandibular tooth set in dental cast.

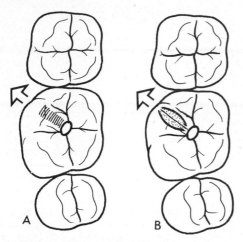

Figure 47–34 Adjustment of Mediotrusive (Balancing) Interference often involves grooving to allow freedom for the opposing cusp movement.

then locate the ICP stops with blue marking paper (two-color method). Often reduction is achieved by grinding new grooves or shallow depressions for the opposing cusp pathway (Fig. 47–34). The effect of the reduction can be checked intermittently by the insertion of Mylar occlusal strips.

Care should be taken, because the complete elimination of mediotrusive interferences may disrupt ICP contact. Therefore, one must weigh the advantages of complete removal of all mediotrusive interferences in relation to the effect of this adjustment on the overall mandibular stability in ICP.

It should be stressed that not all mediotrusive contact is necessarily pathologic. It hardly could be, since the probability of observing a mediotrusive contact on at least one side in healthy young adults is 84 per cent.[17] It is probable that the traumatic potential of mediotrusive interferences is related to *intensity* of contact combined with the lack of adequate cross-arch canine guidance. Thus, correct adjustment of mediotrusive interferences may involve reducing them so that they conform to smooth, interference-free functional contact. A functional chewing test is helpful in making this assessment. The test is conducted as follows: Place a strip of adhesive occlusal registration wax over the mandibular quadrant in question. Give another strip of folded occlusal registration wax to the patient, and instruct him or her to chew the wax on the opposite side three to five times. If there are significant mediotrusive interferences, oblique perforations of the applied wax strip will be observed. Repeat the test following adjustment for comparison and evaluation.

When the mediotrusive interferences have been dealt with on one side, the laterotrusive interferences are adjusted for the opposite side (step 7). Thus, the lateral excursion of one laterotrusive (working) side and its corresponding mediotrusive (balancing) side is completely corrected before the other lateral excursion is treated.

Step 7. Reduce Interferences on the Laterotrusive (Working) Side. *Lateral guidance is dominated by the canine and first premolar teeth (termed the canine segment) in healthy young adults. The canine tooth is most frequently involved in disclusion.*[17, 36] The disclusion scheme is likely to include more posterior teeth with advancing age and accelerated wear. The lack of adequate guidance in the canine area brings on *single-tooth molar interferences* that have traumatic potential during function and parafunction. The first 2 mm of excursive guidance from ICP and RCP are important because maximum force can be applied near the closed position.

The positional availability of teeth as discluders and the periodontal status of all potential discluder teeth should be clinically assessed. Laterotrusive discluding contact should be on the ipsilateral canine and, frequently, on the first premolar, unless these teeth are weakened periodontally. In the case of mobile canines, all the teeth on the laterotrusive side, except the second molar, should assist in lateral guidance. *An attempt should be made to remove or neutralize single-tooth interferences on the molar teeth.* Contact area may be reduced on the canine and premolars if severe surface-to-surface faceting predominates. Existing "lock and key" facets on laterotrusive cusps should be rounded over without shortening the clinical crown.

In lateral function, whether canine segment or group, the discluding angle should be great enough to prevent mediotrusive contact on the contralateral side and a definite separation of the ipsilateral molar teeth (Fig. 47–35). Normally, very little reduction is done on the canine and premolar teeth, as these contacts are considered to be important for disclusion of the molar teeth in lateral movement. *Unrestricted smooth contact movement in laterotrusion is more important than the number of contacts that are brought into lateral function.*

Laterotrusive contacts can be marked with the two-color method described previously. Reshape the inner inclines of the maxillary buccal cusps, if possible, as grinding of the mandibular buccal cusps could interfere with ICP vertical stops. Always grind to the point

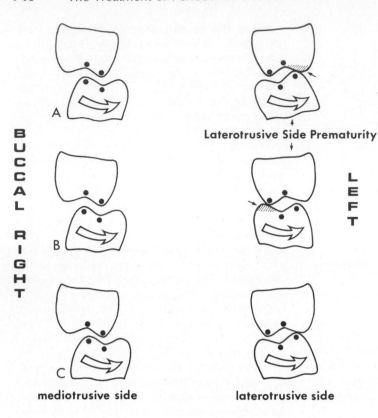

B U C C A L   **R I G H T**

L E F T

Laterotrusive Side Prematurity

mediotrusive side   laterotrusive side

Figure 47–35 Correction of Laterotrusive Interferences (Hatched Areas) on Posterior Teeth to Gain Smooth Contact Movement Patterns. Mandibular movement indicated by arrows. *A,* Laterotrusive interference on buccal cusps. *B,* Laterotrusive interference on lingual cusps. *C,* Unrestricted glide after correction of laterotrusive interferences. Note absence of contact on the mediotrusive side.

of the ICP vertical stop. Never include it in the reduction. Adjustment of the inclines often can be achieved through the process of grooving. All reductions should result in spherical or grooved surfaces. *Avoid creating flat planes.* Check your adjustment using Mylar occlusal strips.

Step 8. Eliminate Gross Occlusal Disharmonies. At this point all occlusal disharmonies involving tooth contact or contact movement will have been removed or lessened. However, other occlusal disharmonies harmful to the periodontal structures may remain; these should be modified. Care should be taken to avoid changing or removing previously attained occlusal contact relationships. Elimination of gross occlusal disharmonies at the beginning of the occlusal adjustment may be tempting, and indeed is permissible. Early gross adjustment should be done only to the extent that tooth contacts important to the future stability of the occlusion are not destroyed in the process.

Extruded Teeth. Extruded teeth are reduced to the level of the occlusal plane by grinding and reshaping within the limits permitted by the position of the pulp. If large areas are exposed by grinding, a dental restoration in conformity with the corrected occlusal relationship is indicated. Extruded unopposed third molars may irritate the mucosa of the opposing jaw, interfere with closure in centric occlusion, and deflect the mandible. Food impaction is also common between extruded third molars and the second molar. Extruded third molars should be extracted or reduced to the occlusal plane and splinted to the second molar.

When an unopposed maxillary third molar is removed, the interdental space between the first and second molars should be watched for evidence of food impaction. Distal thrusts produced on occlusal contact may momentarily break the contact between the maxillary first and second molars and permit impaction of food (Fig. 47–36). At the first sign of such impaction, ICP contacts should be evaluated and adjusted if their incline contact relationships promote distal movement of the second molar. If subsequent adjustment fails to result in closure of the contact, it may be necessary to splint the first and second molars together.

Plunger Cusps. Plunger cusps are cusp points that wedge into the interproximal spaces between opposing teeth and cause food impaction (Fig. 47–37). Distolingual cusps of maxillary molars often are plunger cusps. The cusp points should be rounded and shortened, and

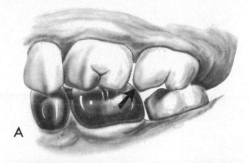

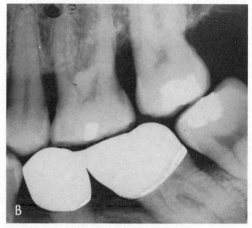

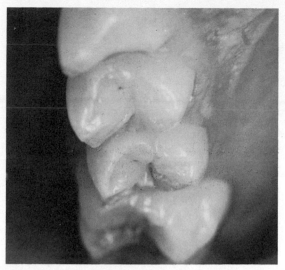

Figure 47–38 Uneven marginal ridges.

Figure 47–36 Displacement of Maxillary Second Molar in the Absence of Distal Support. *A,* Impact of mandibular first molar *(arrow)* leads to displacement of maxillary second molar and creates area of food impaction. Note absence of contact between the mandibular molars. *B,* Radiograph showing accentuated bone loss in area of food impaction on mesial surface of maxillary second molar.

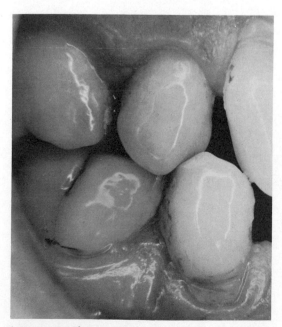

Figure 47–37 Plunger Cusp on the Maxilla. The premolar forces food between the mandibular teeth, causing gingival inflammation.

if this does not suffice, the opposing interproximal space can be protected by splinting the teeth adjacent to it.

Uneven Adjacent Marginal Ridges. Differences in the height of adjacent marginal ridges may cause food impaction and should be corrected by either reducing the height of the comparatively high marginal ridge or increasing the height of the lower one with a restoration (Fig. 47–38). Extreme differences are overcome by using both procedures. In grinding the marginal ridges the natural tooth contour should be preserved. *The marginal ridge should not be reduced if this entails sacrifice of occlusal contact.*

Rotated, Malposed, and Tilted Teeth. Teeth that are rotated or tilted facially or lingually may interfere with functional movement of the mandible and cause food accumulation and impaction. Depending on their severity, such conditions can be corrected by tooth grinding or by orthodontic procedures (see Chapter 48) or restorations that conform to the corrected occlusal and proximal relationship of the dentition (Fig. 47–39).

Facets and Flat Occlusal Wear. Facets are flattened planes produced by wear on a convex tooth surface[44]; they vary in size and outline (Fig. 47–40). They are detected by examination after the teeth have been dried. Study casts are also helpful. Occlusal contact at the periphery of broad facets may create lateral or tipping forces potentially injurious to the periodontium and should be adjusted so that only a small area remains in occlusal contact (Fig. 47–41).

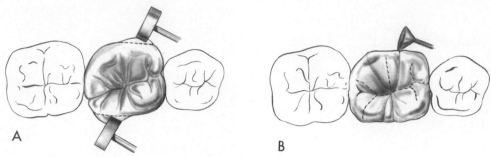

Figure 47–39 Reshaping Slightly Rotated Tooth by Grinding. *A,* Slightly rotated molar. Areas to be removed by grinding indicated by dashed lines. *B,* Occlusal surface recontoured *(dashed lines)* and buccal grooves relocated.

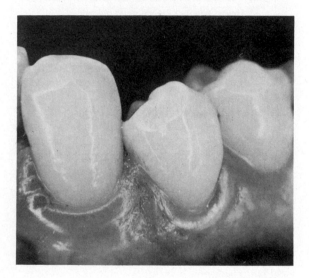

Figure 47–40 Prominent facets on the premolars.

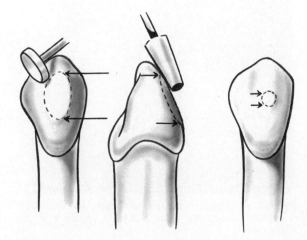

Figure 47–41 Reduction of Facet by Grinding. The dimensions of the facet before and after reduction are indicated by the arrows.

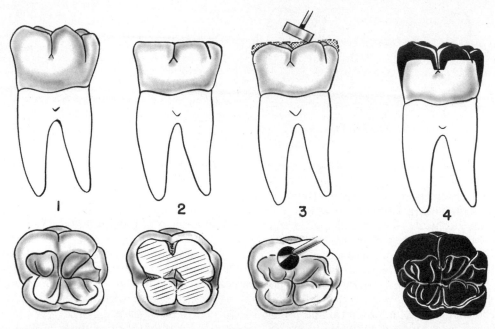

Figure 47–42 Reshaping the Occlusal Surface of a Mandibular Molar Altered by Functional Wear. *1*, The unworn molar crown. *2*, The molar crown altered by wear. *3*, Reshaping the molar crown to reduce the area of the occlusal surface and restore cuspal inclines and marginal ridges. (The outlined stippled area is the portion of the tooth surface removed.) *4*, The use of a restoration to reshape a worn molar crown when correction by grinding is not feasible.

Flat Occlusal Wear. When excessive wear produces broad, flat, or cupped-out occlusal surfaces, forces applied at the periphery are directed outside the confines of the root and may create tipping forces injurious to the periodontium. The occlusal surface is modified by grinding to restore the normal faciolingual and mesiodistal diameters, cuspal anatomy, grooves, and marginal ridges (Fig. 47–42). Proximal contact relationships must be maintained. If the desired correction is not attainable by grinding, the use of a restoration is indicated (Fig. 47–42). Incisal edges flattened by excessive occlusal wear are also reshaped by grinding (Fig. 47–43).

STEP 9. RECHECK TOOTH CONTACT RELATIONSHIPS. Tooth contact relationships in all positions and movements are rechecked to verify that the following *seven* criteria are met:

1. There is no asymmetrical shift from RCP to ICP. If a shift is present, it is smooth, symmetrical, and less than 1 mm in magnitude.

2. The completed adjustments have light contact or none between the incisor teeth and

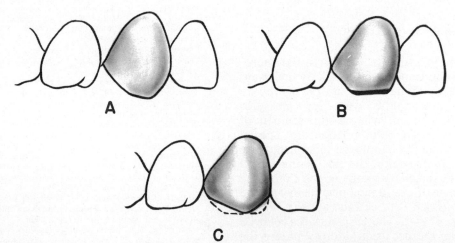

Figure 47–43 Recontouring Canine Altered by Incisal Wear. *A*, Contour of unworn maxillary canine. *B*, Facet frequently seen at incisal edge of canine. *C*, Correction of facet. Areas of tooth removed are indicated by the broken line.

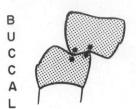
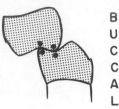

CROSSBITE

Figure 47–44 Crossbite showing reversal of normal buccolingual cuspal relationships. Large black dots indicate the areas of centric maintenance.

firm contact between as many posterior teeth as possible.

3. The patient perceives "even" (bilateral) contact when closing the teeth to ICP.

4. Sharp occlusal sounds are produced when the patient taps slowly and firmly into ICP.

5. Molar excursive interferences are eliminated or significantly reduced so that unrestricted glide paths are available for the posterior cusps.

6. Tooth guidance under lateral and protrusive excursions is smooth and without effort.

7. The displacement of mobile teeth is minimized under closure and gliding movements.

The above criteria also can serve as guidelines to help determine the *feasibility* of achieving a satisfactory result by means of occlusal adjustment. There are many instances when restorative or prosthetic treatments are necessary, sometimes in combination with orthodontic and surgical intervention. In questionable cases, a trial carving of articulated casts is the best means by which to judge the anticipated fulfillment of the foregoing criteria.

STEP 10. POLISH ALL ROUGH OCCLUSAL SURFACES. The occlusal surfaces are smoothed and polished so that they feel "comfortable" to the patient.

Special Problems (Crossbite)

Crossbite is a reversal of the normal buccolingual relationship of the maxillary and mandibular teeth. When only a few teeth are involved, orthodontic corrective measures should be employed. When a large segment of the arch is in crossbite relationship, special techniques must be employed in adjusting the occlusion. In crossbite, the tips of the buccal cusps of the maxillary teeth and the tips of the lingual cusps of the mandibular teeth and the areas into which they occlude are the vertical stops (Fig. 47–44). The cusp surfaces relieved in adjusting the occlusion in crossbite are the reverse of those in patients with a normal buccolingual relationship. The prognosis for achieving a stable postoperative occlusion is less favorable when dealing with crossbite relationships.

Maintenance of Occlusal Stability

There is evidence that the method of occlusal adjustment recommended here will provide stability for the short term. Teeth and dental restorations wear with use, however, and as a result, the occlusion changes over longer periods. No method of occlusal adjustment creates a permanent occlusal relationship. The occlusion must be checked periodically for minor adjustments, and the patient should be advised accordingly.

REFERENCES

1. Arnold, N. R., and Frumker, S. C.: Occlusal Treatment. Philadelphia, Lea & Febiger, 1976.
2. Azarbal, M.: Comparison of myo-monitor centric position to centric relation and centric occlusion. J. Pros. Dent., *38*:331, 1977.
3. Bell, D. H., Jr: Sagittal balance of the mandible. J.A.M.A., *64*:486, 1962.
4. Blaschke, D. D., Solberg, W. K., and Sanders, B.: Arthrography of the temporomandibular joint: review of current status. J. Am. Dent. Assoc., *100*:388, 1980.
5. Clark, T. D., Perachio, A., and Mahan, P.: A neurophysiological study of bruxism in the rhesus monkey. I.A.D.R. Abstracts, No. 1970, p. 190.
6. Clayton, J. A., Kotowicz, W. E., and Zahler, J. M.: Pantographic tracings of mandibular movments and occlusion. J. Prosthet. Dent., *25*:389, 1971.
7. Dawson, P. E.: Evaluation, Diagnosis, and Treatment of Occlusal Problems. St. Louis, C. V. Mosby Company, 1975, p. 56.
8. Farrar, W. B.: Diagnosis and treatment of anterior dislocation of the articular disc. N.Y. J. Dent., *40*:348, 1971.
9. Federick, D. R., Pameijer, C. H., and Stallard, R. E.: A correlation between force and distalization of the mandible in obtaining centric relation. J. Periodontol., *45*:70, 1974.
10. Glickman, I., Pameijer, J. H., Roeber, F. W., and Brion, M. A. M.: Functional occlusion as revealed by miniaturized radio transmitters. Dent. Clin. North Am., *13*:666, 1969.
11. Glickman, I., Smulow, J. B., Vogel, G., and Passamonti, G.: The effect of occlusal forces on healing following mucogingival surgery. J. Periodontol., *37*:319, 1966.
12. Graf, H.: Bruxism. Dent. Clin. North Am., *13*:659, 1969.
13. Grove, C. J.: Trauma produced by occlusion, due to horizontal stress. J. Am. Dent. Assoc., *11*:813, 1924.
14. Haddad, A. W.: The functioning dentition. *In* Kawamura, J. (ed.): Frontiers of Oral Physiology: Physiology of Oral Tissues. Basel, S. Karger, 1976.
15. Ingervall, B.: Retruded contact position of mandilble. A comparison between children and adults. Odontol. Rev., *15*:150, 1964.

16. Ingervall, B.: Retruded contact position of mandible in the deciduous dentition. Odontol. Rev., *15*:414, 1964.
17. Ingervall, B.: Tooth contacts on the functional and non-functional side in children and young adults. Arch. Oral Biol., *17*:191, 1972.
18. James, A. F.: A discussion by correspondence. Dent. Items Int., *45*:584, 1923.
19. Jankelson, B.: Physiology of human dental occlusion. J. Am. Dent. Assoc., *50*:664, 1955.
20. Jankelson, B.: A technique for obtaining optimum functional relationship for the natural dentition. Dent. Clin. North Am. *4*:131, 1960.
21. Jankelson, B., et al.: Neural conduction of the myo-monitor stimulus. A quantitative analysis. J. Prosthet. Dent., *34*:245, 1975.
22. Kantor, M. E., Silverman, S. I., and Garfinkel, M. A.: Centric-relation recording techniques. A comparative investigation. J. Prosthet. Dent. *28*:593, 1972.
23. Karlsen, K.: Traumatic occlusion as a factor in the propagation of periodontal disease. Int. Dent. J., *22*:387, 1972.
24. Krogh-Poulsen, W. G., and Olsson, A.: Management of the occlusion of the teeth. *In* Schwartz, L. S., and Chayes, C. M. (eds.): Facial Pain and Mandibular Dysfunction. Philadelphia, W. B. Saunders Company, 1968.
25. Lund, P., Nishiyama, T., and Moller, E.: Postural activity in the muscles of mastication with the subject upright, inclined, and supine. Scand. J. Dent. Res., *78*:417, 1970.
26. Lundeen, H. C.: Centric relation records: the effect of muscle action. J. Prosthet. Dent., *31*:244, 1974.
27. Möller, E., Sheik-Ol-Eslam, A., and Lous, L.: Deliberate relaxation of the temporal and masseter muscles in subjects with functional disorders of the chewing apparatus. Scand. J. Dent. Res., *78*:478, 1971.
28. Mühlemann, H. R., Herzog, H., and Rateitschak, K. H.: Quantitative evaluation of the therapeutic effect of selective grinding. J. Periodont., *28*:11, 1957.
29. Polson, A. M., Meitner, S. W., and Zander, H. A.: Trauma and progression of marginal periodontitis in squirrel monkeys III. Adaptation of interproximal alveolar bone to repetitive injury. J. Periodont. Res., *11*:279, 1976.
30. Polson, A. M., Meitner, S. W., and Zander, H. A.: Trauma and progression of marginal periodontitis in squirrel monkeys.

IV. Reversibility of bone loss due to trauma alone and trauma superimposed upon periodontitis. J. Periodont. Res., *11*:290, 1976.
31. Ramfjord, S. P.: Occlusion. Indent, *1*:20, 1973.
32. Ramfjord, S. P.: Bruxism, a clinical and electromyographic study. J. Am. Dent. Assoc., *62*:21, 1961.
33. Ramfjord, S. P., and Ash, M. M.: *Occlusion.* 2nd ed. Philadelphia, W. B. Saunders Company, 1971, p. 206.
34. Remien, J. C., and Ash, M. M.: Myo-monitor centric: an evaluation. J. Prosthet. Dent., *31*:137, 1974.
35. Reynolds, J. M.: Occlusal Adjustment. Pamphlet. Augusta, Ga., 1975.
36. Scaife, R. R., Jr., and Holt, J. E.: Natural occurrence of cuspid guidance. J. Prosthet. Dent., *22*:225, 1969.
37. Scharer, P., Butler, J., and Zander, H.: Die heilung parodontaler Knochentaschen bei okklusalar Dysfunktion. Schweiz. Mschr. Zahnheilk., *79*:244, 1969.
38. Schuyler, C. H.: Fundamental principles in the correction of occlusal disharmony, natural and artificial. J. Am. Dent. Assoc., *22*:1193, 1935.
39. Schuyler, C. H.: Factors contributing to traumatic occlusion. J. Prosthet. Dent., *11*:708, 1961.
40. Shore, N. A.: Temporomandibular Joint Dysfunction and Occlusal Equilibration. 2nd ed. Philadelphia, J. B. Lippincott Company, 1976.
41. Solberg, W. K., and Clark, G. T. (eds.): Temporomandibular Joint Problems: Biologic Diagnosis and Treatment. Chicago, Quintessence Publishing Company, 1980. 177 pp.
42. Solberg, W. K., Woo, M. W., and Houston, J. B.: Prevalence of mandibular dysfunction in young adults. J.A.D.A., *98*:25, 1979.
43. Strohaver, R. A.: A comparison of articulator mountings made with centric relation and myocentric position records. J. Prosthet. Dent., *28*:379, 1972.
44. Thomas, B. O. A., and Gallagher, J. W.: Practical management of occlusal dysfunctions in periodontal therapy. J. Am. Dent. Assoc., *46*:18, 1953.
45. Vollmer, W. H., and Rateitschak, K. H.: Influence of occlusal adjustment by grinding on gingivitis and mobility of traumatized teeth. J. Clin. Periodontol., *2*:113, 1975.
46. Watt, D.: A study of the average duration of occlusal sounds in different age groups. Br. Dent. J., *138*:385, 1975.

chapter forty-eight

Minor Orthodontic Movement in Periodontal Therapy

RATIONALE FOR ORTHODONTIC MOVEMENT IN PERIODONTAL THERAPY

Orthodontic procedures to change the position of the teeth are sometimes required in periodontal therapy. The advisability of undertaking orthodontic correction depends upon the following factors: (1) the severity of the periodontal problem and the possibility of improving it by orthodontics, (2) the level of the remaining bone, and (3) the possibility of the periodontal and occlusal conditions worsening without orthodontic correction. It should be understood that there is no correlation between malocclusion and periodontal disease. Therefore, the existence of a malocclusion is not by itself an indication for orthodontic therapy; only if it hinders plaque control or creates significant unfavorable forces is such therapy called for.

The following factors may justify orthodontic movement as a part of periodontal therapy:

REDUCING PLAQUE RETENTION. **Crowded teeth** are frequently very difficult to clean, making the introduction of dental floss and other cleaning devices practically impossible. This occurs most frequently in lower anterior areas of the mouth. **Tipped teeth**, usually in an edentulous area, create plaque accumulation sites that are difficult to clean. In addition, they open the distal contact, creating an area of food impaction. **Malposed teeth** may also create abnormal occlusal relationships that favor trauma from occlusion. The creation of abnormal contacts with the opposing jaw may trigger the development of bruxing habits. **Teeth in lingual version** have enlarged contact surfaces and altered embrasure spaces housing smaller papillae and a soft tissue facial ridge. Flossing is frequently impossible around these teeth.

IMPROVING GINGIVAL AND OSSEOUS FORM. There is an interrelationship between the position of a tooth and the shape of the gingiva and bone that surround it. A typical example would be a lower first or second molar tilted into an edentulous mesial space. This tooth will have a very narrow space between its crown and the bone that will easily become inflamed and where a pocket may develop. Bone reshaping may correct the bony defect, but it will also create a topography inconsistent with a healthy gingival sulcus. Orthodontic therapy may improve the shape of the periodontium and reduce the indications for bone surgery.

FACILITATING PROSTHETIC REPLACEMENTS. The uprighting of tilted abutment teeth may be very important in restorative dentistry. Parallel abutment teeth will require less removal of tooth structure, reduce the chance of pulpal damage, and facilitate better contoured crowns, all of which will benefit the periodontal condition.

IMPROVING ESTHETICS. Migration and diastemata between anterior teeth are relatively frequent features of moderate and advanced periodontal disease. These changes may be due to tongue-thrusting or other habits. Posterior tooth prematurities are usually combined with loss of periodontal support.

INDICATIONS

The most common problems that can be solved by minor orthodontic therapy include the following: (1) crowded teeth, (2) closure of anterior diastemata, (3) mesial tilting of molars, (4) anterior open bite, and (5) open contacts.

In most cases, consultation with an orthodontist and frequently referral to him or her for this particular phase of therapy are in the best interest of the patient. In all phases of orthodontic/periodontal therapy, a close collaboration between the orthodontist and the periodontist is most desirable.

CONTRAINDICATIONS

The only formal contraindication to orthodontic treatment in patients with periodontal disease is the persistence of gingival inflammation in spite of adequate Phase I therapy procedures. The superimposition of tooth movement on inflamed gingiva may worsen the periodontal problem.

Age is not a formal contraindication to orthodontic treatment, although it is generally assumed that bone remodeling processes may occur more slowly in older patients.

WHEN IN THE SEQUENCE OF PERIODONTAL PROCEDURES SHOULD ORTHODONTIC TREATMENT BE PERFORMED?

Orthodontic treatment should not be started until the inflammation of the gingiva has been reduced to a minimum through adequate scaling, root planing, and correction of other irritational factors and the patient is aware of and willing to cooperate with the most fastidious home care technique.

Periodically during the orthodontic treatment, the periodontist should check the condition of the tissues. The reason for this is twofold: (1) since the orthodontic treatment will create forces on the teeth, the reduction or total elimination of inflammation will reduce the chances of a combination of the two effects becoming detrimental to the tissues; and (2) following the elimination of inflammation, teeth frequently change their position.

Major occlusal adjustment and surgical procedures are better performed after the completion of orthodontic therapy. In any case, after orthodontic treatment a final occlusal adjustment should be performed.

Surgical procedures are done after orthodontic treatment because (1) orthodontics may change the shape of the periodontium, reducing the need for or the extent of surgery; and (2) the removal of supracrestal periodontal fibers during surgery will facilitate retention, since new, reoriented fibers will form.

DIFFERENT ORTHODONTIC TREATMENT MODALITIES

The many methods that can be used for tooth movement fall into two basic categories: fixed appliances and removable appliances. Some of the simpler methods of tooth movement will be described here, more as examples of what can be done than as a complete review of the subject. The reader is urged to study some of the textbooks on adult orthodontics and to consult an orthodontist for evaluation and frequently for performance of the methods.

Correction of Pathologic Migration

The following factors should be considered when orthodontic correction of migrated teeth is contemplated:

1. The availability of space for the teeth to be repositioned.

2. The absence of interference from teeth in the opposing arch.

3. The extent to which loss of posterior tooth support, reduced vertical dimension, and accentuated anterior overbite complicate orthodontic movement.

4. The availability of sufficient anchorage from which forces can be applied.

5. Habits that may interfere with the desired tooth movement.

HAWLEY APPLIANCE FOR THE CORRECTION OF PATHOLOGIC MIGRATION. This is a removable tissue-borne appliance with an anterior wire frame extension or labial bow. It may be modified in a variety of ways for moving individual teeth (Fig. 48–1) and is most often used on the maxilla. The tissue-borne portion covers the palate, is usually made of acrylic, and may have clasps on the posterior teeth for added retention. To prevent irritation to the gingiva, it should cover approximately one third of the length of the crowns. The margin of the appliance is cut away when necessary to create space for the desired tooth movement.

The labial bow is embedded in the acrylic and extends through the interproximal spaces between the canines and premolars onto the

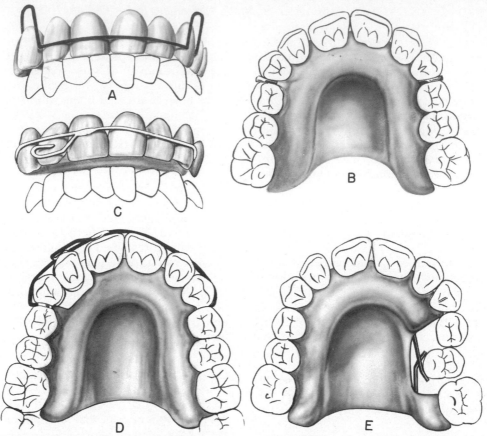

Figure 48–1 The Hawley Appliance. *A*, Hawley appliance with labial bow. *B*, Acrylic tissue-borne portion covers approximately one third of the length of the crowns. *C*, Wire soldered to labial bow to move lateral incisor. The palatal acrylic is used as an anterior bite plate. *D*, Palatal view showing acrylic cut away to provide space for the lateral incisor. *E*, Wire spring embedded in acrylic to move the second premolar buccally. If necessary, the proximal tooth surfaces are stripped to provide space.

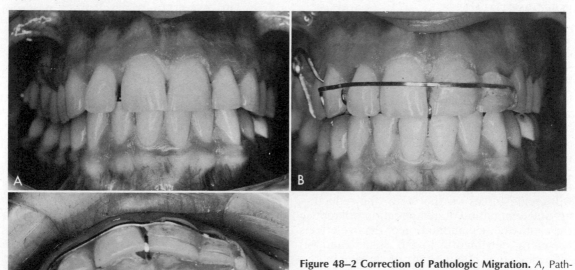

Figure 48–2 Correction of Pathologic Migration. *A*, Pathologic migration of maxillary lateral incisor. *B*, Hawley appliance with wire spring on distal surface of lateral incisor accomplishes desired movement. *C*, Lingual view of labial bow with wire spring to lateral incisor.

facial surfaces of the anterior teeth (Fig. 48–1). When used on the mandible, the tissue-borne portion of the appliance is horseshoe-shaped; it may be made of acrylic or metal, depending on the strength required.

To correct pathologic migration of maxillary anterior teeth, the wire labial bow or rubber dam elastics attached to hooks embedded in the acrylic at the distal surface of each canine are used. The appliance should be worn at all times until the desired movement is effected (Fig. 48–2).

Correction of Mesially Tipped Teeth

When the permanent first molar is extracted and not replaced, a series of events take place (these are described in Chapter 26). The changes include mesial tilting of the second molar, which creates an area difficult to clean.

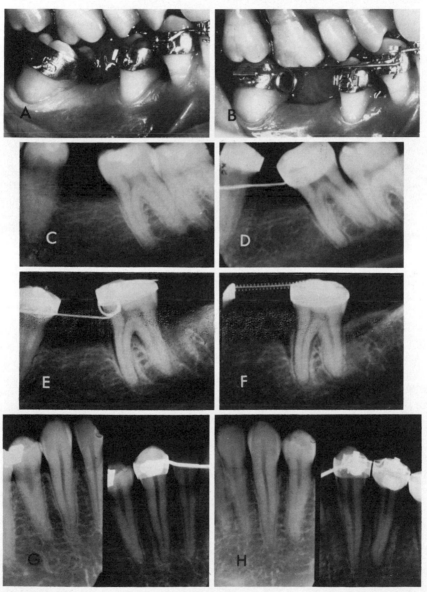

Figure 48–3 Molar Uprighting: Reciprocal Spring. A variety of mechanisms have been devised to upright tipped molars. *A* and *B*, Reciprocal spring formed from a rectangular wire engaged into a horizontal tube on the molars to be uprighted. *C* and *D*, Typical radiographic changes noted as a molar is uprighted. *E*, As the molar begins to move, bone forms on the mesial aspect. *F*, Final tooth position. *G*, Even with proper anchorage, some undesired movement can occur. A shift in root position is observed on the contralateral side of a molar uprighting, and external tooth resorption and change in the position of the root are noted on the ipsilateral side (*H*). (From Swanson, J. C., and Rosenberg, F.: Dent. Clin. North Am., 24:231, 1980.)

A number of methods have been proposed for uprighting molar teeth that have tilted into an edentulous mesial space.[5, 8, 9] Figure 48–3 shows the bone response to uprighting a tipped molar with a reciprocal spring formed from a rectangular wire engaged into a horizontal tube on the molars to be uprighted.

Several authors have found that pockets mesial to uprighted molars are shallower than pockets mesial to control teeth that have not been uprighted. This is apparently due to a reduction in soft tissue height while the bone height remains unchanged. Gingival inflammation does not differ from that around control teeth.[1, 7]

The presence of other discrepancies, such as lingual inclination, necessitates treatment by an orthodontist.

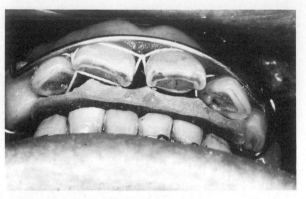

Figure 48–5 Grassline Ligature used in conjunction with bite plate to correct rotated teeth.

Correction of Malposed Teeth

Grassline ligatures and rubber dam elastics[6] are useful for the correction of malposed individual teeth. With grassline ligatures, tooth movement is effected by contraction of the ligature after it absorbs moisture from the mouth. The dry ligature is applied in such a manner that the force created by contraction is in the direction of the desired tooth movement. Particular care must be taken to include a sufficient number of teeth for anchorage (Figs. 48–4 and 48–5). The ligature should be placed close to the contact points, incisal to the cingulum, to prevent slipping and irritation of the gingiva. Ligatures are usually replaced weekly until the desired tooth movement is attained.

Teeth can be moved more rapidly with rubber dam elastics, but the risk of damage to the supporting tissues is greater. Rootward sliding of the band, causing injury to the periodontium and extrusion of teeth, is an infrequent complication of the use of rubber dam elastics.

Correction of Crowded Mandibular Anterior Teeth

Crowded and malposed teeth frequently present a problem from both the periodontal and the orthodontic viewpoints (Fig. 48–6). The gingiva around teeth in labial version is often attached apical to the level on the adjacent teeth. On teeth in lingual version, the labial gingiva is often enlarged and attracts irritating plaque and debris. Orthodontic correction of malposed teeth creates gingival contours more conducive to periodontal health.

A tooth may be extracted to correct crowding (Fig. 48–7), provided the extraction creates

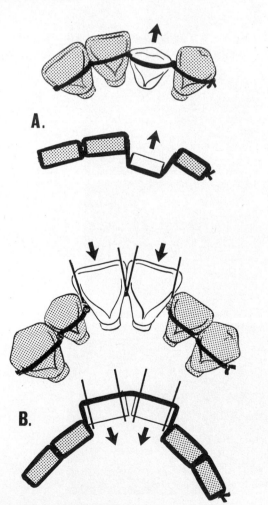

Figure 48–4 Grassline Ligature to Correct Malposition. *A,* Repositioning of lingually placed lateral incisor. *B,* Two labially placed central incisors are brought into proper alignment. The proximal surfaces of the incisors may be trimmed (vertical lines) to fit into available space.

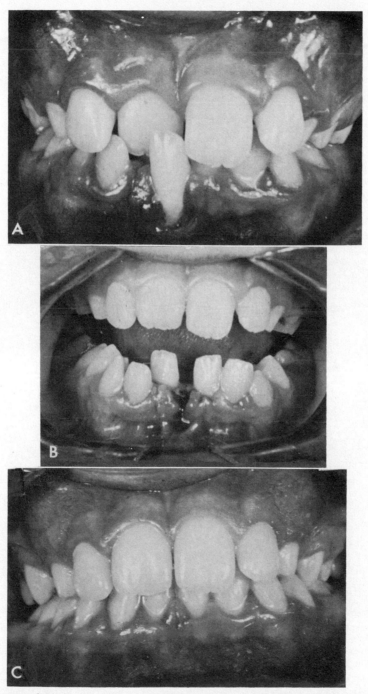

Figure 48–6 Improvement of Gingival Condition Following Correction of Crowding in the Mandibular Anterior Region. *A,* Marked gingival disease associated with malocclusion. *B,* Central incisor removed. *C,* Improved condition of the gingiva associated with improvement in the tooth relationship after orthodontic treatment. (Courtesy of Dr. Coenraad F. A. Moorrees.)

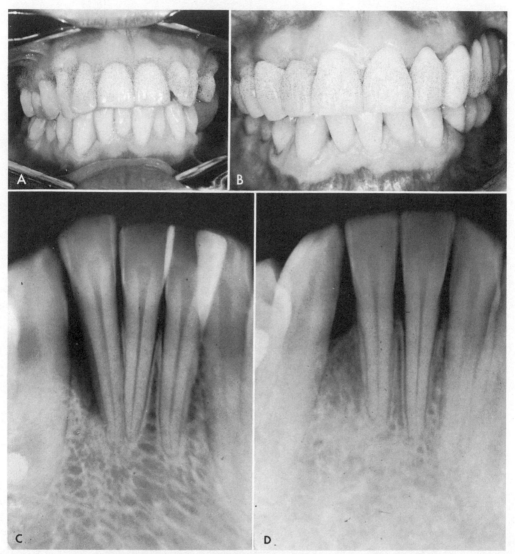

Figure 48–7 Improvement in the Condition of the Bone Following Correction of Anterior Irregularity. *A,* Crowding of mandibular teeth with left central incisor in labial version. *B,* After treatment, which included extraction of the right lateral incisor, alignment of the anterior teeth, and prosthesis. *C,* Before treatment. Note the angular bone defect. *D,* Three years after treatment. Note improvement in the bone. (Restorations by Dr. Philip Williams.)

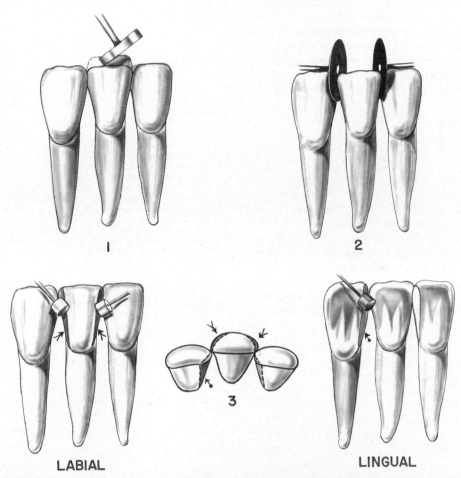

LABIAL   **LINGUAL**

Figure 48–8 Grinding as an Adjunct to the Treatment of Malposed and Extruded Anterior Teeth. *1,* Reduction of the incisal edge of a prominent mandibular anterior tooth. *2,* Grinding of the proximal surfaces of a mandibular tooth in labial version, as well as the proximal surfaces of the adjacent teeth, to provided space for proper alignment. *3,* Where space cannot be provided by grinding the proximal surfaces as illustrated in 2, the mesial and distal aspects of the labial surface of the malposed tooth are reduced, along with the marginal ridges on the lingual surfaces of the adjacent teeth.

sufficient space for proper alignment of the teeth that remain. Another consideration when tooth extraction is being contemplated is the degree of overbite. Normally, the mandibular teeth are "contained within" the maxillary arch. Extraction of a mandibular incisor may result in "closing in" of the arch with an increase in the overbite and the possibility of undesirable periodontal sequelae.

Another consideration when tooth extraction is contemplated is the mechanics required to realign the remaining teeth without proximal tipping. Improper proximal contacts create areas of potential food impaction. When possible, it is preferable to avoid tooth extraction by judicious grinding of the proximal surfaces to create space for the crowded teeth (Fig. 48–8).

Retention

Some type of retention is usually necessary after the desired tooth movement has been completed. Optimally, all the forces that caused the initial displacement of the tooth will have been controlled and, therefore, the retention will be temporary. In most cases, even if all the unfavorable factors have disappeared, a period of retention will be needed until all the bone and ligamentous structures around the tooth have been remodeled to accommodate to the new tooth position. This can be accomplished by continuing the use of the appliance for a longer period in an inactive state. Temporary retention devices should be used 24 hours a day for a period twice as long as it took to bring the tooth to its desired position.

Wire ligatures are often used after elastics or grassline ligatures have been employed. Other types of temporary splinting, as described in Chapter 58, can be used. Permanent retention by means of fixed prostheses is also often used.

REFERENCES

1. Brown, J. S.: The effect of orthodontic therapy on certain types of periodontal defects. I. Clinical findings. J. Periodontol., *44*:742, 1973.
2. Cooper, M. E.: Minor tooth movement in the management of the periodontal patient. *In* Prichard, J. (ed.): The Diagnosis and Treatment of Periodontal Disease. Philadelphia, W. B. Saunders Company, 1979.
3. Edwards, J. G.: A study of the periodontium during orthodontic rotation of teeth. Am. J. Orthod., *50*:441, 1963.
4. Ewen, S. J., and Pasternak, R.: Periodontal surgery, an adjunct to orthodontic therapy. Periodontics, *2*:162, 1964.
5. Hirschfeld, L.: Minor tooth movement in periodontal therapy. *In* Schluger, S., Youdelis, R., and Page, R. C.: Periodontal Disease. Philadelphia, Lea & Febiger, 1977.
6. Hirschfeld, L., and Geiger, A.: Minor Tooth Movement in General Practice. St. Louis, C. V. Mosby Company, 1966.
7. Kraal, J. H., et al.: Periodontal conditions in patients after molar uprighting. J. Prosthet. Dent., *43*:156, 1980.
8. Swanson, J. C., and Rosenberg, F.: Orthodontic movement in periodontal therapy. Dent. Clin. North Am., *24*:231, 1980.
9. Wagenberg, B. D., Eskow, R. N., and Langer B.: Orthodontic procedures that improve periodontal prognosis. J. Am. Dent. Assoc., *100*:370, 1980.

Surgical Phase

The Surgical Phase of Therapy

Although in a strict sense all instrumental therapy can be considered surgical, we will refer here only to those techniques that include the intentional severing or incising of gingival tissue with the purpose of controlling or eliminating periodontal disease. Therefore, scaling and root planing are not included, since these procedures do not intentionally act upon the gingival tissue.

OBJECTIVES OF THE SURGICAL PHASE

The surgical phase of periodontal therapy consists of techniques performed for pocket therapy and techniques performed for the correction of related morphologic problems, namely mucogingival defects. In many cases procedures are combined so that one surgical intervention fulfills both objectives.

The purpose of **surgical pocket therapy** is to eliminate the pathologic changes in the pocket wall; to create a stable, easily maintainable state; and, if possible, to promote periodontal regeneration.

In order to fulfill these objectives, *surgical techniques (1) increase accessibility to the root surface, making it possible to remove all irritants; (2) reduce pocket depth, making it possible for the patient to maintain the root surfaces free of plaque and (3) remodel soft and hard tissues in order to attain a harmonious topography.* In cases in which it is reasonable to expect a restoration of the marginal periodontium, with bone regeneration and reattachment, a surgical approach is the treatment of

choice. In some cases, soft tissue surgery may suffice or bone surgery may be necessary to remove irregular bone contours.

The other objective of the surgical phase of periodontal therapy is the correction of morphologic defects that may favor plaque accumulation and pocket recurrence. These are the mucogingival techniques used to create attached gingiva or to cover denuded roots. They are dealt with in Chapter 56.

SURGICAL POCKET THERAPY

Surgical pocket therapy can be directed to (1) opening up the pocket area to ensure the removal of irritants from the tooth surface or (2) eliminating, or reducing the depth of, the periodontal pocket.

The effectiveness of periodontal therapy is predicated upon success in completely eliminating calculus and plaque from the tooth surface. Numerous investigators have shown that the difficulty of this task increases as the pocket becomes deeper.[2, 4] There are many irregularities on the root surface that increase the difficulty of the procedure. As the pocket gets deeper, the surface to be scaled increases, more irregularities appear on the root surface, and accessibility is impaired[8, 11]; the presence of furcation involvements sometimes creates insurmountable problems (see Chapter 33).

All these problems can be reduced by eliminating or displacing the soft tissue wall of the pocket, thereby increasing the visibility and accessibility of the root surface. The flap ap-

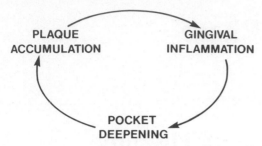

PLAQUE
ACCUMULATION

GINGIVAL
INFLAMMATION

POCKET
DEEPENING

Figure 49–1 Accumulation of plaque leads to gingival inflammation and pocket deepening, which in turn increases the area of plaque accumulation.

proach and the gingivectomy technique attain this result.

The need to eliminate or reduce the depth of the pocket is another important consideration. Pocket elimination consists of reducing the depth of periodontal pockets to that of a physiologic sulcus in order to facilitate access during the procedure and to render the area cleansable by the patient afterward. The presence of a pocket creates areas which are impossible for the patient to keep clean, and therefore the vicious circle depicted in Figure 49–1 is established.

RESULTS OF POCKET THERAPY

A periodontal pocket can be in an active state or in a period of inactivity or quiescence.

An **active pocket** is one under which bone is being lost. It can be diagnosed clinically by bleeding and secretion, either spontaneously or upon probing. After Phase I therapy, the inflammatory changes in the pocket wall subside, rendering the pocket inactive and reducing its depth. The extent of this reduction depends on the depth before treatment and on the degree to which the depth is due to the edematous and inflammatory component of the pocket wall. Whether the pocket remains inactive will depend on its depth and on the individual characteristics of the plaque components and the host response. *Recurrence of the initial activity is very likely*.

Inactive pockets can sometimes heal with a long junctional epithelium. However, this condition is also unstable, and the chance of recurrence and re-formation of the original pocket is always present because the epithelial union to the tooth is a weak one.

Studies have shown that inactive pockets can be maintained for long periods with little loss of attachment by means of frequent scaling and root planing procedures.[5, 7, 9]

A more reliable and permanent result is obtained by transforming the pocket into a **healthy sulcus.** The healthy sulcus can be located where the bottom of the pocket was localized. This results in no gain of attachment; it will expose the area of the root that was previously the tooth wall of the pocket. It should be understood that such a result after periodontal treatment does not cause recession but, rather, uncovers the recession previously induced by the disease. The healthy sulcus can also be located coronal to the bottom of the pre-existent pocket. This is conducive to a **restored marginal periodontium;** the result is a sulcus of normal depth with substantial gain of attachment, although the location of the sulcus may be slightly apical to the cemento-enamel junction. The creation of a healthy sulcus and a restored periodontium means a total restoration of the condition existing before periodontal disease began.

Figure 49–2 shows in schematic form these possible results of pocket therapy.

POCKET ELIMINATION VERSUS POCKET MAINTENANCE

Total pocket elimination has traditionally been considered one of the main goals of periodontal therapy. Elimination was considered vital because of the need to improve the accessibility of the root surfaces for the therapist during treatment and for the patient after healing.

Another viewpoint has emerged in recent years, supported by clinical longitudinal studies.[12] It has been shown that after surgical therapy, pockets of 4 and even 5 mm can be maintained in a healthy state and without radiographic evidence of advancing bone loss. This was accomplished by scaling and root planing, with oral hygiene reinforcement performed at regular intervals of not more than 3 months beginning after pocket therapy. In these cases the residual defect can be penetrated with a thin periodontal probe, but no pain, exudate, or bleeding results; also, no plaque appears to form on the subgingival root surfaces.

These clinical longitudinal studies do not reduce the indications for periodontal surgery, since the results obtained are based on surgical exposure of the root surfaces for a thorough and complete elimination of irritants. They do, however, emphasize the importance of the maintenance phase and of the close monitoring

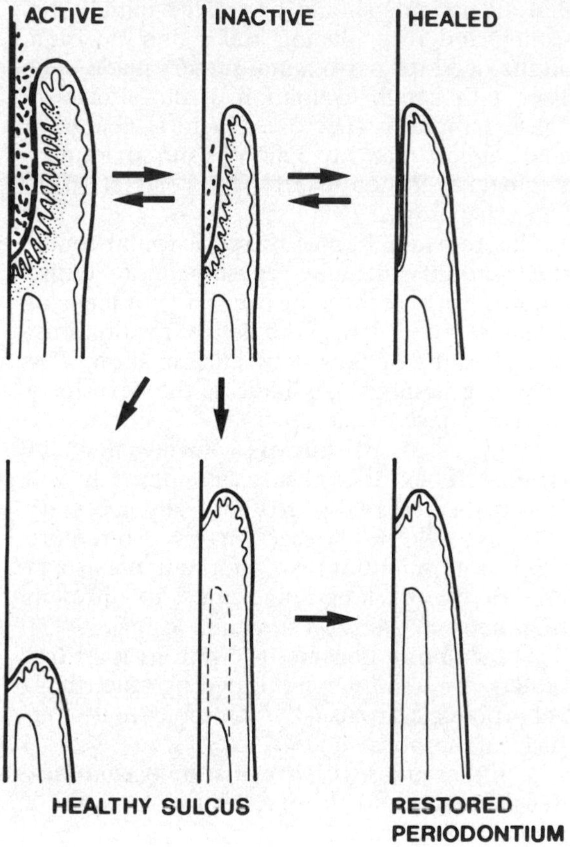

Figure 49–2 Possible Results of Pocket Therapy. An active pocket can become inactive and heal by means of a long junctional epithelium. Surgical pocket therapy can result in a healthy sulcus, with or without gain of attachment. The former may include restoration of bone height, with re-formation of periodontal ligament fibers and layers of cementum.

of both level of attachment and pocket depth, together with the other clinical parameters (bleeding, secretion, and tooth mobility). *The transformation of the initial deep, active lesion into a shallower, inactive, maintainable one requires some form of definitive pocket therapy and constant supervision thereafter.*

Pocket depth is an extremely useful and widely employed clinical parameter, but it must be evaluated together with level of attachment and the presence of bleeding, exudation, and pain. The most important parameter for evaluating whether a pocket (or deep sulcus) is progressive is the **level of attachment,** which is measured in millimeters from the cemento-enamel junction; in the last analysis it is the apical displacement of the level of attachment that places the tooth in jeopardy, not the increase in pocket depth, which may be due to coronal displacement of the gingival margin.

Pocket depth remains an important clinical parameter upon which decisions about treatment selection can in part be based. Lindhe et al.[6] compared the effect of root planing alone and in conjunction with a modified Widman flap on the resultant level of attachment and in relation to initial pocket depth. They re-

ported that scaling and root planing procedures induce loss of attachment if performed in pockets shallower than 2.9 mm, whereas in deeper pockets gain of attachment occurs. The modified Widman flap induces loss of attachment if done in pockets shallower than 4.2 mm but results in a greater gain of attachment than does root planing in pockets deeper than 4.2 mm.

Furthermore, probing depths established following active therapy and healing (approximately 6 months after treatment) can be maintained unchanged or reduced even further during a maintenance care period involving careful prophylaxis once every 3 months.[6]

Ramfjord et al.[9] and Rosling et al.[10] have shown that, regardless of the surgical technique used for pocket therapy, a certain pocket depth will recur. *In the last analysis, therefore, maintenance of this depth without any further loss of attachment becomes the goal.*

INDICATIONS FOR PERIODONTAL SURGERY

Several longitudinal studies carried out in the last two decades have pointed to the fact that all patients should be treated initially by scaling and root planing and a final decision on the need for periodontal surgery made only after a thorough evaluation of the effects of Phase I therapy. The assessment is generally made no less than 1 to 3 months and sometimes as much as 9 months after the completion of Phase I therapy.[1]

This re-evaluation of the periodontal condition should include reprobing the entire mouth, with rechecking for the presence of calculus, root caries, defective restorations, and all signs of persistent inflammation. The following findings may indicate the need for a surgical phase of therapy:

1. In cases of **furcation involvement of Grades II or III,** a surgical approach will ensure the removal of irritants; any necessary root resection or hemisection will also require surgical intervention. No information exists at present on the long-range effect of different treatment methods on furcation lesions.

2. **Infrabony pockets in distal areas of last molars,** frequently complicated by mucogingival problems, are usually unresponsive to nonsurgical methods.

3. Other areas with **irregular bony contours, deep craters,** and so forth may also require a surgical approach.

4. **Deep pockets** on teeth where a complete removal of root irritants is not considered clinically possible may call for surgery.

5. **Persistent inflammation** in areas with moderate to deep pockets may require a surgical approach. In areas with shallow pockets or normal sulci, persistent inflammation may point to the presence of a mucogingival problem that needs a surgical solution.

CRITICAL ZONES IN POCKET SURGERY

There are different techniques for pocket therapy. The criteria for their selection are based on clinical findings in the soft tissue pocket wall, in the tooth surface, in the underlying bone, and in the attached gingiva.

Zone 1. The Soft Tissue Wall

The soft tissue wall of the pocket is inflamed and presents varying degrees of degeneration and ulceration with engorged blood vessels close to the surface, often separated from the contents of the pocket only by a thin layer of tissue debris.

In this zone determine the following:

1. Whether the pocket wall extends in a straight line from the gingival margin or follows a tortuous course around the tooth.

2. The number of tooth surfaces involved by the pocket.

3. The location of the bottom of the pocket on the tooth surface and the pocket depth.

The connective tissue between the pocket wall and the bone should also be explored. This tissue may be soft and friable or firm and bound to the bone. This is a significant consideration in the treatment of infrabony pockets.

Zone 2. The Tooth Surface

Adherent to the tooth are calculus and other surface deposits of varying amounts and textures. The superficial calculus is generally clay-like in consistency, obvious, and easily detached by well-directed instrumentation. However, deep in the pocket the calculus is hard, flint-like, and tenaciously adherent to the surface. In the coronal portion of the root the cementum is extremely thin, and a ledge is often formed at the cemento-enamel junction which must be taken into consideration when the tooth is scaled. The cementum surface may be softened by caries or deformed by adherent cementicles.

In this zone determine the following:

1. The extent and location of deposits.

2. The condition of the tooth surface and the presence of softened, eroded areas.

3. The accessibility of the root surface to the necessary instrumentation.

Phase I therapy should have solved many if not all of the problems on the tooth surface. Further evaluation of the results of Phase I therapy should be done at this time to determine the appropriate pocket elimination method.

Zone 3. The Bone

The shape and height of the alveolar bone next to the pocket wall should be established by careful probing and clinico-radiographic examination. Bony craters, angular bone losses, and other bone deformities are important criteria for the selection of the pocket eradication technique.

Zone 4. The Attached Gingiva

The presence or absence of an adequate band of attached gingiva is a factor to be considered when selecting the pocket eradication method. Diagnostic techniques for mucogingival problems are described in Chapter 56. An inadequate attached gingiva may be due to a high frenum attachment, marked gingival recession, or a deep pocket that reaches the level of the mucogingival junction. All of these possible conditions should be explored and their influence on pocket elimination determined.

METHODS OF POCKET ELIMINATION

An understanding of the underlying pathologic processes is helpful in the treatment of periodontal disease. However, pocket elimination per se is a technical procedure that must be mastered along with the many other techniques of general dentistry. The methods of pocket elimination are classified under three main headings:

1. **Reattachment techniques** offer the ideal result, since they eliminate pocket depth by reuniting the gingiva to the tooth at a position coronal to the bottom of the pre-existing pocket. Reattachment is usually associated with filling in of bone and regeneration of the periodontal ligament and cementum.

2. **Removal of the lateral wall of the pocket** is the most common method. The lateral wall of the pocket can be removed by (a) *retraction* or *shrinkage*, in which scaling and root planing procedures resolve the inflammatory process and the gingiva therefore shrinks, reducing the pocket depth; (b) *surgical removal* performed by the gingivectomy technique; and (c) *apical displacement* with an apically positioned flap.

3. **Removal of the tooth side of the pocket,** which is accomplished by tooth extraction or by partial tooth extraction (hemisection or root resection).

The techniques, what they accomplish, and the factors governing their selection are presented in the next chapters.

Criteria for Method Selection

Scientific criteria to establish the indications for each technique are difficult to determine. Longitudinal studies following a significant number of cases over a significant number of years, standardizing multiple factors and different parameters, would be needed. Clinical experience, however, has suggested the following criteria for selecting the method to be used to eliminate the pocket in individual cases:

1. **Gingival pockets.** Two factors are taken into consideration: (a) the character of the pocket wall, and (b) the pocket accessibility.

The pocket wall can be either edematous or fibrotic. Edematous tissue will shrink after the elimination of local factors, thereby reducing or totally eliminating pocket depth. Pockets having a fibrotic wall will not appreciably reduce their depth after scaling and root planing. After considerably longer periods of adequate plaque control their depth may become somewhat reduced.

Pocket elimination must be based on total elimination of the responsible local factors. Accessibility then becomes an important consideration. The following table will clarify the rationale for the selection of a particular pocket eradication method in gingival pockets:

Pocket Wall / Accessibility	Edematous	Fibrotic
Good	Curettage	Gingivectomy
Poor	Gingivectomy	Gingivectomy

2. **Suprabony pockets.** Two problems must be considered: (a) the presence or absence of an adequate band of attached gingiva, and (b) the presence of bone deformities requiring some type of surgical correction. The following table will summarize the rationale for the selection of a particular treatment technique in suprabony pockets:

Adequate Attached Gingiva		Inadequate Attached Gingiva	
No Bone Deformities	*Bone Deformities*	*No Bone Deformities*	*Bone Deformities*
Closed or open root planing or gingivectomy	Mucoperiosteal apically positioned flap with osseous contouring	Mucosal apically positioned flap or gingival extension with free soft tissue autograft	Mucoperiosteal apically positioned flap with osseous contouring

3. **Infrabony pockets.** Treatment of infrabony pockets may be directed to obtaining bone regeneration and reattachment or to contouring the remaining bone to an acceptable

morphology. The decision depends mainly on the exact shape of the bony defect (number of walls, width, and general configuration). The only way to determine the shape of the bone is by visual inspection. Therefore, the technique indicated for the treatment of infrabony pockets will be the mucoperiosteal flap, with osseous surgery aimed at bone regeneration or bone removal according to the morphology of the defect. This technique may also be combined with mucogingival procedures when an inadequate amount of attached gingiva is present. Other indications for the solution of mucogingival problems will be given in Chapter 56.

REFERENCES

1. Badersten, A., Nilveus, R., and Egelberg, J.: Effect of non-surgical periodontal therapy. II. Severely advanced periodontitis. J. Clin. Periodontol., in press.
2. Bower, R. C.: Furcation morphology relative to periodontal treatment. Furcation root surface anatomy. J. Periodontol., *50*:366, 1979.
3. Davies, W. I. R.: Open curettage and pocket elimination. *In* Shanley, D. (ed.): Efficacy of Treatment Procedures in Periodontics. Chicago, Quintessence Books, 1980.
4. Gher, M. E., and Vernino, A. R.: Root morphology—clinical significance in pathogenesis and treatment of periodontal disease. J. Am. Dent. Assoc., *101*:627, 1980.
5. Hill, R. W., et al.: Four types of periodontal treatment compared over two years. J. Periodontol., *52*:655, 1981.
6. Lindhe, J., et al.: "Critical probing depths" in periodontal therapy. J. Clin. Periodontol., *9*:323, 1982.
7. Pihlstrom, B. L., Ortiz Campos, C., and McHugh, R. B.: A randomized four-year study of periodontal therapy. J. Periodontol., *52*:227, 1981.
8. Rabbani, G. M., Ash, M. M., and Caffesse, R. G.: The effectiveness of subgingival scaling and root planing in calculus removal. J. Periodontol., *52*:119, 1981.
9. Ramfjord, S. P., et al.: Results following three modalities of periodontal therapy. J. Periodontol., *46*:522, 1975.
10. Rosling, B., et al.: The healing potential of the periodontal tissues following different techniques of periodontal surgery in plaque-free dentitions. A 2-year clinical study. J. Clin. Periodontol., *3*:233, 1976.
11. Waerhaug, J.: Healing of the dento-epithelial junction following subgingival plaque control. II. As observed on extracted teeth. J. Periodontol., *49*:119, 1978.
12. Weeks, P. R.: Pros and cons of periodontal pocket elimination procedures. J. Western Soc. Periodontol., *28*:4, 1980.
13. Zamet, J. S.: A comparative clinical study of three periodontal surgical techniques. J. Clin. Periodontol., *2*:87, 1975.

General Principles of Periodontal Surgery

Surgical periodontal procedures are usually performed in the dental office. The indications for performing periodontal surgery in the hospital are given later in this chapter.

All surgical procedures should be very carefully planned. The patient should be adequately prepared both medically and psychologically, as well as for all the practical aspects of the intervention. This chapter will cover the preparation of the patient and the general considerations that are common to all periodontal surgical techniques. Complications that may occur during or after surgery will also be discussed.

OUTPATIENT SURGERY

Preparation of the Patient

RE-EVALUATION AFTER PHASE I THERAPY. Almost every patient is subject to the so-called initial or preparatory phase of therapy, which basically consists of thorough scaling and root planing and the removal of all irritants responsible for the periodontal inflammation. This will (1) eliminate some lesions entirely; (2) render the tissues more firm and consistent, thus permitting a more accurate and delicate surgery; and (3) acquaint the patient with the office and with the operator and his or her assistants, thereby reducing the patient's apprehension and fear.

The re-evaluation phase consists of reprobing and re-examining all the pertinent findings that previously indicated the need for the surgical procedure. Their persistence will confirm the indication. Decisions are made at this time with reference to the number of surgical procedures to be performed, the dates for all the procedures, the expected outcome, and the postoperative care that will be needed. All this is discussed with the patient and a final decision made.

PREMEDICATION. Some patients will need special premedication because of their systemic diseases or because they are apprehensive. The former have been discussed in Chapter 36.

Prophylactic Antibiotic Coverage. Antibiotics should be administered prophylactically in all patients with heart disease, diabetes, and certain other diseases (see Chapter 36).

For patients who do not have any of these special conditions, the value of administering antibiotics routinely after periodontal surgery has not been clearly demonstrated. Ariaudo[3] reported reduced postoperative complications when lincomycin was administered starting 48 hours prior to periodontal surgery and continued for 4 days after surgery. Others using penicillin from the day of surgery have reported a reduction in pain and swelling.[9, 20, 32] The prophylactic use of antibiotics in periodontal patients who are otherwise healthy has been advocated in bone grafting procedures and has been claimed to enhance the chances of reattachment. Although the rationale for such use appears logical, there is no research evidence to support it. In any case, the risks inherent in the administration of antibiotics should be evaluated together with the potential benefits.

Informed Consent

The patient should be informed at the time of the initial visit about the diagnosis, the prognosis, the different possible treatments with their expected results, and all the pros and cons of each approach. At the time of surgery, the patient should again be informed, verbally and in writing, of the procedure about to be performed, and he or she should indicate agreement that the procedure be performed by signing at the appropriate place on the consent form.

Emergency Equipment

The operator, all assistants, and everyone in the office should be trained to handle all the possible emergencies that may arise. Emergency drugs and equipment should be readily available at all times.

The most common emergency is syncope. *Syncope* is a transient loss of consciousness due to a reduction in cerebral blood flow. The most common cause is fear and anxiety. Syncope is usually preceded by a feeling of weakness, and then the patient develops pallor, sweating, coldness of the extremities, dizziness, and slowing of the pulse. The patient should be placed in a supine position with the legs elevated; loosen tight clothes and ensure a wide open airway. The administration of oxygen is useful. Unconsciousness persists for a few minutes.

A history of previous syncopal attacks during dental appointments should be explored before treatment is begun, and, if these are reported, extra efforts to relieve the patient's fear and anxiety should be made.

The reader is referred to other texts[2] for a complete analysis of this important topic.

Sedation and Anesthesia

Periodontal surgery should be painless. The patient should be assured of this at the outset and should be thoroughly anesthetized by means of local block and infiltration injections. Injections directly into the interdental papillae may be helpful.

Apprehensive and neurotic patients require special management. The history, physical condition, and personality of the patient should be taken into consideration in order to determine the medications required, if any. Diazepam (Valium), 10 mg orally before operating, can be used in apprehensive patients. Intravenous sedation with diazepam or inhalation analgesia with nitrous oxide–oxygen is also helpful in some cases. The operator should learn the techniques for administering these agents and understand their indications, contraindications, and risks before attempting to use them in patients.[2] Many of these drugs require that the patient come to the dental office accompanied by a responsible adult who can drive him or her home if necessary.

Tissue Management

1. **Operate gently and carefully.** In addition to being most considerate to the patient, this is also the most effective way to operate. Tissue manipulation should be very gentle. Thoroughness is essential, but roughness must be avoided because it produces excessive tissue injury and postoperative discomfort and delays healing.

2. **Observe the patient at all times.** It is essential to pay careful attention to the patient's reactions. The facial expression indicates whether the patient is in pain; the onset of pallor and perspiration is a warning sign of patient weakness.

3. **Be certain the instruments are sharp.** Instruments must be sharp to be effective; successful treatment is not possible without sharp instruments. Dull instruments inflict unnecessary trauma because of the excess force usually applied to compensate for their ineffectiveness. A sterile sharpening stone should be available on the operating table at all times.

Scaling and Root Planing

Although scaling and root planing will have been performed previously as part of Phase I therapy, all exposed root surfaces should be carefully explored and planed as needed as part of the surgical procedure. In particular, areas of difficult access, such as furcations or deep pockets, often have rough areas or even calculus that went undetected during the preparatory sessions. The assistant, who is separating the tissues and using the aspirator, should also, from a different angle, check for the absence of calculus and the smoothness of each surface.

Hemostasis

An aspirator is indispensable for performing periodontal surgery. It provides the operator with a clear view of each root surface, which is necessary for thorough removal of deposits and planing. Further, it permits an accurate appraisal of the extent and pattern of soft tissue and bone involvement and prevents the seepage of blood into the floor of the mouth and oropharynx.

Periodontal surgery produces profuse bleeding in its initial incisional steps. However, after the existing granulation tissue has been removed, the bleeding disappears or is considerably reduced. Packing with gauze squares and the use of an aspirator are necessary to keep a dry field.

Excessive hemorrhaging after these initial steps may be due to lacerated capillaries and arterioles or to damage to larger vessels caused by surgical invasion of anatomic areas: e.g., the palate halfway from the teeth to the mid-palate, where the palatine arteries run. Bleeding from vessels emerging from the retroincisal foramina or from the inferior alveolar artery is rare. Proper design of the flaps, taking into consideration these anatomic structures, will prevent accidents.

Minor areas of persistent bleeding can be stopped by pressure with gauze for a few minutes. A cotton pellet dipped in ferric subsulfate powder may sometimes be needed.

Thrombin is a drug capable of hastening the process of blood clotting. It is intended for topical use only and is applied as a liquid or a powder.

Oxidized cellulose (Novocell, Oxycel) and absorbable gelatin sponges (Gelfoam) are useful hemostatics in deep wounds. Patients with bleeding disorders should be carefully prepared for surgery, frequently by a hematologist (see Chapter 36).

Periodontal Dressings (Periodontal Packs)

After the surgical periodontal procedures are completed, the area is covered with a surgical pack. In general, dressings have no curative properties; they assist healing by protecting the tissue rather than by providing "healing factors." The pack serves the following functions:

1. Controls postoperative bleeding.
2. Minimizes the likelihood of postoperative infection and hemorrhage.
3. Provides some splinting of mobile teeth.
4. Facilitates healing by preventing surface trauma during mastication and irritation from plaque and food debris.
5. Protects against pain induced by contact of the wound with food or with the tongue during mastication.

Types of Pack

Numerous types of dressings have been proposed for periodontal use. The most common types of dressing are:

ZINC OXIDE–EUGENOL PACKS. These are based on **the reaction of zinc oxide and eugenol.** These include the Wondr-Pak developed by Ward[38] in 1923 and several others that modified Ward's original formula. The addition of accelerators, such as zinc acetate, gives the dressing a better working time. Other substances that have been added include asbestos, used as a binder and a filler, and tannic acid. It has been shown, however, that asbestos can induce lung diseases and that tannic acid may lead to liver damage; therefore, both substances should be avoided. Zinc oxide–eugenol type dressings come in a liquid and a powder that are mixed prior to use. Some of them may be prepared ahead of time, wrapped in wax paper, and frozen for prolonged storage. The presence of eugenol in this type of pack may induce an allergic reaction that produces reddening of the area and burning pain in some patients.

NONEUGENOL PACKS. The reaction between a **metallic oxide and fatty acids** is the basis for Coe-Pak, which is the most widely used type of dressing in the United States. This is supplied in two tubes that are mixed immediately before use until a uniform color is obtained. Fingers should be lubricated with petrolatum (Vaseline). Coe-Pak can be handled and molded 3 to 5 minutes after mixing and remains workable for 15 to 20 minutes. Working time can be shortened by adding a small amount of zinc oxide powder to the pink paste (from the accelerator tube) before spatulating. This dressing does not contain asbestos or eugenol, thereby avoiding the problems associated with these substances.

Other noneugenol packs include the following:

1. **Cyanoacrylates.** *N*-butyl cyanoacrylate is a periodontal dressing which is applied in drops or as a spray and solidifies in 5 to 10 seconds.[5, 6] Polymerization from liquid to solid is catalyzed by moisture, heat, and pressure. The dressing adheres to smooth and irregular surfaces for periods of from 2 to 7 days. *N*-butyl cyanoacrylate has been studied extensively in clinical trials but has not yet been released for general periodontal use.

2. **Zinc oxide and glycol alcohol.** Dressings composed of a powder containing zinc oxide plus rosin, tannic acid, and kaolin and a liquid consisting of ethylene glycol and butyl alcohol are also on the market (Peridres). The same powder can be mixed with eugenol.

3. **Tissue conditioners.** These are methacrylic gels with some modifications to increase their adhesion and rigidity. Antibacterial substances such as chlorhexidine can be added to them.[1]

Retention of Packs

Periodontal dressings are usually kept in place mechanically by interlocking in interdental spaces and by joining the lingual and facial portions of the pack.

In isolated teeth or when there are several missing teeth in an arch, retention of the pack may be difficult. Numerous reinforcements and splints and stents for this purpose have been described.[15, 16] Adhesion to the enamel is a desirable feature of a periodontal dressing.[40] Whereas cyanoacrylates and methacrylic gels have good adhesive properties, other packs show a low level of adhesion.

Antibacterial Properties of Packs

Improved healing and patient comfort[4] with less odor and taste[5] have been obtained by including zinc bacitracin in the pack. Other antibiotics, such as oxytetracycline (Terramycin),[11] neomycin, and nitrofurazone, have also been tried, but all produce hypersensitive reactions.[26] The emergence of resistant organisms and opportunistic infection have been reported.[34]

Allergy

Contact allergy to eugenol and to rosin has been reported.[33]

How to Prepare and Apply the Periodontal Dressing

Zinc oxide packs are mixed with eugenol or noneugenol liquids on a wax paper pad with a wooden tongue depressor. The powder is gradually incorporated with the liquid until a thick paste is formed.

Coe-Pak is prepared by mixing equal lengths of paste from the accelerator and base tubes until the resulting paste is a uniform color. In 2 to 3 minutes the paste loses its tackiness and can be handled with lubricated fingers (Fig. 50–1).

The pack is then rolled into two strips approximately the length of the treated area. The end of one strip is bent into a hook shape and fitted around the distal surface of the last tooth, approaching it from the distal surface (Fig. 50–2*A*). The remainder of the strip is brought forward along the facial surface to the midline and gently pressed into place along the incised gingival margin and interproximally. The second strip is applied from the lingual surface. It is joined to the pack at the distal surface of the last tooth, then brought forward along the cut gingival margin to the midline (Fig. 50–2*B*). The strips are joined interproximally by applying gentle pressure on the facial and lingual surfaces of the pack (Fig. 50–2*C*). For isolated teeth separated by edentulous spaces, the pack should be made continuous from tooth to tooth, covering the edentulous areas. (Fig. 50–3).

The pack should cover the gingiva, but overextensions onto uninvolved mucosa should be avoided. *Excess pack irritates the mucobuccal fold and floor of the mouth and interferes with the tongue.* Overextension also jeopardizes the remainder of the pack because it tends to break off, taking pack from the operated area with it. *Pack that interferes with the occlusion should be trimmed away before the patient is dismissed* (Fig. 50–4). Failure to do this causes discomfort and jeopardizes retention of the pack.

The operator should have the patient move the tongue forcibly out and to each side, and the cheek and lips should be displaced in all directions to mold the pack while it is still soft. After the pack has set, it should be trimmed to eliminate all excess.

As a general rule, the pack is kept on for 1 week after surgery. This guideline is based upon the timetable of healing and clinical experience. It is not a rigid requirement; the period may be extended, or the area may be repacked for an additional week.

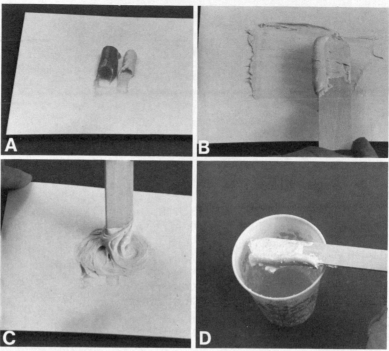

Figure 50–1 Preparing the Surgical Pack (Coe-Pak). *A,* Equal lengths of the two pastes are placed on paper pad. *B,* Mix with a wooden tongue depressor for 2 or 3 minutes until *C,* the paste loses its tackiness. *D,* Paste is placed in a paper cup of water at room temperature. With lubricated fingers it is then rolled into cylinders and placed on the surgical wound.

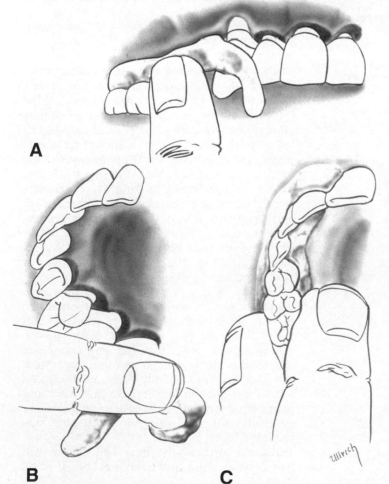

Figure 50–2 Inserting the Periodontal Pack. *A,* Strip of pack is hooked around last molar and pressed into place anteriorly. *B,* Lingual pack joined to the facial strip at the distal surface of the last molar and fitted into place anteriorly. *C,* Gentle pressure on facial and lingual surfaces joins pack interproximally.

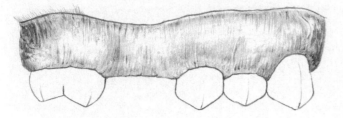

Figure 50–3 Continuous Pack Covers Edentulous Space.

Fragments of the surface of the pack may come off during the week, but this presents no problem. If a portion of the pack is lost from the operated area and the patient is uncomfortable, it is usually best to repack the area. Remove the remaining pack, wash the area with warm water, and apply a topical anesthetic before replacing the pack, which is then retained for 1 week. Patients may develop pain from an overextended margin which irritates the vestibule, floor of the mouth, or tongue. The excess pack should be trimmed away, making sure that the new margin is not rough, before the patient is dismissed.

Instructions for the Patient After Surgery

After the pack is placed, the following printed instructions are given to the patient to be read before he or she leaves the chair:

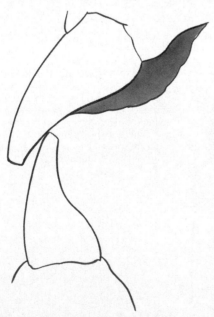

Figure 50–4 The Pack Should Not Interfere with the Occlusion.

INSTRUCTIONS FOR

Mrs. Jane Smith

The operation which has been performed on your gums will help you keep your teeth. The following information has been prepared to answer questions you may have about how to take care of your mouth. Please read the instructions carefully—our patients have found them very helpful.

When the anesthesia wears off, you may have slight discomfort—not pain. Two acetaminophen (Tylenol) tablets will usually keep you comfortable. You may repeat every 4 hours if necessary.

We have placed a periodontal pack over your gums to protect them from irritation. The pack prevents pain, aids healing, and enables you to carry on most of your usual activities in comfort. The pack will harden in a few hours, after which it can withstand most of the forces of chewing without breaking off. It may take a little while to become accustomed to it.

For your benefit the pack should remain in place as long as possible. **Do not remove it.** If particles of the pack chip off during the week, do not be concerned as long as you do not have pain. If a piece of the pack breaks off and you are in pain, or if a rough edge irritates your tongue or cheek, please call the office. The problem can be easily remedied by replacing the pack. The pack will be removed at your next appointment.

For the first 3 hours after the operation avoid hot foods in order to permit the pack to harden. After this, eat anything you can manage without chipping the pack. Eggs, Jell-O, cereals, soups, milk, fish, hamburger, or any semisolid or finely minced foods are suggested. Avoid citrus fruits or fruit juices, highly spiced foods, and alcoholic beverages. They will cause pain. Food supplements and/or vitamins are generally not necessary. We will prescribe them if needed.

Do not smoke—the heat and smoke will irritate your gums and delay healing. If at all possible, use this opportunity to give up smoking. Smokers have more gum disease than nonsmokers.

Rinsing is not part of the treatment, but it will help make your mouth feel refreshed. **Do not rinse today.** Beginning tomorrow, you may rinse as often as you wish with one of the popular, pleasant-flavored mouthwashes. Do not use it in concentrated form; dilute it—⅓ mouthwash to ⅔ warm water.

Clean the parts of your mouth which have been treated in previous weeks using the methods in which you were instructed. The gums most likely will bleed more than they did before the operation. This is perfectly normal in the early stage of healing and will gradually subside. Do not stop cleaning because of it.

Follow your regular daily activities, but avoid excessive exertion of any type. Golf, tennis, skiing, bowling, swimming, or sunbathing should be postponed until 2 days after the operation.

You may experience a slight feeling of weakness or chills during the first 24 hours. This should not be cause for alarm but should be reported at the next visit.

Swelling is not unusual, particularly in areas which required extensive surgical procedures. The swelling generally subsides in 3 or 4 days. If the swelling is painful or appears to become worse, please call the office.

There may be occasional blood stains in the saliva for the first 4 or 5 hours after the operation. This is not unusual and will correct itself. If there is considerable bleeding beyond this, take a piece of gauze, form it into the shape of a U, hold it in the thumb and index finger, apply it to both sides of the pack, and hold it there under pressure for 20 minutes. Do not remove it during this period to examine it. If the bleeding does not stop at the end of 20 minutes, please contact the office. **Do not try to stop the bleeding by rinsing.**

If any other problems arise, please call the office.

The Patient During the First Postoperative Week

Properly performed, periodontal surgery presents no serious postoperative problems. Unfavorable sequelae are the exception rather than the rule; the following may arise in the first postoperative week:

1. *Persistent bleeding after surgery*. The pack should be removed, the bleeding points located, and the bleeding stopped with pressure, electrosurgery, or electrocautery. After the bleeding is stopped, the pack is replaced.

2. *Sensitivity to percussion*. Sensitivity to percussion may be caused by the extension of inflammation into the periodontal ligament. The patient should be questioned regarding the progress of the symptoms. Progressively diminishing severity is a favorable sign. The pack should be removed and the gingiva checked for localized areas of infection or irritation which should be cleaned or incised to provide drainage. Particles of calculus that may have been overlooked should be removed. Relieving the occlusion is usually helpful.

Sensitivity to percussion may also be caused by excess pack which interferes with the occlusion. Removal of the excess usually corrects the condition.

3. *Swelling*. Sometimes within the first 2 postoperative days patients report a soft, painless swelling of the cheek in the area of operation. There may be lymph node enlargement, and the temperature may be slightly elevated. The area of operation itself is usually symptom-free. This type of involvement results from a localized inflammatory reaction to the operative procedure. It generally subsides by the fourth postoperative day, without necessitating removal of the pack. Penicillin, 250 mg every 4 hours for 48 hours, is helpful as a prophylactic measure following the next operation.

4. *Feeling of weakness*. Occasionally patients report having experienced a "washed out," weakened feeling for about 24 hours after the operation. This represents a systemic reaction to a transient bacteremia induced by the operative procedure. It is prevented by premedication with penicillin, 250 mg every 4 hours, beginning 24 hours before the next operation and continuing for a 24-hour postoperative period. Prophylactic chemotherapy is ordinarily not used, except for patients with a history of rheumatic fever, cardiovascular disease, diabetes, or prolonged corticosteroid therapy (see Chapter 36).

Removal of the Periodontal Pack and Return Visit Care

When the patient returns after 1 week, the pack is taken off by inserting a surgical hoe along the margin and exerting gentle lateral pressure (Fig. 50–5). Pieces of pack retained

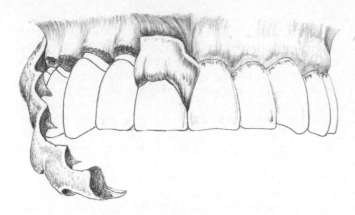

Figure 50–5 Removal of the Periodontal Pack.

interproximally and particles which adhere to the tooth surfaces are removed with scalers. Particles may be enmeshed in the cut surface and should be carefully picked off with fine cotton pliers. The entire area is syringed with warm water to remove superficial debris.

What to Look for at the Time of Pack Removal

The following are the usual findings when the pack is removed.

If a *gingivectomy* has been performed, the cut surface will be covered with a friable meshwork of new epithelium which should not be disturbed. After a *flap operation,* the areas corresponding to the incisions will be epithelialized but may bleed readily when touched; they should not be disturbed. Pockets should not be probed. The facial and lingual mucosa may be covered with a grayish-yellow or white granular layer of food debris that has seeped under the pack. It is easily removed with a moist cotton pellet.

The root surfaces may be sensitive to a probe or to thermal changes, and the teeth may be stained.

Red, bead-like protuberances of granulation tissue persist if calculus has not been completely removed. The granulation tissue is removed with a curette, exposing the calculus so that it can be removed and the root can be planed. Removal of the granulation tissue without removal of calculus will be followed by recurrence.

Fragments of calculus delay healing. Each root surface should be rechecked visually to be certain no calculus is present. Sometimes the color of the calculus is similar to that of the root. The grooves on proximal root surfaces and the furcations are areas in which calculus is likely to be overlooked.

WHEN TO REPACK. After the pack is removed, it is usually not necessary to replace it. However, it is advisable to repack for an additional week for patients with (1) a low pain threshold who are particularly uncomfortable when the pack is removed, (2) unusually extensive periodontal involvement, or (3) slow healing. Clinical judgment will help decide whether to repack the area or leave the initial pack on longer than 1 week.

TOOTH MOBILITY. Tooth mobility is increased immediately after surgery,[8] but by the fourth week it diminishes beyond the pretreatment level.[23]

FINAL CHECK ON SMOOTHNESS OF THE ROOT SURFACES. One week after the pack is removed from the final quadrant, all root surfaces are checked to see that they are smooth and firm. A rubber cup with fine pumice and polishing strips are used for the final smoothing of the root at this time.

Care of the Mouth While Periodontal Surgery Is in Progress

Care of the mouth by the patient between the treatment of the first and the final areas, as well as after surgery is completed, is extremely important. It begins after the pack is removed from the first operation. The patient has been through a presurgical period of instructed plaque control and should be reinstructed at this time.

Vigorous brushing during the first week after the pack is removed is not feasible. However, the patient is informed that plaque and food accumulation will retard healing and is advised **to try to keep the area as clean as possible** by the gentle use of interdental cleansers and dental floss and light water irrigation. Brushing is introduced when healing of the tissues permits; the vigor of the overall hygiene regimen is increased as healing progresses. Patients should be told that there will most likely be more gingival bleeding than before the operation, that it is perfectly normal and will subside as healing progresses, and that it should not deter them from following their oral hygiene regimen.

Chlorhexidine mouthwashes or topical application of chlorhexidine with Q-tips is indicated for the first few postoperative weeks in those countries where its use is permitted.

Management of Postoperative Pain

Periodontal surgery performed following the basic principles outlined here should produce only minor pain and discomfort.[36] However, in some cases severe pain may be present; its control then becomes an important part of patient management.[29]

In general, procedures that involve extensive and/or prolonged bone surgery are more likely to induce postoperative pain than more conservative procedures such as the so-called modified Widman flap or gingivectomy.

A common source of postoperative pain is *overextension of the periodontal pack* onto the soft tissue beyond the mucogingival junction or onto the frena. Overextended packs cause localized areas of edema, usually noticed 1 to 2 days after surgery. Removal of excess pack is followed by resolution in about 24 hours.

When severe postoperative pain is present, the patient should be seen at the office on an emergency appointment. The area should be anesthetized by infiltration or topically, the pack removed, and the wound examined. Postoperative pain related to *infection* will induce localized lymphadenopathy and a slight elevation in temperature. It should be treated with systemic antibiotics and analgesics.

Extensive and excessively prolonged exposure and dryness of bone will also induce severe pain. This may necessitate narcotic analgesics, such as oxycodone compounds (Percodan) or meperidine hydrochloride (Demerol).

Treatment of Sensitive Roots

Root hypersensitivity is a relatively common problem in periodontal practice. It may occur spontaneously when the root becomes exposed owing to gingival recession or pocket formation, or it may appear after scaling and root planing and surgical procedures. It is manifested as pain induced by cold or hot temperatures, more commonly the former; by citrus fruits or sweets; or by contact with a toothbrush or a dental instrument.

It occurs more frequently in the cervical area of the root, where the cementum is extremely thin or sometimes even nonexistent, exposing the dentin. Scaling and root planing procedures remove this thin cementum, inducing the hypersensitivity.

The transmission of stimuli from the surface of the dentin to the nerve endings located in the dental pulp or in the pulpal region of the dentin could occur through the odontoblastic process or owing to a hydrodynamic mechanism by means of displacement of dentinal fluid. The latter process seems more likely and would explain the importance of burnishing desensitizing agents in order to obturate the dentinal tubule.

A very important factor for reducing or eliminating hypersensitivity is adequate plaque control. However, hypersensitivity may prevent plaque control, and therefore a vicious circle may be created.

DESENSITIZING AGENTS. A number of agents have been proposed to control root hypersensitivity. Pattison and Pattison[30] list the following possible mechanisms of action for desensitizing agents: (1) precipitation or denaturing of organic material at the exposed end of the odontoblastic process, (2) deposition of an inorganic salt at the exposed end of the dentinal tubules, (3) stimulation of secondary dentin formation within the pulp, and (4) suppression of pulpal inflammation.

The patient should be informed about the possibility of root hypersensitivity before treatment is undertaken. The following information on how to cope with the problem should also be given:

1. Hypersensitivity appears owing to the exposure of dentin, which is inevitable if calculus and plaque and their products, buried in the tissue, are to be removed.

2. Hypersensitivity will slowly disappear over a few weeks.

3. Plaque control is very important for the reduction of hypersensitivity.

4. Desensitizing agents do not produce immediate relief. They have to be used for several days or even weeks to produce results.

Clinical evaluation of the many agents proposed has proved very difficult, in part because it is difficult to measure and compare different persons' pain, because hypersensitivity disappears by itself after a time, and because desensitizing agents take a few weeks to act.

Desensitizing agents can be applied by the patient at home or by the dentist or hygienist in the dental office.

Agents Used by the Patient. The most common are dentifrices used by the patient for his or her oral hygiene. The following agents in dentifrices have been reported to be useful: strontium chloride (Sensodyne),[7, 35] sodium monofluorophosphate (Colgate),[19] formaldehyde (Thermodent),[10] polyglycol (Protect), and potassium nitrate (Denquel).

An aqueous solution of 2 per cent sodium fluoride can also be used instead of a dentifrice; the patient should be cautioned not to swallow it.

Fluoride rinsing solutions and gels can also be used after the usual plaque control procedures.[37]

Agents Used in the Dental Office. Fluoride solutions and pastes are the agents of choice. In addition to their antisensitivity properties they have the advantage of their anticaries activity, which is particularly important for patients with a tendency to develop root caries.

Fluoride paste consists of equal parts of sodium fluoride, kaolin, and glycerin. This paste is applied as follows:

1. Isolate the tooth or teeth requiring desensitization and dry them with cotton pellets.

2. Burnish the paste with an instrument; leave it for 2 minutes.

3. Remove the paste with warm water and rinse thoroughly.

The patient may feel an initial sensation of cold or pain that may require anesthesia prior to the application of the paste.

Iontophoresis can be used to deliver sodium fluoride into the tooth structure.[12a] The results with this method are controversial.

Other desensitizing agents for office use are zinc chloride, 8 per cent solution; liquid phenol; formaldehyde; ammoniacal silver nitrate; a mixture of sodium carbonate monohydrate, 2.5 grams, and potassium carbonate, 12.5 mg; and sodium silicofluoride.[18, 25] Except for the last two, these agents should not be used on freshly cut dentin.

Corticosteroid hormones have also been used for desensitizing exposed root surfaces.[28] They probably act by reducing the inflammatory reaction of the pulp.

HOSPITAL PERIODONTAL SURGERY

Ordinarily, periodontal surgery is an office procedure performed in quadrants or sextants at weekly or biweekly intervals. Under certain circumstances, however, it is in the best interest of the patient to treat the mouth in one operation with the patient hospitalized.

Indications

PATIENT PROTECTION. There are patients with systemic conditions that are not severe enough to contraindicate elective surgery but that may require special precautionary measures best provided in a hospital. This group includes patients with cardiovascular disease, diabetes, and hyperthyroidism, those undergoing prolonged steroid therapy, and those with a history of rheumatic fever or abnormal bleeding tendencies.

The purpose of hospitalization is to protect patients by anticipating their special needs—not to perform periodontal surgery when it is contraindicated by the patients' general condition. There are patients for whom elective surgery is contraindicated regardless of whether it is performed in the dental office or in the hospital. When consultation with the patients' physician leads to this decision, palliative periodontal therapy, in the form of scaling and curettage if permissible, is the necessary compromise.

THE APPREHENSIVE PATIENT. Gentleness, understanding, and preoperative sedation usually suffice to calm the fears of most patients. For some patients, however, the prospect of a series of surgical procedures is sufficient stress to trigger disturbances that jeopardize the well-being of the patient and hamper treatment. Explaining that the treatment at the hospital will be performed painlessly and that it will be preceded by a depth of sedation that is not practical for ambulatory patients visiting a dental office is an important step toward allaying their fears. The thought of completing the necessary surgical procedures in one session rather than in repeated visits is an added comfort to the patient, because it eliminates the prospect of repeated anxiety in anticipation of each treatment.

With complete-mouth surgery, there is less stress for the patient. It is performed after a night's rest in the hospital and under ample sedation rather than after coming straight from the street into the dental office (sometimes after rushing to be on time for the appointment). The patient is returned to the hospital room after surgery for a check of his physical condition and for a restful postoperative sleep, instead of leaving the dental office and making the trip home.

PATIENT CONVENIENCE. For patients whose occupation entails considerable contact with the public, surgery performed at weekly intervals sometimes presents a special problem. It means that for a period of several weeks, some area of the mouth will be covered by a periodontal pack. With the complete-mouth technique, the pack is ordinarily retained for only 1 week. Patients find this a very acceptable alternative to several weeks of involvement with the pack. For a variety of other reasons, patients may desire to attend to their surgical needs in one session under optimal conditions.

Hospital Admission and Presurgical Medical Examination

If, after consideration of all factors, complete-mouth operation is selected as the procedure of choice, a hospital appointment is made.

The length of the hospital stay is 48 hours. The patient enters early in the afternoon preceding the morning of the operation to allow time for a physical examination, for a hemogram and other laboratory procedures, and for medical consultations.

Preparations are made for special precautionary measures that may be required before, during, or after surgery. For example, diabetics who consider themselves to be "under control" sometimes require a short period of dietary supervision and regulation of insulin before surgery. The medical examination occasionally reveals a disease of which the patient is not aware, as well as conditions which the patient felt were not relevant to his or her dental problem and were omitted from the case history taken in the dentist's office.

Premedication and Anesthesia

PREMEDICATION. Patients should be given a sedative or tranquilizer the night before surgery. Barbiturates may be used, but frequently diazepam, 10 mg orally, is sufficient to ensure a restful night. Another 10-mg tablet of diazepam is administered 1 hour prior to the procedure. If a higher level of sedation is necessary, intravenous diazepam, 10 to 20 mg, together with 25 to 50 mg of meperidine hydrochloride to prolong the sedative effect, is the method of choice. Deeper levels of sedation may be achieved with the use of intravenous barbiturates either alone or in combination with other agents, as in the Jorgensen

technique.[2] Patients undergoing complete-mouth surgery as an outpatient procedure are also usually medicated before and during surgery with oral or intravenous diazepam. Patients with systemic problems (history of rheumatic fever, cardiovascular problems, and so forth) are premedicated as needed (see Chapter 36).

ANESTHESIA. Local or general anesthesia[24] may be used. Local anesthesia is the method of choice, except for especially apprehensive patients. It permits unhampered movement of the head, which is necessary for optimal visibility and accessibility to the various root surfaces. Local anesthesia is utilized in the same manner as for routine periodontal surgery. In those cases in which general anesthesia is utilized, it is important that the patient also receive local anesthesia to ensure reduced bleeding during the procedure.

The Operation

Surgery in the operating room is performed on the operating table with patient's back elevated at an angle of approximately 30° and the head at the level of the operator's elbows. The assistant responsible for the aspirator stands on the side of the table opposite the operator.

When general anesthesia has been utilized, it is wise to delay placing the periodontal dressing until the patient has recovered sufficiently to have a demonstrable cough reflex. Periodontal dressings placed before the end of general anesthesia can be displaced during the recovery period and pose serious risks of being inhaled.

Postoperative Instructions at the Hospital

The patient is returned to his or her room, and the following postoperative instructions are entered in the record:

Cold, semisolid foods only.
Demerol, 50 mg every 4 hours, if necessary.

The patient is discharged from the hospital the morning following the operation, with an appointment scheduled for a week later at the dentist's office.

Postoperative instructions and care for patients after complete mouth periodontal surgery are the same as those outlined previously in this chapter.

First Postoperative Office Visit

The patient is seen at the office 1 week after the operation. The pack is usually removed, and plaque control methods are reviewed. If it appears advisable, one or more areas of the mouth may be repacked for another week.

REFERENCES

1. Addy, M., and Douglas, W. H.: A chlorhexidine-containing methacrylic gel as a periodontal dressing. J. Periodontol., *46*:465, 1975.
2. Allen, G. D.: Dental Anesthesia and Analgesia (Local and General). 2nd ed. Baltimore, Williams & Wilkins, 1979.
3. Ariaudo, A. A.: The efficacy of antibiotics in periodontal surgery. J. Periodontol., *40*:150, 1969.
4. Baer, P. N., Goldman, H. M., and Scigliano, J.: Studies on a bacitracin periodontal dressing. Oral Surg., *11*:712, 1958.
5. Baer, P. N., Summer, C. F., III, and Miller, G.: Periodontal dressings. Dent. Clin. North Am., *13*:181, 1969.
6. Bhaskar, S. N., et al.: Oral surgery–oral pathology conference number 18, Walter Reed Army Medical Center. Oral Surg., *22*:526, 1966.
7. Blitzer, B.: A consideration of the possible causes of dental hypersensitivity: treatment by a strontium-ion dentifrice. Periodontics, *5*:318, 1967.
8. Burch, J., et al.: Tooth mobility following gingivectomy. A study of gingival support of the teeth. Periodontics, *6*:90, 1960.
9. Dal Pra, D. J., and Strahan, J. D.: A clinical evaluation of the benefits of a course of oral penicillin following periodontal surgery. Aust. Dent. J., *17*:219, 1972.
10. Forrest, J. O.: A clinical assessment of three desensitizing toothpastes containing formalin. Br. Dent. J., *114*:103, 1963.
11. Fraleigh, C. M.: An evaluation of topical Terramycin in post-gingivectomy pack. J. Periodontol., *27*:201, 1956.
12. Frisch, J., Levin, M. P., and Bhaskar, S. N.: The use of tissue conditioners in periodontics. J. Periodontol., *38*:359, 1968.
12a. Gangarosa, L.: Iontophoretic application of fluoride by tray techniques for desensitizing multiple teeth. J. Am. Dent. Assoc., *95*:50, 1981.
13. Glendinning, D. E. H.: A method for retention of the periodontal pack. J. Periodontol., *47*:236, 1976.
14. Greenhill, J. D., and Pashley, D. H.: The effects of desensitizing agents on the hydraulic conductance of human dentin "in vitro." J. Dent. Res., *60*:686, 1981.
15. Hirschfeld, A. S., and Wasserman, B. H.: Retention of periodontal packs. J. Periodontol., *29*:199, 1958.
16. Holmes, C. H.: Periodontal pack on single tooth retained by acrylic splint. J. Am. Dent. Assoc., *64*:831, 1962.
17. Holroyd, S. F.: Antibiotics in the practice of periodontics. J. Periodontol., *42*:584, 1971.
18. Hunter, G. C., Jr., Barringer, M., and Spooner, G.: Analysis of desensitization of dentin by sodium silico-fluoride and Gottlieb's solution by use of radioactive silver nitrate. J. Periodontol., *32*:333, 1961.
19. Kanouse, M. C., and Ash, M. M., Jr.: The effectiveness of a sodium monofluorophosphate dentifrice on dental hypersensitivity. J. Periodontol., *40*:38, 1969.
20. Kidd, E. A., and Wade, A. B.: Penicillin control of swelling and pain after periodontal osseous surgery. J. Clin. Periodontol., *1*:52, 1974.
21. Koch, G., et al.: Contact allergy to medicaments and materials used in dentistry. II. Sensitivity to eugenol and rosin. Odontol. Revy, *22*:375, 1971.
22. Koch, G., et al.: Contact allergy to medicaments and materials used in dentistry. IV. Sensitizing effect of eugenol/rosin in surgical dressing. Odontol. Revy, *24*:109, 1973.
23. Majewski, I., and Sponholz, H.: Ergebnisse nach parodontal therapeutischen Massnahmen unter besonderer Berucksich tigung der Zahnbeweglichkeitssung mit dem Makroperiodontometer nach Muhlemann. Zahnaerztl. Rundsch., *75*:57, 1966.
24. Manson, J. D., and Millar-Danks, S.: General anesthesia for periodontal surgery. J. Clin. Periodontol., *5*:163, 1978.
25. Massler, M.: Desensitization of cervical cementum and dentin by sodium silicofluoride. J. Dent. Res., *34*:761, 1955.
26. Meyler, A.: Side Effects of Drugs. Vol. 5. Amsterdam, Excerpta Medica Foundation, 1966.
27. Miller, J. T., Shannon, K. L., Kilyore, W. G., and Bookman, J. E.: Use of water-free stannous fluoride–containing gel in the control of dental hypersensitivity. J. Periodontol., *40*:490, 1969.
28. Mosteller, J. H.: Use of prednisolone in the elimination of postoperative thermal sensitivity. J. Prosthet. Dent., *12*:1176, 1962.
29. Murphy, N. C., and DeMarco, T. J.: Controlling pain in periodontal patients. Dent. Survey, *55*:46, 1979.
30. Pattison, G. L., and Pattison, A. M.: Periodontal Instrumentation. Reston, Va., Reston Publishing Company, 1979.
31. Peden, J. W.: Dental hypersensitivity. J. Western Soc. Periodontol., *25*:75, 1977.
32. Pendrill, K., and Reddy, J.: The use of prophylactic penicillin in periodontal surgery. J. Periodontol., *51*:44, 1980.
33. Romanow, I.: Allergic reactions to periodontal pack. J. Periodontol., *28*:151, 1957.
34. Romanow, I.: Relationship of moniliasis to the presence of antibiotics in periodontal packs. Periodontics, *2*:298, 1964.
35. Ross, M. R.: Hypersensitive teeth: effect of strontium chloride in a compatible dentifrice. J. Periodontol., *32*:49, 1961.
36. Strahan, J. D., and Glenwright, H. D.: Pain experience in periodontal surgery. J. Periodont. Res., *1*:163, 1967.
37. Tarbet, W. J., Silverman, G., Stolman, J. W., and Fratarcangelo, P. A.: A clinical evaluation of a new treatment for dentinal hypersensitivity. J. Periodontol., *51*:535, 1980.
38. Ward, A. W.: Inharmonious cusp relation as a factor in periodontoclasia. J. Am. Dent. Assoc., *10*:471, 1923.
39. Watts, T. A. P., and Combe, E.C.: Periodontal dressing materials. J. Clin. Periodontol., *6*:3, 1979.
40. Watts, T. A. P., and Combe, E. C.: Adhesion of periodontal dressings to enamel *in vitro*. J. Clin. Periodontol., *7*:62, 1980.

Gingival Curettage

The word "curettage" is used in periodontics to mean *the scraping of the gingival wall of a periodontal pocket to separate diseased soft tissue. "Scaling" refers to the removal of deposits from the root surface, whereas "planing" means smoothing the root to remove infected and necrotic tooth substance.* Scaling and root planing may inadvertently include various degrees of curettage. However, they are different procedures, with different rationales and indications, and should be considered as separate parts of periodontal treatment.

Curettage hastens healing by reducing the task of the body's enzymes and phagocytes, which ordinarily remove tissue debris during healing. Also, by removing the epithelial lining of the periodontal pocket, curettage removes a barrier to reattachment of the periodontal fibers to the root surface. It has been reported that bacteria invade the pocket lining and the junctional epithelium in advanced periodontal disease.[22] Curettage removes these areas of bacterial penetration.

Some degree of irritation and trauma to the gingiva is unavoidable in curettage, even if it is performed with extreme care. In such cases, the injurious effects are of microscopic proportion and generally do not significantly affect healing. Overzealous curettage causes postoperative pain and retards healing.

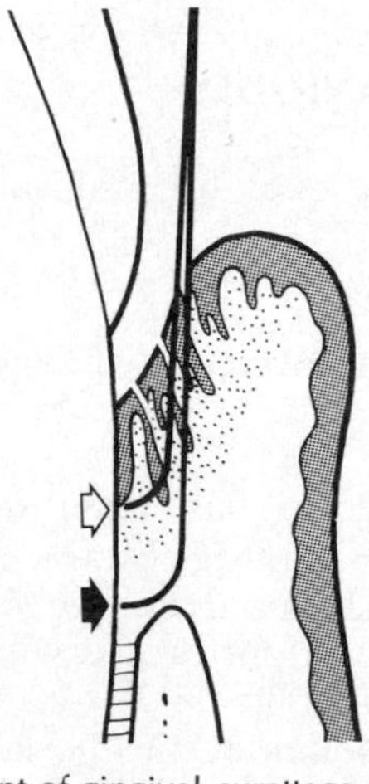

A differentiation has been made between gingival and subgingival curettage (Fig. 51–1). **Gingival curettage** consists of the removal of the inflamed soft tissue lateral to the pocket wall, whereas **subgingival curettage** refers to the procedure that is performed apical to the epithelial attachment, severing the connective tissue attachment down to the osseous crest.

One other point that should be clarified is that some degree of curettage is done unintentionally when scaling and root planing are performed. This is called **inadvertent curettage,** and it is not the topic of this chapter. We shall refer here to the purposeful curettage performed during the same visit as scaling and root planing or as a separate operation; its aim is to reduce pocket depth by enhancing shrinkage and/or reattachment.

INDICATIONS

Curettage is the technique of choice for the following purposes:

1. Elimination of suprabony pockets located in accessible areas and having an inflamed, edematous pocket wall that will shrink to the sulcus depth after treatment. If the pocket wall is firm and fibrous, other surgical procedures will be required to eliminate the pocket, because the fibrous pocket wall will not shrink sufficiently following curettage.

2. Reattachment attempts in moderately deep infrabony pockets located in accessible areas where a type of "closed" surgery is deemed advisable. The presence of tortuous pockets, furcation involvements, or other technical obstacles to a thorough and complete removal of irritants from the root surface and subsequent planing will contraindicate this approach.

Figure 51–1 Extent of gingival curettage (*white arrow*) and subgingival curettage (*black arrow*).

3. Curettage can be done as a nondefinitive procedure in order to reduce inflammation prior to pocket elimination by other methods or in patients in whom more aggressive surgical techniques (e.g., flaps) are contraindicated owing to age, systemic problems, psychologic problems, and so forth. It should be understood that in these patients the goal of pocket elimination is compromised and the prognosis will be impaired. The clinician should resort to this approach only when there is no possibility that the indicated surgical techniques can be performed, and both clinician and patient must have a clear understanding of its limitations.

4. Curettage is also frequently done on recall visits[20] as a method of maintaining areas of recurrent inflammation and pocket depth, particularly where pocket reduction surgery has previously been performed.

RATIONALE

The removal of tissue debris and chronically inflamed granulation tissue accelerates healing and enhances gingival shrinkage, thereby inducing pocket reduction.

By eliminating the junctional epithelium and inflamed areas apical to it, subgingival curettage will also favor reattachment (new attachment) of fibers at a level coronal to that of pre-existent fibers.

Curettage does not eliminate the causes of inflammation, i.e., bacterial plaque and deposits. Therefore, it should always be preceded by scaling and root planing, which are the basic periodontal therapy procedures. Scaling and root planing can be performed in a previous session, followed by a re-evaluation to establish the need for curettage, or they can be done in the same visit as curettage. The former is the ideal sequence of treatment. However, in highly inflamed edematous tissue, inadvertent curettage may disrupt the tissues to such a degree that completion of the curettage at the same appointment is advisable.

BASIC TECHNIQUE

Scaling and root planing have been described in detail in Chapter 43. The use of local infiltrative anesthesia for this procedure is optional. Gingival curettage, on the other hand, always requires some type of local anesthesia.

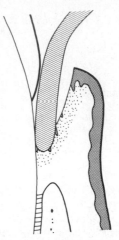

Figure 51–2 Gingival curettage performed with a horizontal stroke of the curette.

The curette is selected so that the cutting edge will be against the tissue: e.g., the Gracey No. 13–14 is used for mesial surfaces and the Gracey No. 11–12 for distal surfaces. The curette is inserted so as to engage the inner lining of the pocket wall and is carried along the soft tissue, usually in a horizontal stroke (Fig. 51–2). The pocket wall may be supported by gentle finger pressure on the external surface. The curette is then placed under the cut edge of the junctional epithelium so as to undermine it.

In subgingival curettage, the tissues attached between the bottom of the pocket and the alveolar crest are removed with a scooping motion of the curette to the tooth surface (Fig. 51–3). The area is flushed to remove debris, and the tissue is partly adapted to the tooth by gentle finger pressure. Sometimes suturing of separated papillae and application of a periodontal pack may be indicated.

OTHER TECHNIQUES

Other techniques for gingival curettage are the following:

Excisional New Attachment Procedure (ENAP)

This technique has been developed and used by the United States Naval Dental Corps.[19, 31, 32] It is a definitive subgingival curettage procedure performed with a knife. The technique is as follows:

1. After adequate anesthesia has been administered, measure pocket depths with a

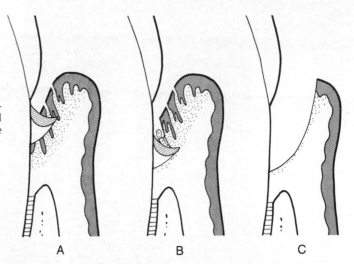

Figure 51–3 Subgingival Curettage. *A,* Elimination of pocket lining. *B,* Elimination of junctional epithelium and granulation tissue. *C,* Procedure completed.

probe and penetrate the gingival tissue at this distance with the probe.

2. With a surgical blade, make an internal bevel incision from the margin of the free gingiva apically to a point below the bottom of the pocket (Fig. 51–4). Carry the incision interproximally on both the facial and the lingual sides, attempting to retain as much interproximal tissue as possible. The intention is to cut the inner portion of the soft tissue wall of the pocket, all around the tooth.

3. Remove the excised tissue with a curette, and carefully root plane all exposed cementum to a smooth, hard consistency. Preserve all connective tissue fibers that remain attached to the root surface.

4. Irrigate with normal saline. Make sure no calculus or large clots are present.

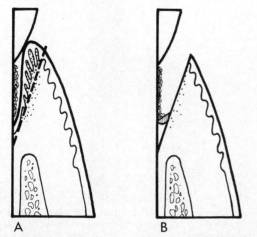

Figure 51–4 Excisional New Attachment Procedure. *A,* Internal bevel incision to point below bottom of pocket. *B,* After excision of tissue, scaling and root planing are performed.

5. Approximate the wound edges; if they do not meet passively, recontour the bone until good adaptation of the wound edges is achieved. Place interproximal interrupted or vertical mattress sutures.

6. Apply pressure for 2 or 3 minutes from both the facial and the lingual aspects with saline-soaked gauze in order to permit only a thin clot between the tissue and the tooth. Place a periodontal dressing.

Ultrasonic Curettage

The use of ultrasonic devices has been recommended for gingival curettage.[16] These instruments are not as effective as hand instruments in removing connective tissue and leaving a smooth pocket wall, but they are better at removing pocket epithelium.[16, 23] However, the bulk of the instruments and the rough tooth surface left by ultrasound curettage contraindicate it for subgingival use.

Caustic Drugs

Since early in the periodontal literature[26, 30] the use of caustic drugs has been recommended in order to induce a "chemical curettage" of the lateral wall of the pocket or even the selective elimination of the epithelium. Drugs such as sodium sulfide, alkaline sodium hypochlorite solution (Antiformin),[5, 9, 10] and phenol[1, 6] have been proposed and discarded after studies showed their ineffectiveness.[2, 8, 10] Moreover, the extent of the tissue destruction with these drugs cannot be controlled, and they may increase rather than reduce the

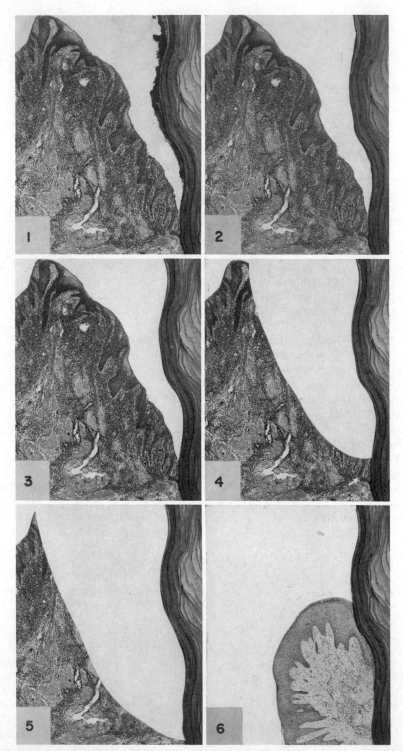

Figure 51–5 Diagrammatic Representation of the Anticipated Tissue Changes in Various Stages of Pocket Eradication Using Scaling and Curettage. *1,* The periodontal pocket with calculus on the root surface. *2,* Calculus removed. *3,* Root surface smoothed. *4,* Pocket wall curetted. Junctional epithelium *(arrow)* not disturbed. *5,* Pocket wall curetted and junctional epithelium removed. *6,* Pocket eradicated.

amount of tissue to be removed by enzymes and phagocytes.

HEALING FOLLOWING SCALING AND CURETTAGE (Fig. 51–5)

Immediately after curettage, a blood clot fills the gingival sulcus, which is devoid of epithelial lining. Hemorrhage is also present in the tissues with dilated capillaries, and abundant polymorphonuclear leukocytes appear shortly thereafter on the wound surface.

This is followed by a rapid proliferation of granulation tissue, with a decrease in the number of small blood vessels as the tissue matures. Restoration and epithelialization of the sulcus generally require from 2 to 7 days,[12, 15, 17, 28] and restoration of the junctional epithelium occurs in animals as early as 5 days after treatment. Immature collagen fibers appear within 21 days. Healthy gingival fibers inadvertently severed from the tooth by scaling, root planing, and curettage[14] and tears in the sulcular epithelium[14, 21] and junctional epithelium are repaired in the healing process.

Several investigators have reported that in monkeys[7, 31] and in humans[29] treated by scaling and curettage, healing results in the formation of a long, thin junctional epithelium with no new connective tissue attachment. Sometimes this long epithelium is interrupted by "windows" of connective tissue attachment.[7]

Opinions differ regarding whether scaling and curettage consistently remove the pocket lining and the junctional epithelium. Some report that scaling and root planing tear the epithelial lining of the pocket without removing either it or the junctional epithelium[14] but that both epithelial structures,[3, 4, 13] sometimes including underlying inflamed connective tissue,[15] are removed by curettage. Others report that the removal of pocket lining and junctional epithelium by curettage is not complete.[24, 27, 28]

CLINICAL APPEARANCE OF THE GINGIVA AFTER CURETTAGE

Immediately after scaling and curettage, the gingiva appears hemorrhagic and bright red.

After 1 week, the gingiva appears reduced in height owing to an apical shift in the position of the gingival margin. The gingiva is also slightly redder than normal, but much less so than in previous days.

After 2 weeks, and with proper oral hygiene by the patient, the normal color, consistency, surface texture, and contour of the gingiva are attained, and the gingival margin is well adapted to the tooth.

REFERENCES

1. Barkann, A.: A conservative technique for the eradication of a pyorrhea product. J. Am. Dent. Assoc., 26:61, 1939.
2. Beube, F. E.: An experimental study of the use of sodium sulphide solution in treatment of periodontal pockets. J. Periodontol., 10:49, 1939.
3. Beube, F. E.: Treatment methods for marginal gingivitis and periodontitis. Texas Dent. J., 71:427, 1953.
4. Blass, J. L., and Lite, T.: Gingival healing following surgical curettage: a histopathologic study. N.Y. Dent. J., 25:127, 1959.
5. Box, K. F.: Periodontal disease and treatment. J. Ontario Dent. Assoc., 29:194, 1952.
6. Bunting, R. W.: The control and treatment of pyorrhea by subgingival surgery. J. Am. Dent. Assoc., 15:119, 1928.
7. Caton, J. C., and Zander, H. A.: The attachment between tooth and gingival tissues after periodic root planing and soft tissue curettage. J. Periodontol., 50:462, 1979.
8. Glickman, J., and Patur, B.: Histologic study of the effect of Antiformin on the soft tissue wall of periodontal pockets in humans. J. Am. Dent. Assoc., 51:420, 1955.
9. Hunter, H. A.: A study of tissues treated with Antiformin citric acid. J. Can. Dent. Assoc., 21:344, 1955.
10. Johnson, R. W., and Waerhaug, J.: Effect of Antiformin on gingival tissue. J. Periodontol., 27:24, 1956.
11. Kalkwarf, K. L., Tussing, G. J., and Davis, M. J.: Histologic evaluation of gingival curettage facilitated by sodium hypochlorite solution. J. Periodontol., 53:63, 1982.
12. Kon, S., et al.: Visualization of microvascularization of the healing periodontal wound. II. Curettage. J. Periodontol., 40:96, 1969.
13. Morris, M. L.: The removal of the pocket and attachment epithelium in humans: a histological study. J. Periodontol., 25:7, 1954.
14. Moskow, B. S.: The response of the gingival sulcus to instrumentation: a histologic investigation. I. The scaling procedure. J. Periodontol., 33:282, 1962.
15. Moskow, B. S.: The response of the gingival sulcus to instrumentation: a histologic investigation. II. Gingival curettage. J. Periodontol., 35:112, 1964.
16. Nadler, H.: Removal of crevicular epithelium by ultrasonic curettes. J. Periodontol., 33:220, 1962.
17. O'Bannon, J. Y.: The gingival tissues before and after scaling the teeth. J. Periodontol., 35:69, 1964.
18. Pattison, G., and Pattison, A. M.: Periodontal Instrumentation—A Clinical Manual. Reston, Va., Reston Publishing Company, 1979.
19. Periodontics Syllabus. NAVED P-5110. U.S. Naval Dental Corps, 1975, pp. 113–115.
20. Ramfjord, S. P., and Ash, M. M., Jr.: Periodontology and Periodontics. Philadelphia, W. B. Saunders Company, 1979.
21. Ramfjord, S. P., and Kiester, G.: The gingival sulcus and the periodontal pocket immediately following scaling of the teeth. J. Periodontol., 25:167, 1954.
22. Saglie, R., Newman, M. G., Carranza, F. A., Jr., and Pattison, G. L.: Bacterial invasion of gingiva in advanced periodontitis in humans. J. Periodontol., 53:217, 1982.
23. Sanderson, A. D.: Gingival curettage by hand and ultrasonic instruments—a histologic comparison. J. Periodontol., 37:279, 1966.
24. Sato, M.: Histopathological study of the healing process after surgical treatment for alveolar pyorrhea. Bull. Tokyo Dent. College, 1:71, 1960.
25. Sorrin, S., and Miller, S. Ch.: The action of sodium sulphide as an epithelial solvent. Dent. Cosmos, 69:1113, 1927.

26. Stewart, H.: Partial removal of cementum and decalcification of tooth in the treatment of pyorrhea alveolaris. Dent. Cosmos, *41*:617, 1899.

27. Stone, S., Ramfjord, S. P., and Waldron, J.: Scaling and gingival curettage—a radioautographic study. J. Periodontol., *37*:415, 1966.

28. Waerhaug, J.: Microscopic demonstration of tissue reaction incident to removal of subgingival calculus. J. Periodontol., *26*:26, 1955.

29. Waerhaug, J.: Healing of the dentoepithelial junction following subgingival plaque control. I. As observed in human biopsy material. J. Periodontol., *49*:1, 1978.

30. Younger, W. J.: Some of the latest phases in implantations and other procedures. Dent. Cosmos, *35*:102, 1893.

31. Yukna, R. A.: A clinical and histological study of healing following the excisional new attachment procedure in rhesus monkeys. J. Periodontol., *47*:701, 1976.

32. Yukna, R. A., et al.: Clinical study of healing in humans following the excisional new attachment procedure. J. Periodontol., *47*:696, 1976.

The Gingivectomy Technique

The term *gingivectomy* means excision of the gingiva. By removing the diseased pocket wall which obscures the tooth surface, gingivectomy provides the visibility and accessibility that are essential for the complete removal of irritating surface deposits and thorough smoothing of the roots (Fig. 52–1). By removing diseased tissue and local irritants, it also creates a favorable environment for gingival healing and the restoration of a physiologic gingival contour.

INDICATIONS AND CONTRAINDICATIONS

The gingivectomy technique is indicated in the following cases[9]: (1) Elimination of supra-bony pockets, regardless of their depth, if the pocket wall is fibrous and firm. Because fibrous gingival tissue does not shrink after scaling and curettage, some form of surgical treatment is necessary to eliminate the pocket. (2) Elimination of gingival enlargements. (3) Elimination of suprabony periodontal abscesses.

The following two findings will contraindicate the gingivectomy technique: (1) The need for bone surgery or even for examination of the bone shape and morphology. (2) The location of the bottom of the pocket apical to the mucogingival junction.

When used for the purposes for which it is intended, the gingivectomy technique is a most effective form of treatment[16] (see Plate VIII).

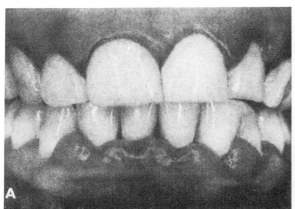 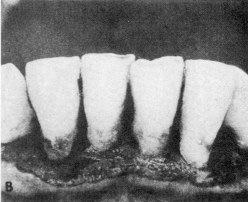

Figure 52–1 Visibility and Accessibility of Calculus. *A,* Gingival enlargement. *B,* Removal of diseased gingiva exposes calculus. (Phase I therapy is sometimes omitted when the indication for a gingivectomy is obvious. It can never be omitted when a flap appears indicated.)

Before   After

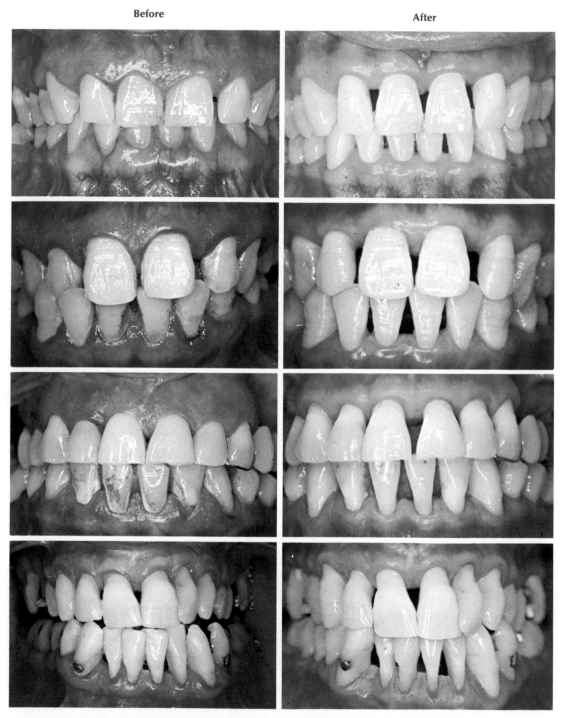

Plate VIII Results Obtained by Treating Suprabony Pockets of Different Depths with Gingivectomy.

A STEP-BY-STEP PROCEDURE FOR PERFORMING THE GINGIVECTOMY

Mark the Pockets

The pockets on each surface are explored with a periodontal probe and marked with a pocket marker. The instrument is held with the marking end in line with the vertical axis of the tooth. The straight end is inserted to the base of the pocket, and the level is marked by pressing the pliers together and producing a bleeding point on the outside surface (Figs. 52–2 and 52–3). The pockets are marked systematically, beginning on the distal surface of the last tooth, then moving to the facial surface, and proceeding anteriorly to the midline. The procedure is repeated on the lingual surface. Each pocket is marked in several areas so as to outline its course on each surface.

Resect the Gingiva

The gingiva may be resected with periodontal knives, a scalpel, or scissors.* The removal of diseased gingiva is an important part of the gingivectomy, but the instrument with which it is done does not affect the outcome of treatment. The choice is based upon individual experience. Periodontal knives are used for incisions on the facial and lingual surfaces and distal to the terminal tooth in the arch. The Orban periodontal knives are used

*The use of electrosurgery will be described later in this chapter.

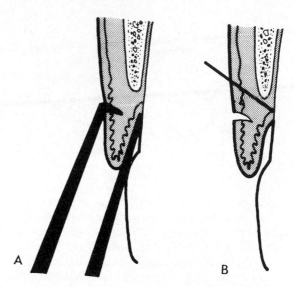

Figure 52–3 Marking the Depth of Suprabony Pocket. *A,* Pocket marker in position. *B,* Beveled incision extends apical to the perforation made by the pocket marker.

for supplemental interdental incisions where necessary, and the Bard-Parker blades No. 11 and No. 12 and scissors are used as auxiliary instruments.

DISCONTINUOUS AND CONTINUOUS INCISIONS. Discontinuous or continuous incisions may be used, depending upon the operator's preference.

The *discontinuous incision* is started on the facial surface at the distal angle of the last tooth and carried forward, following the course of the pocket and extending through the interdental gingiva to the distofacial angle of the next tooth (Fig. 52–4). The next incision is begun where the previous one crosses the interdental space and is carried to the distofacial angle of the next tooth. Individual incisions are repeated for each tooth to be operated.

The *continuous incision* is started on the facial surface of the last tooth and carried forward without interruption, following the course of the pockets (Fig. 52–5).

After the incisions have been made on the

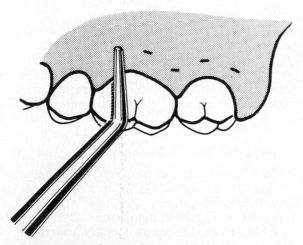

Figure 52–2 Pocket Marker No. 27G Makes Pinpoint Perforations that indicate pocket depth.

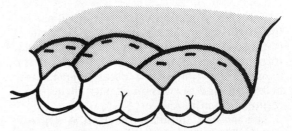

Figure 52–4 Discontinuous Incision apical to bottom of the pocket indicated by pinpoint markings.

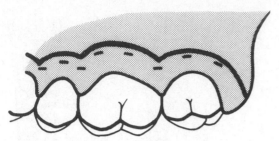

Figure 52–5 Continuous Incision begins on the molar and extends anteriorly without interruption.

facial surface, the procedure is repeated on the lingual surface. To avoid the blood vessels and nerves of the incisive canal, and also to produce a better postoperative gingival contour, the incisions should be carried along the sides of the incisive papilla, not horizontally across it (Fig. 52–6).

THE DISTAL INCISION. After the facial and lingual incisions are completed, they are joined by an incision across the distal surface of the last erupted tooth. The distal incision is made with a periodontal knife inserted below the bottom of the pocket and is beveled so that it blends with the facial and lingual incisions (Fig. 52–7).

HOW TO MAKE THE INCISION. The incision is started apical to the points marking the course of the pockets[30, 37] and directed coronally to a point between the base of the pocket and the crest of the bone. **It should be as close as possible to the bone without exposing it so as to remove the soft tissue coronal to the bone.** Removal of the soft tissue between the bottom of the pocket and the bone is important, because (1) it provides the greatest likelihood of removing the entire junctional epithelium, (2) it ensures the exposure of all root deposits at the bottom of the pocket (Fig. 52–8), and (3) it eliminates excessive fibrous tissue, which may interfere with the attainment of physiologic contour when the gingiva heals (Fig. 52–9). Exposure of bone is undesirable. Should it occur, healing usually presents no problem if the area is adequately covered by the periodontal pack.

Some authors, however, recommend placing the incision 1 to 2 mm coronal to the bottom of the pocket in order to reduce the potential root exposure after healing and to limit the tissue destruction which occurs immediately below the line of incision as part of the tissue response to injury.[33]

The incision should be beveled at approximately 45° to the tooth surface. This is most important where the pocket wall is enlarged

and fibrous, such as on the palatal surface in the molar area (Fig. 52–10). Failure to bevel leaves a broad fibrous plateau which takes more time than ordinarily required to develop a physiologic contour. In the interim, plaque and food accumulation may lead to recurrence of pockets.

The incision should re-create the normal festooned pattern of the gingiva as far as possible, but not if this means leaving part of the pocket wall intact. The diseased pocket wall must be completely removed even if it requires departure from the regular outline of normal gingiva.

The incision should pass completely through the soft tissue to the tooth (Fig. 52–11). Incomplete incisions make it difficult to detach the pocket wall and leave adherent tissue tabs that must be removed with scissors or a periodontal knife.

If in the course of the operation it becomes apparent that the incision is inadequate, it should be modified. The most common error is failure to make the incision close enough to the bone. Very often, deep calculus is revealed after the incision is corrected.

TEETH ADJACENT TO EDENTULOUS AREAS. For pockets on teeth adjacent to an edentulous area, the usual incisions are made on the facial and lingual tooth surfaces. In addition, a single incision is made across the edentulous ridge apical to the pockets on the teeth and close to the bone (Fig. 52–12). Pockets adjacent to edentulous spaces should not be excised as separate units, as this creates gingival troughs that complicate subsequent prosthesis.

Remove the Marginal and Interdental Gingivae

Starting at the distal surface of the last erupted tooth, the gingival margin is detached at the line of incision with surgical hoes and scalers. The instrument is placed deep in the incision in contact with the tooth surface and moved coronally with a slow, firm motion (Fig. 52–13).

Appraise the Field of Operation

After the pocket wall is excised and the field is cleaned, the following features can be observed (Fig. 52–14A):

1. Bead-like granulation tissue.

2. Some calculus remnants that may extend close to where the pocket was attached. Calculus is **dark brown and slate-like in consist-**

Text continued on page 788

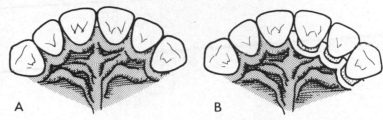

Figure 52–6 Incision Made Lateral to the Incisive Papilla. *A,* Palatal area. *B,* After tissue removal.

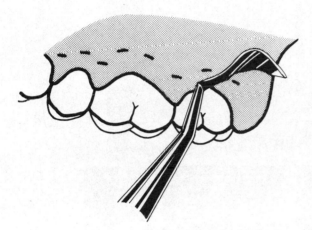

Figure 52–7 Beveled Distal Incision on the Maxilla made with periodontal knife.

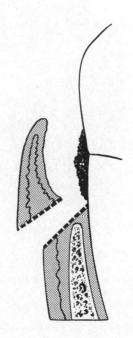

Figure 52–8 Complete Removal of Pocket Wall Assures Exposure of Calculus.

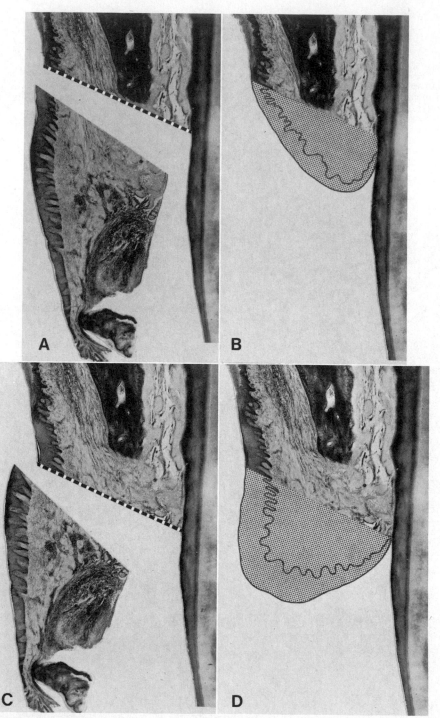

Figure 52–9 Incision Close to Bone Facilitates Healing Which Produces Physiologic Gingival Contour. *A,* Labial incision close beyond the pocket and close to the bone. *B,* Diagrammatic representation of healed gingiva with physiologic contour and normal sulcus. *C,* Incision is close to the bottom of the pocket but not deep enough. It leaves a remnant of epithelial attachment on the tooth and a wide band of inflamed fibrous connective tissue between the bottom of the pocket and the bone. *D,* Diagrammatic representation of bulbous gingiva and wide, deep sulcus formed on incompletely resected inflamed fibrous tissue.

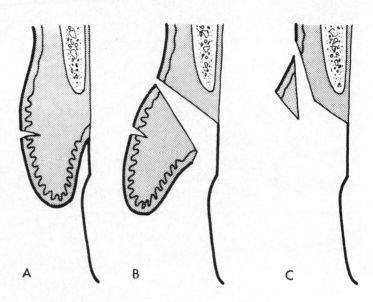

Figure 52–10 Beveled Incision for the Removal of Bulbous Fibrous Palatal Pocket. *A,* Bulbous gingiva on the palatal surface of upper first molar after use of pocket marker to mark pocket depth. *B,* Gingiva resected with a beveled incision. *C,* Corrective second incision is sometimes required to attain a better contour.

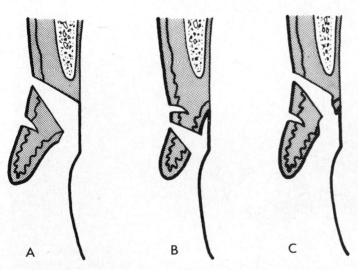

Figure 52–11 Correct and Incorrect Incisions. *A,* **Correct Incision** is apical to the bottom of the pocket, is beveled, and completely penetrates the soft tissue. The notch is made by the pocket marker at the level of the bottom of the pocket. *B,* **Incorrect Incision** is not deep enough, leaves part of pocket behind. *C,* **Incorrect Incision** does not penetrate the soft tissues, leaves adherent tissue tab on tooth.

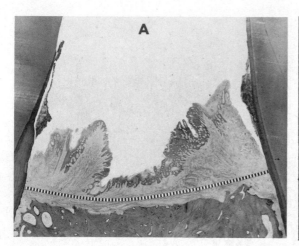

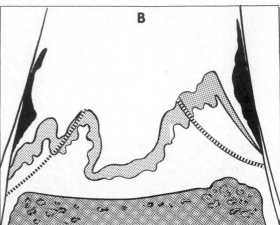

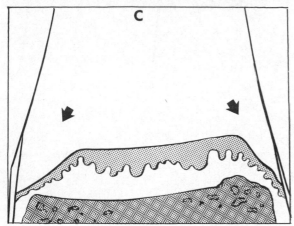

Figure 52–12 Incision Across Edentulous Space. *A,* Periodontal pockets adjacent to fibrous edentulous space. The proper incision is indicated by the dotted line. *B,* Incorrect incisions remove pockets separately, leaving fibrous mucosa intact. *C,* Troughs which result from improper incisions.

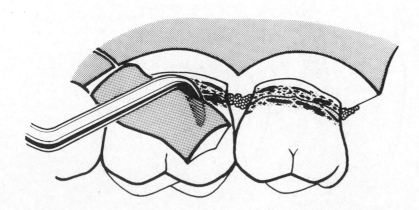

Figure 52–13 Detaching the Gingiva with a Surgical Hoe. When the discontinuous incision is used, the marginal and interdental gingivae are removed as a unit.

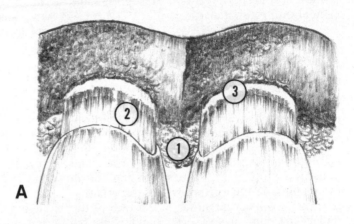

Figure 52–14 After the Pocket Wall is Removed.
A, Field of operation immediately after removing pocket wall. (1) Granulation tissue; (2) calculus and other root deposits; (3) clear space where bottom of the pocket was attached. *B*, Granulation tissue removed with curette to provide clear view of root surfaces. *C*, Root surfaces scaled and planed.

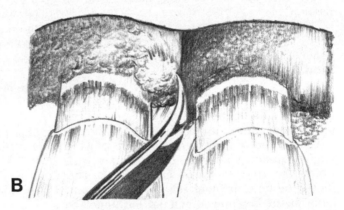

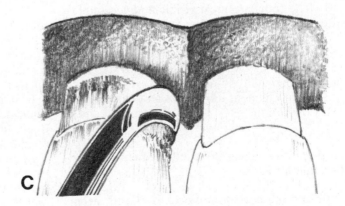

ency, but some particles may be almost the same color as the root.

3. A band-like light zone on the root where the base of the pocket was attached.

Other features that may be noted at this time are softening of the root surface, indentations produced by cellular resorption, and cementum protuberances.

Remove the Granulation Tissue

The granulation tissue is removed before thorough scaling is attempted so that hemorrhage from the granulation tissue will not obscure the scaling operation (Fig. 52–14*B*).

Curettes are used for this purpose. The curette is guided along the tooth surface and under the granulation tissue, separating it from the underlying bone. Removal of the granulation tissue will reveal either the surface of the underlying bone or a covering band of fibrous tissue.

Remove the Calculus and Necrotic Root Substance

The calculus and necrotic cementum are removed and the root surface is smoothed, using scalers and curettes (Fig. 52–14*C*).

The success of the gingivectomy depends in large measure upon the thoroughness with which the root is scaled and planed. This should be done immediately after the granulation tissue is removed and not postponed to a subsequent visit for the following reasons:

1. The roots are most visible and accessible after the granulation tissue is removed.

2. The gingiva cannot heal properly if root deposits are permitted to remain until the next visit, when they will be obscured by the inflamed gingiva.

3. Postponement introduces an unnecessary extra operation.

Hygiene Procedures Before Placement of the Periodontal Pack

Before the periodontal pack is placed, **each surface of every tooth** is checked for calculus or soft tissue remnants, after which the area is washed several times with warm water and covered with a gauze sponge folded in a U shape. The patient is instructed to bite on the sponge, which remains in place until the bleed-

ing stops. Persistent bleeding interferes with adaptation and setting of the periodontal pack. It usually can be traced to a bleeding point partially covered by a clot. The clot is cleaned away with a pledget of cotton saturated with hydrogen peroxide. **Pressure is then applied to the bleeding point with a pledget of cotton.** If the bleeding is interproximal, the cotton is wedged between the teeth.

The Blood Clot

The cut surfaces should be covered by a clot before the pack is applied. The clot protects the wound and provides a scaffolding for the new blood vessels and connective tissue cells formed in healing. The clot should not be too bulky. Excessive clot interferes with retention of the periodontal pack. It is also an excellent medium for bacterial growth and increases the possibility of infection and delays healing. This permits downgrowth of the epithelium onto the root, which limits the height of connective tissue attachment.[20]

The Periodontal Pack

The different types of packs and the technique recommended for their application are described in detail in Chapter 50.

HEALING FOLLOWING GINGIVECTOMY

The initial response after gingivectomy is the formation of a protective surface clot; the underlying tissue becomes acutely inflamed, with some necrosis. The clot is replaced by granulation tissue. After 12 to 24 hours, epithelial cells at the margins of the wound show an increase in glycogen[34] and DNA synthesis and migrate over the granulation tissue to separate it from the contaminated surface layer of the clot. Epithelial activity at the margins reaches a peak in 24 to 36 hours[6]; the new epithelial cells arise from the basal and deeper spinous layers of the wound edge epithelium and migrate over the wound over a fibrin layer that is later resorbed and replaced by a connective tissue bed.[14] The epithelial cells advance by a tumbling action, with the cells becoming fixed to the substrate by hemidesmosomes and a new basement lamina.[15] Surface epithelialization is generally complete after 5 to 14 days. During the first 4 weeks after gingivectomy, keratinization is less than it was prior to surgery.

In experimental animals, the surgically removed junctional epithelium is reconstructed within 2 to 3 weeks.[12, 13, 17] Hemidesmosomes and basement lamina may be absent on the connective tissue side of the junctional epithelium. The outer surface of the gingival margin is healed by 14 days after surgery, but the epithelium of the gingival sulcus requires 3 to 5 weeks to heal.

In the initial 12 hours after gingivectomy, there is a slight reduction in cementoblasts and some loss of continuity of the osteoblastic layer on the outer aspect of the alveolar crest.[6] New bone formation occurs at the alveolar crest as early as the fourth day after gingivectomy,[28] and new cementoid appears in 10 to 15 days.[32]

By 24 hours, there is an increase in new connective tissue cells, mainly angioblasts, just beneath the surface layer of inflammation and necrosis; by the third day, numerous young fibroblasts are located in the area.[29] The highly vascular granulation tissue grows coronally, creating a new free gingival margin and sul-

cus.[25] Capillaries derived from blood vessels of the periodontal ligament migrate into the granulation tissue, and within 2 weeks they connect with gingival vessels.[38] Vasodilation and vascularity begin to decrease after the fourth day of healing and appear to be almost normal by the sixteenth day.[22] The connective tissue is still undergoing repair at the twenty-eighth day.

The flow of gingival fluid in humans is initially increased following gingivectomy and diminishes as healing progresses.[1, 31] The maximum is reached after 1 week, coinciding with the time of maximum inflammation.

The tissue changes that occur in postgingivectomy healing are the same in all individuals, but the time required for complete healing varies considerably, depending upon the area of the cut surface and interference from local irritation and infection. In patients with physiologic melanosis, the pigmentation is diminished in the healed gingiva (Fig. 52–15).

Epithelialization and re-formation of the junctional epithelium and re-establishment of the gingival and alveolar crest fiber system are

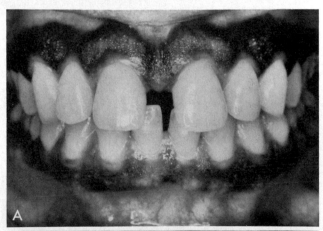
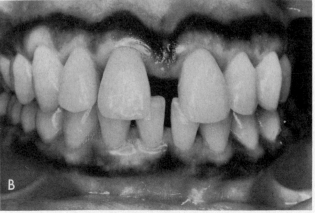

Figure 52–15 Physiologic Melanosis Diminished Following Gingivectomy. *A,* Before treatment—extensive physiologic pigmentation of the gingiva. *B,* One year after gingivectomy. Pigmentation is diminished; periodontal pockets are eliminated, and physiologic gingival contour is restored.

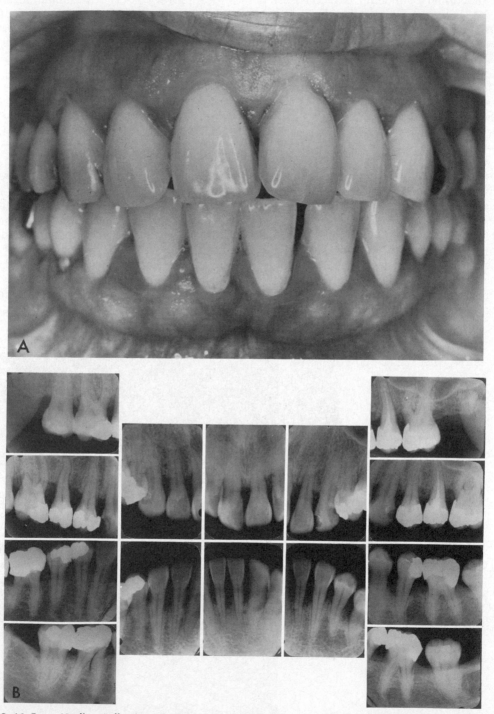

Figure 52–16 Bone Healing Following Gingivectomy. *A,* Generalized periodontal disease in 32-year-old patient. *B,* Extensive generalized bone loss. Note angular bone loss in mandibular incisor area.

Illustration continued on opposite page

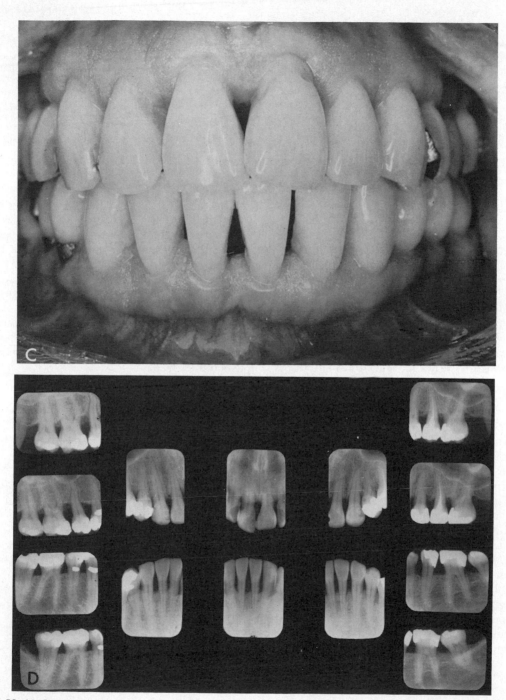

Figure 52–16 *Continued* C, Excellent condition of the gingiva 1 year after gingivectomy. *D*, Radiographs after 1 year showing generalized smoothing of the interdental margins and filling in of bony defect in mandibular incisor area (compare with *B*).

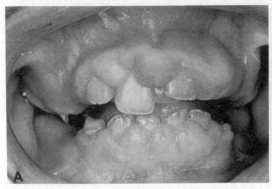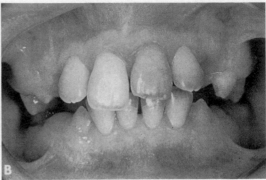

Figure 52–17 Gingival Enlargement in Child. *A,* Gingival enlargement associated with phenytoin therapy treated by complete-mouth gingivectomy. *B,* After healing.

slower in chemically created gingival wounds than in those produced by surgery.[36] Thirty-two days has been estimated as the average time required for complete repair of the epithelium following gingivectomy, and 49 days has been estimated for the connective tissue.[35]

The following time sequence for healing following gingivectomy in humans has also been reported.[3]

Two Days. Clot formed. Bone covered by proliferating connective tissue from the sides of the wound. Numerous leukocytes and fibrin shreds present.

Four Days. A portion of the clot remains adjacent to the tooth surface. Underlying portion of the clot replaced by granulation tissue. Epithelium with rete pegs extends over part of the surface. Dense inflammatory infiltration.

Six Days. Entire wound covered by fairly well differentiated stratified squamous epithelium. There is consolidation of the granulation tissue and some collagen formation. Inflammation present.

Sixteen Days. Epithelium appears mature with new rete pegs. Connective tissue very collagenous. Slight chronic inflammatory exudate still present.

Twenty-one Days. Epithelial rete pegs well developed. Some thickening of the stratum corneum. Hyperplasia and spongiosis of the epithelium. Increased collagenization of the connective tissue. Gingiva clinically normal.

Figure 52–16 shows physiologic bone contouring 1 year after treatment by gingivectomy. Figure 52–17 shows the result of treatment of fibrous gingival enlargement with the gingivectomy technique.

GINGIVECTOMY BY CHEMOSURGERY

Several techniques have been described advocating the use of chemicals rather than a knife to remove the gingiva.

One technique entails the use of 5 per cent paraformaldehyde (trioxymethylene) incorporated in a modified zinc oxide–eugenol paste and placed on the gingival margin and into the pocket.[23] Another technique suggests the use of potassium hydroxide.[18]

These methods have the following disadvantages: (1) their depth of action cannot be controlled, and, therefore, healthy attached tissue underlying the pocket may be injured; and (2) gingival remodeling cannot be accomplished effectively.

GINGIVECTOMY BY ELECTROSURGERY

Indications

The instrument with which the tissue is removed is but one aspect of the gingivectomy technique. The use of electrosurgery for the gingivectomy incision has the following advantages and disadvantages:

Advantages: Electrosurgery permits an adequate contouring of the tissue and controls hemorrhage.[7, 24]

Disadvantages: Electrosurgery cannot be used in patients who have a noncompatible or a poorly shielded cardiac pacemaker. The treatment causes an unpleasant odor. If the electrosurgery point touches the bone, irreparable damage can be done[2, 10, 21, 26]; further, the heat generated by injudicious use can cause tissue damage and loss of periodontal support when the electrode is used close to bone. When the electrode touches the root, areas of cementum burn are produced.[39]

Therefore, the use of electrosurgery should be limited to superficial procedures such as removal of gingival enlargements, gingivoplasty, relocating frenum and muscle attachments, and incising periodontal abscesses and pericoronal flaps. *It should not be used for*

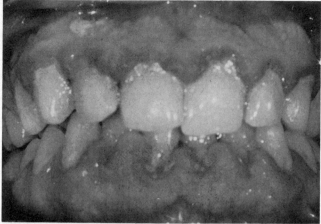

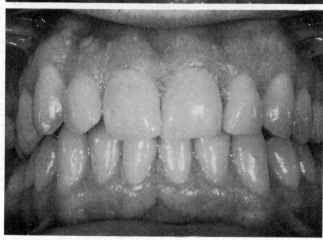

Figure 52–18 Attainment of Desired Gingival Contour by Properly Beveling the Gingivectomy Incision. Before treatment *(above).* Pronounced gingival enlargement consisting of a combination of edematous and fibrous tissue. After treatment *(below).* Gingival contour attained by properly beveling the incision in the regular gingivectomy technique.

procedures that involve proximity to the bone, such as treatment of infrabony pockets, flap operations, or mucogingival surgery.

Technique

The removal of gingival enlargements and gingivoplasty[24] are performed with the needle electrode, supplemented by the small ovoid loop or the diamond-shaped electrodes for festooning. A blended cutting and coagulating (fully rectified) current is used. In all reshaping procedures the electrode is activated and moved in a concise "shaving" motion.

In the treatment of acute periodontal abscesses, the incision to establish drainage can be made with the needle electrode without exerting painful pressure. The incision will remain open because the edges are sealed by the current. After the acute symptoms subside, the regular procedure for the treatment of the periodontal abscess is followed (see Chapter 42).

For hemostasis, the ball electrode is used. Hemorrhage must be controlled by direct pres-sure (air, compress, or hemostat) first; then the surface is lightly touched with a coagulating current. Electrosurgery is very helpful for the control of isolated bleeding points. Bleeding areas located interproximally are reached with a thin, bar-shaped electrode.

Frenum and muscle attachments can be relocated to facilitate pocket elimination, using a loop electrode. For this purpose, the frenum or muscle is stretched and sectioned with the loop electrode and a coagulating current.

For cases of acute pericoronitis, drainage may be obtained by incising the flap with a bent needle electrode. A loop electrode is used to remove the flap after the acute symptoms subside.

Healing Following Electrosurgery

Some investigators report no significant differences in gingival healing following resection by electrosurgery and periodontal knives[5, 19]; others find delayed healing, greater reduction in gingival height, and more bone injury following electrosurgery.[26] There appears to be little difference in the results obtained following **shallow** gingival resection with electrosurgery and periodontal knives. However, when used for **deep resections close to bone,** electrosurgery reportedly can produce gingival recession, bone necrosis and sequestration, loss of bone height, furcation exposure, and tooth mobility, which do not occur with the use of periodontal knives.[10]

GINGIVOPLASTY

Gingival and periodontal disease often produces deformities in the gingiva which interfere with normal food excursion, collect irritating plaque and food debris, and prolong and aggravate the disease process. Gingival clefts and craters, shelf-like interdental papillae caused by acute necrotizing ulcerative gingivitis, and gingival enlargement are examples of such deformities. *Artificially reshaping the gingiva to create physiologic gingival contours is termed gingivoplasty.*[11]

The gingivoplasty technique is similar to the gingivectomy technique; its purpose, however, is different. Gingivectomy is performed in order to eliminate periodontal pockets and includes reshaping as part of the technique. Gingivoplasty is done in the absence of pockets with the sole purpose of recontouring the gingiva.

Gingivoplasty may be done with a periodontal knife, scalpel, rotary coarse diamond stones,[8] or electrosurgery.[7] It consists of procedures that resemble those performed in festooning artificial dentures—namely, tapering the gingival margin, creating an escalloped marginal outline, thinning the attached gingiva, and creating vertical interdental grooves and shaping the interdental papillae to provide sluiceways for the passage of food. Proper beveling of the gingivectomy incision achieves comparable results (Fig. 52–18).

REFERENCES

1. Arnold, R., Lunstad, G., Bissada, N., and Stallard, R.: Alterations in crevicular fluid flow during healing following gingival surgery. J. Periodont. Res., *1*:303, 1966.
2. Azzi, R., Kenney, E. B., Tsao, T. F., and Carranza, F. A., Jr.: The effect of electrosurgery upon alveolar bone. J. Periodontol., *54*:96, 1983.
3. Bernier, J., and Kaplan, H.: The repair of gingival tissue after surgical intervention. J. Am. Dent. Assoc., *35*:697, 1947.
4. Donnenfeld, O. W., and Glickman, I.: A biometric study of the effects of gingivectomy. J. Periodontol., *37*:447, 1966.
5. Eisenmann, D., Malone, W. F., and Kusek, J.: Electron microscopic evaluation of electrosurgery. Oral Surg., *29*:660, 1970.
6. Engler, W. O., Ramfjord, S., and Hiniker, J. J.: Healing following simple gingivectomy. A tritiated thymidine radioautographic study. I. Epithelialization. J. Periodontol., *37*:298, 1966.
7. Flocken, J. E.: Electrosurgical management of soft tissues and restoration dentistry. Dent. Clin. North Am., *24*:247, 1980.
8. Fox, L.: Rotating abrasives in the management of periodontal soft and hard tissues. Oral Surg., *8*:1134, 1955.
9. Glickman, I.: The results obtained with the unembellished gingivectomy technic in a clinical study in humans. J. Periodontol., *27*:247, 1956.
10. Glickman, I., and Imber, L. R.: Comparison of gingival resection with electrosurgery and periodontal knives—a biometric and histologic study. J. Periodontol., *41*:142, 1970.
11. Goldman, H. M.: The development of physiologic gingival contours by gingivoplasty. Oral Surg., *3*:879, 1950.
12. Henning, F.: Healing of gingivectomy wounds in the rat: reestablishment of the epithelial seal. J. Periodontol., *39*:265, 1968.
13. Henning, F.: Epithelial mitotic activity after gingivectomy. Relationship to reattachment. J. Periodont. Res., *4*:319, 1969.
14. Innes, P. B.: An electron microscopic study of the regeneration of gingival epithelium following gingivectomy in the dog. J. Periodont. Res., *5*:196, 1970.
15. Krawczyk, W. S.: A pattern of epithelial cell migration during wound healing. J. Cell Biol., *49*:247, 1971.
16. Lekovic, V., Kenney, E. B., and Carranza, F. A., Jr.: Comparative clinical study of root planing and gingivectomy. Unpublished data.
17. Listgarten, M. A.: Electron microscopic features of the newly formed epithelial attachment after gingival surgery. J. Periodont. Res., *2*:46, 1967.
18. Löe, H.: Chemical gingivectomy. Effect of potassium hydroxide on periodontal tissues. Acta Odontol. Scand., *19*:517, 1961.
19. Malone, W. F., Eisenmann, D., and Kusck, J.: Interceptive periodontics with electrosurgery. J. Prosthet. Dent., *22*:555, 1969.
20. Morris, M. L.: Healing of human periodontal tissues following surgical detachment from vital teeth: the position of the epithelial attachment. J. Periodontol., *32*:108, 1961.
21. Nixon, K. C., Adkins, K. F., and Keys, D. W.: Histological evaluation of effects produced in alveolar bone following gingival incision with an electrosurgical scalpel. J. Periodontol., *46*:40, 1975.
22. Novaes, A. B., Kon, S., Ruben, M. P., and Goldman, H.: Visualization of the microvascularization of the healing periodontal wound. III. Gingivectomy. J. Periodontol., *40*:359, 1969.
23. Orban, B.: New methods in periodontal treatment. Bur, *42*:116, 1942.
24. Oringer, M. J.: Electrosurgery for definitive conservative modern periodontal therapy. Dent. Clin. North Am., *13*:53, 1969.
25. Persson, P. A.: The healing process in the marginal periodontium after gingivectomy with special regard to the regeneration of epithelium (an experimental study on dogs). Odont. T., *67*:593, 1959.
26. Pope, J. W., Gargiulo, A. W., Staffileno, H., and Levy, S.: Effects of electrosurgery on wound healing in dogs. Periodontics, *6*:30, 1968.
27. Prandi, E. C., Blitzer, B., and Carranza, F. A., Jr.: Evaluación biométrica de la técnica de gingivectomia en humanos. Rev. Asoc. Odontol., Argent., *57*:84, 1969.
28. Ramfjord, S., and Costich, E. R.: Healing after simple gingivectomy. J. Periodontol., *34*:401, 1963.
29. Ramfjord, S. P., Engler, W. D., and Hiniker, J. J.: A radiographic study of healing following simple gingivectomy. II. The connective tissue. J. Periodontol., *37*:179, 1966.
30. Ritchey, B., and Orban, B.: The periodontal pocket. J. Periodontol., *23*:199, 1952.
31. Sandalli, P., and Wade, A. B.: Alterations in crevicular fluid flow during healing following gingivectomy and flap procedures. J. Periodont. Res., *4*:314, 1969.
32. Stahl, S. S.: Soft tissue healing following experimental gingival wounding in female rats of various ages. Periodontics, *1*:142, 1963.
33. Stahl, S. S.: Periodontal Surgery: Biologic Basis and Technique. Springfield, Ill., Charles C Thomas, Publisher, 1976.

34. Stahl, S. S., Witkin, G. J., Cantor, M., and Brown, R.: Gingival healing. II. Clinical and histologic repair sequences following gingivectomy. J. Periodontol., *39*:109, 1968.

35. Stanton, G., Levy, M., and Stahl, S. S.: Collagen restoration in healing human gingiva. J. Dent. Res., *48*:27, 1969.

36. Tonna, E., and Stahl, S. S.: A polarized light microscopic study of rat periodontal ligament following surgical and chemical gingival trauma. Helv. Odontol. Acta, *11*:90, 1967.

37. Waerhaug, J.: Depth of incision in gingivectomy. Oral Surg., *8*:707, 1955.

38. Watanabe, Y., and Suzuki, S.: An experimental study in capillary vascularization in the periodontal tissue following gingivectomy or flap operation. J. Dent. Res., *42*:758, 1963.

39. Wilhelmsen, N. R., Ramfjord, S. P., and Blankenship, J. R.: Effects of electrosurgery on the gingival attachment in Rhesus monkeys. J. Periodontol., *47*:160, 1976.

The Periodontal Flap

A periodontal flap is a section of gingiva and/ or mucosa surgically separated from the underlying tissues to provide visibility of and access to the bone and root surface. The flap also allows the gingiva to be positioned in a different location in patients with mucogingival involvement.

The basic steps for the flap technique were described early in the twentieth century by several clinicians[6, 15, 21, 22]; with some modifications and refinements, these steps constitute the techniques utilized today. The flap operation is used in many different situations and varies according to the degree of flap reflection, the amount of tissue reflected, the types of incisions utilized, and the final position of the flap.

CLASSIFICATION OF FLAPS

Periodontal flaps are classified as either full thickness (mucoperiosteal) or partial thickness (mucosal) flaps (Fig. 53–1). In **full thickness flaps,** all of the soft tissue, including the periosteum, is reflected to expose the underlying bone. This complete exposure of and access to the underlying bone is indicated if osseous surgery is contemplated. The full thickness flap is reflected by means of a blunt dissection. A periosteal elevator is used to separate the mucoperiosteum from the bone by moving it mesially, distally, and apically until the desired reflection is accomplished.

The **partial thickness flap** includes only the epithelium and a layer of the underlying connective tissue. The bone remains covered by a layer of connective tissue, including the periosteum. Sharp dissection is necessary to reflect a partial thickness flap. A surgical scalpel (No. 15 or No. 11) is utilized to separate the flap carefully. The partial thickness flap is indicated when the flap is to be positioned apically or when the operator does not desire to expose bone.

There are conflicting data regarding the ad-

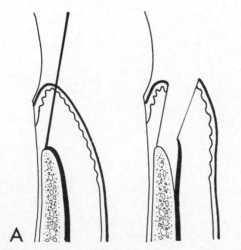 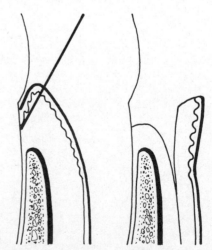

Figure 53–1 *A,* Diagram of the internal bevel incision (first incision) to reflect a full thickness (mucoperiosteal) flap. Note that the incision ends on the bone to allow for the reflection of the entire flap. *B,* Diagram of the internal bevel incision to reflect a partial thickness flap. Note that the incision ends on the root surface to preserve the periosteum on the bone.

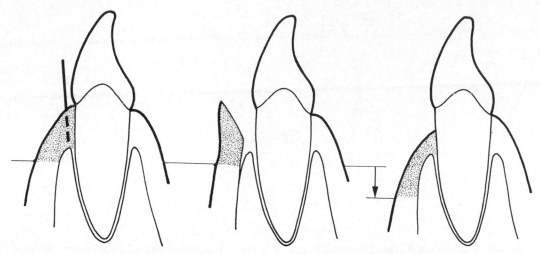

Figure 53–2 The internal bevel incision is placed at the crest of the gingiva in an apically positioned flap to preserve the entire attached, keratinized gingiva. The flap is reflected, and the entire flap is placed in an apical position.

visability of uncovering the bone when this is not actually needed. Some writers have shown that marginal bone loss occurs when bone is stripped of its periosteum and that this loss is prevented when the periosteum is left on the bone.[5] Others have shown results that suggest that the differences may not be clinically significant.[9] Therefore, the use of the partial thickness flap may be necessary only in cases in which the crestal bone margin is very thin and will be exposed when the flap is placed apically. The periosteum left on the bone may also be used in suturing the flap when it is positioned apically.

Flaps can also be classified as (1) repositioned or positioned flaps and (2) unrepositioned flaps, depending on the placement of the flap at the conclusion of the surgical procedure. An **unrepositioned flap** is placed in the position it had before surgery, whereas a **repositioned flap** can be placed apical (Fig. 53–2), coronal, or lateral to its original position. This chapter will present general considerations and techniques for unrepositioned and apically positioned flaps. Coronally and laterally positioned flaps will be dealt with in Chapter 56.

Apically positioned flaps have the important advantage of preserving the outer portion of the pocket wall and transforming it into attached gingiva. They therefore accomplish the double objective of eliminating the pocket and increasing the width of the attached gingiva. Repositioning a flap is made possible by totally separating the attached gingiva from the underlying bone; displacement is then possible owing to the movability of the unattached

portion of the gingiva. Repositioned flaps cannot be done in the palate owing to the absence of nonattached gingiva.

When regeneration of the alveolar crest is expected, unrepositioned flaps should be utilized because they can totally cover the crestal area.

DESIGN OF THE FLAP

The design of the flap will be dictated by the surgical judgment of the operator and may depend on the objectives of the operation. The degree of access to the underlying bone and root surfaces necessary and the final position of the flap must be considered in designing the flap. Preservation of good blood supply to the flap is a very important consideration.

INCISIONS

Periodontal flaps utilize horizontal and vertical incisions. **Horizontal incisions** are directed along the margin of the gingiva in a mesial or a distal direction (Fig. 53–3). Two types of horizontal incisions have been recommended: the internal bevel incision,[8] which starts at a distance from the gingival margin and is aimed at the bone crest; and the crevicular incision, which starts at the bottom of the pocket and is directed to the bone margin. In addition, the interdental incision is performed after the flap is elevated.

The **internal bevel incision** is the incision basic to all periodontal flap procedures. It is

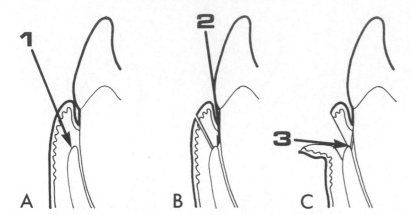

Figure 53–3 The first (internal bevel), second (crevicular), and third (interdental) incisions are the three incisions necessary for flap surgery.

the incision from which the flap will be reflected to expose the underlying bone and root. The internal bevel incision accomplishes three very important objectives: it (1) removes the pocket lining; (2) conserves the relatively uninvolved outer surface of the gingiva, which, if apically positioned, will become attached gingiva; and (3) creates a sharp, thin flap margin for adaptation to the bone-tooth junction. This incision has also been termed the "first incision," since it is the initial incision in the reflection of a periodontal flap, and the "reverse bevel incision," since its bevel is in reverse direction from that of the gingivectomy incision. The No. 15 or No. 11 surgical scalpel is used most commonly. That portion of the gingiva left around the tooth contains the epithelium of the pocket lining and the adjacent granulomatous tissue. It will be discarded after the crevicular (second) and interdental (third) incisions are performed (Fig. 53–3).

This incision starts from a designated area on the gingiva and is directed to an area at or near the crest of the bone (Fig. 53–4). The starting point on the gingiva is determined by whether the flap will be apically positioned or nonrepositioned (Figs. 53–5 and 53–6). For a nonrepositioned flap, the incision is made at or near an area just coronal to the bottom of the pocket (Fig. 53–6). This incision can be accomplished only if there is sufficient attached gingiva remaining apical to the incision. If the incision is made too close to the tooth, it may result in the recreation of a soft tissue pocket caused by the flap's extending beyond the tooth-bone junction. If the incision is too far from the tooth, it may be difficult to cover the bone properly during flap closure. The proper placement of the flap during closure is essential to prevent either recurrent pockets or bone exposure. This is determined by where this

first incision is placed. The internal bevel incision should be scalloped to preserve the interdental papilla. This will allow for better coverage of the bone at both the radicular and the interdental areas.

If the surgeon contemplates osseous surgery, the first incision should be placed in such a way as to compensate for the removal of bone tissue so that the flap will end at the tooth-bone junction.

If the purpose of the surgery is an apically positioned flap, the internal bevel incision should be made as close to the tooth as possible (0.5 to 1.0 mm) (Fig. 53–7A). There is no need to determine where the bottom of the pocket is in relationship to the incision, as one

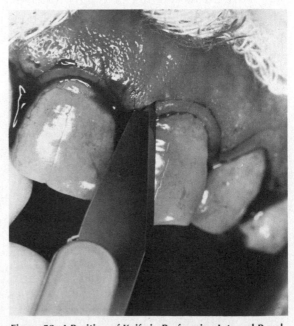

Figure 53–4 Position of Knife in Performing Internal Bevel Incision.

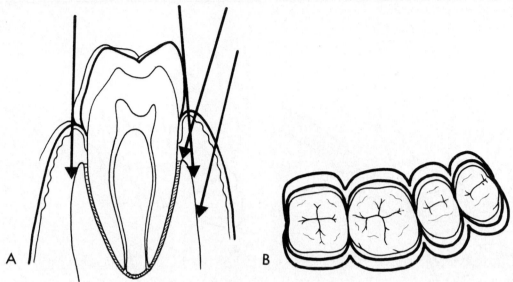

Figure 53–5 *A,* The internal bevel (first) incision can be made at varying locations and angles according to the different anatomic and pocket situations. *B,* An occlusal view of the different locations where the internal bevel incision can be made. Note the scalloped shape of the incisions.

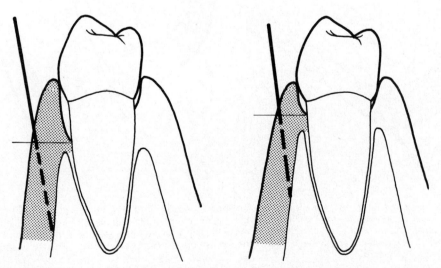

Figure 53–6 The location of the different areas where the internal bevel incision is made in a nonrepositioned flap. The incision is made at the level of the pocket to discard the tissue coronal to it if there is sufficient remaining attached gingiva.

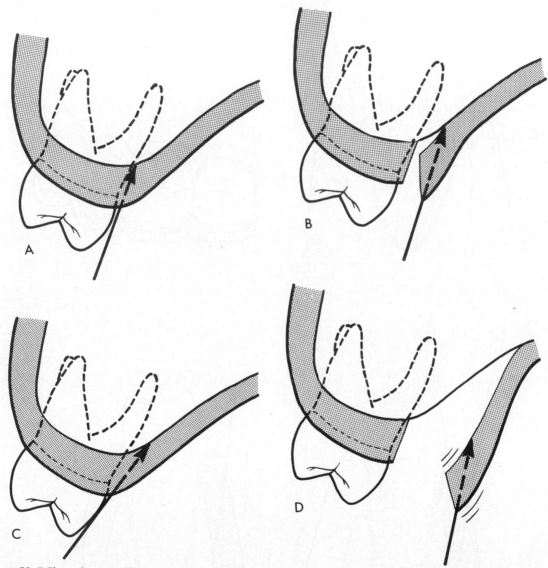

Figure 53-7 These diagrams illustrate the angle of the internal bevel incision in the palate and the different ways to thin the flap. *A,* The usual angle and direction of the incision. *B,* The thinning of the flap after it has been slightly reflected with a second internal incision. *C,* The beveling and thinning of the flap with the initial incision if the position and contour of the tooth allow. *D,* The problem encountered in thinning the flap once it has been reflected. The flap is too loose and free to position and incise properly.

would for the nonpositioned flap, since the purpose of this surgery is to conserve the maximum amount of attached gingiva. The flap will be placed approximately at the tooth-bone junction by apically displacing the flap. Its final position, however, is not determined by the placement of this first incision.

The **crevicular incision,** also termed the "second incision," is made from the base of the pocket to the crest of the bone (Fig. 53–8). This incision, together with the initial reverse bevel incision, will form a V-shaped wedge ending at the crest of bone. The incision is carried around the entire tooth. The beak-shaped No. 12B blade is usually used for this incision.

A periosteal elevator can now be inserted into the initial internal bevel incision and the flap separated from the bone. The most apical end of the internal bevel incision is more exposed and visible. With this access, the surgeon is now able to make the third or **interdental incision** to separate the collar of gingiva which is left around the tooth. The Orban knife is usually utilized for this incision. The incision is made not only around the facial and lingual radicular area but also interdentally, connecting the facial and lingual segments, to completely free the gingiva around the tooth (Fig. 53–9).

These three incisions will now allow the removal of the gingiva around the tooth, i.e,

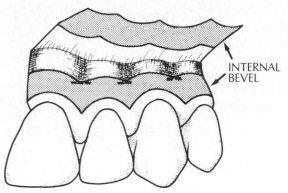

Figure 53–9 After the flap has been elevated, a wedge of tissue remains on the teeth, attached by the base of the papillae. An interdental incision along the horizontal lines seen in the interdental spaces will sever these connections.

the pocket epithelium and the adjacent granulomatous tissue. A curette or a large scaler (U15/30) can be used for this purpose. After removal of the large pieces of tissue, the remaining connective tissue in the osseous lesion should be carefully curetted out so that one can visualize the entire root and the bone surface adjacent to the teeth.

Before the flap is reflected to the final position for scaling and osseous resection, its thickness must be checked. It is best to thin this tissue prior to the complete reflection of the flap, since a free, mobile flap is difficult to hold for thinning (see Fig. 53–7). A sharp, thin papilla positioned properly around the interdental areas at the tooth-bone junction is essential to prevent recurrent soft tissue pockets.

Flaps can be reflected using only the horizontal incision if sufficient access can be obtained by this means and if apical, lateral, or coronal positioning of the flap is not anticipated. If no vertical incisions are made, the flap is called an **envelope flap.**

Vertical or **oblique releasing incisions** can be utilized on either one or both ends of the horizontal incision or on both, depending on the design and purpose of the flap. Vertical incisions at both ends are necessary if the flap is to be repositioned. Vertical incisions must extend beyond the mucogingival line, reaching the alveolar mucosa, to allow for the release of the flap to be repositioned.

As a general rule, vertical incisions in the lingual and palatal areas are avoided. Facial vertical incisions should not be made in the center of an interdental papilla or over the radicular surface of a tooth. Incisions should be made at the line angles of a tooth so as

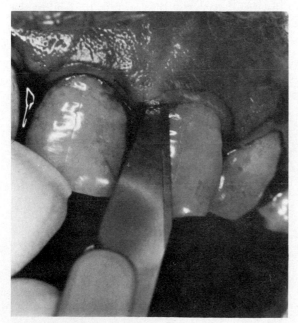

Figure 53–8 Position of Knife in Performing Crevicular Incision.

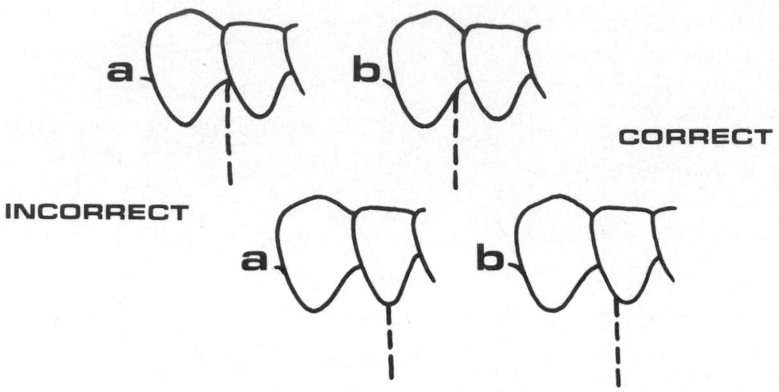

Figure 53–10 The correct and incorrect location of a vertical incision. This incision should be made at the line angles to prevent the splitting of a papilla or incising directly over a radicular surface. *a,* Incorrect incisions. *b,* Correct incisions.

either to include the papilla in the flap or to avoid it completely (Fig. 53–10). The design of the vertical incision should also be such that short (mesial-distal) flaps with long, apically directed horizontal incisions can be avoided, since these could jeopardize the blood supply to the flap.

Several authors[1, 2, 16, 19] have proposed the so-called *interdental denudation procedure,* which consists of horizontal internal bevel non-scalloped incisions to remove the gingival papillae and denude the interdental space. This technique completely eliminates the inflamed interdental areas, which will heal by secondary intention and results in excellent gingival contour. It is contraindicated when bone implants will be used.

DISTAL MOLAR SURGERY

The treatment of periodontal pockets on the distal surface of terminal molars is frequently complicated by the presence of bulbous fibrous tissue over the maxillary tuberosity or prominent retromolar pads in the mandible. Deep vertical defects are also commonly present in conjunction with the redundant fibrous tissue. Some of these osseous lesions may result from incomplete repair after the extraction of impacted third molars (Fig. 53–11).

The gingivectomy incision is the most direct approach in treating distal pockets which have no osseous lesions and adequate attached gingiva. However, the flap approach is less traumatic postsurgically, since it results in a primary closure wound rather than the open secondary wound left by a gingivectomy incision. In addition, it produces attached gingiva and provides access for examination and, if needed, correction of the osseous defect. Operations for this purpose have been described by Robinson[20] and Braden[3] and modified by

several other authors. Some representative procedures are discussed here.

MAXILLARY MOLARS. The treatment of distal pockets on the maxillary arch is usually simpler than the treatment of a similar lesion on the mandibular arch because the tuberosity presents a greater amount of fibrous attached gingiva than does the area of the retromolar pad. Also, the anatomy of the tuberosity extending distally, is more adaptable to pocket elimination than is that of the mandibular molar arch. However, the lack of a broad area of attached gingiva and the abruptly ascending tuberosity sometimes complicates therapy (Fig. 53–12).

The following considerations will determine the location of the incision for distal molar surgery: accessibility, amount of attached gingiva, pocket depth, and available distance from the distal aspect of the tooth to the end of the tuberosity or retromolar pad.

Technique (Fig. 53–13). Two parallel incisions, beginning at the distal portion of the tooth and extending to the mucogingival junction distal to the tuberosity or retromolar pad, are made. The faciolingual distance between these two incisions depends on the depth of the pocket and the amount of fibrous tissue involved. The deeper the pocket, the greater the distance between the two distal incisions. It must be kept in mind that, when the tissue between the two incisions is removed and the flaps are thinned, the two flap edges must approximate each other at a new apical position without overlapping. A transversal incision is made at the distal end of these two incisions so that a long, rectangular piece of tissue can be removed. These incisions are usually interconnected with the incisions for the remainder of the surgery in the quadrant involved. These distal incisions should be confined to the attached gingiva, since bleeding and flap management become problems when

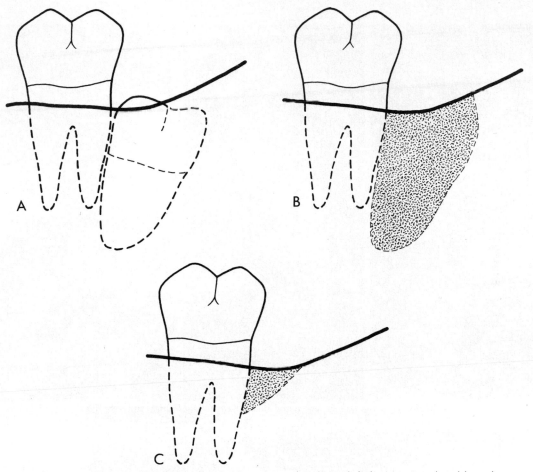

Figure 53–11 *A,* The impaction of a third molar distal to a second molar with little or no interdental bone between the two teeth. *B,* The removal of the third molar creates a pocket with little or no bone distal to the second molar. *C,* This often leads to a vertical osseous defect distal to the second molar.

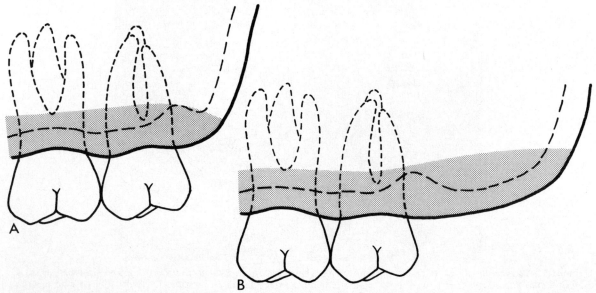

Figure 53–12 *A,* The removal of a pocket distal to the maxillary second molar may be difficult if there is minimal attached gingiva. If the bone ascends acutely apically, the removal of this bone may make the procedure easier. *B,* A long distal tuberosity with abundant attached gingiva is an ideal anatomic situation for distal pocket eradication.

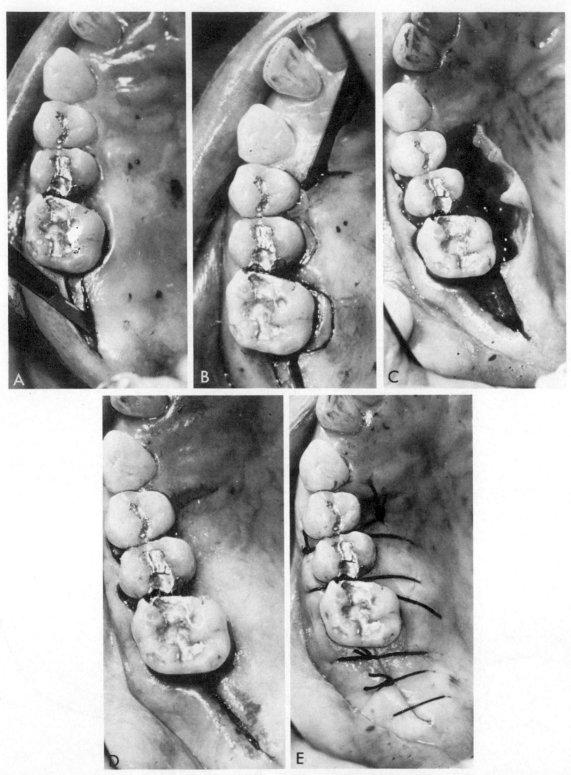

Figure 53–13 *A,* A distal pocket eradication procedure with the incision distal to the molar. *B,* The scalloped incision around the remaining teeth. *C,* The flap reflected and thinned around the distal incision. *D,* The flap in position prior to suturing. It should be closely approximated. *E,* The flap sutured both distally and over the remaining surgical area.

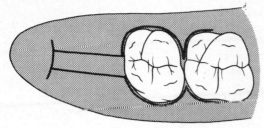

Figure 53–14 A typical incision design for a surgical procedure distal to the maxillary second molar.

the incision is extended into the alveolar mucosa. If access is a problem, especially in cases of short distances from the distal aspect of the tooth to the mucogingival junction, a vertical incision can be made at the end of the mesial-distal incisions.

In treating the tuberosity area, the two distal incisions are usually made at the midline of the tuberosity (Fig. 53–14). In most cases, no attempt is made to undermine the underlying tissue at this point. These incisions are made straight down into the underlying bone, where access is difficult. A No. 12B blade is generally used. It is easier to dissect out the underlying redundant tissue when the flap is partially reflected. When the distal flaps are apposed, the two flap margins should closely approximate each other.

MANDIBULAR MOLARS. Incisions for the mandibular arch differ from those used for the tuberosity owing to differences in the anatomy and histology of the areas. The retromolar pad area does not usually present as much fibrous attached gingiva. The attached gingiva, if present, may not be found directly distal to the molar. The greatest amount may be distolingual or distofacial and may not be over the bony crest. The ascending ramus of the mandible may also create a very short horizontal area distal to the terminal molar (Fig. 53–15). The shorter this area is, the more difficult it is to treat any deep distal lesion around the terminal molar.

The two incisions distal to the molar should follow the area with the greatest amount of attached gingiva (Fig. 53–16). Therefore, the incisions could be directed distolingually or distofacially, depending on which area has more attached gingiva. Before the flap is completely reflected, it is thinned with a No. 15 blade. It is easier to thin the flap before it is completely free and mobile. After the reflection of the flap and the removal of the redundant fibrous tissue, any necessary osseous surgery is performed. The flaps are approximated similarly to those in the maxillary tuberosity area.

Figure 53–15 *A,* Pocket eradication distal to a mandibular second molar with minimal attached gingiva and a close ascending ramus is anatomically difficult. *B,* For surgical procedures distal to a mandibular second molar, abundant attached gingiva and distal space are ideal.

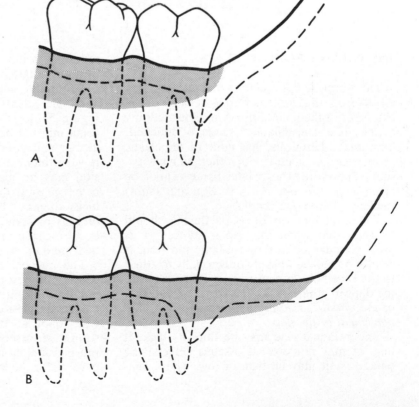

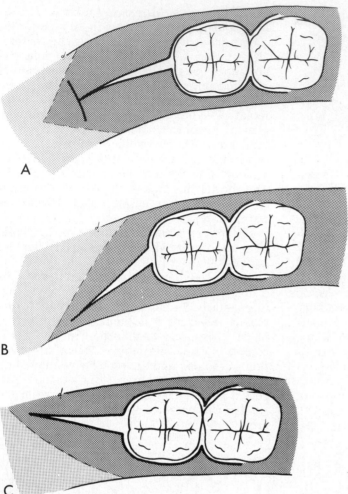

A

B

Figure 53–16 Incision designs for surgical procedures distal to the mandibular second molar. The incision should follow the areas of greatest attached gingiva and underlying bone.

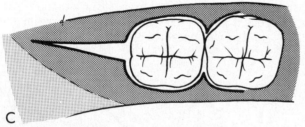

C

THE PALATAL FLAP

The surgical approach to the palatal area differs from that for other areas because of the character of the palatal tissue and the anatomy of the area. The palatal tissue is all attached, keratinized tissue and has none of the elastic properties associated with other gingival tissues. Therefore, the palatal tissue cannot be apically positioned, nor can a partial (split) thickness flap be accomplished.

The initial incision for the palatal flap should be such that when the flap is sutured, it is precisely adapted at the root-bone junction. It cannot be moved apically or coronally to adapt to the root-bone junction, as can be done with the flaps in other areas. Therefore, *the location of the initial incision is important for the final placement of the flap.*

The palatal tissue may be thin or thick; it may or may not present osseous defects; the palatal vault may be high or low. These ana-

tomic variations may require changes in the location, angle, and design of the incision.

The initial incision for a flap varies with the anatomic situation presented. As shown in Figure 53–17, the initial incision may be the usual internal bevel incision, followed by crevicular and interdental incisions. If the tissue is very thick, a horizontal gingivectomy incision may be made, followed by an internal bevel incision that starts at the edge of this incision and ends on the lateral surface of the underlying bone. The placement of the internal bevel incision must be such that the flap will fit around the tooth without exposing the bone.

The purpose of the palatal flap should be considered before the incision is made. If the intent of the surgery is débridement, the internal bevel incision is planned so that the flap will adapt at the root-bone junction when sutured. If osseous resection will be necessary, the incision should be planned so as to compensate for the lowered level of the bone when

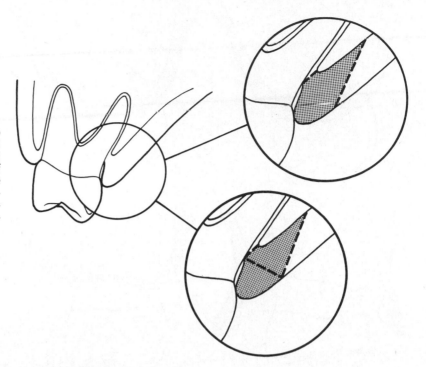

Figure 53–17 Examples of two methods for eliminating a palatal pocket. One incision is an internal bevel incision made at the area of the apical extent of the pocket. The other procedure utilizes a gingivectomy incision, which is followed by an internal bevel incision.

the flap is closed. Probing and sounding of the osseous level and the depth of the infrabony pocket should be used to plan the position of the incision. The apical portion of the scalloping should be narrower than the line angle area since the palatal root tapers apically. A rounded scallop will result in a palatal flap which will not fit snugly around the root. This procedure should be done prior to the complete reflection of the palatal flap, since a loose flap will be difficult to grasp and stabilize for dissection.

It is sometimes necessary to *thin the palatal flap once it has been reflected.* This can be accomplished by holding the inner portion of the flap with a mosquito hemostat or Adson forceps as the inner connective tissue is carefully dissected away with a sharp No. 15 scalpel blade. Care must be taken not to perforate or overthin the flap. The edge of the flap should be thinner than the base; therefore, the blade should be angled toward the lateral surface of the palatal bone. The dissected inner connective tissue is removed with a hemostat. As with any flap, the triangular papilla portion (Fig. 53–18) should be thin enough to fit snugly against the bone and into the interdental area.

The principles for the use of vertical releasing incisions are similar to those for using other incisions. Care must be exercised that the length of the incision is minimal, so as to avoid the numerous vessels located in the palate.

SUTURING TECHNIQUES

There are many types of sutures, suture needles, and materials[7, 13]; the following methods, using a 3/8 circle reverse cutting needle and 3-0 black braided silk, fill most needs in periodontal surgery.

The periodontal flap is closed either with independent sutures or, preferably, with the continuous independent sling sutures. The latter method eliminates the pulling of the buccal and lingual or palatal flaps together and, instead, utilizes the teeth as an anchor for the flaps. There is less tendency for the flaps to buckle, and the forces on the flaps are better distributed.

One may or may not utilize periodontal dressings. Since the flaps are not apically displaced, there is no need to use dressings other than for patient comfort.

INTERDENTAL LIGATION. Two types of interdental ligation can be used; the direct or loop suture and the figure eight suture. They are illustrated in Figures 53–19 and 53–20. In the figure eight suture, there is thread between the two flaps. This suture will therefore be used when the flaps are not in close apposition because of apical positioning or unscalloped incisions. It is simpler to perform than the direct ligation.

The direct suture will permit a better closure of the interdental papilla and should be per-

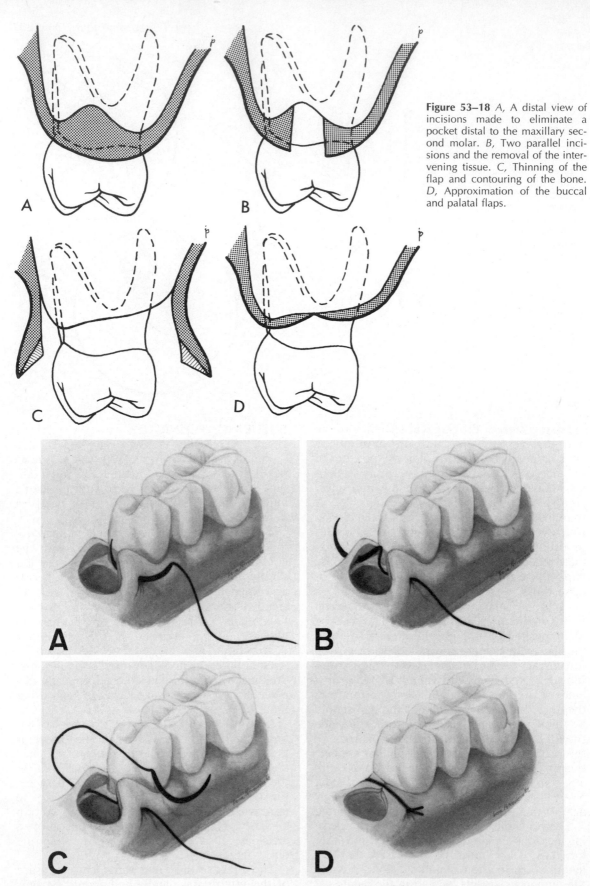

Figure 53–18 *A,* A distal view of incisions made to eliminate a pocket distal to the maxillary second molar. *B,* Two parallel incisions and the removal of the intervening tissue. *C,* Thinning of the flap and contouring of the bone. *D,* Approximation of the buccal and palatal flaps.

Figure 53–19 A simple loop suture is used to approximate the buccal and lingual flaps. *A,* The needle penetrates the outer surface of the first flap. *B,* The undersurface of the opposite flap is engaged, and *C,* the suture is brought back to the initial side, where *D,* the knot is tied.

808

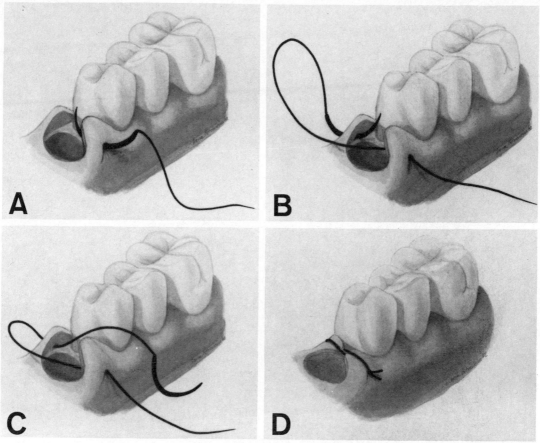

Figure 53–20 An interrupted figure eight suture is used to approximate the buccal and lingual flaps. *A,* The needle penetrates the outer surface of the first flap and *B,* the outer surface of the opposite flap. *C,* The suture is brought back to the first flap, and *D,* the knot is tied.

formed when bone grafts are used or when close apposition of the scalloped incision is required.

SLING LIGATION. The sling ligation can be used for a flap on one surface of a tooth, involving two interdental spaces. It is illustrated in Figure 53–21.

HORIZONTAL MATTRESS SUTURE. This suture is often used for the interproximal areas of diastemata or for wide interdental spaces in order to properly adapt the interproximal papilla against the bone. Two sutures are often necessary. The horizontal mattress suture can be incorporated with continuous independent sling sutures, as shown in Figure 53–22.

The penetration of the needle is done in such a way that the mesial and distal edges of the papilla lie snugly against the bone. The needle enters the outer surface of the gingiva and crosses the undersurface of the gingiva horizontally. The mattress sutures should not be close together at the midpoint of the base of the papilla. The needle reappears on the outer surface at the other base of the papilla and continues around the tooth with the sling sutures.

CONTINUOUS INDEPENDENT SLING SUTURE (Fig. 53–23). This is used when there is both a facial and a lingual flap involving many teeth. The suture is initiated on the facial papilla closest to the midline, since this is the easiest place to position the final knot. A continuous sling suture is laced for each papilla on the facial surface. When the last tooth is reached, the suture is anchored around it to prevent any pulling of the facial sutures when the lingual flap is sutured around the teeth in a similar fashion. The suture is again anchored around the last tooth prior to the final knot. This type of suture does not produce a pull on the lingual flap when the latter is sutured. The two flaps are completely independent of each other owing to the anchoring around both the initial and the final tooth. The flaps are tied to the teeth and not to each other because of the sling sutures.

This type of suturing is especially appropriate for the maxillary arch because the palatal

Text continued on page 817

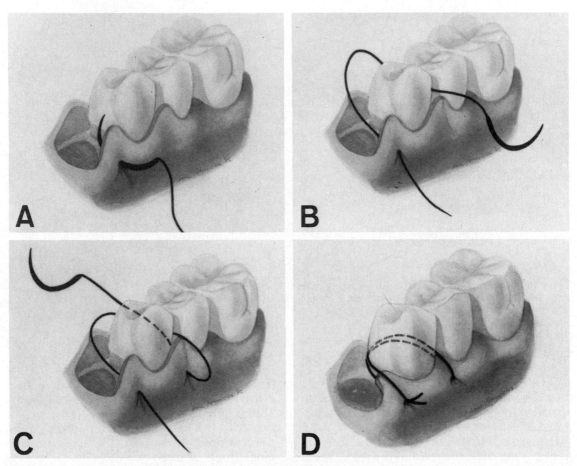

Figure 53–21 A single, interrupted sling suture is used to adapt the flap around the tooth. *A,* The needle engages the outer surface of the flap and *B,* encircles the tooth. *C,* The outer surface of the same flap of the adjacent interdental area is engaged, and *D,* the suture is returned to the initial site and the knot tied.

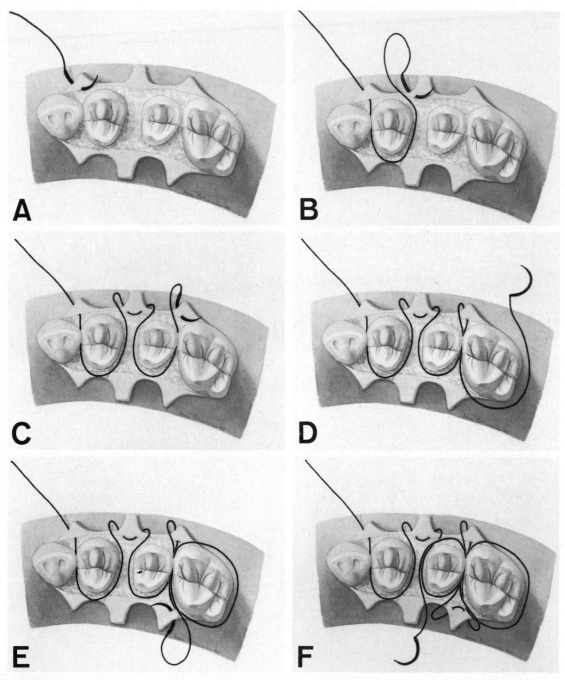

Figure 53–22 A continuous, independent sling suture utilizing a horizontal mattress suture around diastemata or wide interdental areas (*B* and *C*). This mattress suture is utilized on both the buccal (*D*) and the lingual (*E* and *F*) surfaces.

Illustration continued on following page

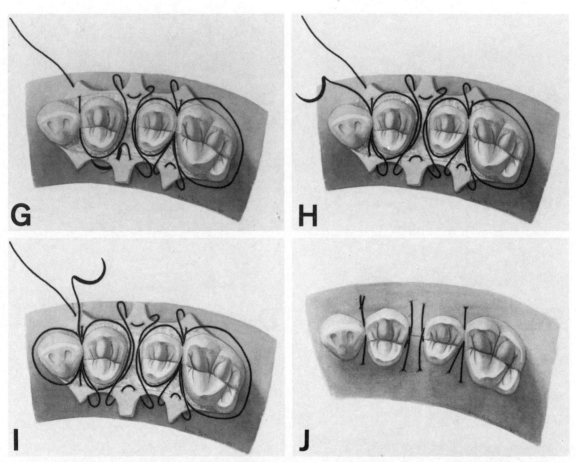

Figure 53–22 *Continued* Continuation of suture on lingual surfaces *(G–I)* and completed suture *(J)*.

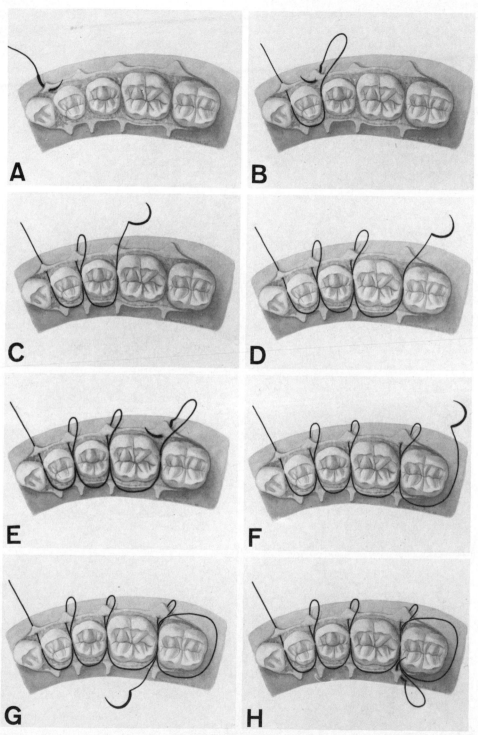

Figure 53–23 The continuous, independent sling suture is utilized to adapt the buccal and lingual flaps without tying the buccal flap to the lingual flap. The teeth are utilized to suspend each flap against the bone. It is important to anchor the suture on the two teeth at the beginning and end of the flap so that the suture will not pull the buccal flap to the lingual flap.

Illustration continued on following page

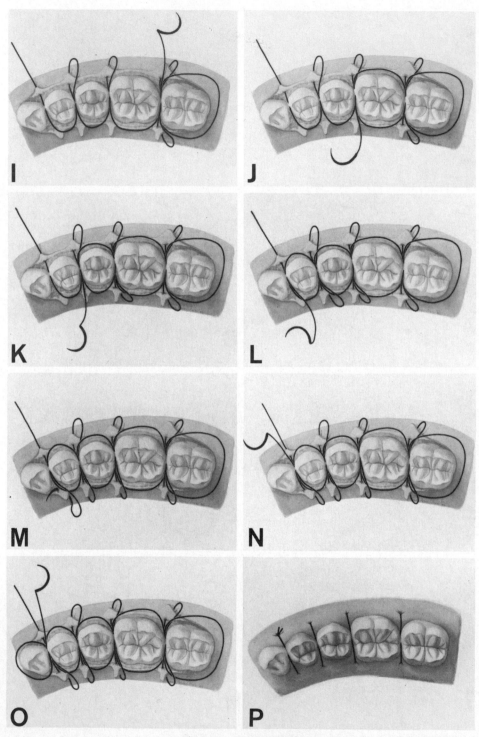

Figure 53–23 *Continued*

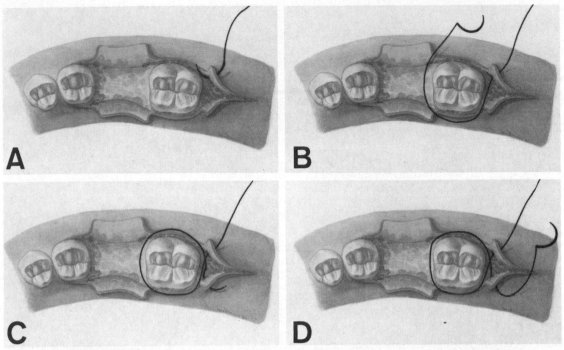

Figure 53–24 The distal anchor suture is utilized to close the flap and to adapt the two closed flaps against the tooth. This suture is used to close flaps which are mesial or distal to a lone-standing tooth.

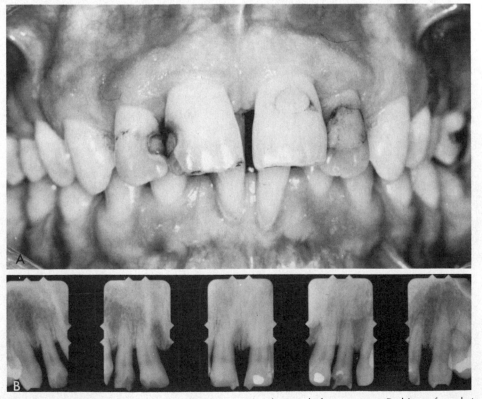

Figure 53–25 The Modified Widman Flap Technique. *A*, Facial view before surgery. Probing of pockets revealed interproximal depths ranging from 4 to 8 mm and facial and palatal depths of 2 to 5 mm. *B*, Radiographic survey of area. Note generalized horizontal bone loss.

Illustration continued on following page

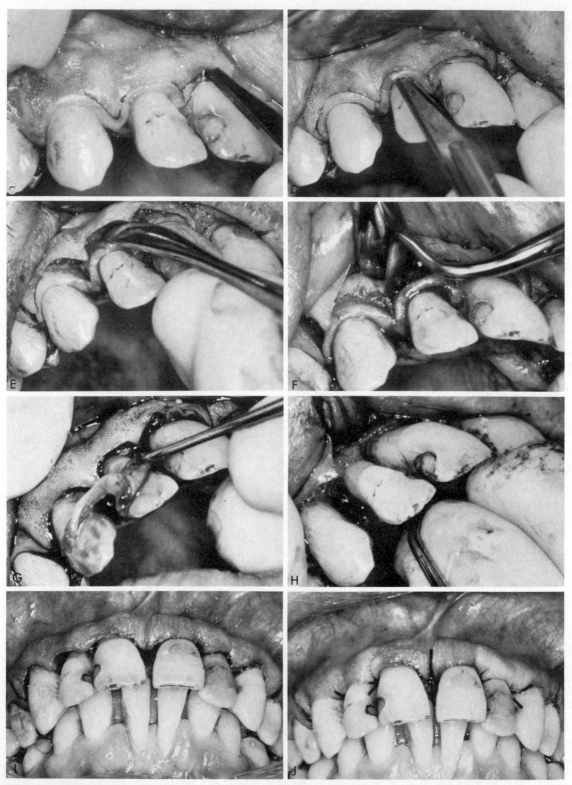

Figure 53–25 *Continued C,* Internal bevel incision. *D,* Crevicular incision. *E,* Elevation of the flap, leaving a wedge of tissue still attached by its base. *F,* Interdental incision sectioning the base of the papilla. *G,* Removal of tissue. *H,* Exposure of root surfaces and marginal bone; root planing and removal of remaining calculus. *I,* Replacement of flap in its original position. *J,* Interdental sutures in place. (Courtesy of Dr. Raul G. Caffesse.)

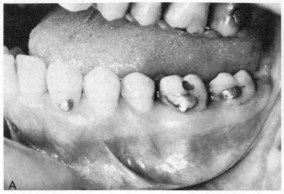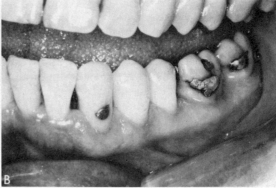

Figure 53–26 A patient before (*A*) and after (*B*) treatment by means of Widman flaps. Note the reduction in gingival height and concomitant pocket depth. (Courtesy of Dr. Raul G. Caffesse.)

gingiva is attached and fibrous, whereas the facial tissue is thinner and mobile.

ANCHOR SUTURE. The closing of a flap mesial or distal to a tooth, as in the mesial or distal wedge procedures, is best accomplished by the anchor suture. This suture closes the facial and lingual flaps and adapts them tightly against the tooth. The needle is placed at the line angle area of the facial or lingual flap adjacent to the tooth, anchored around the tooth, passed beneath the opposite flap, and tied. As indicated in Figure 53–24, the anchor suture can be repeated for each area which requires it.

SURGICAL CURETTAGE (MODIFIED WIDMAN FLAP)

The Widman flap, described early in the modern periodontal literature, has recently been revised with several refinements. Morris in 1965 described it as an "unrepositioned mucoperiosteal flap."[14] He incorporated the internal bevel incision and described the importance of firm apposition of gingival tissue to the root as a prerequisite for success. In 1974, Ramfjord and Nissle described the so-called modified Widman flap,[18] which was investigated in detail in a longitudinal study. The main advantage of this technique over the closed curettage procedure is that it offers the possibility of establishing an intimate postoperative adaptation of healthy collagenous connective tissue and normal epithelium to tooth surfaces.[17] The modified Widman flap provides access for adequate instrumentation of the root surfaces and immediate closure of the area. The following is a step-by-step description of the procedure (Fig. 53–25):

1. The initial incision is a scalloped internal bevel incision to the alveolar crest and 1 to 2 mm away from the gingival margin (Fig. 53–25*C*). Care should be taken to insert the blade in such a way that the papilla is left with a thickness similar to that of the remaining facial flap. Vertical relaxing incisions are usually not needed.

2. The gingiva is reflected with a periosteal elevator (Fig. 53–25*E*).

3. A crevicular incision is made from the bottom of the pocket to the bone, circumscribing the triangular wedge of tissue containing the pocket wall (Fig. 53–25*D*).

4. A third incision is made in the interdental spaces coronal to the bone with a curette or an interproximal knife, and the gingival collar is removed (Fig. 53–25*F* and *G*).

5. Tissue tags and granulation tissue are removed with a curette. The root surfaces are checked and scaled and planed if needed (Fig. 53–25*H*). Residual periodontal fibers attached to the tooth surface should not be disturbed.

6. Bone architecture is not corrected except where it prevents good tissue adaptation to the necks of the teeth. Every effort is made to adapt the facial and lingual interproximal tissue adjacent to each other in such a way that no interproximal bone remains exposed at the time of suturing (Fig. 53–25*I*). The flaps may be thinned to allow for close adaptation of the gingiva around the entire circumference of the tooth and to each other interproximally.

7. Interrupted direct sutures are placed in each interdental space (Fig. 53–25*J*) and covered with tetracycline (Achromycin) ointment and with a periodontal surgical pack.

Ramfjord and co-workers have performed a longitudinal study comparing the Widman procedure, as modified by them, with the curettage technique and the pocket elimination methods that include bone contouring when needed.[17] The techniques were selected at random, and results were analyzed yearly up to 7 years posttherapy. They reported approximately similar results with the three methods tested. Pocket depth was initially similar for all methods but was maintained shallower with the Widman flap (Fig. 53–26); the attachment level remained higher with the Widman flap.

REFERENCES

1. Barkann, L.: A conservative surgical technique for the eradication of pyorrhea pockets. J. Am. Dent. Assoc., *26*:61, 1939.
2. Beube, F. E.: Interdental tissue resection: an experimental study of a surgical technique which aids in repair of the periodontal tissues to their original contour and function. Oral Surg., *33*:497, 1947.
3. Braden, B. E.: Deep distal pockets adjacent to terminal teeth. Dent. Clin. North Am., *13*:161, 1969.
4. Carranza, F. A., Sr.: Tratamiento Quirurgico de la Paradentosis (Piorrea Alveolar). Thesis. University of Buenos Aires, 1935.
5. Carranza, F. A., Jr., and Carraro, J. J.: Effect of removal of periosteum on postoperative result of mucogingival surgery. J. Periodontol., *34*:223, 1963.
6. Cieszynski, A.: Bemerkungen zur radikal-chirurgischen Behandlung der sogennante Pyorrhea Alveolaris. Dtsch. Monatschr. Zahnh., *32*:376, 1914.
7. Dahlberg, W. H.: Incisions and suturing: some basic considerations about each in periodontal flap surgery. Dent. Clin. North Am., *13*:149, 1969.
8. Friedman, N.: Mucogingival surgery: the apically repositioned flap. J. Periodontol., *33*:328, 1962.
9. Hoag, P. M., Wood, D. L., Donnenfeld, O. W., and Rosenfeld, L. D.: Alveolar crest reduction following full and partial thickness flaps. J. Periodontol., *43*:141, 1972.
10. Kirkland, O.: The suppurative periodontal pus pocket: its treatment by the modified flap operation. J. Am. Dent. Assoc., *18*:1462, 1931.
11. Levine, H. L., and Stahl, S. S.: Repair following periodontal flap surgery with the retention of gingival fibers. J. Periodontol., *43*:99, 1972.
12. Matelski, D. E., and Hurt, W. C.: The corrective phase: the modified Widman flap. *In* W. C. Hurt (ed.): Periodontics in General Practice. Springfield, Ill., Charles C Thomas, 1976.
13. Morris, M. L.: Suturing techniques in periodontal surgery. Periodontics, *3*:84, 1965.
14. Morris, M. L.: The unrepositioned mucoperiosteal flap. Periodontics, *3*:141, 1965.
15. Neumann, R.: Die Alveolar-Pyorrhea und ihre Behandlung. Berlin, H. Meusser, 1912.
16. Prichard, J. F.: Present state of the interdental denudation procedure. J. Periodontol., *48*:566, 1977.
17. Ramfjord, S. P.: Present status of the modified Widman flap procedure. J. Periodontol., *48*:558, 1977.
18. Ramfjord, S. P., and Nissle, R. R.: The modified Widman flap. J. Periodontol., *45*:601, 1974.
19. Ratcliff, P. A., and Raust, G. T.: Interproximal denudation: a conservative approach to osseous surgery. Dent. Clin. North Am., *8*:121, 1964.
20. Robinson, R. E.: The distal wedge operation. Periodontics, *4*:256, 1966.
21. Widman, L.: The operative treatment of pyorrhea alveolaris. A new surgical method. Sven. Tandlak. Tidskm. (Special Issue), Dec. 1918.
22. Zentler, A.: Suppurative gingivitis with alveolar involvement. J.A.M.A., *71*:1530, 1918.

Osseous Surgery

The damage resulting from periodontal disease reveals itself in variable destruction of the tooth-supporting bone. Generally, bony deformities are not uniform. They are not indicative of the alveolar housing of the tooth prior to the disease process, nor do they reflect the overlying gingival architecture. Bone loss has been classified as horizontal or vertical. In fact, however, bone loss is most often a combination of horizontal and vertical loss. Horizontal bone loss generally results in a relative thickening of the marginal alveolar bone, since bone tapers as it approaches its most coronal margin.

The effect of this thickening and the development of vertical defects leaves the alveolar bone with countless combinations of bony shapes. If these various topographic changes are to be altered to provide a more physiologic bone pattern, a method for osseous recontouring must be followed.

Osseous surgery may be defined as the procedure by which changes in the alveolar bone can be accomplished to rid it of deformities induced by the periodontal disease process or other related factors, such as exostosis and tooth supraeruption.

Osseous surgery can be either additive or subtractive in nature. **Additive osseous surgery** includes the procedures directed at restoring the alveolar bone to its original level, whereas subtractive methods are designed to restore the form of pre-existing alveolar bone to the level existing at the time of surgery or slightly more apical to it.

Additive osseous surgery brings about the ideal result of periodontal therapy; it implies the re-establishment of the periodontal ligament, gingival fibers, and junctional epithelium at a more coronal level (see Chapter 35). The terms "new attachment" and "reattachment" are used to refer to this concept, the former being preferable. This type of osseous surgery is theoretically possible through grafting, which will be discussed in this chapter,

and through "nongrafting" procedures, which have been discussed in Chapters 35, 51, and 53.

Subtractive osseous surgical procedures provide a surgical alternative to the additive methods and should be resorted to when the latter are not feasible. They will be discussed in this chapter.

SELECTION OF TREATMENT TECHNIQUE

The morphology of the osseous defect will to a great extent determine the treatment technique to be used. One-wall angular defects usually have to be recontoured surgically. Three-wall defects, particularly if they are narrow and deep, can be successfully treated by techniques that aim at reattachment and bone regeneration. Two-wall angular defects can be treated by either method, depending on their depth, width, and general configuration.

Therefore, except for one-wall defects and wide and shallow two-wall defects and craters, pockets are treated with the objective of obtaining optimal repair by natural healing processes.

OSSEOUS RESECTIVE SURGERY

Osseous resective surgery is the most predictable pocket reduction technique. However, to a greater degree than any other surgical technique, osseous resective surgery is performed at the expense of bony tissue and attachment level.[57, 105, 115] This means that its value as a surgical approach is limited by the presence, quantity, and shape of the bony tissues and by the amount of subsequent attachment loss that is acceptable. *The major rationale for osseous resective surgery is centered on the tenet that discrepancies in levels and shapes of the bone and gingiva predispose to the recurrence of pocket depth postsurgi-*

cally.[75] Although this concept is not universally accepted,[42, 64, 116] and despite the fact that the procedure induces loss of radicular bone in the healing phases, *there are cases in which recontouring of bone is the only logical treatment choice.* The goal of osseous resective therapy is reshaping the marginal bone to resemble the alveolar process undamaged by periodontal disease. The technique is accomplished in combination with apically repositioned flaps, and it eliminates periodontal pocket depth and improves tissue contour to provide a more easily maintainable environment. The relative merits of pocket reduction procedures have been discussed in Chapters 35 and 49; here we will provide a discussion of the osseous resective technique and of how and where it may be accomplished.

TERMINOLOGY. Numerous terms have been developed to describe the topography of the alveolar housing, the procedures for its removal, and the resulting correction. These terms should be clearly defined.

Procedures used to correct osseous defects have been classified in two groups: osteoplasty and ostectomy.[38] **Osteoplasty** refers to reshaping the bone without removing tooth-supporting bone. **Ostectomy** (or osteoectomy) includes the removal of tooth-supporting bone. Either or both of these procedures may be necessary to produce the desired result.

Terms that describe the bone form after reshaping can refer to morphologic features or to the thoroughness of the reshaping performed. Examples of morphologically descriptive terms include "negative," "positive," "flat," and "ideal." These terms all relate to a preconceived standard of **ideal osseous form.** Osseous form is considered to be ideal when the bone is consistently more coronal on the interproximal surfaces than on the facial and lingual surfaces. The ideal form of the marginal bone has similar interdental height, with gradual, curved slopes between interdental peaks (Fig. 54–1). The terms "positive architecture" and "negative architecture" refer to the relative position of interdental bone to radicular bone. The architecture is said to be **positive** if the radicular bone is apical to the interdental bone. The bone is said to have **negative architecture** if the interdental bone is more apical than the radicular bone. **Flat architecture** is the reduction of the interdental bone to the same height as the radicular bone. Terms that relate to the thoroughness of the osseous reshaping techniques are "definitive" and "compromise." **Definitive osseous reshaping** implies that further osseous reshaping would not improve the overall result. **Compromise osseous reshaping** indicates a bone pattern that cannot be improved without significant osseous removal that would be detrimental to the overall result. "Compromise" and "definitive" osseous architecture, then, are terms that can be useful to the clinician not as descriptions of morphologic features, but as terms that express expectations of the therapeutic result.

Methods of Osseous Resective Surgery

Osseous resective surgery is an extremely precise, demanding technique. *The reshaping process is fundamentally an attempt to gradualize the bone sufficiently to allow soft tissue structure to follow the contour of the bone.* The soft tissue will predictably attach to the bone within certain specific dimensions. For exam-

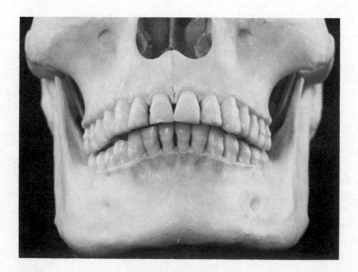

Figure 54–1 Skull Photograph of a Healthy Periodontium. Note the shape of the alveolar bone housing. This bone is considered to have ideal form. It is more coronal in the interproximal areas, with a gradual slope around and away from the tooth.

ple, in the repair of any angular defect there will always be connective tissue as well as junctional epithelium. The length and quality of both are dependent upon numerous factors, including the health of the tissue, the condition of the root surface, and the topography, as well as the proximity of the bone surrounding the tooth. If each of these factors is to be controlled to the best of our ability so as to obtain the optimum result, we must approach osseous surgery in a very precise way.

It will be assumed in this chapter that the gingival tissue has been reflected by the apically repositioned flap, described in Chapter 53. Reshaping of the bone may necessitate selective changes in gingival height. These changes must be calculated and accounted for in the initial flap design. For this reason it is important that the clinician have a presurgical knowledge of the underlying bone tissue prior to flap reflection. One must gain as much indirect knowledge as possible from soft tissue palpation, radiographic assessment, and transgingival probing (called "sounding").

Radiographic examination can reveal the existence of angular bone losses in the interdental spaces; these usually coincide with infrabony pockets. The radiograph will not show the number of bony walls of the defect, nor will it determine with any accuracy the presence of angular bone defects on facial or lingual surfaces. Clinical examination and probing will determine the presence and depth of periodontal pockets on any surface of any tooth and can also give a general sense of the bony topography, but infrabony pockets can go undetected by probing. Both clinical and radiographic examinations can indicate the presence of infrabony pockets when the following are found: (1) angular bone losses, (2) irregular bone losses, and (3) pockets of irregular depth in adjacent areas of the same tooth or adjacent teeth.

The experienced clinician can use **transgingival probing** to predict many features of the underlying bony topography. The information so obtained can change the treatment plan. For example, an area that had been selected for osseous resective surgery may be found to have a narrow defect that was unnoticed in the initial probing and radiographic assessment and is ideal for augmentation procedures. Such findings can and do change the flap design, the osseous procedure, and the result expected from the surgical intervention.

Transgingival probing is extremely useful just prior to flap reflection. It is necessary to anesthetize the tissue locally prior to inserting the probe. The probe should be "walked" along the tissue-tooth interface so the operator can feel the bony topography. The probe may also be passed horizontally through the tissue to provide more information in three dimensions regarding bony contours. This technique can provide information about the thickness, height, and shape of the underlying base. It must be remembered that this information is still "blind," and, though it is undoubtedly better than probing alone, it has significant limitations. Nevertheless, this step is recommended immediately prior to the surgical intervention.

The situations that one can encounter after periodontal flap reflection vary greatly. When all soft tissue is removed around the teeth, there may be large exostoses, ledges, troughs, craters, vertical defects, or combinations of any of these. For this reason, each osseous situation presents uniquely challenging problems, especially if reshaping to the optimum level is contemplated.

In order to handle the multitude of clinical situations, the following sequential steps are suggested (Fig. 54–2 *A* to *D*): (1) vertical grooving, (2) radicular blending, (3) flattening interproximal bone, and (4) gradualizing marginal bone.

Not all steps are necessary in every case, but the sequencing of the steps in the order given is necessary to expedite the reshaping procedure, as well as to minimize the removal of bone.

VERTICAL GROOVING. Vertical grooving is designed to reduce the thickness of the alveolar housing and to provide relative prominence to the radicular aspects of the teeth (Fig. 54–2*B*; see also Fig. 54–13*B*). It also provides continuity from the interproximal surface onto the radicular surface. It is the first step of the resective process because it can define the general thickness and subsequent form of the alveolar housing. This step is usually performed with rotary instruments such as round carbide burs or diamonds. The advantages of vertical grooving are most apparent with thick bony margins, shallow crater formations, or other areas that require maximum osteoplasty and minimum ostectomy. Vertical grooving is contraindicated in areas with close root proximity or thin alveolar housing.

RADICULAR BLENDING. Radicular blending, the second step of the osseous reshaping technique, is an extension of vertical grooving (Fig. 54–2*C*). Conceptually, it is an attempt to

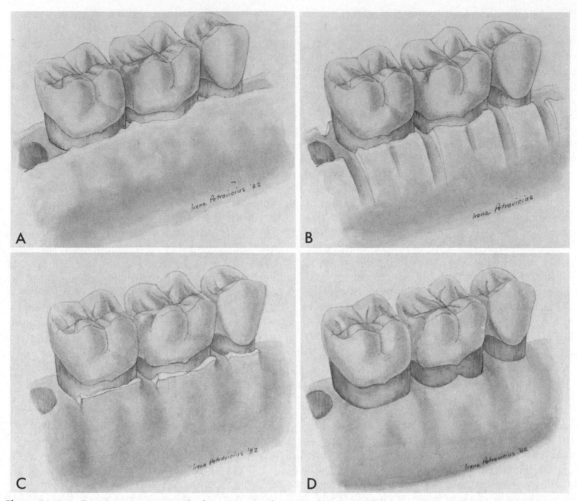

Figure 54–2 *A,* Drawing representing the bony topography in moderate periodontitis, with interdental craters. *B,* Vertical grooving, the first step in correction by osseous reshaping. *C,* Radicular blending and flattening of interproximal bone. *D,* Gradualizing the marginal bone. Note the area of the furcation on the first molar where the bone is preserved.

gradualize the bone over the entire radicular surface to provide the best results from vertical grooving. This provides a smooth, blended surface for good flap adaptation. The indications are the same as for vertical grooving, i.e., thick ledges of bone on the radicular surface where selective surgical resection is desired. Naturally this step is not necessary if vertical grooving is very minor or if the radicular bone is thin or fenestrated. Both vertical grooving and radicular blending are purely osteoplastic techniques that do not remove supporting bone. In most situations they comprise the bulk of osseous resective surgery. Classically, shallow crater formations, thick osseous ledges of bone on the radicular surface, and Class I and early Class II furcation involvements are treated almost totally with these two steps.

FLATTENING INTERPROXIMAL BONE. Flattening of the interdental bone requires the removal of very small amounts of supporting bone (Fig. 54–3). It is indicated when interproximal bone levels vary horizontally. By definition, most of the indications for this step will be one-wall interproximal defects or so-called hemiseptal defects. The omission of flattening in such cases results in increased pocket depth on the most apical side of the bone loss. This step is typically not necessary in classic crater formations or in flat interproximal defects. It is best utilized in defects that have a coronally placed one-wall edge over a three-wall angular defect, and it can be helpful in obtaining good closure and, subsequently, an improved healing process in the three-wall defect. The limitation of this step, as with osseous resective surgical therapy in general, is with the advanced lesion. Large hemiseptal defects would require removal of inordinate amounts of bone to provide a flattened architecture; the operation is too costly in terms of

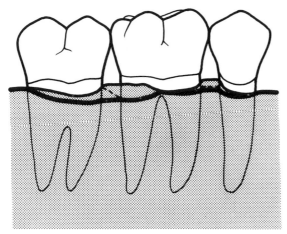

Figure 54–3 Diagrammatic Representation of Bone Irregularities in Periodontal Disease. The thick line is the proposed correction of the defect. Note the flattening of the interproximal bone between the molars and the protection of the furcal bone on the first molar. Facial crest height is reduced in both interproximal areas to the depth of the defect.

bony support. Compromise osseous architecture is the only logical solution.

GRADUALIZING MARGINAL BONE. This final step in the osseous resective technique is also a process of ostectomy. Bone removal is minimal but necessary to provide a sound, regular base for the gingival tissue to follow. The failure to remove small bony discrepancies on the gingival line angles (often called "widow's peaks") allows the tissue to rise to a higher level than the base of the bone loss in the interdental area (see Fig. 54–2C and D). This may make the process of selective recession and subsequent pocket reduction incomplete. This step of the procedure also requires gradualization and blending of the radicular surfaces (Fig. 54–3; see also Fig. 54–13C). The two ostectomy steps should be done with great care so as not to produce niches or grooves on the roots. When the radicular bone is thin, it is extremely easy to overdo this step, to the detriment of the entire surgical effort. For this reason various hand instruments, such as chisels and curettes, are preferable to rotary instruments for gradualizing marginal bone.

Instrumentation for Osseous Resection

A number of hand and rotary instruments have been used for osseous resective surgery. Some excellent clinicians use only hand instruments and rongeurs, whereas others prefer a combination of hand and rotary instruments. Rotary instruments are useful for the osteoplastic steps outlined above, whereas hand instruments provide the most precise and safe results with ostectomy procedures. Neverthe-

less, care and precision are required each step of the way to prevent excessive bone removal or root damage, both of which are irreversible. Figure 54–4A to F illustrates some of the instruments commonly used for osseous resective techniques.

Specific Osseous Reshaping Situations

The osseous corrective procedure that has been described is classically applied to shallow craters with heavy faciolingual ledges (Fig. 54–5). The correction of other osseous defects is also possible; however, careful case selection for definitive osseous surgery is very important.

The correction of one-wall hemiseptal defects requires that the bone be reduced to the level of the most apical portion of the defect. Therefore, great care should be taken to select defects that will not require unmanageable ostectomy on the well-supported tooth (Fig. 54–6). If one-wall defects occur next to an edentulous space, the edentulous ridge is reduced to the level of the osseous defect (Fig. 54–7). Artificial remodeling of bone is not required when one-wall vertical defects are "back to back" on the same interdental septum, since treatment of the pockets without alteration of the bone is generally followed by resorption of the intervening bony septum, which eliminates both one-wall defects (Fig. 54–8).

Other situations that complicate osseous correction are exostoses (Fig. 54–9; Plate IX, D and E), malpositioned teeth, and supraerupted teeth. Each of these situations is best controlled by following the four steps previously outlined. In most situations the unique features of the bony profile will be well managed by prudently applying the same principles (Fig. 54–10; Plate IX).

There are, however, situations that require deviation from the definitive osseous reshaping technique. Examples include dilacerated roots, root proximity, and furcations that would be compromised by osseous surgery.

Summary

There is considerable difference of opinion regarding the wisdom of artificially remodeling bone in the treatment of periodontal disease. The biologic expense of selective recession and attachment loss must be constantly weighed against the benefits of pocket reduction when a patient is considered for osseous resective surgery.

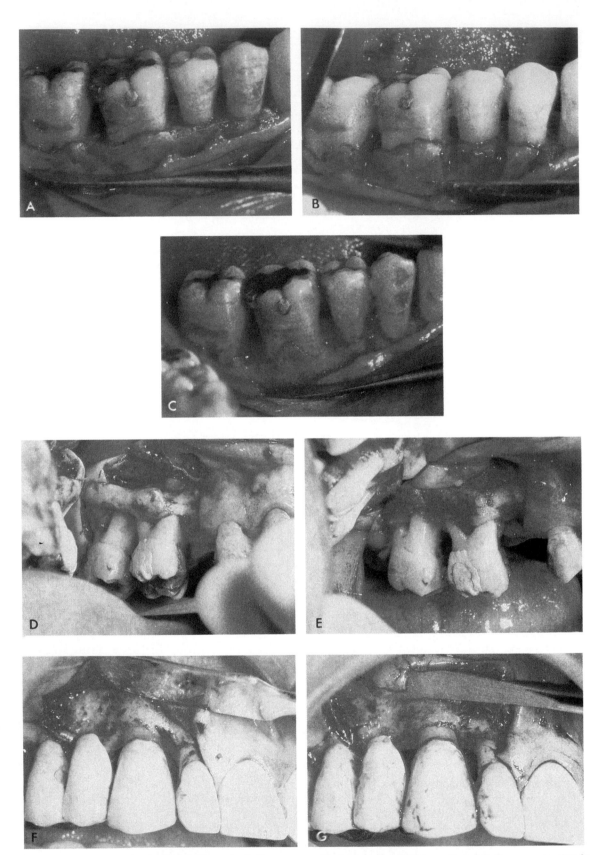

Plate IX Bone Contouring in Flap Surgery *A–C,* Bone contouring in interdental craters. *D* and *E,* Bone contouring in exostoses. *F* and *G,* Bone contouring in one-wall vertical defect.

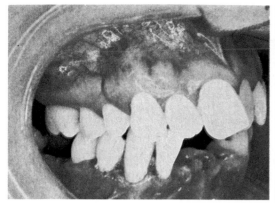

A, Before treatment.

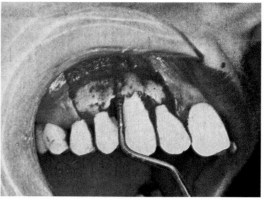

B, Deep three-wall infrabony defect with measuring probe inserted.

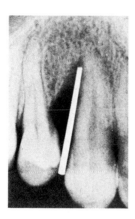

C, Radiograph before treatment indicates angular osseous defect. Gutta percha point extends to base of pocket.

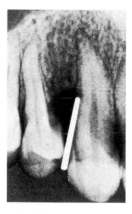

D, Nine months after treatment. Radiograph indicates repair of osseous defect. Gutta percha point shows new level of sulcus.

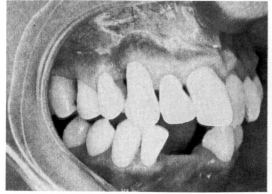

E, Nine months after treatment. Gingiva healed with physiologic contour.

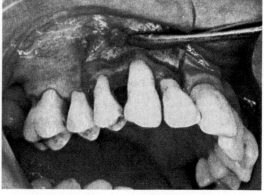

F, Elevation of flap confirms radiographic appearance of repaired bone defect and reattachment of periodontium to tooth.

Plate X Flap Operation for Infrabony Pocket.

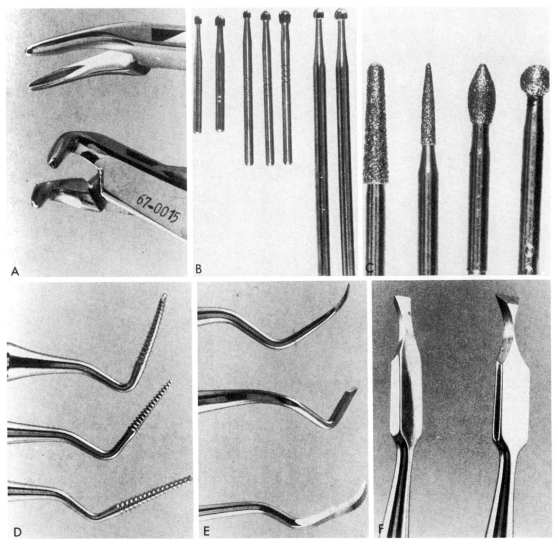

Figure 54—4 Instruments Often Used in Osseous Surgery. *A,* Rongeurs: Friedman and 90° Blumenthal. *B,* Carbide round burs: friction grip, surgical length friction grip, slow-speed handpiece. *C,* Diamond burs. *D,* Interproximal files: Schluger and Sugerman. *E,* Back-action chisels.· *F,* Ochsenbein chisels.

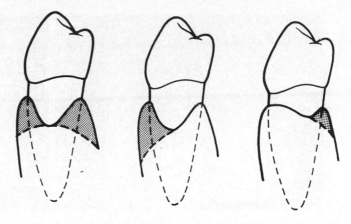

Figure 54–5 Interproximal Craters. The shaded areas illustrate different techniques for the management of such defects. The technique that reduces the least amount of supporting bone is preferable.

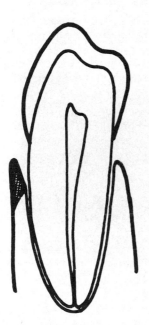

Figure 54–6 A one-wall defect located on the facial surface is reduced by osteoplasty. A one-wall defect located on an interproximal surface requires ostectomy for reduction.

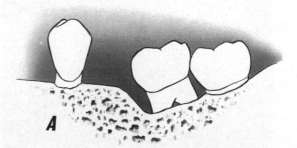

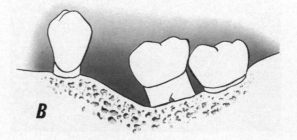

Figure 54–7 Reduction of One-Wall Infrabony Angular Defect. *A*, Angular bone defect mesial to the tilted molar. *B*, Defect reduced by "ramping" angular bone.

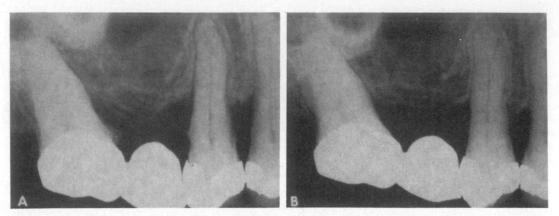

Figure 54–8 Angular Bone Defects Repaired by Healing Without Osseous Surgery. *A,* Angular bone defects under bridge. *B,* Three years after pocket elimination and occlusal adjustment. (Courtesy of Dr. Carl Stoner.)

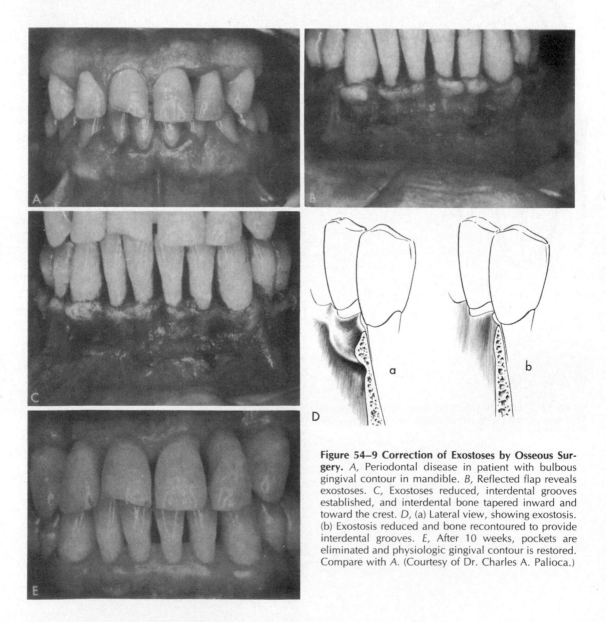

Figure 54–9 Correction of Exostoses by Osseous Surgery. *A,* Periodontal disease in patient with bulbous gingival contour in mandible. *B,* Reflected flap reveals exostoses. *C,* Exostoses reduced, interdental grooves established, and interdental bone tapered inward and toward the crest. *D,* (a) Lateral view, showing exostosis. (b) Exostosis reduced and bone recontoured to provide interdental grooves. *E,* After 10 weeks, pockets are eliminated and physiologic gingival contour is restored. Compare with *A.* (Courtesy of Dr. Charles A. Palioca.)

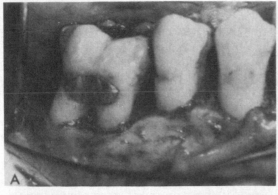

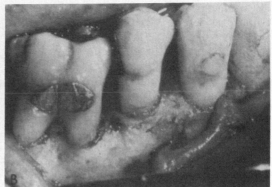

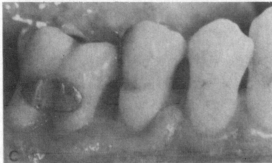

Figure 54–10 *A,* Photograph taken before osseous surgery. *B,* After osseous management. *C,* Results 3 weeks after surgery.

As with all therapeutic procedures used in clinical periodontics, precision of technique and consistent application allow the osseous resection technique to result in its full benefit.

OSSEOUS REGENERATIVE SURGERY

The other major area of osseous surgery is osseous regeneration. This technique is admittedly less predictable than osseous resection, but the rewards include not only the elimination of the periodontal pocket but also the restoration of the periodontal apparatus by filling in the osseous defect and restoring smooth physiologic bone contours (Plate X). Nature reduces the facial and lingual walls of interdental craters while filling in the depressed craters with new bone. The likelihood of obtaining this "bone fill" depends in large measure on the architecture of and the number of bony walls in the defect (see Chapter 16).

The earliest reattachment attempts were carried out using subgingival curettage[93, 113] (see Chapter 51). The shallower pocket obtained following curettage may be due in part to reestablishment of a connective tissue attachment in the bottom of the pocket and in part to shrinkage of the inflamed tissue.[5] Radiographic evidence of bone regeneration has been shown after subgingival curettage.[15, 16, 36, 71, 80, 96]

Reconstructive periodontics can be subdivided into two major areas: *non–graft-associated new attachment and graft-associated new attachment.*

Graft Materials and Procedures

Traditionally, periodontal reconstruction using nongraft material is best accomplished in the three-wall pocket[44] and the periodontal and endodontal abscess.[48, 71] However, the defects left by most periodontal diseases are not of three-wall configuration. Therefore, numerous other therapeutic grafting modalities for restoring these defects have been investigated and attempted. Several authors have advocated that in new attachment attempts employing a flap procedure, bone grafts should be inserted into the angular defects in order to improve bone regeneration and achieve a greater amount of new connective tissue attachment.[18, 50, 69, 70, 86, 87, 99]

Periodontal defects as sites for bone transplantation differ from osseous cavities surrounded by bony walls. Saliva and bacteria may easily penetrate along the root surface, and epithelial cells may proliferate into the defect, resulting in contamination and possible exfoliation of the grafts. Therefore, the principles established to govern transplantation of bone into closed osseous cavities may not be fully applicable to transplantation of bone into periodontal defects.[26]

The considerations that govern the selection of a material have been defined by Schallhorn[96]:

1. Biologic acceptability.
2. Predictability.
3. Clinical feasibility.
4. Minimal operative hazards.
5. Minimal postoperative sequelae.
6. Patient acceptance.

Naturally, it is difficult to find a material with all these characteristics, and to date there is no "ideal" material or technique.

Once the material is placed in the bony defect, it may act in a number of ways. It may have no effect; it may act only as a scaffolding material for the host to lay down new bone; it may actively induce bone formation; or through its own viability it may deposit new bone in the defect.

Graft materials have been developed and tried in many complex forms. To familiarize the reader with various types of graft material, as defined by either the technique or the material used, a brief discussion of each is provided.

Autogenous Bone Grafts

BONE FROM INTRAORAL SITE. In 1923 Hegedus attempted to use bone grafts for the reconstruction of bone defects produced by periodontal disease.[47] The method was revived by Nabers and O'Leary[69] in 1965, and numerous efforts have been made in the last two decades to define its indications and technique.

Sources of bone include that from healing extraction wounds,[86] edentulous ridges,[51] bone trephined from within the jaw without damaging the roots, newly formed bone in wounds especially created for the purpose,[46] and bone removed during osteoplasty and ostectomy.

All the bone grafting techniques require presurgical scaling, occlusal adjustment as needed, and exposure of the defect with a full thickness flap. Incisions must be planned so as to cover the bony area completely after suturing. The use of antibiotics for a few days after the procedure is generally recommended.

Osseous Coagulum. Robinson described a technique using a mixture of bone dust and blood that he termed *osseous coagulum.*[85] The technique uses small particles ground from cortical bone. The advantage of the particle size is that it provides additional surface area for the interaction of cellular and vascular elements.

Sources of the implant material include the lingual ridge on the mandible, exostoses, edentulous ridges, the bone distal to a terminal tooth, bone removed by osteoplasty or ostectomy, and the lingual surface of the mandible or maxilla at least 5 mm from the roots. Bone is removed with a carbide bur, No. 6 or No. 8, at speeds between 5000 and 30,000 rpm. The coagulum formed by mixing the bone particles and blood is placed in a sterile dappen dish or amalgam cloth.

The coagulum is placed in the defect a little at a time, starting at the bottom and packing and drying with moist gauze until there is a considerable excess. The flap is replaced over the coagulum and sutured (Fig. 54–11).

The obvious advantage of this technique is the ease of obtaining bone from already exposed surgical sites. This technique is also very quick to accomplish and can be done in areas without great preparation. In addition, it complements osseous resective techniques needed in the area (Plate IX).

The disadvantages of the technique are centered on its relatively low predictability[36] and on the inability to procure adequate material for large defects. The major criticism of this technique has been its nearly total reliance on cortical bone for graft material. Although notable success has been reported by many individuals, studies documenting the technique's efficacy are still inconclusive.[19, 36, 39, 84]

Bone Blend. Some of the disadvantages of osseous coagulum derive from the inability to use aspiration during accumulation of the coagulum; another problem is the unknown quantity and quality of the bone fragments in the collected material. To overcome these problems, Diem, Bowers, and Moffitt[21] have proposed the so-called bone blend technique.

The bone blend technique uses an autoclaved plastic capsule and pestle (Fig. 54–12). Bone is removed from a predetermined site (extraction socket, exostosis, edentulous area, or region of the defect) by chisels or rongeur forceps. The pestle and bone fragments are placed in the capsule, and a few drops of sterile saline are added. The capsule is closed, wrapped in sterile gauze, and placed in the triturator. The bone is triturated for 60 seconds. A dense mass of bone, such as that removed from an exostosis, may require more blending time. After trituration the bone blend is observed clinging to the walls of the capsule and to the pestle. It is removed from the capsule with a spoon-shaped instrument. Trituration reduces the bone fragments to a workable, plastic-like osseous mass, similar to

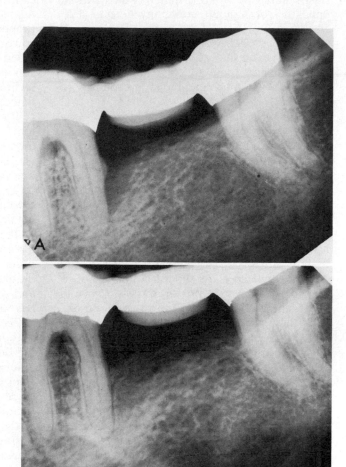

Figure 54–11 Bone Defect on Distal Root of First Molar Treated with Osseous Coagulum Implants. *A,* Before treatment. *B,* One year after treatment. (Courtesy of Dr. R. Earl Robinson.)

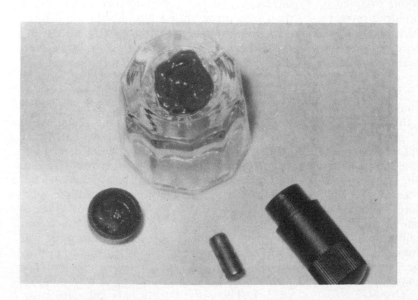

Figure 54–12 The sterile capsule shown below is used to produce the soft, pliable osseous mass present in the top of the dappen dish.

slushy amalgam in consistency, which can be "packed" or molded into bony defects (Fig. 54–12).

Froum and co-workers have studied this technique extensively by comparing it with iliac autografts and open curettage and have found osseous coagulum-bone blend procedures to be at least as effective.[39-41]

Intraoral Cancellous Bone Marrow Transplants. Hiatt and Schallhorn have described the use of cancellous bone obtained from the maxillary tuberosity, edentulous areas, and healing sockets.[51]

The *maxillary tuberosity* frequently contains a good amount of cancellous bone, particularly if the third molars are not present; also, foci of red marrow are occasionally observed. After a ridge incision is made distally from the last molar, bone is removed with a curved and cutting rongeur. Care should be taken not to extend the incision too far distally to avoid sectioning the tendons of the palatine muscle; also, the location of the maxillary sinus has to be analyzed in the radiograph in order to avoid cutting into it.

Edentulous ridges can be approached with a flap, and cancellous bone and marrow are removed with curettes. *Healing sockets* are allowed to heal for 8 to 12 weeks, and the apical portion is utilized as donor material. The particles are reduced to small pieces (Figs. 54–13 and 54–14).

Hiatt and Schallhorn report a mean fill of 3.44 mm in 166 sites studied.

Bone Swaging. Ewen[33] and Ross, Malamed, and Amsterdam[89] proposed bone swaging or contiguous osseous grafts as another intraoral technique for the treatment of angular defects (Fig. 54–15). This technique requires that bone from the edentulous area adjacent to the defect be pushed into contact with the root surface without fracturing the bone from its base. If the transposition can be carried out without interrupting the blood supply, theoretically the graft should remain viable.

This technique is complicated by varying degrees of elasticity of the bone. Bone with a greater cancellous composition is more flexible. Bone without adequate cancellous material tends to fracture from the alveolus, providing a noncontiguous bone graft. Bone swaging is therefore technically difficult, and its use is limited by the need for a substantially cancellous composition of the bone and the presence of an edentulous area adjacent to the defect being grafted.

Bone from Extraoral Sites. *Iliac Autografts.* The use of fresh or preserved iliac cancellous marrow has been extensively investigated. This material has been used by orthopedic surgeons for years. Schallhorn and coworkers[94-99] and others[6, 11, 20, 23-25, 45] have provided data from human and animal studies to support the use of autogenous iliac grafts. This technique has been proved successful in bony defects with various numbers of walls, in furcations, and even supracrestally to some extent. In comparison with other known techniques, it also provides the greatest potential for success. Problems have also been associated with its use, however. Schallhorn has observed postoperative sequelae of infection, exfoliation and sequestration, varying rates of healing, root resorption, and rapid recurrence of the defect.[95] The last two, which of course have the most lasting effects, have also been observed by other authors as well.[11, 25] In addition, problems of increased patient expense and difficulty in procuring the donor material have been noted.[97]

Techniques for Iliac Bone Graft. Numerous authors have described techniques for obtaining bone marrow from both the posterior and anterior iliac crests. Several excellent descriptions of a technique utilizing a modified Turkel trephine needle are available.[23, 32, 109] Briefly, the technique requires the patient to be placed in the supine position or in a lateral decubitus position. The area of the anterior crest is surgically prepared and draped. A point 3 to 4 cm dorsal to the anterior spine and in the center of the iliac crest is the point of entry. This point is anesthetized with a subcutaneous injection of 1 per cent lidocaine. The skin is then punctured with a No. 11 blade to introduce the outer needle and stylet. The cutting tip of the stylet is placed through the skin into the periosteum and rotated to penetrate approximately 2 mm into the bone. This provides a secure rest for the outer needle, which should be parallel to a line from the pubic bone to the anterior iliac spine. The stylet is removed, and the inner needle is inserted. The inner needle is then withdrawn with the cancellous bone in its shaft (Fig. 54–16*A* and *B*). The outer needle remains in place, allowing reentry at various angulations for multiple marrow cores. After the desired number of cores is obtained, the outer needle is removed and a pressure bandage is placed. Suturing is seldom necessary. The biopsied material may then be used fresh or frozen. *Fresh* material has been associated with root resorption[95] (Fig. 54–17). The reason for this is still unknown. Ellegaard concluded that the osteogenic potential of fresh iliac bone marrow cannot be

Text continued on page 836

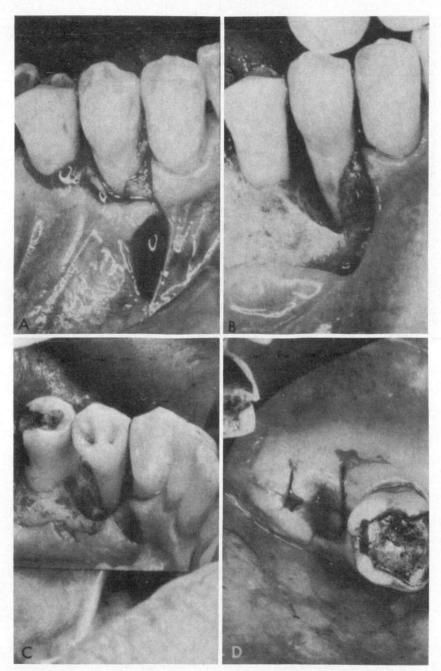

Figure 54–13 Autogenous Bone Transplant from Extraction Site. *A,* Separating mucoperiosteal flap. *B,* Buccal view of angular defect on the distal surface of the first premolar. *C,* Elevating lingual mucoperiosteal flap and view of angular defect. *D,* Bone obtained from 6-week-old extraction site.

Illustration continued on following page

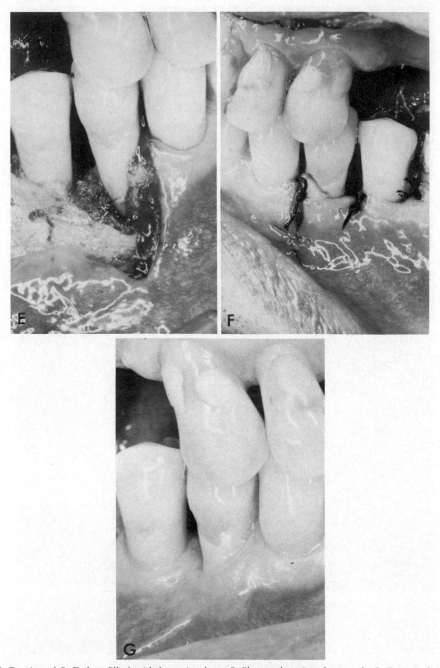

Figure 54–13 *Continued E,* Defect filled with bone implant. *F,* Flap replaced and sutured. *G,* Two and one-half months after treatment. Note excellent gingival contour. (Courtesy of Dr. Edward S. Cohen.)

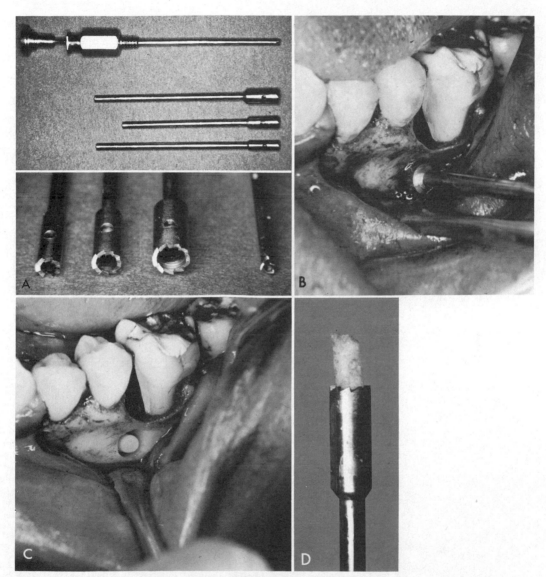

Figure 54–14 Autogenous Bone Transplant Obtained With Trephine. *A,* Trephines. *Top,* Manual trephine. *Center,* Different-sized power trephines No. 2, No. 4, and No. 6. *Bottom,* Orifices of trephines. *B,* Mucoperiosteal flap elevated, showing osseous defect on the mesial surface of the first molar. Trephine inserted into bone distal to the second molar. *C,* Bone separated by trephine. *D,* Bone transplant; the cancellous portion is used, the cortical layer is removed.

Illustration continued on following page

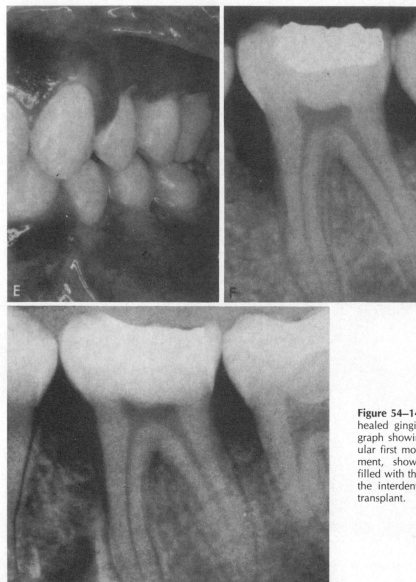

Figure 54–14 *Continued E,* Appearance of healed gingiva after 5 months. *F,* Radiograph showing osseous defect on mandibular first molar. *G,* Six months after treatment, showing osseous defect partially filled with the implant. Radiolucent area in the interdental bone is donor site of the transplant.

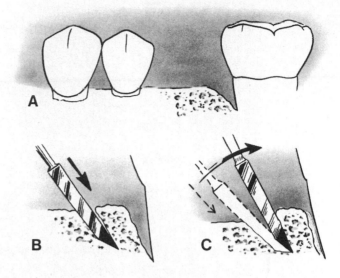

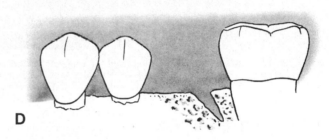

Figure 54–15 Bone Swaging to Fill Infrabony Defect. *A,* Infrabony defect on the mesial aspect of the mandibular molar. *B,* Separate section chiseled. *C,* Bone swaged into infrabony defect *(arrow).* *D,* Infrabony defect filled with bone.

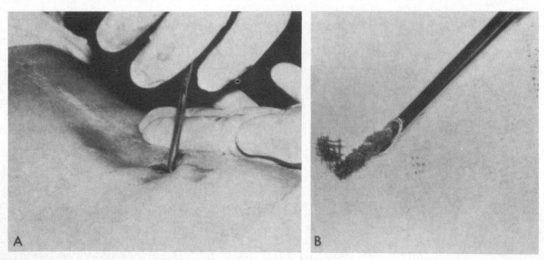

Figure 54–16 *A,* Trephine needle placed in iliac crest. *B,* One cylinder of material obtained. Numerous cylinders of material can be obtained through one skin perforation.

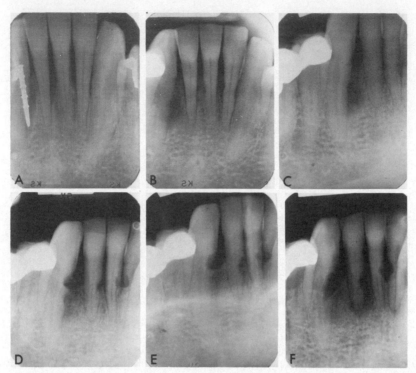

Figure 54–17 *A*, November, 1973. Radiograph of a patient immediately prior to the placement of a fresh iliac autograft. *B*, Two months later, bone repair is evident. Note the early radiolucent areas on the mesial aspect of the canine. *C*, After 7 months bone "fill" is occurring, but obvious root resorption is present. *D*, April, 1975. Root resorption is now apparent on all grafted teeth. Note the obvious degree of "fill" of the original bone defects. *E*, February, 1976. Further involvement. *F*, October, 1977. Four years later, root resorption has progressed into the pulp of the lateral incisor, causing a periosteal-endosteal complication.

utilized in new attachment procedures until methods of preventing root resorption and ankylosis are developed.[26] Therefore, *stored material is usually preferred.*

Various cryopreservation techniques have been discussed by Sottosanti and Bierly.[106] A commonly used method described by Schallhorn, Hiatt, and Boyce requires the storage of marrow in minimum essential medium with glycerol in a refrigerator at 4°C.[99] More elaborate and expensive techniques of programmed freezing also have been developed to maintain cell viability.[4, 8]

Most authors agree that careful case selection and preparation are necessary for the successful placement of the marrow into periodontal defects.[24, 31, 86, 99]

In preparing the implant site, care should be taken to preserve as much covering tissue as possible (Fig. 54–18). A full or partial thickness flap is reflected without an internal bevel incision at the margin. Care must be taken to maintain the blood supply and integrity of the gingival tissue to cover the graft material. This principle applies to all materials or techniques used. The intact gingival tissue is thought to provide nourishment to the grafted material and to prevent intraoral contamination.

After the area is exposed, granulation tissue

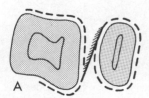 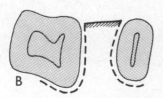

Figure 54–18 Interdental Incisions for Greater Tissue Conservation. *A*, When interdental space permits, a diagonal incision is made across the papillary area. The effective amount of tissue can be increased by beveling the incision (shown by the cross-hatched lines). *B*, If larger interdental areas are available, a "flag"-type incision can be utilized to provide complete interdental coverage.

is removed and the roots are scaled and planed (Fig. 54–19*A, B,* and *C*). The cortical bone in the walls of the osseous defect is perforated with a small round bur in several areas to permit vascularization of the implant.

The cores of marrow and cancellous bone are placed snugly into the defect, which is overfilled if possible (Fig. 54–19*D*). The flaps are returned over the area, sutured, and covered with dry foil and a periodontal dressing. Antibiotics are used prophylactically, beginning the evening before surgery and continuing for several days postoperatively. Healing is usually uneventful, with normal gingival contours restored within 2 months (Fig. 54–19*E, F,* and *G*).

Schallhorn, Hiatt, and Boyce described the results of a clinical study of 182 transplants in 52 patients.[99] Freshly frozen iliac autografts were used in all cases. Evaluations were performed for from 5 to 24 months. The results indicated that the most fill occurred in three-wall defects, but complete fill was obtained in 33 two-wall defects (4.18 mm was the average fill). The overall average of fill was approximately 3.0 mm. In one-wall defects and interradicular lesions, new attachment was obtained to a lesser extent. However, ankylosis and root resorption were noted in some cases. Hiatt and Schallhorn found that iliac marrow grafts result in greater supracrestal bone apposition and fill of furcation defects than do grafts from intraoral sites.[51]

Ellegaard and co-workers compared the effect of fresh iliac crest marrow in new attachment procedures in interradicular and three-wall vertical defects in monkeys.[30, 31] A total of 107 bifurcation defects and 94 vertical defects were created in 17 rhesus monkeys. Eight to 10 weeks after creation of the defects, new attachment attempts were made. Autogenous young cancellous bone and fresh or frozen iliac bone marrow were transplanted into the defects. Regeneration of periodontal tissues took place to the greatest extent with autogenous bone transplants in interradicular lesions, whereas no difference was observed between three-wall vertical defects treated with and without bone grafts. Transplantation of fresh iliac bone marrow resulted in a high degree of bone formation but with ankylosis and resorption of the root surface.

Dragoo and Sullivan provided additional information based on the results of histologic evaluation of four patients treated with iliac bone marrow for one- and two-wall vertical defects and suprabony pockets.[24, 25] They found an average apposition of supracrestal bone of 0.7 mm and an average supracrestal new attachment area of 1.03 mm.

PREVENTION OF EPITHELIAL MIGRATION. Despite the gratifying results achieved with the various autogenic techniques described, the results of bone grafting have not been as predictable as demanded by many therapists. Postoperative inflammation and epithelial migration into the defects have been cited by Ellegaard, Karring, Davies, and Loe as important factors limiting bone augmentation.[29] In an attempt to decrease one of these factors, epithelial migration, Ellegaard et al. developed the following technique[26, 28-30]:

On the facial and lingual aspects of vertical defects, a split flap procedure was performed. Granulation tissue was removed from the defects, and, following transplantation of the autogenous bone grafts, the defects were covered with a free palatal graft (Fig. 54–20) (see Chapter 56). Ellegaard and associates have found a greater degree of connective tissue attachment and less residual pocket formation with this technique than with the standard flap procedure described earlier. This technique is contrary to the carefully engineered primary closure flap technique previously described, and its value is a matter for further investigation.

Allografts and Xenografts

Although most data indicate that autografts of cancellous bone and marrow offer the greatest potential for success,[12, 20, 26] xenografts[1, 9, 60, 104] and allografts[2, 54, 56, 59, 62, 67, 68, 72, 90, 92] have provided some successful results.

Unfortunately, obtaining donor material for autograft purposes necessitates inflicting surgical trauma on another part of the patient's body. Obviously, it would be to the patient's as well as the therapist's advantage if a suitable substitute could be utilized for grafting purposes which would offer similar potential for repair and not require the additional surgical removal of donor material. However, both allografts and xenografts are foreign to the organism and therefore have the potential to provoke an immune response. The principal antigenic component in these grafts seems to be contained in the red marrow, although bone devoid of marrow has also been shown to exert an antigenic effect.[13, 14]

Attempts have been made to suppress the antigenic potential of allografts and xenografts by radiation, freezing, and chemical treatment.[10]

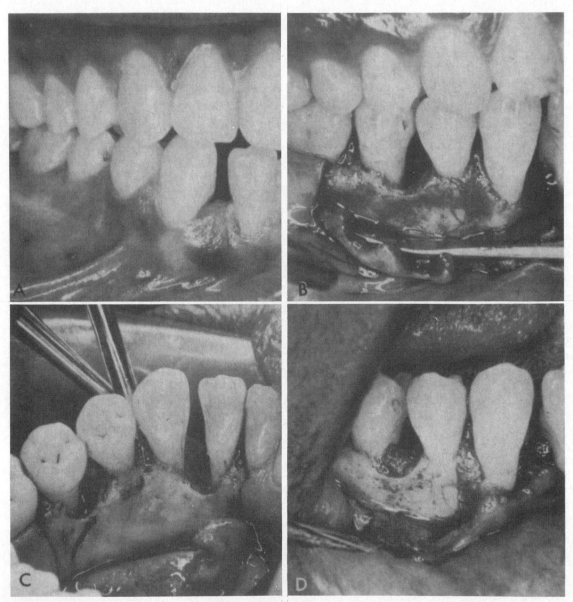

Figure 54–19 Autogenous Hip Marrow Implant. *A,* Before treatment. *B,* Mucoperiosteal flap reveals osseous defect on the second premolar. *C,* Lingual view of infrabony defect revealed by periosteal flap. (Note the defect between the canine and the lateral incisor.) *D,* Hip marrow implant in premolar osseous defect.

Illustration continued on opposite page

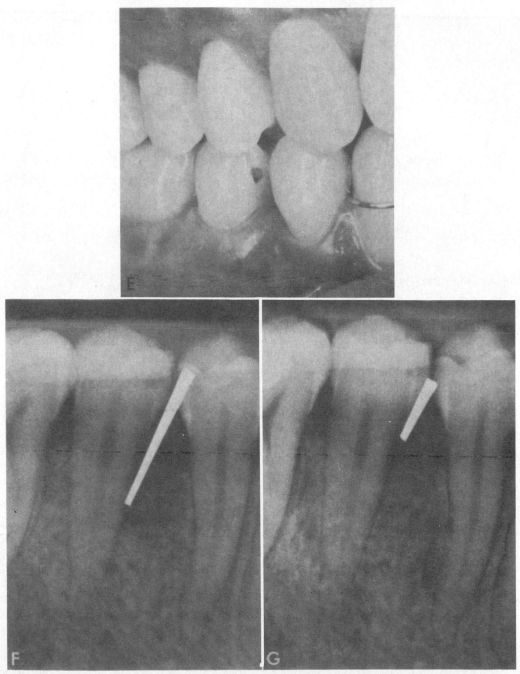

Figure 54–19 *Continued E,* Seven months after treatment. *F,* Osseous defect before treatment. The gutta percha point is at the base of the pocket. *G,* Seven months after treatment. The bone is repaired. The gutta percha point is at the base of the healed sulcus, which is now attached higher on the root. (Courtesy of Dr. Edward S. Cohen.)

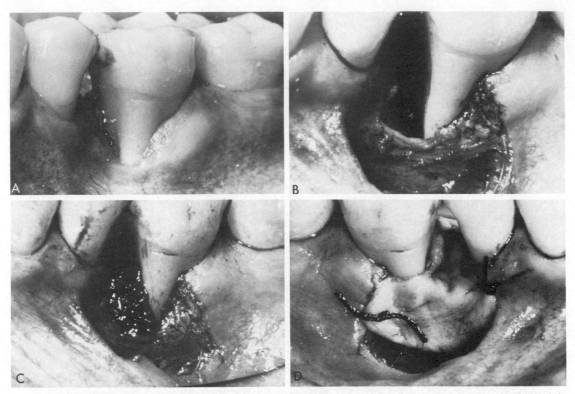

Figure 54–20 Ellegaard's Technique for Preventing Epithelial Migration. *A,* Preoperative photograph illustrates bone defect on mesial aspect of molar. *B,* Area is débrided of connective tissue. *C,* Osseous material is placed in defect. *D,* A free gingival graft is placed over osseous material and secured with interrupted sutures.

Iliac Marrow Allografts. On the basis of studies in dogs,[49] Hiatt and Schallhorn established a rationale and methodology involving the banking and utilization of allogeneic iliac material.[50, 98] Cancellous bone with its marrow was removed from the iliac crests of "living cadavers" being used for major organ transplant therapy following brain death. The material was stored in sterile vials, as with autografts, in minimum essential medium with 15 per cent glycerol as a cryoprotective agent. The vials were then frozen, and the material was tested for sterility. Freezing reduces the antigenic potential of the material, thereby rendering the graft more acceptable to the host.[14, 50, 98]

Patients were selected and matched with recipients for major blood grouping and human lymphocyte antigens (HLA). No more than two compatible donor lymphocyte antigens were present in any materials used. Thus, the rationale for using allografts of bone and marrow is based on immunologic testing parameters and the body of knowledge acquired in organ transplant therapy. A total of 194 sites, including furcations, one-, two- and three-wall defects, and suprabony pockets, in 20 patients were treated by the same technique described for using autografts of human iliac crest material.[98] Although perfect cross-matching was never achieved and 2 of the 20 patients developed cytotoxin antibodies to lymphocyte antigens, no rejection of the allografts was observed. Coronal regeneration of bone was determined by preoperative and postoperative measurements. An average bone apposition of 3.6 mm was found in a total of 121 three-, two-, and one-walled defects. In five furcation defects the average augmentation of bone was 3.3 mm, and in 68 supracrestal defects apposition was 2.06 mm. These results are similar to those obtained by the same investigators in a study using fresh and frozen iliac autografts or autografts from intraoral sites.[51, 52] Though these findings are promising, the theoretic complications of sensitizing recipients to future transplant therapy are of great concern.[97]

Freeze-Dried Iliac Allografts. Promising work on freeze-dried allografts has been undertaken at the Navy Tissue Bank. The material is obtained under sterile conditions from a cadaver that has met the rigid criteria for tissue donation established by the Navy Tissue Bank.[67] The bone is frozen, and the tissue water is removed by lyophilization. This process, commonly referred to as freeze-drying, is carried out under vacuum at a low temperature ($-40°C$). Mellonig et al.[67] reported a longitudinal clinical study involving many periodontists who used freeze-dried crushed cortical bone as a graft material in human periodontal defects. Results of the study indicate that of the 97 defects treated, 23 manifested complete bone regeneration, 39 showed better than 50 per cent regeneration, and 23 showed less than 50 per cent osseous repair. Twelve defects, of which nine were furcation involvements, failed to demonstrate any bony regeneration. This study provides strong evidence that freeze-dried bone allografts may have definite potential as grafting material in certain defects; however, the limitations of the study are obvious, and better-controlled investigations are needed.

A preliminary controlled study in rats showed that freeze-dried fine-particled bone allografts in extraoral sites may induce the differentiation of osteoblasts from host cells under some circumstances.[37] The limitations of this approach include possible antigenicity and the potential of disease transfer from the cadaver.

Xenografts. *Calf bone*, treated by detergent extraction, sterilization, and freeze-drying, has been used to formulate a material (Boplant) for the treatment of osseous defects.[2] Although some studies were promising,[101, 103] Boplant was withdrawn from the market because immunologic complications developed after its use.[52]

Kiel Bone, which is calf or ox bone that is denatured with 20 per cent hydrogen peroxide, dried with acetone, and sterilized with ethylene oxide, has also been studied. However, data are not sufficient for a complete evaluation.

Anorganic bone is ox bone from which the organic material has been extracted by means of ethylenediamine; it is then sterilized by autoclaving. Melcher has used anorganic bone for obtaining new attachment in vertical defects.[65, 66] However, he warned against the use of anorganic bone, because of protracted sequestration of the graft particles and slow resorption.

Nonbone Graft Material

In addition to bone graft materials, many different nonbone graft materials have been tried for restoration of the periodontium. Among them are dura,[29] cartilage,[7, 90, 92] ce-

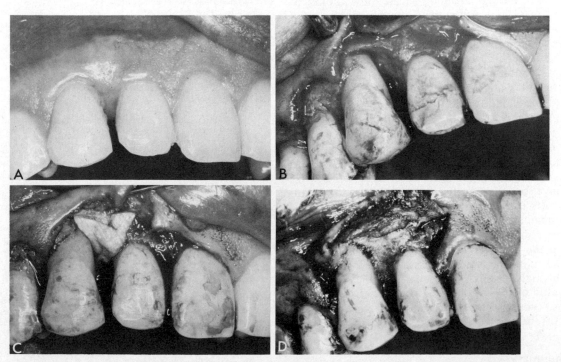

Figure 54–21 *A,* Preoperative photograph of a sclera graft area. *B,* An incision is made to conserve gingival tissue, and the area is débrided. Note the vertical defect on the mesial aspect of the canine. *C,* Sclera is placed over defect. *D,* Re-entry shows apparent remodeling of defect. (Courtesy of Dr. Jules Klingsberg.)

mentum,[91] dentin,[3, 102, 111] plaster of Paris,[58, 104] ceramics,[9, 60, 61, 73] and sclera.[54-56, 76, 110]

Sclera. Klingsberg has promoted the use of sclera as an allogeneic nonbone material to rebuild the attachment to bone and/or gingiva.[55, 56] Sclera was originally utilized in periodontal procedures because it is a dense fibrous connective tissue with poor vascularity and minimal cellularity. This affords a low incidence of antigenicity and other untoward reactions.[53] In addition, sclera may provide a barrier to apical migration of the junctional epithelium and serve to protect the blood clot during the initial healing period.

Utilization of sclera was demonstrated by Klingsberg,[54-56] and the technique for its preparation and preservation was described by Feingold and Chasens.[34]

Although some studies show that sclera is well accepted by the host and is sometimes invaded by host cells and capillaries and replaced by dense connective tissue,[35] it does not appear to induce osteogenesis or cementogenesis.[68, 76, 110] It may, however, be useful for its scaffolding effect (Fig. 54–21). The scientific research available does not warrant its routine use in periodontal therapy.

Cartilage. Cartilage has been used for repair studies in monkeys and for treatment of periodontal defects in humans.[90, 92] It can serve as a scaffolding around which new bone is formed, and some new attachment was obtained in 60 of 70 cases studied. Cartilage has received only limited evaluation.

Plaster of Paris. Although plaster of Paris was found to be useful in one uncontrolled clinical study,[1] others have reported that it does not induce bone formation.[104] Its usefulness, therefore, appears questionable.

Ceramics. Bioceramics, such as tricalcium phosphate and durapatite, have acquired wide popularity through commercial advertising in recent years. Porous ceramics in powder form have been suggested as substitutes for bone grafts in the treatment of periodontal defects. This material seems to be well tolerated by the organism, and bone apposition occurs directly on the ceramic lattice.[61] However, analysis of the clinical effectiveness of these materials through research has been limited.[73, 81, 107] The value of these materials in clinical practice has not been sufficiently tested to warrant their current clinical use.

Summary

In summary, the subject of grafting has received a great deal of attention because of its obvious importance in improving the results of therapy. The clinician should make an effort to differentiate between those materials that have been studied in depth and with acceptable results and others that, although promising, are still experimental. Research papers must be given critical evaluation; the adequacy of controls, selection of cases, methods of evaluation, and long-range postoperative results must be considered.

The following methods can be recommended on the basis of available information: autogenous bone implants obtained from intraoral sites, particularly extraction sockets, edentulous areas, and tuberosity areas; osseous coagulum–bone blend techniques; and frozen iliac bone and marrow autogenous transplants. The clinician should also remember that careful curettage, whether open or closed, has been shown to result in bone regeneration without the use of bone-inducing agents. Caution in the adoption of new, as yet not fully proven, methods is recommended.

REFERENCES

1. Alderman, N. E.: Sterile plaster of Paris as an implant in the infrabony environment: a preliminary study. J. Periodontol., *40*:11, 1969.
2. Arrocha, R., Wittwer, J., and Gargiulo, A.: Tissue response to heterogenous bone implantation in dogs. J. Periodontol., *39*:162, 1968.
3. Bang, G., and Urist, M. R.: Bone induction in excavation chambers in matrix of decalcified dentin. Arch. Surg., *94*:781, 1967.
4. Barkin, M., and Newman, N.: Ultrastructure of bone marrow prior to and after programmed freezing. Oral Surg., *33*:341, 1972.
5. Beube, F. E.: Radiographic and histologic study of reattachment. J. Periodontol., *23*:158, 1952.
6. Bierly, J. A., Sottosanti, J. S., Costley, J. M., and Cherrick, H. M.: An evaluation of the osteogenic potential of marrow. J. Periodontol., *46*:277, 1975.
7. Boyne, P. J., and Cooksey, D. E.: Use of cartilage and bone implants in restoration of edentulous ridges. J. Am. Dent. Assoc., *71*:1426, 1965.
8. Boyne, P. J., and Yeager, J. E.: An evaluation of osteogenic potential of frozen marrow. Oral Surg., *28*:764, 1969.
9. Bump, R. L., Salimeno, T., Hooker, S. P., and Wilkinson, E. G.: Grafting one-wall infrabony pockets with woven ceramic fabric. I.A.D.R. Abstracts, 1974, p. 98.
10. Buring, K., and Urist, M. R.: Effects of ionizing radiation on the bone induction principle in the matrix of bone implants. Clin. Orthop. Rel. Res., *55*:225, 1967.
11. Burnette, W. E.: Fate of the iliac crest graft. J. Periodontol., *43*:88, 1972.
12. Burwell, R. G.: Studies in the transplantation of bone. VII. J. Bone Joint Surg., *46*:110, 1964.
13. Burwell, R. G., and Gowland, G.: Studies in the transplantation of bone. III. The immune responses of lymph nodes draining components of fresh homologous cancellous bone treated by different methods. J. Bone Joint Surg., *44*:131, 1962.
14. Burwell, R. G., Gowland, G., and Dexter, F.: Studies in the transplantation of bone. VI. Further observations concerning the antigenicity of homologous cortical and cancellous bone. J. Bone Joint Surg., *45*:597, 1963.
15. Carranza, F. A., Sr.: A technic for reattachment. J. Periodontol., *25*:272, 1954.

16. Carranza, F. A., Sr.: A technique for treating infrabony pockets so as to obtain reattachment. Dent. Clin. North Am., 4:75, 1960.

17. Carranza, F. A., Sr., and Carranza, F. A., Jr.: The management of the alveolar bone in the treatment of the periodontal pocket. J. Periodontol., 27:29, 1956.

18. Carraro, J. J., Sznajder, N., and Alonso, C. A.: Intraoral cancellous bone autografts in treatment of infrabony pockets. J. Clin. Periodontol., 3:104, 1976.

19. Coverly, L., Toto, P., and Gargiulo, A.: Osseous coagulum: a histologic evaluation. J. Periodontol., 46:596, 1975.

20. Cushing, M.: Autogenous red marrow grafts: potential for induction of osteogenesis. J. Periodontol., 40:492, 1969.

21. Diem, C. R., Bowers, G. M., and Moffitt, W. C.: Bone blending: a technique for osseous implants. J. Periodontol., 43:295, 1972.

22. Donnenfeld, O. W., Hoag, P. M., and Weissman, D. P.: A clinical study in the effects of osteoplasty. J. Periodontol., 41:131, 1970.

23. Dragoo, M. R., and Irwin, R. K.: A method of procuring cancellous iliac bone utilizing a trephine needle. J. Periodontol., 43:82, 1972.

24. Dragoo, M. R., and Sullivan, H. C.: A clinical and histologic evaluation of autogenous iliac bone grafts in humans. Part I. Wound healing after 2 to 8 months. J. Periodontol., 44:599, 1973.

25. Dragoo, M. R., and Sullivan, H. C.. A clinical and histologic evaluation of autogenous iliac bone grafts in humans. Part II. External root resorption. J. Periodontol., 44:614, 1973.

26. Ellegaard, B.: Bone grafts in periodontal attachment procedures. J. Clin. Periodontol., 3:5, 1976.

27. Ellegaard, B., and Löe, H.: New attachment of periodontal tissues after treatment of intrabony lesions. J. Periodontol., 42:648, 1971.

28. Ellegaard, B., Karring, T., and Löe, H.: Retardation of epithelial migration in new attachment attempts in intrabony defects in monkeys. J. Clin. Periodontol., 3:23, 1976.

29. Ellegaard, B., Nielsen, I. M., and Karring, T.: Lyodura grafts in new attachment procedures. J. Dent. Res., 55: Special issue B, B-304, 1976.

30. Ellegaard, B., Karring, T., Davies, R., and Löe, H.: New attachment after treatment of intrabony defects in monkeys. J. Periodontol., 45:368, 1974.

31. Ellegaard, B., Karring, T., Listgarten, N., and Löe, H.: New attachment after treatment of interradicular lesions. J. Periodontol., 44:209, 1973.

32. Ellis, L. D., Jensen, W. N., and Westermann, M. P.: Needle biopsy of bone and marrow. Arch. Intern. Med., 114:214, 1964.

33. Ewen, S. J.: Bone swaging. J. Periodontol., 36:57, 1965.

34. Feingold, J. P., and Chasens, A. I.: Preserved scleral allografts in periodontal defect in man. I. Preparation, preservation and use. J. Periodontol., 48:1, 1977.

35. Feingold, J. P., Chasens, A. I., Doyle, J., and Alfano, M. C.: Preserved scleral allografts on periodontal defects in man. II. Histologic evaluation. J. Periodontol., 48:4, 1977.

36. Freeman, E., and Turnbull, R. S.: The value of osseous coagulum as a graft material. J. Periodont. Res., 8:299, 1973.

37. Freeman, E., and Turnbull, R. S.: Short communication: histologic evaluation of freeze-dried fine particles bone allografts. Preliminary observation. J. Periodontol., 48:288, 1977.

38. Friedman, N.: Periodontal osseous surgery: osteoplasty and osteoectomy. J. Periodontol., 26:257, 1955.

39. Froum, S. J.: Comparison of different autograft material for obtaining bone fill in human periodontal defects. J. Periodontol., 45:240, 1974.

40. Froum, S. J., Thaler, R., Scoop, I. W., and Stahl, S. S.: Osseous autografts. I. Clinical responses to bone blend or hip marrow grafts. J. Periodontol., 46:515, 1975.

41. Froum, S. J., Thaler, R., Scoop, I. W., and Stahl, S. S.: Osseous autografts. II. Histologic responses to osseous coagulum-bone blend grafts. J. Periodontol., 46:656, 1975.

42. Glickman, I., Smulow, J. B., O'Brien, T., and Tannen, R.: Healing of the periodontium following mucogingival surgery. Oral Surg., 16:530, 1963.

43. Goldman, H.: A rationale for the treatment of the intrabony pocket. One method of treatment—subgingival curettage. J. Periodontol., 20:83, 1949.

44. Goldman, H. M., and Cohen, D. W.: The infrabony pocket: classification and treatment. J. Periodontol., 29:272, 1958.

45. Haggerty, P. C., and Maeda, L.: Autogenous bone grafts: a revolution in the treatment of vertical bone defects. J. Periodontol., 42:626, 1971.

46. Halliday, D. G.: The grafting of newly formed autogenous bone in the treatment of osseous defects. J. Periodontol., 40:511, 1969.

47. Hegedus, Z.: The rebuilding of the alveolar process by bone transplantation. Dent. Cosmos, 65:736, 1923.

48. Hiatt, W. H.: Periodontal pocket elimination by combined endodontic-periodontic therapy. J. Periodontol., 1:153, 1963.

49. Hiatt, W. H.: The induction of new bone and cementum formation. III. Utilizing bone and marrow allografts in dogs. J. Periodontol., 4:596, 1970.

50. Hiatt, W. H., and Schallhorn, R. G.: Human allografts of iliac cancellous bone and marrow in periodontal osseous defects. I. Rationale and methodology. J. Periodontol., 42:642, 1971.

51. Hiatt, W. H., and Schallhorn, R. G.: Intraoral transplants of cancellous bone and marrow in periodontal lesions. J. Periodontol., 44:194, 1973.

52. Hjorting-Hansen, E.: Studies on implantation of anorganic bone in cystic jaw lesions. Thesis. Munksgaard. Copenhagen, 1972.

53. Johnson, W., et al.: Transplantation of homografts of sclera: experimental study. Am. J. Ophthal., 54:1019, 1962.

54. Klingsberg, J.: Preserved sclera in periodontal surgery. J. Periodontol., 43:634, 1972.

55. Klingsberg, J.: Scleral allografts in the repair of periodontal osseous defects. N.Y. State Dent. J., 38:418, 1972.

56. Klingsberg, J.: Periodontal scleral grafts and combined grafts of sclera and bone: two year appraisal. J. Periodontol., 45:262, 1974.

57. Knowles, J. N., Burgett, F. G., Morrison, E. C., Nissle, R. R., and Ramfjord, S. P.: Comparison of results following three modalities of periodontal therapy related to tooth type and initial pocket depth. J. Clin. Periodontol., 7:32, 1980.

58. Kornbleuth, J.: Histologic evaluation of plaster as a seal for bone autografts. I.A.D.R. Abstracts, 1972, p. 184.

59. Kromer, H.: Transplantation in Surgical Treatment of Cysts of the Jaw and Periodontal Pockets. Oslo, Oslo University Press, 1960.

60. Levin, M. P., Getter, L., and Cutright, D. E.: A comparison of iliac marrow and biodegradable ceramic in periodontal defects. J. Biomed. Mater. Res., 9:183, 1975.

61. Levin, M. P., Getter, L., Adrian, J., and Cutright, D. E.: Healing of periodontal defects with ceramic implants. J. Periodontol., 1:197, 1974.

62. Libin, B. M., Ward, H. L., and Fishman, L. L.: Decalcified lyophilized bone allografts for use in human periodontal defects. J. Periodontol., 46:51, 1975.

63. Lobene, R., and Glickman, I.: The response of alveolar bone to grinding with rotary diamond stones. J. Periodontol., 34:105, 1963.

64. Matherson, D. G., and Zander, H. A.: An evaluation of osseous surgery in monkeys. I.A.D.R. Abstracts, No. 325, 1963, p. 116.

65. Melcher, A. H.: The use of heterogenous anorganic bone in periodontal bone grafting: a preliminary report. I. Dent. Assoc. So. Africa, 13:80, 1958.

66. Melcher, A.: The use of heterogenous anorganic bone as an implant material in oral procedures. Oral Surg., 15:996, 1962.

67. Mellonig, J. T., et al.: Clinical evaluation of freeze-dried bone allografts in periodontal osseous defects. J. Periodontol., 47:125, 1976.

68. Moskow, B. S., Gold, S. I., and Gottsegen, R.: Effects of scleral collagen upon the healing of experimental osseous wounds. J. Periodontol., 47:596, 1976.

69. Nabers, C. L., and O'Leary, T. J.: Autogenous bone transplants in the treatment of osseous defects. J. Periodontol., 36:5, 1965.

70. Nabers, C. L., and O'Leary, T. J.: Autogenous bone grafts: case report. Periodontics, 5:251, 1967.

71. Nabers, J. M., Meador, H. L., Nabers, C. L., and O'Leary, T. J.: Chronology, an important factor in the repair of osseous defects. Periodontics, 2:304, 1964.

72. Narang, R., and Wells, H.: Bone induction in experimental periodontal bone defects in dogs with decalcified allogenic bone matrix grafts: a preliminary study. Oral Surg., 33:306, 1972.

73. Nery, E. B., and Lynch, K. L.: Preliminary clinical studies

of bioceramic in periodontal osseous defects. J. Periodontol., *49*:523, 1978.

74. Ochsenbein, C.: Osseous resection in periodontal surgery. J. Periodontol., *29*:15, 1958.

75. Ochsenbein, C.: Current status of osseous surgery. J. Periodontol., *48*:577, 1977.

76. Passell, M. S., and Bassada, N. F.: Histomorphologic evaluation of scleral grafts in experimental bony defects. J. Periodontol., *46*:629, 1975.

77. Patur, B., and Glickman, I.: Clinical and roentgenographic evaluation of the post-treatment healing of infrabony pockets. J. Periodontol., *33*:164, 1962.

78. Pennel, B. M., King, K. O., Wilderman, M. H., and Barron, J. M.: Repair of the alveolar process following osseous surgery. J. Periodontol., *38*:426, 1967.

79. Prichard, J. F.: The intrabony technique as a predictable procedure. J. Periodontol., *28*:202, 1957.

80. Prichard, J. F.: Regeneration of bone following periodontal therapy. Oral Surg., *10*:247, 1957.

81. Rabalais, M. L., Yukna, R. A., and Mayer, E. T.: Evaluation of durapatite ceramic as an alloplastic implant in periodontal osseous defects. J. Periodontol., *52*:680, 1981.

82. Ramfjord, S. P., Kerr, D. A., and Ash, M. M.: World Workshop in Periodontics. American Acad. Periodont. and Univ. Michigan, 1966.

83. Ramfjord, S. P., Nissle, R. R., Schick, R. A., and Cooper, H., Jr.: Subgingival curettage versus surgical elimination of periodontal pockets. J. Periodontol., *39*:167, 1968.

84. Rivault, A. F., Toto, P. D., Levy, S., and Gargiulo, A. W.: Autogenous bone grafts: osseous coagulum and osseous retrograde procedures in primates. J. Periodontol., *42*:787, 1971.

85. Robinson, R. E.: Osseous coagulum for bone induction. J. Periodontol., *40*:503, 1969.

86. Rosenberg, M. M.: Free osseous tissue autografts as a predictable procedure. J. Periodontol., *42*:195, 1971.

87. Rosenberg, M. M.: Reentry of an osseous defect treated by a bone implant after a long duration. J. Periodontol., *42*:360, 1971.

88. Ross, S. E., and Cohen, D. W.: The fate of a free osseous tissue autograft: a clinical and histologic case report. Periodontics, *6*:145, 1968.

89. Ross, S. E., Malamed, E. H., and Amsterdam, M.: The contiguous autogenous transplant—its rationale, indications and technique. Periodontics, *4*:246, 1966.

90. Schaffer, E. M.: Cartilage transplants into periodontium of rhesus monkeys. Oral Surg., *11*:1233, 1956.

91. Schaffer, E. M.: Cementum and dentine implants in a dog and a rhesus monkey. J. Periodontol., *28*:125, 1957.

92. Schaffer, E. M.: Cartilage grafts in human periodontal pockets. J. Periodontol., *29*:176, 1958.

93. Schaffer, E. M., and Zander, H. A.: Histologic evidence of reattachment of periodontal pockets. Parodontologie, *7*:101, 1953.

94. Schallhorn, R. G.: The use of autogenous hip marrow biopsy implants for bony crater defects. J. Periodontol., *39*:145, 1968.

95. Schallhorn, R. G.: Postoperative problems associated with iliac transplants. J. Periodontol., *43*:3, 1972.

96. Schallhorn, R. G.: Osseous grafts in the treatment of periodontal osseous defects. *In* Stahl, S. S. (ed.): Periodontal Surgery. Springfield, Ill., Charles C Thomas, 1976.

97. Schallhorn, R. G.: Present status of osseous grafting procedures. J. Periodontol., *48*:570, 1977.

98. Schallhorn, R. G., and Hiatt, W. H.: Human allografts of iliac cancellous bone and marrow in periodontal osseous defects. II. Clinical observations. J. Periodontol., *43*:67, 1972.

99. Schallhorn, R. G., Hiatt, W. H., and Boyce, W.: Iliac transplants in periodontal therapy. J. Periodontol., *41*:566, 1970.

100. Schluger, S.: Osseous resection: a basic principle in periodontal surgery. Oral Surg., *2*:316, 1949.

101. Scoop, I. W., Kassouny, D. Y., and Morgan, F. H.: Bovine bone (Boplant). J. Periodontol., *37*:400, 1966.

102. Scoop, I. W., Kassouny, D. Y., and Register, A. A.: Human bone induction by allogenic dentin matrix. I.A.D.R. Abstracts, No. 105, 1970, p. 100.

103. Scoop, I. W., Morgan, F. H., Dooner, J. J., Fredrics, H. J., and Heyman, R. A.: Bovine bone (Boplant) implants for infrabony oral lesions (clinical trials in humans). Periodontics, *4*:169, 1966.

104. Shaffer, C. D., and App, G. R.: The use of plaster of Paris in treating infrabony periodontal defects in humans. J. Periodontol., *42*:685, 1971.

105. Smith, D. H., Ammons, W. F., Jr., and Von Belle, G.: A longitudinal study of periodontal status comparing osseous recontouring with flap curettage. I. Results after 6 months. J. Periodontol., *51*:367, 1980.

106. Sottosanti, J. S., and Bierly, J. A.: The storage of bone marrow and its relation to periodontal grafting procedures. J. Periodontol., *46*:162, 1975.

107. Strub, J. R., Gaberthal, T. W., and Firstone, A. R.: Comparison of tricalcium phosphate and frozen allogenic bone implants in man. J. Periodontol., *50*:624, 1979.

108. Sugarman, E. F.: A clinical and histological study of the attachment of grafted tissue to bone and teeth. J. Periodontol., *40*:381, 1969.

109. Tarrow, A. B., Turkel, H., and Thompson, M. S.: Infusion via the bone marrow and biopsy of bone marrow. Anesthesiology, *13*:501, 1952.

110. Turnbull, R. S., Freeman, E., and Melcher, A. H.: Histological evaluation of the osteogenic capacity of sclera. J. Dent. Res., *55*:972, 1976.

111. Urist, M. R.: Bone histogenesis and morphogenesis in implants of demineralized enamel and dentin. Oral Surg., *29*:38, 1971.

112. Urist, M. R., et al.: Bone induction principle. Clin. Orthop., *53*:243, 1967.

113. Waerhaug, J.: The gingival pocket. Odont. Tidskr., *60*:suppl. 1, 1952.

114. Wilderman, N. M., and Wentz, F. M.: Repair of a dentogingival defect with a pedicle flap. J. Periodontol., *36*:218, 1965.

115. Zamet, J. S.: A comparative clinical study of three periodontal surgical techniques. J. Clin. Periodontol., *2*:87, 1975.

116. Zander, H. A., and Matherson, D. G.: The effect of osseous surgery on interdental tissue morphology in monkeys. I.A.D.R. Abstracts, No. 236, 1963, p. 117.

chapter fifty-five

Treatment of Furcation Involvement and Combined Periodontal–Endodontic Therapy

The diagnosis, prognosis, and treatment of teeth with furcation involvement (Fig. 55–1) are governed by the general principles applicable to single-rooted teeth. However, in spite of the added stability provided by extra root anchorage, furcated teeth and their surroundings present several anatomic characteristics that make therapy difficult and its results unpredictable.

These anatomic considerations refer to tooth, bone, and gingival interrelationships and will be described after the classification of furcation involvements is discussed.

CLASSIFICATION OF FURCATION INVOLVEMENTS

The classification of the different degrees of furcation involvement allows us to better understand the prognosis of the lesions and their therapy.

Grade I Involvement

This is the incipient or early lesion. The pocket is suprabony, involving the soft tissue; there is slight bone loss in the furcation area (Fig. 55–2). Radiographic change is not usual, since bone loss is minimal (Fig. 55–3).

Grade II Involvement

In these cases, bone is destroyed on one or more aspects of the furcation, but a portion of the alveolar bone and periodontal ligament remains intact, permitting only partial penetration of the probe into the furca. The lesion is essentially a cul-de-sac (Figs. 55–2 and 55–3).

The depth of the horizontal component of the pocket will vary; this determines whether the furcation involvement is early or advanced. There may also be a *vertical* or *apical component* of the pocket that extends into the osseous structure. This infrabony pocket, combined with the horizontal component of tissue destruction, can complicate diagnosis, prognosis, and therapy.

The radiograph may or may not reveal the Grade II furcation involvement. In the mandibular molars, the close proximity of the roots, thick bone remaining between the roots, or the angulation of the x-ray beam can conceal the furcation involvement. The maxillary molars present further problems with diagnosis because the roots overlap each other radiographically from the facial view. A furcation involvement between the two facial roots may not be seen on the radiograph because the palatal root obscures it.

Grade III Involvement

In this type of furcation involvement, the interradicular bone is completely absent, but the facial and/or lingual orifices of the furcation are occluded by gingival tissue. Therefore, the furcation opening cannot be seen clinically, but it is essentially a through-and-through tun-

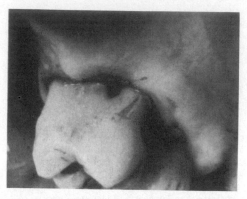

Figure 55–1 Typical Furcation Opening Involving the Distofacial and Palatal Roots of a Maxillary Molar.

nel (Fig. 55–2). There may be an angular lesion in the interradicular area, creating an apical or vertical component along with the horizontal loss of bone. This type of lesion can be present in both the Grade III and Grade IV lesions.

If the radiograph of the mandibular molars is taken at the proper angle and the roots are divergent, these lesions will appear on the radiograph as a radiolucent area between the roots (Fig. 55–3). The maxillary molars present a difficulty in diagnosis similar to the problems encountered with the Grade II involvement owing to the roots overlapping each other.

Grade IV Involvement

As in Grade III lesions, the interradicular bone is completely destroyed, but here the gingival tissue is also receded apically so that the furcation opening is clinically visible. Therefore, these involvements also present tunnels, without the orifices' being occluded by the gingiva.

The radiographic picture is essentially the same as that for Grade III lesions.

ANATOMIC CONSIDERATIONS

The following anatomic features are of importance for the clinical management of furcation lesions.

TOOTH. Three features should be considered:

1. Location of the furcation relative to the cemento-enamel junction. A furcation located near the cemento-enamel junction will become involved early in the disease process. A furcation located at a distance from the cemento-enamel junction will be invaded later but will be more difficult to reach and instrument (Fig. 55–4).

2. Concavity of the inner surface of exposed roots. All the root surfaces facing the furcation present some degree of concavity or depression in an occlusoapical direction.[3, 4] This makes instrumentation for calculus removal and root planing almost impossible at times, even after surgical exposure (Fig. 55–5B) (see Chapter 33).

3. Degree of separation of the roots. Wide separation of the roots facilitates instrumentation and resective therapy (Fig. 55–4).

BONE. Bone shape in the exposed furcation area may be horizontal, or there may be different degrees of vertical bone loss next to the roots or on the furcation side of the facial or lingual bone (Figs. 55–6A and 55–7A). Therefore, not only the horizontal depth, but also the vertical or apical depth, must be considered.

In addition, a thick buccal or lingual bony ledge—for example, in teeth adjacent to an external oblique ridge or a lingual torus—may favor the formation of trough-like vertical lesions in the furcation area. A thin radicular bone, on the other hand, will result in complete loss of the bone, and no vertical lesion will form.

GINGIVA. The presence of sufficient attached keratinized gingival tissue and adequate

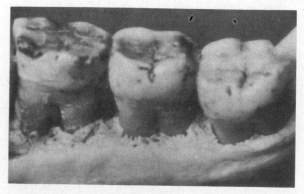

Figure 55–2 Teeth in Skull Demonstrating the Different Degrees of Furcation Involvement. The first molar has a Grade III or Grade IV involvement, the second molar a Grade II lesion, and the third molar a Grade I, or incipient, involvement.

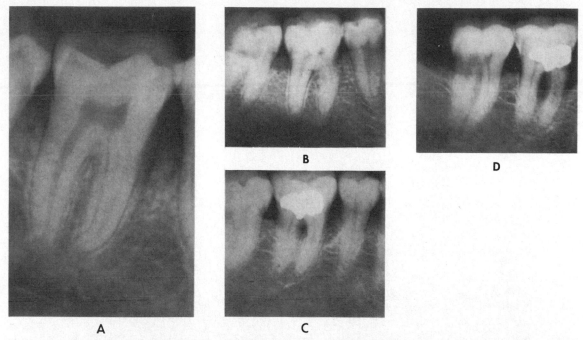

Figure 55–3 Radiographs of Different Degrees of Furcation Involvement. *A,* Grade I, no marked change. *B,* Grade II, small area of radiolucency. *C,* Distinct triangular area of radiolucency. *D,* Pronounced bone loss. The lesions shown in *C* and *D* would be Grade III or Grade IV, depending on whether the furcation is clinically visible owing to gingival recession.

Figure 55–4 Different Anatomic Features That May Be of Importance in Prognosis and Treatment of Furcation Involvement. *A,* Widely separated roots. *B,* Roots are separated but close to one another. *C,* Fused roots (synostosis) separated only in their apical portion. *D,* Presence of enamel projection that may be conducive to an early furcation involvement.

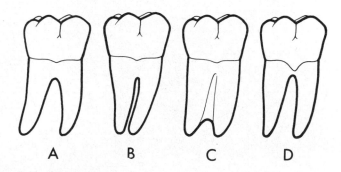

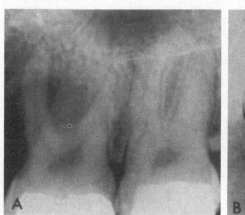

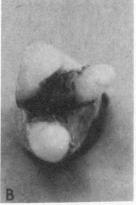

Figure 55–5 *A,* Radiograph of furcation involvement of the maxillary first molar. Note the advanced bone loss around the mesiofacial root and the trifurcation area. *B,* Apical view of the first molar shown in *A,* after extraction. Note the heavy calculus deposits in the trifurcation area.

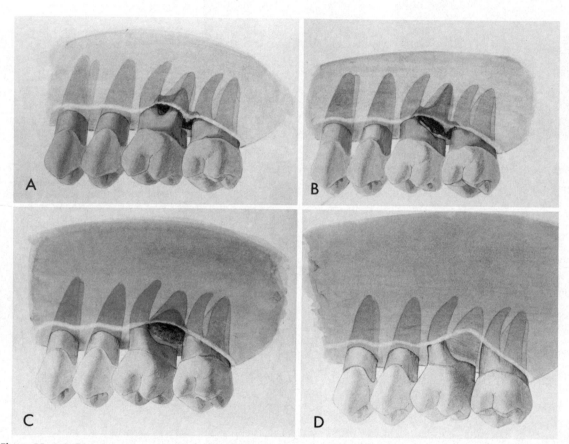

Figure 55–6 *A,* Diagrammatic view of furcation involvement around the distofacial root of maxillary first molar; note the bony lesion with a vertical component. *B,* The root has been resected; note the resultant socket and osseous defect. *C,* Partial "fill" of the socket several months after the resection. *D,* The final osseous contour after osteoplasty of the area.

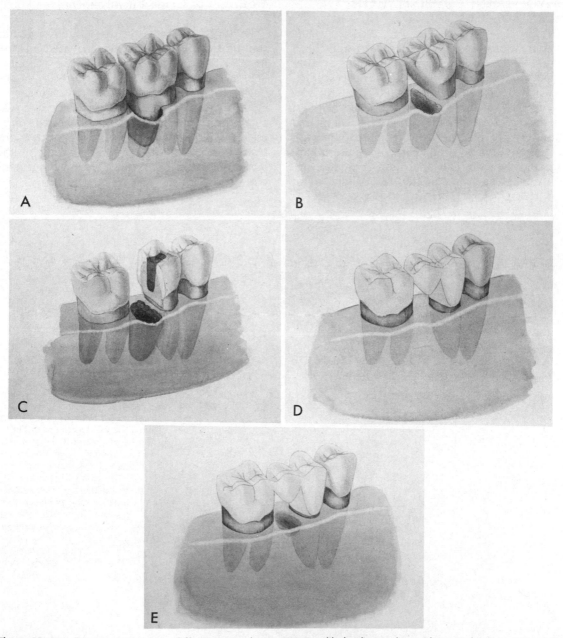

Figure 55–7 *A,* Diagrammatic view of furcation involvement in mandibular first molar, with vertical lesions around the distal root. *B,* After resection of distal root; note the resultant socket. *C,* Another approach, utilizing hemisection of the distal half of the tooth (root and crown). *D,* A temporary bridge is placed while the socket "fills" with bone. *E,* The final result after osteoplasty of the area, several months later.

vestibular depth will facilitate the gingival management of the furcation area.

TREATMENT OF FURCATION INVOLVEMENT COMBINED WITH SUPRABONY POCKETS

Furcations are treated by scaling and curettage, gingivectomy, flap operation, or root resection, depending on the severity of the involvement and the architecture of the destructive process. Suprabony pockets without osseous deformities are treated by scaling and curettage or by gingivectomy; furcations with infrabony pockets and osseous defects are treated with the flap operation. Furcation involvement may be confined to a single tooth,

but very often several teeth are affected. The furcations are treated as they are encountered in the systematic care of the mouth.[4]

Treatment of Grade I Involvement

Each furcation involvement usually presents suprabony pockets, which are treated by scaling and curettage or by gingivectomy, depending on pocket depth and the fibrosity of the pocket walls. Since the destructive process is in its incipient stages, it is not necessary to enter the furcation during the treatment process. Elimination of the pocket is followed by resolution of inflammation and repair of the periodontal ligament and adjacent bone margin.

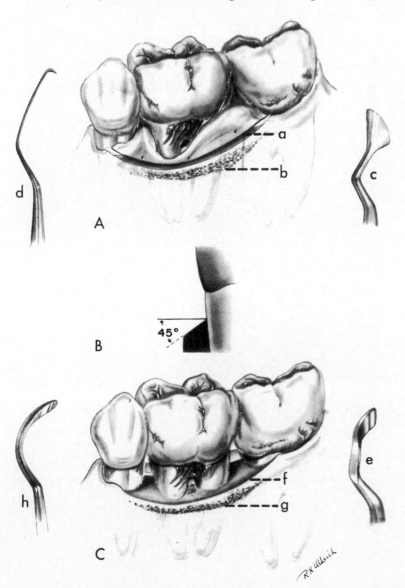

Figure 55–8 Gingivectomy Technique for the Treatment of Furcation Involvement. *A,* Line of incision for removing the gingiva (*a*). The level of the underlying bone (*b*). *B,* The gingiva is cut at a 45° angle to the tooth. *C,* Appearance of the area after the gingival pocket wall has been removed. The cut surface (*f*). The level of the underlying bone (*g*).

Illustration continued on opposite page

In the treatment of early furcation involvements, the facial groove is sometimes eliminated by reshaping the tooth (*odontoplasty*) to reduce posttreatment accumulation of plaque and debris.[5]

Treatment of Grade II Involvement

Under local anesthesia, each tooth surface is probed down to the bone to determine the pattern of periodontal destruction. One aspect of the furcation is intact in Grade II involvement; treatment is performed from the most extensively involved side and is usually gingivectomy or an apically positioned flap.

Figure 55–8 shows diagrammatically a case successfully treated by gingivectomy. A gingivectomy incision is made through the pinpoint markings, conforming to the outline of the underlying bone margin (Fig. 55–8*A*). The incision is made with periodontal knives or a No. 12 Bard-Parker scalpel and is beveled at approximately a 45° angle to the tooth (Fig. 55–8*B*). The resected gingiva is detached, exposing underlying bead-like granulation tissue, which is removed with curettes. The root is scaled and planed.

The area is cleaned with warm water, and strips of periodontal pack are placed on the facial and lingual surfaces and pressed together so that they join interproximally for retention (Fig. 55–8*D*). The pack is removed after 1 week.

When the pack is removed, the area is cleaned and the roots are checked for small particles of calculus and for smoothness. The patient is instructed in plaque control in the

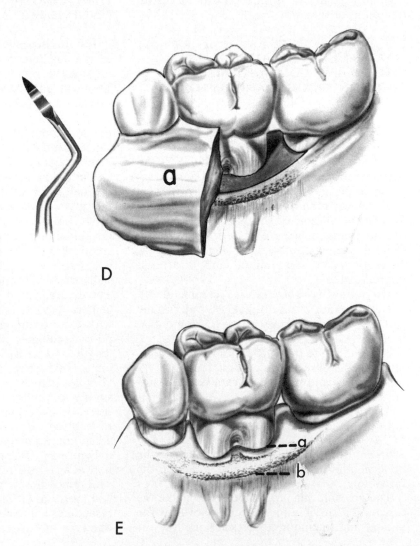

Figure 55–8 *Continued D,* The pack in position (*a*). Part of the field is uncovered to show the relationship of the pack to the furcation. This part is also covered with pack. *E,* The healed lesion, showing the contour of the gingiva (*a*) and the level of the bone (*b*). See the treated cases shown in Figure 55–9.

furcation area. Interdental cleansers such as PROXABRUSH should be used in these areas.

Treatment of Grade III and Grade IV Involvements

In these conditions, interradicular tissue destruction permits a probe to pass freely through the furcation. The gingiva is resected just coronal to the bone or displaced to the same level to provide visibility and access from all directions so that the involved root surfaces may be throughly planed and smoothed without disturbing the bone. The periodontal pack is placed for 1 week except when patient comfort requires repacking for an additional week.

Figure 55–9 shows the posttreatment gingival contour that can be attained with successful treatment of furcations.

TREATMENT OF FURCATION INVOLVEMENT COMBINED WITH INFRABONY POCKETS AND OSSEOUS DEFECTS

When infrabony pockets and osseous defects are part of the clinical picture of furcation involvement, the treatment of choice is the flap operation (see Chapter 53 and 54).

Furcation involvements combined with vertical defects require bone contouring as well as instrumentation of the root surface facing the furcation. Success with regenerative procedures such as autogenous bone grafts has generally been very limited and is at best unpredictable.

The following procedure is recommended:

1. Reflection of a full thickness flap facially and lingually or palatally; removal of granulation tissue (see Chapter 53).

2. Bone contouring to adjust angular bone losses to the base of the existing bone.

3. Scaling and planing of exposed root surfaces.

4. Further recontouring of bone to attain a harmonious osseous topography (see Chapter 54).

5. Suturing of the flap at the level of the bone margin in order to expose and open the furcation.

The goals of this procedure are to make the furcation accessible for plaque removal by the patient and to eliminate vertical bone loss.

OCCLUSAL ADJUSTMENT IN THE TREATMENT OF FURCATIONS WITH INFRABONY POCKETS AND OSSEOUS DEFECTS. Furcation involvement is not of itself indicative of trauma from occlusion; inflammation may be the only responsible destructive factor. However, of all the areas of the periodontium, the furcation is most susceptible to injury from excessive occlusal forces. When furcation involvement is complicated by infrabony pockets and osseous defects, or if the tooth is excessively mobile, checking the occlusion and adjusting it, if necessary, are essential. If the treated teeth are used as abutments for restorations, every effort should be made to align the occlusal forces along the vertical axes of the teeth in order to attain optimal bone repair.

ROOT RESECTION AND HEMISECTION IN THE MANAGEMENT OF FURCATION INVOLVEMENT

The treatment of advanced Grade II and Grade III furcation involvements will often require the removal or resection of a root.[1, 8] This will allow access to the remaining root surfaces for scaling and root planing and for the patient's plaque control. Root resection is the treatment of choice for many of the advanced furcation lesions when positive, definitive results are needed.

The following factors must be considered in the selection of a tooth for root resective therapy: (1) Advanced bone loss around one root with an acceptable level of bone around the remaining root(s), (2) Angulation and position of the tooth in the arch. A molar which is buccally or lingually out of position or mesially or distally tilted cannot be resected, (3) The divergence of the roots. Teeth with divergent roots are easier to resect, whereas teeth with closely approximated or fused roots are poor candidates for root resection. (4) The length and curvature of the roots are also important. Long, straight roots are more favorable than short, conical roots. (5) The feasibility of endodontics and restorative dentistry. If endodontic treatment and/or crown restorations are not possible, the tooth is not a candidate for resective therapy.

Figure 55–7B and C illustrates the difference between a root resection and a hemisection. The removal of a root without the removal of any portion of the crown is termed a **root resection** or **root amputation** procedure. When one root and its corresponding crown portion

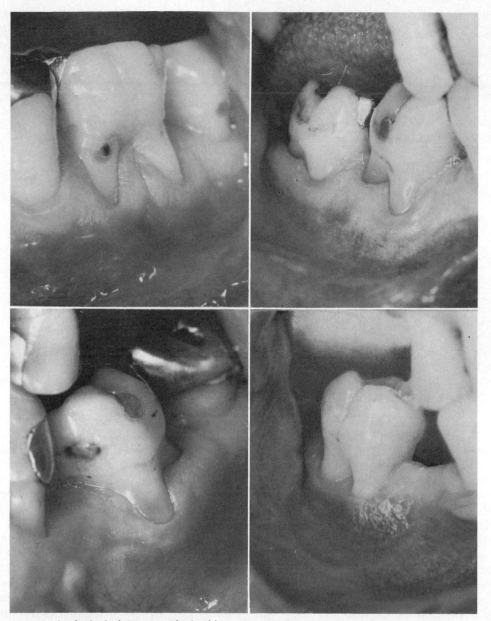

Figure 55–9 Optimal Gingival Contour Obtained by Treatment of Furcation Involvements of Different Severity.

are cut and removed, as in Figure 55–7C, the procedure is called a **hemisection.** This is often done for the mandibular molars and can consist of removal of either the mesial or the distal half depending on which root is involved. A crown and sometimes a fixed bridge are necessary following a hemisection procedure (see Fig. 55–7E).

The maxillary first molar usually presents the most favorable anatomic features for resective therapy (see Fig. 55–6). If the furcation involvement is between the two buccal roots and there are no interdental furcal lesions, the removal of the distal buccal root is the therapy of choice, since this root is usually the smallest in both diameter and length. When other furcal openings become involved, such as the mesial and distal interdental areas of the maxillary molars, the choice of the root to be resected must take into consideration the numerous factors of tooth and bone anatomy discussed earlier. A clinical study[7] has shown that removal of one of the buccal roots of a maxillary molar does not increase the mobility of the tooth in normal function; splinting is not always necessary.

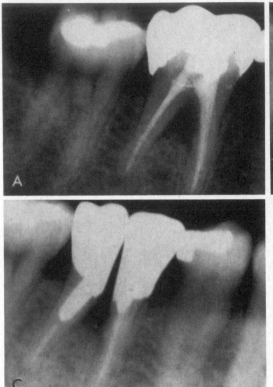

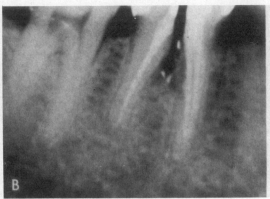

Figure 55–10 The Bisection Technique for Treatment of Furcation Involvements. *A,* Radiograph of a mandibular first molar with a furcation involvement. *B,* Bisection of the molar to eliminate the Class III furcation involvement. *C,* The final result of the bisection procedure, with crowns placed on each root.

The treatment of advanced Grade II or of Grade III furcations of a mandibular molar can also be accomplished by a **bisection** (bicuspidization) procedure if the molar presents the proper anatomic features and stability. Long divergent roots with the bone loss restricted to the furcal area are ideal for this procedure (Fig. 55–10). The molar is simply cut into two separate mesial and distal portions, without the removal of any part of the root or crown. The tunnel-like effect of the furcation involvement is eliminated by creating two separate teeth from the single molar (Fig. 55–10*B*). The two portions of the teeth will require crowns.

In most cases of root resection, the endodontic therapy is accomplished first, in which case the procedure is called **nonvital** root resection. But there are many cases in which the root is resected without endodontic therapy. This is done if one did not anticipate the resection of a root prior to surgery but, during periodontal flap surgery, the furcation involvement becomes visible. Also, many furca-involved teeth are difficult to diagnose by radiographs and probing alone, and one does not want to commit the patient to an endodontic procedure until the furcation area is examined after the flap is reflected. In these cases, the endodontic therapy can be done several days after the periodontal surgical procedure. Root resection without prior endodontic therapy is called **vital** resection therapy.

Another consideration in root resection procedures is the possibility that a second surgical procedure may be necessary several months after the resective therapy. This may occur in cases of close root proximity in which there are extensive osseous lesions around the resected root. The socket left by the removal of the root requires several months to fill and may leave a residual osseous defect close to the remaining roots. This may result in a vertical bone loss next to the adjacent roots (see Fig. 55–6*A*). Attempts to recontour the bone at the time of the initial surgery may result in excessive removal of bone. By allowing the bone to fill the socket, one can later reopen the area for a final, definitive osseous correction of the resected area. If the tooth presents widely divergent roots with good interradicular bone, the socket left by the removal of the root may not affect the remaining roots. In these cases, a second surgical procedure may not be necessary (Fig. 55–11).

Technique for Root Resection

The following steps are recommended:
1. Under local anesthesia, probe the area to determine the extent and outline of alveolar

Figure 55–11 Apical View of Two Maxillary Molars with Different Degrees of Root Proximity. *Left,* Close root proximity. After one root is resected, a defect may form that will require a second intervention. *Right,* Widely separated roots. A second surgical procedure may not be necessary.

LEFT   RIGHT

bone destruction around the root to be removed (Fig. 55–12*A*).

2. Elevate a mucoperiosteal flap (Fig. 55–12*B* and *C*).

3. With a contra-angle handpiece and a cross-cut bur, sever the root where it joins the crown (Fig. 55–12*D*). Remove the root (Fig. 55–12*E*).

4. With a stone or diamond point, smooth the resected root stump and contour the tooth to create an easily cleanable area (Fig. 55–12*F*).

5. Scale and plane the root surfaces, which becomes visible and more accessible when the root is removed. This is a most critical part of the treatment.

6. Clean the area, replace the flap, suture, and cover with a periodontal pack.

Remove the pack and sutures after 1 week. Physiologic gingival contour is usually restored by 2 months after surgery (Fig. 55–12*G*), and bone repair is detectable radiographically by 9 months (Fig. 55–12*H* and *I*).

Hemisection

Hemisection involves the same technique as is used for root resection, except that half the crown is removed along with one of the roots of a mandibular molar. The retained mesial or distal half serves as a useful abutment for a dental restoration (Fig. 55–13; see also Fig. 55–7).

Previous endodontic therapy is mandatory in cases in which the pulp chambers will be opened.

COMBINED PERIODONTAL-ENDODONTIC THERAPY

The periodontium is a continuous unit; pathologic involvement of the periapical area extends into the marginal area and vice versa.

Figure 55–14 diagrams the different ways in which pulpal and periodontal pathologic processes may be interrelated[10]:

1. A periapical lesion originating in a pulpal infection may have a pathway of fistulization from the apex and along the root to the gingiva (Fig. 55–14*A*). This can become secondarily complicated into a so-called retrograde periodontitis.[11] Pulpal infection can also extend through an accessory canal directly to the gingiva or to the furcation area, causing bone loss.[9] Differential diagnosis should consider whether the involved area is the only periodontally diseased part of the mouth and the pulpal and periapical status of the tooth. Isolated furcal radiolucencies in "pulpally suspect" teeth with no pockets may point to a pulpal origin of infection. In these cases endodontic therapy alone or with minimal periodontal treatment may be all that is needed (Fig. 55–15). If a long-standing, primarily endodontic, lesion has become periodontally involved, periodontal therapy may be necessary in addition to the endodontic treatment. However, it is frequently advisable to perform the endodontic therapy first and wait a few months before proceeding with periodontal treatment, as the remaining lesion may be considerably reduced if not totally eliminated after that time (Fig. 55–14*B*).

2. Marginal periodontitis can progress to the apex of a root or to the emergence of an accessory canal and induce a secondary pulpal involvement (Fig. 55–14*C* and *D*). Periodontal therapy is necessary in these cases, and the need for endodontic treatment will depend on tooth vitality. If the tooth is nonvital, either as a result of pathologic involvement of the pulp or because the pulp's blood vessels were severed during periodontal treatment, endodontic therapy will be indicated.

3. A true combined lesion is present when two separate lesions of endodontic and periodontal origin coalesce. In these cases both periodontal and endodontic therapy are indicated (Fig. 55–14*E*).

References follow on page 859

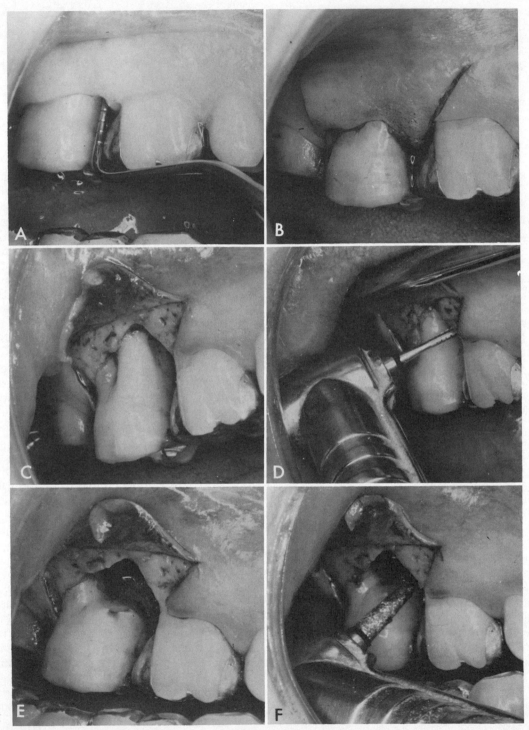

Figure 55–12 Resection of the Mesiofacial Root of a Molar with Furcation Involvement. *A,* Probing the extent of periodontal destruction. *B,* Incisions for a flap. *C,* Mucoperiosteal flap elevated, revealing extensive bone loss and an osseous defect on mesiofacial root. *D,* Root being resected with cross-cut bur. *E,* Root removed; sharp stump remains. *F,* Sharp stump planed and tooth contoured to facilitate cleaning. *G,* Area healed, showing excellent gingival contour where root was removed. *H,* Radiograph taken before treatment, showing extensive bone loss around mesiofacial root. *I,* Radiograph taken 9 months after treatment, showing bone repair where root was removed.

Illustration continued on opposite page

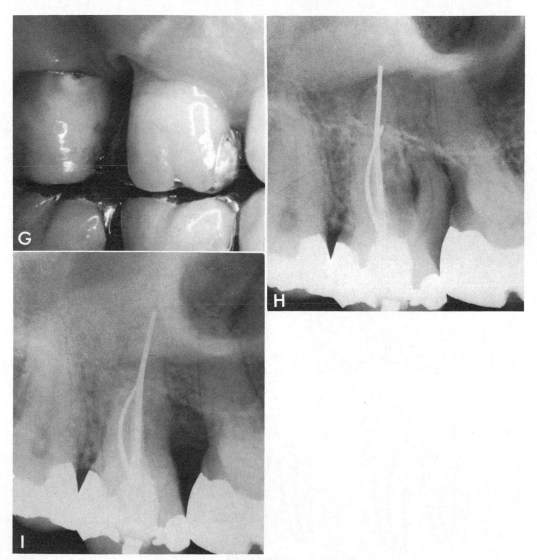

Figure 55–12 *Continued*

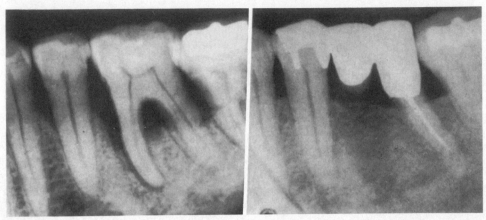

Figure 55–13 Hemisection. *Left,* Bifurcation involvement of first molar. *Right,* Radiograph taken 2 years and 3 months after resection of the mesial half of the first molar. (Courtesy of Dr. John Cane.)

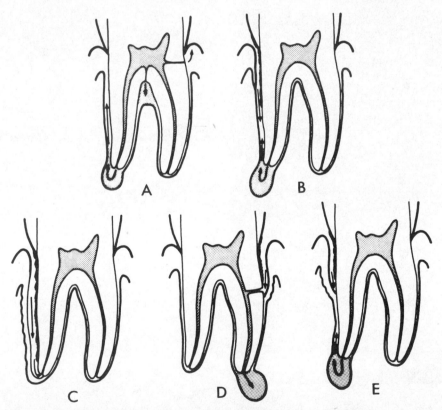

Figure 55–14 Diagrammatic Representation of Different Types of Endo-Periodontal Problems. *A,* An originally endodontic problem, with fistulization from the apex and along the root to the gingiva. Pulpal infection can also spread through accessory canals to the gingiva or to the furcation. *B,* A long-standing periapical lesion draining through the periodontal ligament can become secondarily complicated, leading to a "retrograde periodontitis." *C,* A periodontal pocket can deepen to the apex and secondarily involve the pulp. *D,* A periodontal pocket can infect the pulp through a lateral canal, and this, in turn, can result in a periapical lesion. *E,* Two independent lesions, periapical and marginal, can coexist and eventually fuse with each other. (Redrawn and modified from Simon, J. H. S., Glick, D. H., and Frank, A. L.: J. Periodontol., 43:202, 1972.)

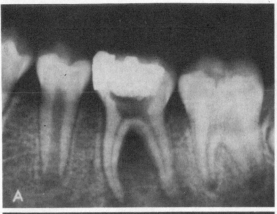

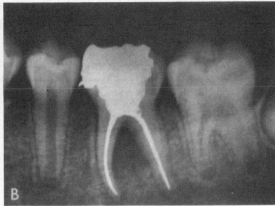

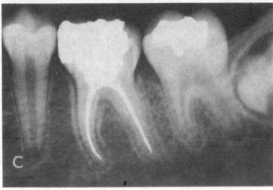

Figure 55–15 *A*, Extensive radiolucent area in furcation, apices, and distal aspect of lower first molar. *B*, Immediately after endodontic therapy. *C*, Complete healing of the lesion. No periodontal treatment was performed. (Courtesy of Dr. John Ingle and the School of Dentistry, University of Washington.)

REFERENCES

1. Amen, C. R.: Hemisection and root amputation. Periodontics, *4*:197, 1966.
2. Bower, R. C.: Furcation morphology relative to periodontal treatment: furcation entrance architecture. J. Periodontol., *50*:23, 1979.
3. Bower, R. C.: Furcation morphology relative to periodontal treatment: furcation root surface anatomy. J. Periodontol., *50*:366, 1979.
4. Ericsson, I., and Nyman, S.: Treatment of molar furcation involvement. Tandlakart., *65*:252, 1973.
5. Goldman, H. M.: Therapy of the incipient bifurcation involvement. J. Periodontol., *29*:112, 1958.
6. Hiatt, W. H.: Periodontic pocket elimination by combined endodontic-periodontic therapy. Periodontics, *1*:152, 1963.
7. Klavan, N.: Clinical observations following root amputations in maxillary molar teeth. J. Periodontol. *46*:1, 1975.
8. Messinger, T. F., and Orban, B. J.: Elimination of periodontal pockets by root amputation. J. Periodontol., *25*:213, 1954.
9. Orban, B. J., and Johnston, H.: Interradicular pathology as related to accessory root canals. J. Periodontol., *3*:21, 1948.
10. Simon, J. H. S., Glick, D. H., and Frank, A. L.: The relationship of endodontic-periodontic lesions. J. Periodontol., *43*:202, 1972.
11. Simring, M., and Goldberg, M.: The pulpal pocket approach: retrograde periodontitis. J. Periodontol., *35*:22, 1964.

Mucogingival Surgery

Mucogingival surgery consists of plastic surgical procedures for the correction of gingivo–mucous membrane relationships that complicate periodontal disease and may interfere with the success of periodontal treatment.

OBJECTIVES

Mucogingival surgery is performed as an adjunct to regular pocket elimination or as an independent procedure for the purpose of widening the zone of attached gingiva when an insufficient amount is present. The width of the attached gingiva varies in different individuals and on different teeth in the same individual (see Chapters 1 and 32). "Attached gingiva" is not synonymous with "keratinized gingiva," since the latter also includes the free gingival margin. The width of the attached gingiva is determined by subtracting the depth of the sulcus or pocket from the distance from the crest of the margin to the mucogingival junction.

The rationale for mucogingival surgery is predicated upon the assumption that a minimum width of attached gingiva is required for optimal gingival health to be maintained. However, several studies have challenged the view that a wide attached gingiva is more protective against the accumulation of plaque than a thin or a nonexistent zone.

No minimum width of attached gingiva has been established as a standard necessary for gingival health. Persons who practice excellent oral hygiene may maintain healthy areas with almost no attached gingiva.

Reduced or absent attached gingiva may be due to several factors:

1. **The base of the periodontal pocket being apical or close to the mucogingival line** (Figs. 56–1 and 56–2). In these cases, some attached gingiva must be created to separate the healed gingival sulcus from the alveolar mucosa and to prevent pockets from recurring. The functional adequacy of the attached gingiva can be predicted by the following *tension test:* Retract the cheeks and lips laterally with the fingers. If such tension pulls the marginal gingiva from the teeth, the attached gingiva is too narrow and should be widened when the pockets are treated.

2. **Frena and muscle attachments that encroach upon periodontal pockets and pull them away from the tooth surface.** Tension from such attachments (a) distends the gingival sulcus and fosters the accumulation of irritants that lead to gingivitis and pocket formation, and (b) aggravates the progression of periodontal pockets and causes their recurrence after treatment (Fig. 56–3). The problem is more common on the facial surface, but it occasionally occurs on the lingual surface (Fig. 56–4).

3. **Recession causing denudation of root surfaces** and creating a functional as well as an

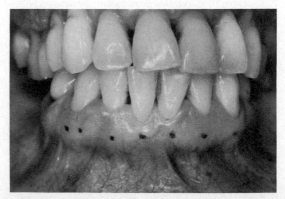

Figure 56–1 Deep Periodontal Pockets Encroach upon Mucogingival Line. Marks inserted to show location of the base of deep periodontal pockets in relation to the mucogingival line.

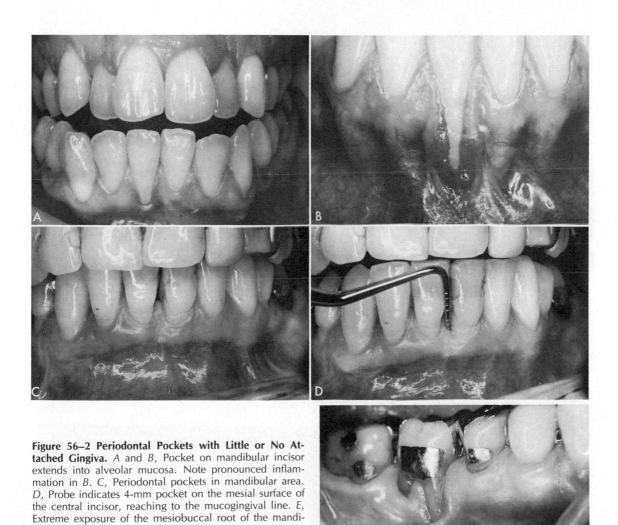

Figure 56–2 Periodontal Pockets with Little or No Attached Gingiva. *A* and *B*, Pocket on mandibular incisor extends into alveolar mucosa. Note pronounced inflammation in *B*. *C*, Periodontal pockets in mandibular area. *D*, Probe indicates 4-mm pocket on the mesial surface of the central incisor, reaching to the mucogingival line. *E*, Extreme exposure of the mesiobuccal root of the mandibular first molar.

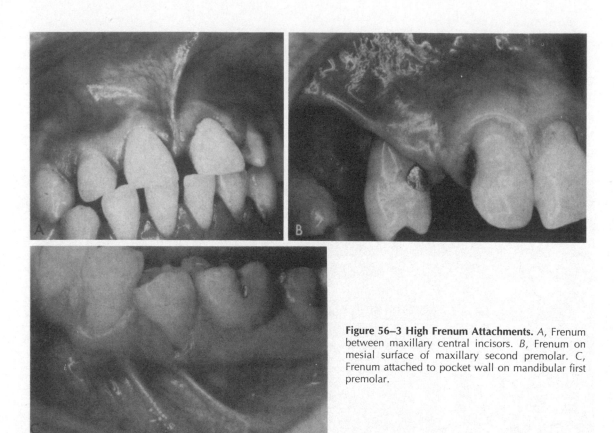

Figure 56–3 High Frenum Attachments. *A*, Frenum between maxillary central incisors. *B*, Frenum on mesial surface of maxillary second premolar. *C*, Frenum attached to pocket wall on mandibular first premolar.

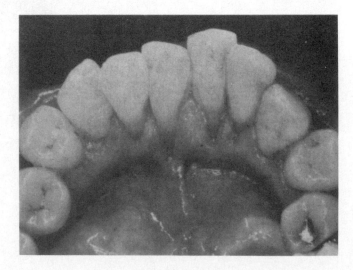

Figure 56–4 Frenum attached to pocket wall on lingual surface of incisor.

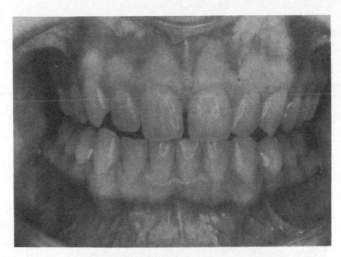

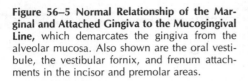

Figure 56–5 Normal Relationship of the Marginal and Attached Gingiva to the Mucogingival Line, which demarcates the gingiva from the alveolar mucosa. Also shown are the oral vestibule, the vestibular fornix, and frenum attachments in the incisor and premolar areas.

esthetic problem. The tension test should also be used in cases of progressive gingival recession to check the effect of soft tissue tension on the gingival margin. Clinical examination and probing will reveal these areas of root denudation.

It should be noted that *deepening of the vestibule is not important in relation to periodontal therapy.*[4] Increasing the depth of the vestibule is very important in the surgical preparation of edentulous ridges.

FACTORS THAT AFFECT THE OUTCOME OF MUCOGINGIVAL SURGERY

Anatomic Structures

The structures involved in mucogingival surgery are the margin and attached gingivae; mucogingival line (junction) (Figs. 56–5 and 56–6); alveolar mucosa; periodontal ligament; cementum; alveolar bone and alveolar periosteum; regional blood vessels, lymphatics, and nerves; muscle and frenum attachments; and fornix of the oral vestibule. The reader is referred to Chapters 1 to 4 for a review of these structures, except for muscle and frenum attachments and the mental nerve, which are discussed here.

MUSCLE ATTACHMENTS. Tension from high muscle attachments interferes with mucogingival surgery by causing postoperative reduction in vestibular depth and width of the attached gingiva. To prevent this, muscle attachments in the operative field must be separated from the bone (Fig. 56–7). The following muscles may be encountered in mucogingival operations:

1. The *mentalis:* Originates on the facial surface of the alveolar process in the incisive

fossa and is inserted into the skin of the chin (Fig. 56–8).

2. The *incisivus labii inferioris:* Originates on the alveolar process close to the border in

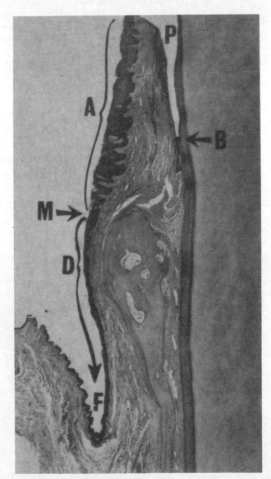

Figure 56–6 Mucogingival Area. Periodontal pocket (P) encroaches upon the mucogingival line (M). The bottom of the pocket is at B. Part of the attached gingiva (A) forms the wall of the pocket. Also note the alveolar mucosa (D) and the vestibular fornix (F).

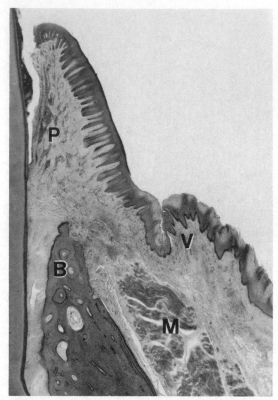

Figure 56–7 Muscle Attachment (M) close to vestibular fornix (V) and crest of the facial bone (B) in an autopsied jaw with periodontal disease. P, periodontal pocket.

the mandibular lateral incisor area and passes to the lower lip.

3. The *depressor labii inferioris:* Originates on the oblique line of the mandible between the symphysis and the mental foramen and passes upward and medially into the lower lip, where it blends with the orbicularis oris and fibers of the opposite side (Fig. 56–8).

4. The *depressor anguli oris (triangularis):* Originates on the oblique line of the mandible to be inserted into the angle of the mouth (Fig. 56–8).

5. The *incisivus labii superioris:* Originates from the alveolar process close to the border in the maxillary lateral incisor area and passes to the upper lip.

6. The *levator anguli oris (caninus):* Arises from the canine fossa below the infraorbital foramen and inserts into the angle of the mouth (Fig. 56–8).

7. The *buccinator:* Attaches along the apical portion of the alveolar process from the maxillary first molar to the posterior portion of the maxilla and on the mandible in the lower end of the retromolar fossa and in the external oblique line (Fig. 56–8).

THE MENTAL NERVE. Trauma to the mental nerve can produce uncomfortable paresthesia of the lip, which recovers slowly. Familiarity with the location and appearance of the mental nerve reduces the likelihood of injuring it. The mental nerve emerges from the mental foramen, located apical to the first and second mandibular premolars, and usually divides into three branches (Figs. 56–9 and 56–10). One turns forward and downward to the skin of the chin. The other two course anteriorly and upward to supply the skin and mucous membrane of the lower lip and the mucosa of the labial alveolar surface.

Irregularity of Teeth

Abnormal tooth alignment is an important cause of gingival deformities that require cor-

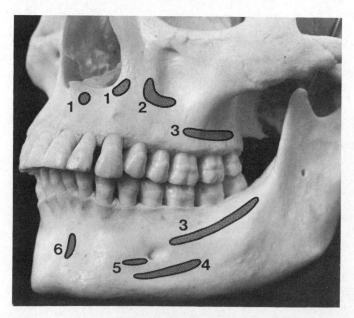

Figure 56–8 Muscle Attachments That May Be Encountered in Mucogingival Surgery. 1, Nasalis; 2, levator anguli oris; 3, buccinator; 4, depressor anguli oris; 5, depressor labii inferioris; 6, mentalis.

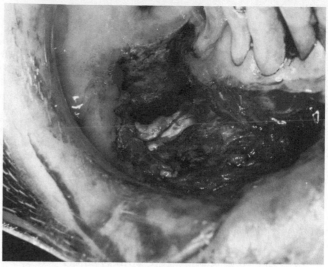

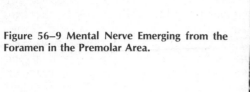

Figure 56–9 Mental Nerve Emerging from the Foramen in the Premolar Area.

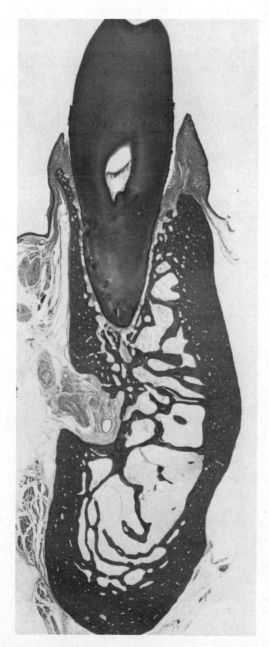

Figure 56–10 Mental Nerve and Blood Vessels in Mental Foramen. Note the relationship of the mental foramen to the apex of the second premolar and the oral vestibule.

rective surgery and is an important factor in determining the outcome of treatment. The location of the gingival margin, the width of the attached gingiva, and alveolar bone height and thickness are all affected by tooth alignment. On teeth that are tilted or rotated labially, the labial bony plate is thinner and located farther apically than on the adjacent teeth, and the gingiva is receded so that the root is exposed.[119] On the lingual surface of such teeth, the gingiva is bulbous and the bone margins are closer to the cemento-enamel junction. The level of gingival attachment on root surfaces and the width of the attached gingiva following mucogingival surgery are affected as much, or more, by tooth alignment as by variations in treatment procedures.

Orthodontic correction is indicated when mucogingival surgery is performed on malposed teeth in an attempt to widen the attached gingiva or to restore the gingiva over denuded roots. If orthodontic treatment is not feasible, the prominent tooth should be ground to within the borders of the alveolar bone, with special care taken to avoid pulp injury.

Roots covered with thin bony plates present a hazard in mucogingival surgery. Even the simplest type of flap (partial thickness) creates the risk of bone resorption on the periosteal surface.[46] Resorption in amounts that ordinarily are not significant may cause loss of bone height when the bony plate is thin or tapered at the crest.

The Mucogingival Line (Junction)

Normally, the mucogingival line in the incisor and canine areas is located approximately 3 mm apical to the crest of the alveolar bone on the radicular surfaces and 5 mm interdentally.[99] In periodontal disease and on malposed disease-free teeth, the bone margin is located farther apically and may extend beyond the mucogingival line.

The distance between the mucogingival line and the cemento-enamel junction before and after periodontal surgery is not necessarily constant. After inflammation is eliminated, there is a tendency for the tissue to contract and draw the mucogingival line in the direction of the crown.[31]

MUCOGINGIVAL OPERATIONS

Descriptions of those operations that have been shown in human and animal studies to be useful, with their accomplishments and limitations, are presented in this chapter. Research findings in some instances are inconclusive or conflicting. This is to be expected for many reasons: subtle differences in the way the same operation is performed by different operators; the difficulty of obtaining histologic material to corroborate what appear to be obvious clinical results; differences between postoperative healing of artificially created and naturally occurring periodontal lesions; differences in tissue response among animal species, between animals and humans, and among different individuals; differences in oral hygiene among humans; and the difference between pretreatment and posttreatment *impressions* gathered from clinical observations and photographs and *facts* based on measurements subjected to statistical analysis.

Initially, the operation that was advocated was a partial thickness flap for the purpose of deepening the vestibular fornix, increasing the width of the attached gingiva, and relocating frenum attachments. Variations of this technique included using a full thickness (mucoperiosteal) flap or a combined full thickness flap in the coronal portion and a partial thickness flap in the apical portion; this modification was based on the assumption that the level to which the bone was denuded would determine the posttreatment width of the attached gingiva (Figs. 56–11 and 56–12).

The postoperative course with these techniques was stormy, sometimes including painful ulcerations or numbness of the lower lip. Moreover, results were not favorable. The increased vestibular depth created with partial thickness operations shrunk during the healing process and practically disappeared in a few months. Increased depths created with full thickness operations tended to be more stable, but a significant marginal bone loss occurred.[20] Combination methods had the disadvantages of both techniques with none of their virtues. From these unsuccessful attempts, however, some of the currently used techniques evolved.

Gingival Extension Procedures

Two types of procedures are currently performed in order to widen the zone of attached gingiva:

1. The *gingival extension operations,* which consist of the surgical deepening of the mucogingival line. In order to prevent the mucogingival line from creeping back coronally during postoperative healing, two methods have

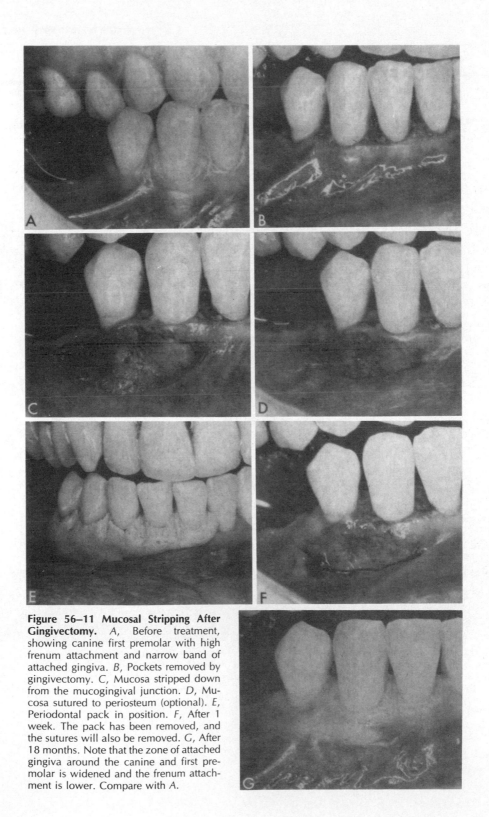

Figure 56–11 Mucosal Stripping After Gingivectomy. *A,* Before treatment, showing canine first premolar with high frenum attachment and narrow band of attached gingiva. *B,* Pockets removed by gingivectomy. *C,* Mucosa stripped down from the mucogingival junction. *D,* Mucosa sutured to periosteum (optional). *E,* Periodontal pack in position. *F,* After 1 week. The pack has been removed, and the sutures will also be removed. *G,* After 18 months. Note that the zone of attached gingiva around the canine and first premolar is widened and the frenum attachment is lower. Compare with *A.*

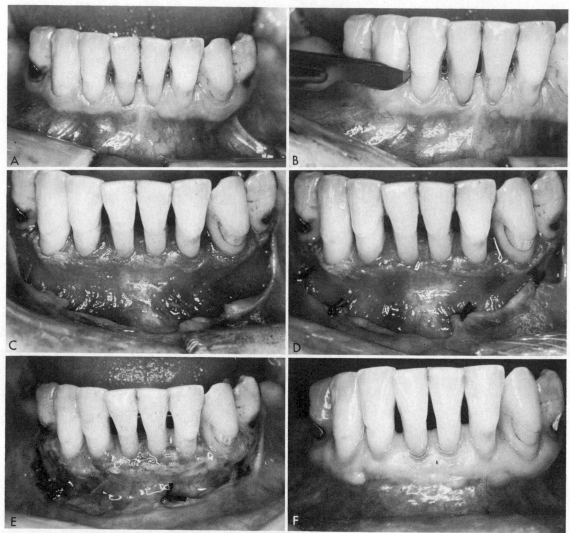

Figure 56–12 Mucosal Stripping with Internal Bevel. *A*, Before treatment, showing periodontal pockets, exposed roots, and narrow band of attached gingiva. *B*, Inner surface of periodontal pockets resected with internal bevel. *C*, Mucosa has been separated away, leaving the bone covered with periosteum. The inner pocket walls have been removed from the teeth, and the roots are scaled. *D*, The mucosa is sutured to the periosteum (optional). *E*, After 1 week, the periodontal pack has been removed, and the sutures will also be removed. *F*, After 8 months. The pockets are eliminated, and there is a widened zone of attached gingiva. Compare with *A*.

proved useful, the placement of a *free mucosal autograft* and the so-called *fenestration procedure.* The former is more predictable and heals with fewer problems, in spite of the two surgical sites needed. It is therefore preferred.

2. The *apical displacement of the existing pocket wall,* which becomes attached to the cementum and/or bone and takes on the appearance and function of attached gingiva.

FREE GINGIVAL AUTOGRAFTS. Free gingival grafts are used to create a widened zone of attached gingiva. They were initially described by Bjorn in 1963[7] and have been extensively investigated in the last two decades.

Procedure. Step 1: Eliminate the Pockets. With a gingivectomy incision, resect the periodontal pockets and scale and plane the root surfaces.

Step 2: Prepare the Recipient Site. The purpose of this step is to prepare a firm connective tissue bed to receive the graft. The recipient site can be prepared by incising at the existing mucogingival junction with a No. 15 Bard-Parker knife to a little more than the desired depth, blending the incision on both ends with the existing mucogingival line. Periosteum should be left covering the bone.

Another technique consists of outlining the recipient site with two vertical incisions from the cut gingival margin into the alveolar mucosa (Fig. 56–13A and B). Extend the incisions to approximately twice the desired width of the attached gingiva, allowing for 50 per cent contraction of the graft when healing is complete. The amount of contraction depends upon the extent to which the recipient site penetrates the muscle attachments. The deeper the recipient site, the greater is the tendency for the muscles to elevate the graft and reduce the final width of the attached gingiva. The periosteum along the apical border of the graft is sometimes penetrated in an effort to prevent postoperative narrowing of the attached gingiva.[13]

Insert a No. 15 Bard-Parker blade along the cut gingival margin and separate a flap consisting of epithelium and underlying connective tissue without disturbing the periosteum. Extend the flap to the depth of the vertical incisions. Suture the flap where the apical position of the free graft will be located.

If a narrow band of attached gingiva remains after the pockets are eliminated, it should be left intact and the recipient site started by inserting the blade at the mucogingival junction instead of at the cut gingival margin.

Prepare the recipient bed for the graft by removing extraneous soft tissue with curved scissors or tissue nippers, leaving a firm connective tissue surface. Control the bleeding with a 2-inch × 2-inch sponge and pressure, and protect the area with a sponge moistened with saline. Make a tinfoil or wax template of the recipient site to be used as a pattern for the graft (Fig. 56–13C and D).

Grafts can also be placed directly on bone tissue. For this technique the flap has to be separated by blunt dissection with a periosteal elevator. Reported advantages of this variant are less postoperative mobility of the graft, less swelling, better hemostasis,[32] and one and one-half to two times less shrinkage[57, 58]; a healing lag is observed for the first 2 weeks, however.[18, 19, 33]

Step 3: Obtain the Graft from the Donor Site. A partial thickness graft is used; the sites from which it is obtained are, in order of preference, attached gingiva, masticatory mucosa from an edentulous ridge, and palatal mucosa. The graft should consist of epithelium and a thin layer of underlying connective tissue. Proper thickness is important for survival of the graft. It should be thin enough to permit ready diffusion of nutritive fluid from the recipient site, which is essential in the immediate posttransplant period. A graft that is too thin may shrivel and expose the recipient site.[68, 78] If the graft is too thick, its peripheral layer is jeopardized because of the excessive tissue that separates it from new circulation and nutrients.[45] Thick grafts may also create a deeper wound at the donor site, with the possibility of injuring major palatal arteries.[109] The ideal thickness of a graft is between 1.0 and 1.5 mm.[50, 68]

Place the template over the donor site, and make a shallow incision around it with a No. 15 Bard-Parker blade. Insert the blade to the desired thickness at one edge of the graft. Elevate the edge and hold it with tissue forceps. Continue to separate the graft with the blade, lifting it gently as separation progresses to provide visibility. Placing sutures at the margins of the graft helps control it during separation and transfer and simplifies placement and suturing to the recipient site.[3]

After the graft is separated, remove loose tissue tabs from the undersurface. Thin the edge to avoid bulbous marginal and interdental contours. Special precautions must be taken with grafts from the palate. The submucosa in the posterior region is thick and fatty and should be trimmed so that it will not interfere with vascularization. Grafts tend to re-estab-

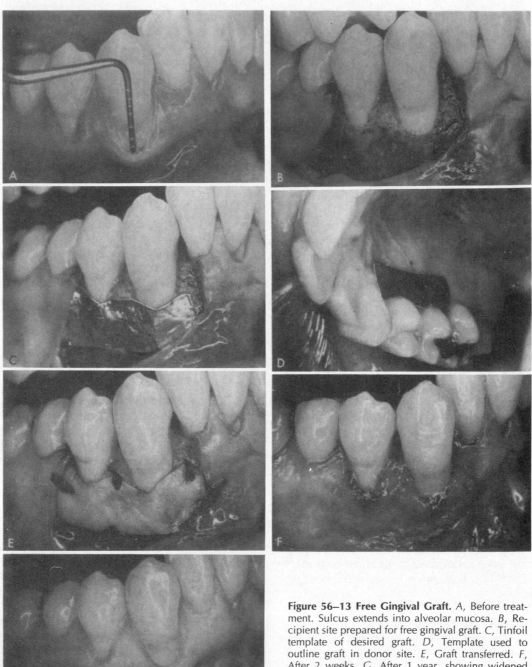

Figure 56–13 Free Gingival Graft. *A,* Before treatment. Sulcus extends into alveolar mucosa. *B,* Recipient site prepared for free gingival graft. *C,* Tinfoil template of desired graft. *D,* Template used to outline graft in donor site. *E,* Graft transferred. *F,* After 2 weeks. *G,* After 1 year, showing widened zone of attached gingiva.

lish their original epithelial structure, so mucous glands may occur in grafts obtained from the palate.

Step 4: Transfer and Immobilize the Graft. Remove the sponge from the recipient site; reapply it, with pressure if necessary, until bleeding is stopped. Clean away excess clot. A thick clot interferes with vascularization of the graft[74]; it is also an excellent medium for bacteria and increases the risk of infection.

Position the graft and adapt it firmly to the recipient site. Space between the graft and the underlying tissue (dead space) will retard vascularization and jeopardize the graft. Suture the graft at the lateral borders and to the periosteum to secure it in position (Fig. 56–13E). Before suturing is completed, elevate the unsutured portion and cleanse the recipient bed beneath it with an aspirator to remove clot or loose tissue fragments. Press the graft back into position and complete the sutures. Be sure the graft is immobilized, because movement interferes with healing. Avoid excessive tension, which will warp the graft and may pull it away from the underlying surface. **Respect for tissue is essential for success.** Use every precaution to avoid injury to the graft. Use tissue forceps delicately to avoid crushing it. Use a minimum number of sutures to avoid unnecessary tissue penetration. The graft can survive some injury, but abuse may damage it beyond recovery.

Step 5: Protect the Donor Site. Cover the donor site with a periodontal pack for 1 week and repeat if necessary (Fig. 56–13F). Retention of the pack on the donor site is sometimes a problem. If facial attached gingiva was used, the pack may be retained by locking it through the interproximal spaces onto the lingual surface. If there are no open interdental spaces, the pack can be covered by a plastic stent wired to the teeth. A modified Hawley retainer is useful to cover the pack on the palate and over edentulous ridges.

The Fate of the Graft. The success of the graft depends upon survival of the connective tissue (Fig. 56–13G). Sloughing of the epithelium occurs in most cases, but the extent to which the connective tissue withstands the transfer to the new location determines the fate of the graft. Fibrous organization of the interface between the graft and the recipient bed occurs within 2 to several days.[96]

The graft is initially maintained by a diffusion of fluid from the host bed, adjacent gingiva, and alveolar mucosa.[41] The fluid is a transudate from the host vessels and provides nutrition and hydration essential for the initial survival of the transplanted tissues. During the first day, the connective tissue becomes edematous and disorganized and undergoes degeneration and lysis of some of its elements. As healing progresses, the edema is resolved and degenerated connective tissue is replaced by new granulation tissue.

Revascularization of the graft starts by the second[12] or third day.[59] Capillaries from the recipient bed and from periodontal ligament included in the recipient site proliferate into the graft to form a network of new capillaries and anastomose with pre-existing vessels.[59] Many of the graft vessels degenerate and are replaced by new ones, and some participate in the new circulation. The central section of the surface is the last to vascularize, but this is complete by the tenth day.

The epithelium undergoes degeneration and sloughing, with complete necrosis occurring in some areas.[17, 93] It is replaced by new epithelium from the borders of the recipient site. A thin layer of new epithelium is present by the fourth day, with rete pegs developing by the seventh day. In skin grafts, the basement membrane remains in situ, disengaged from the overlying epithelium and attached to the underlying connective tissue. New epithelial cells migrate over the basal membrane and appear to be guided by it. The plasma membrane of the cells thickens and forms hemidesmosomes that attach to the basement membrane, and the regenerating epithelium synthesizes new basement membrane.[42]

The fact that heterotopically placed grafts maintain their structure (keratinized epithelium) even after the grafted epithelium has become necrotic and has been replaced from neighboring areas of nonkeratinized epithelium suggests that there exists a genetic predetermination of the specific character of the oral mucosa that is dependent on stimuli that originate in the connective tissue.[61] It has been shown in clinical studies that the width of keratinized gingiva can be extended by means of grafts composed only of connective tissue obtained from areas where it is covered by keratinized epithelium.[14, 30, 37]

As seen microscopically, healing of a graft of intermediate thickness (0.75 mm) is complete by 10½ weeks; thicker grafts (1.75 mm) may require 16 weeks or longer.[44]

The gross appearance of the graft reflects the tissue changes within it. At the time of transplantation the graft vessels empty, and the graft is pale. The pallor changes to an ischemic grayish white during the first 2 days, until vascularization begins and a pink color appears. The plasmatic circulation accumulates and causes softening and swelling of the graft, which are reduced when the edema is removed from the recipient site by the new blood vessels. Loss of epithelium leaves the graft smooth and shiny. New epithelium creates a thin, gray, veil-like surface which develops normal features as the epithelium matures.

Functional integration of the graft occurs by the seventeenth day, but the graft is morphologically distinguishable from the surrounding tissue for months. It may eventually blend with adjacent tissues, but more often, although it is pink, firm, and healthy, it tends to be somewhat bulbous (Figs. 56–14 and 56–15). This ordinarily presents no problem, but if it traps irritating plaque or is esthetically unacceptable, thinning of the graft may be necessary.

Thinning Bulbous Grafts. Paring down the surface will not reduce the bulbous condition, because the surface epithelium tends to proliferate again. The graft should be thinned as follows:

Step 1. With a No. 15 Bard-Parker blade, make vertical incisions along the lateral border of the graft to the gingival margin. If the graft does not extend to the gingival margin, make the incisions along three of the borders.

Step 2. Elevate the graft from the underlying periosteum, and thin it by removing tissue from the undersurface.

Step 3. Replace the graft and suture.

Accomplishments of Free Gingival Grafts. Free gingival grafts effectively widen the attached gingiva. Several biometric studies have analyzed the width of the attached gingiva after the placement of a free gingival graft.[16, 53, 57] James et al.[57] have reported that after 24 weeks, grafts placed on denuded bone shrink 25 per cent, whereas grafts placed on periosteum shrink 50 per cent. The greatest amount of shrinkage occurs within the first 6 weeks.

The placement of a gingival graft, however, does not per se improve the status of the gingiva in comparison with that of the gingiva surrounding contralateral teeth with equal degrees of recession where no graft was placed, provided plaque control is equivalent on both sides.[35, 36, 107] Therefore, the indication for a free gingival graft should be based on the presence of *progressive gingival recession and inflammation*. When recession continues to progress after a period of a few months with good plaque control, a graft can be placed in order to prevent further recession and loss of attached gingiva.

Other materials have been used to replace gingival tissue in gingival extension operations. Attempts with lyophilized dura mater[62, 89] and with sclera[72] have not been satisfactory; the use of irradiated free gingival allografts showed satisfactory results,[87] but further research is necessary before they can be considered for clinical use.

Free Gingival Grafts and Denuded Roots. Grafts placed over exposed roots generally shrink, re-exposing the root.[81] Some degree of success may, however, be expected if the defect is long and narrow.

Since the vascular bed is required for preservation of a free gingival graft, grafts cannot be expected to correct extensive root exposure.[56, 96] However, if the gingival defect is narrow, collateral circulation from the connective tissue around the margins of the recipient site aids survival of the graft over the root.[101] The graft may be firmly adherent and resist separation from the tooth by a periodontal probe,[71] but the extent to which it is reattached to the root by new fibers embedded into new cementum has not been established. Reattachment of free gingival grafts has been reported on artificially exposed roots in animals,[73] but the results in humans are as yet inconclusive.[100, 102]

Free autogenous gingival grafts have been found useful for covering "nonpathologic" dehiscences and fenestrations; "nonpathologic" refers to openings of the bone through the tooth surface not previously exposed to the oral environment and found in the course of flap surgery.[34]

Although in general free gingival grafts placed on denuded roots will shrink and re-expose the root, when placed apical to the denuded area they prevent further recession. Some authors have reported the occurrence of creeping reattachment as 11 to 24 per cent, depending on the recession width.[65, 109]

FENESTRATION OPERATION. This operation is designed to widen the zone of attached gingiva with a minimum loss of bone height.[83-85] It has also been called periosteal separation.[27] It utilizes a partial thickness flap, except in a rectangular area at the base of the operative field, where the periosteum is elevated and the bone is exposed (Fig. 56–16). This is the area of fenestration. Its purpose is to create a scar that is firmly bound to the bone and will prevent separation from the bone and narrowing of the width of the attached zone.

Procedure. *Step 1: Eliminate the Periodontal Pockets.* A gingivectomy incision should be used (Fig. 56–17*B*).

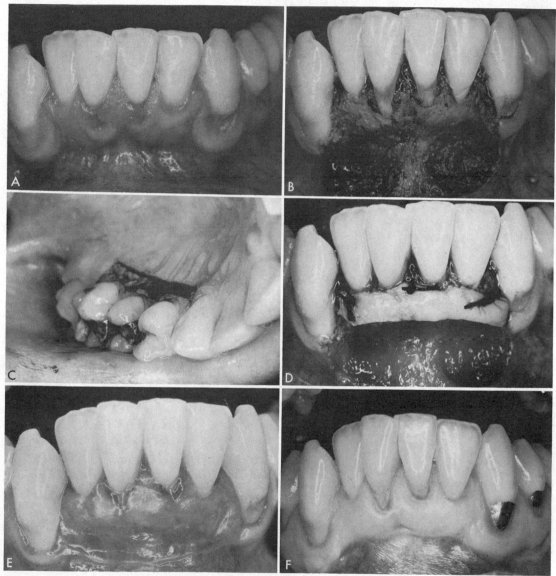

Figure 56–14 Free Gingival Graft (same patient as in Fig. 56–13). *A,* Before treatment. Pockets extend into alveolar mucosa. *B,* Recipient site prepared for graft. *C,* Graft obtained from the palate. *D,* Graft sutured in position. *E,* After 2 weeks. *F,* After 1 year. Note the widened zone of attached gingiva.

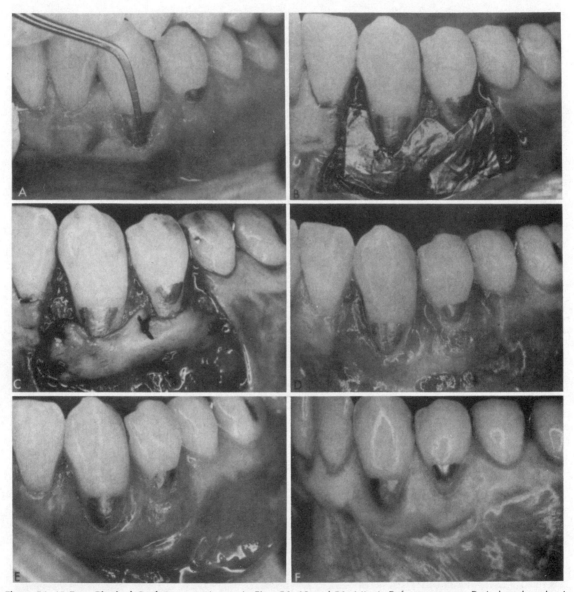

Figure 56–15 Free Gingival Graft (same patient as in Figs. 56–13 and 56–14). *A,* Before treatment. Periodontal pocket in the canine extends into the alveolar mucosa. *B,* Recipient site prepared and template made for desired graft. *C,* Graft sutured in place. *D,* After 2 weeks. *E,* After 9 weeks. *F,* After 1 year. Note the widened zone of healthy attached gingiva. Compare with *A.*

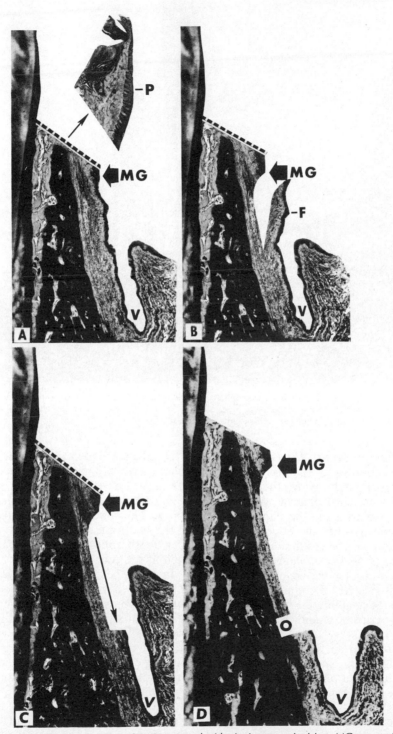

Figure 56–16 Fenestration. *A,* Periodontal pocket (P) resected with gingivectomy incision. MG, mucogingival junction; V, vestibular fornix. *B,* Incision at mucogingival junction separates partial thickness flap (F), leaving periosteum and a layer of connective tissue on the bone. *C,* Partial thickness flap moved apically, deepening the oral vestibule (V). *D,* Fenestration (O) cut through the periosteum, leaving the bone exposed.

Illustration continued on following page

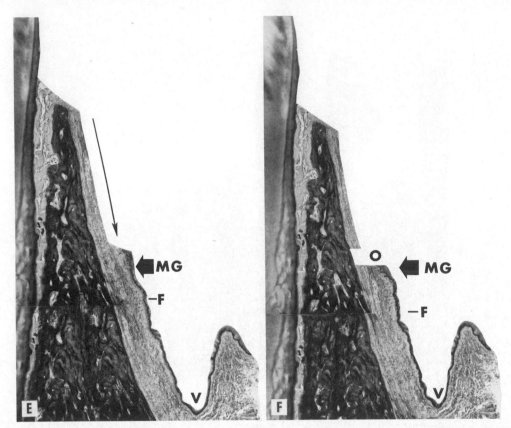

Figure 56–16 *Continued E*, Variation of operation when little or no attached gingiva remains following gingivectomy. Partial thickness flap is separated at the cut gingival margin and moved apically (F), deepening the oral vestibule (V) in the process. *F*, Fenestration (O) cut through the periosteum, exposing the bone.

Step 2: Elevate a Partial Thickness Flap. Extend the dissection apically (Fig. 56–17C) to a level approximately twice the desired width of the new attached gingiva. With scissors, remove irregularities in the flap margin. Slide the flap apically until the edge is at the newly created level of the vestibule.

Step 3: Cleanse the Periosteum. At this stage, there is a wide area of bone covered by periosteum and a thin layer of connective tissue. With scissors, remove all muscle fibers and soft tissue from the periosteum until the surface is smooth and firm.

Step 4: Fenestration. At the deepest level in the vestibule, make an incision through the periosteum to the labial plate along the length of the operative field. Bluntly dissect the periosteum and overlying tissue from the bone (a fenestration) across the operative field (Fig. 56–17C). The margin of the flap may be sutured to the periosteum at the lower border of the fenestrated area, but this is not necessary.

Apply pressure with 2-inch × 2-inch gauze pads until the bleeding stops; remove excess clot, then insert a periodontal pack (Fig. 53–17D). Replace the pack after 2 weeks and twice at weekly intervals if needed. If sutures are used, remove them after 1 week.

Accomplishments of the Fenestration Operation. The fenestration produces an increase in the width of attached gingiva and in vestibular depth approximately one half of that created at the time of operation.

In the fenestration area, a scar forms that ultimately develops microscopic features resembling those of attached gingiva.[77, 84] The scar is initially firmly attached to the underlying bone[23] and prevents narrowing of the new zone of attached gingiva (Fig. 56–17F). The binding effect lasts about 4 weeks. By 3 months the width of the attached gingiva is reduced by approximately 28 per cent[82]; it remains that way for approximately a year, after which the width is usually further reduced. **Post-treatment shrinkage of the attached gingiva is anticipated at the time of operation by providing space for twice the desired width of attached gingiva.**

The tendency of repositioned muscle attachments to return to their original position is an

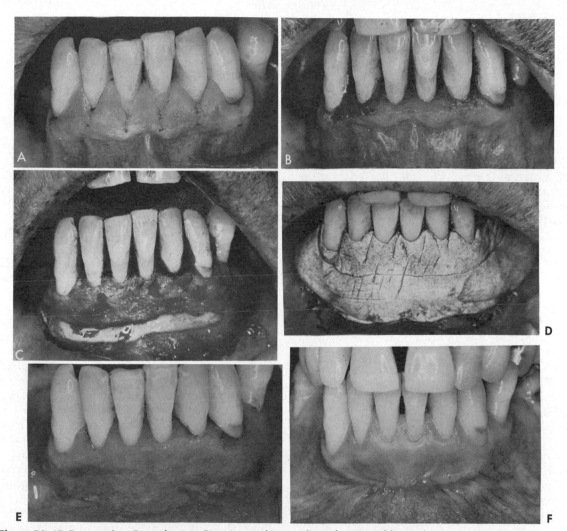

Figure 56–17 Fenestration Operation. *A,* Pinpoint markings indicate location of base of periodontal pockets close to mucogingival line. *B,* After the removal of pockets by gingivectomy. Note the absence of attached gingiva in the lateral incisor and canine area *(left)*. *C,* Flap reflected with periosteum intact. Bone denuded of periosteum in horizontal area at the base of the fornix. *D,* Periodontal pack in place. *E,* Three weeks postoperation. *F,* Five months postoperation. Note the wide zone of attached gingiva with a scar at its base.

important limiting factor in vestibular extension operations. The most lasting results are obtained when minimal invasion of the musculature is required in order to create increased space for attached gingiva.[77] Muscle attachments encountered in the course of deepening the vestibule must be removed to reduce the likelihood of their return. Contraction of the scar also tends to reduce posttreatment vestibular depth.[94]

Other Techniques

THE APICALLY POSITIONED FLAP. Positioned flaps are used to correct mucogingival deformities; they avoid some of the limitations of gingival extension operations and require less extensive surgical interference.[2, 39, 40, 65, 66] This operation utilizes the apically positioned flap, partial thickness or full thickness, for the combined purposes of eliminating pockets and widening the zone of attached gingiva. The partial thickness (mucosal) flap is generally used to avoid exposure of bone and the accompanying risks of bone resorption and aggravation of bone dehiscences and fenestrations.[86, 95] The full thickness (mucoperiosteal) flap is indicated when access to the bone for recontouring purposes is also desired.

A step-by-step description of the surgical technique for apically positioned flaps is given in Chapter 50 and is shown in Figures 56–18 to 56–22.

Accomplishments. The apically positioned full thickness flap operation increases the width of the attached gingiva and relocates the fornix of the vestibule and frena apically. It results in less postoperative discomfort and heals more rapidly than gingival extension procedures. The width of the attached gingiva is increased by approximately half the pretreatment depth of the pockets.[32]

The edge of the flap may be located in three positions in relation to the bone: (1) *Slightly coronal to the crest of the bone.* This location attempts to preserve the attachment of supracrestal fibers; it may also result in thick gingival margins and interdental papillae with deep sulci and may create the risk of recurrent pockets. (2) *At the level of the crest of the labial plate* (Fig. 56–18C). This results in a satisfactory gingival contour, provided the flap is adequately thinned. (3) *Two millimeters short of the crest* (Fig. 56–18D). This position produces the most desirable gingival contour and the same posttreatment level of gingival attachment as is obtained by placing the flap

at the crest of the bone.[40] New tissue will cover the crest of the bone to produce a firm, tapered gingival margin. Placing the flap short of the crest increases the risk of a slight reduction in bone height,[28] but this is compensated for by the advantages of a well-formed gingival margin.

The posttreatment width of the attached gingiva can be estimated before the operation by using the following formula:

Estimated posttreatment width of attached gingiva =

$$\frac{\text{Pretreatment depth of pockets}}{2} + \frac{\text{Pretreatment width of attached gingiva}}{}$$

This is applicable if the flap is positioned at the crest. Since the pocket wall contributes to the increase in attached gingiva, the operation is best suited for patients with deep pockets who require additional attached gingiva. The final width of the attached gingiva may be increased by placing the flap farther apically from the crest (Figs. 56–19 and 56–20).

VESTIBULAR EXTENSION OPERATION. This technique, originally described by Edlan and Mejchar,[38] produces statistically significant widening of attached nonkeratinized tissue. This increase in width in the mandibular area reportedly persists in patients observed for periods of up to 5 years.[38, 88, 108]

Procedure. Step 1: Outline the Operative Field (Fig. 56–23). Starting at the junction of the gingival margin and attached gingiva, make a vertical incision at each end of the operative field, extending approximately 12 mm from the alveolar margin into the vestibule. Join the vertical incisions with a horizontal incision.

Step 2: Reflect a Flap (Fig. 56–23B). Separate a mucosal flap and elevate it to expose the periosteum of the bone.

Step 3: Separate the Periosteum from the Bone (Fig. 56–23C). Starting at the crest of the facial bone, just under the elevated flap, separate the periosteum and attached muscle fibers from the bone and transpose them to the lip.

Step 4: Replace the Mucosal Flap (Fig. 56–23D). Fold the mucosal flap down over the bone and suture it to the inner surface of the periosteum. The fornix of the vestibule is now formed by the junction of the mucosal flap and the transposed periosteum.

Step 5: Suture the Periosteum (Fig. 56–23E). The upper edge of the periosteum is sutured to the mucosa of the lip or vestibule where the

Text continued on page 886

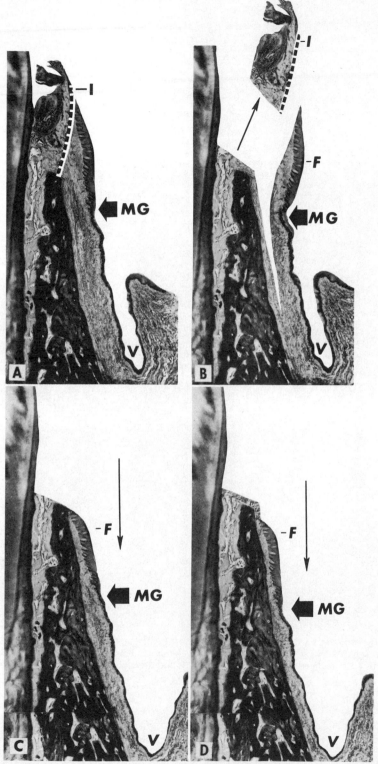

Figure 56–18 Apically Positioned Partial Thickness Flap. *A,* Internal incision (I) separates inner wall of periodontal pocket. MG, mucogingival junction; V, vestibular fornix. *B,* Partial thickness flap (F) separated away, leaving periosteum and layer of connective tissue on the bone. Inner wall of periodontal pocket (I) is removed and the tooth scaled and planed. *C,* Partial thickness flap (F) positioned apically with the edge of the flap at the crest of the bone. Note that the vestibular fornix is also moved apically. *D,* Partial thickness flap (F) positioned apically with the edge of the flap several millimeters below the crest of the bone.

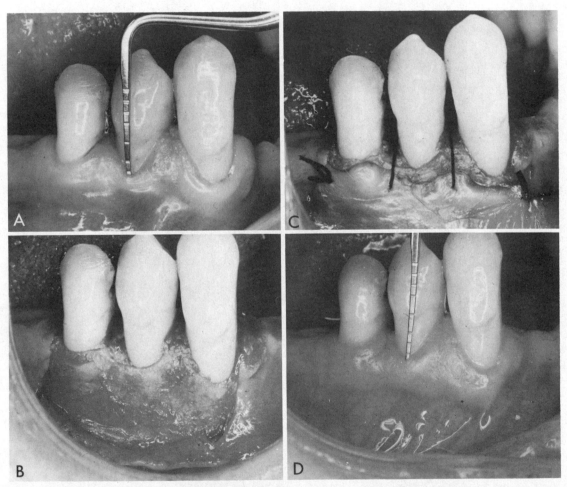

Figure 56–19 Apically Positioned Partial Thickness Flap. *A*, Before treatment, the base of pocket extends to the mucogingival line. *B*, Mucosal flap separated from the periosteum, teeth scaled and smoothed. *C*, Flap replaced below the crest of the bone. *D*, Eight months after treatment. Note the shallow sulcus and the widened zone of attached gingiva. Compare with *A*.

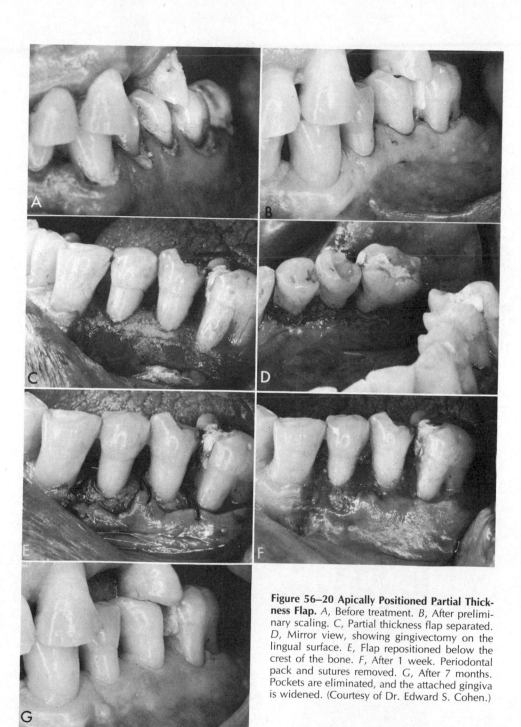

Figure 56–20 Apically Positioned Partial Thickness Flap. *A,* Before treatment. *B,* After preliminary scaling. *C,* Partial thickness flap separated. *D,* Mirror view, showing gingivectomy on the lingual surface. *E,* Flap repositioned below the crest of the bone. *F,* After 1 week. Periodontal pack and sutures removed. *G,* After 7 months. Pockets are eliminated, and the attached gingiva is widened. (Courtesy of Dr. Edward S. Cohen.)

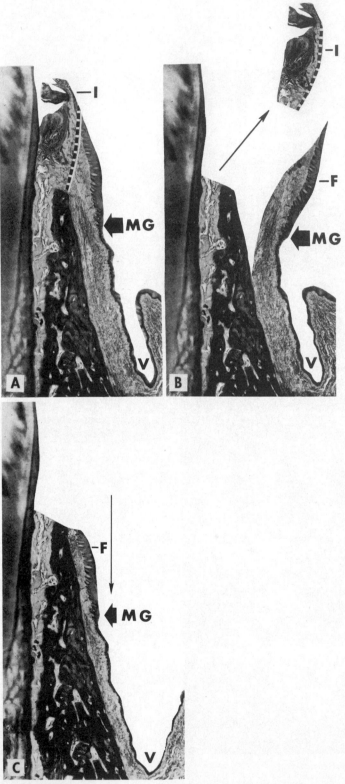

Figure 56–21 Apically Positioned Full Thickness (Mucoperiosteal) Flap. *A,* Internal incision (I) separating inner wall of periodontal pocket. MG, mucogingival junction; V, vestibular fornix. *B,* Full thickness flap (F), including periosteum, is separated from the bone. Inner wall of periodontal pocket removed. Tooth scaled and planed. C, Flap positioned apically on the bone with the edge of the flap at the bony crest.

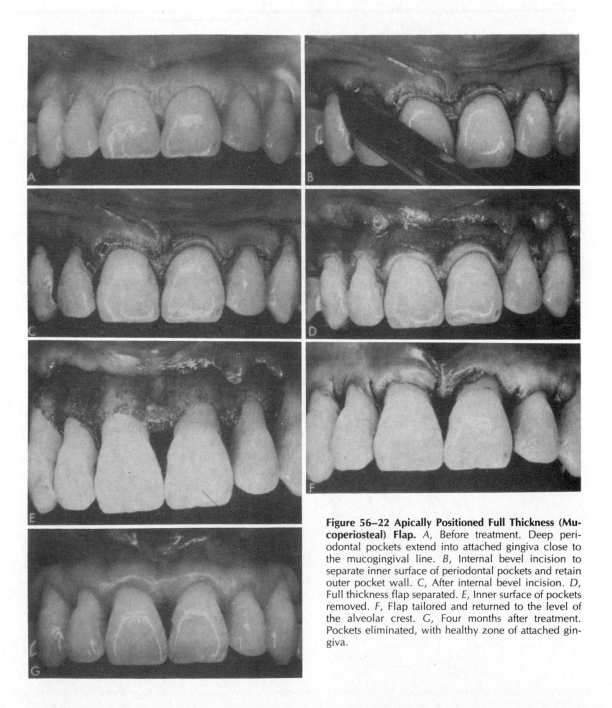

Figure 56–22 Apically Positioned Full Thickness (Mucoperiosteal) Flap. *A,* Before treatment. Deep periodontal pockets extend into attached gingiva close to the mucogingival line. *B,* Internal bevel incision to separate inner surface of periodontal pockets and retain outer pocket wall. *C,* After internal bevel incision. *D,* Full thickness flap separated. *E,* Inner surface of pockets removed. *F,* Flap tailored and returned to the level of the alveolar crest. *G,* Four months after treatment. Pockets eliminated, with healthy zone of attached gingiva.

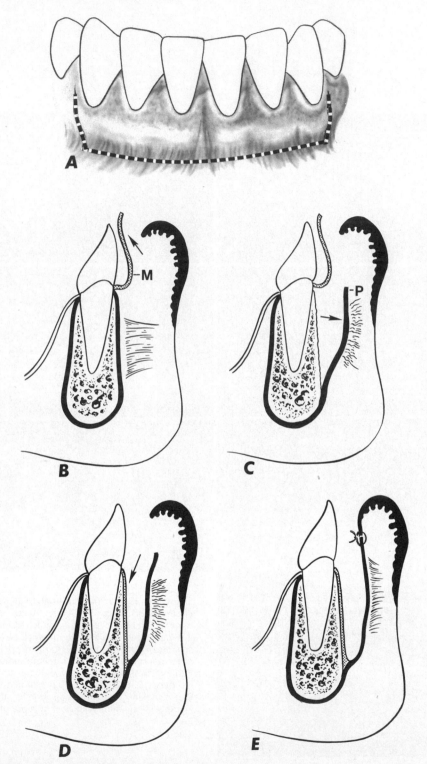

Figure 56–23 Edlan-Mejchar Operation for Vestibular Deepening. *A,* The operative field is outlined by two vertical incisions from the junction of the marginal and attached gingivae to approximately 12 mm from the alveolar margin into the vestibule. The vertical incisions are joined by a horizontal incision. *B,* A mucosal flap (M) is elevated, exposing the periosteum on the bone. *C,* The periosteum (P) is separated from the bone, starting from the line of attachment of the mucosal flap; the periosteum, including muscle attachments, is transposed to the lip. *D,* The mucosal flap is folded down over the bone *(arrow)* and sutured to the inner surface of the periosteum. *E,* The periosteum is transposed to the lip and sutured where the initial horizontal incision was made.

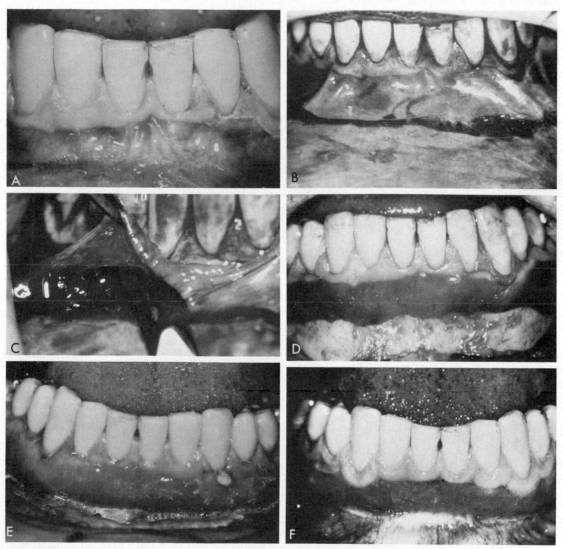

Figure 56–24 Vestibular Extension Operation. *A,* Before surgery. *B,* Horizontal incision in inner side of lip. *C,* Dissection of flap. *D,* After separation of periosteum and muscle fibers, flap is folded down over the bone. *E,* Results 1 week after operation. *F,* Results 1 year after operation. Note the nonkeratinized attached tissue. (Courtesy of Dr. Max O. Schmid.)

horizontal initial incision was made. According to Edlan and Mejchar, the periosteum is covered with epithelium within 7 to 10 days, and the mucous membrane attaches to the bone in 2 to 3 weeks. Figure 56–24 shows the steps in a clinical case.

Operations for Coverage of Denuded Roots

PEDICLE GRAFT: LATERALLY (HORIZONTALLY) POSITIONED FLAP. The purpose of this operation is to cover root surfaces denuded by a gingival defect or by periodontal disease and to widen the zone of attached gingiva.[48, 51]

Procedure. Step 1: Prepare the Recipient Site. Make a rectangular incision, resecting the periodontal pockets or gingival margin around the exposed root (Figs. 56–25 and 56–26B). The incision should extend to the periosteum and include a border of 2 to 3 mm of bone mesial and distal to the root to provide a connective tissue base to which the flap can attach. The rectangle should extend apically a sufficient distance into the alveolar mucosa to provide space for the zone of attached gingiva.

Remove the resected soft tissue without disturbing the narrow zone of periosteum around the root, and scale and plane the root surface (Fig. 56–26C).

Step 2: Prepare the Flap. The periodontium of the donor site should be healthy, with a satisfactory width of attached gingiva and minimal loss of bone and without dehiscences or fenestrations. Malposed or rotated teeth should be avoided. Inflammation should be

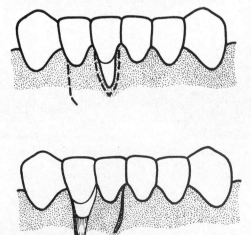

Figure 56–25 Laterally Positioned Flap for Coverage of Denuded Root. *Top,* Incisions removing gingival margin around exposed root and outlining flap. *Bottom,* After gingiva around exposed root is removed, flap is separated, transferred, and sutured.

eliminated before the flap operation is undertaken. A full thickness or partial thickness flap may be used, but the latter is preferable because it offers the advantage of more rapid healing in the donor site[6] and reduces the risk of loss of facial bone height, particularly if the bone is thin or if dehiscence or fenestration is suspected. However, if the gingiva is thin, partial thickness may not be sufficient for flap survival.

With a No. 15 Bard-Parker blade, make a vertical incision from the gingival margin to outline a flap adjacent to the recipient site. Incise to the periosteum of the bone and extend the incision into the oral mucosa to the level of the base of the recipient site (Fig. 56–26D). The flap should be sufficiently wider than the recipient site to cover the root and provide a broad margin for attachment to the connective tissue border around the root. The interdental papilla at the distal end of the flap or a major portion of it should be included to secure the flap in the interproximal space between the donor and recipient teeth.

Make a vertical incision along the gingival margin and interdental papilla. Insert a No. 15 Bard-Parker blade into the incision and, directing the blade apically, separate away a flap consisting of epithelium and a thin layer of connective tissue, leaving the periosteum on the bone. Hold the edge of the flap with tissue forceps, and continue the dissection to the desired depth in the oral vestibule. Tailor the margin of the flap to conform to the recipient site, and thin it if necessary so that it will not be bulbous.

It is sometimes necessary to make a *releasing incision* to avoid tension on the base of the flap, which impairs the circulation when the flap is moved (Fig. 56–26E). To do this, make an oblique incision into the alveolar mucosa at the distal corner of the flap, pointing in the direction of the recipient site (Fig. 56–26F).

Step 3: Transfer the Flap. Slide the flap laterally onto the adjacent root, making sure that it lies flat and firm, without excess tension on the base. Fix the flap to the adjacent gingiva and alveolar mucosa with interrupted sutures. A suspensory suture may be made around the involved tooth to prevent the flap from slipping apically (Fig. 56–26G).

Step 4: Protect the Flap and Donor Site. Cover the operative field with a soft periodontal pack, extending it interdentally and onto the lingual surface to secure it. Remove the pack and sutures after 1 week (Fig. 56–26H), and repack twice at weekly intervals.

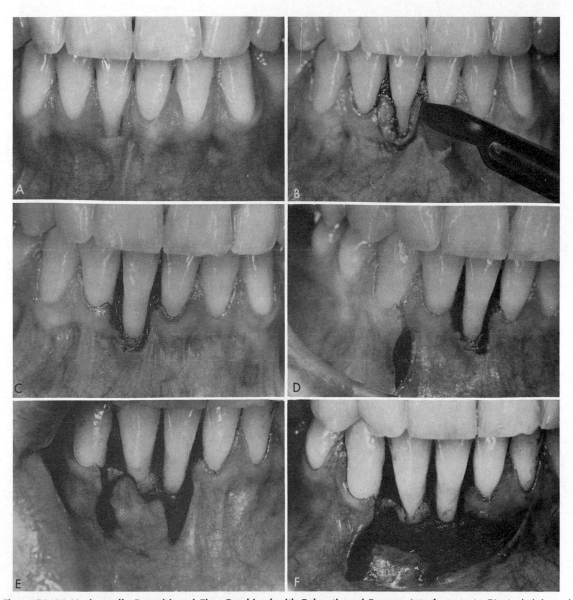

Figure 56–26 Horizontally Repositioned Flap Combined with Relocation of Frenum Attachment. *A*, Gingival defect of central incisor. *B*, Defect incised. *C*, Gingiva removed and tooth scaled and planed. *D*, Vertical incision on canine for sliding flap. *E*, Sliding flap detached. Note high frenum attachment between the central incisors. *F*, Frenum detached and resected to level of vestibular fornix.

Illustration continued on following page

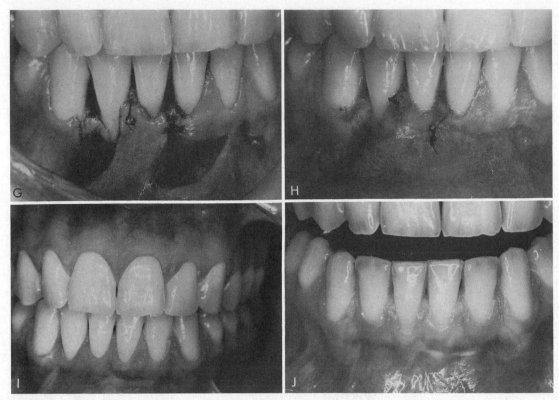

Figure 56–26 *Continued* G, Sliding flap repositioned laterally on central incisor and fixed lateral and suspensory suture. H, One week postoperation. Sutures to be removed. I, Five weeks after operation. J, Seven years after treatment. Note the preservation of gingival position and contour.

Variations. There are many variations in the incisions for this operation. A common one is the use of converging oblique incisions over the recipient site and a vertical or oblique incision at the distal end of the donor site so that the transposed flap is slightly wider at its base. In another modification, the marginal attachment in the donor site is preserved to reduce the likelihood of recession and marginal bone resorption, but this requires a donor site with a wide zone of attached gingiva.[47]

The laterally positioned flap is most often used on single teeth. However, when two adjacent roots are exposed, twin flaps are used to correct the condition. The procedure is the same as that for a single lateral flap, except that there are two teeth in the recipient site and there are two donor sites, one on each side of the involved area. The results are the same as those following laterally positioned flaps on single teeth.

Accomplishments. Attainment of a functionally satisfactory zone of attached gingiva in the recipient site is not a problem (Figs. 56–26 and 56–27). Some cellular degeneration and necrosis are associated with the transfer of the flap, but this is followed by repair. The morphologic features of the transplanted tissues do not change.[90-92]

Coverage of the exposed root surface has been reported to be 61 per cent,[1] 69 per cent,[51] and 72 per cent.[93] Histologic studies in dogs have reported 50 per cent coverage.[25, 115]

The flap attaches to the connective tissue bordering the root and bridges over the formerly denuded root surface. It appears to be attached and may adhere so firmly to the root as to resist insertion of a periodontal probe.[1] There is some shrinkage of the flap with time, but the root remains partially covered. Better results are obtained with narrow, long gingival defects than with broad, shallow ones.

The extent to which the flap "reattaches" to the root with the formation of new cementum and the embedding of new connective tissue fibers has not been settled. Reattachment on artificially denuded roots in experimental animals[116] and in some clinical studies in humans has been reported,[100, 103, 104] but it does not occur consistently enough to be predictable.

In the donor site there is uneventful repair and restoration of gingival health and contours, with some loss of radicular bone (0.5

mm) and recession (1.5 mm) reported with full thickness flaps.

CORONALLY POSITIONED FLAP. The purposes of this operation are (1) to eliminate periodontal pockets and (2) to attempt to obtain reattachment of the gingiva to root surfaces previously denuded by disease.

Procedure. The inner wall of the periodontal pockets is separated from the outer wall, and a mucoperiosteal flap is laid back, exposing the diseased area. The inner walls of the pockets are removed, and the tooth surfaces are scaled free of deposits and planed.

The flap is returned and sutured in place at a level coronal to the pretreatment position. The area is covered with a periodontal pack, which is removed along with the sutures after

1 week. The pack is replaced for an additional week if necessary.

When the denuded tooth has insufficient attached gingiva, the following procedure can be performed:

1. Gingival extension operation with a free autogenous graft. The technique described earlier is performed. This will create several millimeters of attached gingiva apical to the denuded root.

2. Two months after this operation, the area is reoperated as follows: Make an internal bevel incision apical to the defect in the healed free gingival graft. Extend the incision laterally, freeing the flap. Scale and plane the exposed root thoroughly. The use of citric acid, pH 1.0, for conditioning the root surface has

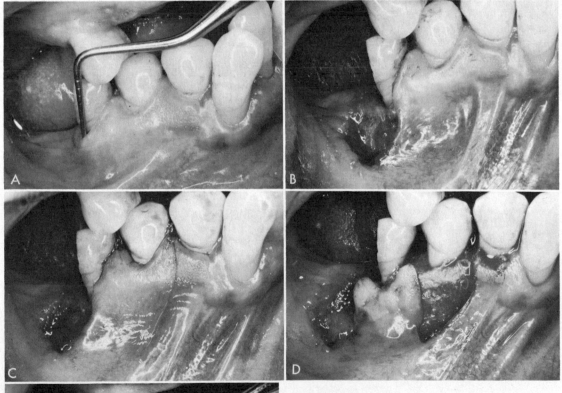

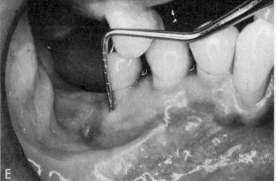

Figure 56–27 Lateral Sliding Partial Thickness Flap. *A,* Before treatment. Periodontal pocket on second premolar extends into the alveolar mucosa. *B,* V-shaped recipient site on second premolar prepared to receive the flap. *C,* Flap outlined on the first premolar. *D,* Partial thickness flap transferred to second premolar. *E,* Seven months after treatment, showing shallow gingival sulcus and widened zone of attached gingiva. Compare with *A.* (Courtesy of Dr. Edward S. Cohen.)

been suggested.[63] Suture the flap at a coronal level, covering the denuded root (Fig. 56–28).

A significant degree of reduction in recession treated by this double-step operation was reported after 2 years by Bernimoulin et al.[5] and confirmed by other authors.[15, 64, 65]

PEDICLE GRAFT (SLIDING PARTIAL THICKNESS FLAP FROM AN EDENTULOUS AREA). The purpose of this operation is to restore attached gingiva on teeth adjacent to edentulous spaces with denuded roots and a small vestibular fornix, often complicated by tension from a frenum.[28] A partial thickness flap of masticatory mucosa from the adjacent edentulous ridge is used.

Procedure. *Step 1: Prepare the Recipient Site.* With a No. 15 Bard-Parker blade, make a V-shaped incision from the gingival margin mesial and distal to the involved tooth into the alveolar mucosa apical to the root apex or apices (Fig. 56–29A and B). Include frenum attachments in the resected area. Elevate the tip of the tissue wedge outlined by the incision with tissue forceps, and dissect away the wedge of tissue with a No. 15 Bard-Parker blade. Leave the periosteum and covering connective tissue on the bone, except in areas where bone is to be recontoured. Remove the loose strands or clumps of tissue from the connective tissue surface to provide a firm base for the transferred flap.

Step 2: Scale and Plane the Root Surfaces.

Step 3: Prepare the Flap. Make an incision along the crest of the edentulous ridge from the proximal tooth surface for a distance equal to or slightly longer than the width of the recipient site. From the end of the incision make a vertical incision from the crest of the ridge into the alveolar mucosa to the level of the base of the wedge-shaped recipient site, outlining a flap that is wider at the base (Fig. 56–29B). Insert a periodontal knife into the incision at the crest of the ridge, and separate away a partial thickness flap of masticatory mucosa, leaving the periosteum on the bone. Continue the separation into the alveolar mucosa.

If the mucogingival junction is high on the edentulous ridge and the buccal masticatory mucosa is narrow, masticatory mucosa from the lingual surface is included in the graft. The initial incision is made on the lingual surface close to, but not at, the mucogingival junction.

Step 4: Transfer the Flap. To facilitate free movement of the flap without stretching or twisting the pedicle and interfering with the circulation, a short, oblique releasing incision may be made at the base in the direction the flap is to be moved. Check the recipient site to be sure bleeding has stopped, and remove excessive clot from the surface.

Move the flap laterally and place it firmly

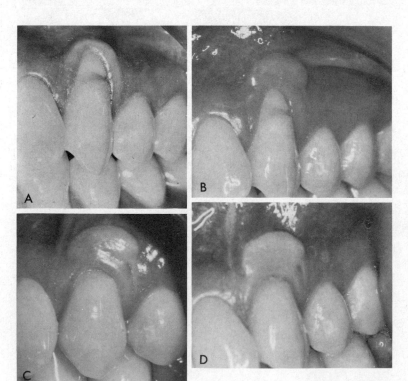

Figure 56–28 Coronally Positioned Flap. *A,* Preoperative view. Note the recession and the thin band of marginal gingiva. *B,* After placement of a free gingival graft. *C,* Six months after coronal displacement of the grafted gingiva. *D,* Two years after coronal displacement of the grafted gingiva. Note the coverage of the receded area. (Courtesy of Dr. Raul G. Caffesse.)

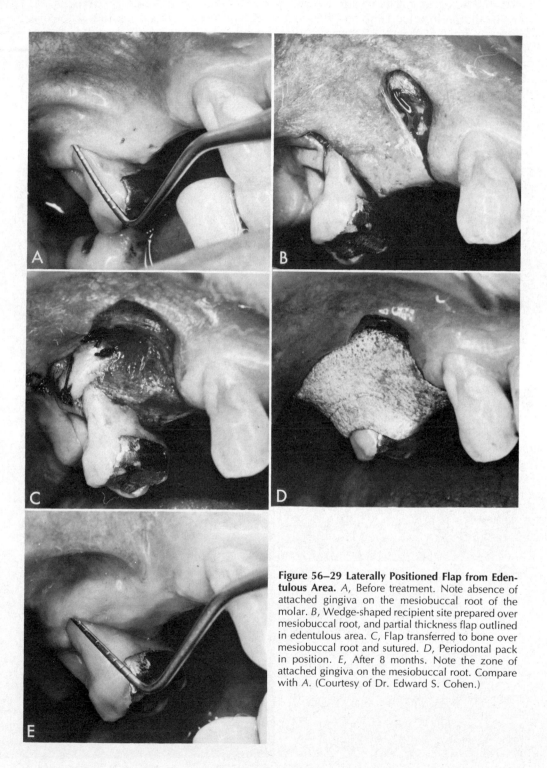

Figure 56–29 Laterally Positioned Flap from Edentulous Area. *A,* Before treatment. Note absence of attached gingiva on the mesiobuccal root of the molar. *B,* Wedge-shaped recipient site prepared over mesiobuccal root, and partial thickness flap outlined in edentulous area. *C,* Flap transferred to bone over mesiobuccal root and sutured. *D,* Periodontal pack in position. *E,* After 8 months. Note the zone of attached gingiva on the mesiobuccal root. Compare with *A.* (Courtesy of Dr. Edward S. Cohen.)

on the recipient surface with the free end at the margin of the bone. Suture one margin of the flap to the adjacent cut tissue surface and the other to the periosteum (Fig. 56–29*C*). A suspensory suture may be made through the free margin of the flap around the tooth to prevent the flap from slipping apically. Cover the area with a periodontal pack (Fig. 56–29*D*), which is removed with the sutures after 1 week. Repack two more times at weekly intervals (Fig. 56–29*E*).

Other Techniques

DOUBLE PAPILLAE POSITIONED FLAPS. The purpose of this operation is to cover roots denuded by isolated gingival defects with a flap formed by joining two interdental papillae. It is recommended when the areas bordering the gingival defect are unsatisfactory for a laterally positioned flap because of insufficient attached gingiva or deep periodontal pockets. These problems are overcome by utilizing the contig-

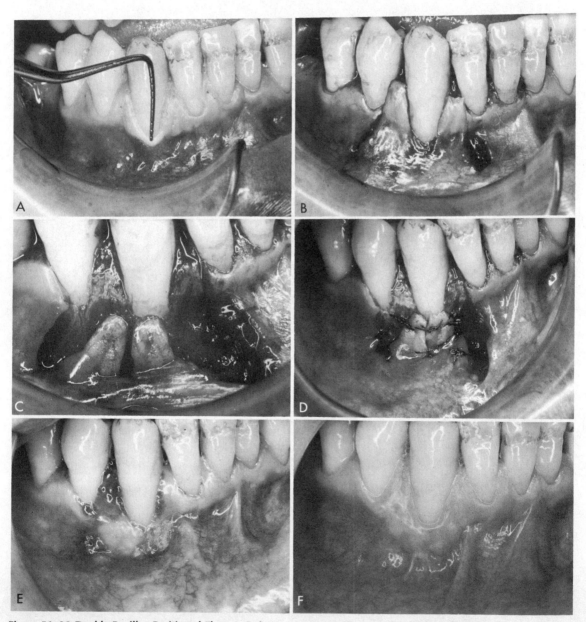

Figure 56–30 Double Papillae Positioned Flap. *A,* Before treatment. Note narrow band of attached gingiva on the canine. *B,* Mesial and distal papillae separated. *C,* Papillae transferred to the canine. *D,* Papillae placed on bony plate and sutured to the periosteum. *E,* After 1 week. *F,* After 7 months. Note the widened zone of attached gingiva. Compare with *A.* (Courtesy of Dr. Edward S. Cohen.)

uous halves of the adjacent interdental papillae.[26, 54] The interdental papillae provide a zone of attached gingiva that is usually wider than that on the radicular surface; these flaps also reduce the risk of loss in radicular bone height because the bone is thicker interdentally than on the roots. Results with this technique, however, are frequently poor, probably because the two flaps are sutured over the root surface. Figure 56–30 shows the procedure.

CORONALLY POSITIONED PEDICLE FLAPS. Of historical interest is an operation developed by Kalmi, Moscor, and Goranov[60] in an effort to improve the appearance of patients with teeth denuded by advanced periodontal disease. It involves covering denuded roots of maxillary anterior teeth by sliding pedicle flaps from adjacent uninvolved gingiva and alveolar mucosa as follows (Fig. 56–31):

Periodontal pockets are resected by gingivectomy, and the roots are scaled and planed. A mucoperiosteal flap as wide as the exposed root surface and outlined by a horizontal incision across the anterior maxilla is elevated from the bone (Fig. 56–31*A* and *B*). The flap is divided in two by a midline V-shaped incision at the frenum, and the two flaps are moved onto the roots and sutured. Reattachment of the flaps to the exposed roots has been reported in experimental animals,[56] but not in humans.[75]

Operations for Removal of Frena

A frenum is a fold of mucous membrane, usually with enclosed muscle fibers, that attaches the lips and cheeks to the alveolar mucosa and/or gingiva and underlying periosteum. *A frenum becomes a problem if its attachment is too close to the marginal gingiva.* It may then pull on healthy gingiva and invite the accumulation of irritants; it may deflect the wall of a periodontal pocket and aggravate its severity; or it may interfere with posttreatment healing, prevent close adaptation of the gingiva and lead to pocket formation, or inhibit proper brushing of the teeth.

FRENECTOMY OR FRENOTOMY. The terms *frenectomy* and *frenotomy* signify operations that differ in degree. *Frenectomy is complete removal of the frenum, including its attachment to underlying bone, such as may be required in the correction of an abnormal diastema between maxillary central incisors. Frenotomy is the incision of the frenum.* Both procedures are used, but frenotomy generally suffices for peri-

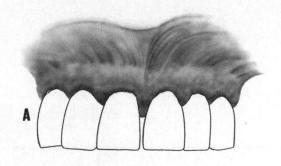

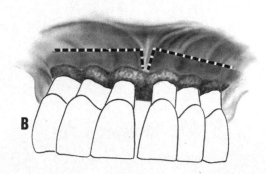

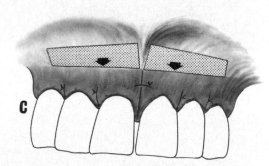

Figure 56–31 Coronally Positioned Pedicle Flap. *A,* Deep periodontal pockets. *B,* Periodontal pockets removed and roots scaled and planed. Mucoperiosteal flaps are outlined by horizontal and vertical incisions indicated by dotted lines. *C,* Flaps drawn down over the root surfaces as indicated by arrows and joined and sutured in position over the roots. The bone in the stippled areas is denuded.

odontal purposes, i.e., relocating the frenum attachment so as to create a zone of attached gingiva between the gingival margin and the frenum. Frenectomy or frenotomy is usually performed in conjunction with other periodontal treatment procedures but occasionally is done as a separate operation.

Frenum problems occur most often on the facial surface between the maxillary and mandibular central incisors and in the canine and

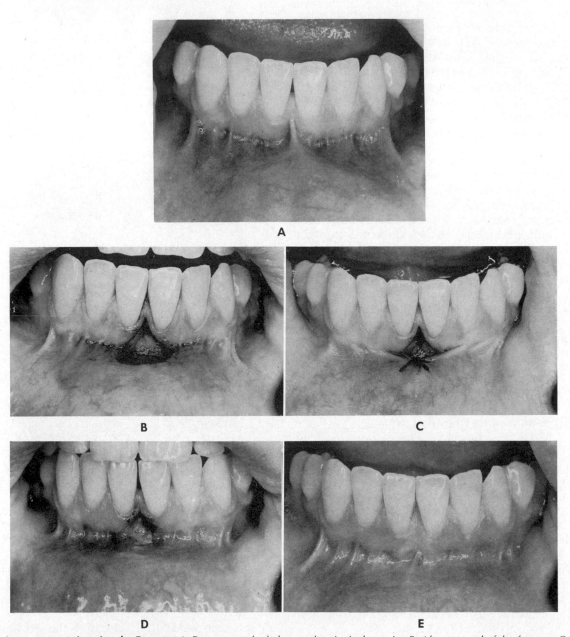

Figure 56–32 Relocating the Frenum. *A,* Frenum attached close to the gingival margin. *B,* After removal of the frenum. *C,* Mucosa sutured in position. *D,* After 1 week, periodontal pack and suture removed. *E,* After 6 months, frenum relocated at the mucogingival line.

premolar areas[113]; they occur less frequently on the lingual surface of the mandible.

Procedure (Fig. 56–32). If the vestibule is deep enough, the operation is confined to the frenum, but it is often necessary to deepen the vestibule to provide space for the repositioned frenum. This is accomplished as follows:

1. Anesthetize the area.

2. Engage the frenum with a hemostat inserted to the depth of the vestibule.

3. Incise along the upper surface of the hemostat, extending beyond the tip.

4. Make a similar incision along the undersurface of the hemostat.

5. Remove the triangular resected portion of the frenum with the hemostat. This exposes the underlying brush-like fibrous attachment to the bone.

6. Make a horizontal incision, separating the fibers, and bluntly dissect to the bone.

7. If necessary, extend the incisions laterally and suture the labial mucosa to the apical periosteum.

8. Clean the field of operation and pack with gauze sponges until bleeding stops.

9. Insert the periodontal pack. First, pack the marginal area, as is ordinarily done following gingivectomy. Then, using the marginal pack as a stable base, add thin strips on the edge to the depth of the incision.

10. Remove the pack after 2 weeks and repack if necessary. One month is usually required for the formation of an intact mucosa with the frenum attached in its new position.

High frenum attachments on the lingual surface are uncommon. To correct these without involving the structures in the floor of the mouth, approximately 2 mm of the attachment is separated from the mucosa with a periodontal knife at weekly intervals until the desired level is reached. The area is covered with a periodontal pack in the intervals between treatments.

CRITERIA FOR SELECTION OF MUCOGINGIVAL TECHNIQUES

Different techniques are available for solving the mucogingival problems outlined in the first part of this chapter (Plate XI). The practitioner must know how to choose among them.

1. **Pockets extending to the mucogingival junction.** Basically two techniques are available, the apically positioned flap and the free gingival graft. Criteria for selection are based on the character of the gingival pocket wall. Thick, manageable pocket walls can be used for an apically positioned flap, and this should be our first choice. This flap does not require a second surgical site and offers the added advantage of exposing the bone as needed. When manageability of the flap is impaired owing to irregular contour or soft, friable tissue, the choice is a gingival extension operation with a free gingival graft.

2. **Absence of attached gingiva with no pocket formation.** The need for any type of surgery should be questioned, since many patients can be adequately maintained with no surgery. However, if there is persistent inflammation and plaque control is difficult, a *free gingival graft* is the technique of choice.

3. **Isolated gingival recession.** The *laterally positioned flap* is the technique of choice; the *coronally positioned flap* displacing a previously placed free gingival graft is the alternative. Both are excellent methods. The laterally positioned flap should be used when sufficient donor tissue is present in a convenient location, since one surgical intervention will solve the problem. The coronally positioned flap requires two surgical interventions, one of which has two surgical sites. It is resorted to when sufficient donor tissue is not present in convenient adjoining locations.

4. **High frenum insertion.** *Frenectomy* is the technique available; it is usually performed together with other pocket elimination methods. The resultant wound can sometimes be covered with a free gingival graft.

COMMENT

New techniques are constantly being developed and are slowly incorporated into periodontal practice. The practitioner should be aware that sometimes new methods are published without adequate clinical research to ensure the predictability of the results and the extent to which they may benefit the patient. Critical analysis of newly presented techniques should guide our constant evolution toward better clinical methods.

Several studies have pointed out that areas with no attached gingiva can be maintained in satisfactory health provided good plaque control is exercised.[35, 36, 67] Furthermore, it has been shown that dentogingival units with wide, narrow, or absent attached gingiva respond to plaque with an inflammatory reaction of the same location and extent.[67, 110, 111] These find-

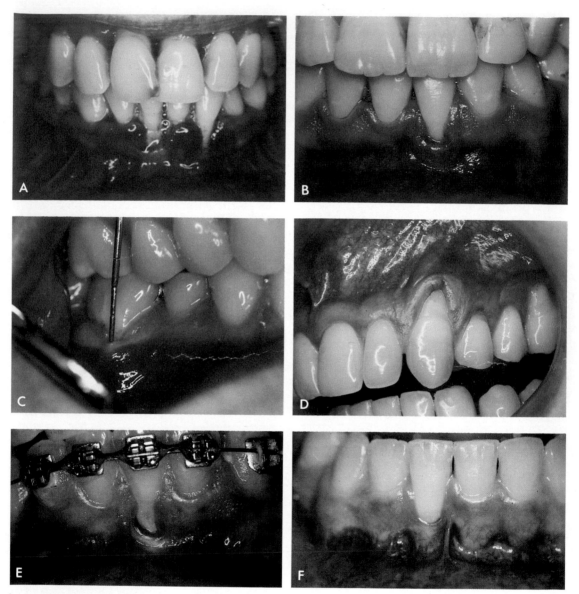

Plate XI Mucogingival Defects
A, Irregular gingival contours, pocket furcations, and recession with severe gingival inflammation.
B, Gingival recession and inflammation. Bottom of pocket is beyond mucogingival junction.
C, Recession on mesiobuccal root of lower first molar. Probe indicates presence of shallow pocket with absence of attached gingiva.
D, Gingival recession and cleft on upper cuspid.
E, Advanced gingival recession and inflammation.
F, After scaling and root planing and adequate plaque control, gingival condition has improved markedly.

ings should reduce the indications for mucogingival surgery to those cases that cannot be
maintained free of inflammation by the patient·
after Phase I therapy. Width measurements of
attached gingiva should not be the sole criterion. This caution refers particularly to free
gingival grafts; indications for other techniques
are clearer.

REFERENCES

1. Albano, E. A., Caffesse, R. C., and Carranza, F. A., Jr.: A
   biometric analysis of laterally displaced pedicle flaps. Rev.
   Asoc. Odontol. Argent., 57:351, 1969.
2. Ariaudo, A. A., and Tyrrell, H. A.: Elimination of pockets
   extending to or beyond mucogingival junction. Dent. Clin.
   North Am., 4:67, 1960.
3. Becker, N. G.: A free gingival graft utilizing a pre-suturing
   technique. Periodontics, 5:194, 1967.
4. Bergenholtz, A., and Hugoson, A.: Vestibular sulcus extension surgery in cases with periodontal disease. J. Periodont.
   Res., 2:221, 1967.
5. Bernimoulin, J. P., Lüscher, B., and Mühlemann, H. R.:
   Coronally repositioned periodontal flap. J. Clin. Periodontol., 2:1, 1975.
6. Bhaskar, S. N., Cutright, D. E., Perez, B., and Beasley, J.
   D., III.: Full and partial thickness pedicle grafts in miniature
   swine and man. J. Periodontol., 42:66, 1971.
7. Björn, H.: Free transplantation of gingiva propria. Sveriges
   Tandlak. T., 22:684, 1963.
8. Bohannan, H. M.: Studies in the alteration of vestibular
   depth. I. Complete denudation. J. Periodontol., 33:120, 1962.
9. Bohannan, H. M.: Studies in the alteration of vestibular
   depth. II. Periosteum retention. J. Periodontol., 33:354,
   1962.
10. Bohannan, H. M.: Studies in the alteration of vestibular
    depth. III. Vestibular incision. J. Periodontol., 34:209, 1963.
11. Bowers, G. M.: A study of the width of attached gingiva. J.
    Periodontol., 34:201, 1963.
12. Brackett, R. C., and Gargiulo, A. W.: Free gingival grafts
    in humans. J. Periodontol., 41:581, 1970.
13. Bressman, E., and Chasens, A. I.: Free gingival graft with
    periosteal fenestration. J. Periodontol., 39:298, 1968.
14. Broome, W. C., and Taggart, E. J., Jr.: Free autogenous
    connective tissue grafting. J. Periodontol., 47:580, 1976.
15. Caffesse, R. G., and Guinard, E.: Treatment of localized
    gingival recessions. Part II. Coronally repositioned flap with
    a free gingival graft. J. Periodontol., 49:358, 1978.
16. Caffesse, R. G., Albano, E., and Plot, C.: Injertos gingivales
    libres en perros: analisis biometrico. Rev. Asoc. Odontol.
    Argent., 60:517, 1972.
17. Caffesse, R. G., Carraro, J. J., and Carranza, F. A., Jr.:
    Injertos gingivales libres en perros: estudio clinico e histolo-
    gico. Rev. Asoc. Odontol. Argent., 60:465, 1972.
18. Caffesse, R. G., Burgett, F. G., Nasjleti, C. E., and Castelli,
    W. A.: Healing of free gingival grafts with and without
    periosteum. Part I. Histologic evaluation. J. Periodontol.,
    50:586, 1979.
19. Caffesse, R. G., Nasjleti, C. E., Burgett, F. G., Kowalski,
    C. J., and Castelli, W. A.: Healing of free gingival grafts
    with and without periosteum. Part II. Radioautographic
    evaluation. J. Periodontol., 50:595, 1979.
20. Carranza, F. A., Jr., and Carraro, J. J.: Effect of removal
    of periosteum on postoperative result of mucogingival sur-
    gery. J. Periodontol., 34:223, 1963.
21. Carranza, F. A., Jr., and Carraro, J. J.: Mucogingival tech-
    niques in periodontal surgery. J. Periodontol., 41:294, 1970.
22. Carranza, F. A., Jr., Carraro, J. J., and Albano, E. A.:
    Mucogingival surgery. In Stahl, S. S. (ed.): Periodontal
    Surgery: Biologic Basis and Technique. Springfield, Ill.,
    Charles C Thomas, 1976.
23. Carranza, F. A., Jr., Carraro, J. J., Dotto, C. A., and
    Cabrini, R. L.: Effect of periosteal fenestration in gingival
    extension operations. J. Periodontol., 37:335, 1966.
24. Carraro, J. J., Carranza, F. A., Jr., Albano, E. A., and Joly,
    G.: Effect of bone denudation in mucogingival surgery in
    humans. J. Periodontol., 35:463, 1964.
25. Chacker, F. M., and Cohen, D. W.: Regeneration of gingival
    tissues in non-human primates. J. Dent. Res., 39:743, 1960.
26. Cohen, D. W., and Ross, S. E.: The double papillae repo-
    sitioned flap in periodontal therapy. J. Periodontol., 39:65,
    1968.
27. Corn, H.: Periosteal separation—its clinical significance. J.
    Periodontol., 33:140, 1962.
28. Corn, H.: Edentulous area pedicle grafts in mucogingival
    surgery. Periodontics, 2:229, 1964.
29. Costich, E. R., and Ramfjord, S. P.: Healing after partial
    denudation of the alveolar process. J. Periodontol., 39:127,
    1968.
30. Donn, B. J., Jr.: The free connective tissue autograft: a
    clinical and histologic wound healing study in humans. J.
    Periodontol., 49:253, 1978.
31. Donnenfeld, O. W., and Glickman, I.: A biometric study of
    the effects of gingivectomy. J. Periodontol., 37:447, 1966.
32. Donnenfeld, O. W., Marks, R., and Glickman, I.: The
    apically repositioned flap: a clinical study. J. Periodontol.,
    35:381, 1964.
33. Dordick, B., Coslet, J. G., and Seibert, J. S.: Clinical
    evaluation of free autogenous gingival grafts placed on alveo-
    lar bone. Part I. Clinical predictability. J. Periodontol.,
    47:559, 1976.
34. Dordick, B., Coslet, J. G., and Seibert, J. S.: Clinical
    evaluation of free autogenous gingival grafts placed on alveo-
    lar bone. Part II. Coverage of non-pathologic dehiscences
    and fenestrations. J. Periodontol., 47:568, 1976.
35. Dorfman, H. S., Kennedy, J. E., and Bird, W. C.: Longi-
    tudinal evaluation of free autogenous gingival grafts. J. Clin.
    Periodontol., 7:316, 1980.
36. Dorfman, H. S., Kennedy, J. E., and Bird, W. C.: Longi-
    tudinal evaluation of free autogenous gingival grafts. A four-
    year report. J. Periodontol., 53:349, 1982.
37. Edel, A.: Clinical evaluation of free connective tissue grafts
    used to increase the width of keratinized gingiva. J. Clin.
    Periodontol., 1:185, 1974.
38. Edlan, A., and Mejchar, B.: Plastic surgery of the vestibulum
    in periodontal therapy. Int. Dent. J., 13:593, 1963.
39. Friedman, N.: Mucogingival surgery: the apically reposi-
    tioned flap. J. Periodontol., 33:328, 1962.
40. Friedman, N., and Levine, H. L.: Mucogingival surgery:
    current status. J. Periodontol., 35:5, 1964.
41. Gargiulo, A. W., and Arrocha, R.: Histo-clinical evaluation
    of free gingival grafts. Periodontics, 5:285, 1967.
42. Giacometti, L., and Parakkal, P. F.: Skin transplantation:
    orientation of epithelial cells by the basement membrane.
    Nature, 223:514, 1969.
43. Glickman, I., Smulow, J. B., Ellinger, H. A., and Foulke,
    C. N.: Healing of apically positioned mucosal flaps and free
    gingival grafts. I.A.D.R. Abstracts, No. 468, 1971, p. 169.
44. Gordon, H. P., Sullivan, H. C., and Atkins, J. H.: Free
    autogenous gingival grafts. II. Supplemental findings—his-
    tology of the graft site. Periodontics, 6:130, 1968.
45. Gottsegen, R.: Frenum position and vestibule depth in rela-
    tion to gingival health. Oral Surg., 7:1069, 1954.
46. Grant, D. A.: Experimental periodontal surgery: sequestra-
    tion of alveolar bone. J. Periodontol., 38:409, 1967.
47. Grupe, H. E.: Modified technique for the sliding flap oper-
    ation. J. Periodontol., 37:491, 1966.
48. Grupe, H. E., and Warren, R. F., Jr.: Repair of gingival
    defects by a sliding flap operation. J. Periodontol., 27:92,
    1956.
49. Guinard, E. A., and Caffesse, R. G.: Localized gingival
    recessions. I. Etiology and prevalence. J. Western Soc.
    Periodontol., 25:3, 1977.
50. Guinard, E. A., and Caffesse, R. G.: Localized gingival
    recessions. II. Treatment. J. Western Soc. Periodontol.,
    25:10, 1977.
51. Guinard, E. A., and Caffesse, R. G.: Treatment of localized
    gingival recessions. Part I. Lateral sliding flap. J. Periodon-
    tol., 49:351, 1978.
52. Hall, W. B.: The current status of mucogingival problems
    and their therapy. J. Periodontol., 52:569, 1981.
53. Hangorsky, V., and Bissada, N. F.: Clinical assessment of
    free gingival graft effectiveness on the maintenance of peri-
    odontal health. J. Periodontol., 51:274, 1980.

54. Harvey, P. M.: Management of advanced periodontitis. Part I. Preliminary report of a method of surgical reconstruction. N.Z. Dent. J., *61*:180, 1965.
55. Hattler, A. B.: Mucogingival surgery—utilization of interdental gingiva as attached gingiva by surgical displacement. Periodontics, *5*:126, 1967.
56. Hawley, C. E., and Staffileno, H.: Clinical evaluation of free gingival grafts in periodontal surgery. J. Periodontol., *41*:105, 1970.
57. James, W. C., and McFall, W. T., Jr.: Placement of free gingival grafts on denuded alveolar bone. Part I. Clinical evaluations. J. Periodontol., *49*:283, 1978.
58. James, W. C., McFall, W. T., Jr., and Burkes, E. J.: Placement of free gingival grafts on denuded alveolar bone. II. Microscopic observations. J. Periodontol., *49*:291, 1978.
59. Janson, W. A., et al.: Development of the blood supply to split-thickness free gingival autografts. J. Periodontol., *40*:707, 1969.
60. Kalmi, J., Moscor, M., and Goranov, Z.: The solution of the aesthetic problem in the treatment of periodontal disease of anterior teeth: gingivoplastic operation. Paradentologie, *3*:53, 1949.
61. Karring, T., Ostergaard, E., and Löc, H.: Conservation of tissue specificity after heterotopic transplantation of gingiva and alveolar mucosa. J. Periodont. Res., *6*:282, 1971.
62. Köster, H. D., and Flores de Jacoby, L.: Vergleicheride Untersuchungen von Schleimhant-transplantaten und lyophilisierter Dura. Dtsch. Zahnaertzl. Z., *28*:1229, 1973.
63. Liu, W. J., and Solt, C. W.: A surgical procedure for the treatment of localized gingival recession in conjunction with root surface citric acid conditioning. J. Periodontol., *51*:505, 1980.
64. Matter, J.: Free gingival graft and coronally repositioned flap. A 2-year follow-up report. J. Clin. Periodontol., *6*:437, 1979.
65. Matter, J., and Cimasoni, G.: Creeping attachment after free gingival grafts. J. Periodontol., *47*:574, 1976.
66. Maynard, J. B.: Coronal positioning of a previously placed autogenous gingival graft. J. Periodontol., *48*:151, 1977.
67. Miyasato, M., Crigger, M., and Egelberg, J.: Gingival conditions in areas of minimal and appreciable width of keratinized gingiva. J. Clin. Periodontol., *4*:200, 1977.
68. Mörmann, W., Schaer, F., and Firestone, A. R.: The relationship between success of free gingival grafts and transplant thickness. J. Periodontol., *52*:74, 1981.
69. Nabers, C. L.: Repositioning the attached gingiva. J. Periodontol., *25*:38, 1954.
70. Nabers, C. L.: When is gingival repositioning an indicated procedure? J. Western Soc. Periodontol., *5*:4, 1957.
71. Nabers, C. L.: Free gingival grafts. Periodontics, *4*:243, 1966.
72. Neacy, K.: The use of allogenic sclera and autogenous gingiva as free gingival grafts. Thesis, University of California at Los Angeles, 1978.
73. Oliver, R. C., and Woofter, C.: Healing and revascularization of free mucosal grafts over roots. I.A.D.R. Abstracts, No. 469, 1971, p. 170.
74. Oliver, R. C.., Löe, H., and Karring, T.: Microscopic evaluation of the healing and revascularization of free gingival grafts. J. Periodontol., *3*:84, 1968.
75. Patur, B., and Glickman, I.: Gingival pedicle flaps for covering root surfaces denuded by chronic destructive periodontal disease—a clinical experiment. J. Periodontol., *29*:50, 1958.
76. Pennel, B. M., King, K. O., Wilderman, M. H., and Barron, J. M.: Repair of the alveolar process following osseous surgery. J. Periodontol., *38*:426, 1967.
77. Pennel, B., King, K. O., Higgason, J. D., Towner, J. D., Fritz, B. D., and Sadler, J. F.: Retention of periosteum in mucogingival surgery. J. Periodontal., *36*:39, 1965.
78. Pennel, B. M., Tabor, J. C., King, K. O., Towner, J. D., Fritz, B. D., and Higgason, J. D.: Free masticatory mucossa graft. J. Periodontol., *40*:162, 1969.
79. Pfeifer, J. S.: The reaction of alveolar bone to flap procedures in man. Periodontics, *3*:135, 1965.
80. Ramfjord, S. P., and Costich, E. R.: Healing after exposure of periosteum on the alveolar process. J. Periodontol., *39*:199, 1968.
81. Rateitschak, K. H., Egli, U., and Fingeli, G.: Recession: a four-year longitudinal study after free gingival grafts. J. Clin. Periodontol., *6*:158, 1979.
82. Redondo, V. F., Bustamante, A., and Carranza, F. A., Jr.: Evaluación biometrica de la tecnica de extensión gingival con fenestración periostica. Rev. Asoc. Odontol. Argent., *56*:346, 1968.
83. Robinson, R. E.: Periosteal fenestration in mucogingival surgery. J. Western Soc. Periodontol., *9*:107, 1961.
84. Robinson, R. E., and Agnew, R. G.: Periosteal fenestration at the mucogingival line. J. Periodontol., *34*:503, 1963.
85. Rosenberg, M. M.: Vestibular alterations in periodontics. J. Periodontol., *31*:231, 1960.
86. Roth, H.: Some speculations as to predictable fenestrations prior to mucogingival surgery. Periodontics, *3*:29, 1965.
87. Rubinstein, H. S., Ruben, M. P., Levy, C., and Peiser, C.: Evidence for successful acceptance of irradiated free gingival allografts in dogs. J. Periodontol., *46*:195, 1975.
88. Schmid, M. O.: The subperiosteal vestibule extension—literature review, rationale and technique. J. Western. Soc. Periodontol., *24*:89, 1976.
89. Schoo, W. H., and Copes, L.: Use of palatal mucosa and lyophilized dura mater to create attached gingiva. J. Clin. Periodontol., *3*:166, 1976.
90. Simaan, G.: Histology study of the so-called attached gingiva following the deepening of the vestibulum by the mucosal flap technique. Czas. Stomat., *69*:91, 1969; Periodont. Abstracts, *17*:116, 1969.
91. Smith, R. M.: A study of the intertransplantation of alveolar mucosa. Oral Surg., *29*:328, 1970.
92. Smith, R. M.: A study of the intertransplantation of gingiva. Oral Surg., *29*:169, 1970.
93. Smukler, H.: Laterally positioned mucoperiosteal pedicle grafts in the treatment of denuded roots. J. Periodontol., *47*:590, 1976.
94. Spengler, D. E., and Hayward, J. R.: Study of sulcus extension wound healing in dogs. J. Oral Surg., *22*:413, 1964.
95. Staffileno, H.: Palatal flap surgery: mucosal flap (split thickness) and its advantages over the mucoperiosteal flap. J. Periodontol., *40*:547, 1969.
96. Staffileno, H., and Levy, S.: Histologic and clinical study of mucosal (gingival) transplants in dogs. J. Periodontol., *40*:311, 1969.
97. Staffileno, H., Levy, S., and Gargiulo, A.: Histologic study of cellular mobilization and repair following a periosteal retention operation via split thickness mucogingival flap surgery. J. Periodontol., *37*:117, 1966.
98. Staffileno, H., Wentz, F., and Orban, B.: Histological study of healing of split thickness flap surgery in dogs. J. Periodontol., *33*:56, 1962.
99. Strahan, J. D.: The relation of the mucogingival junction to the alveolar bone margin. Dent. Practit. Dent. Record, *14*:72, 1963.
100. Sugarman, E. F.: A clinical and histological study of the attachment of grafted tissue to bone and teeth. J. Periodontol., *40*:381, 1969.
101. Sullivan, H. C., and Atkins, J. H.: Free autogenous gingival grafts. I. Principles of successful grafting. Periodontics, *6*:5, 1968.
102. Sullivan, H. C., and Atkins, J. H.: The role of free gingival grafts in periodontal therapy. Dent. Clin. North Am., *13*:133, 1969.
103. Sullivan, H. C., Carman, D., and Dinner, D.: Histological evaluation of the laterally positioned flap. I.A.D.R. Abstracts, No. 467, 1971, p. 169.
104. Sullivan, H. C., Dinner, D., and Carman, D.: Clinical evaluation of the laterally positioned flap. I.A.D.R. Abstracts, No. 466, 1971, p. 169.
105. Tavtigian, R.: The height of the facial radicular alveolar crest following apically positioned flap operations. J. Periodontol., *41*:412, 1970.
106. Tisot, R. J., and Sullivan, H. C.: Evaluation of the survival of partial thickness and full thickness flaps. I.A.D.R. Abstracts, No. 470, 1971, p. 170.
107. Trey, E., and Bernimoulin, J. P.: Influence of free gingival grafts on the health of the marginal gingiva. J. Clin. Periodontol., 7:381, 1980.

108. Wade, A. B.: Vestibular deepening by the technique of Edlan and Mejchar. J. Periodont. Res., *4*:300, 1969.

109. Ward, V. J.: A clinical assessment of the use of the free gingival graft for correcting localized recession associated with frenal pull. J. Periodontol., *45*:78, 1974.

110. Wennstrom, J., Lindhe, J., and Nyman, S.: Role of keratinized gingiva for gingival health. J. Clin. Periodontol., *8*:311, 1981.

111. Wennstrom, J., Lindhe, J., and Nyman, S.: The role of keratinized gingiva in plaque-associated gingivitis in dogs. J. Clin. Periodontol., *9*:75, 1982.

112. West, T. L., and Bloom, A.: A histologic study of wound healing following mucogingival surgery. J. Dent. Res., *40*:675, 1961.

113. Whinston, G. J.: Frenotomy and mucobuccal fold resection utilized in periodontal therapy. N.Y. Dent. J., *22*:495, 1956.

114. Wilderman, M. N.: Repair after a periosteal retention procedure. J. Periodontol., *34*:487, 1963.

115. Wilderman, M. N.: Exposure of bone in periodontal surgery. Dent. Clin. North Am., *8*:23, 1964.

116. Wilderman, M. N., and Wentz, F. M.: Repair of a dentogingival defect with a pedicle flap. J. Periodontol., *36*:218, 1965.

117. Wilderman, M. N., Wentz, F. M., and Orban, B. J.: Histogenesis of repair after mucogingival surgery. J. Periodontol., *31*:283, 1960.

118. Wood, D. L., Hoag, P. L., Donnenfeld, O. W., and Rosenfeld, L. D.: Alveolar crest reduction following full and partial thickness flaps. J. Periodontol., *43*:141, 1972.

119. Woofter, C.: The prevalence and etiology of gingival recession. Periodont. Abstracts, *17*:45, 1969.

chapter fifty-seven

Treatment of Gingival Enlargement

Treatment of gingival enlargement is based upon an understanding of the etiology and underlying pathologic changes (see Chapter 10). Enlargements caused by inflammation alone can be treated effectively by local procedures. When systemic or unknown conditions are partly or entirely responsible, local treatment will only reduce the enlargement by the extent to which inflammation contributes to it. Because gingival enlargements differ in etiology, their treatment is best considered under separate headings.

TREATMENT OF CHRONIC INFLAMMATORY GINGIVAL ENLARGEMENT

SCALING AND CURETTAGE. Chronic inflammatory enlargements, which are soft and discolored and are caused principally by edema and cellular infiltration, are treated by scaling and curettage, provided the size of the enlargement does not interfere with complete removal of deposits from the involved tooth surfaces.

GINGIVECTOMY. Since most chronic inflammatory gingival enlargements include a significant fibrotic component that will not undergo shrinkage following scaling and curettage or are of such size that they obscure deposits on the tooth surfaces and interfere with access to them, gingivectomy (see Chapter 52) is the treatment of choice (Plate XII). **The location and bevel of the incision are particularly critical.** The following procedure is used:

After the area is anesthetized, the junction of the enlarged gingiva with the adjacent mucosa is probed and outlined with pinpoint markings (Fig. 57–1A). The incision is made **apical to the markings and sufficiently close to the bone to assure complete removal of the enlarged tissue and complete exposure of all**

root deposits. No extraneous fibrous tissue should be left on the bone, because it interferes with the attainment of normal gingival contour. The mucosa adjacent to the enlargement should be tapered by beveling the incision (Fig. 57–1B). The teeth are scaled and planed, and a periodontal pack is inserted for 1 week.

Tumor-like Inflammatory Enlargement. Tumor-like inflammatory enlargements are treated by gingivectomy as follows:

Under local anesthesia the tooth surfaces beneath the mass are scaled to remove calculus and other debris. The lesion is separated from the mucosa at its base with a No. 12 Bard-Parker blade. If the lesion extends interproximally, the interdental gingiva is included in the incision to ensure exposure of irritating root deposits. After the lesion is removed, the involved root surfaces are scaled and planed and the area cleansed with warm water. A periodontal pack is applied and removed in a week, at which time the patient is instructed in plaque control.

TREATMENT OF THE GINGIVAL ABSCESS

In contrast to a periodontal abscess, which involves the supporting periodontal tissues, the *gingival abscess is a lesion of the marginal or interdental gingiva, usually produced by an impacted foreign object.* It is treated as follows:

Under topical anesthesia the fluctuant area of the lesion is incised with a Bard-Parker blade, and the incision is gently widened to permit drainage. The area is cleansed with warm water and covered with a gauze pad. After bleeding stops, the patient is dismissed for 24 hours and instructed to rinse every 2 hours with a glassful of warm water.

When the patient returns, the lesion is generally reduced in size and symptom-free. A

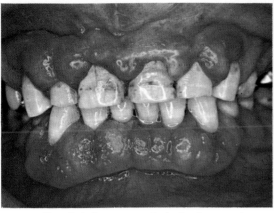

A, Chronic inflammatory gingival enlargement.

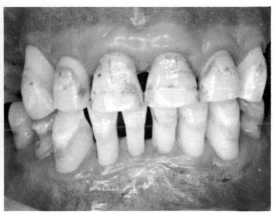

B, After treatment.

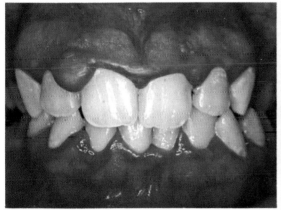

C, Chronic inflammatory enlargement associated with mouth breathing.

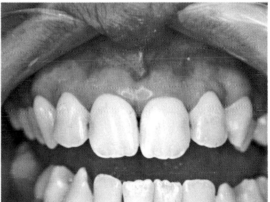

D, After treatment.

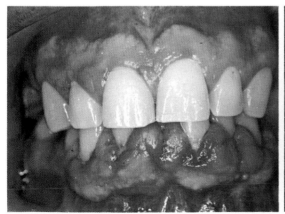

E, Gingival enlargement associated with phenytoin therapy.

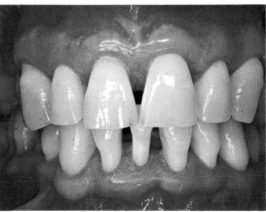

F, After treatment.

Plate XII

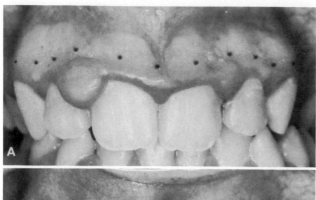

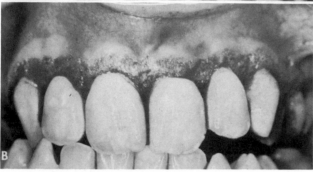

Figure 57–1 Gingivectomy Incision for Gingival Enlargement. *A,* Chronic inflammatory gingival enlargement with tumor-like area. Pinpoint markings outline extent of the enlargement. *B,* Enlarged gingiva removed. Note the beveled incision. (For the pre- and posttreatment appearance see Plate XII *C* and *D*.)

topical anesthetic is applied, and the area is scaled and curetted. If the residual size of the lesion is too great, it is removed surgically.

TREATMENT OF GINGIVAL HYPERPLASIA ASSOCIATED WITH PHENYTOIN (DILANTIN) THERAPY

Gingival enlargement does not occur in all patients receiving phenytoin; when it does occur, it may be of three types:

Type I. **Noninflammatory hyperplasia caused by the phenytoin** (Fig. 57–2*A*). Discontinuing the phenytoin is the only method of eliminating it. When this is done, the enlargement disappears after a few months. The feasibility of discontinuing the drug should be discussed with the neurologist. Except in cases of severe disfigurement, persisting after periodontal

treatment and creating psychologic problems, the existence of moderate or severe hyperplasia is not reason enough to discontinue the use of phenytoin.[8] There may be, however, neurologic indications for discontinuing the use of the drug that may occur.[8] In most instances, though, the administration of phenytoin must continue, and other periodontal treatments to control hyperplasia have to be used (see Type III).

Type II. **Chronic inflammatory enlargement entirely unrelated to the phenytoin** (Fig. 57–2*B*). The enlargement is caused entirely by local irritants and resembles inflammatory enlargement in patients not receiving phenytoin. It can be treated successfully, without recurrence, by gingivectomy and fastidious plaque control.

Type III. **Combined enlargement is a combination of hyperplasia caused by phenytoin**

NON-INFLAMMATORY HYPERPLASTIC ENLARGEMENT	INFLAMMATORY ENLARGEMENT	COMBINED ENLARGEMENT
A	**B**	**C**

Figure 57–2 Types of Gingival Enlargement in Patients Under Phenytoin Therapy. *A,* Noninflammatory hyperplastic enlargement caused by the phenytoin. *B,* Inflammatory enlargement caused by local irritation without phenytoin-induced hyperplasia. *C,* Combined enlargement that results from inflammation superimposed upon phenytoin-induced hyperplasia.

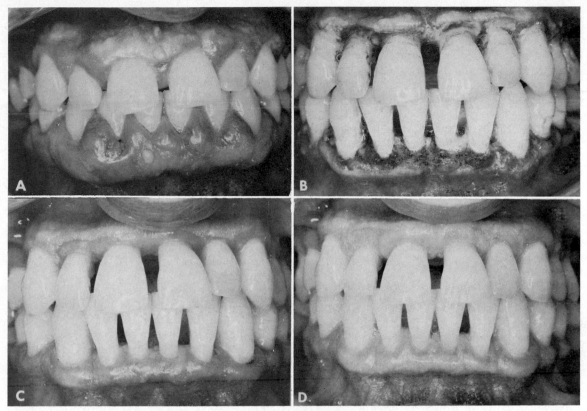

Figure 57–3 Combined Type of Gingival Enlargement Associated with Phenytoin Therapy. *A,* Enlargement caused by phenytoin combined with superimposed inflammation. *B,* Appearance at time of pack removal, 1 week after complete mouth gingivectomy. *C,* After 4 months. *D,* After 5 years. There is some hyperplasia caused by the phenytoin, but its size has been kept to a minimum by periodic scalings and diligent plaque control, which prevent inflammation from recurring.

and inflammation caused by local irritation (Fig. 57–2). *This is the most common type of enlargement in patients treated with phenytoin* (Fig. 57–2*C*). It is treated by gingivectomy or flap surgery and elimination of all sources of local irritation, plus fastidious plaque control by the patient.

The initial treatment of combined enlargement presents no difficulty; the problem is with recurrence. Recurrence can be kept to a minimum by periodic scaling and diligent plaque control by the patient[6] (Plate XII). A hard natural rubber fitted bite guard worn at night sometimes assists in the control of recurrence.[1, 2]

Local treatment is very effective; it keeps patients comfortable and without disfigurement for years,[3, 5, 7] but does not keep them entirely free of enlargement.[9, 10] It prevents the return of that part of the enlargement caused by inflammation (Fig. 57–3); it does not usually prevent the recurrence of the hyperplastic component of the enlargement caused by the phenytoin, although it has been reported to do so in some cases.[4, 6] In patients treated with

phenytoin whose gingival enlargement is caused by local irritation alone, with no drug-induced hyperplasia, recurrence is totally preventable by local measures.

TREATMENT OF LEUKEMIC GINGIVAL ENLARGEMENT

Leukemic enlargement occurs in acute or subacute leukemia and is uncommon in the chronic leukemic state. The medical care of leukemic patients is often complicated by gingival enlargement with superimposed painful acute necrotizing ulcerative gingivitis, which interferes with eating and creates toxic systemic reactions. The bleeding and clotting times and platelet count of the patient are checked and the hematologist consulted before periodontal treatment is instituted. (see Chapter 36).

Treatment of acute gingival involvement is described in Chapter 41. After the acute symptoms subside, attention is directed to correction of the gingival enlargement. The rationale is to remove the local factors in order to control the inflammatory component of the enlargement.

The enlargement is treated by scaling and curettage carried out in stages under topical anesthesia. The initial treatment consists of gently removing all loose accumulations with cotton pellets, superficial scaling, and instruction in oral hygiene procedures for plaque control. Oral hygiene is extremely important in these cases and should be performed by the nurse, if necessary.

Progressively deeper scalings are carried out at subsequent visits. Treatments are confined to a small area of the mouth to facilitate control of bleeding. Antibiotics are administered systemically the evening before and for 48 hours after each treatment to reduce the risk of infection.

TREATMENT OF GINGIVAL ENLARGEMENT IN PREGNANCY

Treatment requires elimination of all local irritants that are responsible for precipitating the gingival changes in pregnancy. *Elimination of local irritants early in pregnancy is a preventive measure against gingival disease, which is preferable to treatment of gingival enlargement after it occurs.*

Marginal and interdental gingival inflammation and enlargement are treated by scaling and curettage (see Chapters 43 and 51). Treatment of **tumor-like gingival enlargements** consists of surgical excision and scaling and planing of the tooth surface. *The enlargement will recur unless all irritants are removed.* Food impaction is a frequent factor.

WHEN TO TREAT. *The lesion should be treated as soon as it is detected. It should not be permitted to remain until the pregnancy terminates, on the assumption that it will disappear spontaneously.* This invites the possibility of increased growth of the lesion during pregnancy, with added patient discomfort. It also misleads the patient into thinking that parturition will solve her gingival problem. **Gingival enlargements do shrink after pregnancy, but they do not disappear**. There is a residual area of local irritation and inflammation which, if untreated, may cause progressive destruction of the periodontal tissues.

In pregnancy the emphasis should be upon (1) preventing gingival disease before it occurs, and (2) treating existing gingival disease before it becomes worse. All patients should be seen as early as possible in pregnancy. Those without gingival disease should be checked for potential sources of local irritation and should be instructed in plaque control procedures (see Chapter 44). Those with gingival disease should be treated promptly, before the conditioning effect of pregnancy upon the gingiva becomes manifest. Precautions necessary for periodontal treatment of pregnant women are presented on p. 568.

Every pregnant patient should be scheduled for periodic dental visits, and their importance as a preventive against serious periodontal disturbances should be stressed.

TREATMENT OF GINGIVAL ENLARGEMENT IN PUBERTY

Gingival enlargement in puberty is treated by scaling and curettage, removal of all sources of irritation, and plaque control. Gingivectomy may be required in severe cases. The problem in these patients is recurrence due to poor oral hygiene.

DRUGS IN THE TREATMENT OF GINGIVAL ENLARGEMENT

Gingival enlargement can be reduced by escharotic drugs, but this is not a recommended form of treatment. The destructive action of the drugs is difficult to control; injury to healthy tissue and root surfaces, delayed healing, and excessive postoperative pain are complications that can be avoided when the gingiva is removed with periodontal knives and scalpels or by electrosurgery. Removal of the enlarged gingiva by any method must be accompanied by elimination of local irritants.

RECURRENCE OF GINGIVAL ENLARGEMENT

Recurrence following treatment is the most common problem in the management of gingival enlargement. Residual local irritation and systemic or hereditary conditions that cause noninflammatory gingival hyperplasia are the responsible factors.

Recurrence of chronic inflammatory enlargement immediately after treatment indicates that all irritants have not been removed. Contributory local conditions, such as food impaction and overhanging margins of restorations, are factors that are commonly overlooked. If the enlargement recurs after healing is complete and normal contour is attained, inadequate plaque control by the patient is the most common cause.

Recurrence during the healing period is manifested as red, bead-like granulomatous masses which bleed upon slight provocation. This is a proliferative vascular inflammatory response to local irritation, usually a fragment of calculus on the root. The condition is corrected by removing the granulation tissue and planing the root surface.

Familial, hereditary, or *idiopathic* gingival enlargement recurs after surgical removal even if all local irritants have been removed. The enlargement can be maintained at minimal size by preventing secondary inflammatory involvement.

REFERENCES

1. Aiman, R.: The use of positive pressure mouthpiece as a new therapy for Dilantin gingival hyperplasia. Chron. Omaha Dent. Soc., *131*:244, 1968.
2. Babcock, J. R.: The successful use of a new therapy for Dilantin gingival hyperplasia. Periodontics, *3*:196, 1965.
3. Bergmann, C. L.: Dilantin: its effect on the gingival tissue. Dent. Digest, *73*:63, 1967.
4. Ciancio, S. G., Yaffe, S. J., and Catz, C. C.: Gingival hyperplasia and diphenylhydantoin. J. Periodontol., *43*:411, 1972.
5. Ginwalla, T. M., et al.: Management of gingival hyperplasia in patients receiving Dilantin therapy. J. Indian Dent. Assoc., *39*:124, 1967.
6. Hall W. B.: Dilantin hyperplasia: a preventable lesion. J. Periodont. Res., *4*:36, 1969.
7. Miller, F. D.: Multipronged attack against Dilantin gingival hyperplasia. Dent. Survey, *42*:51, 1966.
8. Reynolds, N. C., Jr., and Kirkham, D. B.: Therapeutic alternatives in phenytoin-induced gingival hyperplasia. J. Periodontol., *51*:516, 1980.
9. Russell, B., and Bay, L.: The effect of toothbrushing with chlorhexidine gluconate toothpaste on epileptic children. J. Dent. Res., *54*(Suppl. A):L114, 1975. (abstract).
10. Staple, P. H., Reed, M. J., Mashimo, P. A., Sedransk, N., and Umemoto, T.: Diphenylhydantoin gingival hyperplasia in *Macaca arctoides*. Prevention by inhibition of dental plaque deposition. J. Periodontol., *49*:310, 1978.

Part VI

Reconstructive Phase

chapter fifty-eight

Restorative-Periodontal Interrelationships

Dental restorations and periodontal health are inseparably interrelated. Technical excellence is important in restorative dentistry. The adaptation of the margins, the contours of the restoration, the proximal relationships, and the surface smoothness fulfill critical biologic requirements of the gingiva and supporting periodontal tissues. Dental restorations therefore play a significant role in maintaining periodontal health.

Gingival and periodontal disease must be eliminated before restorative procedures are begun for the following reasons:

Tooth mobility and pain interfere with mastication and function of restorative dentistry.

Inflammation of the periodontium impairs the capacity of abutment teeth to meet the functional demands of restorative dentistry. Restorations constructed so as to provide beneficial functional stimulation to a healthy periodontium become a destructive influence when superimposed upon existing periodontal disease, shortening the life of the teeth and the restoration.

The position of teeth is frequently altered in periodontal disease. Resolution of inflammation and regeneration of periodontal ligament fibers following periodontal treatment cause the teeth to move again, often in the direction of their original position. Restorations designed for teeth before the periodontium is treated may produce injurious tensions and pressures on the treated periodontium.

Partial prostheses constructed on casts made from impressions of diseased gingiva and edentulous mucosa will not fit properly when periodontal health is restored. When the inflammation is eliminated, the contour of the gingiva and adjacent mucosa is altered (Fig. 58–1). Shrinkage creates spaces beneath the pontics of fixed bridges and the saddle areas of removable prostheses. Resultant plaque accumulation leads to inflammation of the mucosa and gingiva of the abutment teeth.

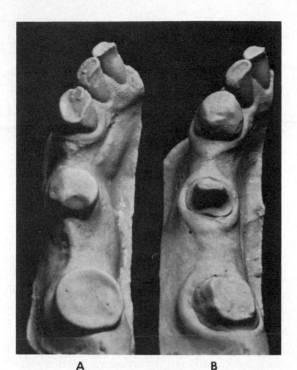

Figure 58–1 Change in Contour of Edentulous Mucosa Following Resolution of Inflammation. *A,* Before treatment. Note the pyramidal contour of the edentulous mucosa. *B,* After resolution of inflammation. The teeth are in process of preparation.

To locate the gingival margin of restorations properly, the position of the healthy gingival sulcus must be established before the tooth is prepared. Margins of restorations hidden behind diseased gingiva will be exposed when the inflamed gingiva shrinks following periodontal treatment.

PREPARATION OF THE PERIODONTIUM FOR RESTORATIVE DENTISTRY

In patients with mutilated dentitions and extensive periodontal disease, the usual treatment sequence is changed, and a temporary prosthesis is constructed before the periodontal pockets are eliminated. The teeth are prepared with provisional margins, which are relocated after the tissues heal. This provides improved occlusal relationships and splinting during the healing period. Approximately 2 months after periodontal treatment, when gingival health is restored and the location of the gingival sulcus is established, the preparations are modified to relocate the margins in proper relation to the healthy gingival sulcus, and a final restoration is constructed.

The aims of periodontal treatment are not limited to the elimination of periodontal pockets and the restoration of gingival health. *Treatment should also create the gingival mucosal environment necessary for the proper function of fixed and removable partial prostheses. Preparation of the mouth for restorative dentistry consists of soft tissue corrective measures performed as part of periodontal treatment.*

Phase I Therapy

The procedures contained in Phase I therapy are directed toward one specific goal, i.e., the control of active dental disease (see Chapters 43 and 44). Therefore, when initial therapy is completed, patients should be in a state of dental health with active caries no longer occurring and with active destruction of the periodontium under control. This will result in elimination of the acute inflammatory response associated with periodontal destruction. Thus, the status of the gingival tissues should be such that further restorative procedures of a more complex nature can be carried out without undue detrimental effects from unhealthy gingiva.

In some patients, periodontal surgery will be necessary. These periodontal surgical procedures should be carried out with due regard for the restorative needs of the patient. Therefore, the final level of the periodontium should allow good access to all restorative marginal regions, and any necessary increase in clinical crown length should be obtained by the postsurgical positioning of the periodontal tissues. If restorative procedures will necessitate the resolution of mucogingival inadequacies, the appropriate surgical procedure should be completed before the restorative therapy is begun.

Obtaining control of periodontal inflammation during Phase I therapy will result in restorative procedures of a much higher quality than what they would be if they were carried out in an environment of gingival inflammation. The presence of an acute inflammatory response in the gingiva results in ulceration of the epithelium that lines the gingival pocket and in an increase of vascularity and edema of the tissues immediately under this epithelium. There is a possibility of continual bleeding and exudation of inflammatory tissue fluid into the gingival crevice and into the environment where restorative dental procedures are carried out. Therefore, it is of utmost importance that all areas of the gingiva that show hemorrhage and significant amounts of inflammatory exudate be brought to an improved state of health before any restorative procedures other than emergency control of dental caries are carried out.

The removal of etiologic factors causing gingival inflammation will result in a return to a more healthy state of the gingiva within 1 or 2 weeks. Thus, plaque control, calculus removal, and the removal of any inadequate dental restorations in the gingival environment should be important first-order procedures in initial therapy.

Periodontal Surgery

The routine procedures of periodontal surgery aimed at the correction of periodontal and mucogingival defects are described in previous chapters. However, there are some surgical procedures which are modified because restorative dentistry or prosthodontic therapy is combined with the periodontal surgical procedure.

POCKETS ADJACENT TO EDENTULOUS REGIONS. Periodontal pockets frequently occur on the proximal surface of teeth adjacent to edentulous regions. Correction of these periodontal defects should occur before any fixed

or removable prosthodontic appliance is placed in these areas. The general principles involved in pocket elimination are similar to those used in other areas, but some special procedures are necessary in order to take into account the special needs of the edentulous space.

Periodontally involved teeth adjacent to edentulous spaces present two problems, which must be treated together: (1) elimination of the pockets and (2) management of the edentulous mucosa. Inflammation from the periodontal pockets extends for varying distances into the adjacent edentulous mucosa (Fig. 58–2) and alters its color, consistency, and shape. The edentulous mucosa affected by inflammation may present various degrees of discoloration and edema with a smooth, glistening surface, depending upon the relative predominance of cellular and fluid exudate or fibrosis. If principally fibrotic, the mucosa is pink, firm, and enlarged, with a lobulated surface.

The contour of the edentulous mucosa and gingiva is affected by mechanical factors as well as by inflammation from adjacent pockets. The edentulous mucosa may conform to the shape of the underlying bone, it may be swollen and rounded faciolingually, or lateral pressure from the tongue and cheek and food excursion may cause a pyramiding of the mucosa to form an elongated triangular ridge (Fig.

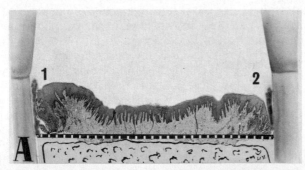

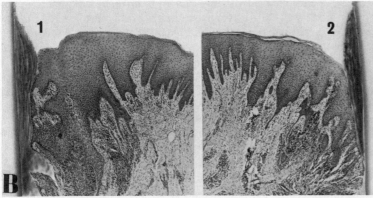

Figure 58–2 Preparation of the Mouth for Prosthesis. *A,* Edentulous mucosa with periodontal pockets (1 and 2) on the adjacent teeth. The location of the necessary incision is indicated by the dotted line. *B,* Inflammation from the periodontal pockets (1 and 2) extends into the edentulous mucosa.

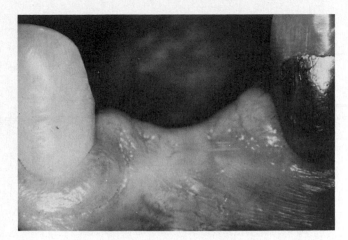

Figure 58–3 "Pyramiding" of Edentulous Mucosa and Adjacent Gingiva. The gingiva and mucosa are contoured by pressure from the tongue and food excursion.

58–3). Because of the absence of the normal protective action of the embrasure, the gingiva is often similarly deformed.

The deformed edentulous mucosa reduces the vertical height available for prosthetic replacements. It does not provide a reliable base for the support of saddle areas or for the proper design of pontics. The triangular mucosa is unsatisfactory for the placement of pontics. In an effort to overcome the problem, short pontics with a deep V-shaped base, which straddles the ridge, are used. These are unsatisfactory, because food wedges between the mucosa and the pontics and the accumulation of plaque causes inflammation that jeopardizes retention of the bridge (Fig. 58–4).

MANAGEMENT OF POCKETS AND EDENTULOUS MUCOSA. The area is prepared for the prosthesis with the following objectives:

1. To establish a healthy gingival sulcus. The pontics adjacent to the natural teeth can be designed to create the gingival embrasure necessary for preservation of gingival health.

2. To eliminate extraneous mucosal tissue so as to permit adequate vertical space for the replacements.

3. To provide a firm, healthy mucosal base for placement of saddles or pontics.

In some situations, when pocket depth occurs in areas adjacent to edentulous areas, a *gingivectomy* may be used to eliminate these pockets and at the same time provide a maintainable contour of the edentulous ridge region (Fig. 58–5). The gingivectomy incision is continued from the gingival tissues into the edentulous area in such a way that the resulting tissue contour will form a firm, thin band of keratinized tissue across the saddle areas. This incision should be made so that the final contour of the saddle areas blends into the adjacent gingival contours and the edentulous ridge has a rounded, smooth contour. The procedure

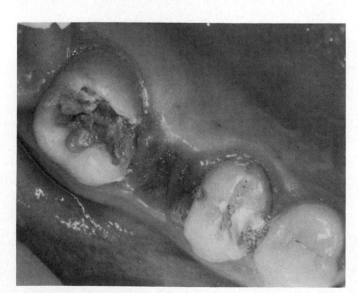

Figure 58–4 Chronic Inflammation of Edentulous Mucosa under bridge with ridge-lap type of pontic.

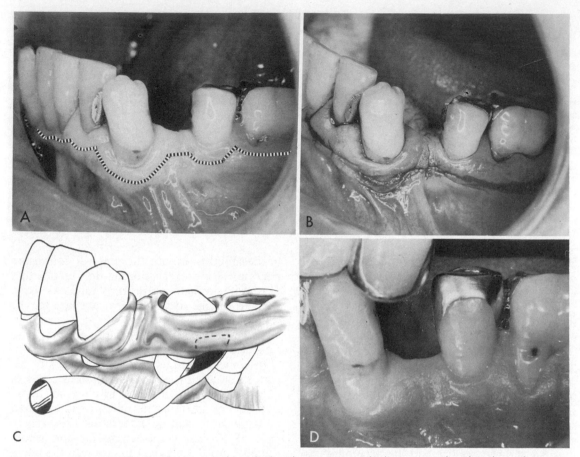

Figure 58–5 Preparation for Prosthesis. *A,* Deformed edentulous mucosa and adjacent periodontal pockets. The incision is indicated by the dotted line. *B,* The incision. *C,* Inflamed gingiva and edentulous mucosa removed. *D,* Mucosa and gingiva healed with deformity corrected.

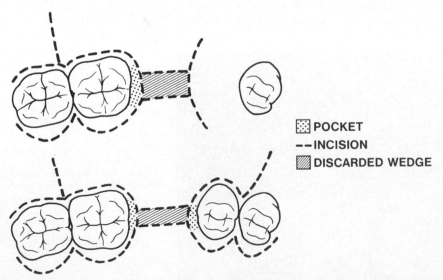

Figure 58–6 Flap Surgery in Edentulous Areas. Incisions for pockets adjacent to edentulous regions. The dotted lines mark the initial incisions. Vertical incisions may be used at the interproximal spaces, or the excision may be continued as an envelope flap design.

will also result in the removal of inflamed tissues in the submucosa so that the final tissue will have a thin yet dense submucosa bound tightly to the periosteum and covered by an intact keratinized epithelium.

Because of the importance of maintaining a keratinized epithelium over the edentulous area, the gingivectomy procedure cannot be used in places where it would result in the complete removal of all keratinized tissue. In these situations, when the gingivectomy would result in the nonkeratinized oral mucosa forming the edentulous ridge or marginal gingival area, a *flap procedure* is indicated. In those areas where the pockets on the proximal surfaces of the teeth adjacent to the edentulous area are of the infrabony type, a flap procedure is also needed. The incisions normally made around the adjacent teeth are carried into the edentulous area in the form of parallel buccal and lingual incisions that run across the crest of the ridge so that an adequate band of keratinized gingiva is maintained on both the buccal and the lingual portions of the flap. These incisions across the edentulous area are made so that the flap is undermined (Fig. 58–6). The inflamed tissue between the buccal and lingual incisions is removed. The undermining of the buccal and lingual flaps leaves a thin band of tissue that will lie close to the underlying bone once the flap is sutured back into position on completion of the operation. The

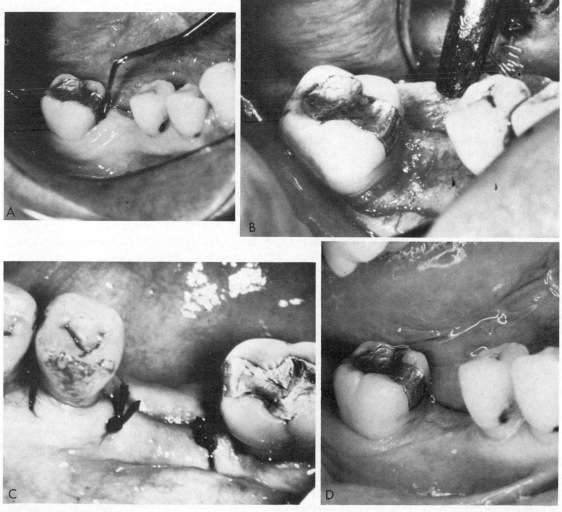

Figure 58–7 Flap Surgery in Edentulous Areas. *A,* Pockets adjacent to edentulous region. There is a 6-mm pocket on the mesial aspect of the lower second molar, and additional crown length is required for abutment preparation. *B,* Wedge-shaped tissue removed. The exposed tooth surfaces are root planed, and any necessary osseous recontouring is carried out. *C,* Closure of flaps. Lingual view of interrupted sutures used to close the flaps and to hold tissue in an apical position. *D,* Three months postoperation. The gingival tissue is established at a more apical level on the tooth. Pocket depth is now 2 mm on mesial aspect of second molar. Additional crown length is available for abutment preparation.

undermining and subsequent repositioning of the flap will result in an apical positioning of the soft tissue covering the edentulous area.

By means of the parallel incisions over the edentulous area, access is obtained to any osseous defects on the adjacent teeth. These periodontal osseous defects can be recontoured in order to eliminate the pockets. The flaps will provide tissue to cover these corrected osseous defects completely so that the healing that follows will be uneventful and of short duration (Fig. 58–7).

MANAGEMENT OF MUCOGINGIVAL PROBLEMS. It is often necessary to carry out a free soft tissue autograft in patients who have a mucogingival defect associated with gingival inflammation and require a dental restoration in the immediate environment of the gingiva (Fig. 58–8). The procedure for carrying out this free soft tissue autograft has been covered in Chapter 56 and need not be further discussed here. Mucogingival surgery should be carried out at least 2 months prior to the completion of the dental restoration. This will allow time for mature tissue to be formed in the gingival margin so that restorative procedures will not cause a return of clinical inflammation. Augmentation of keratinized gingiva provides stability of the free gingival margin and surrounding gingival tissues so that the dental restoration can be placed in an environment where gingival health can be maintained.

CROWN-LENGTHENING PROCEDURES. In situations when a small clinical crown is present on the tooth and this is deemed inadequate for the retention of a required cast restoration, it is necessary to increase the size of the clinical crown using periodontal surgical procedures. These crown-lengthening procedures will enable the dentist performing the restoration to develop an adequate area for the crown retentive requirements without extending the crown margins deep into the periodontal tissues. Although in some cases it may be possible to achieve lengthening of the crown by the use of gingivectomy procedures, it is generally necessary to use a flap procedure to establish a new level for the gingival margin. Frequently the amount of increased length required means that it is necessary to remove some alveolar bone in order to ensure that the exposed crown is of sufficient length for the required restoration (Fig. 58–9). Once the level of apical extension of the crown margin is decided upon, this level is used as a guide to whether osseous surgery is indicated. It is essential that there be at least 3 mm between the most apical extension of the crown margin and the alveolar bone crest. This space will allow sufficient room for the supracrestal collagen fibers that are part of the periodontal support mechanism, as well as allowing for a gingival crevice of 2 to 3 mm. If this guideline is used, the margin of the crown will finally be positioned at its correct level at approximately half way down the gingival crevice. Failure to allow sufficient space between the crown margin and the alveolar crest height means that the finished restoration will be positioned deep in the periodontal tissues and will result in increasing inflammation and pocket formation (Fig. 58–10).

PERIODONTAL ASPECTS OF FIXED AND REMOVABLE PROSTHESES

In addition to esthetics, the purposes of fixed and removable prostheses include the improvement of masticatory efficiency and the prevention of tilting and extrusion of teeth with resultant disruption of the occlusion and food impaction.

Occlusal Adjustment Before Prosthesis

Traumatic occlusal relationships should be eliminated before restorative procedures are begun, and restoration should be constructed in conformity with the newly established occlusal patterns. If this is not done, the prosthesis perpetuates occlusal relationships injurious to the periodontium.

The harmful effects of occlusal trauma are not confined to the teeth involved in the restoration and their antagonists. Other areas of the dentition are secondarily affected by an occlusal disharmony created or perpetuated by an inlay or bridge. Delaying occlusal adjustment until the restorations are inserted often necessitates grinding through the occlusal surface of the newly constructed restorations.

The occlusion must be checked at regular intervals after a prosthesis is inserted. Occlusal relationships change with time as the result of wear of restorative materials and setting of saddle areas of removable prostheses, especially those without distal support.

Tooth Preparation in Relation to the Gingival Margin

The first requirement for proper location of the gingival margin of a crown or other resto-

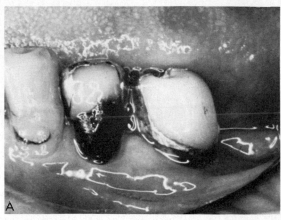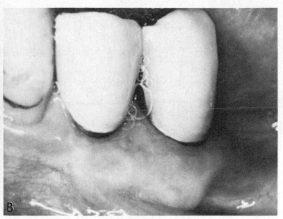

Figure 58–8 Mucogingival Problems. *A,* Preoperative mucogingival problem. There is inadequate gingiva in the region where a crown margin is to be placed. The presence of a plaque-enhancing margin necessitates the development of an adequate band of gingiva. *B,* Postoperative soft tissue autograft 6 months after mucogingival surgery and placement of restoration. Note the adequate band of gingiva.

ration close to the gingiva is a healthy gingival sulcus. Preparation is not complete until the gingiva is healthy and its position on the root has been established. Periodontal pockets should not be permitted to remain undisturbed for the ostensible purposes of "keeping the root covered" or "hiding the margins of the restorations." When the gingiva is treated, as it eventually must be, the denuded root and margins of the restoration that were "hidden" by the inflamed gingiva become visible. In the interim, the patient has suffered unnecessary destruction of the periodontium, and the longevity of the tooth and restoration has been jeopardized.

Treatment of the gingiva, final tooth preparation, and impression taking should not be attempted in one operation, for this does not allow time for the gingiva to heal, and the location of the margin of the restoration in relation to the healed gingival sulcus can only be estimated.

Dental restorations should be kept away from the gingiva whenever possible. Extension of cavity margins into the gingival sulcus should only occur in those situations when there is a definite indication for introducing restorative materials into the subgingival environment. If the restorative margin is placed subgingivally, it is more difficult for the patient's oral hygiene procedures to control the bacteria that colonize this area.

There are some clinical situations in which it is advisable to carry the margin of the restoration into the gingival sulcus, e.g., the existence of a previous restoration extending

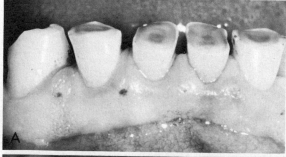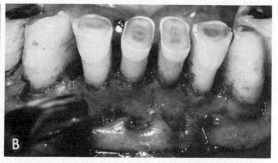

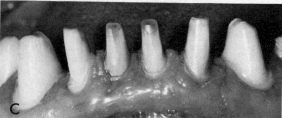

Figure 58–9 Crown Lengthening Using Flap Surgery. *A,* Before treatment there are short clinical crowns with inadequate crown length for retention of full crown restorations. *B,* Osseous recontouring has been carried out, with the alveolar crest now positioned apical to original level. *C,* Healing at 6 weeks showing sufficient clinical crowns for preparation of artificial full crowns. (Courtesy of Drs. R. Vandersloot and I. Logan.)

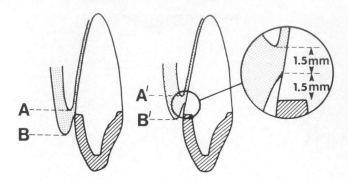

Figure 58–10 Guidelines for Crown-Lengthening Procedure. *A*, alveolar crest; *B*, gingival margin; *A'*, level of alveolar crest after surgical crown lengthening; *B'*, level of gingival margin after surgical crown lengthening. Note that crown margins are positioned in middle of gingival sulcus. Enlargement shows crown margin 1.5 mm coronal to base of gingival crevice. Alveolar crest is 1.5 mm apical to base of gingival crevice.

into the gingival area, the presence of rampant caries or caries that extends apically into the gingival environment, the need for apical extension in order to obtain adequate retention of the restoration, and the advantage of placing the restoration subgingivally on the labial surface of upper anterior teeth in those patients to whom appearance is of primary importance. In *all* other cases, dental restorations should be kept away from the gingival third of the tooth.

Once a decision has been made to place restorative dental materials into the gingival crevice, the level at which the margin should be placed is of critical importance. It is advisable to keep the restorations in the coronal half of the gingival crevice. Thus, all subgingival margins should be placed within 1 to 2 mm of the free gingival margin wherever possible (Fig. 58–11). This allows access to the margin for oral hygiene procedures and will give better access for refining the margin during cavity preparation and impression taking. The coronal half of the gingival sulcus has a much thicker protective layer of epithelium (the oral sulcular epithelium) than does the apical half of the sulcus, where the junctional epithelium is just a few cells thick. This coronal region therefore has better resistance to the toxic products of dental plaque than does the region of the junctional epithelium.

It should be recognized that placing a margin in the gingival crevice at the time of completion of a restoration does not guarantee that this relationship of the gingiva to the margin will maintain itself. There is no reliable way to predict accurately what the movement of the gingival margin over time will be. In patients with an adequate level of oral hygiene associated with a nontraumatic toothbrushing technique, there is much less risk of apical migration of the gingival margin than there is in patients with ineffective and/or traumatic oral hygiene techniques utilizing hard toothbrushes. All clinical signs of gingival inflam-

mation should be resolved before restorations are placed, as the shrinkage associated with the resolution of gingival inflammation will frequently cause the healthy gingival margin to be positioned apical to its location when the gingiva was inflamed.

"Avoid the Gingival Third"

The full crown is extremely useful because it fulfills requirements that can be met by no

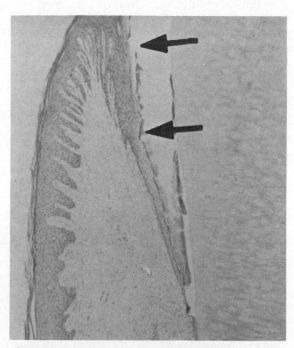

Figure 58–11 Position of Gingival Margins. In those cases in which subgingival margins are indicated, the ideal position for the margin is the coronal half of the gingival sulcus (*arrows*). In this region the thick band of oral sulcular epithelial cells provides a better barrier to penetration of bacterial products than does the narrow junctional epithelium found in the apical half of the sulcus. Cavity preparation, impression taking, and cementation of restorations are all more likely to be ideal when good access to the margin is made possible by positioning it in the coronal half of the gingival sulcus.

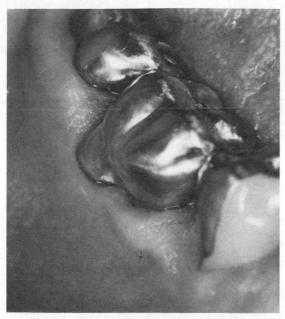

Figure 58–12 Tooth Contour Restored by Crown. Note the excellent condition of the gingiva in the bifurcation area.

other type of restoration (Fig. 58–12). However, even when ideally constructed in relation to the gingival sulcus, the full crown introduces the risk of gingival inflammation. Crowns substitute a foreign substance, such as gold, acrylic, or porcelain, for the natural tooth wall of the gingival sulcus. The materials themselves are not irritating, but plaque can accumulate on these surfaces, and this irritates the gingiva. If not removed within 24 to 48 hours, this plaque may undergo calcification and develop into calculus. The junction of the crown and the tooth also presents a problem. Even with a perfect marginal fit, an extremely thin cement line, which attracts plaque,[59] is unavoidable.

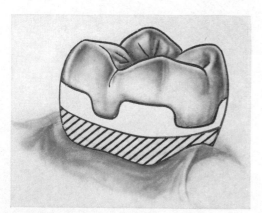

Figure 58–13 "Avoid the Gingival Third." Inlay constructed without involving the gingival third of the crown

The risk of irritation to the gingiva is reduced by restorations that terminate coronal to the gingival margin,[59] encroaching upon the gingival third of the tooth (Fig. 58–13).[63] Wherever possible, inlays,[58] pinledges, and three-quarter crowns should be used as individual restorations and retainers for fixed prostheses. This is not a matter of substituting other restorations for purposes that can only be fulfilled by crowns. However, when there is a choice and high caries incidence is not a problem, the gingival third of the tooth should not be involved in the restoration.

Gingival Retraction for Taking Impressions

When using elastic impression materials, it is often necessary to retract the gingiva to gain access to the gingival margin of the preparation. Several methods of accomplishing this are described below. These are methods for retracting healthy gingiva. They are not for the removal, displacement, or shrinkage of inflamed, swollen gingival tissue. The gingiva must be healthy and its position on the tooth established before the impression is taken.

METHODS OF RETRACTING THE GINGIVA. *Surgery.* Surgical resection of the gingiva is the preferred method for providing access to the margin of the preparation. Under local anesthesia the gingiva is excised apical to the margin of the preparation with periodontal knives or a No. 11 Bard-Parker blade (Fig. 58–14). Bleeding is controlled with pressure from a cotton pellet, moistened with epinephrine if necessary. The gingiva will regenerate and be restored to its normal position, provided it was healthy when the preparation was started. If the gingiva is diseased when the tooth is prepared, resection of the gingiva or inadvertent removal of plaque and calculus during tooth preparation would effect shrinkage in the pocket well and lead to exposure of tooth surface beyond the margin of the preparation (Fig. 58–15). The recession is sometimes erroneously attributed to the surgery.

Electrosurgery. The gingiva may also be retracted by electrosurgery; this avoids the problem of bleeding. Electrosurgery may be used for gingival retraction in some situations in which access to margins is required. It should be carried out so as to minimize tissue damage, and the current should be adapted so that electrosection is used rather than coagulation. The use of equipment that provides a fully rectified current and an undamped wave

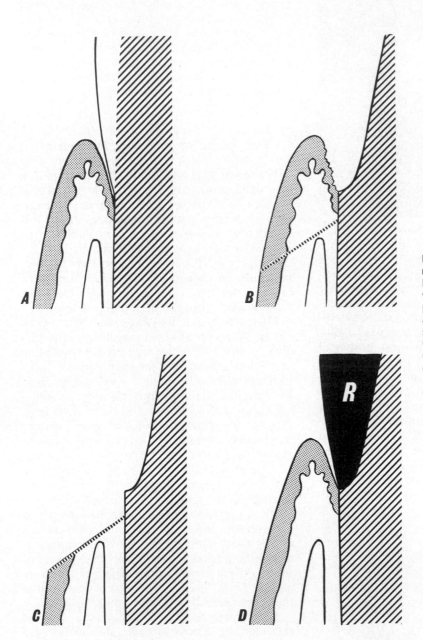

Figure 58–14 Marginal Gingiva Removed to Provide Access for Taking Impressions. *A,* Normal dentogingival relationship before tooth is prepared. *B,* Chamfer-type tooth preparation. The gingival margin is slightly lacerated during preparation. Gingiva incised at dotted line. *C,* Gingival margin removed by periodontal knife or electrosurgery. *D,* Restoration (R) in position at the base of the healed gingival sulcus.

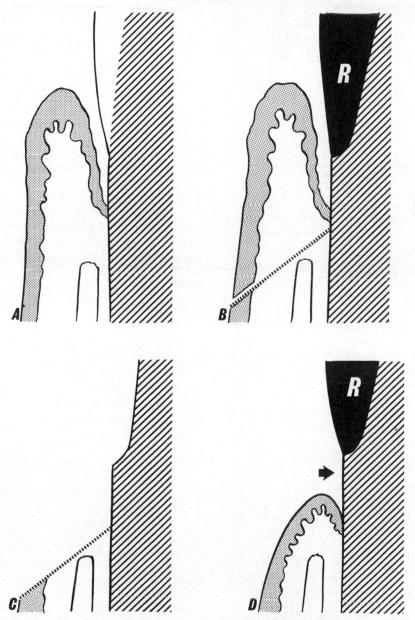

Figure 58–15 Recession Following Restoration of Tooth with Untreated Periodontal Disease. *A,* Periodontal pocket present before tooth preparation. *B,* Restoration (R) erroneously inserted in tooth with untreated periodontal pocket. Dotted line shows incision required for elimination of pocket. *C,* Diseased gingiva removed. *D,* Gingiva heals, revealing the root surface (*arrow*), which had been denuded by periodontal disease before restoration was inserted.

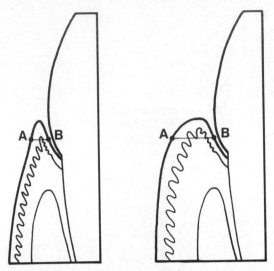

Figure 58–16 Electrosurgery for Retraction. The use of electrosurgery in patients in whom the gingival tissue is thin buccolingually (i.e., A-B on the left diagram) will result in destruction of almost all the gingival tissue, causing postoperative gingival recession. In these situations retraction cords are the method of choice for obtaining access to the gingival margins. When a thick covering of gingiva is present (i.e., A-B on the right diagram), it is possible to use electrosurgical techniques for gingival retraction.

form results in the least amount of tissue damage.[31] Several studies have shown that the careful use of electrosurgery in the superficial part of the gingival crevice results in little if any residual damage to the gingiva.[10, 19] Reports have emphasized the dangers of electrosurgery when the cutting instrument is allowed to be in close proximity to the base of the crevice and cementum.[42, 71] In patients in whom there is a thin covering of gingiva and alveolar bone over the root, electrosurgery should not be used, as the loss of tissue from the internal or crevicular surface can result in gingival recession.[54] In these patients the gingiva should be retracted with retraction strings (Fig. 58–16).

Retraction Strings. Strings impregnated with chemicals are used for gingival retraction. Among the types of chemicals used for this purpose are vasoconstrictors (8 per cent racemic epinephrine),[21] which cause rapid transient elevation in blood pressure and blood sugar and are contraindicated in patients with coronary disease, hyperthyroidism, or diabetes. They also produce local ischemia, which may be injurious to the gingiva. Also used are corrosives (8 per cent zinc chloride, 10 per cent tannic acid, and 10 per cent trichloroacetic acid) and astringents (14 per cent aluminum sulfate).

Impregnated strings will cause the gingiva to wilt away from the tooth and expose the margin of the preparation. The gingiva will ordinarily return to its proper position, provided it was healthy at the outset and the string is not permitted to keep the gingiva separated long enough to permit disease-producing plaque to accumulate in the sulcus. Impregnated strings should not be used on diseased gingiva; pocket walls temporarily retracted from the root will return and jeopardize the tooth and restoration (Fig. 58–17). Because the effects of the chemicals cannot be controlled, pressure retraction of the gingiva with chemical-free strings or other methods of retraction are preferred.

The use of retraction strings can result in tissue tearing and inflammation if the strings are kept dry.[2] The epithelial lining of the gingival sulcus adheres to the dry string and is torn when the string is removed prior to taking impressions. It is advisable to moisten impression retraction strings with saline while they are placed in the gingival crevice, in order to limit tearing of the epithelium. Tearing of the epithelium will make taking an accurate impression difficult or even impossible, as it will result in immediate hemorrhage into the area of the gingival sulcus (Fig. 58–18).

There have been reports of periodontal abscesses associated with impression material left in the gingival environment following the taking of impressions for fixed prosthodontic appliances.[42, 50] Immediately after an impression is removed from the mouth, it should be carefully checked to make sure that no pieces have been torn from it and left in the gingival environment. The gingival sulcus should also be carefully inspected to ensure that no residual pieces of impression material are left in the gingival tissues.

Even with extreme care the gingiva is often lacerated in the course of tooth preparation. If the gingiva is healthy before the restoration is started, it will regenerate and return to its previous position on the tooth,[24, 25] provided the area to which it was attached is not cut away and included in the preparation.

Temporary Coverage

Temporary restorations are often a cause of periodontal inflammation and gingival recession.[14] All temporary restorations should be constructed so that they minimize the damage done to the gingiva during the time they are

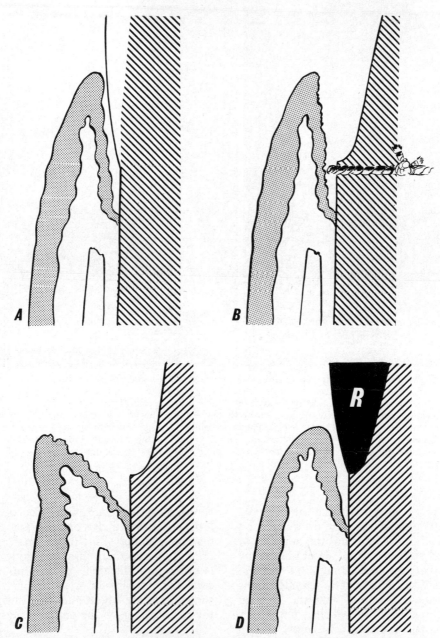

Figure 58–17 Periodontal Pocket Persisting After Retraction *A,* Periodontal pocket present before tooth is prepared. *B,* Tooth prepared, retraction string placed to retract diseased gingiva. *C,* Diseased gingiva temporarily retracted to provide access to tooth for impression. *D,* Restoration (R) inserted. The periodontal pocket has returned.

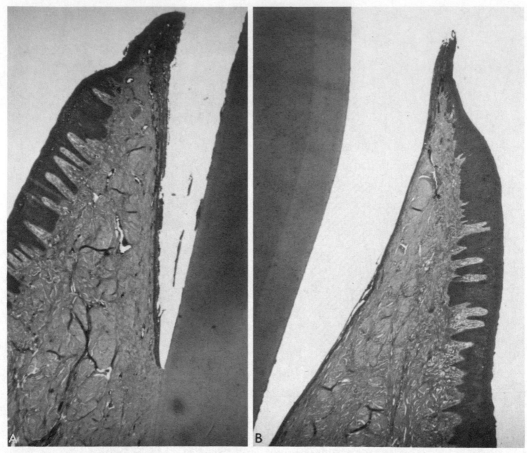

Figure 58–18 Gingival Response to Retraction Strings. *A,* Photomicrograph of gingival sulcus region of a dog after removal of gingival retraction cord that had been placed in the sulcus for 7 minutes. In this case the cord was dried prior to placement, and the sulcus was air dried during the time the cord was in place. Note the tearing of the sulcular epithelium and the initial acute inflammatory reaction in the connective tissue of the gingiva, with dilatation of blood vessels. There is evidence of bleeding into the gingival crevice. *B,* Photomicrograph of gingival sulcus region of a dog after removal of gingival retraction cord that had been placed in the sulcus for 7 minutes. In this case the cord was moistened with saline prior to placement, and the gingival sulcus was bathed with saline during the time the cord was in place. Note the intact epithelium, the absence of acute inflammation, and the lack of hemorrhage.

in the mouth. It is important that the marginal integrity of temporary restorations be as good as is technically possible, and the surfaces of these temporary restorations should be highly polished so that plaque accumulation on them is minimized. The contour of these restorations should also be compatible with the gingival tissues. In those cases in which a temporary restoration is to be in place for more than a few days, the requirements of contour, polish, and fit should be the same as for the final restoration. Such long-term restorations should not be called temporary but should be regarded as **provisional or treatment restorations** that may remain in place for many months. Provisional or treatment restorations allow the dentist to assess the effect of the final restoration on the periodontium. The

contour of the restorations, the occlusal pattern, and the patient's oral hygiene procedures may be modified while provisional restorations are in place so that optimal periodontal health is obtained. The final restorations can duplicate the provisional restorations, providing some certainty about the long-term effect of the restorations on the periodontium (Fig. 58–19).

The Embrasures

When teeth are in proximal contact, the spaces that widen out from the contact are known as embrasures. The interdental space is divisible into a facial and a lingual embrasure (Fig. 58–20), an occlusal or incisal embrasure

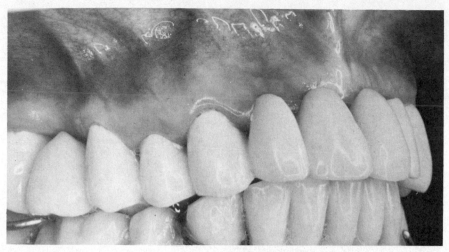

Figure 58–19 Provisional Restorations. Provisional restorations provide an opportunity to evaluate the patient's response to the final restorations. The esthetics can be modified, but, more importantly, the contour of the restorations can be changed so that the gingival tissues can be kept healthy. When previous restorations have caused gingival inflammation, a provisional restoration can become a treatment restoration as it provides an environment for the gingiva to return to health. These restorations should be made of heat-cured acrylic, should have accurate marginal adaption, and should be contoured and polished so as to duplicate the form of the natural teeth. (Courtesy of Dr. John Flocken.)

that is coronal to the contact area (Fig. 58–21*A*) and a gingival embrasure, which is the space between the contact area and the alveolar bone.[5, 70] The gingival embrasure is filled with soft tissue, but in periodontal disease (Fig. 58–21*B*) spaces are created in the gingival embrasure.

THE GINGIVAL EMBRASURE. Embrasures are critical considerations in restorative dentistry. Proximal surfaces of dental restorations are important because they create the embrasures essential for gingival health (Fig. 58–22). From the periodontal viewpoint, the gingival embrasure is the most significant. Periodontal disease causes tissue destruction, which reduces the level of the alveolar bone, increases the size of the gingival embrasure, and creates open interdental space. Restorations may be constructed so as to preserve the morphology of the crown and root and retain the enlarged embrasure and the open interdental space (Fig. 58–23*A* and *B*), or the teeth may be reshaped by the restorations so as to relocate the gingival embrasure close to the new level of the gingiva.

This is accomplished by changing the contour of the proximal surfaces and locating the contact areas more apically (Fig. 58–23*C*). The interdental gingiva will assume its normal shape by filling the new embrasure provided for it, which must be adequate in all dimensions.

The following dimensions of the gingival embrasure are important to the preservation of gingival health:

Height. The distance between the contact area and the bone margin (Fig. 58–24*A*). When the contact area is too close to the cervical line of the tooth, the embrasure is shortened.

Width. The distance mesiodistally between the proximal surface (Fig. 58–24*B*).

Depth. The distance faciolingually from the contact area to a line joining the proximofacial or proximolingual angles (Fig. 58–24*C*).

The proximal surfaces of crowns should taper away from the contact area—facially, lingually, and apically. Excessively broad proximal contact areas and inadequate contour in

Figure 58–20 Occlusal View of Mandibular Molars showing facial (F) and lingual (L) embrasures.

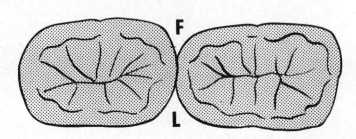

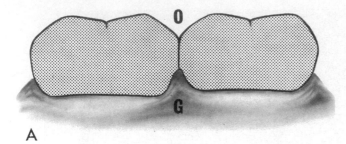

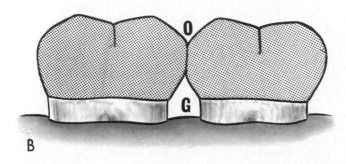

Figure 58–21 Occlusal (O) and Gingival (G) Embrasures. *A,* Interdental gingiva fills gingival embrasure (G). *B,* Open gingival embrasure (G) in patient with periodontal disease.

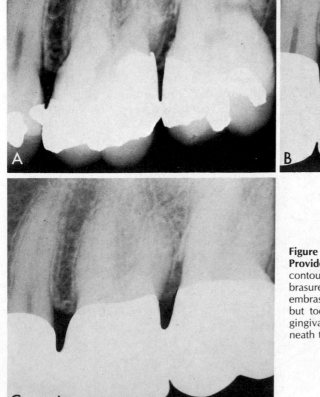

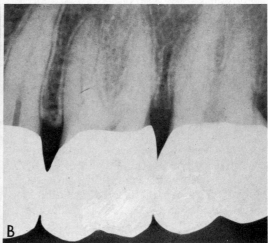

Figure 58–22 Contour of Restoration Corrected to Provide Proper Gingival Embrasures. *A,* Improperly contoured restorations on the molars; the gingival embrasure is too narrow. *B,* New restorations; the gingival embrasure between the molars is now wider at its base but too narrow beneath the contact area. *C,* Proper gingival embrasure created by widening the space beneath the molar contact area.

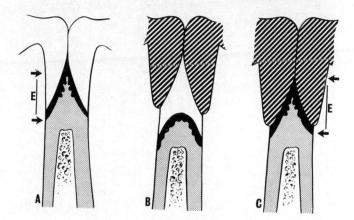

Figure 58–23 Relocation of the Gingival Embrasure. *A,* Normal gingival embrasure (E) filled with gingival tissue. *B,* Space created in gingival embrasure by periodontal disease and restorations constructed to retain the space. *C,* Restorations constructed so as to move the gingival embrasure (E) close to the gingiva by recontouring the proximal surfaces and locating the contact area further apically.

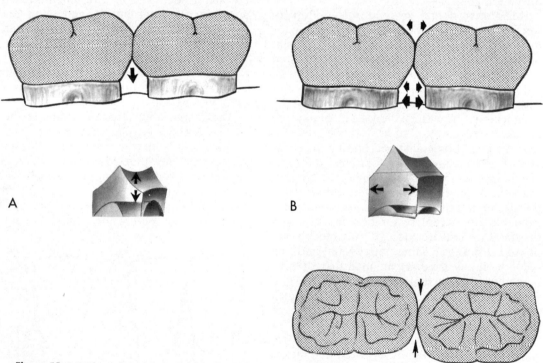

Figure 58–24 Dimensions of the Gingival Embrasure (indicated by arrows). *A,* Height. *B,* Mesiodistal width. *C,* Faciolingual depth.

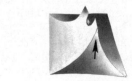

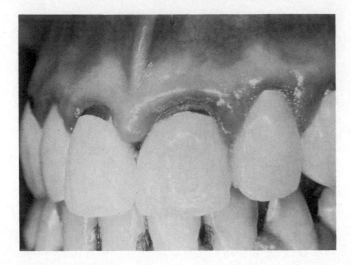

Figure 58–25 Inadequate gingival embrasures lead to gingival disease.

the cervical region crowd out the facial and lingual gingival papillae. The prominent papillae lead to gingival inflammation and pocket formation (Fig. 58–25).

Restorative dental procedures too often result in the restorative material taking up space that is normally occupied by the interdental papilla. This problem has been accentuated since the advent of restorations in which metal is bonded to porcelain. The problem begins with underpreparation of the tooth, so that the technician is left with no choice except to place an excessive amount of restorative material into the interproximal space. During the preparation of dies for cast restorations, the technician first removes all the replicated gingival tissue in order to gain access to the margins; thus it is impossible to visualize the space available for dental restoration in the interproximal embrasure area. If two models are poured from the same impression and the second one is used as an indicator of how much space is currently occupied by the gingival tissues, the technician can have a much better understanding of what the contour of the final restorations should be.

Overcrowding of the interdental space results in a narrowed embrasure area that makes oral hygiene difficult. The space available for gingival tissues is reduced also, so that a thin strand of collagen is often all that can occupy this space. This reduction in the space available for gingiva means that the ability of the collagen to form an efficient seal in association with the junctional epithelium is diminished. This increases the risk of periodontal destruction and will eventually lead to pocket formation and destruction of the support of the tooth (Fig. 58–26).

In fixed bridgework the soldered joint is frequently carried too far in an apical direction and so invades the embrasure space from its coronal aspect. This also results in inadequate space for the interdental gingiva and leads to inflammation and destruction of periodontal tissues (Fig. 58–27). For those patients who require increased strength in a soldered joint, it is best obtained by extending the soldered joint buccally and lingually, rather than coronally and apically.

The responsibility for determining the size of the soldered joint should rest with the dentist, not with the technician. Frequently the technician will decide the position and size of the soldered joint without being aware of how much gingival tissue is present in the interproximal embrasure. The problem of the interproximal embrasure space being en-

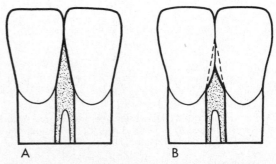

Figure 58–26 Interproximal Crown Contours. Overcontouring of crowns in the interdental region results in encroachment upon the space available for gingival tissue. *A*, Normally available space. *B*, Excess mesio-distal width of crowns and excess length of contact points result in compression of gingival tissue and predilection to inflammation. Access for oral hygiene is also much more difficult when embrasure spaces are overfilled with restorative materials.

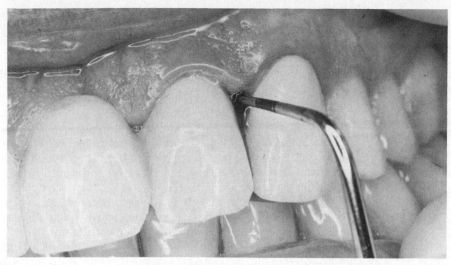

Figure 58–27 Excessive Contact Area. Soldered joint carried too far apically. The periodontal probe is at the apical level of the soldered joint. There is a 7 mm pocket in the adjacent interproximal periodontium.

croached upon by restorative materials is maximized in those patients whose gingival tissue fully occupies the embrasure space. In patients in whom periodontal surgery or gingival recession has resulted in recession of the interdental papilla, the problem of encroachment into the space is minimized. The principles that determine the size and form of the soldered joint apply equally to the size and form of contact points associated with all interproximal restorations (Fig. 58–28).

Contours of Restorations

The facial and lingual contours of restorations are also important in the preservation of gingival health.

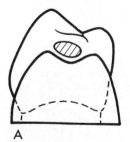
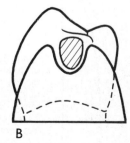

A   B

Figure 58–28 Size and Shape of Contact Areas. *A,* Correct shape of soldered joint or contact area. *B,* Incorrect shape with excessive apical extension of soldered joint or contact area. This results in the gingival col being disrupted, and the interproximal tissue is forced to take on a morphology in which the buccal and lingual portions of the papilla are split. This interproximal tissue is less able to remain healthy because of its form and because of the inaccessibility of the midproximal gingival sulcus region to oral hygiene procedures.

The most common error in re-creating the contours of the tooth in dental restorations is overcontouring of the facial and lingual surfaces. In one study approximately 80 per cent of full gold crowns were wider than the tooth they were replacing, and all porcelain-bonded-to-metal crowns were too wide buccolingually.[46] This overcontouring generally occurs in the gingival third of the crown and results in an area where oral hygiene procedures are unable to control plaque accumulation. Consequently, plaque bacteria accumulate in the gingival area and the gingiva becomes inflamed.

Overcontouring of restorations is a result of the mistaken belief that all natural teeth have a pronounced supragingival bulge in the gingival third of the clinical crown. In fact, much of the bulge that is present on natural teeth occurs in the area of the gingival crevice and does not have the function normally ascribed to it, i.e., deflecting food away from the gingiva. Apparently, undercontouring is not nearly as damaging to the gingiva as overcontouring. Evidence from studies in animals and humans demonstrates that overcontouring is a significant factor in gingival inflammation,[31, 34, 47, 55, 73] but undercontouring has little if any effect on gingival health[29, 47] (Fig. 58–29).

Overcontouring on the buccal or labial surfaces frequently occurs in metal-bonded-to-porcelain crowns owing to the technician's attempt to obtain a thickness of porcelain adequate to mask the underlying metal and provide the most esthetic appearance for the crown. Frequently the technician has no choice

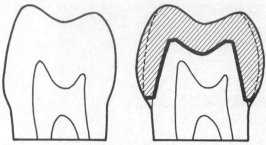

Figure 58–29 Buccolingual Crown Contours. Overcontouring of crowns in the buccolingual dimension is frequently due to inadequate removal of dentin during cavity preparation. The original contour of the tooth in the left diagram cannot be reproduced in the crown (shaded area in the right diagram) because there is not enough space for porcelain and metal in the gingival third.

but to put excess porcelain in this area, as removal of tooth material in the crown during cavity preparation has been inadequate. It is important to remove enough tooth material to allow adequate width for the metal and porcelain so that the resulting crowns will not bulge beyond the space normally occupied by the anatomic crown of the tooth. A minimum space of 2 mm is required.

In those patients in whom periodontal destruction or periodontal surgery causes the gingival margin to be in a much more apical position than it was during health, the facial and lingual contours become even more significant. In these cases the bulge on the facial contour of the crown, which normally would be subgingival, now appears supragingivally. This makes the portion of the exposed root immediately apical to the bulge less accessible for oral hygiene, with resultant plaque accu-

mulation and periodontal inflammation. In these cases it is frequently necessary to recontour existing restorations or even existing natural crowns to facilitate oral hygiene procedures. This problem is especially important in the area of the facial furcations of upper and lower molars and in the area of the lingual furcations of lower molars (Fig. 58–30).

In those situations in which the furcation has been exposed by periodontal surgical procedures or by gingival recession, it is important that the crown be contoured in such a way as to facilitate access for oral hygiene. In these cases it is important to emphasize the midfacial groove of the crown so that this groove is confluent with the furcation. It is equally important to remove the apical bulge of the crown, thereby eliminating any plaque traps apical to the cemento-enamel junction. These crown contours should be mirrored in the contours of the underlying bone in those cases in which osseous surgery is carried out. Thus the midfacial groove that runs apically in the bone, covering the molar roots, is continued in a groove running occlusoapically in the crown preparation and in the area of the furcation in the completed restoration (Fig. 58–31).

The Occlusal Surface

Occlusal surfaces should be designed so as to direct forces along the long axis of the teeth. They should restore occlusal dimensions and cuspal contours in harmony with the remainder of the natural dentition—after occlusal abnor-

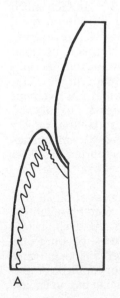
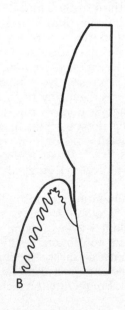
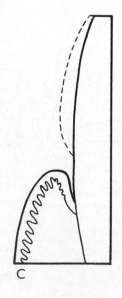

A   B   C

Figure 58–30 Facial Contour of Crowns in Relation to Gingiva. *A,* The gingival margin is normally coronal to the facial bulge of the anatomic crown. *B,* When the gingiva recedes, it is overprotected by the contour of the crown, so plaque accumulation is facilitated. *C,* The crown of the tooth is reshaped so that the gingiva is accessible for proper oral hygiene procedures. This should be carried out in areas where gingival recession is associated with gingival inflammation.

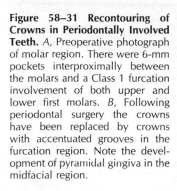
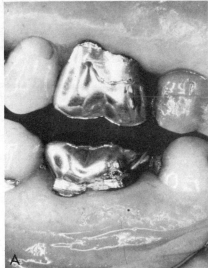
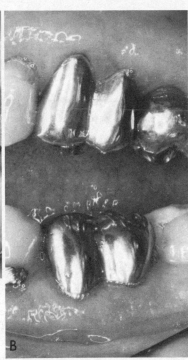

Figure 58–31 Recontouring of Crowns in Periodontally Involved Teeth. *A,* Preoperative photograph of molar region. There were 6-mm pockets interproximally between the molars and a Class 1 furcation involvement of both upper and lower first molars. *B,* Following periodontal surgery the crowns have been replaced by crowns with accentuated grooves in the furcation region. Note the development of pyramidal gingiva in the midfacial region.

malities have been eliminated by occlusal adjustment. The occlusal surfaces of the teeth should not be arbitrarily narrowed. Proper occlusal relationships are more important than the width of the occlusal table in the attainment of physiologic occlusal forces. The anatomy of the occlusal surface should provide well-formed marginal ridges and occlusal sluiceways to prevent interproximal food impaction.

The Effect of Surface Finish of Restorative Materials on the Periodontium

The surface of restorations should be as smooth as possible in order to limit plaque accumulation. Roughened tooth surfaces and roughened surfaces in the subgingival region result in increased plaque accumulation and increased gingival inflammation.[30, 60, 67]

In the clinical situation, porcelain, highly polished gold, and highly polished acrylic all result in similar plaque accumulation.[8, 28, 49] There is evidence that porcelain may accumulate less plaque than gold in dogs, and it has been suggested that this is due to differences in the inherent properties of these materials, but the surface roughness of these materials seems to be the most important factor in

humans.[8] The surface roughness of vacuum-fired porcelain is 1.262 microinches, that of highly polished gold 1.085 microinches, and that of highly polished acrylic 1.015 microinches.[8] (Fig. 58–32). This compares with a surface roughness of 4.0 microinches on amalgam restorations polished with xxx silex and tin oxide[7] and a surface roughness of 4.7 and 3.8 microinches for dentin polished with pumice and zircate, respectively.[64] Composite restorative materials have a much rougher surface of 8.0 microinches, and polishing and finishing of these restorations result in an even rougher surface of 40.0 microinches with pumice and 28.0 microinches with aluminum oxide.[69] Plaque accumulation occurs very quickly on composite restorations that have a rough surface due to finishing procedures.

The exact relationship between the degree of surface roughness and plaque accumulation is as yet undetermined. There is evidence that the amount of plaque accumulating in patients with relatively poor oral hygiene is not affected to a significant degree by minor changes in root surface configuration.[53] In patients with rough dental restorations, however, one can expect that the surface configuration may play an important role in plaque accumulation.[32, 69] Therefore, all restorative materials placed in the gingival environment should have as high a polish as is possible on their surface.

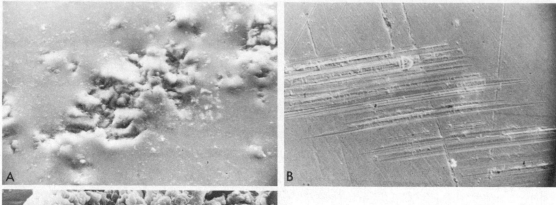

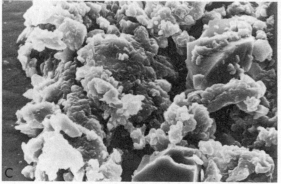

Figure 58–32 Surface of Restorations. *A,* Scanning electron micrograph of surface of vacuum-fired porcelain (× 1100). Note the irregular surface with roughness of approximately 1 microinch. *B,* Scanning electron micrograph of cast gold restoration (× 1100). The surface was given a final polish with rouge on a felt wheel. The surface irregularities are approximately 1 microinch. *C,* Scanning electron micrograph of composite restoration (× 1100). Note the extreme irregularity of the surface, which would facilitate plaque accumulation.

Pontics

A pontic should meet the following requirements: it should (1) be esthetically acceptable, (2) provide occlusal relationships that are favorable to the abutment teeth and opposing teeth and the remainder of the dentition, (3) restore the masticatory effectiveness of the tooth it replaces, (4) be designed to minimize accumulation of irritating dental plaque and food debris and to permit maximum access for cleansing by the patient, and (5) provide embrasures for the passage of food.

Plaque, which causes inflammation of the mucosa under pontics and the gingiva around abutment teeth, tends to accumulate around fixed prostheses because special effort is required to keep them clean. The health of the tissues around fixed prostheses depends primarily upon the patient's oral hygiene; the materials of which pontics are constructed appear to make little difference, and pontic design is important only to the extent that it enables the patient to keep the area clean. Plaque accumulates to an equal degree upon pontics made of glazed and unglazed porce-

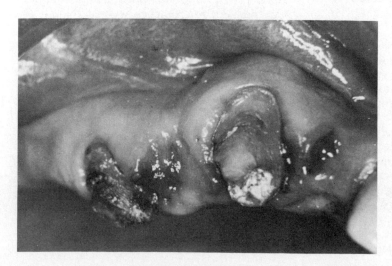

Figure 58–33 Poor Pontic Design. Chronic inflammation of edentulous mucosa under bridge with ridge-lap type of pontic.

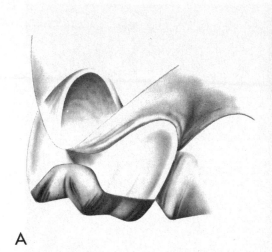

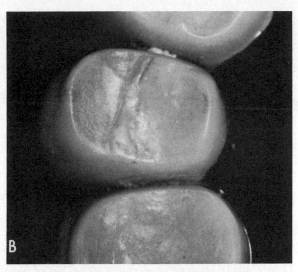

Figure 58–34 Saddle-Type Pontics. *A,* Diagrammatic view of saddle-type pontic in position. *B,* Undersurface of saddle-type pontic. Note the irregularities that conform to the surface of the underlying mucosa and trap food debris.

lain,[23] polished gold, and polished acrylic resin,[50, 62] despite the finding that the surfaces of the latter two are smoother.[8]

The principles of contours of crowns apply equally to pontics, but with pontics there is an additional concern associated with the contour of the tissue-facing surface. In general, this surface should be kept as convex as possible, and all concavities should be eliminated. The convexity of the tissue surfaces of pontics allows oral hygiene procedures to be effective in keeping the tissue of the edentulous ridge healthy. Concavities in the tissue surfaces of pontics result in plaque trap areas where accumulation of dental bacteria will lead to inflammation of the adjacent edentulous tissues (Figs. 58–33 to 58–36).

The bullet-shaped spheroidal pontic (Fig. 58–37) is the most hygienic next to the sanitary type (Fig. 58–38). The proximal surfaces are tapered to create spaces between adjoining pontics for self-cleansing passage of food and stimulation of the edentulous mucosa by food excursion and for cleansing with toothbrush and dental floss. Tapering should also re-create spaces adjacent to the abutment teeth that approach the shape and dimension of the natural embrasure to protect the marginal gingiva (see Fig. 58–36). A pontic no larger than a premolar may be cantilevered off the end of a multiunit bridge to prevent extrusion of the opposing teeth. Proper contour of such terminal pontics is especially important (see Fig. 58–36*E*), because the absence of protection

Figure 58–35 Replacement of Saddle-Type Pontics by Bullet-Shaped Pontics Leads to Resolution of Mucosal Inflammation. *A,* Bullet-shaped pontics inserted in area previously covered by saddle-type pontics. Note the inflammation where the saddle-type pontics had been. *B,* After several months, note the excellent condition of the mucosa under the bullet-shaped pontics.

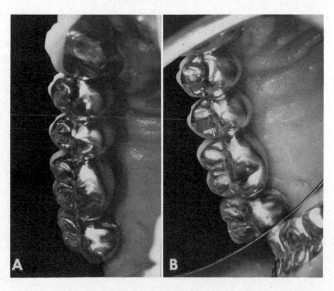

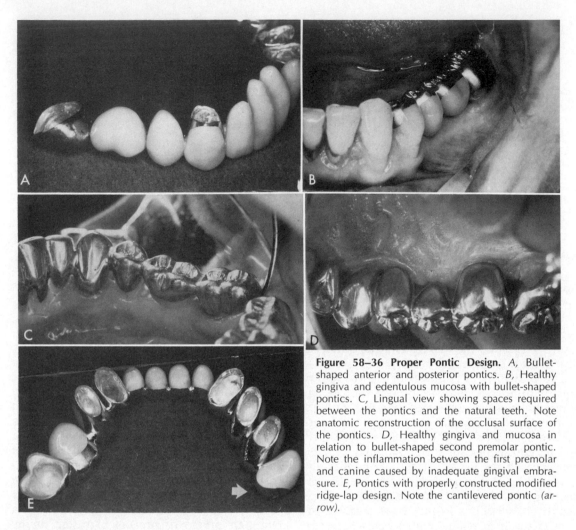

Figure 58–36 Proper Pontic Design. *A,* Bullet-shaped anterior and posterior pontics. *B,* Healthy gingiva and edentulous mucosa with bullet-shaped pontics. *C,* Lingual view showing spaces required between the pontics and the natural teeth. Note anatomic reconstruction of the occlusal surface of the pontics. *D,* Healthy gingiva and mucosa in relation to bullet-shaped second premolar pontic. Note the inflammation between the first premolar and canine caused by inadequate gingival embrasure. *E,* Pontics with properly constructed modified ridge-lap design. Note the cantilevered pontic *(arrow).*

from a proximal tooth increases the risk of food accumulation under the pontic.

In the posterior segments of the mouth, the bullet-shaped pontic is the most appropriate. In the anterior segments, where esthetics is a

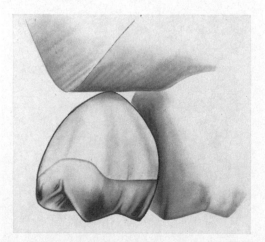

Figure 58–37. Bullet-Shaped Spheroidal Type of Pontic.

primary consideration, the modified ridge-lap design may be used (Fig. 58–39). This pontic design should have a convex surface on its tissue-facing surface, and the tip of the pontic should just barely contact the edentulous mucosa. Casts should not be scraped or scored in an attempt to seat the pontic into the mucosa, as this creates a depression around the pontic that makes it very difficult to gain access for plaque removal. The pontic follows the facial contour of the ridge to the crest where it joins the lingual surface. The lingual surface of the pontic should follow the normal tooth form for a distance of approximately half its occlusogingival length, then taper in a convex line to meet the facial portion at the crest of the ridge.[72]

The least damaging pontic design is the sanitary or hygienic pontic. This pontic should be designed so that there is at least a 3-mm space between the undersurface of the pontic and the edentulous ridge; this allows the tongue and cheeks to remove any food parti-

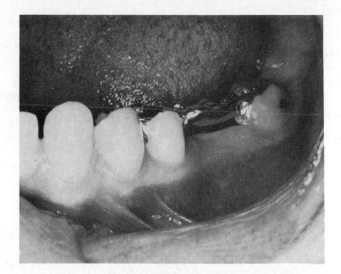

Figure 58–38 Sanitary-Type Fixed Bridge with Healthy Gingiva and Edentulous Mucosa.

cles that may lodge in this area. It is often necessary to use a design other than the hygienic pontic for esthetic reasons.

Saddle-type pontics, which straddle the ridge and have a concave tissue-facing surface, are the least desirable type of pontic design and should be avoided. Saddle-type pontics make it impossible for the patient to control plaque and inevitably result in inflammation of the tissues with which they are in contact.

The natural teeth should guide the design of the occlusal surface of pontics. The width of the occlusal surface should not be narrowed to less than that of the tooth being replaced. The assumption that reduced occlusal width pro-

vides occlusal forces more favorable to the periodontium of the abutment teeth has not been proved.

Narrowing the proximal contact areas of posterior teeth causes recession and inflammation of the interdental gingiva. Restoring the width of the contact area leads to resolution of the inflammation and keratinization of the interdental gingiva. Abnormally shaped spaces between narrowed pontics and broad proximal surfaces of adjacent natural teeth create food impaction problems (Fig. 58–40). Occlusal width is also necessary to shunt the food laterally so that it is not forced into the tissue around the base of the pontic; the gin-

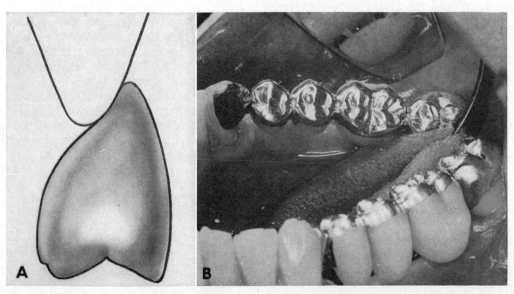

Figure 58–39 Modified Ridge-lap Pontic for Esthetics. *A,* Bullet-shaped pontic extended onto the facial aspects of the edentulous ridge. *B,* Modified ridge-lap type of pontic replacing the first molar. The premolars are bullet shaped. Note the excellent condition of the mucosa made possible by adequate spaces for food passage.

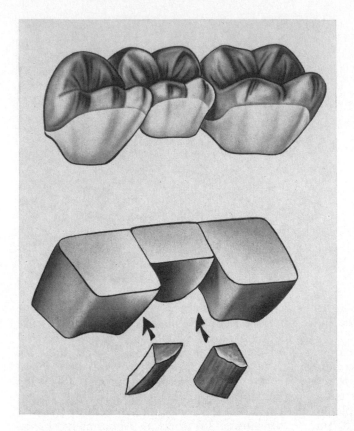

Figure 58–40 Occlusal Width of Pontics. *Above,* Pontic with narrow occlusal width creates food impaction problems. *Below,* Occlusal width required to provide proper proximal relations between pontic and adjacent teeth.

giva of abutment teeth is especially vulnerable to inflammation and pocket formation.[16]

The functional relationships of the cusps are the most critical consideration in the design of the occlusal surface of pontics. The cusps should be in harmony with the functional pattern of the entire dentition. Abnormal occlusal relationships jeopardize the opposing teeth and the remainder of the dentition, as well as the periodontium of the abutment teeth.

Cementation

Retained cement particles irritate the gingiva and should be removed. Removal of cement from the interproximal joints of pontics and abutments can be facilitated by coating the exterior surfaces of the prosthesis with mineral oil prior to cementation.

During cementation it is important that the restoration be sealed as close to the tooth preparation as possible. This will minimize the cement line, which enhances plaque formation. Crowns may be more closely adapted to the tooth if a constant axial force is applied at the time of cementation, together with a vibratory movement applied buccolingually.[43]

The dentition should be evaluated periodontally, and which teeth are to be included

in the prosthesis should be determined before it is designed. Permanent cementation should not be postponed indefinitely for the ostensible purpose of "testing" questionable teeth.

Failure to finalize cementation of prostheses is contraindicated for several reasons:

1. It interferes with adaptation of the gingiva to the margin of the restorations.

2. Seepage under temporarily cemented restorations may lead to caries and pulp involvement that escape detection, particularly if patients do not adhere to the schedule of periodic removal and recementation.

3. It encourages diagnostic indecision.

4. It is an unnecessary burden to the patient, who is never finished with treatment; meanwhile, the dentist is repeatedly confronted with a problem case.

5. The technical excellence required for a permanent restoration is often unwittingly compromised by the thought that needed corrections can be made "the next time."

ROOT RESECTIONS

There has been an increasing use of root resections for treating periodontally involved upper and lower molars over the past few years (see Chapter 55). In lower molars the

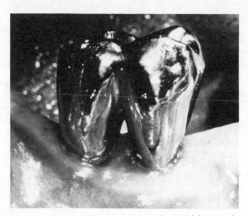

Figure 58–41 Bisection of Lower Molar with Retention of Both Roots. Separate full crown preparations have been made on each root. The gold crowns are splinted together with sufficient space between them for interproximal plaque control.

most dependable way to carry out this procedure is to use the hemisection approach, in which the tooth is cut in half through the crown. Root canal therapy is necessary on the retained portions of the molar. In some situations it is possible to retain both portions of the hemisected tooth, whereas in other situations one half will need to be extracted because of advanced periodontal destruction. In situations in which both parts of the tooth are to be retained, it is essential that an adequate embrasure space be created between the two halves of the tooth. All too often when teeth are hemisected the resulting restoration is detrimental to periodontal health because the embrasure space is too narrow. It is therefore important when hemisected teeth are prepared for crown and bridge procedures that adequate tooth material is removed in the areas between the roots, so that a wide embrasure space is constructed, which will allow passage of an

oral hygiene device (Fig. 58–41). The two segments of the hemisected lower molar should be regarded as much the same as two premolar teeth; thus, adequate space must be created between their roots for an interdental papilla and functional periodontal fibers.

When a **lower molar** is hemisected and one portion is extracted, the remaining portion will often serve as an abutment for a three-unit bridge (Fig. 58–42). It is important when the root is sectioned that care be taken to eliminate any remnants in into the furcation areas of the resected roots. The contour of the final restoration should be a smoothly flowing line from the contact area down to the most apical portion of the tooth preparation. Frequently the teeth are sectioned improperly, so that a small amount of the furcation remains on the retained root. This provides a plaque trap which makes the maintenance of periodontal health very difficult after the final restoration is placed.

Root-resective techniques in the **upper molar** region have applications entirely different from those seen in the lower molars. Whereas it is possible to maintain the vitality of many root-resected upper molars by placing a pulp-capping medicament over the exposed pulp canal, most root-resected upper molars eventually receive endodontic therapy. The use of endodontic therapy in these teeth provides two major advantages: first, it ensures that there will be no pulpal inflammation and patient discomfort subsequent to the resective technique; second, it allows for recontouring of the crown so that plaque control is simplified in the area where the root has been resected. *Failure to recontour the crown in the area of the resected root frequently results in an accumulation of plaque and a return of the periodontal defect because of the patient's inability*

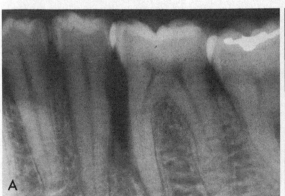
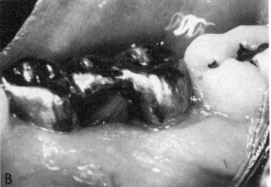

Figure 58–42 Hemisection of Lower Molar with Retention of One Root. *A,* Radiograph showing localized osseous defect on mesial root of first molar. *B,* Lingual view of fixed bridge utilizing distal root of first molar; note access for plaque control.

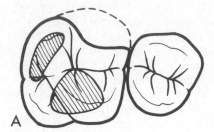
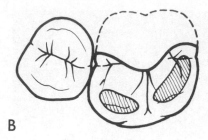

Figure 58–43 Crown Contours for Root-Resected Upper Molars. *A,* Mesiobuccal root amputation. Distobuccal and palatal root areas are shaded; original crown contours are shown by dotted line. The modified crown contours allow access for oral hygiene while maintaining the contact area. *B,* Palatal root amputation. Note that the contour of the palatal surface is modified to allow adequate plaque control.

to clean around the space where the root has been removed. Crowns that are placed on upper molars which have undergone root resection must be contoured in a specific way to ensure that the patient has access for oral hygiene (Fig. 58–43). This means that there is a dramatic change from the normal anatomic crowns seen on these teeth. When a mesiobuccal or distobuccal root has been resected, it is necessary to hollow out the crown contours in the area coronal to the area where the root was removed, so that adequate access is available for oral hygiene procedures (Fig. 58–44). In situations when a palatal root has been resected it is important that the crown be recontoured over the area where the palatal root was previously present. This will result in a much thinner crown buccopalatally, with emphasis on a groove running in the midpalatal surface. In other words, the crown form of this tooth with a palatal root resection would be somewhat similar to that seen in a narrow lower molar (Fig. 58–45). The crown recon-

touring that is associated with root-resected upper molars can occasionally be carried out on the natural tooth, but there are limitations as to how much recontouring can be done because of the risk of exposing vital dentin. The advantage of endodontic therapy is that the final cast restoration reduces the possibilities of crown fracture and is the best way to ensure that appropriate contours can be obtained.

REMOVABLE DENTURE PROSTHESES

At the present time, available clinical data show that even with advanced periodontal disease and extensive tooth loss, fixed bridges combined with periodontal therapy, including vigorous maintenance therapy, can result in periodontal health.[41]

From the periodontal viewpoint, fixed prostheses are the restorations of choice for replacement of missing teeth, but there are some

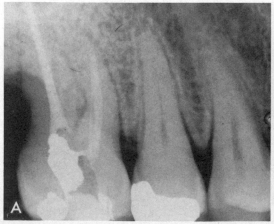
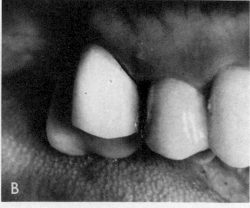

Figure 58–44 Root Resection of Upper Molar. *A,* Radiograph showing localized defect on distal buccal root of upper first molar. *B,* Following root resection the molar has been restored with modifications of crown contour to facilitate plaque control.

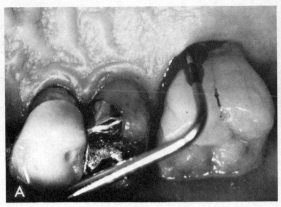 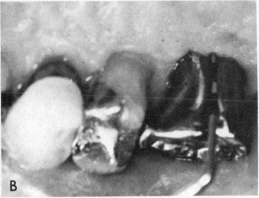

Figure 58–45 Palatal Root Resection. *A*, Preoperative view showing deep periodontal defect on palatal root. *B*, Postoperative view showing gold crown narrowed in buccopalatal dimension following resection of palatal root.

clinical situations when removable partial prostheses are the only possible way to restore the lost function of the dentition. There have been studies on the effect of removable prosthetic appliances on gingival and periodontal health.[6, 56, 66] It has been shown that the teeth that are included in the design of a partial denture have significantly more periodontal destruction than those teeth that are not included in the design.[6] It has also been shown that those patients who have removable prosthetic appliances have worse periodontal health than their counterparts who have a similar dental situation but whose missing teeth have not been replaced.[56] There is increased caries and increased mobility associated with teeth used as abutments for removable prosthodontic appliances.[6, 56] The detrimental effects of caries and periodontal destruction are accentuated in those patients who have poor oral hygiene; therefore, it is unwise to consider a removable partial denture in patients whose oral hygiene is inadequate. A major part of the treatment plan for patients requiring removable partial prostheses is the establishment of a satisfactory level of oral hygiene.[56] The presence of a partial denture may increase plaque formation around the remaining teeth,[1] so oral hygiene must receive great emphasis in these patients.

From the periodontal viewpoint, a fixed prosthesis is the restoration of choice, but a removable partial prosthesis may also be extremely effective. Its usefulness in the total treatment of periodontal problems should not be minimized.[18] The periodontal implications of removable partial prostheses must be understood so that the device will benefit the periodontium and not cause periodontal destruction and tooth mobility.[15, 37, 43, 56]

Design

To provide maximum stability for removable partial prostheses, every effort should be made to retain posterior teeth for the distal support of the saddle areas.

Some partial denture designs include the use of metal plates as connectors; these plates are positioned so that they cover the gingival tissues.[34, 35] Other designs leave the gingival tissues uncovered as part of the partial denture design and use bars as the major connectors.[13] The advocates of covering the gingiva suggest that this minimizes food impaction and calculus formation on the tooth surface. Those who suggest leaving the gingiva free point out the advantages of access to the gingiva by the tongue and muscles of mastication. There is no experimental evidence to support either point of view, and the question of whether the gingiva should be covered is unanswered at this time.

The relationship of the partial denture framework to the distal surface of abutment teeth in a bilateral distal extension partial denture is also an area of controversy. There is some support for the practice of having the metal framework tightly adapted to the distal surface and the gingiva of this tooth,[34, 35] whereas others suggest that this area should be relieved of pressure and that no impingement of the denture framework should occur here.[13]

A recent clinical study[4] has shown that the I-bar type of removable partial denture can be utilized by many patients with little or no detrimental effect on periodontal health. This particular design utilizes an I-bar infrabulge clasp, mesially positioned occlusal rests, and metal guide planes; it emphasizes the need for

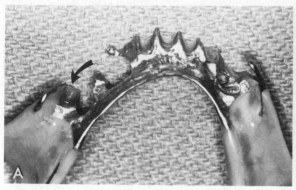
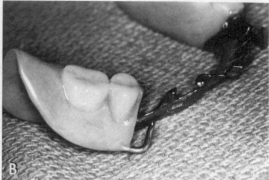

Figure 58–46 I-Bar Design for Removable Partial Denture. *A,* Tissue surface of a removable partial denture for a lower bilateral edentulous patient. Note metal extension that fits tightly against distal surface of distal abutment tooth (*arrow*). *B,* Same removable partial denture showing I-bar clasp and occlusal rest placed in mesial part of abutment tooth.

intraoral adjustment of the denture framework to minimize undue torque on the abutment teeth.[65] This particular design of removable prostheses has also been shown to provide more favorable loading of abutment teeth than that seen with a circumferential clasp design[36] (Fig. 58–46).

Clinical research has shown that many patients who were previously treated with removable prosthodontic appliances, e.g., those with bilateral edentulous areas, can be treated with fixed appliances using multiple cantilevered pontics.[41] This controversial approach to the treatment of edentulous areas in patients with advanced periodontal disease has been carefully documented and followed in many patients over a period of 6 years. There seems to be no doubt that, if patients are treated for periodontal destruction and then placed on a strict oral hygiene program, distally extending cantilevered pontics can be used in conjunction with fixed prosthodontic appliances. In these cases the occlusal pattern was established by an intraoral technique for developing a functionally generated path over a period of many months in provisional restorations. This type of occlusal pattern is apparently the least destructive to the abutment teeth when they are used as supports for multiple pontics.

CLASPS. It has been generally accepted that clasps should be passive and exert no force on

the teeth when the denture is at rest.[61] Research shows that the use of a suprabulge or circumferential clasp exerts a great deal of force on the abutment tooth[9]—force beyond that required for orthodontic movement even when a wrought wire clasp is used. Such nonfunctional force against the tooth causes the increased mobility that has been reported following the insertion of removable partial dentures. Apparently, after a period of 18 months to 2 years, the abutment teeth either move or are able to develop a stronger periodontal support so that their mobility often returns to the denture level of mobility.[51] It has been suggested that the use of an infrabulge or I-bar clasp may alleviate the traumatic forces associated with circumferential clasps.[34, 61, 65] However, in one laboratory study the I-clasp design resulted in more movement of abutment teeth than did circumferential and back-action clasps. In the clinical situation, the use of guide planes and I-clasps is associated with a modification of fitting surfaces so that there is equilibration of forces in the abutment teeth—this may result in less force being applied to these teeth. The I-bar clasp has the advantage of producing a minimal change in the buccal surface of the tooth on which it is placed as compared with the circumferential clasp, which affects the buccal contour of the entire surface.[34, 35] The overcontouring of the buccal

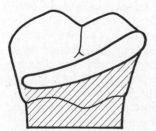
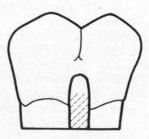

Figure 58–47 Effect of Clasp Design. The amount of gingiva affected by the change in tooth contour associated with a circumferential clasp is much greater than that associated with an I-bar infrabulge clasp.

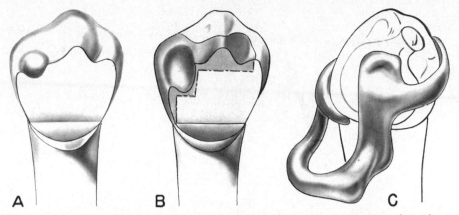

Figure 58–48 Occlusal Rests in Line with Vertical Axis. *A,* Properly constructed lug rest in a premolar without a restoration. *B,* Properly constructed lug rest in a restoration in a premolar. *C,* Clasp in position on a premolar with a lug rest in a restoration. (After Dr. Irving R. Hardy.)

surface associated with a circumferential clasp on the tooth surface may result in increased gingival inflammation in much the same way as does overcontouring of artificial crowns (Fig. 58–47).

Stress breakers, which connect the retainer and saddle areas by flexible and movable joints, are sometimes used to prevent excessive occlusal forces on abutment teeth. However, comparisons have revealed no advantage of stress breakers over rigid connectors in this respect.[3] With rigid connectors between clasps and saddle areas, the resilience of the mucosa acts as a stress breaker. It permits controlled movement of the prosthesis so that the tissue-borne sections take the initial occlusal stress and prevent sudden impact on the periodontium of the natural teeth.

OCCLUSAL RESTS. Occlusal rests should be designed to direct the forces along the vertical axis of the tooth. To accomplish this, the rest is seated in a spoon-shaped preparation in the abutment tooth with the floor inclined so that the deepest point is toward the vertical axis of the tooth[27] (Fig. 58–48). This purpose is also accomplished by extending occlusal rests beyond the central zone of the occlusal surface of premolars or by covering the occlusal surface overlying one of the roots of the molars.[48]

Lug rests on inclined lingual surfaces of anterior teeth tend to be spread by occlusal forces so that the denture settles. The facial and lingual arms of the clasp then impinge upon the gingiva, and the connecting bar digs into the lingual mucosa. Pockets form, and the roots are denuded (Fig. 58–49). Spreading of lug rests on anterior teeth can be prevented by constructing a restoration on the abutment teeth with a horizontal ledge on the lingual

surface into which the clasp fits (Fig. 58–50). The floor of the ledge should be sloped so as to direct the forces axially. An incisal stop will also prevent settling of clasps (Fig. 58–51). The notch is cut for a slight distance into the tooth substance, at a point approximately one third from the distoincisal angle. The incisal rest fits into the notch and is tapered to terminate in a point on the facial surface.

Removable partial prostheses should always be constructed with occlusal rests. Rests are sometimes omitted for the ostensible purpose of reducing axial load on teeth with weakened periodontal support. Such dentures jeopardize the teeth because they settle and cause gingival and periodontal disturbances.

PRECISION ATTACHMENTS. Precision attachments are used for esthetic reasons and to direct occlusal forces axially rather than laterally. There are many types of precision attachments, and advantages have been demonstrated for some.[26] They cause greater stress and displacement on the abutment teeth of free-end saddle prostheses than is produced by conventional back-action clasps.[57] More evidence is required to establish the relative merits of precision attachments and clasps in terms of their effects upon the periodontium.

MULTIPLE ABUTMENTS. Multiple abutments reduce injurious lateral and torsional stresses on abutment teeth and should be standard procedure in patients with reduced periodontal support. Multiple abutments are made by connecting inlays or crowns or by clasping abutment and adjacent teeth in sequence. When the terminal tooth is periodontally weak, more than one adjacent tooth should be used for added support. Joining a weakened tooth to a strong one is just as likely

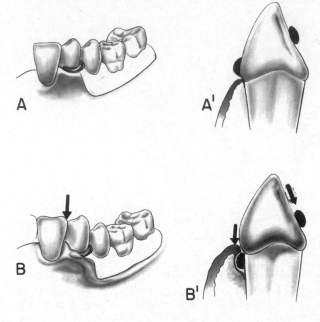

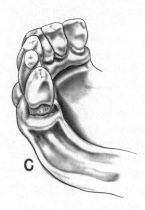

Figure 58–49 "Settling" of a Lingual Bar with an Inadequate Lug Rest on the Canine. *A*, Lingual bar in position. *A'*, Labiolingual view showing cross section of labial and lingual arms of the clasp. *B*, Lingual bar settles in direction indicated by arrow. *B'*, Labial arm digs into gingiva; lingual arm slides down along inclined plane of lingual surface. *C*, View of distal surface of canine showing recession of gingiva and marginal gingival disease resulting from settling of partial denture.

Figure 58–50 A Method of Preventing Settling of a Clasp on the Mandibular Canine. *A*, Restoration is made for canine, including ledge on lingual surface. *B*, Lingual arm of clasp fits into ledge on lingual surface.

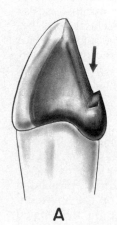
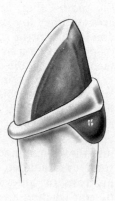

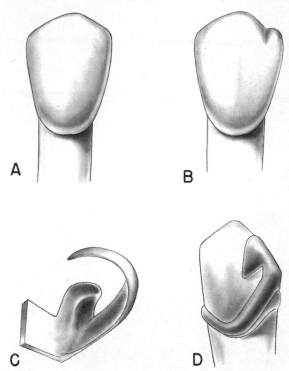

Figure 58–51 Incisal Stop on Anterior Tooth. *A,* Mandibular canine. *B,* Notch is cut in incisal edge. *C,* View of clasp with incisal rest. *D,* Clasp in position on tooth. (After Dr. Irving R. Hardy.)

to weaken the strong tooth as it is to strengthen the weak one (Fig. 58–52). It is always advisable to consider whether the long-term interest of the patient would be better served by extracting the prospective weak abutment tooth and making a multiple abutment of two adjacent teeth that are relatively well supported. In patients who have had generalized periodontal involvement, all teeth should be joined together by the partial denture, either by clasping or by inclusion in continuous clasps.

Combined Fixed and Removable Partial Prostheses

Isolated teeth with reduced periodontal support are particularly vulnerable to periodontal injury and loosening when used as abutments in removable partial prostheses. They lack mesial and distal buttressing action to assist in withstanding the forces transmitted by the denture. In such cases, fixed and removable prostheses should be combined. The isolated teeth should be joined to their nearest neighbors by a fixed bridge (Fig. 58–53) and can then be used as abutments for removable prostheses.

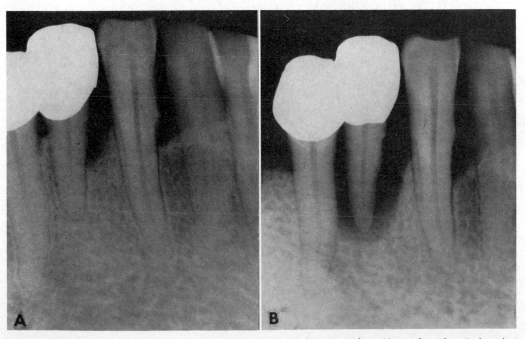

Figure 58–52 Weakened Tooth Splinted to Single Firm Tooth. *A,* First premolar with weakened periodontal support splinted to firm second premolar. *B,* After 3 years, periodontal condition is worse, second premolar is also denuded of bone, and both premolars are mobile.

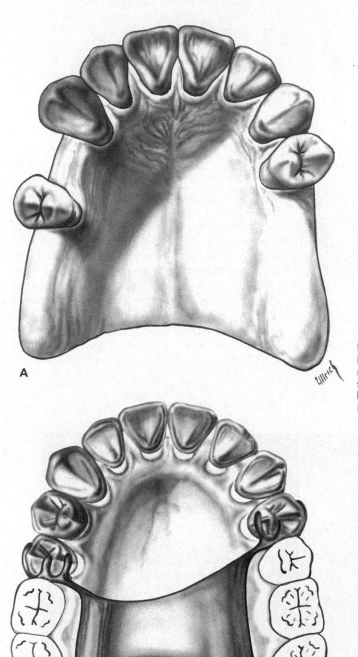

A

B

Figure 58–53 Combined Fixed and Removable Partial Prosthesis. *A,* Prosthesis is required for mouth with isolated second premolar. *B,* Isolated second premolar included in fixed prosthesis before palatal bar is constructed. First premolar is replaced by a pontic.

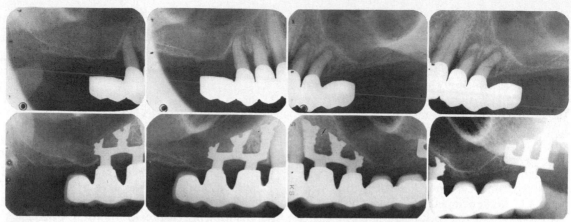

Figure 58–54 Endo-osseous Blade Implant Used as Distal Abutment for Fixed Prosthesis. *Top,* Before restoration. Radiographs showing periodontal and periapical involvement of maxillary premolars with cantilevered distal pontics. *Bottom,* Endo-osseous blade implants replacing two premolars *(left)* and replacing two premolars and providing a distal abutment for the fixed prosthesis *(right)*. The entire restoration is a single unit.

The use of **blade implants** as a distal abutment in patients whose natural molars are totally missing has had relatively wide clinical acceptance (Fig. 58–54). However, when reproducible methods are used to follow these cases, it is found that the use of such a therapeutic approach must be regarded as experimental at this time. There is evidence that the design of many of the blade implants used will prevent the detection of destruction of the tissues surrounding the posts when a periodontal probe is used clinically, even though large amounts of destruction can be detected histologically and radiographically.

Overdentures

The ability to maintain some teeth in the dental arch for use as abutments for an over-denture has had wider application in recent years. This procedure has three obvious advantages for the patient. First, there is increased retention and stability of the denture base. Second, there is evidence that the proprioceptive capacity of a patient with a full denture utilizing some teeth as abutments is dramatically improved over that seen with a conventional full denture design.[39, 45] Third, the presence of teeth under a full denture provides a reduced amount of stress on the edentulous ridges, resulting in less bone resorption over time.[12] Because many of the teeth which are utilized for overdenture abutments have had periodontal involvement, it is important that appropriate periodontal considerations be part of the treatment planning and therapy provided for these areas. The presence of an adequate zone of keratinized gingiva around these abutment teeth is of critical im-

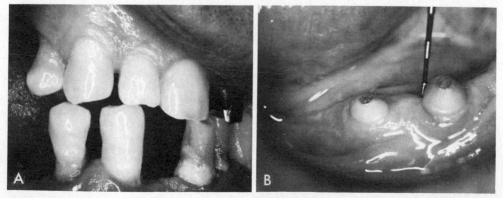

Figure 58–55 Preparation of Teeth for Overdenture. *A,* Preoperative view. Lower canine and first premolar have periodontal involvement and unfavorable crown-to-root ratio. *B,* After periodontal flap surgery and endodontic therapy, these teeth have been prepared with dome-shaped contours as abutments for a full lower overdenture. Note reduced crown-to-root ratio.

portance. It is also essential that remaining residual periodontal defects be treated in much the same way as they would be around any periodontally involved tooth prior to the final restoration. One great advantage that the overdenture concept has for periodontally involved teeth is that it is possible to improve the crown-root ratio dramatically. This results in a great diminution in the excessive forces which will be applied to the remaining root. The preparation of the root surface for an overdenture can be carried out utilizing four major approaches. The simplest is to provide a small, dome-shaped amalgam restoration over the area of the root facing the oral cavity (Fig. 58–55). Also, a cast post and coping can be applied over the root surface. Another alternative is the use of a precision- or semi-precision-type attachment placed on the root and then mated with an analogous attachment inside the denture. And, finally, it is possible to utilize a bar joining two retained roots together in order to provide a sharing of the load between these two roots. It appears that the domed amalgam restoration results in the least amount of traumatic forces to the retained roots and therefore should be the method of choice in most cases.[68] The major disadvantage of this doming procedure is that it provides the least amount of retention for the denture compared with other procedures. In those cases in which denture retention is of critical importance, the use of a bar or of attachments may be indicated. However, it should be recognized that these bar prostheses complicate the oral hygiene necessary to maintain the periodontal tissues; therefore, they should be used only in those patients who have demonstrated an adequate level of, and dedication to, plaque control. In situations in which

recurrent caries is an important consideration, the post and coping technique may be used where a cast restoration with subgingival margins protects the exposed root surface from root caries.

PERIODONTAL SPLINTING

A splint is an appliance for the immobilization or stabilization of injured or diseased parts. Teeth may be splinted as part of Phase I therapy, before periodontal surgery, utilizing temporary or provisional splints. Permanent splints utilizing cast restorations may be placed as part of the restorative phase of therapy.

Splinting of periodontally involved teeth should not be the sole method of obtaining tooth stability. One must always determine the etiology of the increased tooth mobility or the pathologic migration of the teeth. Frequently the cause is an abnormal occlusal pattern, i.e., a deflective occlusal contact resulting in nonaxial forces on teeth and/or excessive occlusal forces associated with parafunction (Fig. 58–56). It is imperative that occlusal stability and control of excessive occlusal forces be obtained first, before splinting is applied. Frequently the modification of occlusal forces will eliminate the need for a splint, as the teeth will become less mobile and more stable in their position.

Occlusal forces applied to splints are shared by all teeth within the splint even if the force is applied only to one section of the splint.[20] The rigidity of a splint allows it to act as a lever, so that the forces applied to some teeth in the splint may be much greater than before splinting.[20] Therefore, the inclusion of a mobile tooth in a splint does not completely relieve it

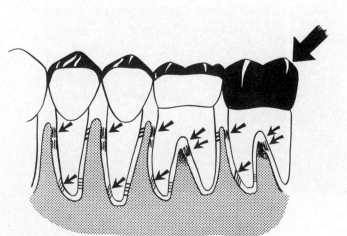

Figure 58–56 Transmission of Forces in a Splint. Excessive occlusal force applied only to second molar *(large arrow)* injures periodontium of all splinted teeth in comparable locations. Small arrows indicate areas of injury. Location of injury depends upon direction of occlusal force.

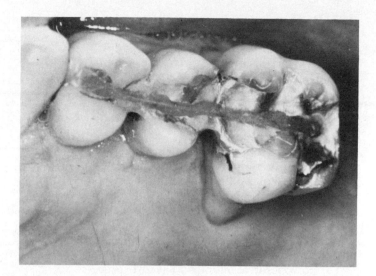

Figure 58–57 Posterior Splint. Wire and acrylic splint. This splint is used for temporary or provisional splinting in posterior teeth with existing amalgam restorations.

of the burden of occlusal forces, nor does it guarantee against injury from excessive occlusal forces. If one tooth in a splint is in a traumatic occlusal relationship, the periodontal tissues of the remaining teeth may also be injured (see Fig. 58–52). Therefore it is of primary importance to stabilize the occlusion prior to splinting.

The use of splinting in periodontal therapy is controversial.[37] There is little evidence to support the much-quoted rationale that the splinting of mobile teeth enhances resistance to further periodontal breakdown and improves the healing response.[11, 40] Therefore, the indications for splinting are more limited than many authors believe. *Splinting in almost all cases should be of a temporary or provisional type, and permanent splints should be used only where they are necessary for obtaining occlusal stability or for replacing missing*

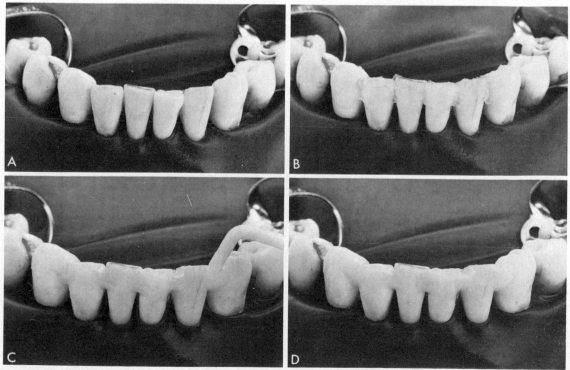

Figure 58–58 Anterior Splint. Technique for acid etch splint. *A,* Teeth are thoroughly scaled and polished to remove all deposits. *B,* Enamel surface is etched with an acid gel for 2 minutes. *C,* Polymerizing resin restorative material is placed on prepared teeth. *D,* Complete splint.

teeth. Permanent splinting does not necessarily reduce the effect of damaging forces on mobile teeth, nor does it predictably reduce mobility.[52]

The two major indications for periodontal splinting are:

1. To immobilize excessively mobile teeth so that the patient can chew more comfortably.

2. To stabilize teeth in their new position after orthodontic movement.

Although there is no agreement as to what degree of tooth mobility is pathologic, the use of splints to make patients comfortable when chewing should be considered only for teeth with mobility of 2 or more on a scale of 3. Immediately after periodontal surgery, there is an increase in mobility, which may necessitate the use of a provisional splint during the first 6 postoperative months. The two procedures of most significance for temporary or provisional stabilization are:

1. The wire and acrylic splint for use in posterior teeth (Fig. 58–57).

2. The acid etch–resin splint for use in anterior teeth (Fig. 58–58).

The introduction of splints into the dental arch generally makes oral hygiene procedures more complex. Therefore, it is important that patients receive special instruction in the techniques required for control of interproximal plaque (see Chapter 44). When an interdental papilla completely fills the embrasure space, the best method of interdental plaque removal is the use of dental floss together with a threader. When the interdental papilla does not fill the embrasure space, the best method for plaque removal is the use of an interdental brush.[17]

REFERENCES

1. Addy, M., and Bates, J. F.: The effect of partial dentures and chlorhexidine on plaque accumulation in the absence of oral hygiene. J. Clin. Periodontol., 4:41, 1977.
2. Al Hamadane, K. K., and Crabb, H. S. M.: Marginal adaptation of composite resins. J. Oral. Rehabil., 2:21, 1975.
3. Barkann, L.: The case for metal ligatures in periodontia. J. Sec. District D. Soc. (N.Y.), 31:341, 1945.
4. Benson, D., and Spolsky, V. W.: A clinical evaluation of removable partial dentures with I bar retainers. J. Prosthet. Dent., 41:246, 1979.
5. Bryan, A. W.: Some common defects in operative restorations contributing to the injury of the supporting structures. J. Am. Dent. Assoc., 14:1486, 1927.
6. Carlsson, G., Hedegard, B., and Koivumaa, K.: Final results of a 4 year longitudinal investigation of dentogingivally supported partial dentures. Study IV. Acta Odontol. Scand., 23:443, 1965.
7. Charbeneau, G. T.: A suggested technique for polishing amalgam restorations. J. Michigan State Dent. Assoc., 47:320, 1965.
8. Clayton, J. A., and Green, E.: Roughness of pontic materials and dental plaque. J. Prosthet. Dent., 23:407, 1970.
9. Clayton, J. A., and Jaslow, C.: A measurement of clasp forces on teeth. J. Prosthet. Dent., 25:21, 1971.
10. Coelho, D. H., Cavallaro, J., and Rothschild, E. A.: Gingival recession with electrosurgery for impression making. J. Prosthet. Dent., 33:422, 1975.
11. Cross, W.: The importance of immobilization in periodontology. Paradontologie, 8:119, 1954.
12. Crum, R. J., and Rooney, G. E.: Alveolar bone loss in overdentures: a 5 year study. J. Prosthet. Dent., 40:610, 1978.
13. Derry, A., and Bertram, U.: A clinical survey of removable partial dentures after 2 years usage. Acta Odontol. Scand., 28:581, 1970.
14. Donaldson, D.: Gingival recession associated with temporary crowns. J. Periodontol., 44:691, 1973.
15. Fenner, W., Gerber, A., and Mühlemann, H. R.: Tooth mobility changes during treatment with partial denture prosthesis. J. Prosthet. Dent., 6:520, 1956.
16. Fröhlich, E., von: Zahnfleischrand und Künstliche Krone in pathologisch-anatomischer Sicht. Dtsch. Zahnaertzl., 22:1252, 1967.
17. Gjermo, P., and Flotra, L.: The effect of different methods of interdental cleaning. J. Periodont. Res., 5:230, 1970.
18. Glickman, I.: The periodontal structures and removable partial denture prostheses. J. Am. Dent. Assoc., 37:311, 1948.
19. Glickman, I., and Imber, T.: Comparison of gingival resection with electrosurgery and periodontal knives. J. Periodontol., 41:142, 1970.
20. Glickman, I., Stein, R. S., and Smulow, J. B.: The effect of increased functional forces upon the periodontium of splinted and nonsplinted teeth. J. Periodontol., 32:290, 1961.
21. Goransson, P., and Nyman, L.: Review of methods for exposing the gingival margin. Sci. Ed. Bull. Int. Col. Dent., 2:24, 1969.
22. Hamp, S. E., Nyman, S., and Lindhe, J.: Periodontal treatment of multirooted teeth. Results after five years. J. Clin. Periodontol., 2:126, 1975.
23. Henry, P. J., Johnston, J. F., and Mitchell, D. F.: Tissue changes beneath fixed partial dentures. J. Prosthet. Dent., 16:937, 1966.
24. Hildebrand, G. Y.: The problem of the cervical preparation. Proc. Swed. Dent. Soc., 1927, S.T.T., p. 14.
25. Hildebrand, G. Y.: Studies in Dental Prosthetics. Stockholm, Aktiebolaget Fahlcrantz Boktryckeri, 1937, p. 226.
26. Homma, S., Homma, M., and Nakamura, Y.: Dynamic study of attachments. J. Dent. Res., 40:228, 1961 (abstract).
27. Ito, H., Inoue, Y., and Yamada, M.: Three dimensional photoelastic studies on the clasp-rest and tooth extraction. J. Dent. Res., 38:203, 1959 (abstract).
28. Kaqueler, J. C., and Weiss, M. B.: Plaque accumulation on dental restorative materials. I.A.D.R. Abstracts, 1970, No. 615, p. 202.
29. Karlsen, K.: Gingival reactions to dental restorations. Acta Odontol. Scand., 28:895, 1970.
30. Keenan, M. P., Shillingburg, H. T., Duncanson, M. G., and Wade, C. K.: Effects of cast gold surface finish on plaque retention. J. Prosthet. Dent., 43:168, 1980.
31. Kelly, W. J., and Harrison, J. D.: Laboratory experimental evaluation of efficiency of clinical electrosurgical techniques. In Oringer, M. J. (ed.): Electrosurgery in Dentistry. 2nd ed. Philadelphia, W. B. Saunders Company, 1975.
32. Knowles, J. W., and Snyder, D. T.: The effect of roughness on supragingival and subgingival plaque formation. I.A.D.R. Abstracts, 1970, No. 345, p. 135.
33. Koivumaa, K. K., and Wennstrom, A.: A histologic investigation of the changes in gingival margins adjacent to gold crowns. Sart. U. R. Odont. Tska, 68:373, 1960.
34. Kratochvil, F. J.: Influence of occlusal rest position and clasp design on movement of abutment teeth. J. Prosthet. Dent., 13:114, 1963.
35. Kratochvil, F. J.: Maintaining supporting structures with a removable partial prosthesis. J. Prosthet. Dent., 26:167, 1971.
36. Kratochvil, F. J., and Caputo, A. A.: Photoelastic analysis of pressure on teeth and bone supporting removable partial dentures. J. Prosthet. Dent., 32:52, 1974.
37. Krogh-Poulsen, W.: Partial denture design in relation to occlusal trauma and periodontal breakdown. Int. Dent. J., 4:847, 1954.
38. Langer, B., Stein, S. D., and Wagenberg, B.: An evaluation

of root resections. A ten year study. J. Periodontol., *52*:719, 1981.

39. Loiselle, R. J., Crum, R. J., Rooney, G. E., Jr., and Stuever, D. H., Jr.: The physiologic bases for the overlay denture. J. Prosthet. Dent., *28*:4, 1972.
40. McCune, R. J., Phillips, R. W., Swartz, M. L., and Mumford, G.: The effect of occlusal venting and film thickness on the cementation of full cast crowns. J. South. Cal. Dent. Assoc., *39*:36, 1971.
41. Nyman, S., Lindhe, J., and Lundgren, D.: The role of occlusion for the stability of fixed bridges in patients with reduced periodontal support. J. Clin. Periodontol., *2*:53, 1975.
42. O'Leary, T. M., Standish, S. M., and Coomer, R. S.: Severe periodontal destruction following impression procedures. J. Periodontol., *44*:43, 1973.
43. Oliveira, J. F., Ishikiriama, A., Vieira, D. T., and Mondelli, J.: Influence of pressure and vibration during cementation. J. Prosthet. Dent., *41*:171, 1979.
44. Osborne, J., Brills, N., and Lammie, G. A.: Partial dentures. Int. Dent. J., *7*:26, 1957.
45. Pacer, F. G., and Bowman, D. C.: Occlusal force discrimination by denture patients. J. Prosthet. Dent., *33*:602, 1975.
46. Parkinson, C. F.: Excessive crown contours facilitate endemic plaque niches. J. Prosthet. Dent., *35*:424, 1976.
47. Perel, M.: Axial crown contours. J. Prosthet. Dent., *25*:642, 1971.
48. Plitzner, J.: Role of occlusal rest lug as transmitter of masticating stress. Dent. Reform., *42*:77, 1938.
49. Podshadley, A. G.: Gingival response to pontics. J. Prosthet. Dent., *19*:51, 1968.
50. Price, C., and Whitehead, F. J. H.: Impression material as foreign bodies. Br. Dent. J., *133*:9, 1972.
51. Rateitschak, K. H.: The therapeutic effect of local treatment on periodontal disease assessed upon evaluation of different diagnostic criteria. I. Changes as to mobility. J. Periodontol., *34*:540, 1963.
52. Renggli, H. H.: Splinting of teeth an objective assessment. Helv. Odontol. Acta, *15*:129, 1971.
53. Rosenberg, R., and Ash, M. M.: The effect of root roughness on plaque accumulation and gingival inflammation. J. Periodontol., *45*:146, 1974.
54. Ruel, J., Schuessler, P. J., Malamet, K., and Morl, D.: Effect of retraction procedures on the periodontium in humans. J. Prosthet. Dent., *44*:508, 1980.
55. Sacket, B. P., and Gildenhuys, R. R.: The effect of axial crown overcontour on adolescents. J. Periodontol., *47*:320, 1976.
56. Seemann, S. K.: Study of the relationship between periodontal

disease and the wearing of partial dentures. Aust. Dent. J., *8*:206, 1963.
57. Shohet, H.: Relative magnitudes of stress on abutment teeth and different retainers. J. Prosthet. Dent., *21*:267, 1969.
58. Shooshan, E. D.: A pin-ledge casting technique—its application in periodontal splinting. Dent. Clin. North Am., *4*:189, 1960.
59. Silness, J.: Treated with dental bridges. III. The relationship between the location of the crown margin and the periodontal condition. J. Periodont. Res., *5*:225, 1970.
60. Sotres, L. S., Van Huysen, G., and Gilmore, H. W.: A histologic study of gingival response to amalgam silicate and resin restorations. J. Periodontol., *40*:543, 1969.
61. Steffel, V. L.: Clasp partial dentures. J. Am. Dent. Assoc., *66*:803, 1963.
62. Stein, R. S.: Pontic-residual ridge relationship: a research report. J. Prosthet. Dent., *16*:251, 1966.
63. Stein, R. S., and Glickman, I.: Prosthetic considerations essential for gingival health. Dent. Clin. North Am., *4*:177, 1960.
64. Taylor, S. M.: The polishing effectiveness of zircate, silex, and pumice on curetted root surfaces. Thesis. Ann Arbor, University of Michigan School of Dentistry, 1967.
65. Thayer, H. H., and Kratochvil, F. J.: Periodontal considerations with removable partial dentures. Dent. Clin. North Am., *23*:357, 1980.
66. Tomlin, M., and Osborne, J.: Cobalt-chromium partial dentures: a clinical survey. Br. Dent. J., *110*:307, 1961.
67. Waerhaug, J.: Effect of rough surfaces upon gingival tissues. J. Dent. Res., *35*:323, 1956.
68. Warren, A. B., and Caputo, A. A.: Load transfer to alveolar bone as influenced by abutment designs for tooth supported dentures. J. Prosthet. Dent., *33*:137, 1975.
69. Weitman, R. T., and Eames, W. B.: Plaque accumulation on composite surfaces after various finishing procedures. J. Am. Dent. Assoc., *91*:101, 1975.
70. Wheeler, R. C.: A Textbook of Dental Anatomy and Physiology. 3rd ed. Philadelphia, W. B. Saunders Company, 1958, pp. 64–65.
71. Wilhelmsem, N. R., Ramfjord, S. P., and Blankenship, J. R.: Effects of electrosurgery on the gingival attachment in rhesus monkeys. J. Periodontol., *47*:160, 1976.
72. Wing, C.: Pontic design and construction in fixed bridgework. Dent. Prac. Dent. Rec., *12*:390, 1962.
73. Yuodelis, R. A., Weaver, J. D., and Sapkos, S.: Facial and lingual contours of artificial complete crowns and their effect on the periodontium. J. Prosthet. Dent., *29*:61, 1973.

Part VII

Maintenance Phase

chapter fifty-nine

Maintenance Care

Rationale for Maintenance Therapy	Recurrence of Periodontal Disease
The Maintenance Program	Classification of Posttreatment Patients
Examination and Evaluation	Referring Patients to the Periodontist
Checking Plaque Control	
Treatment	

Preservation of the periodontal health of the treated patient requires as positive a program as does the elimination of periodontal disease. After Phase I is completed, patients are placed on a schedule of periodic recall visits for maintenance care to prevent recurrence of the disease (Figs. 59–1 and 59–2).

Transfer of the patient from active treatment status to a maintenance program is a definitive step in total patient care that requires time and effort on the part of the dentist and staff. Patients must be made to understand the purpose of the maintenance program, with emphasis on the fact that preservation of the teeth is dependent upon it. Patients who are not maintained in a supervised recall program subsequent to active treatment will show obvious signs of recurrent periodontitis.[1] In fact, one study has found that tooth loss in treated patients is three times as great in patients who do not return for regular recall visits as in those who do.[5] It is meaningless simply to inform patients that they are to return for periodic recall visits without pinpointing their significance and without describing what is expected of the patient between visits.

The maintenance phase of periodontal treatment starts immediately after the completion of Phase I therapy (see Figs. 59–1 and 59–2). While the patient is in the maintenance phase, the necessary surgical and restorative procedures are performed. This will ensure that all areas of the mouth will retain the degree of health attained after Phase I therapy.

RATIONALE FOR MAINTENANCE THERAPY

Studies have shown that even with appropriate periodontal therapy some progression of disease may continue.[4, 17, 23] The most likely explanation for the recurrence of periodontal disease is incomplete subgingival plaque removal.[32] If subgingival plaque is left behind during scaling, it will lead to regrowth within the pocket. The regrowth of subgingival plaque is a slow process compared with that of supragingival plaque. During this period of (perhaps) months, the subgingival plaque may not induce inflammatory reactions which can be discerned at the gingival margin. The clinical diagnosis may be further confused by the introduction of adequate supragingival plaque control, because the inflammatory reactions caused by the plaque in the soft tissue wall of the pocket are not likely to be manifested clinically as gingivitis. Thus, inadequate subgingival plaque control can lead to continued loss of attachment even without the presence of clinical gingival inflammation.

Another possible explanation for recurrence of periodontal disease is the nature of the histologic healing of the dentogingival unit following periodontal treatment. Histologic studies have shown that periodontal procedures usually do not result in the formation of new connective tissue attachments to root surfaces.[2, 26, 28] What is usually seen in histologic sections is a long, tight junctional epithelium. Since connective tissue reattachment does not

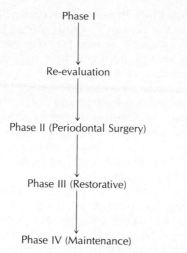

Phase I

↓

Re-evaluation

↓

Phase II (Periodontal Surgery)

↓

Phase III (Restorative)

↓

Phase IV (Maintenance)

Figure 59–1 Incorrect sequence of periodontal treatment phases. Maintenance phase should be started immediately after the re-evaluation of Phase I.

usually occur, it has been speculated that inflammation will rapidly separate long junctional epithelial attachments. Thus, treated periodontal patients are predisposed to recurrent pocket formation if optimal maintenance care is not performed.

Subgingival scaling has been shown to alter the microflora of periodontal patients.[15, 20, 25] A single session of scaling and root planing in patients with chronic periodontitis resulted in significant changes in the subgingival microflora. The following alterations were reported: (1) a decrease in the proportion of motile rods for 1 week, (2) a marked elevation in the proportion of coccoid cells for 21 days, and (3) a marked reduction in the proportion of spirochetes for 7 weeks.

Another study reported that subgingival bacteria had not returned to pretreatment proportions after 3 to 6 months.[25] However, the rate

of return of the pretreatment microbial flora was variable from patient to patient.

These findings indicate that mechanical débridement produces a relatively long-lasting effect on the microbial flora and that the proportions of different groups of microorganisms return to their baseline values after varying time periods.

In one study, the proportion of spirochetes obtained in baseline samples of subgingival flora was highly correlated with clinical periodontal deterioration over a period of 1 year.[11] More research is required to confirm the usefulness of culturing subgingival microflora. In the meantime, *there is a sound scientific basis for recall maintenance, since subgingival scaling alters the subgingival microflora for variable but relatively long periods.*

THE MAINTENANCE PROGRAM

Periodic recall visits form the foundation of a meaningful long-term prevention program. The interval between visits is initially set at 3 months but may be varied according to the patient's needs.

Periodontal care at each recall visit comprises three parts (Table 59–1). The first is concerned with examination and evaluation of the patient's current oral health. The second part of the recall appointment includes the necessary maintenance treatment and oral hygiene reinforcement. The third part involves scheduling the patient for the next recall appointment, further periodontal treatment, or

TABLE 59–1 MAINTENANCE RECALL PROCEDURES

Part I: Examination (approximate time, 17 minutes)[24]
  Medical history changes
  Oral pathology examination
  Oral hygiene status
  Gingival changes
  Pocket depth changes
  Mobility changes
  Occlusal changes
  Dental caries
  Restorative and prosthetic status
Part II: Treatment (approximate time, 35 minutes)[24]
  Oral hygiene reinforcement
  Scaling
  Polishing
  Chemical irrigation
Part III: Schedule next procedure (approximate time, 1 minute)[24]
  Schedule next recall visit
  Schedule further periodontal treatment
  Schedule or refer for restorative or prosthetic treatment

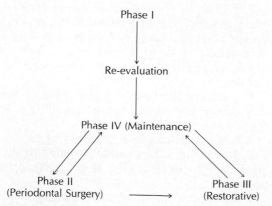

Phase I

↓

Re-evaluation

↓

Phase IV (Maintenance)

Phase II (Periodontal Surgery) ——→ Phase III (Restorative)

Figure 59–2 Correct sequence of periodontal treatment phases.

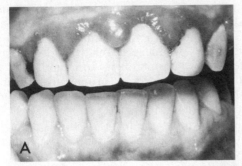

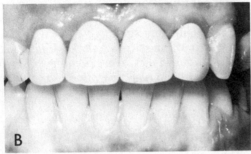

Figure 59–3 *A,* Hyperplastic gingivitis related to crown margins and plaque accumulation in a 27-year-old woman. *B,* Four months following treatment, there is significant improvement. However, there is still some inflammation around crown margins which cannot be resolved without replacing the crowns.

restorative dental procedures. The time required for patients with multiple teeth in both arches is approximately 1 hour.[24] This 1-hour slot includes greeting the patient, set-up time, and cleanup.

EXAMINATION AND EVALUATION. (Figs. 59–3 and 59–4). The recall examination is similar to the initial evaluation of the patient discussed in Chapter 32. However, since the patient is not new to the office, the dentist will primarily be looking for changes that have occurred since the last evaluation. Analysis of the current oral hygiene status of the patient is essential. Updating of changes in the medical history and evaluation of restorations, caries, prostheses, occlusion, tooth mobility, gingival status, and periodontal pockets are important parts of the recall appointment. The oral mucosa should be carefully inspected for pathologic conditions.

A complete series of intraoral radiographs is taken every 2 to 4 years, depending on the initial severity of the case and the findings at the recall visit. These are compared with previous radiographs in order to check the bone height, repair of osseous defects, signs of trauma from occlusion, periapical pathology, and caries.

CHECKING PLAQUE CONTROL. Plaque control in the patient's mouth should be checked with disclosing agents (see Chapter 44). Patients should perform their hygiene regimen immediately before the recall appointment so that effectiveness can be assessed. Plaque control must be reviewed and corrected until the patient demonstrates the necessary proficiency, even if it requires additional instruction sessions. Patients instructed in plaque control have less plaque and gingivitis than uninstructed patients.[1, 30, 31]

TREATMENT. The required scaling and root planing are performed, followed by an oral prophylaxis (see Chapter 44). Irrigation with antimicrobial agents, such as stannous fluoride (1.64%),[14] is performed in maintenance patients with remaining pockets.[10, 14, 24]

RECURRENCE OF PERIODONTAL DISEASE

Occasionally, lesions may recur. This can usually be traced to inadequate plaque control on the part of the patient. It should be understood, however, that it is the dentist's responsibility to teach, motivate, and control the patient's oral hygiene technique and that the patient's failure is our failure. Surgery should not be undertaken unless the patient has shown proficiency and willingness to cooperate by performing adequately his or her part of therapy.[29]

Other causes for recurrence are the following:

1. Inadequate or insufficient treatment that has failed to remove *all* the potential factors favoring plaque accumulation. Incomplete calculus removal in areas of difficult access is a common source of problems.

2. Inadequate restorations placed after the periodontal treatment was completed.

3. Failure of the patient to return for periodic checkups. This may be due to the patient's conscious or unconscious decision not to continue treatment or to the dentist and staff not having emphasized the need for periodic examinations.

4. Presence of some systemic diseases that may affect host resistance to previously acceptable levels of plaque.

A failing case can be recognized by:

1. Recurring inflammation revealed by gingival changes and bleeding of the sulcus upon probing.

2. Increasing depth of sulci, leading to the recurrence of pocket formation.

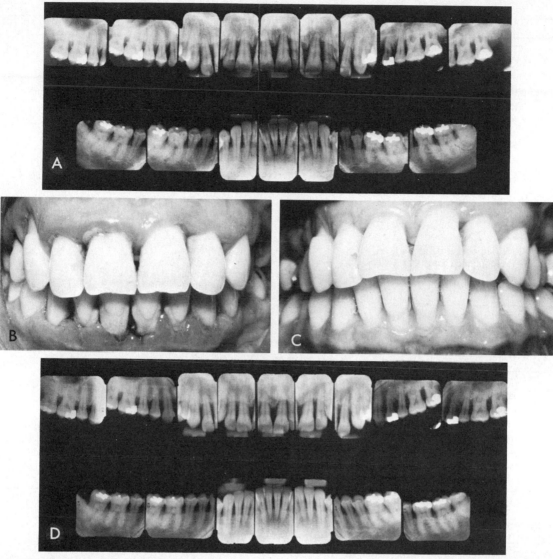

Figure 59–4 *A,* The patient was 38 years old in 1976 when these original radiographs were taken. Because of the advanced bone loss, the maxilla was treated with subgingival curettage, whereas the mandible was treated with a combination of surgical and nonsurgical therapy. This patient is a classic C maintenance patient. *B,* Pretreatment photographs taken in 1976. Note the inflammation and heavy calculus deposits. *C,* Photographs taken in 1980. The gingiva is not clinically inflamed. *D,* The radiographic results are as good as can be expected in such a severe case. There has been no bone loss between 1976 and 1980.

3. Gradual increases in bone loss, as determined by the radiograph.

4. Gradual increases in tooth mobility as ascertained by clinical examination.

The decision to re-treat a periodontal patient should not be made at the preventive maintenance appointment but should be postponed for 1 to 2 weeks.[3] Often the mouth will look a great deal better at that time, owing to the resolution of edema and the resulting improved tone of the gingiva. A summary of the symptoms of recurrence of periodontal disease and their probable causes can be found in Table 59–2.

CLASSIFICATION OF POSTTREATMENT PATIENTS

The first year following periodontal therapy is important in terms of indoctrinating the patient in a recall pattern and reinforcing oral hygiene. In addition, it may take several months to evaluate the results of some peri-

TABLE 59–2 SYMPTOMS AND CAUSES OF RECURRENCE OF DISEASE

Symptom	Possible Causes
Increased inflammation	Poor oral hygiene Subgingival calculus Inadequate restorations Deteriorating or poorly designed prostheses Systemic disease modifying host response to plaque
Recession	Toothbrush abrasion Inadequate keratinized gingiva Frenum pull Orthodontic therapy
Increased mobility with no change in pocket depth and no radiographic change	Occlusal trauma due to lateral occlusal interference Bruxism High restoration Poorly designed or worn-out prostheses Poor crown-to-root ratio
Increased pocket depth with no radiographic change	Poor oral hygiene Infrequent recall Subgingival calculus Poorly fitting partial denture Mesial inclination into edentulous space Failure of new attachment surgery Cracked teeth Grooves in teeth New periodontal disease
Increased pocket depth with increased radiographic bone loss	Poor oral hygiene Subgingival calculus Infrequent recall visits Inadequate or deteriorating restorations Poorly designed prostheses Inadequate surgery Systemic disease modifying host response to plaque Cracked teeth Grooves in teeth New periodontal disease

odontal surgical procedures accurately. Consequently, some areas may have to be retreated because the results are not optimal. Furthermore, the first-year patient will often present etiologic factors that may have been overlooked and that may be more amenable to treatment at this early stage. For these reasons, the recall interval for first-year patients should not be longer than 3 months.

The patients who are on a periodontal recall schedule are a most varied group. Table 59–3 lists several categories of maintenance patient and a suggested recall interval for each. One must realize that patients can improve or relapse to a different classification with the reduction or exacerbation of periodontal disease. When one dental arch is more involved than the other, the patient is classified by the arch that is in the worse condition.

In summary, maintenance care is a critical phase of therapy. The long-term preservation of the dentition is closely associated with the frequency and quality of recall maintenance.

REFERRING PATIENTS TO THE PERIODONTIST

The majority of periodontal care of the population belongs in the hands of the general dentist. This is because of the overwhelming number of patients with periodontal disease and the intimate relationship between periodontal disease and restorative dentistry.

For various reasons, an ever greater number of periodontal patients are expected in future years. For one thing, the number of caries per capita has dwindled in the last 20 years by about 50 per cent, and there is some evidence that the decline will continue.[24] The reason for this is the development of fluorides. As more people retain their teeth throughout their lifetime, and as the proportion of older people in the population increases, more teeth will be at risk of periodontal disease. Hence, the prevalence of periodontal disease is likely to increase in the future.

This expected increase in the number of

periodontal patients will necessitate a greater understanding of periodontal problems and an increased level of expertise for their solution on the part of the general practitioner of dentistry. However, there will always be a need for specialists to treat particularly difficult cases, patients with systemic health problems, and situations in which a complex prosthetic construction requires absolute assurance of reliable results.

Where to draw the line between the cases to be treated in the general dental office and those to be referred to a specialist will vary for different practitioners and for different patients. The diagnosis will indicate the type of periodontal treatment required. If the periodontal destruction necessitates surgery on the distal surfaces of second molars, extensive osseous surgery, or involved bone grafting, the patient will usually be best treated by a specialist. On the other hand, patients who require localized areas of gingivectomy or flap curettage can usually be treated by the general dentist.

It will be immediately obvious that some patients should be referred to a specialist, whereas most patients will clearly have problems that can be treated by a general dentist.

TABLE 59–3 RECALL INTERVALS FOR VARIOUS CLASSES OF RECALL PATIENTS

Classification	Characteristics	Recall Interval
First year	First-year patient—routine therapy and uneventful healing	3 months
	or	
	First-year patient—difficult case with complicated prosthesis, furcation involvement, poor crown-to-root ratios, questionable patient cooperation	1 to 2 months
Class A	Excellent results maintained well for 1 year or more Patient displays good oral hygiene, minimal calculus, no occlusal problems, no complicated prostheses, no remaining pockets, and no teeth with less than 50 per cent of alveolar bone remaining	6 months to 1 year
Class B	Generally good results maintained reasonably well for 1 year or more, but patient displays some of the following factors: 1. Inconsistent or poor oral hygiene 2. Heavy calculus formation 3. Systemic disease that predisposes to periodontal breakdown 4. Some remaining pockets 5. Occlusal problems 6. Complicated prostheses 7. Ongoing orthodontic therapy 8. Recurrent dental caries 9. Some teeth with less than 50 per cent of alveolar bone support	3 to 4 months (decide on recall interval on the basis of the number and severity of negative factors)
Class C	Generally poor results following periodontal therapy and/or several negative factors from the following list: 1. Inconsistent or poor oral hygiene 2. Heavy calculus formation 3. Systemic disease that predisposes to periodontal breakdown 4. Remaining pockets 5. Occlusal problems 6. Complicated prostheses 7. Recurrent dental caries 8. Periodontal surgery indicated but not performed for medical, psychologic, or financial reasons 9. Many teeth with less than 50 per cent of alveolar bone support 10. Condition too far advanced to be improved by periodontal surgery	1 to 3 months (decide on recall interval on the basis of the number and severity of negative factors; consider re-treating some areas or extracting the severely involved teeth)

However, for a third group it will be difficult to decide whether treatment by a specialist is required. Any patient who does not plainly belong in the second of these categories should be a candidate for referral to a specialist.[18]

The decision as to whether a patient's periodontal problem should be treated in a general practice should be guided by the degree of risk that the patient will lose a tooth or teeth for periodontally related reasons. The most important factors in the decision are the extent and location of the periodontal deterioration present. Teeth with pockets of 5 mm or more, measured from the cemento-enamel junction, may have a prognosis of rapid decline. The location of the periodontal deterioration is also an important factor in determining the risk of a tooth being lost. Teeth with furcation lesions may be at risk even when there is more than 50 per cent bone support remaining. Therefore, cases in which strategic teeth fall into these categories are usually best treated by specialists.

An important question remains: Should the maintenance phase of therapy be performed by the general practitioner or by the specialist? This should be determined by the amount of periodontal deterioration present. Class A recall patients should be maintained by the general dentist, whereas Class C patients should be maintained by the specialist (Table 59–3). Class B patients fall into the gray area in between and can alternate recall visits between the general and specialty offices. The rule suggested is that the patient's disease should dictate whether the general practitioner or the specialist should perform the maintenance therapy.

REFERENCES

1. Axelsson, P., and Lindhe, J.: The significance of maintenance care in the treatment of periodontal disease. J. Clin. Periodontol., 8:281, 1981.
2. Caton, J. G., and Zander, H. A.: The attachment between tooth and gingival tissues after periodic root planing and soft tissue curettage. J. Periodontol., 50:462, 1979.
3. Chace, R.: Retreatment in periodontal practice. J. Periodontol., 48:410, 1977.
4. Hirschfeld, L., and Wasserman, B.: A long-term survey of tooth loss in 600 treated periodontal patients. J. Periodontol., 49:225, 1978.
5. Lietha-Elmer, E.: Langsfristgie Ergebnisse reglemassig betreuter und unbetreuter Parodontosepatienten. Schweiz. Mschr. Zahnheilk., 87:613, 1977.
6. Lightner, L. M., O'Leary, J. T., Drake, R. B., Crump, P. O., and Allen, M. F.: Preventive periodontic treatment procedures: result over 46 months. J. Periodontol., 42:555, 1971.
7. Lindhe, J., and Koch, G.: The effect of supervised oral hygiene on the gingiva of children. J. Periodont. Res., 1:260, 1966.
8. Lindhe, J., and Koch, G.: The effect of supervised oral hygiene on the gingiva of children. Lack of prolonged effect of supervision. J. Periodont. Res., 2:215, 1967.
9. Lindhe, J., and Nyman, S.: The effect of plaque control and surgical pocket elimination on the establishment and maintenance of periodontal health. A longitudinal study of periodontal therapy in cases of advanced disease. J. Clin. Periodontol., 2:67, 1975.
10. Lindhe, J., Heijl, L., Goodson, J. M., and Socransky, S. S.: Local tetracycline delivery using hollow fiber devices in periodontal therapy. J. Clin. Periodontol., 6:141, 1979.
11. Listgarten, M. A., and Hellden, L.: Relative distribution of bacteria at clinically healthy and periodontally diseased sites in humans. J. Clin. Periodontol., 5:115, 1978.
12. Listgarten, M. A., and Levin, S.: Positive correlation between the proportions of subgingival spirochetes and motile bacteria and susceptibility of human subjects to periodontal deterioration. J. Clin. Periodontol., 8:122, 1981.
13. Listgarten, M. A., Lindhe, J., and Hellden, L: Effect of tetracycline and/or scaling on human periodontal disease. J. Clin. Periodontol., 5:246, 1978.
14. Mazza, J. E., Newman, M. G., and Sims, T. N.: Clinical and antimicrobial effect of stannous fluoride on periodontitis. J. Clin. Periodontol., 8:213, 1981.
15. Mousques, T., Listgarten, M. A., and Phillips, R. W.: Effect of scaling and root planing on the composition of human subgingival microbial flora. J. Periodont. Res., 15:144, 1980.
16. Nyman, S., Rosling, B., and Lindhe, J.: Effect of professional tooth cleaning on healing after periodontal surgery. J. Clin. Periodontol., 2:80, 1975.
17. Oliver, R. C.: Tooth loss with and without periodontal therapy. Periodont. Abstracts, 17:8, 1969.
18. Parr, R. W., Pipe, P., and Watts, T.: Periodontal Maintenance Therapy. Berkeley, Calif., Praxis Publishing Company, 1974.
19. Ramfjord, S. P., Knowles, J. W., Nissle, R. R., Burgett, F. G., and Shick, R. A.: Results following three modalities of periodontal therapy. J. Periodontol., 46:522, 1975.
20. Rosenberg, E. S., Evian, C. I., and Listgarten, M. A.: The composition of the subgingival microbiota after periodontal therapy. J. Periodontol., 52:435, 1981.
21. Rosling, B., Nyman, S., and Lindhe, J.: The effect of systematic plaque control on bone regeneration in infrabony pockets. J. Clin. Periodontol., 3:38, 1976.
22. Rosling, B., Nyman, S., Lindhe, J., and Jern, B.: The healing potential of the periodontal tissues following different techniques of periodontal surgery in plaque-free dentitions. J. Clin. Periodontol., 3:233, 1976.
23. Ross, I. F., Thompson, R. H., and Galdi, M.: The results of treatment: a long term study of one hundred and eighty patients. Parodontologie, 25:125, 1971.
24. Schallhorn, R. G., and Snider, L. E.: Periodontal maintenance therapy. J. Am. Dent. Assoc., 103:227, 1981.
25. Slots, J., Mashimo, P., Levine, M. J., and Genco, R. J.: Periodontal therapy in humans. I. Microbiological and clinical effects of a single course of periodontal scaling and root planing, and of adjunctive tetracycline therapy. J. Periodontol., 50:495, 1979.
26. Stahl, S. S.: Repair potential of the soft tissue–root interface. J. Periodontol., 48:545, 1977.
27. Stahl, S. S., and Froum, S. J.: Human clinical and histologic repair responses following the use of citric acid in periodontal therapy. J. Periodontol., 48:261, 1977.
28. Stahl, S. S., et al.: Gingival healing. IV. The effects of home care on gingivectomy repair. J. Periodontol., 40:264, 1969.
29. Sternlicht, H. C.: Evaluating long-term periodontal therapy. Texas Dent. J., 92:4, 1974.
30. Suomi, J. D., West, J. D., Chang, J. J., and McClendon, B. J.: The effect of controlled oral hygiene procedures on the progression of periodontal disease in adults: radiographic findings. J. Periodontol., 42:562, 1971.
31. Suomi, J. D., Greene, J. C., Vermillion, J. R., Doyle, J., Chang, J. J., and Leatherwood, E. C.: The effect of controlled oral hygiene on the progression of periodontal disease in adults: results after the third and final year. J. Periodontol., 42:152, 1971.
32. Waerhaug, J.: Healing of the dento-epithelial junction following subgingival plaque control. J. Periodontol., 49:119, 1978.
33. Withers, J. A., et al.: The relationship of palatogingival grooves to localized periodontal disease. J. Periodontol., 52:41, 1981.

chapter sixty

Results of Periodontal Treatment

Treatment and Prevention of Gingivitis	Treatment of Loss of Attachment
Prevention and Treatment of Loss of Attachment	**Tooth Mortality**
Prevention of Loss of Attachment	

The prevalence of periodontal disease and the high tooth mortality due to this disease raise an important question: Is periodontal treatment effective in preventing and stopping the progressive destruction of periodontal disease? Evidence that periodontal therapy is effective in preventing the disease, slowing the destruction of the periodontium, and reducing tooth loss is now overwhelming.

TREATMENT AND PREVENTION OF GINGIVITIS

For many years, the belief that good oral hygiene is necessary for the successful prevention and treatment of gingivitis has been widespread among periodontists. In addition, worldwide epidemiologic studies have confirmed a close relationship between the incidence of gingivitis and lack of oral hygiene.[4, 5]

Conclusive evidence on the relation of oral hygiene and gingivitis in healthy dental students was shown by Löe and co-workers.[13, 28] After 9 to 21 days without oral hygiene, experimental subjects with previously excellent oral hygiene and healthy gingiva developed heavy accumulations of plaque and generalized mild gingivitis. When oral hygiene was reinstituted, the plaque in most areas disappeared in 1 or 2 days, and the gingival inflammation in these areas disappeared 1 day after the plaque had been removed. Gingivitis is therefore reversible and can be resolved by daily effective plaque removal.

A number of long-term studies have shown that gingival health can be maintained by a combination of effective oral hygiene and dental scaling.[1, 2, 7, 9, 15, 26, 27]

A 3-year study on 1248 General Telephone workers in California was conducted to determine whether the progression of gingival inflammation is retarded in an oral environment in which high levels of hygiene are maintained.[26, 27] Experimental and control groups were computer matched on the basis of periodontal and oral hygiene status, past caries experience, age, and sex. During the study period, several procedures were instituted to ensure that the oral hygiene status of the experimental group was maintained at a high level. They were given a series of frequent oral prophylaxis treatments, combined with oral hygiene instruction. Subjects in the control groups received no attention from the study team except for annual examinations. They were advised to continue their usual daily practices and accustomed visits for professional care. After 3 years, the increase in plaque and debris in the control group was four times as great as that in the experimental group. Similarly, gingivitis scores were much higher in the control subjects than in the matching experimental group. **It is therefore an established fact that chronic marginal gingivitis can be controlled by good oral hygiene and dental prophylaxis.**

PREVENTION AND TREATMENT OF LOSS OF ATTACHMENT

Although periodontal therapy has been employed for more than 100 years, it is only within the last 15 years or so that a number of studies have been conducted to determine the effect of treatment on reducing the progressive loss of periodontal support for the natural dentition.

Prevention of Loss of Attachment

A longitudinal investigation to study the natural development and progression of periodontal disease was conducted by Löe and co-workers.[14] The first group was established in Oslo, Norway, in 1969 and consisted of 565 healthy male nondental students and academicians between 17 and 40 years of age. The principal reason for selecting Oslo as a study site was that this city had had a preschool, school, and postschool dental program offering systematic preventive, restorative, endodontic, orthodontic, and surgical therapy on an annual recall basis for all children and adolescents, complete with a documented attendance record, for the last 40 years. This study population represents a group that has had maximum exposure to conventional dental care throughout their life. A second group was established in Sri Lanka in 1970 and consisted of 480 male tea laborers between 15 and 40 years of age. They were healthy and well built by local standards, and their nutritional condition was clinically fair. The workers had never been exposed to any programs relative to the prevention or treatment of dental diseases. Toothbrushing was unknown.

The results of this study are quite interesting. The Norwegian group, as the members approach 40 years of age, has a mean individual loss of attachment of slightly above 1.5 mm, and the mean annual rate of attachment loss is 0.08 mm for interproximal surfaces and 0.10 mm for buccal surfaces. As the Sri Lankan approaches 40 years of age, the mean individual loss of attachment is 4.50 mm, and the mean annual rate of progression of the lesion is 0.30 mm for interproximal surfaces and 0.20 mm for buccal surfaces. Figure 60–1 gives a graphic interpretation of the difference between the two groups. This study suggests that without interference the periodontal lesions progress at a relatively even pace and that progress is continuous.

In the previously discussed study of General Telephone workers in California, loss of attachment was measured clinically, whereas alveolar bone loss was measured radiographically.[26, 27] After 3 years, the control group showed loss of attachment at a rate more than three and one-half times that of the matching experimental group during the same period (Fig. 60–2). In addition, subjects who received frequent oral prophylaxis and were instructed in good oral hygiene practices showed less bone loss radiographically after 3 years than did the control subjects. **It is clear that loss of attachment can be reduced by good oral hygiene and frequent dental prophylaxis.**

Treatment of Loss of Attachment

Thus far, the studies cited involved treatment of populations without extensive periodontal disease. A longitudinal study of patients with moderate to advanced periodontal disease, conducted at the University of Michigan, showed that the progression of periodontal disease can be stopped for a period of 3 years postoperatively regardless of the modality of treatment.[19, 21, 22] Even for long-term observations, the average loss of attachment was only 0.3 mm over 7 years.[22] These results indicated a more favorable prognosis for treatment of advanced periodontal lesions than previously assumed.

Another study was conducted on 75 patients with advanced periodontal disease to determine the effect of plaque control and surgical pocket elimination on the establishment and maintenance of periodontal health.[11] This study showed that no further alveolar bone loss occurred during the 5-year observation period. The meticulous plaque control practiced by the patients in this study was consid-

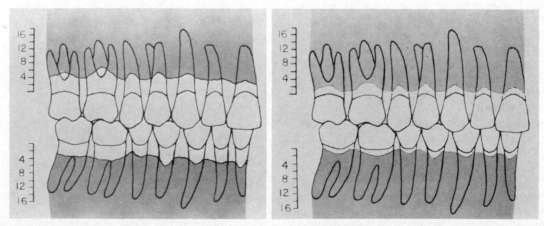

Figure 60–1 *Left,* Mean periodontal support of teeth of Sri Lankan tea laborers at approximately 40 years of age. *Right,* Mean periodontal support of teeth of Norwegian academicians at approximately 40 years of age. (From Löe, H., et al.: J. Periodontol., *49:*607, 1978.)

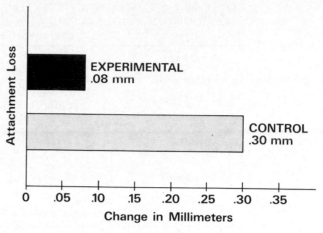

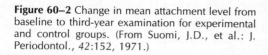

Figure 60–2 Change in mean attachment level from baseline to third-year examination for experimental and control groups. (From Suomi, J.D., et al.: J. Periodontol., 42:152, 1971.)

ered a major factor in the excellent results produced.

None of these studies used a control group, since leaving periodontal patients untreated cannot be justified. However, in a study in private practice,[3] an effort was made to find and evaluate patients with diagnosed moderate to advanced periodontitis who did not follow through with recommended periodontal therapy. Thirty patients ranging in age from 25 to 71 years were found and evaluated after periods ranging from 18 to 115 months. All of these untreated patients had progressive increases in pocket depth and radiographic evidence of progressive bone resorption. Comparing this study[3] with others,[19, 21, 22] **it is logical to conclude that treatment is very effective in reducing loss of attachment.**

TOOTH MORTALITY

The ultimate test for the effectiveness of periodontal treatment is whether the loss of teeth can be prevented. There are now enough studies from both private practice and research

institutions to document that loss of teeth is retarded or prevented by therapy.

The combined effect of subgingival scaling every 3 to 6 months and controlled oral hygiene was evaluated over a 5-year period.[15] Tooth loss was significantly reduced for all patients. This study showed that frequent subgingival scalings will reduce tooth loss even when oral hygiene is "not good" (Table 60–1).

In the previously mentioned longitudinal study conducted at the University of Michigan, 104 patients with a total of 2604 teeth were included.[19, 21, 22] After 1 to 7 years of treatment, 53 teeth were lost for various reasons (Table 60–2). Thirty-two teeth were lost during the first and second years after initiation of treatment. The remaining 21 teeth were lost in a random pattern over the next 6 years. The loss of teeth due to advanced periodontal disease following treatment was, therefore, minimal (2 per cent).

Another study was undertaken to test the effect of periodontal therapy in cases of advanced disease.[11] The subjects were 75 patients who had lost 50 per cent or more of their periodontal support (Fig. 60–3). Treatment

TABLE 60–1 AVERAGE LOSS OF TEETH DURING FIVE-YEAR PERIOD AS COMPARED WITH "NORMAL" LOSS OF TEETH IN 1428 MEN AND WOMEN AGED 20 THROUGH 59

	Grade of Oral Hygiene		
	Good	Fairly Good	Not Good
"Normal" loss of teeth. Estimate based on the data recorded at the initiation of the period.	1.1	1.4	1.8
Actual loss of teeth during the five-year period	0.4	0.6	0.9

From Lovdal, A., et al.: Acta Odontol. Scand., 19:537, 1961.

TABLE 60–2 TOOTH MORTALITY FOLLOWING TREATMENT OF ADVANCED PERIODONTITIS IN 104 PATIENTS WITH 2604 TEETH TREATED OVER A 10-YEAR PERIOD

Teeth Lost	Reason
2	Pulpal disease
3	Accidents
4	Prosthetic considerations
14	One patient wanted a maxillary denture for cosmetic reasons
30	Periodontal
53 total	**All reasons**

2 per cent of the teeth were lost during the study period.

Adapted from data in Ramfjord, S. P., et al.: J. Periodontol., *44*:66, 1973.

consisted of oral hygiene, scaling, extraction of untreatable teeth, periodontal surgery, and prosthetics where indicated. After completion of periodontal treatment, there followed a 5-year period during which none of the patients showed any further loss of periodontal support. No teeth were extracted in the 5-year posttreatment period. It should be pointed out that the patients in this study were selected because of their capacity to meet high requirements of plaque control following repeated instruction in oral hygiene techniques. This fact does not detract from the validity of the study, but tends to show the etiologic importance of bacterial plaque. The results show that periodontal surgery coupled with a detailed plaque control program not only will temporarily cure the disease but also will prevent further progression of periodontal breakdown—even in patients with severely reduced periodontal support.

There have been several studies in private practice that have attempted to measure tooth loss following periodontal therapy. In one study, 180 patients who had been treated for chronic destructive periodontal disease were evaluated.[24] The average age of the patients before treatment was 43.7 years. From the beginning of treatment to the time of the survey, the majority of patients lost no teeth (Fig. 60–4). A total of 141 teeth were lost. Three patients of 180 (1.7 per cent) lost 35 teeth, or approximately 25 per cent of the teeth lost. Twelve additional patients lost 46 teeth, or 32.6 per cent of the teeth lost. Many patients in the study had advanced alveolar bone loss, including extensive furcation involvements. A relatively small number (141) of the teeth were lost in the study group of 180 patients between the beginning of periodontal treatment and the time of the study. The teeth were lost for several reasons, including periodontal disease as well as caries and other nonperiodontal causes. The length of time after treatment varied from 2 to 20 years, with an average of 8.6 years. Of considerable significance is the fact that a large number of teeth (81 teeth, or 57.5 per cent) were lost by a few patients (15 patients, or 8.4 per cent). Even when this group is considered with the

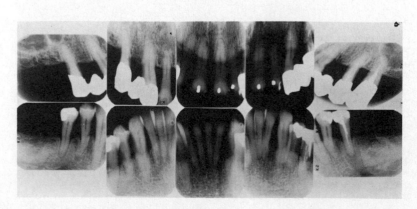

Figure 60–3 Radiographs Taken 5 Years After Typical Periodontal Treatment. Note the advanced bone loss, in spite of which teeth were retained in a healthy condition for the duration of the study. (From Lindhe, J., and Nyman, S.: J. Clin. Periodontol., 2:67, 1975.)

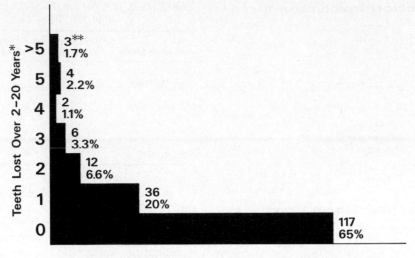

Number of Patients (n=180) with Percentage of Total

*Average of 8.6 years.
**3 patients lost 35 teeth.

The average tooth lost per patient
was 0.9 per 10 years.

Figure 60–4 Tooth Mortality. (Adapted from Ross, I.F., Thompson, R.H., and Galdi, M.: Parodontologie, 25:125, 1971.)

remaining 165 patients, it may be seen that the periodontal care provided helped to retain most teeth, as the average patient lost slightly less than one tooth (0.9) over 10 years following treatment.

In another study, all the patients in a practice who had been treated 5 or more years previously and had received regular preventive periodontal care since that time were included.[17, 18] There were 442 patients included, with an average length of time since treatment of 10.1 years. Two thirds of the patients were over 40 at the time of treatment. These patients had been seen every 4.6 months, on the average, for their preventive periodontal care, which consisted of oral hygiene instruction and prophylaxis (Figs. 60–5 and 60–6).

The total tooth loss due to periodontal disease was 178 of just over 11,000 teeth available for treatment. More important, 78 per cent of the patients did not lose a single tooth following periodontal therapy, and 11 per cent lost

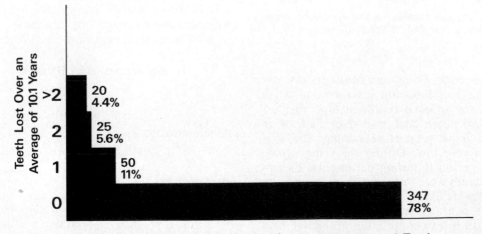

Number of Patients (n=442) with Percentage of Total

Figure 60–5 Tooth Mortality in 442 Periodontal Patients Treated over a Period of 10 Years. (Courtesy of Dr. R.G. Oliver.)

Furcation Involvement

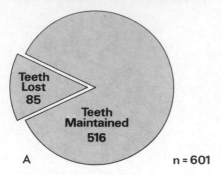

A   n = 601

One-half Bone Lost

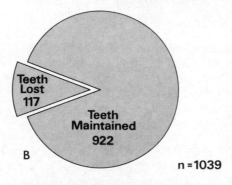

B   n = 1039

Guarded Prognosis

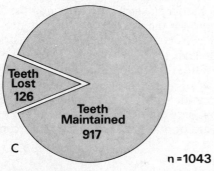

C   n = 1043

Figure 60–6 Tooth Mortality in 442 Periodontal Patients Treated over a Period of 10 Years. (Courtesy of Dr. R.G. Oliver.)

TABLE 60–3 TOOTH MORTALITY IN STUDIES IN PRIVATE PRACTICE

Author of Study	Average Number of Teeth Lost per 10 Years with Periodontal Treatment
Hirschfeld and Wasserman[6]	1.0
McFall[17]	1.4
Oliver[18]	0.72
Ross et al.[24]	0.9

(11 per cent) of 1039 teeth with half or less of the bone remaining were lost. Of the teeth listed as having a guarded prognosis for any reason by the clinician performing the initial examination, only 126 (12 per cent) of 1043 were lost over this 10-year average period. When one looks at these figures from the standpoint of the average tooth mortality per patient, one finds that 0.72 teeth are lost per patient per 10 years.

In a third study in private practice, 600 patients were followed over a period between 15 and 53 years after periodontal therapy (Table 60–3; Figs. 60–7 and 60–8).[6] The majority (76.5 per cent) had advanced periodontal disease at the start of treatment. There were 15,666 teeth present, an average of 26 teeth per patient. During the follow-up period (average, 22 years), a total of 1312 teeth were lost owing to all causes. Of this number, 1110 were lost for periodontal reasons. The average tooth mortality per patient was 2.2 teeth; when this is converted to a 10-year rate, an average of one tooth was lost per 10 years in each patient. During this period of observation, 666 teeth with a questionable prognosis were lost, out of a total of 2141. This means that 31 per cent of the teeth with a questionable prognosis were lost over 22 years of treatment. A total of 1464 teeth with furcation involvement were

only one tooth. When one considers that over 600 teeth had furcation involvements at the time of the original treatment and that well over 1000 teeth had less than half of the alveolar bone support remaining, the tooth loss was very low. During the same average 10-year period following periodontal therapy, only 45 teeth were lost through caries or pulpal involvement. Even more surprising are the statistics over an average 10-year period for teeth with less than optimum prognoses.

Only 85 (14 per cent) of a total of 601 teeth with furcation involvement were lost, and 117

Status at Start

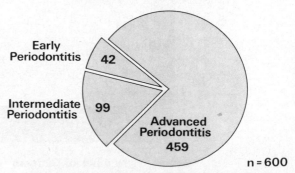

n = 600

Figure 60–7 Data from 600 Periodontal Patients.

Tooth Mortality

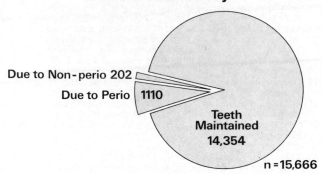

Figure 60–8 Data from 600 Periodontal Patients.

Due to Non-perio 202

Due to Perio 1110

Teeth Maintained 14,354

n = 15,666

After 15 - 53 years. Average of 22 years.

treated, and 31.6 per cent were lost during the period of study. Eighty-three per cent of the patients lost fewer than three teeth over the 22-year average treatment period and were classified as well maintained. The remaining 17 per cent of the patients were divided into two groups, identified as either downhill (four to nine lost) or extreme downhill (10 to 23 teeth lost). This 17 per cent of the patients studied accounted for 69 per cent of the teeth lost owing to periodontal causes. This study also showed that relatively few teeth are lost following periodontal therapy. In addition, relatively few of the guarded prognosis teeth, including teeth with furcation involvement, are lost. And, finally, a small percentage of patients are losing most of the teeth.

Comparison of these tooth mortality studies with other epidemiologic surveys is hazardous, since few involve treatment and few are longitudinal. Marshall-Day and associates reported an average tooth loss due to all causes of 5.2 teeth per 10 years after the age of 35.[16] In patients over 40, the rate increased to 6 teeth per 10 years. The United States Public Health Service surveys indicate that about 4.3 teeth are lost per 10 years after the age of 35 in the general population.[5, 10] It is obvious from such studies that tooth loss in the general population far exceeds that in the treated periodontal patients.

In a previously discussed study in private practice,[3] an effort was made to find and evaluate patients with diagnosed moderate to advanced periodontitis who did not follow through with recommended periodontal therapy. Patients with untreated periodontal disease were losing teeth at a rate greater than 0.61 teeth per year (6.1 per 10 years). A total of 83 teeth were lost in 30 patients, but the authors excluded one patient who had lost 25

teeth. Including this patient would have increased the tooth loss in untreated patients to an even higher rate.

In summary, the prevalence of periodontal disease and the high tooth mortality due to the disease have raised the need for effective treatment. Treatment is now available that is effective in preventing the disease and in stopping the progression of bone destruction once periodontitis is present. In addition, there is overwhelming evidence that periodontal therapy greatly reduces tooth mortality. Every dental practitioner should be familiar with the philosophy and techniques of periodontal therapy. Failure to diagnose and treat or make periodontal treatment available to our patients will cause unnecessary dental problems and tooth loss.

REFERENCES

1. Axelsson, P., and Lindhe, J.: Effect of controlled oral hygiene procedures on caries and periodontal disease in adults. Results after 6 years. J. Clin. Periodontol., 8:239, 1981.
2. Bay, I., and Møller, I. J.: The effect of a sodium monofluorophosphate dentifrice on the gingiva. J. Periodont. Res., 3:103, 1968.
3. Becker, W., Berg, L., and Becker, E. B.: Untreated periodontal disease: a longitudinal study. J. Periodontol., 50:234, 1979.
4. Greene, J. C.: Periodontal disease in India: report of an epidemiological study. J. Dent. Res., 39:302, 1960.
5. Greville, T. N. E.: United States Life Tables by Dentulous or Edentulous Condition, 1971, and 1957–58. Dept. of Health Education and Welfare, Publication No. (HRA) 75–1338, August, 1974.
6. Hirschfeld, L., and Wasserman, B.: A long-term survey of tooth loss in 600 treated periodontal patients. J. Periodontol., 49:225, 1978.
7. Hoover, D. R., and Lefkowitz, W.: Reduction of gingivitis by toothbrushing. J. Periodontol., 36:193, 1955.
8. Ladavalya, M. R. N., and Harris, R.: A study of the gingival and periodontal conditions of a group of people in Chieng Mai province. J. Periodontol., 30:219, 1959.
9. Lightner, L. M., O'Leary, J. T., Drake, R. B., Crump, P. P., and Allen, M. F.: Preventive periodontic treatment procedures: results over 46 months. J. Periodontol., 42:555, 1971.

10. Linder, F. E., et al.: Decayed Missing and Filled Teeth in Adults. United States—1960–1962. Public Health Service Publication No. 1000, Series 11, No. 23, February, 1967.

11. Lindhe, J., and Nyman, S.: The effect of plaque control and surgical pocket elimination on the establishment and maintenance of periodontal health. A longitudinal study of periodontal therapy in cases of advanced disease. J. Clin. Periodontol., *2*:67, 1975.

12. Löe, H., and Silness, J.: Periodontal disease in pregnancy. I. Prevalence and severity. Acta Odontol. Scand., *21*:533, 1976.

13. Löe, H., Theilade, E., and Jensen, S. B.: Experimental gingivitis in man. J. Periodontol., *36*:177, 1965.

14. Löe, H., Anerud, A., Boysen, H., and Smith, M.: The natural history of periodontal disease in man. J. Periodontol., *49*:607, 1978.

15. Lovdal, A., Arno, A., Schei, O., and Waerhaug, J.: Combined effect of subgingival scaling and controlled oral hygiene on the incidence of gingivitis. Acta Odontol. Scand., *19*:537, 1961.

16. Marshall-Day, C. D., Stephens, R. G., and Quigley, L. F.: Periodontal disease: prevalence and incidence. J. Periodontol., *26*:185, 1955.

17. McFall, W. T., Jr.: Tooth loss with and without periodontal therapy. Periodont. Abstracts, *17*:8, 1969.

18. Oliver. R. C.: Personal communication, 1977.

19. Ramfjord, S. P., and Nissle, R. R.: The modified Widman flap. J. Periodontol., *45*:601, 1974.

20. Ramfjord, S. P., Nissle, R. R., Shick, R. A., and Cooper, H.: Subgingival curettage versus surgical elimination of periodontal pockets. J. Periodontol., *39*:167, 1968.

21. Ramfjord, S. P., Knowles, J. W., Nissle, R. R., Burgett, F. G., and Shick, R. A.: Results following three modalities of periodontal therapy. J. Periodontol., *46*:522, 1975.

22. Ramfjord, S. P., Knowles, J. W., Nissle, R. R., Shick, R. A., and Burgett, F. G.: Longitudinal study of periodontal therapy. J. Periodontol., *44*:66, 1973.

23. Ross, I. F., and Thompson, R. H.: A long-term study of root retention in the treatment of maxillary molars with function involvement. J. Periodontol., *49*:238, 1978.

24. Ross, I. F., Thompson, R. H., and Galdi, M.: The results of treatment. A long term study of one hundred and eighty patients. Parodontologie, *25*:125, 1971.

25. Russell, A. L.: Some epidemiological characteristics of periodontal diseases in a series of urban populations. J. Periodontol., *28*:286, 1957.

26. Suomi, J. D., West, J. D., Chang, J. J., and McClendon, B. J.: The effect of controlled oral hygiene procedures on the progression of periodontal disease in adults: radiographic findings. J. Periodontol., *42*:562, 1971.

27. Suomi, J. D., Greene, J. C., Vermillion, J. R., Doyle, J., Chang, J. J., and Leatherwood, E. C.: The effect of controlled oral hygiene on the progression of periodontal disease in adults: results after the third and final year. J. Periodontol., *42*:152, 1971.

28. Theilade, E., Wright, W. H., Jensen, S. B., and Löe, H.: Experimental gingivitis in man. II. J. Periodont. Res., *1*:1, 1966.

INDEX

Note: Pages numbers in *italic* type refer to illustrations; (t) indicates a table. The expression "vs." denotes differential diagnosis from.

ABRASION, dental, 498, *499*
Abscess(es), gingival, 122, *125*
  etiology of, 125
  histopathology of, 125
  treatment of, 900
  vs. periodontal abscess, 265
  periapical, vs. periodontal, 264
  pericoronal, 163
  periodontal, 125, 259–265, *260–264*
    acute, 259, *261, 262*
      incision of, *655*
      treatment of, 654
    chronic, 259, *261, 262, 264*
      treatment of, 654–659
    classification of, 259
    clinical features of, 259
    complicating furcation involvement, *251*
    diagnosis of, 264
    flap operation for, 656–659, *658*
    gingivectomy for, 654, *656*
    treatment of, 654–659
    vs. gingival abscess, 265
    vs. periapical abscess, 264
  suprabony, gingivectomy for, 779
Abutment(s), multiple, 937
Acid base balance disturbances, 457
Acromegaly, 460
Acrosclerosis, and diffuse scleroderma, 183
Actinomycosis, 189–190
Acute herpetic gingivostomatitis, 157–161, *157–160*
  antibody titrations in, 159
  biopsy in, 159, *160*
  communicability of, 161
  diagnosis of, 159–161
  etiology of, 157
  fever in, 158
  histopathology of, 158–159
  history of, 158
  in children, 296
  isolation of virus in, 159
  signs and symptoms of, 157–158
    oral, 147, 157, *157, 158*
    systemic, 158
  smears in, 159
  treatment of, 653

Acute herpetic gingivostomatitis *(Continued)*
  vesicles of, 159
  vs. acute necrotizing ulcerative gingivitis, 153(t)
  vs. aphthous stomatitis, 160, *160*
  vs. bullous lichen planus, 160
  vs. desquamative gingivitis, 160
  vs. erythema multiforme, 160
  vs. Stevens-Johnson syndrome, 160
Acute necrotizing ulcerative gingivitis (ANUG), 146–157, *147–148, 150–151*
  antibiotics in, 649
  bacteria as causes of, 154
  bacteria seen in, 149–151, *150*
  carcinoma and, 155
  chronic gingival disease and, 154
  classification of, 146
  clinical course of, 149
  clinical features of, 146–149
  connective tissue changes in, 149
  differential diagnosis of, 152–153
  epidemiology of, 155–156
  epithelial changes in, 149
  etiology of, 152
  factors predisposing to, 154
  gingival bleeding in, 148
  gingival connective tissue changes in, 149
  gingival zones in, 149–150
  healing of, gingival changes with, 646
  histopathology of, 149
  history of, 148
  in children, 296
  in leukemic patient, 152
  incubation zones in, 154
  metal intoxication and, 155
  noncommunicability of, 155
  nutritional deficiency and, 154
  nutritional supplements in, 649
  pericoronal flaps and, 652
  prevalence of, 155–156
  psychosomatic factors in, 155
  sequelae of, 650
  symptoms and signs of, extraoral, 148
    oral, *147*, 148

Acute necrotizing ulcerative gingivitis (ANUG) *(Continued)*
  treatment of, 643–646
    drugs in, 647, 649(t)
    gingival contouring after, *648*
    gingival healing after, *648*
    initial response to, *645, 646*
    nutritional supplements in, 649
    reattachment of gingiva after, *647*
    surgical, 647
  ulcerative colitis and, 155
  vitamin C deficiency and, 154
Acute ulceromembranous gingivitis, 147–157. See also *Acute necrotizing ulcerative gingivitis.*
  vs. acute herpetic gingivostomatitis, 153(t)
  vs. agranulocytosis, 152
  vs. chronic desquamative gingivitis, 153(t)
  vs. chronic destructive periodontal disease, 149
  vs. chronic periodontal disease, 153(t)
  vs. diphtheria, 153(t)
  vs. gonococcal stomatitis, 152
  vs. streptococcal gingivostomatitis, 152
  vs. syphilis, 153(t)
  vs. Vincent's angina, 152
Adaptation, diseases of, 472–474
Addison's disease, melanin oral pigmentation in, 111, *112*
Adjustment, occlusal. See *Occlusal adjustment.*
Adolescents, periodontitis in, 196, *198.* See also *Puberty.*
Adrenal insufficiency, manifestations of, 567(t)
  periodontal treatment and, 567
Age(ing), alveolar bone and cementum changes with, 83
  and gingival keratinization, 14
  and severity of gingivitis, 328–333
  and severity of periodontal disease, 328–333
  effects on periodontium, 82–86
  gingival and mucosal changes with, 82